Saving Lives, Training Caregivers, Making Discoveries

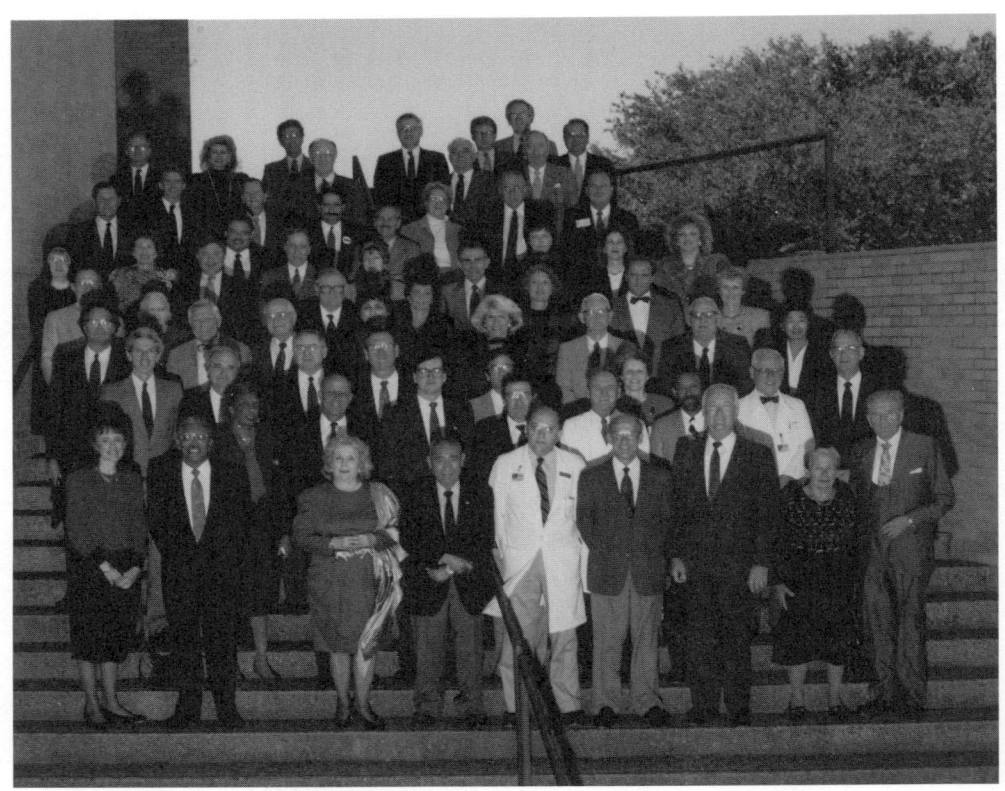

Centennial Planning Commission.

SAVING LIVES, TRAINING CAREGIVERS, MAKING DISCOVERIES

A Centennial History of the University of Texas Medical Branch at Galveston

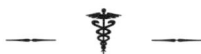

BY CHESTER R. BURNS

Texas State Historical Association
Austin

Library of Congress Cataloging-in-Publication Data

Burns, Chester R.
   Saving lives, training caregivers, making discoveries : a centennial history of the University of Texas Medical Branch
at Galveston / Chester R. Burns.
              p. cm.
Includes bibliographical references and index.
    ISBN 0-87611-187-8
    1. University of Texas Medical Branch at Galveston--History. 2. Medical colleges--Texas--Galveston--History. I. Title.
    R746.T4 B87 2003
    610'.71'1764139--dc21

                                                      2003004111

5   4   3   2   1   03   04   05   06   07

Published by the Texas State Historical Association in cooperation with the Center for Studies in Texas History at the
University of Texas at Austin.

∞ The paper used in this book meets the minimum requirements of the American National Standard for Permanence
of Paper for Printed Library Materials, z39.48—1984.

Book design by Holly Zumwalt Taylor. Dustjacket design by David Timmons.

The University of Texas Medical Branch at Galveston and Old Red are trademarks of the University of Texas System.

"We live forward, we understand backwards."
—William James

"The past is always with us, never to be escaped; it alone is enduring."
—William Osler

This book is dedicated to the memory and honor of Doctors Truman Graves Blocker Jr. and Virginia Irvine Blocker. Their devotion, dreams, and tireless energies propelled UTMB to new peaks of excellence.

Contents

Acknowledgments   viii

Preface   xi

Introduction   1

Chapter 1: Beginnings and Early Years   9

   The City's Rich Medical Heritage   9

   Texans Select Galveston   13

   Ten Years to Start   15

   The First Decade   21

Chapter 2: Political Networks and Executive Leaders   41

   First Relocation Frenzy   42

   Edward Randall, John Spies, and Revolution   46

   Chauncey Leake: Order and Progress   54

   John Truslow: Planning and Reflexibility   61

   The Blocker–Levin Boom Eras   63

   Thomas N. James: A Research Focus   70

Chapter 3: Economic Resources and Business Offices   75

   Operating Income and Business Personnel: 1901–1940   75

   Operating Income and Business Personnel: 1941–1968   80

   Operating Income and Business Personnel: 1969–1991   90

Chapter 4: Campus Development: Buildings and Caretakers   103

   The Carter Era   105

   Edward Randall and the Sealy & Smith Foundation   107

   Federal Dollars for Campus Buildings   109

   Chauncey Leake's Dreams   110

   John Truslow, Don Walker, and Comprehensive Planning   114

   Blocker's Boom Years   116

   Levin's Boom Years   121

   Tom James's Imprints   126

   Campus Caretakers   128

   A Centennial Year Walk   131

Chapter 5: Caring and Curing   137

   From Acute to Chronic Diseases, 1901–1940   138

   From Penicillin to Home Dialysis, 1941–1968   144

   From Medicare to AIDS, 1969–1991   159

Chapter 6: Learning and Teaching 181
   The School of Medicine 181
   The School of Pharmacy 205
   The School of Nursing 206
   The School of Allied Health Sciences 219
   The Graduate School of the Biomedical Sciences 226
   The Institutes 232
Chapter 7: Inquiry and Research 239
   Before Chauncey Leake, 1900–1942 240
   Between Leake and Blocker, 1942–1964 247
   From Blocker to James, 1964–1991 259
Chapter 8: Identities, Rituals, Images—On Campus 275
   Patients: Bonds of Suffering and Relief 276
   Corporate Executives: Bonds of Power and Money 278
   Teachers: Bonds of Authority 281
   Students: Bonds of Metamorphosis 287
   Support Staff: Bonds of Jobs 309
   Storytellers: Bonds of Time and Meaning 313
Chapter 9: Identities, Rituals, Images—Off Campus 317
   Alumni: Bonds of Loyalty and Reputation 317
   Professional Networks: Bonds of Leadership and Reputation 332
   Peer Reviews: Bonds of Accountability and Reputation 346
   Storytellers: Bonds of Time and Meaning 352
Chapter 10: A Centennial Perspective 357
   Quarter-Century Landmarks 358
   The Centennial Years 373
   Facing the Twenty-first Century 376
Appendices 389
Notes 471
Bibliography 609
Index 625
About the Author 660

Acknowledgments

In 1985 Ronald A. Carson, director of the Institute for the Medical Humanities (IMH) at the University of Texas Medical Branch at Galveston (UTMB), invited William C. Levin, president of UTMB, to sponsor the preparation of a centennial history of UTMB. I am profoundly grateful to Ron Carson and Bill Levin for their unswerving advocacy of this writing project. Thomas N. James, Levin's successor, offered encouragement, advice, and additional financial support. John D. Stobo, UTMB's current president, wholeheartedly affirmed the endeavor. I am also grateful to Jere Pederson and Richard Moore for providing space and other measures of support.

During the first ten years of the project, I was privileged to receive the help of some outstanding research assistants. After retiring as director of UTMB's Public Information Office, Myles Knape devoted five years to this project, focusing especially on campus development and oral history interviews. A Ph.D. graduate in history from Rice University, Megan Seaholm studied the evolution of student life, giving special attention to the experiences of women students.

John Swann, a Ph.D. graduate in the history of pharmacy and history of science from the University of Wisconsin, organized the project's research files and meticulously investigated the development of scientific research at UTMB, including the evolution of graduate programs in the biomedical sciences. While working on her master's degree in history at Rice University, Annette Scarpitta gathered valuable information from local newspapers. The most important social outcome of the research phase of this project was the marriage of Annette and John, and their collaboration in the creation of Matthew Swann, who is now a seven-year-old with a brown belt (first degree) in tae kwon do.

While doctoral candidates in the IMH graduate program, Cheryl Vaiani gathered many details about the history of the School of Nursing and Patricia Jakobi analyzed financial records to provide much of the data presented in chapter three. Brian Dirck, several medical students (Joseph Acosta, Rhonda Capps, Doug Christie, Susan Dozier, Karen Guillory, Darcey Kobs, III, David Larned, Michael Lifshen, Ted Margo, Diana Ochoa, and Michael O'Malley), and six IMH graduate students (Janet Beasley, Dale Gorell, Patricia Jakobi, Suzanne Peloquin, Claudia Rappaport, and Sydney Singer) obtained useful information from the *Galveston Daily News* and some medical journals. Heather Campbell, another IMH graduate student, offered valuable suggestions after reading the original draft of the entire manuscript and a revised draft.

Librarians and custodians of institutional records provided much aid. In the UT Board of Regents' office in Austin, Arthur Dilly, Margaret Glover, and others provided invaluable assistance and guidance. At the Center for American History in Austin, Don

Carleton, Ralph Elder, and others helped in so many ways. Staff members at the Rosenberg Library in Galveston answered questions and located source materials; these included Jane Kenamore, Lisa Lambert, Casey Greene, Julia Dunn, and Margaret Schlankey. Employees at the Moody Medical Library were especially helpful. As administrators, Emil Frey, Brett Kirkpatrick, and Larry Wygant provided constant encouragement. In the Blocker Collections, Inci Bowman, Sarita Oertling, and Margaret Dutton cheerfully honored countless requests for assistance. Mary Donna Piazza and Nick Marr prepared the streaming audio files of the oral history interviews (see bibliography). Larry Wygant, my friend and fellow student of the medical history of Texas, prepared the index to this book.

Some professors at UTMB offered helpful suggestions after reading certain chapters. These included George Bryan, Armond Goldman, Ellen More, Adrian Perachio, and Mel Schreiber. Vernie Stembridge, a graduate of UTMB's medical school in 1948, offered several suggestions that improved chapter nine. Some UTMB employees provided unique assistance. John Glowczwski helped select the photographs and Steve Schuenke prepared the campus schematics.

Secretarial help was spectacular. For almost ten years, Betty Grefenstette, the project's full-time secretary, never failed to provide exceptional support to me, the research assistants, and other typists. I am especially saddened by the fact that she did not live to see the project completed. But she never lost her faith and hope that it would be completed. Nina Fox, my IMH secretary for ten years, devoted many hours to typing research notes. Her cheerful attitude resurrected my tired spirit on many occasions. Others who provided typing services at various times included Lucy Enriquez, Kathleen Modd, and Denise Morris. Michelle McCall has been my secretary for five years. Her computer skills and "merry sunshine" made the completion of this book a joyful endeavor.

Collaboration with the Texas State Historical Association (TSHA) has been a rewarding experience. The anonymous referee for the manuscript offered incisive criticisms and many valuable suggestions. Holly Taylor and George Ward displayed meticulous editorial care in transforming my manuscript into a polished and readable volume. Ron Tyler has been a masterful director of the TSHA for almost seventeen years. I am profoundly grateful for his unflinching endorsement of this project.

I would also like to acknowledge the career-long support I have received from Dr. John P. McGovern of Houston and from the trustees of the Rockwell Fund in Houston. Jack McGovern has been a friend and fellow student of medical history for more than three decades. His personal gifts and encouragement have heartened my spirit many times during these years. Truman Blocker Jr. obtained the initial endowment from the trustees of the Rockwell Fund that established the James Wade Rockwell Professorship in Medical History, which I have been privileged to enjoy for more than three decades. This honor and the additional gifts of the trustees of this fund have sustained me more than once during my tenure of service at UTMB.

When I started this project almost eighteen years ago, I had no inkling that it would take such a long time to complete it. I alone am responsible for the decision to move slowly and carefully in crafting this history. For me, the project was always a part-time endeavor that was sandwiched between other expectations about teaching, service, and writing. I apologize to anyone who has been overly distressed with my plodding ways.

While working on this book, I have ridden many emotional roller coasters, experiencing both the depths of despair and the highs of glorious insight. Without the skillful assistance of two superb clinical psychologists, Harold Russell and Larry Micheletti, I would not have completed this book. My wife Ann and our family (daughter Christine with husband Todd Krause and three daughters, Amy, Megan, and Charlotte; and son Derek with wife Susan Hines) have provided the love and care that enabled perseverance and endurance. My gratitude to all is as boundless as the waves that daily caress the shores of Galveston Island.

CHESTER R. BURNS
Galveston, Texas
April 2003

Preface

Any uninformed stranger visiting the east end of Galveston Island today will marvel at the large complex of buildings and the many people scurrying between and within these buildings associated with the University of Texas Medical Branch at Galveston (UTMB). I was one of those strangers when I visited the campus in April 1969 as a prospective member of the faculty in the School of Medicine. President Truman Blocker Jr. and Dean Joe White gave me a role as a teacher of medical history that I have enjoyed to this day.

UTMB's seventy-fifth anniversary history had been published two years earlier and I learned much from its contents. In preparing this centennial history, however, I decided to reexamine UTMB's entire development and not just update the seventy-fifth anniversary history.

I did not attempt to write a "definitive" or encyclopedic history of UTMB. I chose to write a comprehensive "introduction" to UTMB's past that discusses the major groups that propelled its evolution and includes a representative sample of major players in those groups. I emphasize the complex interplay between groups and individuals in the development of UTMB. There are many people who were and are associated with UTMB who are not mentioned in this book. I alone am responsible for the final selections, as no one exerted any untoward influences on the book's contents.

Three goals motivated my persistence with this project. First, I wanted to pay tribute to those whose voices are now stilled, but whose devotion to UTMB still echoes in our memories. In considering their contributions, I focus on the ways their roles shaped the policies and practices of the groups that constituted the institution as a whole.

Crucial decisions of the founders are traced in the initial chapter that describes UTMB's origins and first decade. In the next eight chapters, I focus on major features of growth and development during the twentieth century. Events associated with power, money, and campus development are described in chapters two, three, and four. The central missions of caregiving, teaching, and research are depicted in chapters five, six, and seven. "On-campus" cultures are the focus of chapter eight, whereas "off-campus" cultures are the focus of chapter nine.

I never claim that the features described in these chapters are isolated from each other in the daily development of UTMB. I do believe that we can acquire a better understanding of UTMB's overall history by focusing—one at a time—on the development of each major component of the institution.

My second goal involves a hope that the contents of this history will reduce the bewilderment of those who participate in UTMB's daily life. I have watched many "strangers" encountering UTMB for the first time—new students attending their first classes, professors beginning new jobs, patients seeking relief from suffering, and employees eager for steady jobs. Newcomers (and old-timers) make decisions every day about ways to adapt to the social circumstances at UTMB, a complex institution that can be bewildering.

I believe that historical knowledge can reduce this bewilderment by providing individuals with a view of the social contexts within which their daily choices occur. I do not believe that UTMB's past rigidly determines the nature of these daily decisions. I do believe that these decisions are always made within social contexts that have evolved through time. I believe that daily choices can be more rational and effective if the person making them has a bountiful appreciation of these contexts. I also hope that this historical perspective will foster mutual respect, trusting empathy, and cheerful cooperation among those who maintain and enrich the institution.

My third goal is to encourage others to study UTMB's past. In chapter ten, I remind the reader that histories of UTMB have, in varying ways, always accompanied the growth and development of the institution. I want to encourage others to tell more stories about UTMB's legacies. In this book, I do not trace the entire career of any individual, nor do I depict any as mythic heroes or scoundrels. I hope that others will write biographies of deserving individuals associated with UTMB. In this book, I do not trace the evolution of a particular department in a particular school or hospital. Instead I offer an overview of each school, hoping that others will write histories of departments. In concluding this book with a brief perspective on UTMB's march toward the twenty-first century, I signal opportunities for future storytellers. I hope that this book and its archival resources will provide some guidance for their efforts.

Introduction

The University of Texas Medical Branch at Galveston (UTMB) emerged as an academic medical center in the last decade of the nineteenth century. It was the institutional product of two cultural dreams: the triumph of Galveston as the largest and wealthiest city in Texas and the reform of medical education in the United States. Transforming these dreams into reality involved decades of human endeavor.

Galveston was the major port of entry for the Republic of Texas. After Texas became a state in 1845 its population grew rapidly, from more than two hundred thousand in 1850 to more than six hundred thousand by 1860. About three hundred people lived in Galveston when the city incorporated in 1839. Approximately four thousand people resided in Galveston by 1850, seven thousand by 1860, and fourteen thousand by 1870. A hub of migrant activity and the largest port in the Gulf of Mexico west of New Orleans, Galveston became the largest city in Texas by the mid-1870s. In 1876, America's centennial year, about twenty thousand "permanent" residents lived in Galveston, together with a varying number of seamen, railroad laborers, and other transients. Two years later, Galveston received national praise as "one of the cleanest cities in the United States."[1] Galvestonians were as proud of this recognition as they were of their longstanding tradition for reputable hospital care.

Between 1865 and 1881, years of post-Civil War Reconstruction and Democratic restoration in Texas, Galveston's destiny became inextricably entwined with hospital care and medical education. Galveston's physicians treated patients in homes and local hospitals, supported medical societies, taught medical students, examined candidates for licensure, organized an effective board of health, and edited the state's earliest medical journals. No other city in Texas could claim such extensive professional activities by its physicians.[2]

These social and professional legacies prompted the voting citizens of Texas to locate their first university medical school more than two hundred miles from the university's main campus in Austin. After ten years of vigorous struggles led by T. C. Thompson, J. F. Y. Paine, George Sealy, and Walter Gresham, UTMB finally opened to great acclaim in October 1891. An extraordinary sharing of power and money from private, city, and state interests enabled its birth. Dollars from private sources were essential to the establishment and evolution of the new academic medical center. By the early 1890s Galveston was the leading cotton shipping port in the United States and the "richest city in Texas," with "forty-one millionaires to its credit."[3] Galvestonians were the first Texans to enjoy electricity, gas lights, and telephones. At its birth, UTMB was the latest addition to Galveston's identity as the "flagship" city of Texas.

The other cultural dream was the reform of American medical education. Of the 127 American medical schools listed in the directory of the Association of American Medical Colleges for 1990–1991, 50 were established before 1891. Many of the more than sixteen thousand graduates of these schools migrated westward, some settling in Texas. Of the 167 physicians with biographical entries in the original *Handbook of Texas*, 95 practiced in Texas before the Civil War ended in 1865. Twenty graduated from sixteen medical schools in the east and south, and nineteen others attended such schools but probably did not graduate. Greensville Dowell, a graduate of Jefferson Medical College in Philadelphia, came to Galveston in 1863 as a surgeon in the Confederate Army.[4] He became the ramrod for the two proprietary medical schools that existed in Galveston between 1865 and 1881. Dowell and others in Galveston viewed themselves as colleagues to those practitioner-educators throughout the United States who wanted to reform the standards and policies of medical schools.

As Ken Ludmerer documented so well, the changes in American medical education that occurred during the last half of the nineteenth century were directly connected to profound changes in the meanings of scientific knowledge and the policies of university educators. American educators interested in reforming higher education adopted the ideals and methods of German universities. America's physicians did the same for their medical schools. Those who studied in the labs and clinics of Berlin and Vienna—like William Welch, Franklin Mall, Henry Bowditch, Russell Chittenden, and George Dock—returned to their home states determined to introduce the newer patterns of scientific research, laboratory education, and specialty practice they had observed among their German-speaking mentors. After two years of study in Germany, Dock returned to his alma mater, the University of Pennsylvania, as an assistant in clinical pathology. In 1888 he left Philadelphia to become professor of pathology and clinical medicine at the proprietary school in Galveston that had been revitalized by local physicians frustrated by delays in opening UTMB. Dock's presence in Galveston signaled a tenacious commitment to educational reform among several practitioner-teachers in the port city.[5]

Regional, national, and international values influenced both the regents who selected UTMB's founding professors and the professors they selected. Their dreams courageously transcended provincial sensibilities in a state that was far more rural than urban during the 1890s. The founding professors quickly adopted new therapies and improved techniques for the care of patients, such as diphtheria antitoxin and X-rays. They developed UTMB into a multi-school (medical, pharmacy, nursing) enterprise, repeatedly revising admission and curricular policies to maintain high standards. A few began to do experimental research. Most participated regularly in more than one professional society; some in local, state, regional, national, and international groups.

Neither high standards nor "flagship" regard, though, could have protected Galveston from the hurricane that destroyed much of the city on September 8, 1900. During what was probably a Category Four hurricane on the Saffir-Simpson scale, Galveston was transformed from "the commercial emporium of the state to the nation's most tragic and demoralized city." An estimated six thousand residents died and four thousand houses and stores were destroyed, leaving an estimated twenty thousand people homeless. Electrical, telegraph, and telephone lines were destroyed, and the four bridges (railroad and wagon) to the mainland were damaged or destroyed. Galveston's resilience and resurrection were astonishing. Within five days a telegraph line to Houston was working, within nine days some telephone service was restored, and within thirteen days a Santa Fe train came across a repaired railroad bridge. The nation's response was astonishing. Clara Barton, the seventy-eight-year-old president of the American Red Cross, and her co-workers arrived in Galveston on September 17. By November 15, when Barton left, the city was well on its way to recovery.[6]

On that same day, UTMB began its tenth annual session. The buildings associated with the institution had been seriously damaged, but dollars from the Sealy family, the UT Board of Regents, and the state's legislators enabled the restoration of the John Sealy Hospital, the Medical College Building, University Hall, and the Nurses' Home. Beauregard Bryan, one of the regents, had exclaimed: "The University of Texas stops for no storm!" Galveston's Central Relief Committee even gave more than $20,000 for the construction of a new "Negro Hospital" on the UTMB campus. Galveston and UTMB had survived the worst natural disaster in the history of the United States.[7]

Yet city officials knew that Galveston's future depended on finding ways to prevent this tragedy from occurring again. In September 1901 Galvestonians initiated a new approach to municipal government that exerted much influence throughout the United States. Working carefully with county and state officials, city commissioners oversaw three major projects designed to improve their city's safety. Between 1903 and 1912, engineers and laborers constructed a seawall to protect the city from the onslaught of gulf waters, raised the height of the sandy land that supported homes and buildings, and established better transportation links with the mainland. By 1912 Galveston was again the leading cotton shipping port in the United States and, among America's port cities, second only to New York City in the total value of imports and exports.[8]

Galveston's wealthy families became richer. The Sealy family continued to spend its wealth for maintaining and improving the John Sealy Hospital, UTMB's clinical teaching facility. By 1910 UTMB was one of the ten American medical schools with the largest budgets because tax and private dollars formed its bedrock of financial support.[9] Although the citizens of Texas and their political representatives had established UTMB as a state institution, private dollars catalyzed its creation and expansion. Establishment of the Sealy & Smith Foundation for the John Sealy Hospital in 1922 secured UTMB's future. UTMB was both a public and a private trust. To honor and maintain these trusts, UTMB evolved as a complex corporate enterprise. Effective hierarchies were essential for obtaining political support, securing dollars, constructing buildings, caring for patients, teaching students, searching for new knowledge, and participating in committees and organizations, on and off campus. An expanding bureaucracy was a central feature of UTMB's first century.

A second feature was adaptation to unprecedented scientific and technological changes, and their impact on medical practice and health care services. By 1930 there were safe blood transfusions, some vitamins, insulin and other hormones, Pap smears, and iron lungs for polio victims. By 1965 there were more vitamins, several antibiotics, tranquilizing drugs, polio and measles vaccines, laser surgery, ultrasound, electron microscopes, kidney transplants, artificial heart valves, and pacemakers. By the 1990s there were other organ transplants (liver, lung, pancreas, cochlea), body scans (CAT, PET, MRI), artificial hearts, drugs that destroyed some cancers, human babies that originated as embryos in laboratory dishes, recombinant gene therapies, and a host of specific drugs, including AZT (for AIDS patients) and Viagra.[10] These changes gave America's physicians and other health care professionals enormous power.

Academic health centers, including UTMB, became central to the institutionalization of this power. They conducted much of the research that led to the improved therapies, produced the physicians and other health care professionals who used the new treatments, and provided medical services to many people, especially the elderly and the indigent. By 1983 there were 123 academic health centers in the United States, eight in Texas. UTMB and Baylor were the only medical schools in Texas in 1940. After World War II both schools experienced enormous changes as they adapted to competition from other academic medical centers. By 1979 the eight schools in Texas admitted 1,180 students compared to the 408 that had been admitted by four schools eleven years earlier. This growth was necessary to provide enough doctors for the rapidly growing number of Texans who wanted the benefits of modern medical science.[11]

During the twentieth century the demand for these benefits and the costs of providing them skyrocketed. As early as 1929 Blue Cross and Blue Shield emerged to help teachers in Dallas meet the costs of medical care at Baylor University Hospital. In the 1960s Medicare and Medicaid became part of President Lyndon B. Johnson's "Great Society." Private and government health insurance programs wrought revolutionary changes in the delivery of medical services and the functions of academic health centers. By the 1980s UTMB and other academic medical centers struggled to adapt to unprecedented social, educational, and scientific demands.[12]

A third feature of UTMB's first century was adaptation to remarkable social and cultural changes in Galveston. By mid-twentieth century, for example, Galveston was described as a "Free State," a "Pleasure Island," controlled by "old plantation paternalism and powerful modern benevolent gangsterism." But Galvestonians rejected the gangsters and redesigned their city's image. By the 1980s they were intensely involved in building new hotels and restaurants, preserving historic homes, and developing cultural activities that would attract families and conventioneers. In 1991 the editors of *Money* magazine ranked the attributes of three hundred cities as "best places to live" in the United States and Galveston was ranked thirteenth.[13]

UTMB was a mainstay of the city. By the last decade of its first century, UTMB was Galveston County's largest employer. UTMB attracted a "resident population of educated, urbane, and affluent citizenry that [was] far larger than the average town of 62,000 could expect to attract." Its employees, students, and their families provided the city with a "rich cultural stew" and "an international aura."[14] By 1991 more than thirty thousand inpatients and three hundred thousand outpatients annually obtained medical services in its seven hospitals and eighty-five clinics. More than six hundred full-time faculty and sixteen hundred students participated in the instructional programs of its four schools (medical, nursing, allied health, biomedical sciences) and two institutes (marine biomedical and medical humanities).

One institute, some student services, and the anatomical dissection lab were located in the original Medical College Building that was listed in the National Register of Historic Places as the Ashbel Smith Building and known by UTMB devotees as Old Red. A painting of Old Red graced the front cover of the September 11, 1991, issue of the *Journal of the American Medical Association*, an issue honoring UTMB's centennial. Old Red is the only surviving medical school building west of the Mississippi River that was constructed before 1900. But the popular belief that Old Red housed the first university medical school west of the Mississippi River is incorrect. UTMB did not include the first medical school, pharmacy school, or nursing school established in the United States west of the Mississippi River. UTMB did include the first university-based medical school, pharmacy school, and nursing school established in Texas. Nearly everything that happened at UTMB during the 1890s comprised "firsts" for academic medicine in Texas. Nationally, the School of Nursing captured two "firsts." When it became part of the University of Texas in 1896, it was the first American nursing school directly affiliated with a state university. The UT regents also gave its director, Hanna Kindbom, an appointment to the UTMB faculty as clinical instructor of nursing. This was the first appointment of a professional nurse to the faculty of an academic institution in the United States.[15]

Other "firsts" accompanied UTMB's evolution. The Galveston State Psychopathic Hospital was the first of its kind located on the campus of an academic medical center in Texas (1931). The Department of Neurology and Psychiatry initiated the first residency program in psychiatry in the Southwest (1933). UTMB's hospitals began the first training programs for physical therapists in the Southwest (1943). The first child psychiatric unit in a public hospital in Texas began at UTMB (1964). The first Shriners Burns Institute in the South began at UTMB in 1966. The Marine Biomedical Institute (1969) and the Institute for the Medical Humanities (1973) were the first of their kind in the United States. The School of Allied Health Sciences was the first school of its kind in the Southwest (1978). When it opened in 1983, the Texas Department of Criminal Justice Hospital was the only prison hospital in the world located on the campus of an academic institution.

Various storytellers have noted some of these "firsts" in their histories about UTMB. Though important, such "firsts" are only a small part of the rich legacies associated with

UTMB's first century. Moreover, historic "firsts" are not automatically personal or institutional "bests." As the stories in this book demonstrate, the quest for excellence never ends for those devoted to an institution's integrity and destiny. As long as UTMB endures, storytellers will write histories about its activities. Such histories can be evidence-based stories with plausible explanations and interpretations, or fiction-filled accounts rooted in faulty memories, raging prejudices, imaginative embellishments, or politicized imperatives. Whatever their characteristics, these stories become essential components of UTMB's identity and destiny.

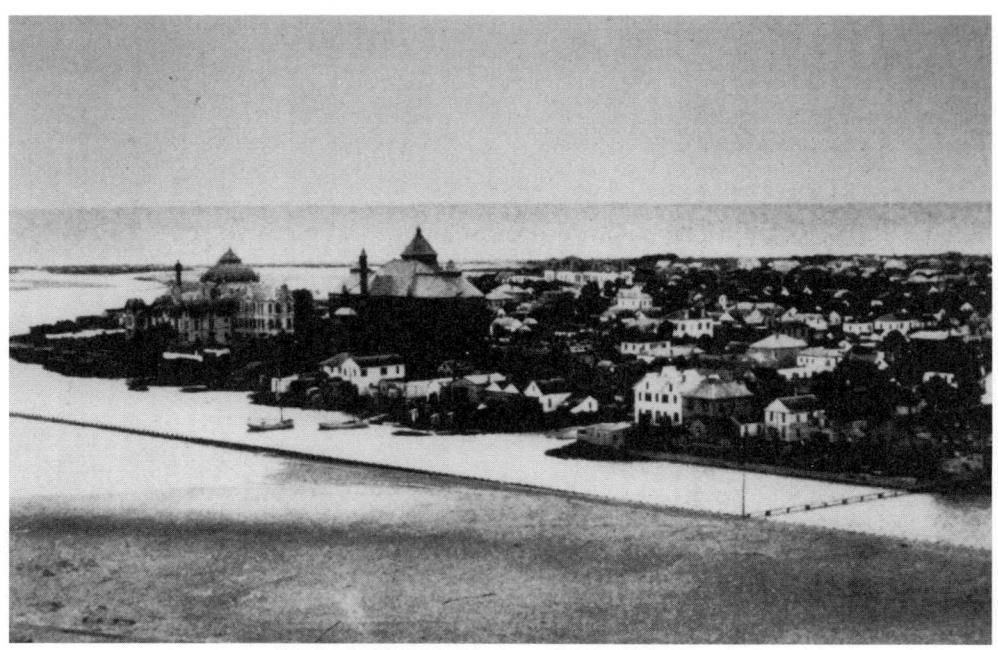

UTMB campus, c. 1895. *Photograph courtesy the Truman G. Blocker Jr. Collections, Moody Medical Library, UTMB. All photographs in this book, unless otherwise noted, are from the Blocker Collections.*

— 1 —

Beginnings and Early Years

"Be it enacted by the Legislature of the State of Texas, that there be established in this State, at such locality as may be determined by a vote of the people, an institution of learning, which shall be called and known as the University of Texas. The medical department of the university shall be located, if so determined by a vote of the people, at a different point from the university proper, and as a branch thereof: and the question of the location of said department shall be submitted to the people and voted on separately from the propositions for the location of the main university." (March 30, 1881)[1]

In October 1891, the University of Texas (UT) opened its Medical Department at Galveston, an institution known today as the University of Texas Medical Branch at Galveston (UTMB). A little more than ten years earlier, the Texas legislature had invited the citizens of the Lone Star State to determine where the state's new university would be located. Because their decisions would alter the state's constitution, all qualified voters in the state were eligible to cast their choices.[2] Why did Texans choose Galveston and not Austin for the medical branch of their new university? Answers and details about the plebiscite are described in the first two sections of this chapter. After the vote was decided, ten years elapsed before instruction began at UTMB. The third section of this chapter analyzes the reasons for this delay. The fourth section of this chapter is a description of the major features that emerged during UTMB's first decade. Political and financial decisions; campus development; care of patients; activities of teachers, students, and alumni; and peer evaluations are described. These features became the foundations for the institution's growth and development during the twentieth century.

THE CITY'S RICH MEDICAL HERITAGE

Galvestonians provided hospitals for sick transients and indigents. Completed in 1845 on Block 668 at Ninth and Strand, the main building of the City Hospital housed many patients during its first three decades. In the summer of 1869 the Sisters of Charity of the Incarnate Word reopened their "Charity Hospital" as St. Mary's

9

Infirmary. By the mid-1870s, about fifty physicians treated residents and visitors when they were sick or injured. Some attended patients admitted to the two new hospital buildings constructed in 1875 and 1876. In use by October 1875, the one hundred-bed, three-story City Hospital cost $18,000. The Sisters of Charity authorized construction of a three-story, $30,000 brick hospital building that opened in May 1876, which allowed St. Mary's to accommodate 250 patients.[3] Galvestonians provided medical care for all people who needed assistance.

Some of Galveston's doctors were members of the Galveston County Medical Society (GCMS) and the Texas State Medical Association (TSMA). The GCMS hosted the TSMA's annual meeting in April 1877. In welcoming about seventy-five doctors, Greensville Dowell's civic pride soared when he declared that Galveston

is situated on a beautiful island, between gulf and bay; and from the top of our new Tremont Hotel you can see all over our city, and view ships sailing many miles out at sea. We have a beach of thirty miles, that on the wettest, dryest or windiest day can be ridden or driven over without mud or dust. We have three railroads running out of the city to all parts of the United States, and ships sailing to all parts of the world. We have wealthy and enterprising merchants and bankers; many very able and distinguished lawyers; wise and prudent physicians; able and devout ministers; large and beautiful churches, and, what is better, large and intelligent congregations. Of newspapers I believe we have three or four—the best in the State, if not equal to any in the United States. The health of our city is equal to any in the world, and still improving. . . . It is no stretch of the imagination to say that the State of Texas will hold and support 40,000,000 of people and not be as thickly inhabited as France or Belgium. That Galveston will be as large as New York is now, and railroads will carry coffee and sugar from here to Alaska by our projected railroads, almost on a straight line, and bring gold and silver from those distant regions. We will have others going to the City of Mexico and the Pacific Ocean. We certainly have a bright future before us.

Dowell's booster spirit accurately reflected the whirl of commercial and cultural activities in Galveston. Because Texans had adopted standard-gauge tracks, cars could move from the docks in Galveston to any city served by American railroads. With Galveston's future looking brighter than ever, TSMA members elected W. D. Kelley of Galveston as their new president.[4]

Establishing a medical school was as important to Galveston's doctors as supporting hospitals and establishing medical societies. Between 1865 and 1881 they supported two medical schools through sixteen annual sessions. Three hundred and eighty-one students, mostly Texans, matriculated at these schools. One hundred and fifty-two (40 percent) graduated. In Texas, formal medical education occurred only in Galveston. Organized as an integral component of Soule University (a Methodist college), the Galveston Medical College began instruction in November 1865.[5] Greensville Dowell was its principal leader. Other faculty members included N. N. Allen, Jesse Boring, W. H. Gantt, D. P. Smythe, Charles Trueheart, John L. Watkins, and John H. Webb. These "professors" were private practitioners who supplemented their income with fees derived from lectures and demonstrations. Their income depended on the number of students and the expenses of operating the school.[6] To graduate, students were required to attend all of the lecture courses given during an annual term from November through March; pass examinations in anatomy, chemistry, physiology, obstetrics, medicine, and surgery; and (with their doctor-preceptors) attend patients in offices, homes, and local hospitals. With written certificates, these mentors testified that their apprentices displayed morally satisfactory characters and technically satisfactory skills.[7] These requirements reflected the educational standards of physicians who had graduated from reputable medical schools and wanted to honor these same standards in Galveston. Students, many lacking suitable preparatory education, struggled with these requirements. Only about one-third of each year's thirty or so matriculates graduated during the early years.[8]

In 1870 Dowell petitioned the state legislature for funds to support the college. The legislators provided no money, but they did charter the Galveston Medical College Hospital on May 31, 1871. This charter established a managing board of trustees, permitted the faculty to oversee clinical instruction of students, and allowed any county court in Texas to send its indigent sick to this hospital for a charge of not more than one dollar per person per day. Dowell and the faculty admitted numerous patients. During 1872, for example, the Galveston County Commissioners paid $1,799.75 to the Galveston Medical College Hospital for indigent care.[9] After Soule University experienced financial difficulties and Methodists in Texas shifted their allegiance to Southwestern University, which opened at Georgetown in 1872, Dowell decided to forego ties with any university. He obtained a new charter, dated March 29, 1873, which established an independent corporation named the Texas Medical College and Hospital (TMCH).[10] There was no interruption in instruction. Dowell and his colleagues viewed the latter school as the natural outgrowth of the former, and even more promising than its predecessor.

During negotiations for the new charter, Dowell had urged legislators to pay one dollar per day for each indigent Texan outside of Galveston County who would receive care at the TMCH. The legislators balked, realizing that this could cost the state $20,000 or more per annum and set a precedent for demands from other localities. "While it may be true," they said, "that the city of Galveston receives over her share of the poor unfortunates of the State, it must be borne in mind that it is by the influx of the citizens of the State within the city limits, for business and pleasure, that the city of Galveston derives her thrift and profit; and while it is the duty, under the law, for each county to provide for the poor and destitute in their limits, they see no special reason why the State should relieve the city and county of Galveston of this charge."[11] But they could not deny Galveston's reputation as a haven for the state's "poor unfortunates" who were sick. The legislators agreed to such payments provided there were state funds "not otherwise appropriated" and provided that the state would never be liable for more than five thousand dollars.[12] Dowell made such demands on the legislators because he believed that the state should pay for the medical care of its indigents, just like the state had been paying for the care of its insane, blind, and deaf citizens for more than a decade.[13]

The failure to obtain state dollars did not impede the TMCH, though. A board of trustees, composed of physicians from various parts of the state and a few non-physicians, governed the institution. Some of the trustees constituted a board of examiners who tested all candidates for professorships in the school. In 1876 J. M. Haden became president of the board and Ashbel Smith, the doyen of the state's physicians, presided over the examining board. The faculty included M. B. Brown as professor of anatomy, Sam Burroughs as professor of chemistry and toxicology, J. M. Callaway as dean and professor of obstetrics and diseases of women and children, Greensville Dowell as professor of surgery, William Penny as professor of the institutes of medicine, J. D. Rankin as professor of theory and practice of med-

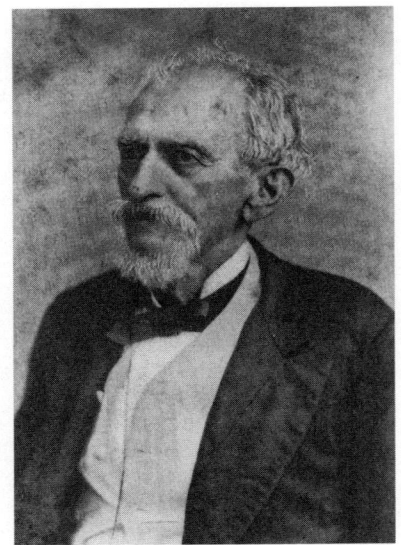

Ashbel Smith

icine, and Hamilton A. West as professor of materia medica and therapeutics. During the following year, A. W. Fly replaced Brown, J. F. Y. Paine replaced Callaway, and George Wise replaced West.[14]

Believing that they were part of the mainstream of national efforts to improve medical education, the TMCH faculty displayed high expectations. In recognition of medicine's cherished past, they used Latin for the diplomas of the thirteen students who graduated on March 15, 1876.[15] When conferring degrees at the commencement ceremonies for eight students on March 16, 1877, and for ten students on March 6, 1878, Ashbel Smith even spoke the Latin language that he had known so well when he graduated from Yale University's School of Medicine fifty years earlier.[16]

The TMCH professors emphasized the future more than the past. In an address to the graduates in 1877, Sam Burroughs praised the new Association of American Medical Colleges (AAMC), a group dedicated to reforming the standards and policies of American medical schools. In June of the previous year, thirty representatives (mostly deans) of twenty-two medical colleges had met in Philadelphia to create a "Provisional Association of American Medical Colleges." Dowell had sent a letter to the organizers expressing full support for the new association. Thirty-six delegates from twenty-six schools attended the second annual meeting in Chicago and renamed themselves as the American Medical College Association (AMCA). Dowell sent a report about the TMCH to those at this meeting, and he attended the meetings in Atlanta (1879) and New York City (1880).[17] The TMCH professors trumpeted AMCA standards, though they believed that reform of the existing schools would occur gradually.[18]

Seventy-four-year-old Ashbel Smith, president of the TMCH trustees, wanted more rapid change. In early March 1880 the TMCH held commencement ceremonies for eight graduates at the Artillery Hall. The Opera House orchestra "discoursed operatic airs in profusion," and Smith proclaimed lofty challenges in profusion. "A state medical college on a grander scale located at Galveston is imperatively needed, as the present one is felt to be deficient in some respects," Smith exclaimed. He noted certain deficiencies. More than one hundred students from Texas attended medical colleges outside of the state. The number of matriculates and graduates at the TMCH had been small and the City Hospital building was not fully adequate as a medical college building. The TMCH had been unable to obtain any state funds for the care of the steadily increasing number of indigent patients.[19] Anticipating obvious queries about the costs of his dream, Smith pleaded for local responsibility: "Cut down the monstrous incomes, revenues or perquisites of your city and county officials to reasonable compensation; require all surplus to be paid into your city treasury; and you will have sufficient money for legitimate and important public uses; erect suitable buildings and make needful appropriations for a purpose vital to the prosperity of this goodly commercial emporium of the herculean state of Texas."[20] Galveston—the wealthiest, largest city in the Lone Star state—should be the medical Hercules for Texas, willing to bear the burdens of indigent medical care and willing to develop a "state medical college on a grander scale." Decisive actions in the following year began to transform Smith's dream into institutional reality.

TEXANS SELECT GALVESTON

On March 30, 1881, the Seventeenth Legislature authorized the establishment of the University of Texas and selected September 6 as the day for the referendum that would determine the location of this university. Texans could situate its medical school in a city that was different from the one they selected for the main campus. James B. Stubbs, senator from Galveston, had persuaded fellow legislators to include this choice in the authorization bill. Stubbs probably encountered little resistance. The TMCH professors were finishing their annual session of lectures for medical students. Cary Wilkinson, physician-in-chief at St. Mary's Infirmary, edited *The Texas Medical and Surgical Record*, the state's only medical journal.[21] As emphasized previously, no other city could claim such remarkable accomplishments in the development of medicine as a reputable profession in Texas.

A few days after the legislative authorization, Galveston's boosters lobbied for the endorsement of fellow physicians who assembled in Waco for the thirteenth annual meeting of the TSMA. Wilkinson chaired a TSMA committee that enthusiastically supported his hometown because it "possessed advantages in the matter of population, healthfulness, clinical material and subjects for anatomical study, to be obtained in no other city in the State." Some TSMA members feared the dangers of hurricanes in Galveston, lobbied for Waco, or expressed strong objections to the separation of the medical school from the main campus. Wilkinson noted that the fear of bad weather had not inhibited the development of outstanding medical schools in Boston, New York, Philadelphia, and Baltimore, all port cities. About to become president of the TSMA, Ashbel Smith argued forcefully for adoption of the committee's report. After three hours of passionate debate, however, the TSMA adopted no formal resolutions.[22] Smith and Wilkinson undoubtedly realized that Galveston's medical legacies and prospects might not be sufficient to carry the vote in September.

Meanwhile, Austin's boosters had started their lobbying efforts. A. P. Wooldridge, the thirty-four-year-old president of the first public school board in Austin, became chair of the "Locating Committee." Fourteen men constituted its executive committee, but a subcommittee of four—Wooldridge, Judge A. W. Terrell, Walter Tips, and John Dickenson—did most of the work. They prepared newspaper announcements, distributed circulars, and gave many speeches about the climatic, geographical, cultural, and political advantages of Austin as the site for the entire university. A schism occurred in this subcommittee in May: Judge Terrell told the editor of the *Houston Post* that Austin did not want the medical branch of the new university. Surprised and distressed, the committee's other members later learned that Terrell thought it would be politically expedient to let Galveston and Houston compete for the medical school, a tactic that might assure Austin of support from both Galvestonians and Houstonians for the main campus.[23]

Citing values of efficiency, economy, and local pride, most of Austin's boosters repeatedly denounced efforts to separate the medical campus and the main campus. The *Dallas Weekly Herald* for June 16, 1881, arrayed quotes from fifteen newspapers in Texas—all supporting the location of the entire university in Austin. But, two weeks later, the same newspaper published a lengthy letter from some "Citizens of Galveston" who argued forcefully for the location of the medical school in Galveston. These anonymous citizens presented the same arguments that had been made previously. Medical students needed to learn anatomy by dissection, pathology by performing autopsies, and clinical medicine by caring for numerous patients with different diseases. In Galveston, there was an ample supply of bodies for dissections and autopsies and a sufficient number of hospitalized patients for bedside teaching. Galveston could furnish "by far" the best facilities for "practical instruction."[24]

By early July Wooldridge realized that Texans would be swayed by these arguments in favor of Galveston, even though reasons for keeping the new university in one location were valid. Senator Stubbs of Galveston wanted to know if Austin's Locating Committee still favored Austin over Galveston. Stubbs declared that Galvestonians would oppose Austin as the site of the main university if Austin did not support Galveston for the medical school. After agonizing deliberation, the committee told Stubbs that Austin was not a candidate for the medical school. Houston and Galveston competed for the medical campus. Waco and Tyler, among others, competed with Austin for the main campus. Even though this was a time of economic retrenchment in Texas led by the state's anti-government, anti-urban, anti-Yankee, and anti-black farmers and landowners, competition for the state's new university was as intense as the heat from the long summer days.[25]

Wooldridge shrewdly recognized that the fate of Austin's claims depended on the way the ballot was designed. Those who went to the polls were invited to decide whether or not they approved the separation of the medical school from the main university, and in which city they would place the entire university, or the main university, or the medical school. How they marked the ballot was important. A few weeks before the election, Wooldridge inquired about the method that would be used to canvass the ballots. The canvassing board consisted of Gov. Oran Roberts, Att. Gen. J. H. McLeary, and Secretary of State T. H. Bowman. On August 19 they issued a divided opinion, with the governor and the secretary of state agreeing and the attorney general dissenting. If the people approved division of the university into a main and a medical branch, Roberts and Bowman declared that the place receiving the most votes for the main university and for the entire university would be selected for the main campus. The one receiving the largest vote for the medical department would be the place selected for its location. McLeary did not agree. If division won, he believed that only those votes for the main campus should be counted and not those for the entire university.

On September 6, 56,480 Texans made their choices, but the results were not announced until October 17. Separation carried: 38,117 were for separation; 18,363 against (67.49 percent of the total). Austin received 16,306 votes for the main university and 14,607 for the entire university, a total of 30,913. Tyler received 18,420 for the main university, but only 554 for the entire university, a total of 18,974. Using the criteria Roberts and Bowman had stipulated, Texans chose Austin for the main campus. For the medical department, Houston received 12,586 votes whereas Galveston received 29,741 votes (70.26 percent of the total). Texans chose Galveston for the medical campus.[26]

TEN YEARS TO START

The first Board of Regents met in Austin on November 15 and 16, 1881. Electing seventy-six-year-old Ashbel Smith as president, the regents established ten academic departments, adopted a plan for the main building on the Austin campus, appointed a committee to ascertain what buildings would be needed for UTMB, and discovered that they had much less money to spend than they had expected. Instruction began in Austin two years later, but not in Galveston until ten years later. Competing political priorities, scarce economic resources, and dedication to superlative educational ideals were the main reasons for the delay. During the first two years, the regents experienced considerable turmoil because of resignations, deaths, and strongly expressed viewpoints. Enormously frustrated about available monies, they allocated some for constructing the main building and for the salaries of the seven professors who constituted the faculty when the university opened in September 1883.[27]

Possibly responding to some newspaper allegations that Smith and Thomas Wooten (a physician-regent from Austin) were quarrelling about UTMB's fate, in September 1883 the regents set aside $15,000 in a reserve fund for the medical school. Eight months later a subcommittee reported "no progress" in developing plans for UTMB The regents decided that it was impractical to establish UTMB at that time because the university's impoverished financial situation made it impossible to establish a good school with high standards.[28]

Financial resources were meager for operating the university. Lands and bonds had been used to capitalize the university—these constituted the Permanent University Fund. Fees received from land sales and interest received on bonds and land sales became pooled income known as the Available University Fund.[29] The regents paid the costs of operating the university with dollars from four sources: the Available University Fund, biennial legislative appropriations from the general revenues of the state, matriculation and laboratory fees from students, and gifts from private donors. After the first biennium had passed, the regents knew that the university would survive, but expansion in Austin or Galveston was impossible without more money.

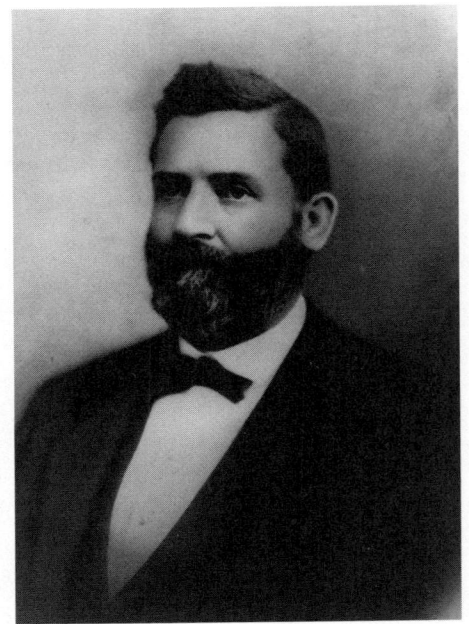

John Sealy I

In December 1886 the regents sent a prodding report to the governor and the legislature. The central message was simple: if the state of Texas wanted a "university of the first class" and a new medical school, the governing authorities must allocate more money. Though sentiments about the disadvantages of separate campuses still surfaced, the regents emphasized the need for money to support growth and adequate maintenance. Based on information sent by the presidents of Vanderbilt University and the University of Virginia, the regents estimated that it would cost $180,000 to begin UTMB.[30] The die was cast: a medical school in Galveston would be a costly enterprise. Did the state really want it?

Fearing a negative answer, incensed Galvestonians interpreted this report as an attempt to scuttle UTMB. On January 22, 1887, the Galveston City Council adopted resolutions that urged legislators to "carry out the provisions of the law" that authorized the establishment of the university's medical branch. The councilmen reaffirmed their willingness to lease the former City Hospital buildings and grounds to the state for the medical school and to marshal the financial resources of the city in support of the school. In a letter to the city council about three weeks later, George Sealy pledged $50,000 from the estate of his deceased brother, John Sealy I, for a new city hospital.[31] Sealy and others asked the councilmen to donate Block 668 and the buildings thereon to the state as the site for the new medical school building and for the new hospital to be named in honor of his brother. Responding favorably on February 21, 1887, the councilmen distributed six thousand copies of their resolution to "the Governor & heads of State Departments & to the individual members of the Legislature, the Regents, & the

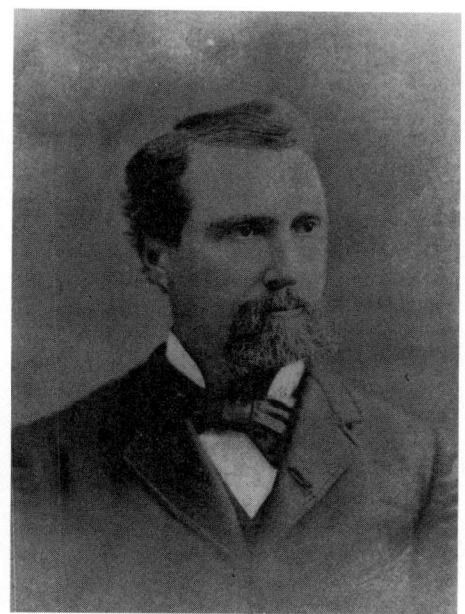

T. C. Thompson. *Photograph courtesy Rosenberg Library, Galveston.*

Physicians of the State."[32] Galvestonians really wanted the medical branch of the University of Texas.

Five days later, forty-seven-year-old T. C. Thompson of Galveston became a regent. In the establishment of UTMB, no event was more fortuitous. A native Texan, Thompson had attended Baylor University and the University of North Carolina. He received a medical degree from Jefferson Medical College in 1861 and was a surgeon in the Confederate army. After practicing in Matagorda and Columbus, Thompson opened a drug store in Galveston and became an influential and popular citizen. Thompson and Wooten shared similar dreams for the medical school.[33] They became close allies, as Wooten rallied professional colleagues in a blistering address to about one hundred doctors assembled in Austin in April 1887 for the TSMA's nineteenth annual meeting. Wooten, president of the Board of Regents, claimed that successive legislatures had stolen at least 10 million dollars of land from the university, and that the donation of 1 million acres of worthless West Texas lands by the legislature in 1883 was merely a token gift of "chips and whetstones."[34] These lands were worthless to the university, argued Wooten, because they did not produce desperately needed revenue.

In contrast to the University of Virginia ($90,000), the University of California ($103,000), and the University of Michigan ($148,000), income for UT that year was only $47,552.54, an amount scarcely enough to maintain the campus in Austin. Wooten urged fellow physicians to help change the attitudes of the state's legislators and his plea stimulated responses, first in Galveston, then in Austin. Some of Galveston's physicians resurrected the TMCH that had closed in 1881 after Dowell's death. They renovated the former City Hospital building and begin instruction in October 1888. If the state ever established UTMB, they would close TMCH and donate supplies and equipment to UTMB.[35] One way or another, Galveston would have a medical school.

The regents and Walter Gresham, the legislative representative from Galveston who was chair of the House Finance Committee, finally agreed on a bill that would provide money for UTMB. On May 17, 1888, the Twentieth Legislature assigned $125,000 to UT, which included $50,000 designated for a medical school building. More than six years had elapsed since the first meeting of the regents. More than three additional years passed before the faculty began teaching medical students. Planning and construction details required much time. The regents accepted the land and buildings the city offered, including the promised hospital, and they authorized three members, Thompson, T. M. Harwood, and Seth Shepard, to have architectural plans prepared for constructing the school's main building, known today as Old Red. The regents held their first meeting in Galveston in early September 1888. They accepted Nicholas Clayton's plans for Old Red, but realized that Block 668 was not large enough for both buildings. In search of more territory, Thompson began negotiating with private landowners.[36]

Further delays involved territorial claims, a need for more money, sorting political duties, and changes in building design. It took Thompson a year to acquire the lots on Block 669 that became the site for Old Red. In the spring of 1889 the Twenty-first Legislature agreed to designate $25,000 of general revenue for the purchase of additional land if Galveston's councilmen would donate an additional $25,000 to the entire project, which they did. Negotiating political obligations was tricky, as the state and the city had to determine who was responsible for managing the daily operations of the hospital. Moreover, someone must have wanted a building that was larger than the one Clayton had designed a year earlier because in September 1889 the regents asked Clayton to revise the plans for Old Red and authorized the preparation of a lease with the city involving the new hospital.[37]

The final agreement, dated October 7, 1889, contained seventeen sections. The Galveston City Council agreed to lease the hospital from the state for one dollar per year for twenty-five years. They would furnish and equip the hospital, provide salaries for all employees (except the physician-professors), maintain the buildings, and name two councilmen to a Board of Managers for the hospital.[38] The state could use all facilities for the instruction of medical students, and the state had a right "to the special conduct of the treatment of all charity patients" admitted to the hospital.

Ten years earlier the councilmen had relinquished their interests in maintaining a new city hospital building because of increasing costs. Now they were willing to maintain a much larger and far more expensive building as well as provide equipment and recurring salaries. The state would provide salaries and supplies only for the physician-professors, and the state could add buildings, but was under no obligation to do so. The governing officials of Galveston agreed to pay for everything else needed to operate the hospital. Galvestonians were giddy with Gilded Age exhilaration. They knew that they lived in the wealthiest city in Texas and the cultural center of a rapidly expanding state. Almost anything was possible.[39]

In November 1889, about six weeks after the hospital lease was signed, workers began constructing Old Red.[40] Less than two months later, the John Sealy Hospital opened on January 10, 1890. During the first three weeks, doctors treated ninety inpatients and twenty-two outpatients. Inadequate nursing care was the major problem. Led by Mrs. George Sealy, a group of Galveston's women organized the John Sealy Hospital Training School for Nurses, which began functioning in March 1890 with a director and eighteen students, who learned their skills as they provided care to patients. By the

DEAR SIR: GALVESTON, Texas, May 5, 1891.

The Texas Medical College will soon be replaced by the Medical Branch of the University of Texas. An appropriation was made by the last legislature to finish, furnish and equip the magnificent building, now nearly completed. The Faculty will be elected at an early day. The institution will be first-class in every respect. The fees will be moderate. The advantages will be such that no Texas medical student can afford to leave the State. The announcement will be issued as soon as practicable, and the session begin about 1st October next.

H. A. WEST, M. D.
Dean Texas Med. College

Postcard ad, May 5, 1891.

fall of that year, doctors and nurses had treated one thousand inpatients and more than four hundred outpatients.[41]

The basic structure of Old Red was in place by December 1890, but the regents told the governor and legislators that the medical school could not open until the new building had been equipped and furnished at an estimated cost of $34,000. It would also cost $33,000 to hire seven professors, or twice that amount for the first two years. Thus, the regents wanted an additional $100,000 to place the school in operation.[42]

Meanwhile, a few medical students were learning their skills at the bedsides of patients admitted to John Sealy Hospital. Faculty of the reorganized TMCH instructed both medical and nursing students. Two medical students received diplomas during commencement ceremonies held in the hospital on March 20, 1891.[43] These students received good training, but not under the official auspices of the University of Texas.

By mid-April 1891, no equipment had been purchased for Old Red and no faculty members had been selected. Thompson and Wooten expected the legislature to designate $30,000 for "finishing the Medical College," but that had not yet happened. Thompson was willing to purchase the equipment when money was available, and he offered suggestions to Wooten about the faculty. Soon thereafter, the Twenty-second Legislature appropriated the money for the furnishings and equipment, but only $22,000 "for the support and maintenance of the medical branch" during each year of the biennium 1891–1893. The regents had requested $100,000; they received $74,000, the first of many economic seesaws yet to come. Nevertheless, the legislators had assigned these dollars from the general revenues of the state. No one could now doubt the state's desire for a viable medical school in Galveston.[44]

Thompson expressed considerable frustration a few days later. He told Wooten: "To go out to the building and contemplate the many and various items required for furnishing it is certainly appalling and the question arises does the supplying of all this depend upon me alone?"[45] Thompson and Wooten finally met in early May to decide how to apportion the dollars for the utilities, furniture, equipment, and supplies. Optimism replaced frustration and H. A. West, dean of the TMCH, sent postal cards throughout the state advertising the new school.

In June the regents decided that the school's first session would begin October 1 and end April 30. They specified salaries for eight professorial chairs and filled two: J. F. Y. Paine as professor of obstetrics and gynecology ($2,500) and H. A. West as professor of the theory and practice of medicine and diseases of children ($2,500). Both Paine and West were TMCH faculty members. The regents solicited candidates for the other professorships by advertising in medical journals. In late August the regents met in Galveston again and adopted a set of regulations for governing UTMB.[46] They created the office of provost, whose incumbent would serve as the registrar, bookkeeper, personnel manager, and business officer for the institution. They permitted the professors to select someone from their group as dean, but he would not receive any special reimbursement for exercising this role. The dean would administer all of the regents' policies; prepare budgets and written reports; recommend all appointments, promotions, and terminations; monitor all aspects of instruction; preside at faculty meetings; and attend to the needs of students. The professors were responsible for developing the "method and system of instruction," and they could adopt rules governing themselves.

The medical staff of the John Sealy Hospital would include the professor of obstetrics and gynecology, the professor of medicine, and the professor of surgery. These three could appoint other teachers and assistants. They were obligated to teach medical students and provide care to indigent patients who had been hospitalized by proper authorization. They would receive no additional fees for providing this care, but they were not restricted from earning unlimited fees from the care of private patients. They could appoint lecturers and purchase equipment. The professors and dean were expected to submit reports to the regents after each annual session ended.

During this meeting, the regents appointed seven additional faculty members and designated annual salaries. These were J. M. T. Finney of Baltimore as professor of surgery ($3,000); A. G. Clopton of Jefferson as professor of physiology and hygiene ($3,000); Seth M. Morris of Austin as professor of chemistry and toxicology ($2,000); William Keiller of Edinburgh, Scotland, as professor of anatomy ($2,500); Edward Randall of Galveston as professor of materia medica and therapeutics ($2,400); Allen J. Smith of Philadelphia as professor of pathology, histology, and bacteriology ($2,000); and George H. Lee of Galveston as demonstrator of anatomy ($1,000). Finney declined his appointment, whereupon the regents selected James E. Thompson, then resident surgeon at the Manchester (England) Royal Infirmary. Resisting parochial pressures, the regents courageously chose a remarkable mix of four doctors from Galveston (all TMCH

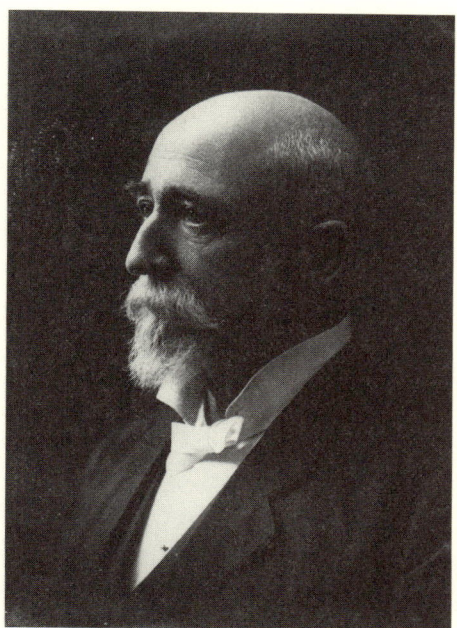

John Fannin Young Paine, c. 1895.

professors), two from other cities in Texas, one from Philadelphia, and two from Great Britain.[47] At its birth, the medical department of the University of Texas was a tributary from the mainstreams of American and British medical education.

THE FIRST DECADE

The opening of John Sealy Hospital in 1890 and Old Red in 1891 added enormous prestige to the Oleander City. Galveston— "backed by her charms of climate, her matchless social and educational advantages, her splendid churches, hospitals, public and private buildings, her incomparable beach, her growing manufacturing interests, her gigantic jetty works . . . her million-bushel elevator, her unlimited wharfage, her prospective bridges to the mainland, her proposed new railroads, her undisputed prestige as a health resort"—is now the site of the state university's only center for training physicians and nurses, proclaimed a Houston physician a few days before UTMB officially opened. Expectations were extremely high. UTMB was expected to be "on the same plane" as Harvard, the College of Physicians and Surgeons in New York City, and the University of Pennsylvania. As well as the foremost school in the foremost city in Texas, UTMB would also be a national treasure.[48]

The school's faculty basked in these expectations. They selected fifty-one-year-old John Fannin Young Paine as their dean and CEO (Appendix A and Appendix B). Tall, balding, bearded, experienced, and imposing, Paine sounded a dean's trumpet during the opening ceremonies on October 5, 1891. "We are in the dawn of a new era in the history of medical education in this country," he proclaimed, "and our regents imbued with a spirit of patriotism, professional pride and progress, and in the light furnished by the experience of similar institutions, have organized this school upon a plan that is in line with the leading medical colleges of the United States and we here register the solemn edict: its standards shall never trail in the dust."[49] A graduate of Tulane, Paine had practiced in Galveston for fifteen years.

Fellow teachers shared his optimism, though they evinced considerable diversity in age, experience, and heritage. Sixty-three-year-old Albert Gallatin Clopton, the oldest, was also a graduate of Tulane, as was George Henderson Lee, the twenty-nine-year-old demonstrator of anatomy. A graduate of the University of Louisville, forty-two-year-old Hamilton Atchinson West had served with Paine on the original as well as the reorganized TMCH faculty. The University of Pennsylvania's School of

Medicine had trained thirty-one-year-old Edward Randall and twenty-eight-year-old Allen John Smith. Seth Mabry Morris, the youngest at twenty-four years, had recently graduated from the College of Physicians and Surgeons in New York City. William Keiller and James Thompson had studied at several institutions in Great Britain and Europe. When they arrived in Galveston, Keiller was thirty years old, Thompson twenty-nine.[50] The political dynamics of UTMB's beginnings revolved around the deliberations and actions of these mostly young, talented, strong-willed, and idealistic physicians.

Policy conflicts emerged between the professors and the regents during the first faculty meeting on September 29, 1891. The regents had assumed the right to select the "lecturers" as well as the professors. Lecturers were local practitioners who volunteered to give lectures on special subjects or consult about the care of charity patients with special problems. The professors wanted this power. When Thompson opposed the faculty's demand for such authority, Clopton traveled to Austin to confer with his friend, Wooten. The regents decided to retain the power of appointing lecturers, but assured the faculty that none would be appointed without considering their recommendations.[51] Centralization of power and authority was the regents' dominant administrative style.

Another political problem involved the selection of the demonstrators who were assistants to the professors. In late December 1891 Keiller delighted the students by changing the time of anatomical dissection from evening to daytime hours. George Lee, the regent-appointed demonstrator of anatomy, was distressed because this change interfered with his schedule for attending private patients. Lee resigned and Keiller hired Thomas Flavin, the first of numerous graduates who became teachers at their alma mater.[52] The regents gave the professors the power to employ instructional assistants. Effective centralized control also required appropriate delegation of power and authority.

It was not easy to discover effective patterns of centralized control and decentralized delegation. UTMB operated in a labyrinth of political networks that included governors, legislators, regents, executive officers (e.g., president, dean, provost), the John Sealy Hospital boards, chairs of academic departments, faculty with their committees, and students. Decisions within each of these networks during the 1890s established the foundations for UTMB's political and financial history. Governors and legislators were always involved in decisions about how much money would be allocated to state institutions. How these persons valued UTMB was extremely important in securing political and economic support. How a governor viewed UTMB, for example, could make a substantial difference in the outcome, since governors could veto line items in appropriation bills.[53]

Governors nominated regents, who began six-year terms after senate confirmation. The regents determined general policies, appointed corporate executives, and delegated authority to these executives and their assistants for solving certain problems and accomplishing certain goals.[54] The regents adopted explicit rules governing behavior in the university. The first set of "Rules and Regulations" was adopted in 1891. Such rules shaped final decisions, though a significant feature during the early years was the relative absence of rules and, during all years, the ever-present choice of altering any rules

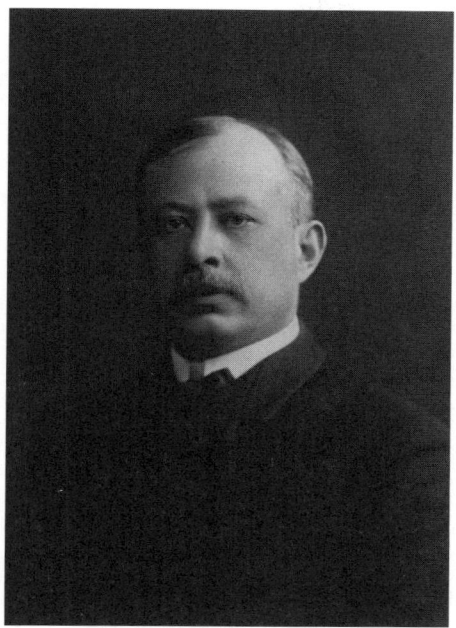

Allen Smith, c. 1897.

that had been adopted previously.[55] The desires of regents, executive officers, and faculty were usually more important than rules.

UTMB progressed steadily because two Galvestonians were regents: T. C. Thompson (1887–1898) and Frank Spencer (1898–1903).[56] Each was a member of a subgroup of regents (usually three) charged with monitoring policies and decisions directly affecting UTMB (Appendix C).

Regent Thompson wanted a pharmacy school and the faculty wanted assistants who would help with teaching and the care of charity patients, thereby permitting them to engage in research or attend more private patients.[57] In June 1893 the regents approved a pharmacy school and permitted the professors of medicine, surgery, and obstetrics and gynecology to appoint "clinical assistants" if two-thirds of the entire medical faculty agreed on the nominated candidates. The faculty wanted more students, so the regents eliminated tuition fees. By the spring of 1894, 116 medical students and 11 pharmacy students had enrolled, prompting Dean Paine to request funds for enlarging laboratory and hospital facilities.[58]

To help deal with irrepressible expansionist sentiments, the regents adopted conservative fiscal policies and delegated executive authority to a full-time academic leader. In July 1896 they hired George Winston, then president of the University of North Carolina, to be UT's CEO and the direct liaison between the faculty and the regents (Appendix D). Winston became an informed and aggressive advocate for the entire university. He believed that UTMB would become the "largest, as well as the best and most prominent medical school in the South and West" if the legislature continued its liberal support. Hoping to encourage this generosity, students and faculty fed oysters to legislators when they visited UTMB early in 1897. But their capacity for support was curtailed as Americans in general experienced economic setbacks that year. Because the legislators appropriated only $38,500 of the requested $55,766.66, anxious regents absorbed the deficit by reducing operating expenses, not faculty salaries.[59]

UTMB survived this period of economic stringency, but not without major political changes. The regents authorized Winston, not Paine, to present all items about UTMB for their consideration. The regents authorized Winston, not Paine, to oversee $3,000 of repair work on Old Red. Clopton and West resigned, the first members of the original faculty to leave. When the regents met in Galveston in September, they accepted Paine's resignation and appointed Allen Smith as the new dean and CEO.[60] To replace

Clopton and West, they appointed twenty-eight-year-old William S. Carter as professor of physiology and fifty-seven-year-old J. W. McLaughlin as professor of medicine. Carter had been teaching at the University of Pennsylvania, his and Smith's alma mater. McLaughlin, a graduate of Tulane, had been a prominent general practitioner in Austin since 1869. Though the regents maintained a balance between "outsiders" and "insiders," between youth and experience, they withdrew the original privilege that had permitted the professors to elect a dean from their own group.[61]

Smith's first appointment as dean lasted only eight months, as struggles about political control continued. Claiming that it infringed on their prerogatives, the regents rejected a new "Constitution of the Medical Faculty" that was dear to Smith's

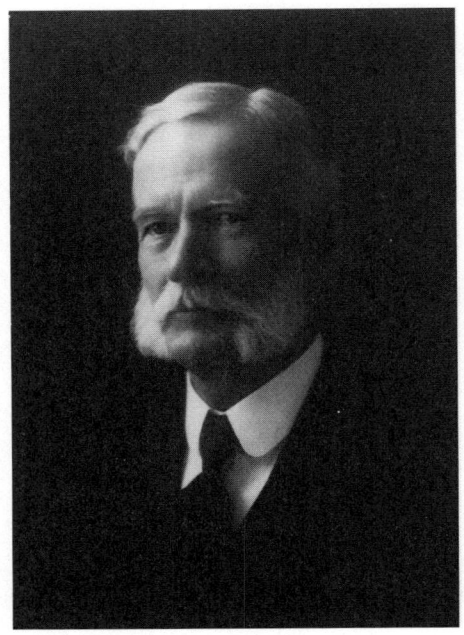

Henry P. Cooke

heart. He protested by resigning in May 1898.[62] Henry P. Cooke became the new dean and CEO. Cooke had practiced in Galveston for twelve years and had served as lecturer in pediatrics for six years. The regents had granted three lecturers (Cooke, Hall, and Lee) the same voting privileges as the professors, even though they were unsalaried private practitioners.[63] This was a risky decision that might have alienated other local private practitioners who were not selected as lecturers as well as the regular faculty members whose political powers were seemingly diluted. Selecting a former lecturer as the new dean also added a frosting of more fears to a peculiar political cake. Perhaps to appease the faculty and certainly to give them more influence in shaping hospital policies, the regents appointed Cooke to the John Sealy Hospital Board of Managers.

These hospital boards were probably the most powerful centers in the political networks before 1941 (Appendices E and H). They authorized and monitored the hospital's budgets that enabled numerous jobs. They appointed the administrative director of the hospital and the director of the nursing service, who was also the director of the nursing school (Appendix F). They controlled the nurses and nursing students, the graduate physicians who provided services to patients, and other hospital personnel.[64] With some members selected by the regents and others by Galveston's councilmen, these boards occupied center stage in any drama produced by the conflicting demands of private, city, and state interests produced. Such power struggles loomed large after 1900.

The other political networks involved faculty and students. Regents and administrators expected faculty to teach, engage in research or other scholarly endeavors, serve on committees, and influence "beneficially students and citizens in various extra-curricular ways." Ranked according to years of experience and evidence of accomplishments, members of the faculty included professors, associate professors, and assistant professors. "Instructors" later became the fourth and lowest rank of the full-time appointments. Administrators organized faculty into departments in the medical and pharmacy schools, but not in the nursing school. Regents appointed one professor as the head or chair after that person had been nominated by the president, who had previously consulted with the dean (Appendix G).[65] A chair presided at meetings of departmental faculty, appointed new faculty or terminated ineffective members, prepared the department's biennial budgets, and wrote annual reports about the department's activities.

Four faculty committees emerged: Executive Committee, Library Committee, Committee on Entrance Examinations for Admission to the School of Pharmacy, and Committee on the School of Nursing (Appendix H). In 1898 the professors delegated most of their power to the Executive Committee. At the beginning of each academic year the faculty constituted this committee by electing two of its members to serve with the dean (*ex officio*). This committee prepared and monitored budgets, established and supervised the curricula of the medical and pharmacy schools, prepared annual catalogs for publication, and enforced regulations governing students. Between 1899 and 1914, only eight faculty members served on this committee (Appendix I). The political style of centralization also appealed to the professors.

In 1894 students began wielding more power because medical and pharmacy (but not nursing) students organized a Students' Council (Appendix H). This council was a politically effective lobby. Students did not want to take exams in the evenings or on Saturday afternoons. The faculty honored these wishes after receiving a petition from the council in 1895. In 1896 the council organized a successful campaign to keep Allen Smith from accepting a professorial position at his alma mater. The council organized athletic and social events, managed the student honor system, and prepared sections about UTMB for the *Cactus*, the UT yearbook.[66]

In 1895 the council began publishing a monthly journal titled *University Medical*. This journal included scientific articles by faculty and students, and many news items submitted by student editors, a group that included nursing school representatives by 1899. In this journal, students regularly chided the state legislature for inadequate appropriations to UTMB and urged students and alumni to support requests for increased funding.[67]

The rhythms of state financing caused the regents to be cautious about the allocation of dollars. They used Available University Fund income for new construction, $40,000 for adding an east wing to the main building in Austin, for example. Because legislators usually did not appropriate the full amounts requested for salaries and operating expenses, the regents also used Available University Fund income for these maintenance obligations.[68] Moreover, no one could predict exactly how much money the legislature would assign the university until the appropriations bill had been signed by the governor, usually in late spring or early summer of odd-numbered years. Because of these political uncertainties, changes in personnel (resignations, deaths, new employees), unexpected emergencies, changes in rank or salary for teachers, and decisions about new programs or special requests, the regents frequently readjusted operating budgets as they negotiated with CEOs and CBOs.

James P. Johnson was UTMB's provost or chief business officer (CBO) during the first decade (Appendix J). To handle operating expenses, Johnson depended on several sources of income. These included fees of matriculating students, money from the state's treasury, donations from the Sealy family, gifts from other citizens, contributions from the city for the care of indigent patients, and payments from private patients (Appendices K, L, and M).

The John Sealy Hospital attracted private patients whose payments for hospital care ranged between $2,500 and $4,500 annually during the first decade. John Burke, Galveston County's physician, believed that between one-third and one-half of the inpatients were non-residents of Galveston, many pay patients. "Often the hospital is so crowded that city patients can not obtain entrance," William Gammon commented.[69] Whether indigent or pay, patients came to a teaching hospital that revolved around the presence of physician-professors who were financially dependent on the state. Every biennium the regents pleaded for more money to support and develop UTMB. In February 1899, for example, they requested $54,919.16 for fiscal year 1900 and $46,249.16 for fiscal year 1901. When legislators appropriated only $35,500 for each year, the regents trimmed operating expenses instead of salaries and they initiated unsuccessful lobbying with the governor to obtain additional state funds. Unsuccessful, in part, because formal education, especially higher education, was still suspect by what one newspaper reporter called the "forks of the creek folks" in the legislature. Even those who did favor university studies bickered jealously when one college received more than another school.[70]

Legislators apportioned tax revenues among several state agencies and institutions. Finding judicious balances was a challenge, but anyone examining the appropriations bill for the biennium beginning March 1, 1899, and ending February 28, 1901, would have understood the distresses of UT and UTMB advocates.[71] In each of the two years, the legislators assigned $40,000 to UT Austin and $35,500 to UTMB. They gave the state's eleemosynary institutions (blind, deaf, retarded, insane) $674,355 for the first year and $520,795 for the second year. To the state's courts and judiciaries, they allocated $689,990 for the first year and $689,540 for the second. The custodial institutions and the courts accounted for half of the total state budget (first year: $2,669,568.92; second year: $2,250,387.20). The University of Texas and its Medical Branch each received slightly more than 1 percent.

This was enough to sustain but not expand UTMB, an institution that included four buildings on a four-acre campus by the end of the century (Appendix N). The oldest building was a three-story frame structure that had been used originally as the City Hospital from 1875 until 1879. Afterward it was the site of the TMCH from 1879 to 1881, a public school building, and again the home of the TMCH during its

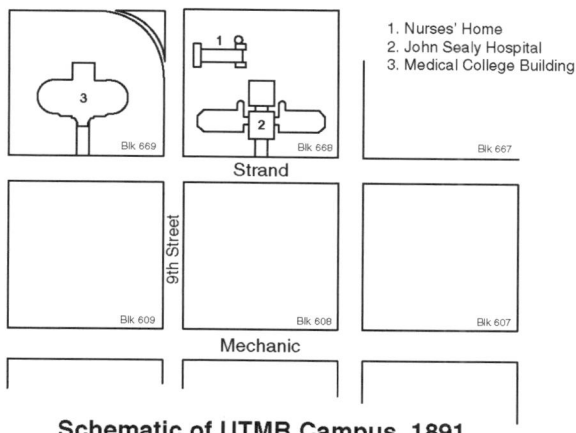

1. Nurses' Home
2. John Sealy Hospital
3. Medical College Building

Schematic of UTMB Campus, 1891

reincarnation between 1888 and 1891. After becoming a component of UTMB, it housed black adults and children, the students who provided nursing services, and, later, white children.[72]

University Hall was the newest building. Hoping to encourage prospective women students, Regent George Brackenridge donated $41,000 to construct a residential hall for women attending the schools of pharmacy and medicine. White Gonzalez brick and terracotta were used to construct this three-story building across the Strand from the hospital. Students began using the building in the summer of 1898. University Hall was "a beautiful tribute to the noble womanhood of Texas" and the only building added during the first decade.[73]

The centerpieces of the campus were the Medical College Building (Old Red) and the John Sealy Hospital. Cedar Bayou pressed brick, red sandstone, and red Texas granite were used in constructing Old Red's round arches, pilasters, circular buttresses, and arcade of windows. Texas pine and cypress were used for the interior, including the grand staircase that supported the students and faculty as they walked to the lecture and laboratory courses in rooms in the basement and the three upper floors. The top floor dissecting room contained many specimens in the anatomical and pathological museums. The other floors contained three lecture amphitheaters; laboratories for chemistry, physiology, histology, pathology, and bacteriology; a library; and offices for the professors.[74]

The John Sealy Hospital included four separate pavilions: a three-story pavilion in the center, two two-story ward pavilions (east and west, with twenty-four beds each), and a separate structure behind the central pavilion that housed the kitchen, dining rooms, boiler room, and laundry. The first floor of the central pavilion housed a reception area, examining rooms, and offices for doctors and administrative personnel. The second floor of the central pavilion contained twelve beds for private patients and the third floor contained the operating amphitheater with seats for 150 students. The first floor of the west

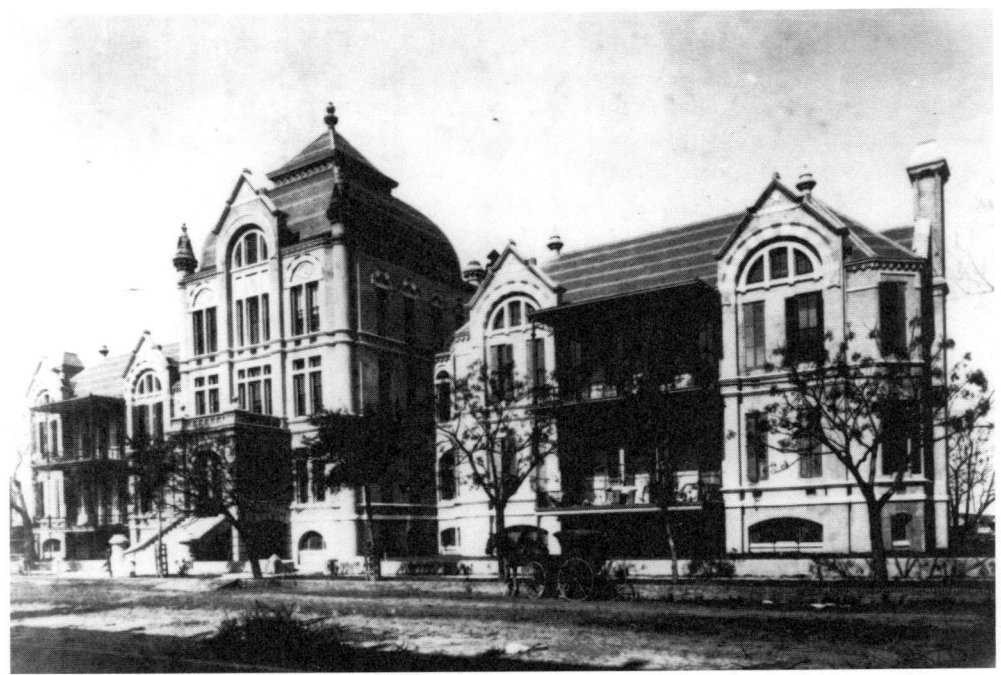

John Sealy Hospital, c. 1898.

pavilion housed male medical patients; the second floor male surgical patients. The first floor of the east pavilion housed female medical patients; the second floor female surgical patients. The basement of the west pavilion contained a waiting room and five outpatient clinic areas. The basement of the east pavilion housed the pharmacy and storerooms. Altogether the hospital contained 108 beds for inpatients.[75]

The professional staff included physicians, one graduate nurse, nursing students as ward or clinic nurses, and one pharmacist. The hierarchy of physicians included the clinical professors; the lecturers, who handled specialized cases; the house surgeon, who was also director of the hospital; and interns.[76] In 1891, for example, the clinical professors and lecturers included H. A. West (physician), J. E. Thompson (surgeon), J. F. Y. Paine (obstetrician and gynecologist), H. P. Cooke (pediatrician), Allen J. Smith (neurologist and pathologist), R. C. Hodges (ophthalmologist), G. P. Hall (otolaryngologist), and George H. Lee (dermatologist). Others included T. L. Kennedy as pharmacist, C. Josephine Durkee as director of the nursing school, J. P. Hendrick as director of the hospital, and T. T. Jackson and William Gammon as interns.

These professionals treated outpatients in the small clinics in the basement of the John Sealy Hospital. During 1891 they attended six hundred outpatients. During the 1890s altogether, they attended more than twenty-two thousand outpatients.[77] Outpatients were admitted to the second and third floor wards as needed or, if black, sent to the Nurses' Home. During a twelve-month period beginning March 1, 1893, for example, 1,129 charity patients and 57 private patients were admitted.[78] The total number of inpatients remained about the same during each of the first six years, then increased thereafter (Appendix O).

A few women came for birthing. "Cured" pregnancies numbered fifteen in 1895 and twenty-eight in 1900. Between January 1890 and January 1901, 252 women gave birth in the hospital.[79] Most women still delivered in their homes.

More sick children were admitted after 1895.[80] Of the children admitted in 1900, 54 percent were treated for infections.

Infectious diseases were the most common medical problems: 64 percent of those admitted to the medical wards in 1895 and 61 percent in 1900. Tuberculosis, malarial fevers, typhoid fever, scarlet fever, tetanus, and diphtheria afflicted patients, as did infections with intestinal worms.[81]

Infectious diseases were also prevalent on the surgical and gynecological wards. Skin ulcers were common and lesions caused by traumatic injuries became sites of microbial growth. Forty-eight patients with traumatic wounds were admitted in 1895; seventy-five in 1900. Doctors drained abscesses, lanced carbuncles and buboes, and resected or amputated gangrenous and chronically infected bones. They treated several women who had endometritis, salpingitis, and vaginitis.[82]

During the 1890s doctors performed more than nine hundred gynecological operations and more than twenty-five hundred general surgical operations, including those for tumors and congenital anomalies of the face and neck, empyema, umbilical hernia, appendicitis, hepatic tumors, kidney diseases, anal fistulae, and popliteal aneurisms.[83] Ether and chloroform were used as general anesthetics. Cocaine and morphine were used as local anesthetics.[84] In 1896 and 1897, X-rays were first used to visualize fractures and to locate bullets in bones.[85]

Though therapeutic approaches were less sophisticated than today, most patients responded favorably to treatment. In 1893 West treated eighteen patients with typhoid fever. Two died of peritonitis, but the others recovered after receiving milk and animal broths, bismuth subnitrate as an intestinal antiseptic, and pepsin and hydrochloric acid to stimulate digestion. In April 1895 Thompson removed the left kidney of a thirty-six-year-old-male who weighed 96 pounds. The kidney contained calculi and was severely infected. In 1897 the patient weighed 166 pounds and did a "heavy day's work at his trade." Using the newly developed diphtheria antitoxin, Gammon successfully treated two children after membranes had begun to form in their throats.[86]

Altogether UTMB's professionals attended more than twelve thousand inpatients during the 1890s, with a death rate that ranged from 5.8 to 8.5 percent. Doctors discharged between 80 and 88 percent of the inpatients as cured or improved, results generally recognized as quite successful. A symbol of wealth, science, charity, and progress, the John Sealy Hospital beckoned patients, professors, and pupils.

The professors were responsible for admitting, instructing, and graduating students who demonstrated their readiness for professional careers. The first medical students enrolled in October 1891; the first pharmacy students in October 1893. The first group of nursing students started training in March 1890, though they were not under UT auspices until May 1896. During the 1890s, 913 men and 83 women matriculated in these three schools. The physician-professors designed the first curriculum for medical students and they supervised those graduates who continued training as interns in the John Sealy Hospital. With the professor of pharmacy, they also designed the curriculum for the pharmacy students and, with the superintendent of the Training School for Nurses, they designed the curriculum for the nursing students. Although the physician-professors formally and informally taught all three groups of students, and although effective care of patients was the goal of all three professions, a separate curriculum emerged for each school.[87]

When the School of Medicine began, its professors wanted to train competent general practitioners who, among many other things, could deliver babies, perform appendectomies, set fractures, and prescribe drugs for diseases experienced by children, women, and men.[88] To accomplish this, the professors fashioned a three-year curriculum and they admitted twenty-two students in the fall of 1891: fourteen first-year, five second-year, and three third-year.[89]

The first-year curriculum included anatomy, physiology, chemistry and physics, drugs and therapeutics, and pathology. The schedule of lecture and laboratory courses included eight hours of instruction every weekday, and anatomical dissection every night except Saturday and Sunday. Only nine of the fourteen first-year students survived this rigorous schedule.[90]

The second-year curriculum included lectures in anatomy, physiology, chemistry, drugs and therapeutics, pathology, medicine, surgery, obstetrics, and medical jurisprudence, and laboratory work in anatomy, pathology, and chemistry. Students attended clinics in medicine, surgery, gynecology, and ophthalmology. Clinics and classes were scheduled from 8 A.M. to 6 P.M. every weekday and dissection followed from 7:30 to 10 P.M. every evening from Monday through Friday. There were clinics and operative gynecology on Saturday mornings and a chemistry lab on Saturday afternoons. Only William Gammon and Thomas Terrell Jackson completed this second-year curriculum.[91]

Third-year students received clinical instruction in the wards, operative amphitheater, or clinics every morning, Monday through Saturday. They listened to lectures from 11 A.M. to 6 P.M., Monday through Friday, except for an hour's break on four of those five days. The lecture subjects included drugs and therapeutics, all of the clinical specialties, and medical jurisprudence. There was also additional laboratory training in pathology. Jesse P. Hendrick, Houston T. Quinn, and Thomas Flavin became the first class of physician graduates on April 22, 1892.

During that commencement, Dean Paine praised the "industrious and harmonious" faculty.[92] Regent Thompson expressed much satisfaction with the faculty, the teaching program, and the budgetary situation. The regents boastfully proclaimed success: "The course of instruction prescribed in the curriculum of the School of Medicine at Galveston is of the very highest grade. It is framed to meet the enlightened demands of the age in the matter of medical education, and in this respect it takes the lead of all the medical schools in the Southern States."[93] Texans had finally produced some rigorously trained homegrown doctors.

Keeping UTMB in a leadership position became a formidable challenge. After the regents eliminated tuition fees in 1893, the number of students increased dramatically and the faculty faced the problem of sustaining quality while accommodating massive growth. They added more teachers, tightened admission procedures, and changed some curricular policies.

Academic departments materialized as professors added demonstrators. Keiller and George Lee first taught anatomy; then Keiller and Thomas Flavin (class of 1892). Clopton hired David Cerna as a demonstrator of physiology. Smith hired William Gammon (class of 1893) as a demonstrator of histology. Morris added Louis Magnenat (class of 1895) as a demonstrator of chemistry. The clinical professors also added demonstrators. Paine selected two graduates from the class of 1895: W. F. Starley Jr. as demonstrator of obstetrics and Thomas L. Kennedy as demonstrator of gynecology. Thompson added Robert L. McMahon (class of 1896) as a demonstrator of surgery. West added John T. Moore (class of 1896) as a demonstrator of medicine. By 1900 six of the ten departments functioned with more than one teacher.[94]

The faculty tightened admission procedures. They used challenging entrance exams for those who had no diplomas or degrees. In 1893 they rejected five applicants because of "insufficient academic preparation" and twelve of thirteen applicants who had studied at eight different medical colleges but could not pass the entrance exams. They also stopped admitting medical students to the third- and fourth-year classes and enthusiastically supported efforts to improve high school and college education in Texas.[95]

The professors changed some curricular policies and practices. Large classes were subdivided for laboratory and clinical teaching. In 1894, for example, Morris created sections for the chemistry course because there were 176 medical and pharmacy students attending the course but only forty-four desks in the laboratory. In the fall of 1895 West divided the second- and third-year classes of sixty students into three sections for their inpatient rotations. In 1896 the third-year class was divided into sections for their rotations through the outpatient clinics. Using both inpatients and outpatients made it possible for each student to receive 560 hours of clinical instruction, substantially more than that at many medical schools.[96]

The professors also increased the length of the annual terms from seven to eight months, and they increased the total number of required years from three to four, beginning with the class entering in October 1897.[97]

The lecture courses, lab courses, and clinical exercises were arranged in a sequential order for these four years. They began with courses about the "normal" structures and functions of the human body, continued with courses about the "abnormal" structures and functions, and ended with courses about dietary, pharmacological, surgical, and other therapeutic approaches to the management of human ills. Students learned thousands of particulate facts, needing this knowledge for class recitations, ward rounds, and formal examinations. By the late 1890s students were required to pass three exams in

Table 1: Lady Board of Managers, John Sealy Hospital Training School for Nurses, 1890

Mrs. Bertrand Adoue	Mrs. John C. (Nellie Ball) League
Mrs. William F. Ladd	Mrs. Joseph G. (Ella Willis) Goldthwaite
Mrs. S. Hartley	Mrs. Charles (Mary Jane Booth) Fowler
Mrs. Robert B. Hawley	Mrs. J. F. Roeck
Mrs. J. H. Hutchings	Mrs. George (Magnolia Willis) Sealy
Mrs. Andrew G. (Lucy Ballinger) Mills	Mrs. George Mann
Mrs. T. (Isabella Dyer) Kopperl	Mrs. Louis (Emma) Fellman
Mrs. Aaron (Cecile) Blum	Mrs. W. (Anne) Ziegler
Mrs. John (Rebecca) Sealy	Mrs. T. J. Groce
Mrs. Robert Irvine	Miss Rebecca Brown
Mrs. Peter J. Willis	Miss Hetty L. Wells

each course before they could be promoted to the next year of the first three years. During the senior year each student was required to pass oral and written exams in eight clinical areas.[98]

Although the professors reported significant improvements in the teaching exercises and in the competencies of the students by fiscal year 1899, only 37 percent of the medical school matriculates actually graduated during the first decade (Appendix P). By 1900 the school had graduated 182 men and four women as physicians.[99]

James Kennedy, UTMB's professor of pharmacy, admitted eleven first-year students when the School of Pharmacy began functioning. The two-year pharmacy curriculum included lecture and laboratory courses in chemistry, botany, drugs, and pharmacy. The chemistry lab was in the basement of Old Red; the pharmacy lab was on the first floor.[100] Students learned the origins and chemical compositions of drugs and how to recognize and prepare them. To earn a Graduate of Pharmacy degree (Ph.G.), students were required to attend both years of the curriculum (392 hours of lectures and 672 hours of labs), satisfactorily complete exams in all subjects, and write a thesis. Only two of the original eleven graduated.

After replacing Kennedy, who died of tuberculosis in 1895, R. R. D. Cline dropped the thesis requirement and changed one of the admission requirements from a first-grade teacher's certificate to a second-grade teacher's certificate. When necessary, he used the same entrance exams as the medical school professors, and he required two letters of reference, preferably from reputable pharmacists. "Daddy" Cline, known for his swallow-tailed dress coat, taught botany and pharmacy, Edward Randall taught drugs and therapeutics, and Seth Morris taught chemistry.[101]

The number of new students enrolling each year increased from eleven in 1893 to thirty-four in 1900, as did the number of graduates, from two in 1895 to thirteen in 1900. Only 38 percent of those admitted during the school's first eight years actually graduated, however (Appendix P). Licensure requirements for pharmacists in Texas did not include graduation from a professional school. Many students attended the school for a year and then passed the licensure exam. By 1900 seventy-six men and six women had received Ph.G. degrees after completing both years.[102]

The nursing school had started in March 1890 as a private venture, spearheaded by a group of energetic women who constituted a Lady Board of Managers (Table 1).[103] After almost five years of toil collecting the $15,000 needed to keep the school afloat, this board asked the regents to request $1,500 from the legislature to help defray these expenses. They agreed to do that, noting the "great advantages" of the school. After an "elegant luncheon" in Galveston on May 15, 1895, the board informed the regents that Governor Culberson had vetoed their request. Wishing to keep the school viable, the regents appropriated $1,200 from the Available University Fund for the salary of Josephine Durkee, the school's director (Appendix B). One year later, on May 15, 1896, the regents assumed official control of the School of Nursing "as a department of the Medical College." Dean Paine proudly declared that "our pupil nurses are doing more work for smaller wages" than those in the other 150 nursing schools in the United States.[104]

The hospital's Board of Managers established all policies affecting the nursing students, except the curriculum. Hanna Kindbom, superintendent of nurses and clinical instructor of nursing, and two medical school professors (Hamilton West and Allen Smith) constituted the Committee on Instruction for the School of Nursing (Appendix Q). Thirteen physician-professors were lecturers.[105]

This superintendent had exclusive authority for admitting students for one month of probationary experience (later two months, then four months). As part of this experience, students were examined in "reading, penmanship, simple arithmetic, and English composition." If they performed satisfactorily, they became "pupil nurses" for two years, uniformed in blue ankle-length dresses, with white linen cuffs, white bibs and aprons, and white caps.[106] They were expected to reside in the Nurses' Home and work on the wards during their first year. During their second year, the superintendent could assign ward work or "private duty" at a home in Galveston.

During both years, the student nurses attended many lectures and bedside demonstrations given by the physician-professors and the superintendent, who also gave numerous written and oral examinations. The subjects included anatomy, physiology, pathology, drugs and therapeutics, principles of nursing, surgical nursing, nursing care of children and pregnant women, nursing care of patients with specific diseases, management of emergencies, preparation of diets, hygiene, and the administration of baths, massage and other forms of physical therapy.[107]

Though students learned much from these lectures and demonstrations, they learned even more from their bedside experiences of caring for sick patients. The inpatients depended on these "pupil nurses," who ordinarily worked twelve-hour shifts (7 A.M. to 7 P.M.). Three or four rotated on night duty, assisted by an orderly. Even with this rigorous curriculum and work routine, the number of matriculates remained rather constant between 1896 and 1900. Seven students graduated during ceremonies in Old Red on March 20, 1897. By 1900, fifty-four of the fifty-seven new matriculates (95 percent) had graduated (Appendix P). Kindbom believed that the School of Nursing was "one of the best arranged and most perfectly operated schools of its kind."[108]

Research was not a part of the School of Nursing and School of Pharmacy. The School of Medicine's physician-professors assigned two meanings to "research." Clinical professors believed that they engaged in research by attending to all aspects of the diagnosis and treatment of a sick patient. Every time a doctor prescribed a drug or a surgeon performed an operation, a therapeutic "experiment" took place. A "scientific" physician could prepare reports of experiences, successful or not, in treating patients.

The clinical professors and lecturers prepared many of these reports. West reviewed the diagnosis and treatment of malaria, tuberculosis, typhoid fever, and pneumonia. Thompson published reports of operative procedures involving intestinal perforation, chronic joint disease, genito-urinary cysts, hepatic neoplasms, and cleft palate. Paine wrote mostly about managing the problems of pregnant women. Cooke analyzed rheumatic fever, typhoid fever, and chicken pox. George Lee, R. C. Hodges, and George Hall published reports about treating various conditions affecting the skin, the eye, and the ear, nose, and throat.[109] These doctors hoped that their clinical case reports would help improve the diagnostic and therapeutic skills of fellow practitioners, in Texas and elsewhere.

The professors assigned another meaning to "research." Researchers could experimentally alter the bodily parts and functions of animals (non-human and human) and collect observations about the results of these alterations. Such results could lead to more precise and predictable measures of control. As the nineteenth century evolved, such experimental manipulations had radically transformed "truths" about the functions of organs and tissues, healthy and diseased.[110] Those who taught at UTMB during its first decade understood this philosophy of experimental medicine, but only two professors conducted experimental research.

David Cerna was teaching physiology at the University of Pennsylvania, his alma mater, when Albert Clopton visited in 1892 and Clopton hired Cerna as a demonstrator. In Galveston Cerna taught medical students and did much experimental research. He and Edward Randall co-authored a paper about chloroform, an anesthetic that sometimes produced unexpected deaths.[111] They wanted to determine if the drug caused death by paralyzing the nervous system, the heart, or the lungs. At least fifteen dogs inhaled the anesthetic until death occurred. With careful measurements, the investigators concluded that respiratory functions ceased before cardiovascular ones.

Collaborating with Dean Carter, Cerna studied the toxicity of phenacetin given to dogs in large quantities, and he studied the effects of large doses of apolysin on at least eleven dogs. Chemically similar to phenacetin, this drug was used clinically as an antipyretic and an analgesic. In moderate doses, the drug did no harm to the animals; in large doses, their circulatory systems collapsed. Carter also studied the effects of thyroidectomy or parathyroidectomy in more than twenty dogs, concluding that the glands were "separate and distinct" in structure and function.[112] But Carter did very little experimental research. After becoming dean in 1897, his days were filled with the

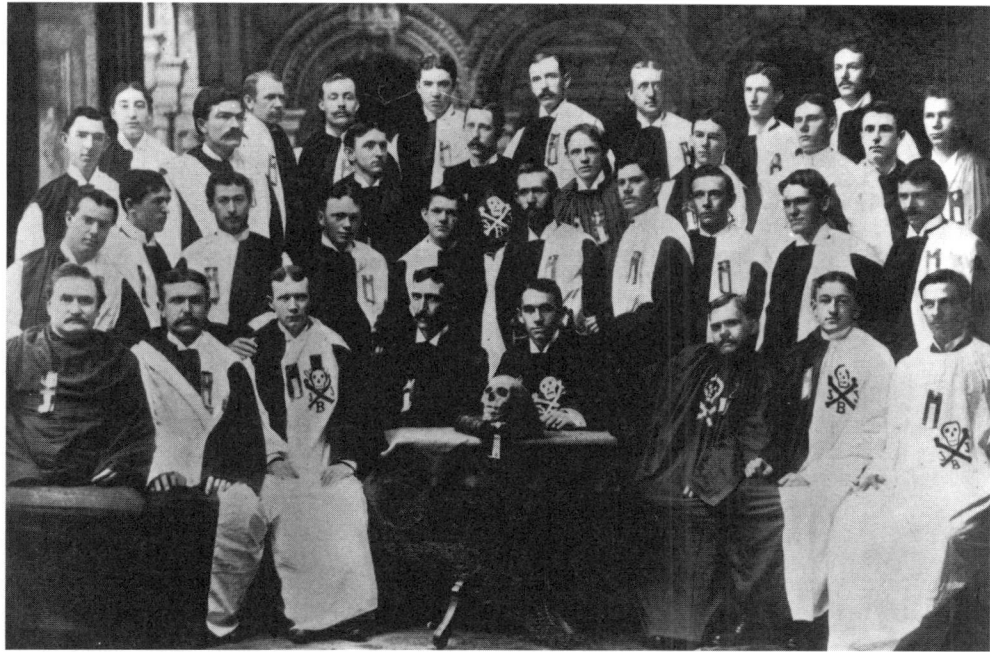

Jolly Bone Jugglers, 1897.

details of a "chief executive officer" responsible for guiding the entire institution with its various groups and distinctive cultures.

Professors wanted promotions, increased salaries, and assistants. In 1894, for example, the regents promoted Seth Morris to full professor and increased his salary. They permitted Allen Smith to employ William Gammon as demonstrator of histology. They increased the salaries of William Keiller, Thomas Flavin, and Provost Johnson. They also returned a portion of student fees to each department for laboratory and teaching materials.[113] Regents and executive officers rewarded outstanding teachers with titles, promotions, assistants, and more money. These were the perks of an academic culture.

The earliest student culture was mostly Texan, Caucasian, and masculine. All medical, pharmacy, and nursing students were Caucasian and most were born in Texas.[114] All nursing students were female and most medical and pharmacy students were male. During the first decade, eighteen women enrolled in the medical school and eight in the pharmacy school (Appendix P). Elements of a female culture gradually percolated through the dominant male culture. Student editors of *University Medical* commented about the daily "spectacle of beautiful young ladies circulating among the other students." The female students added unmistakable cultural leavening. A few students were married.[115]

Students displayed remarkable initiative and self-sufficiency, especially in meeting the costs of lodging and meals. During 1899–1900, for example, 196 male students lived at seventy-four different addresses. Thirty-eight (19 percent) lived alone. Most lived in rooming houses with other students, some of which provided board. In 1899 the students organized a Dining Club that provided three daily meals for twelve dollars a month at tables situated on the first floor of University Hall, the only place on campus where a large number of students—130 in 1900—could gather.[116]

Classes organized themselves with officers, colors, mottoes, and yells. Sophomore and freshmen medical students displayed keen rivalries. The freshman class of 1898 proclaimed its dignity:

Though our outward appearance may look tough,
beyond all doubt we are 'the stuff.'
As from little acorns grow big trees,
so from us freshmen grow MDs.

Strong bonds from shared experiences melded classes and interclass groups, though these bonds did not insulate the matriculates from the high attrition rate.[117]

Students persistently commented on the difficulties of their studies. "Many, many are the nights we have burned midnight oil trying to absorb something contained in those great, big textbooks." The devil of failure was a constant companion, setting the mood for every class, especially when the class prepared a brief history for the *Cactus*. The medical graduates of 1897 declared: "Eighty-four strong, this class began its career in October, '94. Since that time more than one half have fallen by the wayside." Though meeting admission requirements, many students were poorly prepared for a professional education. Some transferred to other schools.[118]

Even with the high attrition rate, students wanted to play as well as study. The Sigma Ribbon Society and the Jolly Bone Jugglers were both organized in 1896 as local fraternities without national affiliation. UTMB's chapter of Alpha Mu Pi Omega, a national medical fraternity, was organized in 1898. Students also organized athletic groups, glee clubs, a college orchestra, a chapter of the YMCA, and pre-professional associations.[119]

In addition to fraternity parties, students entertained themselves by attending UT football games, horse shows, and theatrical productions, and by merry-making in rooming houses and even in classrooms. One of Keiller's classes ended with a display of clog dancing by some students from West Texas. Less constructive displays were not uncommon, especially towel fights in the labs. The faculty posted notices urging students to "refrain from chewing tobacco and expectorating" in the classrooms and labs.[120]

Special student-faculty rituals occurred during opening ceremonies usually held in October and commencement ceremonies usually held in May or June. The opening ceremonies were formal events with exhortative speeches given by faculty or guests. Beginning in 1898, all students graduated together. These ceremonies usually included prayers, music, and an address by a faculty member or a visiting dignitary together with the presentation of diplomas.[121] These rituals affirmed new professional identities for graduating physicians, pharmacists, and nurses.

These professionals served patients throughout Texas and elsewhere. Among the nurse graduates in 1898, for example, four remained in Galveston; one each went to Victoria, Houston, and Sherman; and one served with the Second Division of the Seventh Army Corps in Savannah, Georgia. Many of the pharmacists resided in larger towns or cities.

Several physicians located in the larger cities, but many established practices in smaller towns. These included Eagle Pass, Sweetwater, Montgomery, Eddy, Marfa, Plantersville, Normanna, Barstow, Corrigan, Cooper, Nada, Maxwell, Meridian, Dublin, Alvin, Cleburne, Thomaston, Colorado, Crowley, Elmont, Forreston, Swan, Moulton, Childress, Melissa, Nelsonville, Leesville, Ballinger, Teneha, Round Timbers, Caldwell, Rockwood, De Soto, Elmendorf, Jefferson, Cuero, Rocket, Coperas Cove, Somerville, Carthage, and Oscar. Several School of Medicine graduates became county health physicians or railway surgeons. A few practiced in other states. More than forty graduates (thirty-seven medical, six pharmacy, four nursing) served in military units during the Spanish-American War.[122]

To craft images of loyalty, continuity, and support, the medical and pharmacy alumni established a formal organization. William Gammon led a group that met during the week of commencement ceremonies in May 1894 to plan the first formal meeting for 1895. The Alumni Association held its second meeting in Old Red on Saturday, May 16, 1896. Jesse Hendrick of Huntsville gave the presidential address and members elected W. F. Starley Jr. of Galveston as incoming president. Eleven members and thirteen graduating seniors (seven medical, six pharmacy) attended the third annual meeting on May 15, 1897. The members elected Marie Delalondre, the first female physician graduate, as first vice president. Twenty-five new members attended the fourth meeting on May 13, 1898, and heard E. P. Becton emphasize the economic impact of UTMB on Galveston's economy with his estimate that students and staff were spending more than $100,000 annually in the city. Later that day the association sponsored a public lecture by UT President George Winston. During commencement week in May 1899 the Alumni Association sponsored a reception in University Hall. After commencement ceremonies in June 1900, the alumni sponsored a sumptuous banquet. Thus, medical and pharmacy graduates planned and enjoyed six annual meetings in Galveston during the first decade.[123]

Alumni, faculty, and students were active in various local, state, regional, national, and international networks of professionals. The extent of their participation is remarkable because it required travel to other cities, states, and countries using time-consuming modes of transport such as horses and carriages, trolleys, railroads, and ships. Teachers and alumni supported medical institutions and organizations in Galveston. Most of the clinical professors were members of the visiting staff at St. Mary's Hospital. Keiller, for example, treated ninety-five marine patients admitted to St. Mary's in 1899.[124] Thompson, Randall, Keiller, Cooke, and others attended private patients at St. Mary's. They were also staunch supporters of the Galveston County Medical Society (GCMS). In 1893–1894 members elected Keiller president, Thompson second vice president, and Cerna secretary. Every year, some professors gave papers during meetings and members elected some professors as officers.[125]

Teachers and alumni exerted major influences in the development of the state's professional organizations. When the TSMA held its twenty-fifth annual meeting in Galveston in 1893, eleven of its thirty-seven new members lived in Galveston. Six professors exercised official roles: West as secretary; Randall as chair of the section on obstetrics and diseases of children; Smith as chair and Cerna as secretary of the section on microscopy and pathology; and West, Paine, and Cooke as members of the publications committee. Other professors were officers, chairs of various sections, or members of committees.[126] Teachers and graduates wrote forty-five of the papers published in the *Transactions of the Texas State Medical Association* during this decade.

Professors and alumni also supported a statewide organization that advocated more scientific research. On January 9, 1892, fourteen persons met in the chemistry lecture room on the UT Austin campus to organize the Texas Academy of Science (TAS).[127] Edgar Everhart, professor of chemistry at UT Austin, became president. A week later, members elected Seth Morris, Allen Smith, and James Thompson as TAS Fellows. Five to ten members met each month in the spring of 1892. During the meeting in Galveston on New Year's Eve (a Saturday) in 1892, Thompson and Charles Gwyn gave papers and Keiller, Cerna, and Flavin were elected members.

UTMB's teachers were very active in the TAS during the next five years. With Cerna as vice president, the TAS held its thirty-seventh regular meeting in Old Red in 1895. Thompson, Keiller, and Cline gave papers, and Paine was elected a fellow. President Bruce Halsted, professor of mathematics at UT Austin, thought UTMB was "the most successful department of the state university," and its medical school was "second to none south of John Hopkins University." Cerna was re-elected vice president in 1896, but not in 1897. Keiller was defeated in the election for council in 1898 and as a candidate for vice president in 1899. Interest in the TAS began to wane as alumni and faculty became more involved with strictly medical organizations, including regional organizations such as the South Texas Medical Association. West gave a paper at its Houston meeting in 1896 and fifty doctors attended the second annual meeting in Galveston in 1897. Cerna, Thompson, and West gave papers, and Morris demonstrated an X-ray machine. Thompson and West gave papers during the fifth semi-annual meeting in December 1898.[128] The group changed its name to the South District Medical Association (doctors from fifteen counties in South Texas).

The professors participated in international meetings and societies. Thompson attended meetings in Great Britain during the summers of 1892, 1893, and 1894. Keiller also visited Great Britain in 1893. Morris studied in German chemistry labs during the summers of 1892 and 1893. Seventeen Texans, including Cerna, Randall, Smith, Thompson, and West, attended the first Pan-American Medical Congress in Washington, D.C., in 1893. Gammon journeyed to Paris in 1896 to study bacteriology, microscopy, and pathology for twenty months, and Cerna attended the second Pan-American Medical Congress in Mexico City. Hanna Kindbom visited fifteen hospitals in the United States, Great Britain, and Europe during the summer of 1898 to observe their training programs for nurses.[129]

Throughout the first decade, faculty, students, and alumni were quite concerned about their international, national, state, and local reputations. After the graduation of only two students in 1893, J. R. Briggs, the physician-editor of *The Texas Health Journal* ascended to the heights of nastiness with his comments. "Tucked off in one corner of the state in a third rate town," UTMB was a "huge joke upon the commonwealth and a sniggering burlesque on our boasted institutions of learning," Briggs exclaimed. "Not only this, but it means that thousands and thousands of dollars are thrown away annually to buy tooth-pick shoes and silk stockings for a little coterie of foreigners who are no more fitted to teach medicine than is the razor-back hog fitted for Heaven—we mean no disrespect to the hog," he added. In contrast, the editors of the *Texas Sanitarian* captured the sentiments of the majority of doctors in Texas when they noted that UTMB required "the same high standard that is required by all the other first class schools in this country, and that is saying a great deal."[130]

At the time of the first commencement in 1892, Dean Paine placed the School of Medicine among the better schools committed to the nation's highest standards. The deans of these schools had organized two associations dedicated to these standards: the Association of Southern Medical Colleges (ASMC) and the Association of American Medical Colleges (AAMC). Initially, UTMB faculty did not participate in the AAMC, but they were among the founding members of the ASMC.[131]

In 1892 representatives from seventeen southern medical schools assembled in Louisville to organize the ASMC. Thompson represented UTMB. ASMC members wanted to "elevate the standard of medical education by requiring a more thorough preliminary training, and an increased length of time of medical study." However, UTMB did not send a representative to the ASMC meetings in 1898 or 1899.[132]

Perhaps the professors were riding high with pride and felt no further need for regional acclaim. UTMB attracted only a few students during its first two years, but by 1894 UTMB ranked thirty-sixth nationally in total number of medical students, twenty-sixth by 1895. Moreover, this growth in numbers did not dilute the quality of the educational experience. During the first four years, only one student who had studied at another medical school passed UTMB's admission exams, whereas those leaving UTMB to study elsewhere successfully passed admission exams. The School of Medicine also ranked competitively with the best schools in terms of the ratio of graduates to matriculates. Pride was seemingly justified, though students from Texas continued attending other medical schools, especially those in Louisiana, Tennessee, and Kentucky.[133]

In 1895, the year after he had started the Alumni Association, Gammon crafted the first historical overview of UTMB. He recounted the origins of the institution as a combined private, city, and state endeavor, described the three campus buildings, listed the names of personnel, and celebrated the "inestimable benefits" to patients, professors, students, and citizens of Galveston.[134] Gilded Age pride suffused the spirits of Gammon and others who believed that they were fulfilling the high expectations surrounding the first university medical center in Texas.

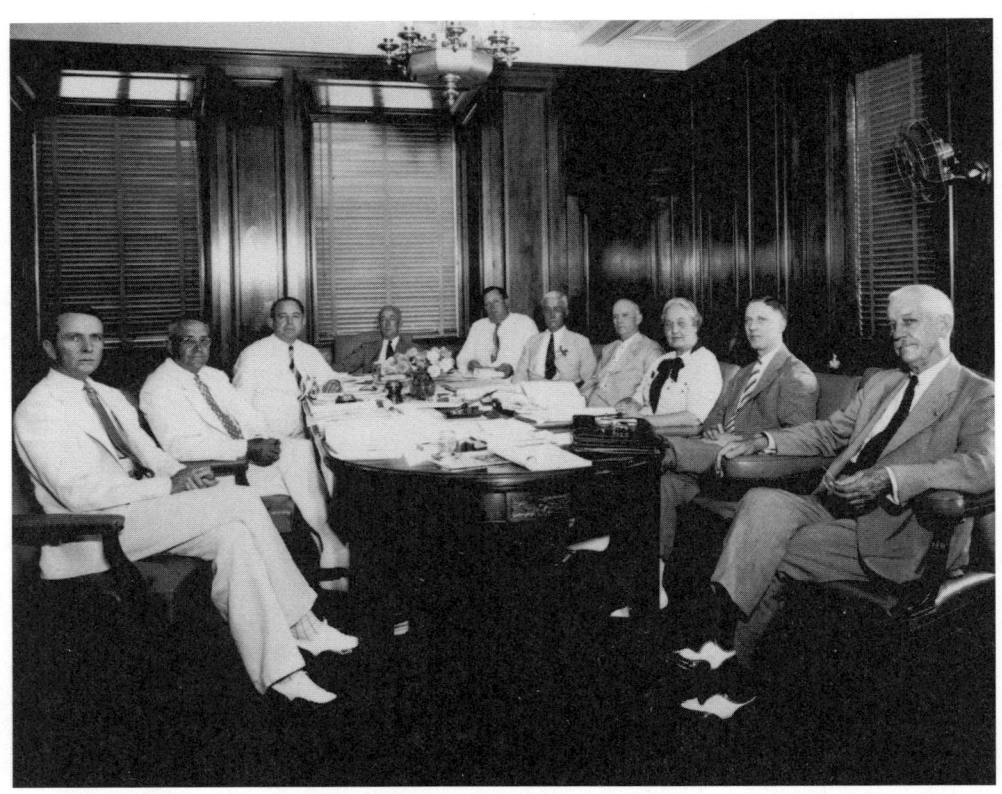

University of Texas Board of Regents, 1937. From left, J. R. Parten (vice chairman), H. J. Lutcher Stark, E. J. Blackert, J. W. Calhoun (UT president), H. H. Weinert, K. H. Aynesworth, Leslie Waggener, Mrs. I. D. Fairchild, Leo C. Haynes (secretary), and Edward Randall (chairman).

— 2 —

Political Networks and Executive Leaders

"Lots of people think for example that I am entirely too optimistic and cheerful. It may be the only defense I have against being so tremendously depressed that I simply couldn't take it any longer. All my life I have tried to promote a feeling of optimism and cheer with expressions of kindliness and goodwill to other people. It really gets to be a sort of a habit, and I am glad of it, because it has helped keep me sane in what is really a very unpleasant world. We can take our choice of looking at things pleasantly or in a depressed way. After all, it is a lot more fun to see interesting and cheerful things in the world than to see these things otherwise. But it does take a direct effort of will to try always to have equanimity and generosity."—Chauncey D. Leake, February 13, 1952[1]

UTMB originated within deliberately created interpersonal networks of political power and authority. The founders designed these networks and subsequent leaders sustained and changed them. How each led colleagues and subordinates depended on specific hierarchical networks, the administrator's personality and style of management, the values embedded in the institution's policies, the issues associated with each daily problem or decision, and the social challenges of a particular era. UTMB's twentieth-century political dynamics are traced in this chapter by focusing on the ways each CEO functioned in the political networks.

After Dean Allen Smith returned to Philadelphia in 1903, William Carter became dean and CEO, and Waverley Smith (Jennie Sealy's lawyer-husband) replaced Spencer as a regent. Smith was one of eight Galvestonians who served as regents between 1903 and 1942 (Appendix C).[2] These and other regents played key roles in responding to those who remained disgruntled about the location of UTMB in Galveston. This chapter begins with a description of Carter's management of the first relocation frenzy.

The next section features the political revolution that occurred at UTMB during the late 1930s and early 1940s. The dual governance of boards of regents and boards of hospital managers created recurring problems. Because Edward Randall controlled so many transactions in these boards and other networks, political war erupted when John Spies torpedoed this power.

Chauncey Leake replaced the disorder of this revolution with stability and progress, though he struggled mightily with the university's leaders in Austin. Events associated with the conservative reflexibilities of John Truslow are presented next, followed by the years of fantastic growth under the leadership of Truman Blocker and Bill Levin. The chapter concludes with a focus on Tom James and the events proximate to UTMB's centennial years.

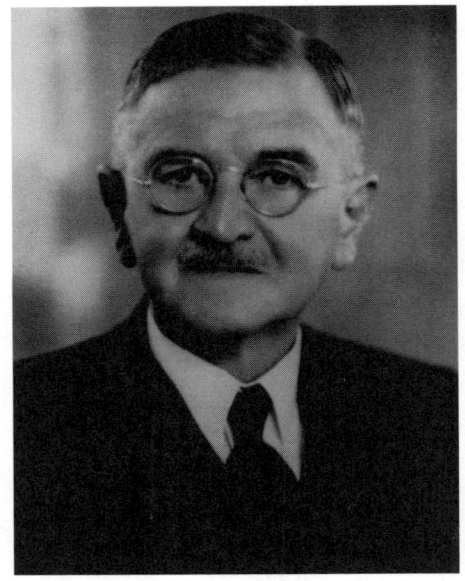

William S. Carter

First Relocation Frenzy

Carter persevered for nineteen years in his first incarnation as CEO.[3] His greatest political struggle involved the persistent legacy of negative sentiments against Galveston as the location of UTMB. The desires of UT presidents who wanted a single campus in Austin, the anxieties of Galveston's officials about the costs of caring for sick indigents, and the need to renegotiate the city's lease of the John Sealy Hospital initiated the first relocation frenzy that lasted from 1911 to 1920.

Many questioned the propriety of living in Galveston after the devastating hurricane of 1900. Although the seawall, grade-raising, and new bridges did improve the city's safety, population growth remained relatively static while that of other cities, especially Houston and Dallas, grew significantly. Those loyal to UT posed a not unreasonable question: should UTMB, site of the state university's only schools of medicine, pharmacy, and nursing, be moved to a larger city where even more sick Texans could receive state-supported medical care? Although UT presidents Winston and William Prather had supported UTMB's existence in Galveston, their successors had serious doubts about UTMB's future in a city so far from the main campus and so vulnerable to recurring storms.[4]

After Abraham Flexner visited Galveston in November 1909, he agreed with the UT presidents. He believed that the decision to locate UTMB away from the main university had been a "regrettable mischance." "Were it placed at Austin," he declared, "it would apparently gain in every way: the town is as large, and various state institutions there would strengthen its clinical opportunities; it would be easier to attract and to hold outsiders in teaching positions; the stimulus of the university would assist the growth of a productive spirit. Whether at Galveston the school will ever be creative is a question; should it become so, isolation increases the liability to slip back into an unproductive groove. Perhaps it is not yet too late for the people of the state to concentrate their state institutions of higher learning in a single plant." But there was no

Sealy family in Austin who could provide the dollars needed for new buildings to house a hospital and medical school.[5]

Carter wanted expansion in Galveston. He persistently requested funds for a new laboratory building, a pavilion to house contagious patients, additional quarters for sick women and children, and a new residence for nursing students. But the regents had no money for construction in Galveston because they assigned scarce Available University Fund resources to the Austin campus and because general revenue funds appropriated by the legislatures to the regents could not be used for construction in Austin or Galveston. Although regents and presidents acknowledged the needs, they were unwilling to allocate Available University Fund money for expansion in Galveston. "There is no question of the need, but I had hoped that we might be able to bring at least a portion of the Medical Department to Austin," declared President Mezes to Regent George Brackenridge, "and have not for that reason considered that much addition to the plant there would be necessary or desirable for the present." Mezes wanted UTMB in Austin.[6]

Galveston's officials periodically balked at the idea of spending so much city money for indigents. In 1911 Mezes informed Regent Chair Clarence Ousley, a former Galvestonian, that Mayor Lewis Fisher wanted to reduce the city's annual contribution to the hospital. Fisher claimed that non-residents received more hospital care than the city's residents. Fisher was mistaken. Legal residents of Galveston constituted the majority of inpatients (71 percent in 1908, 74 percent in 1909) and charity patients constituted the largest number of these (91 percent in 1908, 88 percent in 1909). Carter quickly persuaded the city commissioners to continue their annual contribution of $30,000.[7]

The need to renegotiate the city's lease of the John Sealy Hospital provided another opportunity to deal with relocation or expansion. Carter, Marvin Graves, and Edward Randall urged the regents to support expansion in Galveston. In a carefully orchestrated spree of cooperation, the regents, Jennie Sealy Smith, and John Sealy II negotiated an agreement with the city commissioners. If the commissioners renewed the hospital's lease before October 1914 and pledged to continue their annual contribution of $30,000, the Sealy siblings would donate $50,000 for a new women's hospital and the regents would contribute $50,000 for a new nurses' home. In January 1913 the commissioners accepted this proposal and signed a new twenty-five-year lease.[8] The same mix of private, city, and state dollars that started UTMB now supported growth that made it much more difficult to relocate the institution.

The new hospital attracted more patients and costs escalated. Though Carter convinced UT President Robert Vinson and the regents that the state should completely manage the hospital, legislators were unwilling to provide dollars for hospital expenses for the biennium 1919–1921. Moreover, Sealy did not want the hospital to become a fully state-funded institution. Not only would he and his family lose prestige and power with such an arrangement, but Galveston's sick poor could be displaced if too many non-residents were admitted and if St. Mary's Infirmary negotiated a less expensive contract with the city for treating indigents.[9] Sealy preferred to honor his father's legacy with periodic donations that would keep the hospital financially solvent.

This first frenzy about relocation became very intense in 1919 and 1920. In 1919 John Rockefeller gave $20 million to the General Education Board (GEB) for distribution to medical schools who wished to improve their facilities. Carter invited Flexner, the board's secretary, to visit Galveston so they could discuss the possibility of acquiring some Rockefeller money for the construction of a laboratory building needed for teaching and research in the basic sciences.[10]

In January 1920 Flexner and others visited Baylor Medical School in Dallas and UTMB. Citizens in Dallas had raised half a million dollars for Baylor's school and Baylor University had pledged $1 million for the school. This impressed Flexner and the GEB gave $300,000 to Baylor. In Galveston, Flexner again expressed considerable doubt about the future of UTMB.[11] He did not believe that a "big medical school" could develop "in a small place," unless it controlled its own hospital. He thought that Dallas and Houston were more appropriate cities for the state's medical school. The GEB did not give any money to UTMB.

The distress of this predicament worsened when Galveston's city commissioners reduced their hospital appropriation for fiscal year 1921 from $30,000 to $10,000. Vinson and the regents agreed that "the entire present plant of the Medical Branch must in the very near future be abandoned." The attitudes of the city commissioners greatly distressed Sealy, Carter, and Randall. Sealy was not willing "to continue the help for the institution" which he had previously given. "The predicament of our hospital is acute and alarming," proclaimed Randall, who realized that Galveston would lose UTMB if John Sealy Hospital closed, because there were other cities in Texas clamoring for the state's only health professional schools.[12]

Regent W. R. Brents wanted UTMB moved to Houston. "Houston offers many advantages which cannot be secured in Galveston," Brents told Vinson. Regent W. H. Dougherty of Gainesville thought that the development of Baylor's medical school in Dallas would eventually "kill" the institution in Galveston. "Galveston is dead," declared Dougherty.[13]

In June 1920 Gov. William Hobby appointed a legislative committee to determine whether or not UTMB should be moved to a larger city. During the summer and fall of 1920, claims, counterclaims, investigations, and negotiations occurred in the struggles between university officials, hospital managers, city commissioners, state legislators, and passionate citizens. After numerous organizations in Galveston protested the relocation of UTMB, the city commissioners relented and allocated $30,000 for the new fiscal year.[14]

Statewide competition became fierce, however. Citizen-physician groups lobbied for Dallas and Houston. Even more troubling, N. P. Colwell, the prestigious secretary of the AMA's Council on Medical Education and Hospitals, believed that removal of UTMB to a larger city would enable it to develop more satisfactorily.[15] The governor's committee held two days of hearings in Galveston in early November 1920. Vinson

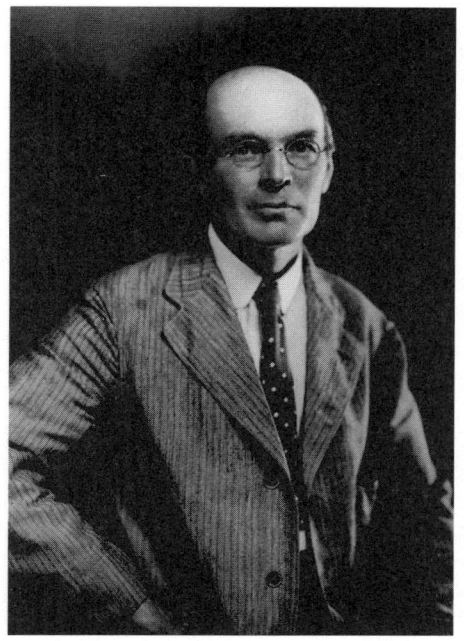

William Keiller

testified that UTMB's physical campus was "utterly inadequate"; that there had been a serious decline in the number of inpatients, which jeopardized clinical teaching; and that there had been too many difficulties negotiating with the city commissioners. He had "no desire to be President of a third-class, jackleg medical college." Among others, Mart Royston, Edward Randall Sr., Marvin Graves, A. O. Singleton, and John Sealy II lobbied for UTMB.[16]

The committee released its report in December. Because there had been considerable agitation about moving the main campus in Austin, the committee decided that no decision about UTMB should be made until a final decision had been made about the main campus.[17] The committee did recommend that John Sealy Hospital become a fully funded state hospital and that the physical plant be upgraded. Because of the power and diplomacy of Carter and Randall, and the fluke of a simultaneous relocation dither about the Austin campus, this first frenzy about relocating UTMB disappeared until the persisting political and economic tensions ignited a second one about twenty-five years later.

After receiving a leave of absence that allowed him to serve the Rockefeller Foundation by developing medical schools in other countries, Carter left Galveston in late February 1922. During the next sixteen years, the regents and the next four UT presidents selected professors at UTMB to be CEOs (Appendix A). They appointed William Keiller as Carter's replacement. Sixty-year-old Keiller had served the school as professor of anatomy for thirty-one years. Keiller gave special attention to the School of Pharmacy, noting that its status as "an appendage of the Medical College" placed UTMB "altogether behind the times." Keiller pleaded for a new pharmacy building in Galveston and courted officers of the Texas Pharmaceutical Association who were willing to solicit donations for such a building. But these donations did not materialize. Keiller continued as dean until the spring of 1926, when the bacteria that cause tuberculosis reappeared in his sputum, prompting his resignation.[18]

As Keiller's successor, the regents selected Henry Hartman, a 1907 graduate, who had been chair of the Pathology Department for thirteen years. In 1927 the School of Pharmacy moved to Austin, a relocation prompted by the desires of its dean for a larger and nationally acceptable school, a need for more laboratory and classroom space because of more students, and the recommendation of the Texas Pharmaceutical Association. Galveston's Chamber of Commerce blamed politics and "foreign influences" for the

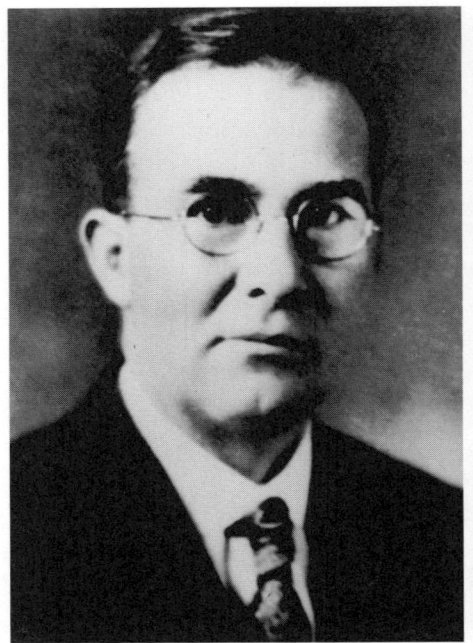

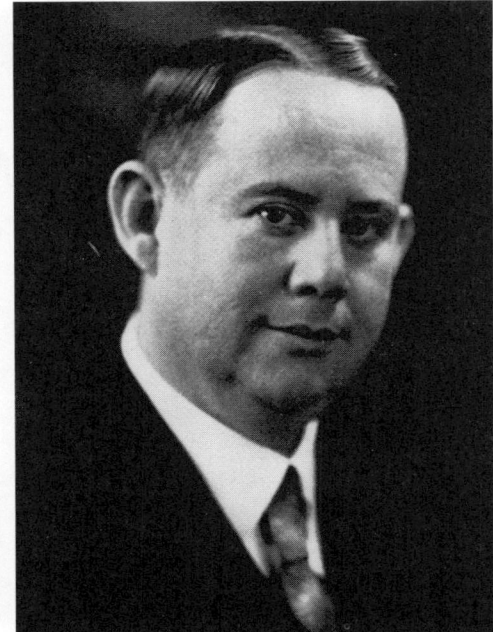

Henry Hartman   George Bethel

move. Hartman resigned the following year. Thirty-four-year-old George Bethel, a 1917 graduate, succeeded Hartman. Bethel had taught anatomy for a short time before becoming director of the health service at UT Austin. He moved to Galveston in early August and was dean and CEO for seven years.[19]

EDWARD RANDALL, JOHN SPIES, AND REVOLUTION

Like Keiller and Hartman, Bethel struggled with imbalances in the political networks. The Executive Committee still wielded foremost powers. Though Randall claimed that this committee was only advisory to the president through the dean, Bethel thought that it acted as if its decisions were "final in certain cases." Randall's omnipotence intimidated Bethel. In response to one of Randall's power moves in 1933, Bethel exclaimed, "I do not like to be a rubber stamp, but I have had to be on many occasions in this institution, and it looks like it is not going to be the last time that I will have to be one."[20] Although Bethel resented Randall's dominance, he knew that remarkably little had happened at UTMB without Randall's imprint.

Randall had received a medical degree from the University of Pennsylvania in 1883 and had begun practice in Galveston in 1886. From 1891 to 1928 he was professor of materia medica and therapeutics. He was the major player in UTMB's political networks for many years. He was a member of the Executive Committee for twenty-five years (1898–1899; 1903–1905; 1906–1928); a member of the John Sealy Hospital Board of Managers for thirty-nine years (1902–1941) and president for thirty-two of those years (1909–1941); charter member and president of the Sealy & Smith

Foundation for twenty-two years (1922–1944); and a member of the UT Board of Regents for eleven years (1929–1940).[21]

When Bethel died in 1935, Randall suggested that sixty-seven-year-old William Carter, who had retired from the Rockefeller Foundation, be invited to serve again as CEO. Carter returned in August. The regents appointed Carter as chair of both the Executive Committee and the John Sealy College of Nursing Committee, and "Dean of Student Life at Galveston."[22] The Executive Committee transacted business between general faculty meetings, approved faculty appointments, advised the dean about budgets, planned changes for the campus, admitted students, and handled decisions of the Student Honor Council.

The John Sealy College of Nursing Committee recommended faculty candidates for the nursing school and determined curricular policies for the nursing students. The regents authorized a Student Social Organization Committee (three faculty members appointed by the president after nomination by the Executive Committee) to oversee student organizations, including fraternities.[23] They also authorized a Library Committee to consult with the librarian regarding the work and growth of the library. Though these three committees acknowledged the existence and importance of nurses, students, and librarians, their deliberations evinced more symbolic than real power. After more than four decades of institutional evolution, political governance of faculty and students still remained structurally centralized within the wills of a small number of individuals (the Executive Committee) and functionally dominated by the desires of only two professors: Edward Randall and A. O. Singleton.

An assessment of UTMB's national reputation catalyzed revolutionary changes. Members of the AMA's Council on Medical Education visited Galveston in January 1936 to inspect UTMB as part of a national survey of medical education project. Carter received their seventy-page report in the summer of 1937.[24]

Although the report's evaluation did not jeopardize UTMB's standing as a first-class school, and although the site visitors acknowledged that an "unusually high type of teaching" was being done at UTMB, graphs in the report exerted tremendous influence on the regents. These graphs ranked the facilities and programs of sixty-six approved four-year medical schools in the United States. UTMB's graph indicated that its reputation had fallen considerably from that of previous years. Only in terms of income (because of the Sealy & Smith Foundation), dean's office administration (because of Carter), and the Department of Anatomy (because of its museum and teachers), did UTMB rank in the upper 20 percent of American medical schools. Many of its ranks were in the middle percentiles, though this was true of other reputable schools because of widespread standardization among all schools between 1925 and 1935.[25] In terms of adequate personnel and physical facilities for some of the basic science departments and for pediatrics, UTMB ranked in the lowest 30 percent.

This situation alarmed the three regents who served on the committee overseeing UTMB (Appendix C). They chanted a need for reforms after Carter left in the summer of 1938. These included seventy-seven-year-old Randall; sixty-four-year-old K. H.

Aynesworth, a Waco surgeon who had graduated from UTMB in 1899; and forty-one-year-old J. R. Parten, a Houston oil man who wanted to "search widely and investigate intensively before any person is selected" as the new dean.[26]

Aynesworth aggressively trumpeted a need for improvement. "I have one heartache always," he remarked, "and that is that our own section of the country has not kept pace; we have spent too much time making excuses and proclaiming our excellency, which after all is whistling to keep up our courage as we go through the cemetery." Aynesworth wanted new departments, especially a Department of Public Health, more money for the school, and "men of the highest calibre" who would be productive as scientific researchers. The regents wanted an "outsider" who would undertake the unspecified "drastic reforms" needed to place UTMB back among the top American medical schools.[27]

This subcommittee of regents, a separate committee of UTMB alumni, and another committee of UTMB faculty considered several candidates, including two brothers, John and Tom Spies. These brothers were native Texans who had earned bachelor's degrees from UT Austin and medical degrees from Harvard. After postgraduate training in surgery, John taught and practiced at Yale, the Peking Union Medical College, and a cancer hospital in Bombay, India (1935–1938). Tom became an academic internist and nutritional researcher, who demonstrated in 1937 that nicotinic acid cured patients with pellagra.[28]

Thirty-eight-year-old Tom was attractive because he was a nationally renowned researcher and could be both dean and professor of public health, a linkage firmly established in the minds of the three regents. But Tom wanted to spend at least a third of his dean's time at the Hillman Hospital in Birmingham continuing his research, which was unacceptable to Randall. Moreover, UT President John Calhoun, who had first recommended the Spies brothers, thought it might be possible to make Tom a dean after his arrival at UTMB, but that he would not be one when he arrived. Thus, everyone was intrigued with Tom's suggestion that his forty-one-year-old brother, John, would make a better dean than he would. Tom assured everyone that he would accept the deanship if John refused.[29]

Randall opposed the local candidate, Edward Schwab, a part-time UTMB internist strongly endorsed by both alumni and faculty committees, and was enthralled with John Spies as a prospect. Randall met John in New York City and invited him to be dean without consulting anyone or without gathering more information. On Spies's first visit to Galveston in October 1938, Randall informed the search committees (during a luncheon) that Spies was the new dean. Nearly everyone was furious with Randall, but the die had been cast. Aynesworth, Parten, and Calhoun decided to support Spies. The regents appointed John Spies as dean and CEO and Tom as a salaried distinguished professor of medical research who could begin work in Galveston whenever he was ready.[30]

In January 1939 John Spies began his new job in Galveston. Within nine months, UTMB was embroiled in a nasty civil war. Regent Chair Parten urged Spies to assume

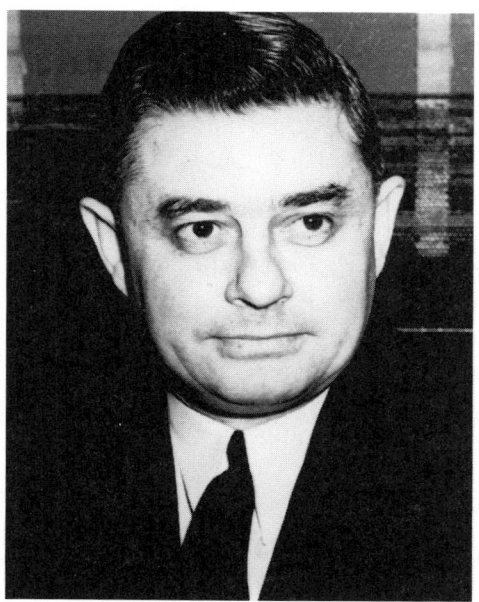

John Spies, 1942.

authoritative control at UTMB. Supporting Spies, UT President Homer Rainey persuaded the regents to amend their rules, thereby reducing the longstanding power of the Executive Committee. Spies supported Aynesworth, who blocked the appointment of three highly valued teachers to distinguished professorships. Spies publicly labeled hospital administrator Lucius Wilson a "liar," and recommended dismissal of the entire nursing faculty and three highly respected professors, including Edward Schwab. Spies also prepared a thirty-page report about several faculty members that was sent to Rainey a few days before six regents conducted a three-day investigation in early October. Testimony given and documents displayed during these hearings in Galveston generated more than a thousand pages of evidence that depicted a political revolution occurring at UTMB.[31]

Three major problems existed. One was the monopoly of power Edward Randall held because of his multiple roles in the political networks. The second involved the legacy of political control that had been vested in the Executive Committee for more than forty years. The old rules permitted the faculty to elect members of the Executive Committee. The new rules allowed the president to appoint members after conferring with the dean. The old rules allowed the Executive Committee to control the affairs of the institution; the new rules transformed this group into a committee that was "advisory" to the dean. Randall attacked Aynesworth as the person responsible for the changes, claiming that he was usually "stirring up trouble." The third problem involved the legacy of the hospital's Board of Managers, a governing arrangement that caused multiple conflicts, particularly with the nursing students and the outpatient clinics. The director of the nursing school was also the "director of nurses" in the hospital and frequently served as the director of the hospital until Lucius Wilson acquired that role in 1928 (Appendix F). Spies claimed that Dora Mathis, then director of nursing, inappropriately dismissed a nursing student because that authority resided with the director of the hospital or with him as the dean of student life. Spies also argued that the John Sealy College of Nursing Committee included unauthorized members and that he, not Mathis, was chair of this committee, which should function as an "advisory" committee to him and not as an "executive" committee for the nursing school. When Randall proclaimed that "The duty of the School of Nursing is to supply nurses to the hospital," Spies retorted, "the students in the College of Nursing are not there to supply nurses to the John Sealy Hospital, but they are there to be educated in nursing."[32] Spies really wanted improvements in the academic status of the nursing school.

Similar conflicts about political control affected decisions about a proposed cancer clinic. Spies wanted to develop a clinic that would involve collaboration between surgeons, radiologists, and pathologists as they attended patients, taught students, and conducted research. The American College of Surgeons had published a list of hospitals that had adopted some standards for operating such clinics. This list identified only three in Texas: Baylor's teaching hospital in Dallas and two hospitals in Temple. Randall commented: "You know, Gentlemen as well as I do that hospitals can get themselves listed in publications such as that very easily with a minimum amount of work; and as for Baylor setting up a first class Clinic, I don't believe that for a second." A few minutes later, Randall declared that if members of the American College of Surgeons came to Galveston, "they would give us just as much credit as those. I don't know anything about Baylor."[33] Randall's credibility waned.

Randall and Singleton obstinately opposed a new cancer clinic, in part because they feared that Spies would use the clinic to attract private patients who they would otherwise treat. Singleton would not allow Spies to be a faculty member in the Department of Surgery, thereby blocking access to patients for Spies. Said Spies: "I am blocked. I can't get any chance to see cancer patients or to organize a Cancer Clinic or nothing. I don't want to talk about myself, but I am the only Dean in the United States that has been trained in cancer work, yet we are doing less here than any other place. There was a report showing that the Federal Government has approved nineteen centers for training people in cancer research, yet I can't get a thing done here." Spies wanted a "State Cancer Institute" at UTMB.[34]

Regent Leslie Waggener sympathized with Singleton: "A man does not care how many full professorships he has in a department provided they all run to him and he has the last word and what he says goes and they do what he says to do; but he can't conceive of that situation with Dr. Spies in his department, and he does not want to give up control of his department." Regent Chair Parten addressed Singleton: "It seems cruel that you can't use him [Spies]." Singleton responded: "Don't you think it is kind of cruel to promise the Dean certain things without knowing whether it will interfere with other people?" Parten replied: "I grant you that but I was led into that, but I think this Board is under obligation to him, and I doubt if Dr. Spies will stay here if he is denied permanently the right to put his hand in surgery." Singleton responded: "If Dr. Spies claims to be a surgeon, then I can't see why he would not make plans to go on in surgery rather than to go into deaning and public health service. He has been accepted here as Professor of Public Health and Dean, and his interests are not in any of these things; he is interested in surgery." Singleton's concerns were substantial.[35]

Singleton had been very distressed about the way Spies became dean. Randall admitted that he had had no understanding of Spies's work as a surgeon. "It transpires," declared Randall, "that he knows very little about public health. He is a research worker in cancer. The whole propaganda was conducted by Tom Spies, his distinguished brother, at a meeting of the Board of Regents of the University of Texas, when they were looking for a Dean." When Spies visited Galveston, Randall added, "He never said anything about being a surgeon or his ambition to be a surgeon. He was not elected surgeon. I freely confess to you it never occurred to me that he wanted to be on the surgical staff. It never occurred to me that he had other ambitions. I thought that he wanted to be Dean of the Medical School and Professor of Public Health and stop there, but his ambition has carried him far, and you have given autocratic powers, and he is asserting autocratic powers." "Now," concluded Randall, "looking back I realize that Dr. Spies was elected by the committee and by me, as Chairman, without the proper investigation, and if a man ever sweat [sic] blood over that question, I have."[36] Randall would ever regret the tactic he used in appointing Spies.

The three days of hearings left Parten, fellow regents, and UTMB faculty exhausted and demoralized. D. Bailey Calvin, associate professor of biochemistry, succinctly captured the essence of the political moment at UTMB: "We have had a dictator, if you please, now we are in danger of having another dictator. I don't know which would be the worst of the two."[37] The worst was yet to come as three more years of power struggles shattered the institution's public reputation.

In the early months of 1940 Rainey continued his support for Spies, including approval of a peculiar arrangement for reorganizing the top administrative structures at UTMB that sustained the dominant powers of Spies and Rainey. The regents, however, began to question their support of Spies and Rainey. Regent Stark proposed that Spies be given "a perpetual leave of absence." Although the motion was not seconded, it signaled a divisiveness that would become more intense during the ensuing months.[38]

Resignations and personnel changes occurred. Randall resigned as regent, but continued as president of the Sealy & Smith Foundation Board. The regents appointed A. J. Peterson and L. E. Dowd to the John Sealy Hospital Board of Managers, replacing Randall and Mart Royston, whose terms had expired.[39] Singleton resigned as a member of this board. Lucius Wilson resigned as the hospital's director, prompting public controversies between Wilson, George Sealy Jr., and Randall.[40]

In November 1940 Gov. W. Lee "Pappy" O'Daniel assured Spies of his support for a major increase in state dollars if UTMB acquired complete control of the John Sealy Hospital complex. Between mid-November 1940 and mid-March 1941 the Galveston City Commissioners of Galveston, the John Sealy Hospital Board, and the Sealy & Smith Foundation Board negotiated a dissolution of the hospital board and the transfer of complete authority for operating the hospital complex to the regents.[41] This was the most significant change in UTMB's power networks since the institution's establishment.

The controversies and struggles intensified during the summer of 1941. In July Rainey announced that Spies would not be reappointed as dean, but would continue as professor of preventive medicine and public health and as director of a new cancer research program that had received $500,000 from the legislature. This announcement generated a two-week maelstrom of public debate that revealed extraordinary support for Spies. In addition to some faculty, students, and alumni, these pro-Spies advocates included the Galveston County Medical Society, the Texas State Medical Association, the Texas State Board of Medical Examiners, some key legislators (including Rep. Arthur Cato of Weatherford, who had submitted the cancer research hospital bill), George Sealy Jr., and Dan Kempner. These boosters cast Spies as an educational progressive who had wrested control of UTMB from a small clique of reactionary conservatives. Spies had expanded clinical services, had garnered more support for faculty research than ever before, had supported the development of a four-quarter medical school curriculum that trained more doctors, and had obtained massive increases in funds from the Forty-seventh Legislature. After twenty-six people testified at their meeting on July 26, 1941, the regents reappointed Spies as dean and CEO for two years.[42]

Important pendulum shifts occurred during the following weeks. Bolstered by the regents' reversal, Spies became more imperious. Recognizing an impasse that was destroying their institution, UTMB's professors finally rose from four decades of political sleep and demanded "the intelligent, informed, and constructive participation of the entire faculty" in the governing process. When the faculty adopted a "Statement of Policy" in early September that requested a reconstitution of the Executive Committee and the delegation of proper authority to departments, Rainey became so threatened that he asked the regents to abandon the Medical Branch subcommittee that had monitored UTMB for fifty years. The regents denied Rainey's bid for exclusive authority after hearing testimony from eighteen professors who wanted a newly empowered Executive Committee.[43] The regents were now listening to the professors.

Buoyed by these events, the professors circulated a sixteen-page document to alumni that contained many specific accusations. Spies violated university rules, intimidated younger faculty, admitted improperly qualified students, urged departments to pass students who had failed, and did not dismiss failing students. "The Faculty has utterly no confidence in the Dean's willingness and ability to maintain high standards of scholarship, teaching and research work." This petition circulated in mid-November, just before the regents' monthly meeting. During that meeting, the regents considered changes in their rules that would brake Rainey's quest for absolute power, dilute Spies's authority in Galveston, and support the professors' desires for more self-governing authority.[44]

In December the regents approved these changes. The Executive Committee, though remaining "advisory," now consisted of three clinical and three pre-clinical professors who had been nominated by the entire faculty. The president appointed faculty committees from recommendations submitted by the faculty without a need for the dean's approval. The new rules also permitted the dean to admit only those students who the Executive Committee had approved. Before this meeting ended, fellow regents rejected a motion by Aynesworth to eliminate the Medical Branch subcommittee and another motion by Aynesworth to conduct a new investigation of UTMB. Aynesworth had lost his power and Rainey and Spies had lost Aynesworth's influence.[45]

Because Spies was labeled a Nazi sympathizer, the Texas House of Representatives established a Committee on Un-American Activities to investigate UTMB. In mid-February 1942 a hurricane of accusations was made against Spies during two days of hearings in Galveston. Spies had never revealed that he had been discharged from Peking's Union Medical College in 1935. Spies had employed a professor who was an imposter and continued supporting him for eighteen months despite serious objections by the faculty.[46] Spies diverted funds from a UTMB research grant to the pockets of his brother, who still worked in Birmingham. Spies kept a "spy book" about faculty and used teachers, students, and technicians as spies throughout the campus. He recorded conversations with faculty and others via a dictograph hidden in his office. He was accused of intimidating and threatening students, and of appearing in public drunk.[47] Spies was thoroughly discredited.

Less than a week after the hearings, the legislative committee released its thousand-page transcript of testimony and conclusions.[48] They found no "un-American" activity at UTMB except a "failure to devote full efforts to training and production of doctors." They recommended that Spies be dismissed and that Rainey be vested with "full power and responsibility" to operate UTMB. They thought that the regents were "grossly negligent in permitting the present conditions to grow and exist" and that the regents were "primarily responsible for the decline and the disrepute of the Medical Branch." Statewide reputation was at stake. AAMC representatives who had inspected UTMB in January agreed with this committee. The AAMC's Executive Council recommended that its members place UTMB on probation during the AAMC annual meeting later that year. National accreditation was now at stake. Rainey's back was against the wall. The first public sign of a major rift between Rainey and Spies occurred in April, when Rainey supported Houston as the site for the university's cancer hospital and refused to name Spies as its administrator. Spies knew that he had lost Rainey's support completely.[49]

In May the AMA's Council on Medical Education sent inspectors to UTMB to determine if the council should also recommend probation. During the week of this site visit, Spies realized that his days as dean were numbered. Publicly and privately Spies attempted to shift blame to Rainey and the regents. "At all times," he declared," I am subject to instructions from my superior, President Homer P. Rainey of the University of Texas, and it is my understanding that the Board of Regents should issue directions to me through him in the usual manner adopted by University administrations. So far as I know I have at all times adhered to the above. Therefore, if anybody has any fault to find with the administration of the Medical Branch in Galveston, he should remember that same is the responsibility of the President and the Board of Regents as above described and not that of the Dean. Thus, the responsibility should be placed where it belongs, and I am willing to assume mine as a subordinate who carries out instructions."[50] Spies remained a martyr to the bitter end.

On June 5, after a two-week meeting in Galveston, the regents announced that they would appoint an "Executive Vice President of the Medical Branch of the University" who would be responsible to the regents through the president. Spies's power was officially curtailed and Rainey was expected to oversee UTMB until the new CEO was employed.[51]

A political revolution had occurred at UTMB between 1939 and 1942. Spies curtailed the formidable powers of two part-time clinicians, Edward Randall and A. O. Singleton. Randall resigned as a regent. Randall and Singleton resigned from the John Sealy Hospital Board of Managers and that board dissolved in 1941. With Spies at the helm, the regents assumed complete control of the hospital and a sizable increase in state funds became available for hospital operations. During Spies's tenure there was more support for medical education by UT officials than ever before and more state dollars for the entire institution than ever before.

As important were Spies's influences on nursing education and research. Spies wanted improved academic status for the School of Nursing and better education for the nursing students. He hired several research scientists as professors, and he truly believed that basic science and clinical research should be primary goals of the School of Medicine faculty. Although he did not conduct much research in Galveston and he could not forego the power dramas to become manager of a major cancer research program, Spies set the stage for an extraordinary change in corporate leadership.[52]

CHAUNCEY LEAKE: ORDER AND PROGRESS

With his wife, Elizabeth, and two teenage sons, forty-six-year-old Chauncey Leake motored from San Francisco to Galveston in September 1942.[53] Leake was ready to begin his twentieth year as a professor and his first as a CEO. He had earned a Ph.D. from the University of Wisconsin in 1923 and then taught pharmacology, physiology, and the history of science there until 1928, when he moved to San Francisco to establish a Department of Pharmacology for the University of California's School of Medicine. Titled executive vice president and dean, Leake became the only non-physician to serve as UTMB's CEO during its first century (Appendix A).

Leake had accepted an extraordinary political challenge. Rainey and the regents expected him to reorganize UTMB, but they offered no plan for that reorganization. Eager to control Rainey, the regents decided that Leake should report directly to them. But Leake knew that he had to establish a good working relationship with Rainey, who had, without the regents' approval, offered Leake a carrot of authority for administering an expanded program of health care professional education under the auspices of the University of Texas.[54] Even before Leake left San Francisco, the regents assumed control of the Texas Dental College at Houston and began planning other units for a proposed Texas Medical Center.

Like the waves cascading on Galveston's shores, events and decisions steadily challenged Leake, who quickly became aware of the geographical and cultural differences between San Francisco and Galveston. "Couldn't be a greater contrast than that between San Francisco and Galveston," he told a friend. "Galveston is flat, hot and quite quaint. Whatever cultural activities exist must be from within. It is a proud place." Leake appeared to thrive in the new setting. "So far it's been nothing but heat, hard work, and confusion here," he wrote to another friend. "However, I am enjoying it immensely and I am finding the opportunity very challenging." "Believe me," he

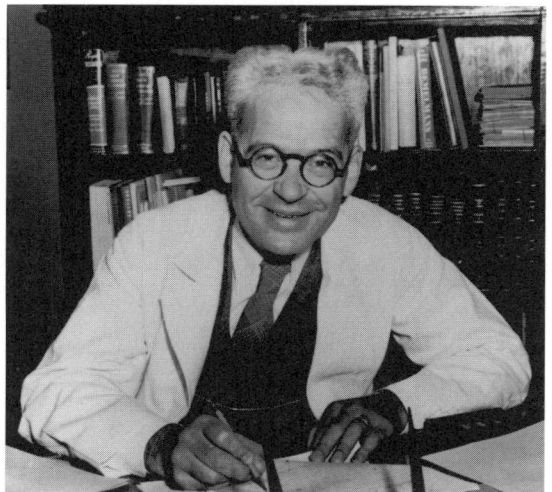

Chauncey Leake Jr., October 1942.

exclaimed, "it's something when 'the eyes of Texas are upon you.'" During the fall of 1942 his correspondence was so extensive that three secretaries prepared his letters and reports.[55]

Leake skillfully reintroduced faculty participation in policy decisions. He invited an advisory committee of alumni and faculty to make recommendations regarding facilities and programs. He invited the chairs of the five major clinical departments in the medical school (obstetrics and gynecology, pediatrics, medicine, surgery, and neuropsychiatry) to function as a committee in developing policies about patient care. He engineered two changes in the regents' rules to give more support to Marjorie Bartholf, the new dean of the John Sealy College of Nursing. One established a liaison committee between the medical and nursing schools, and the other permitted Bartholf to become an *ex-officio* member of the Executive Committee, now named the Faculty and Admissions Committee.[56]

Leake and the faculty were soon ready for re-accreditation inspections. AAMC representatives visited UTMB in May 1943 and AMA representatives visited in September. Both organizations removed UTMB from probationary status in November, an important step in boosting morale throughout the entire institution.[57]

Leake supported the expansion of UT medical units. On New Year's Day 1943 the *Dallas Morning News* published his full-page statement about UT's health education programs. Leake acknowledged the outstanding accomplishments of the dental school and the M. D. Anderson Institute for Cancer Research, both in Houston. He acknowledged the efforts of the Hogg Foundation to improve mental hygiene and he characterized UTMB as "the University Center for basic instruction in medicine, nursing, public health, and auxiliary fields." He hoped that UT would develop a School of Public Health, an Institute for Geographic Medicine, and an Institute for Geriatrics. He fully supported the development of Baylor's institutions in Houston and those of the Southwestern Medical Foundation in Dallas.[58] Leake fearlessly grasped the size and potential of the Lone Star State.

Satisfied with Leake's accomplishments and bubbling with future dreams, the regents began a process of evaluating the university's entire medical education program. During their first review session in November 1943, a discussion of the possibility of moving UTMB to Austin set the stage for the second relocation frenzy, which was centered in Rainey's quest for total political control.[59]

During the next six months Rainey prepared a ninety-four-page report on the future of the University of Texas. He argued that UT Austin had made great strides in its development during the preceding twenty-five years, especially as an institution for research and graduate study. UT Austin was one of four universities in the South that was part of the Association of American Universities. In contrast, UTMB had "simply not kept pace with the development of the rest of the University" and continued "to lag far behind."[60] Rainey recommended a major overhaul of UT's health professional schools, beginning with the relocation of UTMB and the new dental school in Houston. He claimed that these schools could be operated more economically and efficiently in Austin.

After listening to Rainey's arguments in July 1944, the regents invited remarks from Leake, who began by refuting Rainey's claims that UT's schools exhibited "glaring deficiencies." Leake thought it was unfair to claim that the "present health education situation is poorly coordinated and uneconomical, or difficult to administer." Ideally, "perhaps," the various schools should be together, but "the fact is they are not all together," Leake added. "The good people of Texas decided that long ago." He then named six private medical schools and six state university medical schools whose medical campuses were separate from the main campus, separations that created no special problems for these schools. Leake then emphasized that the primary problem in the UT program was not location, but adequate financial and political support. He thought it was desirable to establish more than one center for health professional education in the "big" state of Texas. Unlike Rainey, Leake understood the virtues of diffusing UT power and money.[61]

Leake searched for ways to dance through these political fireworks without serious injury. He was distressed about Rainey's misleading statements and especially about the way Rainey handled relationships with the regents. The regents had asked Rainey to work with Leake and dental school Dean Fred Elliott to prepare the report about the university's statewide program. Without conversing with anyone, Rainey presented his recommendations to the regents. Moreover, violating the regents' requests, Rainey released his report to the press and distributed ten thousand copies to various Texans. Leake firmly disagreed with Rainey's belief that public controversy was a way to gather support for the university.[62]

Leake and Rainey had parted political company, though they were never fireside buddies. In late August Leake captured the circumstances well in a comment to Ashley Montagu: "The President of the University has gotten ants in his pants. He wants to move the School away from Galveston to satisfy a pet peeve he's had for a number of years about some of the men on the staff. It's very annoying to me, but there isn't much I can do about it."[63] But Leake had done much about it. He defended progress at UTMB, he refuted erroneous claims Rainey made about UTMB, and he argued forcefully for a multi-center approach in the development of UT's health institutions.

The dramas of this second relocation frenzy occurred throughout the summer of 1944. The regents received many letters and testimonials about UTMB. Officers of the Galveston County Medical Society told the regents that Homer Rainey's statements about UTMB were "incorrect and untrue." In a letter to Regent Chair John H. Bickett Jr., Ray Bowen, president of the Galveston Chamber of Commerce, and A. D. Simpson, president of the Houston Chamber of Commerce, emphasized the extent of UT investments in Galveston and Houston. The Galveston Chamber of Commerce also established a special committee to lobby against Rainey's proposal. Led tirelessly and cleverly by I. H. "Ike" Kempner, this committee hired Sen. Carl Lovelady as a lobbyist and sent telegrams and letters to many individuals.[64]

The regents sided with Leake. On September 29, 1944, the regents declared that UTMB should remain in Galveston and that "further agitation about removing the Medical School from Galveston should stop as it is a detriment to the school." They also recommended acceptance of an offer of $2 million from the Sealy & Smith Foundation to construct a new teaching hospital and they recommended the construction of a laboratory building, a dormitory for women medical students, a gymnasium-auditorium, and an addition to the Rebecca Sealy Nurses' Home. They wanted to reopen the State Psychopathic Hospital, which had been closed by hurricane damage. They wanted to support the Department of Pediatrics by enlarging the Children's Hospital and remodeling the Stewart Convalescent Home for Children. The regents also supported further development of the M. D. Anderson Cancer Hospital and the dental school in Houston. Leake was ecstatic: "The Austin meeting was exciting. The Regents rejected all the President's proposals and put me on the spot by adopting as a policy what I had recommended!"[65] Rainey's credibility with the regents had disappeared.

About a month later the regents fired Rainey and appointed Theophilus S. Painter, a renowned professor of biology at UT Austin, as acting president. Regents Bickett, Hilmer H. Weinert, and Dan J. Harrison resigned. Leake interpreted the situation quite accurately: "The split has finally come between the Regents and the President. The President detailed to the faculty some sixteen instances which he considers to be violations of the proper relationships between a governing board and the President. While he attempts to make the issue one of academic freedom, it is quite apparent that it is really whether or not he is to be allowed to run things as he pleases without any control whatsoever. I still believe the whole matter is a build up for a political campaign for the Governorship!"[66]

Within two weeks Gov. Coke Stevenson appointed five senators to an "Investigating Committee" that began two weeks of hearings about these controversies.[67] The committee heard testimony from five regents, six professors from UT Austin and two from UTMB, Rainey, J. R. Parten, and a few others. Much of the testimony about UTMB involved the turbulence of the Spies years.

Regent Orville Bullington thought that removing UTMB from Galveston would ignore the traditions and generosity of the citizens of Galveston and would "militate against any plan of making it [UTMB] the medical center of Texas as it should be." Regent D. F. Strickland believed that Rainey entertained "as much hatred and ill will against the people of the Medical School as any man I ever saw." Rainey claimed that UTMB was "a mediocre school, always would be a mediocre school if it remained in Galveston, always had been, is now and always would be." But Strickland had obtained evidence that indicated that UTMB was "way above the average of the Medical Schools of the country." Strickland thought that Rainey's assertions about UTMB had insulted not only the students currently in training but the "thousands of doctors in Texas" who had been trained there. Strickland, like other regents, concluded that UTMB could never prosper under Rainey's administration. J. R. Parten testified about his experiences as a regent between 1935 and 1941, and called for Rainey's reinstatement, claiming that his courage would stand as an "everlasting monument" in the history of American education.[68]

The regents did not reinstate Rainey when they met on January 26, 1945. They continued to support Painter as the UT's new CEO. In early August Painter spent a week in Galveston to do "a little fishing," eat "a little seafood," and "get acquainted with the Medical School situation" so that he could be helpful to Leake and the faculty "in making the institution better and better with the passing of the months."[69] Painter was uncomfortable, however, because Leake acted as if he still had the same freedom that he had exercised during Rainey's administration and because Painter believed that the future of medical education in Texas involved the development of the Texas Medical Center in Houston.

But Painter underestimated the rugged determination of Galvestonians who supported UTMB, especially that of Sen. William Stone of Galveston and Ike Kempner, who had chaired the Galveston Chamber of Commerce's Medical College Committee for more than twenty years. Supported by donations from local businesses, Kempner's committee fought valiantly and successfully against a bill to relocate UTMB that had received a favorable vote by a senate committee in the spring of 1945. Both Stone and Kempner challenged Galvestonians to provide strong financial support for improvements at UTMB.[70]

With Stone, Kempner, and other boosters elevating his spirit, Leake persistently requested increases in UTMB's budget. As a way of controlling Leake's demands, imposing more order on the budgetary process, and reasserting the authority of the regents, Painter resurrected the budgetary authority of the Faculty and Admissions Committee, functions that had disappeared under Spies. After informing Leake about this decision, Painter told the Medical Committee of the regents that he felt much better about the general situation: "At the same time, you know and I know that I will still have to reach up every few weeks and pull Chauncey back down to earth."[71] Leake thought that such gravitational exercises were real slaps to his face.

By July 1946 Leake was telling some friends that "the new President turns out to be very stiff, and is cutting our budget to the point where we can't maintain the pretense of trying to be a first class institution. I am frankly discouraged and ready to quit this administration if I can get a job somewhere in teaching and research." The proposed UTMB budget for 1947 had been cut below the operating funds that had been used for fiscal year 1946 and Leake expected resignations and a loss of morale. "We are very depressed over the opposition of the University administration to the development of the Medical Branch," declared Leake in a letter to Ella Sealy Newell.[72] Less than four years after his arrival, Leake's exhilaration about UTMB was waning rapidly.

In 1947 Leake experienced another major change in administrative status. He had energetically supported the development of other UT health institutions. In December 1942, only a few months after his arrival in Texas, Leake approved the transfer of four UTMB professors to Houston as the initial group of researchers for the M.D. Anderson Hospital for Cancer Research, and Leake participated in ceremonies dedicating this new institution in February 1944. In March 1945 the regents reaffirmed their commitment to the development of this hospital, announced plans to construct a new building for the dental school, and declared their interest in establishing a School of Public Health and other institutions in Houston. In July 1947 the regents agreed that "it was neither reasonable nor fair" to impose upon Leake the responsibilities of administering the UT health units at Houston.[73] After five years of successful efforts in a role that he enjoyed, Leake was relieved of responsibilities for the expansion of UT health institutions.

In spite of this change, the continuing budgetary seesaws, and the uncomfortable strokes from the political brush of Painter, Leake's spirit remained positive until the advent of the UT System in 1950. To accommodate their decision to reorganize the university's central administration, the regents adopted new rules and regulations in April 1950. The regents appointed two principal administrators: a chancellor as CEO of the UT System, and a vice president and comptroller as the system's chief business officer. Ten component units comprised the UT System. The six health professional units included UTMB, the University of Texas Dental Branch (Houston), the University of Texas M. D. Anderson Hospital for Cancer Research (Houston), the University of Texas School of Public Health (Houston), the University of Texas Post-Graduate School of Medicine (Houston), and the University of Texas Southwestern Medical School (Dallas).[74] Each of these components would have two principal administrators: a chief executive officer and a chief business officer.

In becoming a system, UT's executives wanted to create more effective balances of centralized and decentralized powers between the administration in Austin and the component institutions. This new system was a response to a great increase in enrollment at UT Austin, the growth and expansion of UTMB, the establishment of five new component institutions between 1940 and 1950, the growth of the UT budget from $4 million in 1940 to almost $16 million in 1950, and the growing involvement of the federal government in higher education. Chancellors would be liberated from administrative details now delegated to the CEOs of the separate institutions. Chancellors could oversee matters of general policy and coordination as well as university transactions involving private organizations, state government, and the federal government. In July 1950 the regents named James P. Hart, associate justice of the Texas Supreme Court, as the first chancellor.[75] The system became functional on September 1, 1950, and Leake became accountable to Hart.

Leake's relationship with Hart was cordial until the fall of 1953 when, contrary to Leake's wishes, Hart and the regents selected George A. W. Currie as UTMB's new hospital administrator.[76] Currie challenged Leake's administrative organization. Leake had developed a fairly simple administrative structure, with eight individuals accountable to him for managing the business, hospital, and academic affairs of the institution (Appendix R). These included a business manager, an administrator for the hospitals, a director of the medical services curricula (the early label for what later became the allied health sciences), a dean of the nursing school, an associate dean who monitored the work of graduate students, a dean of the medical faculty, a dean for students and curriculum, and a librarian. Currie complicated Leake's administrative style by adding new accountabilities in the management matrix for the hospitals.

Financial troubles also plagued Leake. With the opening of the new John Sealy Hospital in 1954, expenses were greater than ever. The legislature, however, failed to appropriate the funds needed to operate the institution adequately and Leake became exceedingly frustrated. He told F. J. L. Blasingame that UTMB was "in a serious plight now."[77]

Another reorganization of the UT System added unbearable stress to Leake's spirit. The regents had employed the Texas Research League to conduct a thorough study of the current organizational arrangements of all system institutions. Staff members of the league identified numerous problems with the system in general and with UTMB in particular. Using their recommendations, the regents eliminated the label of chancellor and re-instituted the label of president for the CEO of the UT System, appointing Logan Wilson to that position on October 1, 1954.[78]

Two months later the regents reorganized many administrative roles in the component institutions, including several at UTMB. Under the new arrangements, only three individuals now reported to Leake: the dean of the nursing school (Bartholf), the dean of the medical school (Blocker), and the hospital and facilities administrator (Currie). One strikingly peculiar outcome of the reorganization was a flip-flop arrangement for Edgar Capplemann and George Currie. Capplemann, UTMB's CBO, who had worked effectively with Leake for nine years, now reported to Currie, who had been the hospital administrator for only one year. Another consequence of the rearrangement was the titular demotion of D. Bailey Calvin from dean of students to associate dean of students. Disorder and distress were compounded when Truman Blocker Jr. resigned as dean of the medical faculty in January 1955.[79]

In that same month, Wilson sent a memo to all employees in the UT System declaring that communications with legislators and other state officials should always be channeled through him and the regents. Exercising more centralized authority toward Leake than either Painter or Hart had displayed, Wilson altered Leake's "semi-autonomous" status as a power hitter for UTMB. In February Leake sent a letter of resignation to Wilson, who hurried to Galveston in early March to calm the faculty's fears. Leake interpreted the reforms as regental authoritarianism.[80] The scope and extent of centralized control was still a major political issue in UT's governance.

In June Leake accepted an offer to establish a Department of Pharmacology at the Ohio State University School of Medicine in Columbus. He functioned as acting executive director from February until his departure from Galveston in August 1955. To manage UTMB until a new executive director could be employed, the regents appointed an "Interim Executive Officer and Executive Committee," consisting of George Currie, Donald Duncan, Raymond Gregory, Titus Harris, Robert Moore, Charles Stone, and Truman Blocker Jr. as chair.[81]

JOHN TRUSLOW: PLANNING AND REFLEXIBILITY

In December 1955 Wilson and the regents selected forty-three-year-old John Truslow as UTMB's new CEO. The Faculty Advisory Committee had recommended Truslow, who was dean of the Medical College of Virginia. Truslow met with the Interim Committee in January 1956 and began full-time work on the first of April.[82]

Truslow developed new administrative networks. He received the regents' support for readjusting some of the awkward arrangements that had been adopted in response to the recommendations of the Texas Research League. The director of physical plant operations and the business manager both reported to the hospital director, for example. Truslow wanted each directly accountable to him. Truslow created a Hospital Advisory Committee that examined all aspects of hospital management. He expected the Dean's Advisory Committee (the renamed Faculty and Admissions Committee) to examine all aspects of managing the medical school. To coordinate policies for the entire institution, he chaired an Administrative Council that included Edwin Troutman (assistant dean) and Warren G. Harding (registrar and assistant to the executive director), Don Walker (chief business officer), Dan Bobbitt (acting hospital administrator), D. Bailey Calvin (dean of students), Marjorie Bartholf (nursing schoool dean), and Truman G. Blocker Jr. (faculty representative).[83]

Spurred by Wilson and Melvin Casberg, the realities of continued growth in the UT System, and some difficulties with John McCullough, president of the Sealy & Smith Foundation Board, Truslow adopted a strategy of comprehensive planning for campus development.[84] Between 1956 and 1959 Casberg was the system's first vice president for medical affairs. Casberg believed that "his principal role was to advise President Logan Wilson about the development of programs in the UT medical units." This role placed Casberg in direct and recurring communications with the CEOs of each health unit. Shortly after assuming his new role on July 1, 1956, Casberg visited UTMB.[85]

Casberg urged Wilson to discuss the following with Truslow: appointment of a dean for the medical school, ways to improve teaching effectiveness, development of a clinical salary augmentation program, and better plant utilization. In June 1957 Wilson urged Truslow to appoint a dean because he feared that Truslow would experience burnout "in trying to cope with too many big problems at the same time." Truslow was indecisive and exceptionally fearful about sharing authority.[86] Fostered by his compulsiveness, the demands on Truslow's energies and time became extraordinary. Later that summer he took a nine-week vacation to recover from physical and mental exhaustion.

A few months after returning from vacation, Truslow became more fearful about developments in Houston, including a proposal for another UT nursing school. He labeled the Texas Medical Center a "monstrosity," a product of "some fine and fundamental yearnings of people who never had the benefit of discipline and experienced direction." Truslow believed that some of those units (the postgraduate school and the graduate programs at the M. D. Anderson Hospital) should be administratively incorporated into UTMB, even though that would "add an almost intolerable administrative burden" to his responsibilities.[87] In addition to the reflexes of fear that impeded his willingness to share administrative authority, Truslow was really threatened by prospects of expansion in Houston and elsewhere.[88]

Reluctantly, Truslow made important personnel changes during the summer and fall of 1958. He shifted D. Bailey Calvin from dean of students to director of an office of research grants and contracts, and he appointed Kenneth Earle as assistant dean (undergraduate) and Stephen Lewis as assis-

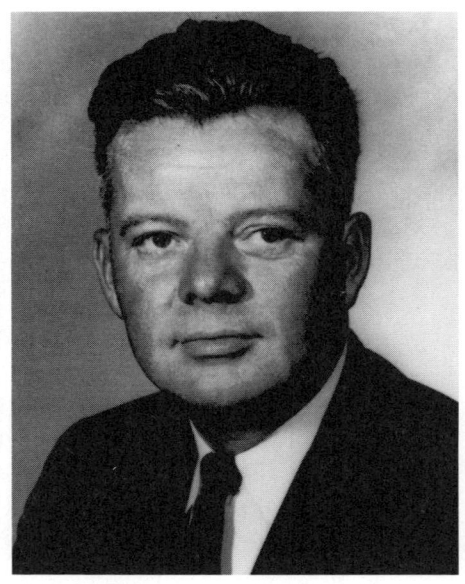

John Truslow

tant dean (graduate and postgraduate). Truslow named H. Frank Connally Jr. as the assistant executive director for UTMB, though Casberg was concerned that Truslow would not delegate responsibilities to Connally. After a visit with Truslow in November 1958, Casberg told Wilson that Truslow was "attempting to be all things to all people," thereby failing to delegate responsibilities to subordinates. Casberg also noted that Don Walker was becoming increasingly dissatisfied with his status because of salary inequities and conflicts with the hospital administrator. Nevertheless, Wilson, Casberg, and the regents publicly affirmed Truslow's leadership even though the UT Committee of 75 had reported an unsatisfactory status for the medical school at UTMB.[89]

Major changes occurred in the spring of 1959. Daniel Bobbitt became director of the hospitals, Kenneth Earle became dean (part-time) of the medical school, Warren G. Harding became director of admissions, Don Walker became comptroller for fiscal affairs, and Edwin Troutman became assistant director of planning. Truslow chaired meetings of the Administrative Council and the hospital's Executive Committee. Earle chaired meetings of the medical school's Executive Committee (department chairs). Both Truslow and Earle attended monthly meetings of the two executive committees.[90]

By early 1960 Truslow was proud of certain improvements at UTMB. The education budget had increased from $1.4 million (1956–1957) to $2.1 million (1959–1960). Faculty salaries in the School of Medicine had increased almost 50 percent and no part-time clinical faculty received salaries. Research grant support had doubled and faculty publications had increased. Several labs were modernized and three electron microscopes had been purchased. The admission, curriculum, and promotion policies for medical students had been revised substantially.[91] To coordinate and distribute information on and off campus, a Public Information Office had been established.

In May 1960 Logan Wilson became chancellor of the UT System and Harry Ransom became president of UT Austin. In September 1960 the regents made tentative decisions about a ten-year development program for the physical plants of all UT components. For UTMB this included seven projects, whose costs were estimated at more than $13 million. The regents pledged more than $3 million in new Permanent University Fund bonds and more than $1 million in Available University Fund income for these projects, extraordinary and unprecedented pledges.[92]

After Wilson's resignation, Ransom became UT's CEO in 1961. He persuaded the regents to end the legacy of relocation sentiments that had infected the development of UTMB from its beginning. They agreed "that the present location be considered permanent and all uncertainty on that point be eliminated in current planning for the future," and "that sincere effort be made to produce an outstanding medical school at Galveston."[93] Ransom really wanted UTMB to thrive in the city of his birth.

Administrative instability reappeared, however, in 1962, when Earle resigned and Truslow found it impossible to function as both executive director and dean. "To put it bluntly," Truslow told Ransom, "I have no intention of continuing indefinitely in a situation in which not any part of Saturday's or Sunday's is my own." During the ensuing months Ransom and the regents periodically expressed concerns about Truslow's style of leadership.[94] In April 1964 the regents announced that Truslow would become a consultant to the chancellor on September 1, 1964. Truman Blocker Jr., then chair of the Department of Surgery, would succeed Truslow as executive dean and director.[95]

The Blocker–Levin Boom Eras

Unlike Leake and Truslow, Truman Blocker knew UTMB from the inside out. A physician graduate in 1933, he had exercised several administrative roles after becoming a member of the faculty in 1936. These roles included chief of the division of plastic and maxillofacial surgery in the Department of Surgery (1944–1960); director of the postgraduate division (1946–1950); director of the special surgery unit (1948–1954); director of hospitals (1950–1953); dean of the medical faculty (1953–1955); chair of the interim governing committee for UTMB (1955–1956); and chair of the Department of Surgery (1960–1964). Blocker was CEO for ten years (1964–1974). When he assumed that role in 1964, the fifty-five-year-old surgeon was described as a "firm, active good natured man" who "smokes a lot of cigarettes and enjoys reading through a pair of gold-rimmed glasses."[96] Blocker claimed: "I know I'm going to make some mistakes, but at the same time, right or wrong, I plan to make lots of decisions." And so he did.

Unlike Truslow, Blocker was eager to share authority and delegate duties. A committee of professors soon made recommendations that Blocker transformed into a new administrative arrangement, which the regents approved in October 1964. He named two coordinating committees. One was the Executive Council, which included himself, Don Walker (associate director), and Warren Harding (assistant director and dean of student affairs). The other was the Administrative Advisory Committee, which included the Executive Council plus Dan Bobbitt (director of university hospitals), William J. McGanity (part-time medical school dean), Betty Rudnick (full-time nursing school dean), and Donald Duncan (director of graduate education). The former reviewed all institutional policies; the latter focused on academic programs and patient care.[97]

To accommodate the roles of new personnel and his vision for institutional improvements, Blocker periodically changed administrative titles and relationships. When Walker left in 1965 to become the UT System's director of facilities, planning and construction, Harding became UTMB's associate director. The Executive Council was eliminated; a new role of assistant direc-

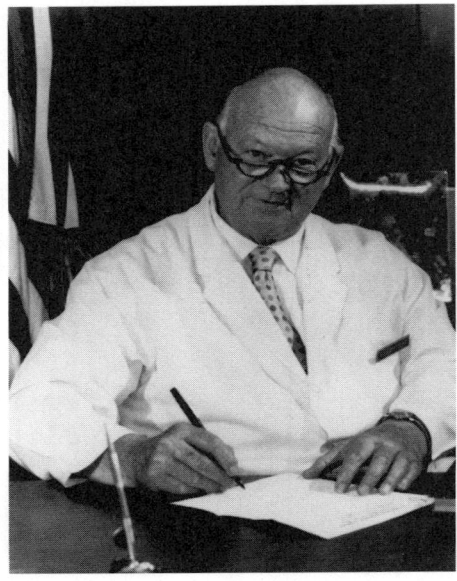

Truman G. Blocker Jr.

tor and coordinator of sponsored research was added; and the title of general director of hospitals was changed to general administrator of university hospitals. The Administrative Advisory Committee was renamed the Administrative Council and included Spencer Thompson as the new assistant director and coordinator of sponsored research.[98] Blocker unceasingly searched for administrative stability and trustworthy managers as he adapted to local conditions and the new statewide expectations of the mid-1960s.

In 1965 the legislature transformed the Texas Commission on Higher Education into the Coordinating Board of the Texas College and University System, a group that would oversee the development of higher education in the entire state. Wanting to prevent unnecessary duplication, the legislators expected this board to approve or disapprove all requests for new programs submitted by university administrators.[99] Responding to this situation, Chancellor Ransom asked Charles "Mickey" LeMaistre, a professor of medicine and associate dean at UT Southwestern, to orchestrate a system-wide study of the "potential of the University of Texas for the training of health professionals for the State of Texas." After reviewing the self-studies, LeMaistre prepared a list of recommendations for all UT health care units.[100] In 1966 the regents invited LeMaistre to become vice chancellor for health affairs and assume responsibility for transforming these recommendations into expanded health programs for the UT System.

In response to LeMaistre's request, Blocker had orchestrated UTMB's first comprehensive self-study, a process that renewed the esteem on the Galveston campus that had been waning for a decade.[101] Blocker demonstrated a remarkable grasp of the intersections between external (off-campus) events and internal (on-campus) change. Unlike Truslow, Blocker viewed new system initiatives as opportunities for institutional progress.

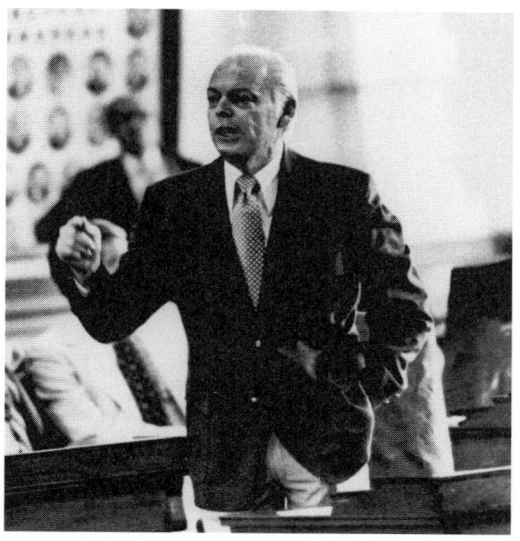

Aaron "Babe" Schwartz, c. 1974.

In 1967 Blocker became UTMB's first "president" when the regents reorganized the UT System hierarchy of top-level administrators. Approving Blocker's recommendations, the regents named Harding as vice president for hospitals and V. E. (Jack) Thompson Jr. as vice president for business affairs. Blocker and LeMaistre proposed additional changes early in 1968 and the regents approved a new administrative arrangement. In June 1968 Joseph M. White became the first full-time dean of the School of Medicine and the first vice president for academic affairs, responsible for overseeing all academic and research programs.[102] In the fall of 1968 Blocker changed Harding's title to that of vice president for health services.

Blocker's executive team included Thompson, White, and Harding. Thompson selected Jim Swinnea as his principal assistant. White appointed Joe Tupin as associate dean (curricular affairs) and Spencer Thompson as associate dean (sponsored research). Harding relied on one administrator and six assistant administrators to manage hospital activities.[103]

Blocker, Thompson, and White met at least once a week and more often as needed. White had regular meetings with his staff and deans every Thursday. Though White felt supported by Blocker, he thought that he had an "arms length relationship" with Thompson. White had little to do with the hospital as a business organization and Thompson was accountable to Don Walker and Blocker.[104] Their staff meetings were lively affairs as these administrators had ample power and money to make substantial changes in the institution.

Together with the regents, Ransom, and other system administrators, LeMaistre had persuaded elected officials to support a tremendous increase in the level of state funding for UT health units in 1967. Frank Erwin, who was a regent between 1963 and 1975 and chair from 1966 to 1971, played an extremely powerful role in these events. During these years, UTMB's legislative fate depended on the goodwill and support of Aaron Robert "Babe" Schwartz. By 1969 Schwartz was a member of the Senate Finance Committee, Conference Committee, and Legislative Budget Board. He was a member of the Finance Committee from 1969 until 1981 and he served on every conference committee for every appropriation bill that was passed during those years. By the late 1960s Blocker and Schwartz had established a mutual regard and trust that augured well for UTMB. Schwartz's esteem for Blocker and UTMB enabled him to provide extraordinary support in obtaining more money and political support than UTMB had ever experienced.[105]

Other important changes occurred in the UT System in 1969 and the early 1970s. LeMaistre became deputy chancellor (1969–1970), chancellor-elect (July 1970–December 1970), and chancellor (1971–1978). To provide some continuity in managing the UT health units, LeMaistre appointed Bill Knisely as vice chancellor for health affairs in 1970. Knisely did not have a "line authority" role, a reality that created some tensions during Knisely's five years of service. Blocker and the other CEOs wanted to deal with LeMaistre and not Knisely.[106]

LeMaistre expected Knisely to establish more patterns of cooperation and communication among the health components in the UT System. Knisely accomplished this by orchestrating monthly meetings of the Health Affairs Council, the CEOs of all UT health care institutions. Knisely also met regularly with local leaders and he established a number of system-wide committees that discussed such matters as library support, animal care facilities, teaching medical history, AHEC programs, insurance and malpractice policies, and allied health programs.[107] Knisely facilitated considerable communication among administrators and others, though local CEOs often viewed him as a "outside party" among key players.

In 1972 the regents reorganized the UT health units into health sciences centers and made all deans of local schools accountable to a local president (except for the nursing schools, which were functioning in their own system-wide network). Like Blocker, all presidents were now accountable to Chancellor LeMaistre.[108] Knisely fervently supported this reorganization because he believed it fostered a better balance of centralized and decentralized power in the UT System.

Other important changes occurred between 1970 and 1974. After Harding resigned in 1970, Blocker assigned responsibilities for managing the health care units to Thompson as vice president for business affairs and hospital services and David Hoxie as administrator of hospitals. In 1970 Ed Brandt Jr. became the first "dean" of the Graduate School of Biomedical Sciences. In 1972 Brandt became associate dean for clinical affairs and in 1973, acting dean of medicine when White resigned. Blocker, Thompson, and Brandt frequently met in the mornings during Blocker's "mail opening sessions."[109] These meetings recurred until Blocker's retirement as president in 1974.

Six feet-four inches tall and approximately 250 pounds, Blocker was an imposing, persuasive, and skillful negotiator. He displayed extraordinarily effective interactions with governors, legislators, UT regents and system administrators, and officers of private foundations, especially those in Galveston. His energies were prodigious, as he also performed surgery on some patients, taught residents and clinical fellows, provided counsel about research projects, and participated in several professional organizations. To handle these roles, he traveled almost every week. In 1970, for example, he took fifty-six trips, all on official business.[110]

During Blocker's tenure UTMB became the largest employer in Galveston, with a yearly payroll that increased from less than $10 million in 1964 to almost $37 million in 1974. The addition of eleven new buildings dramatically changed the campus. Blocker supported the creation of a new school (the School of Allied Health Sciences)

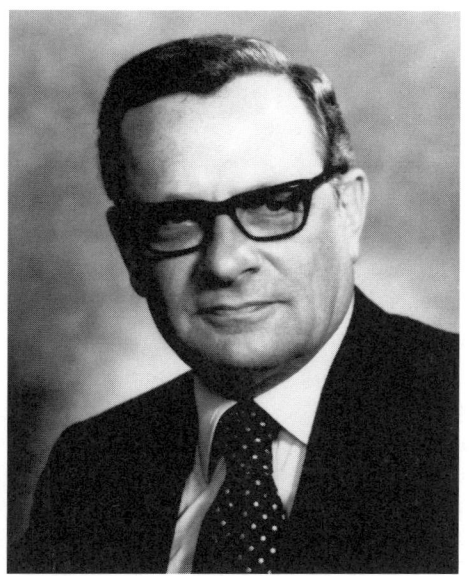

William C. Levin

and two institutes (the Marine Biomedical Institute and the Institute for the Medical Humanities). He developed the rare book and historical collections in the Moody Medical Library. He supported the development of a Department of Family Medicine in the School of Medicine, and other new programs in audiology and speech pathology, home dialysis, renal transplants, early health education, and hyberbaric medicine. In 1974 Blocker was aptly described as "the pivotal force" in UTMB's "phenomenal rise toward a position of preeminence among the world's teaching medical centers." After Blocker died in 1984, Bill Levin eulogized him as a man of "superlative intellect, energy, insight, imagination, and enthusiasm."[111] By then, Levin had emulated his mentor by exercising his own superlative skills as CEO for ten years.

In September 1974 fifty-seven-year-old William C. Levin became UTMB's second president and fourteenth CEO. A physician graduate in 1941 and a member of the faculty for thirty years, Levin became director of the hematology division of the Department of Internal Medicine and medical director of the hospital's blood bank in 1946, director of the Clinical Research Center in 1962, and president-designate in February 1974. Levin wanted to strengthen the family medicine program, develop a cancer center, and establish new programs in environmental medicine. He also wanted to continue some clinical research and attend selected patients. Declared Levin, "I believe I can be a better administrator if, as a physician, I stay abreast of some of the nitty-gritty." However, the nitty-gritty of the CEO role became so demanding that Levin eventually ceased working as a researcher and limited his clinical services to a few private patients. Like Blocker, he worked tirelessly and passionately as an advocate for improvements at UTMB, experiencing what he thought was something akin to religious zeal.[112]

Also like Blocker, Levin whirled in the political networks that included elected state officials, regents, UT System officers, and UTMB administrators. Levin worked directly with governors and legislators. He met with Bill Clements in Austin. Dolph Briscoe and Mark White visited him in Galveston. He made arrangements with clinical faculty to provide health care needed by any elected official. He invited legislators to visit UTMB. For example, more than two hundred state legislators and their spouses toured the new Texas Department of Criminal Justice Hospital during a weekend visit to Galveston in March 1983. With the help of Don Stevens and others, Levin hosted two more weekend visits of Texas legislators in 1985 and 1987.[113] Levin also participated in hearings about annual operating budgets and biennial budget requests, as well as meetings with the coordinating board.

Levin interacted personally and directly with the regents, usually inviting each new regent to Galveston for a dinner and tour of UTMB. He spoke with system administrators almost daily and some visited UTMB. In April 1976, for example, LeMaistre participated in an all-day meeting with administrators who wanted to chart directions for UTMB's future. Though governors, legislators, regents, and system administrators had varying agendas, Levin believed that most wanted UTMB to flourish and most wanted to support Levin in achieving UTMB's goals.[114]

In Galveston Levin was the fulcrum for managerial networks and a switchboard for conversations with other executives. He talked, on the phone or in person, almost daily with Thompson, whose team of business executives included eleven people. Levin held weekly luncheons with the Administrative Council, whose members served as advisors about all UTMB policies. He also spoke regularly with Ed Brandt, who was dean of medicine between 1974 and 1977. In 1974 Levin named Brandt as chair of a newly created Academic Council that initially included the Graduate School of the Biomedical Sciences dean (Saunders), the School of Allied Health Sciences dean (Bing), the Director of the Marine Biomedical Institute (Wolf), and the director of the Institute for the Medical Humanities (Bean). Brandt viewed this council as a replacement for the previous position of vice president for academic affairs.[115]

UTMB's executives also adapted to changes in system administration. In late July 1977 Don Walker replaced LeMaistre as UT's CEO. Levin and the other UT presidents enthusiastically endorsed Walker. In 1977 Walker invited Brandt to become vice chancellor for health affairs, hoping that Brandt could provide more coordination of the four UT health units. Replacing Brandt as dean, George Bryan worked fearlessly with Levin to initiate important changes in personnel and roles. After becoming associate dean for graduate medical education and medical director of the UTMB hospitals in 1977, Al LeBlanc established a cooperative relationship between hospital services and academic departments that had not existed previously at UTMB. In 1977 William Schottstaedt became associate dean for continuing education, UTMB's first full-time coordinator of continuing education programs for the medical school. In 1980 Levin named LeBlanc as associate vice president of university hospitals and Thompson as executive vice president for administration and business affairs.[116]

Because Walker and Brandt had former ties to UTMB, communication between Levin, his executive team, and system administrators proceeded smoothly during the late 1970s. Revitalizing regular meetings of the Health Affairs Council, Brandt nurtured more cooperation between UT's academic health centers, focusing especially on equalization of salaries at the four centers, improved communication with the State Board of Medical Examiners, and regular interactions with the TMA's legislative committee. Brandt did not have a line authority position to the presidents of the four institutions, meaning that each president experienced formal accountability to Walker, not Brandt. This created frustrations and frictions at times, but Walker and Brandt worked well together.[117]

Expansion and growth in the UT System was phenomenal during the 1970s. By 1981 the fourteen component institutions of the system (eight general, six health) included more than eight hundred classroom and research buildings containing more than $3 billion of furniture and equipment used by nine thousand faculty members instructing more than 110,000 students and more than thirty-two thousand non-teaching personnel.[118] To deal with these circumstances, the regents made two important policy changes involving vice chancellors and strategic planning.

The regents assigned more control to the vice chancellors of the system; they believed that re-centralization was necessary to help the CEOs of component institutions cope with fiscal constraints, relate more effectively with the coordinating board, and deal more constructively with regulatory agencies.[119] After Brandt became assistant secretary of health in 1981, Charles B. Mullins became executive vice chancellor for health affairs. In the search for effective balances of power between system executives and component CEOs, the regents expected Mullins to exert more centralized control over UT's health units. Levin and the other presidents became accountable to Mullins. Levin could continue to approach legislators and regents directly as long as he informed Mullins and Walker about these interactions.

In June 1981 the regents adopted a "strategic" planning process recommended by system administrators who wanted a comprehensive plan for all UT units. Each component institution was expected to develop a six-year plan with clear objectives and strategies designed to attain those goals. The academic years 1983–1989 constituted the initial six-year cycle. Every two years the regents would review accomplishments and prospective plans for the subsequent two years, which would make the planning process a continuous one for the entire system. In February 1982 the regents emphasized their commitment to strategic planning and delegated authority to the local CEOs for designing and implementing planning tactics for each unit.[120]

In adapting to these strategic planning initiatives, Bryan and Charles Tandy developed a schema for UTMB. Appointed as assistant to the president for planning, Tandy chaired a steering committee of twelve faculty members, who prepared the first strategic plan. This committee recommended that seventeen programs receive additional emphasis between 1983 and 1989. After Levin gave a report about this planning process to the regents in April 1983, Mullins praised Levin for his "excellent presentation" and lauded UTMB for its leadership in fashioning a model plan.[121] Levin then became a member of a planning policy committee that coordinated efforts throughout the system during the next three years. By early 1986 UT institutions had developed exemplary "role and scope" tables, "mission" statements, and planning processes. The University of Texas displayed more comprehensive coordination than ever before.[122]

UTMB also enjoyed a functionally efficient administrative network. To achieve even more comprehensive coordination of its academic programs, Levin named Bryan as vice president for academic affairs in 1983. This executive position made the deans of the other three schools and directors of the two institutes accountable to Bryan for both academic and research programs (Appendix S). As vice president, Bryan selected new

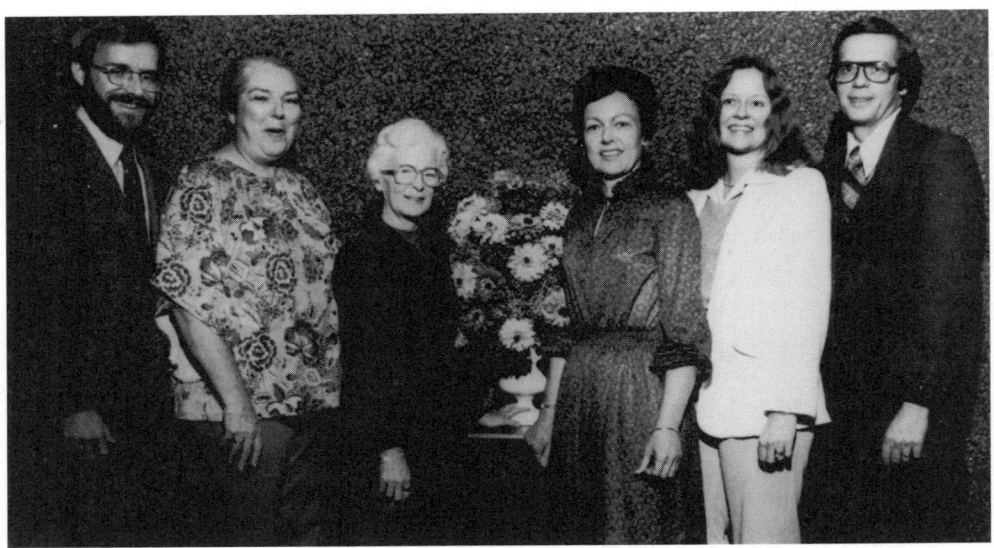

Support staff for Dean George Bryan, 1979. From left, Charles W. Tandy, Bettylu Fitzsimmons, Peggy Brenkus, Jean Neal, Liz Hermann, and Dan J. Oldani.

deans for three schools and a director for one institute. As dean, he selected new chairs for fifteen School of Medicine departments during the years of Levin's tenure as CEO. To achieve better coordination of clinical services, Levin named Jim Guckian as vice president for medical professional affairs and director of UT-MED, the faculty group practice plan, in 1985.[123]

Levin retired as president in August 1987.[124] During his thirteen years as CEO, Levin, together with Bryan, selected a cadre of new leaders for nearly all of the top administrative positions. He reorganized the Development Office. He fostered the adoption of a master space allocation plan and an affirmative action plan. He established an Alumni Advisory Committee on Minority Affairs, an Affirmative Action Office, and an Affirmative Action Advisory Committee. Levin presided during years of extraordinary growth and development that included a fantastic increase in financial support, a transformation of the campus with the renovation or addition of thirteen major buildings, and the addition of many new programs in patient care, education, and research.

THOMAS N. JAMES: A RESEARCH FOCUS

In September 1987 Thomas N. James, then almost sixty-two years of age, became UTMB's third president and fifteenth CEO (Appendix A). Regent Chair Jess Hay thought that James would bring a "new perspective" to UTMB, including "an appreciation for quality, an understanding of the essential role of basic and clinical research, and an intense motivation to train excellent physicians." Hay predicted that UTMB would have "an exciting and innovative future" under his leadership.[125]

Shortly after arriving in Galveston, James emphasized his commitment to all three of UTMB's missions: patient care, education, and research. He planned to continue his

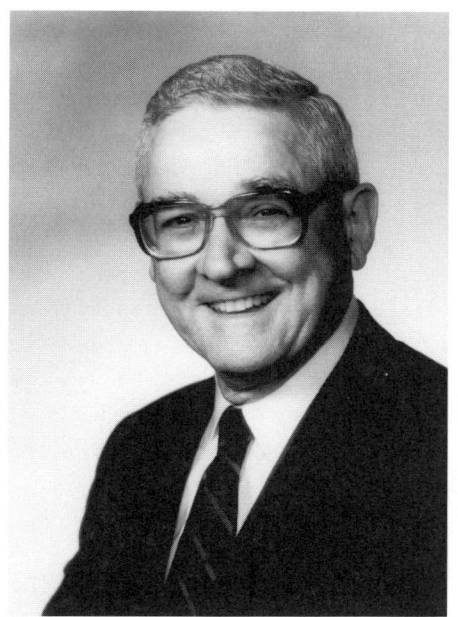

Thomas N. James, 1987. *Photograph courtesy Heinz Kugler Photography, Inc.*

own research involving anatomical studies of the heart and do all that he could to enhance research capabilities at UTMB. "An academic center," James proclaimed, "should provide new concepts of patient care and theories in medical science rather than depending entirely upon someone else's words. We are an academic center, which means we have to generate some of these new concepts and theories ourselves." James—in legacy and prospect—symbolized a research focus for UTMB's immediate future.[126]

James whirled on the same political merry-go-rounds as Blocker and Levin. He established styles of engagement with legislators, regents, system officers, and UTMB administrators, attending regularly scheduled meetings according to specific institutional calendars and participating in many other meetings with a variety of individuals in these political networks. James met several times with legislators elected to represent Galveston, sometimes at his initiative and sometimes in response to their requests.[127] In 1989 and 1991 James, Pederson, and others attended meetings of the Legislative Budget Board to present UTMB's budget. James attended meetings of the coordinating board as needed, particularly to lobby for the Medical Research Building and the doctoral program for the School of Nursing.

James attended UT System meetings that included bimonthly meetings of the regents and quarterly meetings of the System Council and the Council of Health Institutions (formerly named the Health Affairs Council). As needed, James discussed programs with the chancellor and vice chancellor for health affairs, determined strategies for approaching the regents with requests for new buildings and programs, and provided the system's administrators with strategic plans and other reports.[128]

In Galveston, James hosted a luncheon meeting every other Wednesday for the Administrative Council, which included the two assistants to the president (Judy Slocumb and Don Stevens), the executive vice president for administration and business affairs (Jere Pederson), four vice presidents (LeBlanc, Bryan, Guckian, and Lemone Yielding), the deans of the four schools (Bryan, Yielding, John Bruhn, and Mary Fenton), the directors of the two institutes (Bill Willis and Ron Carson), and the directors of certain institutional offices. This group discussed specified agenda items that affected the entire institution. Votes seldom occurred, though consensus was not unusual. The participants functioned as "advisers" to each other and, especially, to Pederson and James, who established a trusting and cordial relationship. Pederson chaired meetings of this council when James was absent, and they "shared" ultimate responsibilities for the overall operations of UTMB.[129]

Between 1987 and 1991 James delegated most business responsibilities to Pederson. By 1990 five vice presidents reported to James and Pedersen: Bryan (academic affairs), Yielding (research), Richard Moore (business affairs), James Arens (clinical affairs), and Fred Wichlep (external affairs). James supported several important changes in the academic and hospital administrative networks.[13]

As mentioned earlier, the regents expected James to expand UTMB's research capabilities. The research budget increased from about $10 million in 1987, the year when James became CEO, to nearly $32 million in 1991. During centennial-year commencement ceremonies, Charles Mullins presented James with the Nicholas and Katherine Leone Award for Administrative Excellence. "While directing our focus on the development of world-class scientific accomplishment and academic excellence, Dr. James has not lost sight of state and local concerns, including our mission of patient care," Mullins declared.[131] James accepted this award with his typical mild-mannered, soft-spoken grace.

Throughout these hundred years, the power matrices of UT and UTMB created a "slow moving bureaucracy" that was like "working in a bed of molasses."[132] To avoid entrapment in these beds, CEOs and other executive administrators needed the help of an extraordinary group of assistants, mostly women, who provided clerical, secretarial, and administrative services. In the CEO offices, these included Florence Magnenat, Addie Hill, Ruth Humphrey, Leah Zinn, Esther Massin, Mary Jane Steding Rogers, Marjorie Watson, Dee Weston, Camille King, Joydelle Wolfram, Patricia Pomeroy, Betty Ray, Jeanne Schaub, Doreen Tipple, Pat Perez, Gale Backe, Claire Donovan, Liz Hermann, Bettylu Fitzsimmons, Patsy Tyler, Lana Meunier, Jean Neal, Kathy Austin, Judy Slocumb, Judy Loney, and Jandee Christensen.[133] These people played key roles in fulfilling UTMB's missions, especially in setting daily tones of interpersonal harmony or dissonance throughout the entire institution.

As demonstrated more than once in this chapter, UTMB's executives appreciated the intimate reciprocities between power politics, pleas for dollars, and the expansion of a campus that would provide more space for the increasing number of patients, faculty, and students. Prominent features of UTMB's economic history are reviewed in the next chapter. Prominent features of campus development are examined in chapter four.

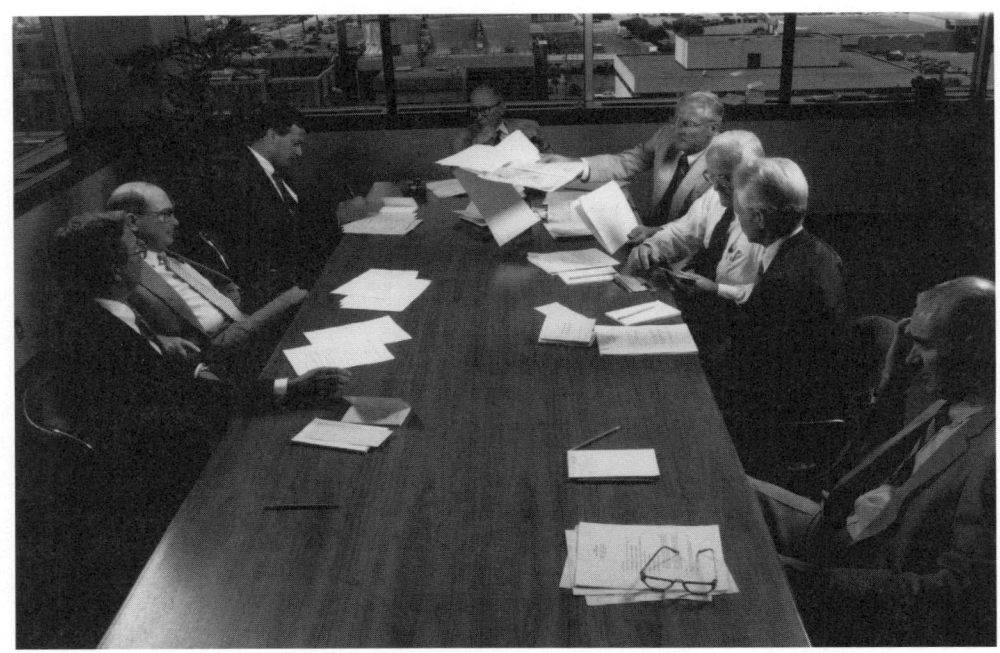

The Sealy & Smith Foundation Trustees, 1991. Left to right: J. Fellman Seinsheimer III, Charles R. Worthen, John W. Kelso, Ballinger Mills Jr., Marc Cuenod (executive director), George Sealy III, Joe C. Blackshear, and John Eckel. *Photograph courtesy the Sealy & Smith Foundation.*

— 3 —

Economic Resources and Business Offices

"I'll be damned if it comes out of the Available Fund of the University!"—Theophilus Painter, 1946[1]

Working carefully with the CEOs, the chief business officers (CBOs) and their assistants acquired, guarded, and spent the dollars needed for daily operations and long-term growth. Evolving financial dynamics during the twentieth century are described in this chapter together with an analysis of sources of income for operating expenses. Some mix of private, city, county, state, and federal dollars provided the economic sustenance for academic and hospital operations, but the percentage share from each source varied considerably as the decades evolved. These variations are depicted for three periods: 1901–1940, 1941–1968, and 1969–1991. These divisions reflect the impact of major turning points in UTMB's financial history that included affirmation by legislators and regents after the 1900 hurricane, full control of the hospitals by the state after 1941, and more federal dollars beginning in the late 1960s. Each section of this chapter also includes a description of the business offices and their development.

OPERATING INCOME AND BUSINESS PERSONNEL, 1901–1940

Three CBOs served UTMB before 1940: James P. Johnson (1891–1903), Thomas H. Nolan (1903–1921), and John C. Nolan (1921–1945) (Appendix J).[2] These individuals collaborated with the CEOs to solicit dollars for the schools, monitored all accounts involving income and expenditures, and supervised their assistants and other employees, such as those who maintained the campus facilities, excluding the hospitals. Hospital accounts and maintenance were handled by individuals employed by the hospital's boards.

The business officers and hospital accountants safeguarded the dollars that came to UTMB during these four decades, especially the private dollars. Had the Sealys not been so generous with their munificence, it is highly probable that UT executives would have succeeded in moving UTMB to Austin during the first relocation frenzy described in the preceding chapter.[3] Troubled by these relocation sentiments and the difficulties of securing adequate funds from the city government for operating the hospital, John Sealy II visited the Rockefeller Foundation offices in New York City to learn about endowing foundations. In 1922 he and his sister, Jennie Sealy Smith, established the Sealy & Smith Foundation for the John Sealy Hospital. Interest from the endowment could be used only in support of whatever was needed for direct patient care, especially for indigents. From 1926 through 1940, the foundation's directors gave more than $2 million to UTMB.[4]

Other private dollars came to UTMB during these years. The women of Galveston repeatedly solicited dollars for the hospitals. Responding to an appeal of the Lady Board of Advisors to the Sealy Hospital Board, churchgoers contributed $3,000 in 1910. By 1915 the Hospital Aid Society, another group of women volunteers, had donated approximately $12,000. On February 27, 1915, for example, they sold 11,510 red, white, and blue pencils at ten cents each to raise funds for the Children's Hospital. These women also sold Red Cross Christmas Seals and valentines to acquire dollars for furnishings, linens, repairs and renovations, staff salaries, clothes, toys, and food for the children. By 1938 the Hospital Aid Society had donated more than $50,000 to UTMB.[5]

These fundraisers and the Sealy legacy accounted for 28 percent of the hospital's operating income from 1890 through 1940. Fees collected from paying patients accounted for approximately 50 percent of the hospital's income through 1940 (Appendices K, L and U).

Private dollars were also important in the development of the schools. From 1891 through 1940, 10 percent of the operating income for the schools came from student fees and 3 percent from benefactors who assigned their dollars to academic programs (Appendices K, M, and V). In 1903 the Women's Club of San Antonio donated funds for scholarships for female students. In addition to periodic contributions for repairs of University Hall, George Brackenridge donated funds for teaching fellowships and loans for female students. In 1921 and 1922 Marvin Graves gave $3,800 to establish three junior positions in the Department of Medicine. In 1930 alumnus B. O. Thrasher bequeathed $10,000 to UTMB and Will C. Hogg assigned $25,000 of his estate to a loan fund for students. Mrs. H. L. Ziegler of Galveston gave $2,000 to be distributed to the "most needy" members of the graduating classes of 1934 and 1935. The earliest grants for research came from the American Medical Association to W. A. Selle in 1931 and 1932 and from Mead, Johnson, and Company to Meyer Bodansky in 1938.[6]

In addition to private dollars, the care of patients in John Sealy Hospital depended on dollars from the city's tax coffers. From 1890 through 1940 about 22 percent of the hospital's operating income came from the city government (Appendices K and U). These dollars honored the political legacy crafted by the Sealy family, city officials, and UT regents at the hospital's birth. The wishes of John Sealy I were safeguarded with the dollars the Sealy family and the city gave to the hospital. As the vicissitudes of pleading for city dollars during the first relocation frenzy demonstrated, sustaining this dual legacy was not easy.

Members of the Sealy family and their friends protected both legacies by acquiring specific roles in governance structures. George Sealy, the brother of John Sealy I, was a member of the hospital's board until his death in 1901 (Appendix E). John Sealy II served on this board from 1901 until his death in 1926, then Jennie Sealy Smith served until her death in 1938. I. H. (Ike) Kempner became the city's treasurer in 1899, served as the commissioner of finance between 1901 and 1916, and was mayor between 1917 and 1919. Fiercely loyal to UTMB, he also served on the hospital's board for ten years (1901–1909; 1911–1913). George Sealy Jr. (son of the brother of John Sealy I) was a city commissioner for four years (1915–1919). At various times, John Sealy II; Jennie Sealy Smith; her husband, Waverley Smith; and George Sealy Jr. were directors of the Sealy & Smith Foundation (Appendix T). These and others carefully monitored the terms of financial support extended by the city, the Sealys, and the foundation's directors.

This legacy of local government support for indigent care was complex and unique. The state's constitution of 1845 actually made county governments responsible for the care of paupers. Before 1900 Galveston County Commissioners did assign some dollars to the Galveston City Hospital and St. Mary's Hospital for this care. However, the Sealy family and the city commissioners assumed the major financial burdens of medical care for local indigents. Beginning in the 1920s the county commissioners allocated a few dollars for this care to John Sealy Hospital, but other indigents from the county received care at UTMB without any reimbursement from the county commissioners.[7] Between 1901 and 1940 the state did not contribute any dollars directly to UTMB for the medical care of indigents. Indirectly, though, the state's support of the schools made such care possible.

Legislators and regents viewed UTMB as the state's premier institution for educating physicians, nurses, and pharmacists. Before 1900, however, financial support had been minimal. In responding to the tragedy wrought by the hurricane in September 1900, legislators and regents became more generous. By mid-November the regents had authorized $57,364 for repairs and new furnishings. In their budget proposals to the legislature for the biennium 1901–1903, they requested $60,000 to cover the expenses of restoration, and $45,000 per year for salaries and operating expenses. The legislators granted the request for repairs and $40,000 of the requested $45,000.[8] Though disappointed about not receiving the full request, the regents did not complain because they knew that legislated amounts from the state's general revenues had increased from $22,000 for fiscal year 1892 to $40,000 for fiscal year 1902.

Between 1901 and 1940 approximately 87 percent of the income needed for operating the schools came from the state's general revenues (Appendix V). Legislated appropriations could be used only for "maintenance and support," whereas Available University Fund dollars could be used for "the erection and repair of buildings and the maintenance and support of the University and its branches." Legislators did assign some tax dollars for construction and maintenance of two eleemosynary institutions on the campus: the State Hospital for Crippled and Deformed Children and the Galveston State Psychopathic Hospital.[9]

UT and UTMB leaders incessantly competed with officials of other state agencies for these dollars. As political fevers mounted during the first relocation frenzy, for example, legislators visited the campus to explore salient issues. In January and February 1911 some met with Dean Carter and others to discuss "the wretched conditions of the outdoor clinics and the nurses' home and the overcrowded wards of the John Sealy Hospital." Some were in favor of more support, but one thought that UTMB should "get on in the future upon the amounts used in the past." The senators who inspected UTMB in February 1913 thought that everything was satisfactory except the nurses' home and inadequate laboratory space. In December 1917, when John Sealy II was chair of the regents' Medical College Committee, three legislators (I. E. Clark, Leonard Tillotson, and Oscar Davis) came to Galveston and solicited testimonies from various faculty members about conditions and needs.[10] It was easier for UTMB's executives to persuade legislators to allocate dollars if they could demonstrate local conditions.

Developing effective patterns of persuasion was an omnipresent challenge, as the number of legislators and state agencies increased, and as another bureaucratic entity—the State Board of Control—entered the fray in 1919.[11] This board prepared biennial budgets for all state institutions and served as the purchasing authority for these institutions. When this board began its work, members knew that the state had received more than $28,000,000 during fiscal year 1919 and had expended slightly more than $27,000,000. The net balance in the state's treasury on September 1, 1919, was more than $4 million. Taxes on oil resulted in receipts of more than $40,000,000 for fiscal year 1920.[12]

Competition for these dollars became intense, especially among educational and custodial institutions. By the 1920s state revenues supported more than seven thousand common school districts, about one thousand independent school districts, almost six hundred classified high schools, more than two thousand unclassified rural schools, fifteen colleges and universities, three penal, and seventeen eleemosynary institutions. For the biennium 1919–1921, the Thirty-sixth Legislature appropriated more than $5 million for the eleemosynary institutions and more than $8 million for the educational ones. Recognizing windfalls in the state's treasury, educational administrators requested almost $40 million for the biennium 1921–1923. The board recommended less than $26 million. UTMB's administrators requested $315,556; the board recommended $265,100. This was a tiny fraction of the total, though a bit more than the previous biennium (Appendix V).[13]

UTMB's executives and professors regularly trekked to Austin to appear before the Board of Control and the finance committees of the Senate and the House to defend requests for appropriations. In March 1929, for example, George Bethel, Edward Randall, and A. O. Singleton pleaded UTMB's case before the House Appropriations Committee.[14]

By the mid-1930s ninety-nine agencies managed 131 separate units in the administrative hierarchy of the state of Texas and each competed for its share of the state's financial pie.[15] Each developed patterns of communication and negotiation with members of the Board of Control; representatives, senators, and their staffs; and governors and their staffs. Each juggled budget figures repeatedly as the vicissitudes of the depression years exacted their painful tolls.

In March 1934 members of the Board of Control met with UTMB's Executive Committee to discuss the sparse appropriations and the rigid rules governing purchases in the state's bureaucracy. Bethel and Nolan were especially distressed by budget cuts in fiscal year 1934 that resulted in a nearly 28 percent reduction of the salaries of fourteen janitors. Nolan thought it "deplorable that the salaries of the lowest paid members of our staff should have thus been reduced, but there is nothing that can be done about it at this time."[16] Professors and others also experienced salary cuts during these years.

As recovery occurred during the late 1930s, leaders of state agencies pleaded for more dollars to underwrite salary increases and expansion of staff positions. The regents, Rainey, and Spies aggressively urged legislators to provide more financial support for UT and UTMB. Rainey repeatedly claimed that UTMB was not first class; Spies persistently argued that UTMB was understaffed and lacked appropriate teaching and research facilities. These pleas worked, as legislators approved increased budgets for fiscal years 1940 and 1941.[17]

Though relying mostly on private, city, and state dollars before 1941, UTMB did receive some federal dollars, first for patient care, then for construction of hospital facilities. In fiscal year 1921, for example, the U.S. Public Health Service contributed $32,316 for the care of its employees and merchant marine families. New Deal dollars from the Public Works Administration were used for partial funding of two new hospitals that opened in 1937. Announced in January 1936, the PWA grant of $128,319 for the new Negro Hospital was touted then as the largest federal grant ever received by an institution in Texas.[18]

UTMB's business offices evolved in support of the academic enterprise. A small portion of income was used for salaries, equipment, and office supplies for the CBOs and their assistants. In 1903, for example, Provost Johnson "supervised" five assistants: a librarian and stenographer (Florence Magnenat), an engineer and mechanic (Michael Little), a janitor (John Carlson), and two workers who helped with the anatomy and pathology labs (August Elbert and Alfred Beverly).[19]

When John Nolan succeeded his father in October 1921, Leah Zinn was his administrative secretary and Kate Feuille was the librarian. The physical plant personnel then included Michael Little as the chief mechanic, two assistant mechanics, and eight "janitors and lab attendants."[20]

By fiscal year 1940, Nolan (earning $300 a month) managed the business duties of the academic enterprise with one assistant ($200 a month) and one secretary ($100 a month). In fiscal year 1941, UTMB's total administrative expenses were less than $100,000.[21] Though income was sufficient for maintenance and some growth during UTMB's first half-century, its business officers were not yet "big business" managers.

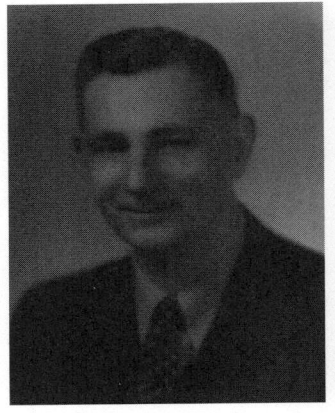 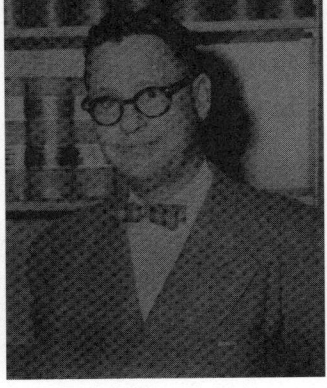 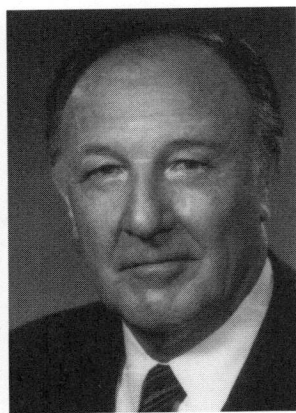

John Nolan   Edgar "Cap" Capplemann   Don Walker

OPERATING INCOME AND BUSINESS PERSONNEL, 1941–1968

Five people were CBOs between 1941 and 1968 (Appendix J). In 1945 Edgar N. "Cap" Capplemann succeeded John Nolan and Capplemann managed both schools and hospitals for ten years. Don Walker was CBO for ten years; Warren Harding for three years. In 1967 Vernon E. "Jack" Thompson became UTMB's first vice president for business and hospital affairs.[22]

To meet expenses between 1941 and 1968, the CEOs and CBOs solicited and received dollars from state, city, county, private, and federal sources. Key struggles and events associated with each source are now reviewed.

Approximately 56 percent of the operating income for the schools and about 42 percent of the operating income of the hospitals came from the state's tax dollars (Appendices W and X). After the regents acquired complete control of the hospitals in March 1941, Rainey and Spies urged expansion and improvements, especially the establishment of a hospital for cancer patients. Legislators responded generously by increasing income for fiscal years 1942 and 1943, including $500,000 for a cancer hospital. However, the political strife with Rainey and Spies caused the legislators and regents to support Houston as the site for the cancer hospital.[23] As the state's new medical institutions appeared in Houston and Dallas during the 1940s and early 1950s, legislators and regents also became more fiscally conservative toward UTMB.

Leake responded by aggressively trumpeting a need for more money to sustain and enhance the quality of academic programs and clinical services. His efforts were successful, as the legislators and regents increased UTMB's income for the 1943–1945 biennium. Leake also persuaded the Sealy & Smith Foundation directors to give $60,000 for indigent care during 1943.[24]

After World War II ended, income from student fees diminished considerably as the Texas legislature offered free tuition to all veterans. There was also a loss of federal dollars as army and navy programs disbanded. To offset these losses, Leake asked UT

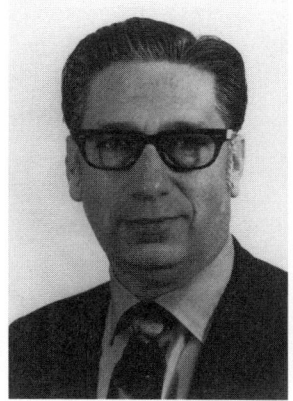

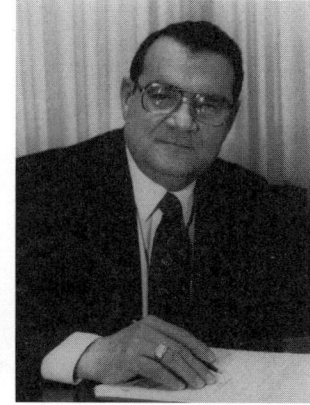

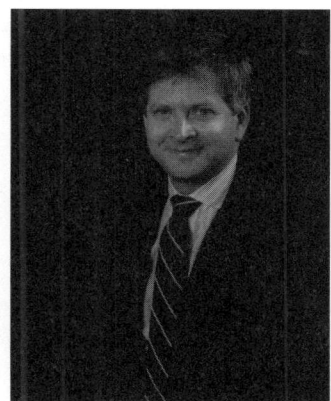

Warren Harding   Vernon "Jack" Thompson   E. J. "Jere" Pederson

President Painter to assign some Available University Fund dollars for UTMB's operating expenses. Painter anticipated a $87,500 shortfall for UTMB's fiscal year 1947 budget and exclaimed to the regents: "I'll be damned if it comes out of the Available Fund of the University!"[25] Painter wanted to use money from that fund for construction on the main campus.

Painter was annoyed with Leake's recurring pleas for more money and he was skeptical about UTMB's future in Galveston. "Another angle to the Medical School situation that should be thoroughly worked out," argued Painter, "is the plan for the future of the Medical School. . . . The establishment of the Medical Center in Houston, I suspect, sets the pattern for the future of the Medical School. In fact, whether we like it or not, it will be futile for us to attempt to develop at Galveston a competing Medical Center. What I think is going to happen in future years is this, that more and more of the time of the men at Galveston, in the clinical years, is going to be spent in Houston, where clinical material is abundant. The result will be that the plant at Galveston will be more largely concerned with the pre-clinical years, and that our primary considerations so far as buildings at Galveston is concerned, will be to provide an adequate laboratory and class building so as to take care of the teaching needs." Painter, like many of his predecessors, believed that the future of medical education in Texas was not in Galveston.[26]

Leake did not believe that the future of Galveston and UTMB was that bleak and he battled fervently for political and financial support. In March 1946 Leake and Capplemann submitted a budget request to the Board of Control for the biennium beginning September 1, 1947. They argued that salaries for faculty must be raised if Texans really wanted a first-class institution. The salaries proposed in his budget were only "in accordance with the second and third rate medical schools" and "not in the same range as such first-class medical schools as Michigan, Minnesota, Wisconsin, Illinois, or California." Unless these salaries were "progressively raised," Leake emphasized, "Texas will have to be satisfied with a second or third rate school, since the quality of a medical school depends largely on the quality of its professional personnel."[27] Leake and Capplemann knew how to massage Texas pride.

There were limits, however. Painter became distressed again when UTMB experienced an operating deficit of $198,000 in the summer of 1946. Painter believed that the hospitals were the "source of most of our trouble," with the deficit reflecting the costs of caring for so many charity patients. The regents loaned UTMB $75,000 to meet urgent expenses, increased room rate charges for the hospitals, and froze the budget for 1946–1947. At Painter's prompting, Leake and others also pleaded with the city commissioners, who approved an increase in their annual appropriation from $40,000 to $75,000, effective July 1, 1946.[28]

Painter and Leake were delighted, but Leake knew that this increase would not be sufficient. Migrants seeking jobs in Texas's industries, military personnel returning from overseas, and a baby boom caused the total number of patients and hospital employees to expand dramatically during the postwar years. More dollars were needed for salaries for residents, nurses, and technicians as well as new faculty. As was true throughout the nation, the costs of supplies and foodstuffs rose signficantly. Leake persisted with bulldog ferocity and the regents responded favorably.

Regent Chair D. K. Woodward Jr. and his wife visited Galveston in late October 1946. Woodward was impressed with the attitude of UTMB's employees. "What struck me as forcibly as anything else," said Woodward, "was the attitude of the people whom I saw and met on the campus, from the kitchen help to the highest officials. I didn't see anyone loafing on the job. All of them appeared to be interested and alert and so far as I could detect they feel that they are engaged in worthwhile employment." Though viewing Leake as an "absolute perfectionist," employees and faculty displayed high regard for him. "Striving for the best is sometimes disconcerting," added Woodward, "as it is always highly expensive, but it never results in standards being lowered." Woodward also experienced cordial cooperation with the directors of the Sealy & Smith Foundation. The regents requested substantial increases in operating income that the legislators granted for the 1947–1949 biennium.[29]

Though revenues increased, UTMB's financial challenges continued. In early 1948, for example, Painter became distressed about the continued use of Available University Fund income for repairs at UTMB, especially on hospital buildings. "If we allow ourselves to be inveigled into repairing and maintaining the hospital," declared Painter, "we will embark on a course which can easily be disastrous for it will be like sinking money in a bottomless pit." Painter thought it was appropriate to use Available University Fund income for repairing and improving buildings devoted to teaching and research (e.g., an elevator for Old Red), but not for hospital buildings (e.g. remodeling ward kitchens). He wanted Sealy & Smith Foundation dollars used for hospital repairs.[30]

Painter and Leake were delighted that the Board of Control recommended an increase of more than $3.5 million for the next biennium. To lobby for this increase, UTMB's officials staged dinners for the legislators. Twenty-one representatives and thirty-one senators came to Galveston in March 1949 and many acknowledged UTMB's accomplishments. A few weeks later, UTMB's leaders felt betrayed when they discovered that their budget request had been changed substantially by both the Board of Control and the Senate Finance Committee. Instead of the requested $5,135,000, the Board of Control recommended $4,143,000 and the Senate Finance Committee recommended only $2,652,000. Most of the cuts involved the hospitals.[31]

Apparently someone had told the legislators that additional state dollars were not necessary because Available University Fund dollars could be used to repair and maintain the hospitals, a belief that had caused the cuts in the budget request. Woodward was incensed. He thought that much political damage had occurred and he chastised Painter for letting this happen. Exclaimed Woodward: "For more than four years, the Board of Regents has been trying to make it plain to the Administration that the policy suggested is contrary to law, as well as contrary to our established policy."[32] Woodward reiterated his belief that the Available University Fund was intended for the educational activities of the university and not for hospital care of indigents. Woodward criticized Painter and Painter criticized Leake.

Painter reminded Leake that the finance committees of both House and Senate were "faced with so many calls for funds" that it was quite understandable that they would look to university funds for money to meet expenses of the hospitals. Painter reminded Leake that he and the regents had been attempting to obtain adequate funds for repairs at the hospitals from the general funds available to the legislators. Painter also chastised Leake for confusing the legislators with direct requests. "I believe that if we pull together from here on out and are very careful about what we say so that none will be charged with 'double talk,' we can get adequate support for the Medical School, but the Medical Branch will pay a high price if the waters are muddied by irresponsible people," added Painter. Muddied or not, the legislative waters surged forth as UTMB received an increase of more than $2 million in state funds for the biennium 1949–1951.[33]

As UTMB's growth escalated during the early 1950s, Leake became even more aggressive. In 1951 his pleas met with much resistance by the Legislative Budget Board (LBB), which recommended a total that was more than $3 million less than the amount Leake requested.[34] For three months UT and UTMB executives struggled valiantly to obtain the original request of more than $8 million for the biennium 1951–1953. They testified at hearings in Austin and they orchestrated visits to Galveston by legislators who wanted to obtain firsthand evidence about UTMB's needs. Ike Kempner and the Medical College Committee of the Galveston Chamber of Commerce hosted the legislators. Sen. Jimmy Phillips negotiated with fellow legislators, who eventually approved the original request.[35]

After the new John Sealy Hospital, the Waverley Smith Pavilion, and the Ziegler Hospital began functioning in 1954, UTMB had a deficit of $500,000 by the summer of 1955. Regents used Available University Fund income to absorb this deficit. They also increased room charges for pay patients and invited local communities to assume a minimum portion of the costs of care of their indigent patients. Regent Chair Tom Sealy and Logan Wilson declared that the legislature "did not appropriate sufficient funds to permit the University to continue to take care of large numbers of indigent patients from virtually every county of the state." The Sealy & Smith Foundation supplemented the hospital's operating income for fiscal years 1956 and 1957, and the Galveston City Commissioners began contributing $75,000 annually for health care for indigent patients living in Galveston County.[36]

John Truslow wanted more from the city. About a month after he became CEO he met with Mayor George Clough, the city commissioners and UT officials. In December 1956 Clough appointed a committee to study UTMB's request for more money. Chamber of Commerce officials recommended a tax levy that would require a voter referendum. After Galvestonians approved this levy in 1957, the commissioners increased their contributions to $200,000 each year.[37] Between 1941 and 1968 the city contributed about 2 percent of the operating income for UTMB hospitals (Appendix W).

Exercising the power often accorded a new CEO, Truslow requested a substantial increase—more than $2 million—in state funding for the biennium 1957–1959, primarily for salary increases and new positions. Gov. Price Daniel supported an increase for UTMB because he wanted to place three hundred additional hospital beds in operation. The Fifty-fifth Legislature (1957) granted most of the requests and the regents approved salary raises for faculty and staff, an event some referred to as "Christmas in June."[38]

During the fall of 1958 Truslow and Wilson challenged Governor Daniel and members of the LBB to support capital improvements at UTMB or to move the school elsewhere. After they responded favorably, in 1960 the regents pledged $13 million for campus development at UTMB. During the late 1950s and early 1960s, Truslow also pressed for more operating dollars and UTMB's appropriations increased somewhat during the biennia 1959–1961 and 1961–1963 (Appendix W and X).[39]

Operating income from the state increased significantly after Blocker became CEO. Gov. John Connally's support of education, increased legislative appropriations, and the continuing goodwill of the regents made this possible. On May 27, 1966, for example, the regents assigned $718,000 from the Available University Fund for support of new buildings and renovations at UTMB.[40] The regents were truly honoring their pledge to support capital improvements; UTMB was now receiving more tangible support from state government than ever before.

Private dollars were especially important during these years. Between 1941 and 1968, approximately 53 percent of the operating income for the hospitals came from paying patients (and their insurance carriers), and 3 percent came from the Sealy & Smith Foundation and other corporate or individual gifts (Appendix W).[41] Approximately 2 percent of the operating income for the schools came from student fees, 8 percent from sales and rentals of items and services, and 13 percent from gifts from private donors, which included individuals, foundations, and corporations (Appendix X). These dollars were used for student loan funds, faculty research projects, and improvements in teaching and patient care services, as the following exemplify.

In 1941 the Galveston County Medical Society Auxiliary held card parties to raise dollars for student loan funds. In 1942 the W. K. Kellogg Company donated $10,000 for medical student loans and $4,000 for nursing student loans. The Varsity Club, another women's group in Galveston, staged dances during the late 1940s to raise money for scholarships for nursing students.[42]

Drug companies, private foundations, and individual citizens supported research during the 1940s. Five pharmaceutical companies provided modest funds for studies Jules K. Lamar and Joseph T. Roberts conducted. Drug companies and private citizens supported the research endeavors of Edgar Poth and George Herrmann. In 1943 the National Research Council gave Joseph Roberts $3,600 for research on the blood supply of nerves. The John and Mary R. Markle Foundation supported Eric Ogden with grants for his research on the renal pressor system. Other groups contributing dollars for research included the Sugar Research Foundation, the International Cancer Research Foundation, the National Foundation for Infantile Paralysis, the Houston Endowment, and the Texas Division of the American Cancer Society.[43]

More substantial improvements in research, teaching, and patient care were made possible by a vast increase in dollars from local and national foundations during the 1950s and 1960s. The W. K. Kellogg Foundation gave $61,000 to the School of Nursing for the development of a nursing service administration course and the National Fund for Medical Education awarded several grants for improvements in teaching strategies with medical students.[44]

The James W. McLaughlin Fellowship Fund for the Study of Infection and Immunity was an extremely important boost to research. In January 1952 Andrew McLaughlin died in Los Angeles. McLaughlin's father was James McLaughlin, who had been UTMB's professor of medicine between 1897 and 1905. To honor his father, Andrew bequeathed $1 million to UTMB for an endowment that would support research fellowships in immunology and infectious diseases. The first awards were made in 1954 and the fund had provided more than $700,000 by 1968.[45]

UTMB's CEOs and CBOs regularly interacted with the Sealy & Smith Foundation directors, and they gave special attention to three other foundations in Texas: the Hogg Foundation for Mental Health, the Harris and Eliza Kempner Fund, and the Moody Foundation.

During the 1950s UTMB faculty received eleven grants from the Hogg Foundation. These dollars supported a child guidance clinic; research projects in the departments of anatomy, physiology, and neurology and psychiatry; and a full-time medical sociologist for the School of Nursing. This foundation granted more than $125,000 to UTMB between 1941 and 1968.[46]

In 1947 the Kempner family in Galveston established a charitable trust named the Galveston Fund, renamed in 1950 as the Harris and Eliza Kempner Fund. During subsequent years UTMB received various gifts from the directors of this fund, as well as some separate endowments from members of the family. A clause in Dan Kempner's will (probated in 1957) honored his wife, Jeane Bertig Kempner, by establishing a fund at UTMB for student scholarships and fellowships.[47] In 1958 trustees of the Kempner Fund established a lectureship in honor of Dan Kempner. Two pathbreaking grants occurred in 1967 and 1968: one endowing the I. H. Kempner Professorship in Human

Genetics and the other supporting the Daniel W., R. Lee, and Stanley E. Kempner Laboratory of Human Genetics. These donations were very important measures of support by a highly respected Galveston family.[48]

In 1942 William L. Moody Jr. established the Moody Foundation.[49] After his death in 1954 the foundation received about $440 million from his estate. Moody's will stipulated that his daughter, Mary Moody Northen, would direct the foundation. Northen withstood several lawsuits from other family members and the foundation began its philanthropic programs in 1960. Harry Ransom encouraged the foundation's directors to award grants to state-supported educational institutions. In 1964 the Moody Foundation initiated its contributions to UTMB with a million-dollar gift for construction of the Moody Medical Library. Between 1966 and 1968 the Moody Foundation awarded grants for three other projects at UTMB.[50]

In addition to nurturing cordial relationships with the directors of these foundations, Blocker also initiated more systematic efforts to attract the financial support of UTMB alumni. During the year before he became CEO, 602 alumni contributed a little more than $46,000 to UTMB. Blocker wanted to increase that total. In 1967 he established a University of Texas Medical Branch Foundation, a group that renamed itself the Foundation Advisory Council (1968), then the Development Board (1971). In 1968 Blocker set the stage for a new era in private philanthropy for UTMB by appointing Charles Chadwick as the institution's first development officer.[51] Their success is described in the next section of this chapter.

The federal government was the other major source of dollars during these years. Between 1943 and 1968 about 21 percent of the operating income for the schools came from federal tax dollars (Appendix X). These dollars supported students and teaching, research activities, construction and reconstruction of buildings, and the care of patients.[52] Consider some examples.

Federal dollars were available for medical students who were trainees in the army and navy during the war years. In 1942, for example, UTMB received $20,000 from the federal government for loans to medical students. To encourage the enrollment of more nursing students, the U.S. Public Health Service (USPHS) gave $10,570 to the John Sealy College of Nursing in 1942 and 1943. Twenty years later, UTMB's professors successfully competed for health service grants available for teaching programs. In 1966, for example, the School of Medicine received $107,381 and the School of Nursing received $40,332.[53]

There was a massive increase in federal dollars for research during these years. In the mid-1940s, various agencies provided grants to Chester Frazier for studies on penicillin and Wendell Gingrich for studies on malaria. UTMB's professors received $92,195 of the $19,259,821 awarded by the USPHS in its initial group of postwar National Institutes of Health grants made between January 1, 1946, and August 31, 1948. Research-minded faculty secured grants and contracts from federal agencies that surpassed a million dollars in 1962, reaching a total of $16,590,466 by the end of 1968.[54]

Federal matching grants for the construction and renovation of teaching facilities became available for the first time with the passage of the "Health Professions Educational Assistance Act of 1963."[55] UTMB, for example, secured a grant authorized by this law for the renovation of the John W. McCullough Outpatient Clinic.

During the late 1960s enormous amounts of federal dollars became available for the care of patients. On July 30, 1965, President Lyndon Johnson approved Public Law 89-97, which added Title XVIII and Title XIX to the Social Security Act. The former became known as Medicare and the latter as Medicaid. Medicare provided federal dollars for medical care to Americans sixty-five years of age or older. Medicaid provided federal grants to states for medical care to old age assistance recipients, blind and disabled persons, and indigent families with dependent children.[56] The passage of these laws resulted in an immediate increase in income for UTMB's hospitals, with dramatic increases beginning in 1969 (Appendices W and Y).

In summary, major changes in financial support occurred between 1941 and 1968 when UTMB needed more dollars than ever to support growth and expansion. The state and the city increased their allocations, especially for patient care services. Private endowments and federal agencies provided most of the dollars needed for expanded research endeavors in the laboratories and wards. Federally funded dollars for the care of the aged and the poor dramatically changed UTMB's treasury and clinical programs.

During these years, the steadily expanding programs of clinical care, teaching, and research required a significant enlargement of business offices and support services. The CBOs needed salaries for new executive assistants and their secretaries. Marvin Hawkins became the first assistant business manager in 1947, serving in that role until 1958. Others included Henry Benecke (1958–1960), Julius Weeks (1961–1962), and Harvey Hall (1962–1968). Charles Richardson was business manager for two years (1968–1970). Salaries and office expenses for executive personnel in the business offices exceeded $1 million by fiscal year 1953 and $4 million by fiscal year 1968.[57]

During the 1940s the business offices added more personnel. In 1941 four people assisted John Nolan in the business office on the first floor of Old Red. Tony Smith, the white-haired bookkeeper, wore a green visor as he stood before a tall desk to handwrite entries in the ledger books. Dorothy Lynn McCoy handled vouchers; Annie Framer and Shirley Hubely performed clerical and secretarial chores. Capplemann, Hawkins, and others hired new accountants, secretaries, cashiers, clerks, typists, and technicians. The physical plant staff expanded considerably. The hospitals expanded older divisions such as nursing services, housekeeping, laundry, dietary, and general stores, and added new ones such as the blood bank.[58] A sizeable group of clerks and technicians now served the seventeen academic departments of the medical school and those of the nursing school.

Academic, hospital, and business departments expanded even more during the 1950s. By the mid-1950s A. P. Freund, Karl Schuster, and Albert Brautigan constructed equipment for research labs in the technical apparatus shop in the basement of the Keiller Building. By 1954 Bill Vanacek directed a print shop that included a secretary and two operators for the shop's three multilith offset presses. Replacing a watchman system, the office of campus police was organized in 1948. By 1954 this office included eleven members plus a campus fire marshal. Bill Schmidt had two assistants when he became director of the Medical Photography Department in 1948 and by 1955 this department included Schmidt, five other photographers, and a secretary.[59]

In 1941 Vurtis Johnston organized the first central receiving room and general stores in a small room in the basement of John Sealy Hospital. Capplemann organized a purchasing department in 1947 and appointed Johnston as purchasing agent in 1948. By 1954 an assistant purchasing agent, two secretaries, and two clerk-typists assisted Johnston. Fitz Ripley managed the general stores when it moved into Storage Building No. 1 and, later, into Storage Building No. 2 (adjacent to the business offices in the early 1950s) and Storage Building No. 3 (adjacent to the Woman's Hospital). By 1954 eleven employees handled the acquisition and distribution of items used in UTMB's offices.[60]

In 1946, A. S. "Buster" Critchfield organized the first post office and assumed responsibility for managing the telephone service. The PBX switchboard was located in the entrance of the John Sealy Hospital before September 1, 1947, and on the first floor of the Keiller building for many years thereafter. In February 1955 the post office moved to the east end of Old Red.[61]

International Business Machines (IBM) equipment came to the campus in 1948 and 1949. A punch-card machine unit for tabulating hospital statistics was acquired in 1948.[62] During the 1950s personnel used various machines, including a sorter, key-punch machine, verifier, 405 tabulator, collator, and reproducer, which were replaced as faster and more advanced machines were created. By 1954 the tabulating department included four key-punch operators who transferred data from equipment inventory records, payroll earnings records, salary ledger sheets, and hospital records to IBM punched cards that could be processed by various machines to generate statistical data.

In 1954 Capplemann and Hawkins supervised business personnel who worked in eighteen specialized offices, such as the bursar's office, the auditor's office, and the personnel office (Appendix R). The bursar's office handled cash and insurance transactions involving patients. When this office moved to the lobby of the John Sealy Hospital in December 1956, Bursar William Harmon supervised a dozen employees, who acquired new National Cash Register accounting machines. Ten employees worked in the vouchering division of the auditor's office in the fall of 1957. Before any checks were issued to companies selling goods to UTMB, these employees verified that invoices, purchase orders, and receiving reports matched properly.[63]

In September 1953 UTMB became the second institution in the UT System to establish a personnel office. James K. Barrett was the director and Dorothy Girardeau was the first full-time personnel interviewer. Initially this office was rather unpopular with the faculty, who had been allowed to select employees independently for more than fifty years. Jim Jannasch became director of this office when Barrett left in

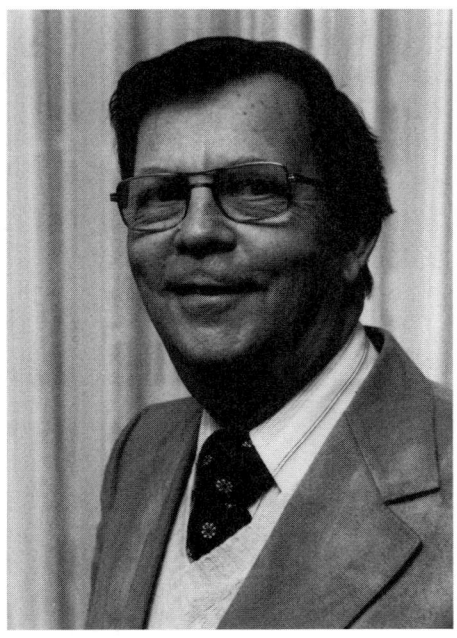

James Jannasch

March 1954.[64] Jannasch changed perceptions about the office by talking with department chairs about their needs for employees and by establishing a faculty committee that helped develop policies for employing new personnel.

Jannasch assigned specialized roles to his staff, expecting individual employees to prepare job descriptions, set wage and salary standards for specific jobs, oversee benefits for all employees, and maintain accurate records. In 1957 Jannasch hired Billy Kimbrough to develop training programs for UTMB employees, including administrative development courses for secretaries. In 1961 Jannasch initiated a national survey of hospital and medical school salaries to determine if UTMB was satisfactorily competitive within the U.S. market. Using data from those surveys, administrative officials developed nationally competitive salary ranges for numerous occupational roles at UTMB during subsequent years.[65]

Don Walker initiated significant improvements in automation capabilities during the early 1960s. Electronic data processing improved considerably in 1961 when a RAMAC 305 computer began handling patient accounts. This machine could receive data from 125 punch cards per minute. Steve Schultz supervised the data processing center then. In 1966 this center was renamed the Service Computation Center. By the following summer, the center's twelve programmers eagerly welcomed a new computer, the IBM System 360/Model 40. Though significantly enhancing the institution's efficiency, these machines increased general administrative expenses during the 1960s, expenses that totaled almost $100,000 in fiscal year 1941 and more than $4 million in fiscal year 1968.[66]

Business-related offices were scattered throughout the campus. During the late 1940s Leake and his secretary, Mary Jane Rogers, had an office in the southeast corner of the Graves building and later moved to the first floor of Old Red. Cappelmann and Marvin Hawkins had offices in one of the barracks buildings and Calvin's office was in the Keiller Building. In the summer of 1950 about fifty employees moved to a new building that housed the business offices.[67]

When Truslow became CEO, administrative offices were consolidated in the old Woman's Hospital building with Truslow and Mary Jane Rogers on the east end of the third floor, and Walker and Bonnie Rickelman on the west end of the third floor.[68] Often Rogers, Rickelman, and Jannasch would work until 11 P.M. or 1 A.M. to complete projects, such as preparing a docket for the monthly meeting of the regents.

In 1967, when Thompson became CBO, there were no dollars for building repairs or capital expenditures, and barely enough money to pay the light bills.[69] With the increase in funds described in the next section, Thompson accumulated surpluses that were invested in new equipment, building restorations, and new buildings, including one that provided a more consolidated environment for the business offices.

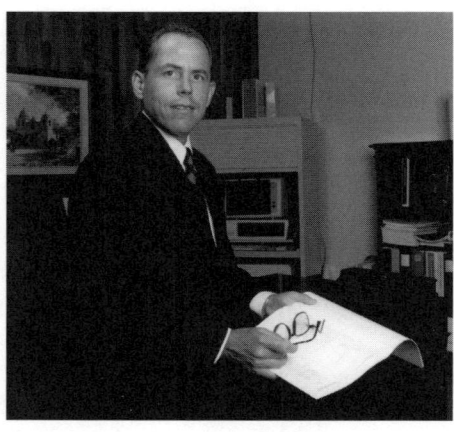

Richard Moore

OPERATING INCOME AND BUSINESS PERSONNEL, 1969–1991

Thompson was CBO for nineteen years during which he interacted with Blocker and Levin almost daily. In 1986 Levin recruited E. J. "Jere" Pederson as Thompson's successor (Appendix J). In 1989 James named Pederson as executive vice president. In September 1990 Pederson appointed Richard Moore as vice president for business affairs.[70] These CBOs witnessed stupendous increases in income from private, federal, county, and state sources during these years. These changes are now described for each of these four sources.

Approximately 57 percent of the operating income for the hospitals came from patients and their insurance carriers (including commercial and federally supported), and about 2 percent came from the Sealy & Smith Foundation and other private entities (Appendix Y).[71] For these same years, approximately 1 percent of the income for the schools came from student fees, 8 percent from sales and rentals of items and services, and 5 percent from gifts and grants from private donors (Appendix Z).[72]

Dollars from local foundations were especially important in providing stability and growth during these years. The Sealy & Smith Foundation provided $19,269,791 for patient care services, especially those given in the Jennie Sealy Hospital and the R. Waverley Smith Pavilion. Preston Shirley, who was a director of this foundation for twenty years, believed that Blocker was "one of the most effective, stubborn, hard-headed bulldogs on getting money from the Sealy-Smith Foundation of anybody who ever lived. . . . Over the years when he was president, he was able to convince the board with his excellent presentations, his hard work and, incidentally, common sense, to get appropriations of slightly in excess of $50 million." Levin and James continued Blocker's legacy of productive relationships with the foundation's directors.[73]

Levin, in particular, urged them to support endowments for professorial chairs. By 1986 the foundation had contributed $2 million to endow four chairs: pediatrics (1978), internal medicine (1984), surgery (1985), and anesthesiology (1986). Levin also persuaded the directors to establish the John Sealy Memorial Endowment Fund for Biomedical Research (1986). Between 1987 and 1991 this endowment fund supported eighty-three grants, worth more than $3 million, to professors.[74]

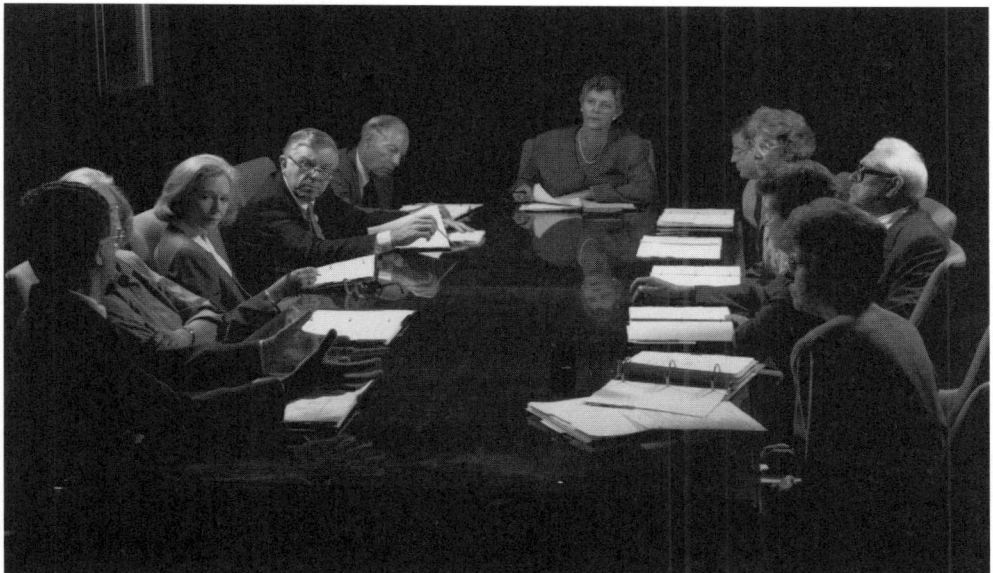

The Kempner Fund Trustees, 1991. Left to right: E. R. "Tim" Thompson Jr., Ann O. Hamilton, Hetta T. Kempner, John T. Currie, Harris K. Weston (vice-chair), Lyda Ann Quinn Thomas (chair), Robert L. K. Lynch (secretary-treasurer), Barbara W. Sasser, Arthur M. Alpert, Leonora K. Thompson (chair emeritus), and Elaine R. Perachio (executive director). *Photograph courtesy the Kempner Fund.*

James strongly supported these innovative approaches by the Sealy & Smith Foundation. As part of the Centennial Campaign he persuaded the directors to establish five additional chairs. These were the Rebecca Sealy Centennial Chair in the School of Nursing, the John Sealy Centennial Chair in the Department of Radiation Therapy, the John Sealy Centennial Chair in Cardiology for the Department of Medicine, the John Sealy Centennial Chair in Rehabilitation Sciences, and the John Sealy Centennial Chair in Neonatology.[75] James also persuaded these directors to endow some Sealy centers for research.

Between 1969 and 1991 funds from the Hogg Foundation, the McLaughlin Fund, the Kempner Fund, and the Moody Foundation also provided extremely important support for the faculty's research efforts. The Hogg Foundation contributed almost $500,000 for behavioral and social studies related to mental health and the McLaughlin Fund donated more than $6.6 million for research support. The Kempner Fund trustees allocated more than $2.5 million for forty-nine distinctive projects between 1957 and 1991. The Moody Foundation donated more than $12 million.[76]

Energized by Blocker's enthusiasm, UTMB's Development Board and staff members in the development office secured more private dollars for institutional growth and development. The Development Board established the President's Club in 1970, a noteworthy group of individuals who gave $5,000 or more. By 1976 there were 108 members in this club. In 1971 the development office initiated a systematic program of annual requests for donations.[77]

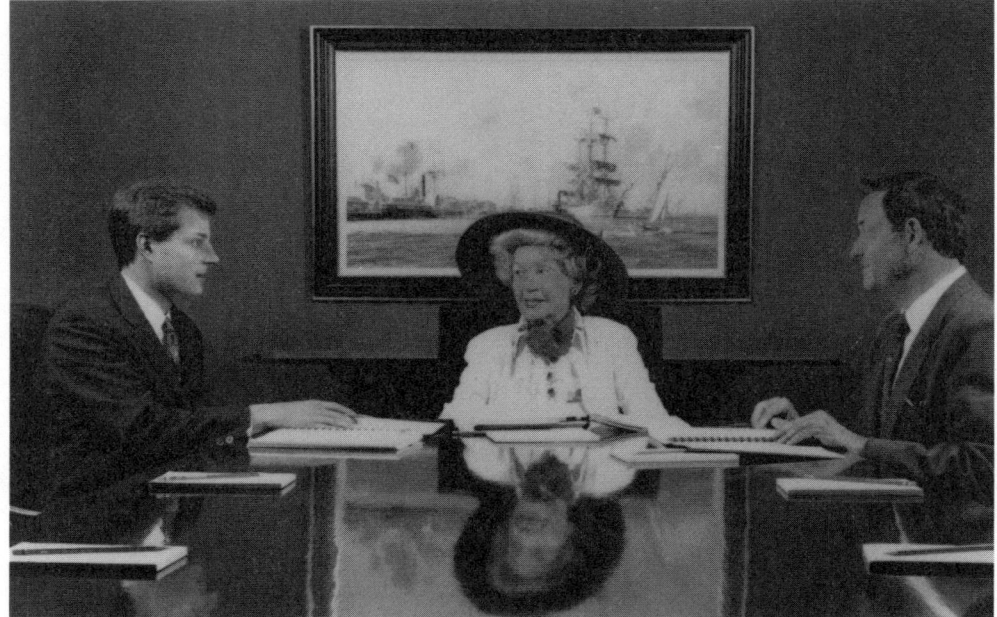

The Moody Foundation Trustees, 1991. Left to right: Ross Moody, Mrs. Frances Moody Newman, and Robert Moody. *Photograph courtesy the Moody Foundation.*

Blocker, Levin, and their development officers expended considerable energy in soliciting private funds for endowed lectureships, professorships, and departmental chairs. By 1981 there were thirty-two lectureships, sixteen professorships, five chairs. By 1982 private donations had established fifty-four separate endowments that were used for scholarships, fellowships, special purchases, and special awards. Levin gave special attention to the Development Board, which usually held annual meetings on a Saturday in January. By the mid-1980s this forty-member board had helped secure more than $16 million of endowments that supported ten named chairs, twenty-one named professorships, and thirty-six named lectureships. As development office directors Gary Merritt, Curtis Lambert, and James P. Daniel assisted Levin in countless ways.[78]

Levin also nurtured the interests of Florence and Marie Hall, widow and daughter of Granville T. Hall (class of 1906), who established the Florence and Marie Hall Endowment for the Improvement of Medical Education. First available in 1979, income from this endowment was used to support the projects of faculty who wanted to improve the quality of teaching. Nine projects were funded in fiscal year 1983, for example.[79]

To extend the extraordinary legacies of private giving Blocker and Levin orchestrated, James established a Centennial Capital Campaign Committee in 1989 with H. L. "Shrub" Kempner Jr. as chair. The committee hoped to acquire $254 million for UTMB's "Second Century." By the end of August 1991, $212 million had been obtained or pledged.[80]

In addition to the prodigious growth of private support, a massive inflow of federal dollars catalyzed important changes between 1969 and 1991. Federal dollars flowed to academic medical centers via the Health Professions Educational Assistance Act (1963), Medicare and Medicaid (1965), the Health Manpower Act (1968), and the Comprehensive Health Manpower Training Act (1971). Dollars for research grants from agencies of the United States Public Health Service escalated. As subsequent chapters indicate, administrators and professors in the schools at UTMB used these dollars to expand and change many programs of teaching and research.

The combination of Medicare and Medicaid plus the expansion of commercial insurance also resulted in a steady increase of income for the hospitals at UTMB in every year between 1969 and 1991 (Appendix Y). This increase in income catalyzed the establishment of institutional trust funds in UT health units, known at UTMB as the Medical Service Research and Development Plan (MSRDP). Administrators and faculty used these dollars to improve salaries and fringe benefits that enabled the recruitment and retention of outstanding faculty. Dollars in these trust funds continued to increase; for example, total MSRDP income for fiscal year 1981 was more than $14 million.[81]

Blocker, Levin, and James strongly encouraged the faculty to compete for federal research dollars. Between 1968 and 1977, for example, professors submitted 304 new grant applications to the National Institutes of Health. More than 60 percent were approved and half of those were eventually funded during years of somewhat diminished federal research support throughout the nation. Of the 129 renewal applications submitted during these same years, 43 percent were approved and funded. U.S. Public Health Service research grants and contracts to the faculty between 1969 and 1991 totaled more than $232 million.[82] Federal dollars provided approximately 15 percent of the total income for the schools during these years (Appendix Z).

As spectacular as the changes were in private and federal support, another revolutionary change occurred in Galveston when the financial challenges of tax-supported medical care for indigents shifted from city government to county government in the 1960s. During the 1940s and 1950s the county's indigents continued to receive care at both St. Mary's Hospital and John Sealy Hospital. After the county commissioners opened the Mainland Hospital in April 1952, they continued to send indigents to UTMB and St. Mary's. They permitted the majority of indigents to go to UTMB hospitals, including those approved by the Galveston County Welfare Department. Ike Kempner, chair of the Medical College Committee of the Galveston Chamber of Commerce, chastised the county commissioners about their lack of financial support for indigent care at UTMB. Kempner was disturbed by the commissioners' policy of deflecting county indigents from their Mainland Hospital to UTMB without paying any costs of their care. In 1962 Kempner and Truslow urged a change in this policy.[83]

Four years later the commissioners established a committee to study this problem. In December 1966 this committee recommended that the commissioners assume full responsibility for the care of the county's indigents beginning January 1, 1969, thereby relieving the city of its $200,000 annual burden. In April 1967 the commissioners accepted this recommendation and negotiated annual agreements with UTMB officials. The city then stopped its payments to UTMB. Between 1969 and 1991 the county commissioners assigned almost $10 million to UTMB for indigent care, slightly less than 1 percent of the operating income for the hospitals.[84]

Beginning in the late 1980s UTMB's officials negotiated agreements with other counties and hospital districts for care of their indigents. In fiscal year 1987, eight counties (Angelina, Aransas, DeWitt, Jasper, Madison, Orange, San Augustine, and Waller) contributed almost $370,000. In fiscal year 1991, sixteen counties (including Galveston) and three hospital districts contributed slightly less than $5,800,000 for indigent care. For services to about two thousand patients from Galveston County alone in fiscal year 1991, UTMB received $1.7 million.[85] These dollars helped UTMB handle some of the burdens of providing care for the steadily growing indigent population, though their total amounts were small when compared to revenue from federal and state sources.

Between 1969 and 1991 about 71 percent of operating income for the schools and about 40 percent of operating income for the hospitals came from state tax dollars (Appendix Y and Z). The same social rhythms that characterized the acquisition of state dollars in previous years continued during these years. These rhythms were always influenced by the vagaries of Texas politics and by the vicissitudes of the state's economy. Although players and rules changed, the cycles of pleading, justifying, altering, and adapting remained constant.

After the School of Allied Health Sciences had been functioning a few years, for example, Blocker told Babe Schwartz that he was having difficulties obtaining dollars for the school and asked Schwartz to add a $6 million line item to UTMB's budget for this school. Schwartz recalled his astonishment: "Truman, how can I tell the legislature that you developed a $6 million line item without me telling them about it? Much less you telling them about it?" Blocker responded: "Aw, you'll figure out a way to do it. Go get 'em, boy." And Schwartz did, knowing that Blocker's passion for UTMB would never flinch. The regents approved a total of $49,329,141 for UTMB's budget during fiscal year 1973, reflecting a 9.3 percent increase in the educational and general budget and an 8.9 percent increase in general revenue funds appropriated by the legislature.[86]

Like other academic medical centers in the state, UTMB benefited from significant increases in state revenues during the 1970s and from legislative decisions to assign substantial portions of these increases to institutions of higher education. For example, state revenues increased from $4.4 billion in fiscal year 1973 to $7.4 billion in fiscal year 1977, a 68 percent increase. Between fiscal years 1973 and 1979, 55.1 percent of the increased appropriations of all funds by the Texas legislature went to education. Biennial appropriations for medical education in Texas from general revenue and federal revenue sharing between 1972 and 1979 increased 251.4 percent (from $167,041,522 to $586,962,357).[87] In these remarkable circumstances, Blocker and Schwartz worked financial wonders for UTMB. Underlying these wonders, though, was a new plateau of work demands for the business offices.

TABLE 3.1: UT SYSTEM CALENDAR FOR PREPARING 1988–1989 BUDGET
REQUESTS TO LBB

June 2, 1986	Five draft copies of Legislative Budget Requests (bound) due to system administration.
June 16–27, 1986	Budget hearings with system administration.
July 1, 1986	Thirty copies of first submission Legislative Budget Requests (unbound) due to system administration for binding.
July 11, 1986	Filing date—first submission of Legislative Budget Requests.
August–September, 1986	Hearings with staffs of Legislative Budget Board and Governor's Office of Management and Budget.
September 24, 1986	Forty-five copies of second submission Legislative Budget Requests (unbound) due to system administration for binding.
October 3, 1986	Filing date—second submission of Legislative Budget Requests.

The CBOs and their assistants ran on time-specific and rule-specific treadmills as they prepared zero-based biennial budget requests. To exemplify these treadmills, consider the budget request procedures for the 1977–1979 biennium. The Legislative Budget Board staff and the executive budget and planning staff from the governor's office sent Thompson a fifty-eight-page set of instructions for preparing appropriation requests for fiscal years 1978 and 1979. These pages included details about the design of tables, proper coding, establishment of priorities, and the structure of the narrative that included program decision packages. A program was defined as "each item of appropriation in the General Appropriations Bill for the 1976–1977 biennium." UTMB's executives were required to prepare funding requests at one of four levels for each program. They were required to declare the advantages and disadvantages associated with each level, and to place them within the framework of UTMB's objectives and priorities for the 1978–1979 biennium.[88]

UTMB's 475-page budget request dated October 15, 1976, begins with a fifteen-page summary of objectives and the amounts that totaled $99,666,301 for fiscal year 1978 and $104,848,134 for fiscal year 1979.[89] Thompson emphasized certain features of the institution. UTMB was the oldest medical school in the state and had provided either medical school or postgraduate training for one third of the state's practicing physicians. UTMB was a major resource for the continuing education of physicians in Texas. UTMB was a major research center for the application of new discoveries to the treatment of disease. UTMB's schools were associated with the only university-owned and operated general referral hospital for all Texans. The Child Health Center had opened in 1976 and the new John Sealy Towers (then under construction) would contain 528 single-bed rooms that would establish a "one-class" service for both staff and private patients.

TABLE 3.2: UT SYSTEM OPERATING BUDGET CALENDAR FOR 1987–1988

August, 1987	UT Board of Regents' Approval of Policies and Continuing Resolution Document.
August 10, 1987	Five draft copies (bound) of budgets due to system administration (including five copies of supplemental data).
August 17–28, 1987	Budget hearings with system administration.
September 8, 1987	Fifteen copies of budgets (bound) due to system administration (with five copies of adjusted supplemental data as applicable).
September 28, 1987	Budget mailed to the UT Board of Regents.
October 8–9, 1987	UT Board of Regents' Budget Meeting.
October 16, 1987	Forty-five copies of budgets (unbound) due to system administration for binding.

Continued excellence at UTMB depended on competitive wages to qualified and dedicated employees. Thompson requested salary step increases of 10.2 percent for the first year of the biennium and 6.8 percent for the second year of the biennium with merit increases for 50 percent of UTMB's personnel in each year of the biennium. Though UTMB did not receive all the money that had been requested, the final appropriations were $84,426,004 for fiscal year 1978 and $86,032,823 for fiscal year 1979.

These financial cycles of budget requests and responses never ceased for the business officers and their colleagues, though important changes in the budgeting process occurred with the advent of strategic planning mandated by the regents in 1981. This approach to goal-setting by each institution allowed system officers to streamline the presentation of institutional budgets to the legislature and governor, adding an element of coordinated rationality for the entire UT System. After this strategy was in place, the regents seldom approved a program innovation or new building unless it appeared in an institution's strategic plan. With the adoption of this approach, the budgeting process became more routine during the 1980s, though different institutional activities occurred during even-numbered and odd-numbered years. For example, consider the years 1986, 1987, 1988, and 1989.

In March 1986 the Governor's Budget Office and the Legislative Budget Board jointly issued instructions to state agencies about budget preparations. The regents and system officers transformed these instructions into guidelines and a calendar for component institutions (Table 3.1). In April UTMB officials began preparing a budget proposal for the biennium that would begin on September 1, 1987, and end on August 31, 1989. After receiving the final appropriations bill adopted by the legislature in 1987, the regents and system officers issued another calendar (Table 3.2) that guided officials in preparing and defending an operating budget for the upcoming fiscal year (September 1, 1987, through August 31, 1988).[90] Knowing what had been appropriated in the

TABLE 3.3: UT SYSTEM OPERATING BUDGET CALENDAR FOR 1988–1989

February 11, 1988	UT Board of Regents' Approval of Budget Policies and Limitations.
April 1, 1988	Seven draft copies (bound) of budgets due to system administration (including five copies of supplemental data).
April 18–19, 1988	Budget hearings with system administration.
May 9, 1988	Ten copies of budgets (bound) due to system administration (with five copies of adjusted supplemental data as applicable).
May 27, 1988	UT Board of Regents' Budget Meeting.
June 24, 1988	Fifty copies of budgets (unbound) due to system administration for binding.

spring of 1987, the regents and system officers followed another calendar (Table 3.3) in approving the operating budget for the second year of the biennium (September 1, 1988, through August 31, 1989).

To create the budget for this second year, departmental chairs, directors, and deans presented their requests to George Bryan during December 1987 and January 1988. Executives then combined this academic budget request with the one from the hospitals and submitted a final budget request in April 1988. Between April and June they met with UT System administrators and staff to review and revise the budget proposal. In June the regents reviewed and approved all system budget proposals for fiscal year 1989, including those for UTMB.

Concurrently during 1988 UTMB officials were also preparing and defending a budget request for the biennium 1990–1991 that would receive legislative action in the spring of 1989. In March 1988 the Governor's Budget Office and the Legislative Budget Board jointly issued guidelines to all state agencies for preparing these requests for operating dollars for fiscal years 1990 and 1991. After reviewing these guidelines, the regents adopted a calendar and UTMB's administrators prepared budget proposals during the spring of 1988.

The system officers then submitted the entire UT System budget to the Legislative Budget Board in June. The board's staff interviewed representatives from UTMB and other component institutions during the summer. Reflecting adjustments made in response to these conversations and adjustments reflecting expenditures during the fiscal year that ended on August 31, 1988, UTMB sent a revised budget to the board in October. Using these revised budgets, the governor's staff and the budget board prepared separate budget recommendations that were available when the legislators convened in January 1989.[91]

During the early months of 1989 the appropriate committees of the legislature conducted hearings with representatives of UT institutions to review budgetary requests.

These committees included the Higher Education Committee of the House, the House Appropriations Committee, and the Senate Finance Committee. After these hearings the house and senate prepared appropriation bills, which went to a joint conference committee for adjustments. The conference committee report was then submitted to the house and senate as the unified appropriations bill that was passed on May 25, 1989. This provided a budget of about $264 million for UTMB's ninety-ninth year and about $266 million for its centennial year.[92]

As growth catapulted during the 1960s, 1970s, and 1980s, the business offices expanded more than ever. Overseeing a $26 million budget in fiscal year 1969, for example, Thompson and his colleagues monitored 110 departmental accounts (schools and hospitals), 375 sponsored research accounts, 450 restricted fund accounts, and 31 student loan accounts. Directors of eleven departments assisted Thompson. These included C. R. Richardson (business manager), John E. Larson Jr. (bursar), Charles King (purchasing agent), Edgar M. Belcher Jr. (data processing), Harvey H. Hall (system development), Louis C. Gilliam (physical plant), Jim Jannasch (personnel), Marvin Hawkins (auxiliary enterprises), John Burr (sponsored research), Maurice Harr (security and traffic), and Jim Swinnea Jr. (buildings).[93]

As the years evolved the CBOs made structural and personnel changes, hiring new assistants and reassigning responsibilities to existing ones, which often involved new titles. In 1970, for example, Thompson delegated new responsibilities to John Poretto as director of fiscal services and to Jim Swinnea Jr. as director of general services. By 1972 nine administrative officers reported to Thompson. In September 1977 he created a new structure for business and hospital administration, appointing Poretto as assistant vice president for hospital affairs. By 1984 eleven executive managers reported to Thompson: one vice president, three assistant vice presidents, two executive directors, three directors, the budget officer, and the chief of the campus police.[94]

Thompson retired in August 1986 after nineteen years as CBO. He praised the employees in the business offices: "The middle management people, the department heads, the clerks and secretaries, those are the ones who make us look good." Thompson was happy to leave the institution "in good shape."[95]

The most important change that affected all business offices during Thompson's years involved the steady expansion of computerization. In January 1973 the hospital's admitting office could access patient accounts because of a new link with the patient finance office. By 1976 the Service Computation Center had added an information system for students and a system for appointments in the outpatient clinics. Using a $2.55 million grant from the Sealy & Smith Foundation, UTMB acquired hardware in 1977 that greatly expanded the institution's data processing capabilities.[96]

Housed on the fourth and fifth floors of the Administration Building in 1980, this center managed more than fifty systems that served administrative, financial, academic, and health care functions. Hardware capabilities were enhanced in 1981 when the center added an IBM 3033 computer. Other equipment added in the early 1980s enhanced the record management system of both hospital administration and business

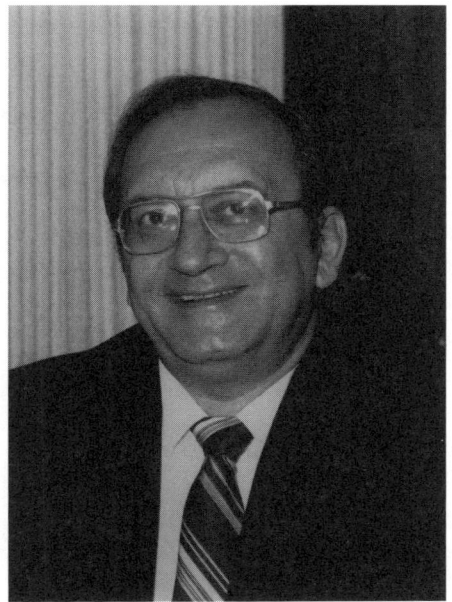

John Kusnerik

administration offices. In 1984 more than two hundred employees learned how to use a new computer system in the new Department of Materials Management (a combination of central supply, general stores, and general receiving). In 1986 the purchasing department became fully computerized and automated. By that year, about one thousand computer workstations were configured in the UTMB 3081 network.[97]

Important planning, structural, personnel, and policy changes occurred in the late 1980s and early 1990s. James and Pederson made a special effort to increase UTMB's support of local businesses. In fiscal year 1990, purchases from local firms amounted to more than $1 million, an increase of 141 percent over fiscal year 1989.[98]

Pederson and his executive team created a formal plan for all business departments. A steering committee shepherded these efforts to streamline and enhance the work of more than 475 employees in twenty-one business departments.[99] After Jannasch retired in 1987, for example, the Personnel Office was renamed the Department of Human Resources. Kathy Shingleton, its director, subdivided this department into seven major areas: hiring, compensation, training, benefits, employee relations, and employee assistance. Pederson, Moore and their colleagues organized financial support services into seven departments accounting; asset management; cash management; cost reimbursements; financial analysis and reporting; and payroll. In 1991 they distributed a manual to administrators and faculty that explained the services offered by all twenty-six business departments.[100]

These efforts in planning and communication vitalized a new sense of respect for business-related services, though their implementation did involve new expenditures.

Administrative expenses for supporting the business offices expanded drastically during the boom years between 1969 and 1991. From about $5 million in fiscal year 1969, they surpassed $11 million in fiscal year 1975; $25 million in fiscal year 1980; $50 million in fiscal year 1986; and $63 million in fiscal year 1991[101]

Throughout its first century UTMB progressed as a business institution because of the stewardship and talents of business professionals like John Kusnerik, who retired in 1991 after thirty-four years of service. He began his career in 1958 as an accountant in the auditor's office and retired as associate vice president and comptroller. "Totally unflappable;" a "pillar of strength and stability;" "loyal and dedicated to his colleagues;" and "one of the most devoted and effective members of the administrative staff" were phrases used to characterize Kusnerik at that time.[102]

UTMB had also progressed as a business institution because of the stewardship and talents of secretaries and administrative assistants who performed countless tasks of daily assistance for the CBOs and other business officers between 1969 and 1991. These included Sheila Simmons, Bonnie Rickelman, Maria Mancuso Tabaracci, June Thomas, Linda Billiot, Linda Corbett, Laura Ford, Cindy Mann, and Michelle Acosta. Like Kusnerik, some of these served UTMB for many years. Maria Mancuso Tabaracci, for example, began as a secretary in the CBO office in 1971 and became Jack Thompson's administrative assistant in 1978.[103] In 1980 Thompson promoted her to assistant to the vice president for administration and business affairs. She became assistant to the executive vice president after Pederson assumed that role in 1986. In

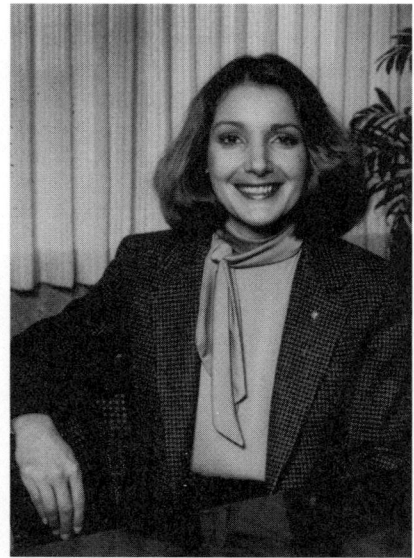

Maria Mancuso Tabaracci

1991 she was promoted to the role of assistant to the executive vice president and director of institutional programs.

Kusnerik and Tabaracci symbolized the values of loyalty, competence, and humaneness that were so important and necessary for institutional excellence during UTMB's first century.

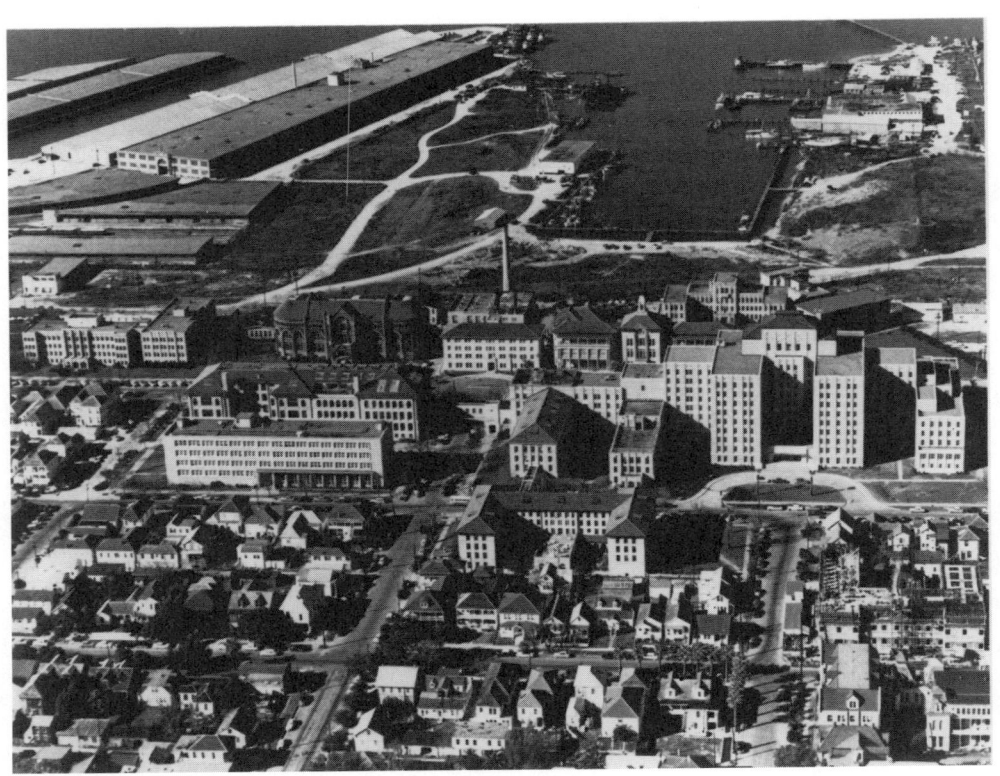
UTMB campus, 1954.

— 4 —

Campus Development: Buildings and Caretakers

"I am authorized to bring your medical school the heartiest congratulations from the Association of American Medical Colleges. Every one of the 74 other sister medical schools on this continent is delighted with the increased facilities that are now provided at the University of Texas for medical education."— Louis B. Wilson, 1932[1]

Each CEO and each CBO attended to campus development, usually hoping to add one or more new buildings that would improve the care of patients, enhance the teaching environment, provide research capabilities, or house students and personnel. These leaders shepherded campus reformation by interacting with regents, other executive officers, planning personnel, office assistants, construction company workers, and campus caretakers. Glimpses of these interactions occur in the following paragraphs, which are organized according to the CEO sequences presented in chapter two. Details indicate the extraordinary amount of time and effort required for adding a new building and remodeling an existing one. Roles of campus caretakers are also described. A centennial year walk concludes this chapter.

Silhouetted in these paragraphs are the drawings of numerous architects and draftsmen who designed these buildings and the sweat of countless men who constructed them: pile drivers, iron and steel workers, concrete workers, bricklayers, plumbers, electricians, masonry workers, and painters. Their meticulous attention and muscular stamina transformed the dreams of powerbrokers, business guardians, and loyal faculty into a campus whose forms are now reviewed in developmental perspective.

By 1902 the buildings included the John Sealy Hospital Old Red, a remodeled Nurses' Home, University Hall, and the new Negro Hospital (Appendix N). After the hurricane of 1900 the old City Hospital building, which had been used for housing black patients, was moved from the west to the east end of the hospital block and restored as a dormitory for nursing students, who occupied it in the spring of 1902.[2]

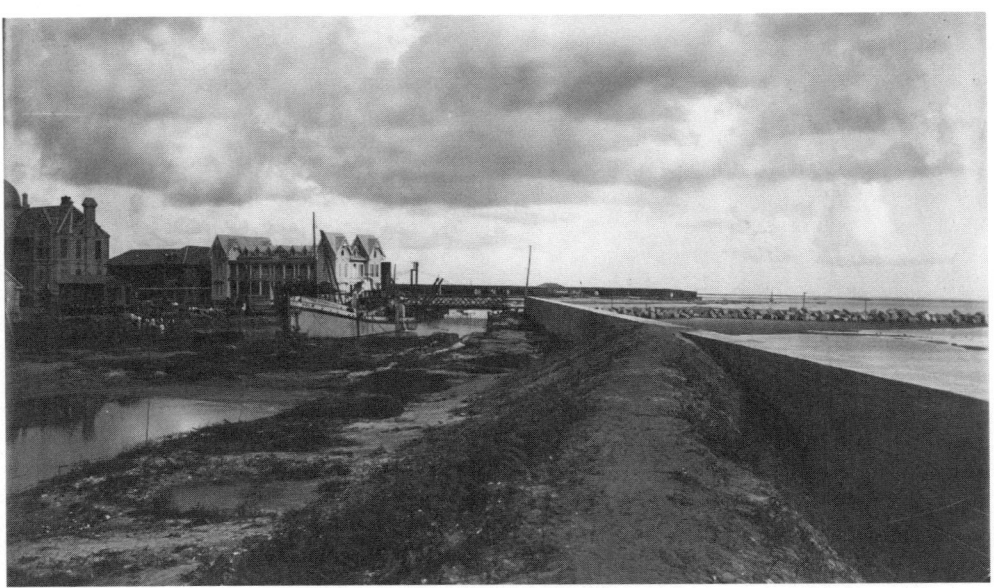

A dredge boat in a canal next to the east border of UTMB's campus during Galveston's grade-raising, 1904 or 1905. Above: Left to right, a portion of John Sealy Hospital, Negro Hospital, Nurses' Home, and the east end of the seawall. Below: Left to right, Strand, Old Red barely visible, John Sealy Hospital, Negro Hospital, Nurses' Home. *Photographs courtesy the Peabody Essex Museum, Salem, Mass.*

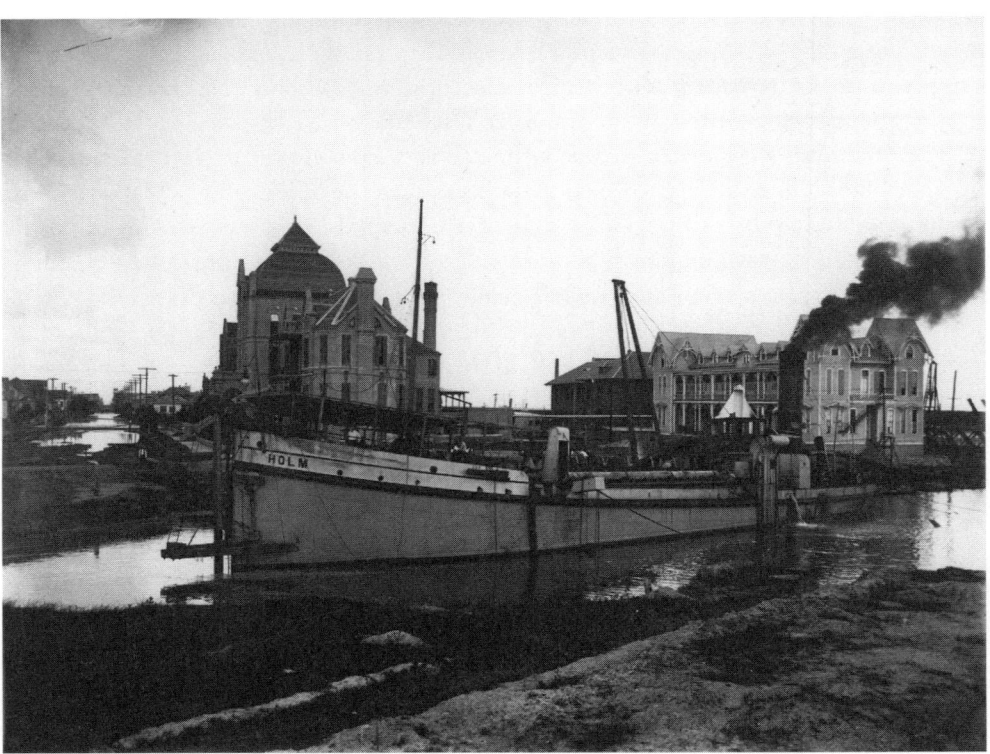

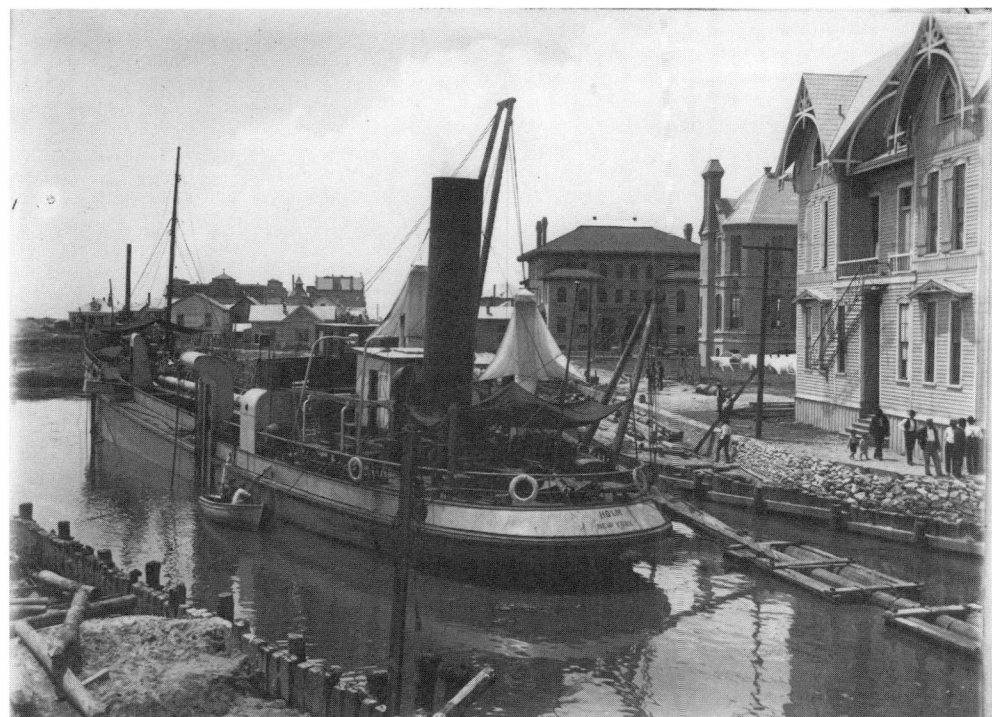

A dredge boat in a canal next to the east border of UTMB's campus during Galveston's grade-raising, 1904 or 1905. Left to right: St. Mary's Infirmary, far distant; University Hall, right center across the street from John Sealy Hospital; Nurses' Home at far right. *Photograph courtesy the Peabody Essex Museum, Salem, Mass.*

Also opening in 1902, the Negro Hospital was the only building added during the second decade. New York City's Chamber of Commerce had donated $18,000 for relief work after the 1900 hurricane. Galveston's Central Relief Committee added $3,500 and the total was used to construct a red brick structure with cream-colored trimmings that contained a few private rooms and two wards with about sixty beds.[3] Though sustaining the era's cultural segregation, this facility was far superior to the rooms used for black patients in the old Nurses' Home.

THE CARTER ERA

Remodeling occurred during the third decade. The Negro Hospital attracted more black patients, who also came to the outpatient clinics in the basement of the John Sealy hospital. Supplies in this basement's storage area were moved to a new storeroom that was added to the back of the John Sealy Hospital in 1911. Afterward, the segregated outpatient waiting rooms were enlarged. In 1915 and 1916 John Sealy II allotted $262,000 for a complete remodeling of the John Sealy Hospital.[4]

New construction also occurred. Between 1912 and 1922 the regents approved the addition of seven buildings: three hospital facilities, one dormitory for nursing students, and three structures for teaching and research.

UTMB had long needed a pavilion for isolating patients with contagious diseases. Tents were used during a meningitis epidemic in 1912 and an exploding stove in one tent caused the death of a patient, providing Carter with a strong case for a more adequate facility. The Thirty-second Legislature assigned $13,000 from a dormant state quarantine fund and the regents added $4,500 of Available University Fund income to pay the costs of constructing the thirty-bed isolation pavilion later that year.[5] This was the first time that the regents used income from that fund for a new building at UTMB.

The Walter Colquitt Memorial Children's Hospital opened in January 1913. The preceding year, when Carter was its president, the Texas Anti-Tuberculosis Association gave $13,000 for the construction of a hospital for children with tuberculosis of the bones. Named in memory of Walter B. Colquitt, son of incumbent Gov. Oscar Colquitt, the Sealy Hospital's board operated this thirty-five-bed hospital. This arrangement continued after the association transferred the hospital to the state during the winter of 1915. Legislators then renamed it as the State Hospital for Crippled and Deformed Children.[6]

On May 31, 1915, Regent George McReynolds participated in ceremonies dedicating two new buildings: a facility for sick women and a dormitory for nurses. Though a separate building, the Woman's Hospital was connected to the John Sealy Hospital by an enclosed passageway. Containing ten private rooms and fifty ward beds restricted to white women, this hospital had a private operating room and a fourth-floor open-air pavilion. John Sealy II and Jennie Sealy Smith contributed $135,000 for this hospital, much more than the $50,000 pledged in their agreement with the city commissioners and the regents in 1913.[7]

The John Sealy Hospital Board also managed the Woman's Hospital and the first Rebecca Sealy Nurses' Home, which could accommodate fifty-five nursing students. This dormitory cost the state $90,500 instead of the $50,000 pledged in the agreement with the city commissioners and the Sealy siblings in 1913. The legislature appropriated $65,000 and the regents contributed the remainder from Available University Fund income.[8] The city commissioners gave $4,000 to furnish the dormitory, which was named in honor of Mrs. John Sealy.

Responding to the research and teaching needs of the professors, the regents next authorized construction of three small buildings. In the fall of 1915 workers built a hollow tile structure, 24 feet wide and 132 feet long, north of Old Red. This "Laboratory of Experimental Medicine" contained an animal care area, a laboratory for experimental surgery, and an autopsy room. In the early 1920s two lath-and-cement buildings were added. One housed the laboratory of chemistry for the pharmacy school, and the department of physiology and the department of pharmacology created labs in the other building. Carter hoped they would attract a new professor of pharmacology who would be an experimental pharmacologist. After Carter left in 1922 Keiller persuaded the regents to appropriate $12,500 for a two-story frame building that housed a laboratory for clinical pathology, a large lecture room, and the EKG lab.[9]

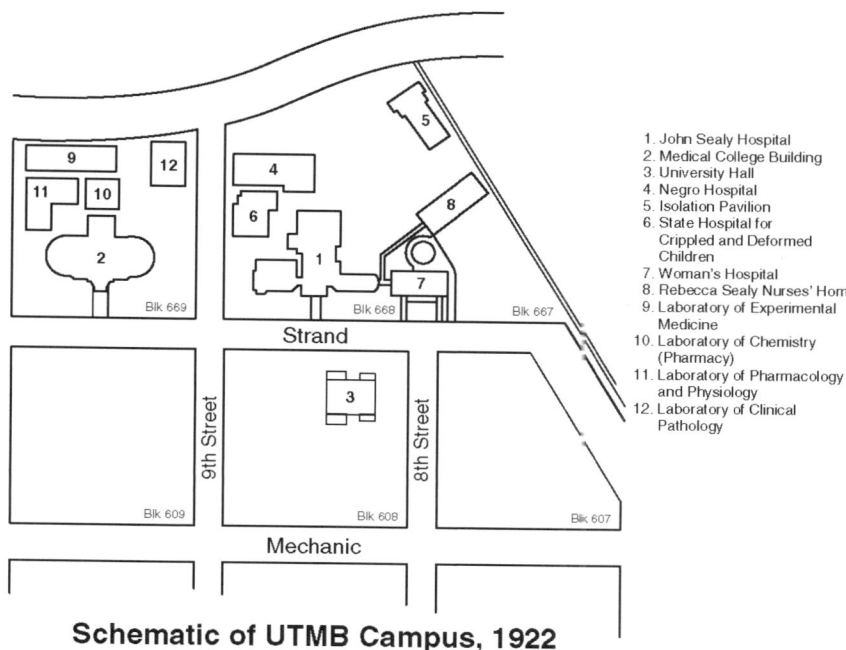

1. John Sealy Hospital
2. Medical College Building
3. University Hall
4. Negro Hospital
5. Isolation Pavilion
6. State Hospital for
   Crippled and Deformed
   Children
7. Woman's Hospital
8. Rebecca Sealy Nurses' Home
9. Laboratory of Experimental
   Medicine
10. Laboratory of Chemistry
    (Pharmacy)
11. Laboratory of Pharmacology
    and Physiology
12. Laboratory of Clinical
    Pathology

Schematic of UTMB Campus, 1922

Altogether between 1915 and 1922, the regents used Available University Fund income to build four academically oriented structures ($52,811), contributed $25,500 to the nurses' home project, and added a new boiler room to heat the Medical College building ($23,396). By the end of fiscal year 1922, the estimated value of the campus surpassed $1 million.[10]

EDWARD RANDALL AND THE SEALY & SMITH FOUNDATION

Keiller's persistence with the regents, the establishment of the Sealy & Smith Foundation, and Edward Randall's powerful presence as president of this foundation after 1908 and as a regent after 1929, heralded significant changes for the campus. Between 1923 and 1942, when other medical centers were less fortunate because of the economic depression, seven new buildings were added to the campus: four hospital facilities, one dormitory, a power plant and laundry, and one academic edifice.[11]

The latter is today's Keiller Building, initially called the Laboratory Building when the west half opened in the summer of 1925. Students first used its labs in the fall of 1925. For more than twenty years, Carter, Keiller, and others had repeatedly expressed a need for this building to house the library, the collections of anatomical and pathological specimens, teaching laboratories, and administrative offices. The regents contributed $328,807, the largest amount of Available University Fund income they had ever allocated for a building at UTMB.[12]

Though Keiller continued to indulge in "those dreams which are essential to progress" and lobbied aggressively for an extension to the Laboratory Building, an enlargement of

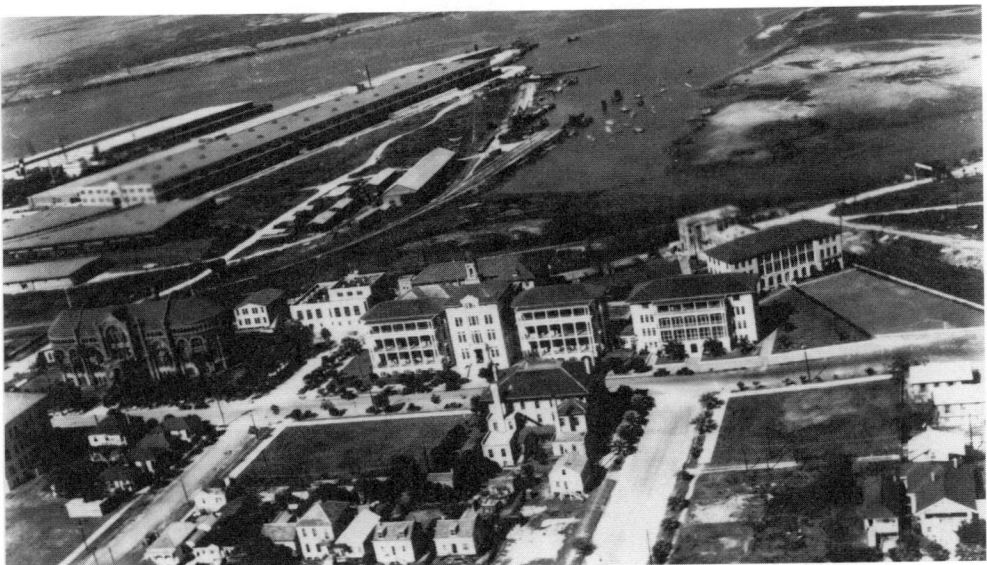

UTMB campus, 1929.

the nurses' home, an extension to the Negro Hospital to accommodate children and pregnant women, and a new outpatient clinic building, none of these dreams came true during his four years as CEO. By the mid-1920s, however, income began to accumulate from the investments of the Sealy & Smith Foundation and the regents began acquiring more income from the university's oil-producing properties.[13] Some of Keiller's dreams did become realities as these dollars made possible a flurry of construction projects.

The Outpatient Clinic Building opened in October 1930; the Sealy & Smith Foundation contributed $500,000 and the regents allocated $50,000 for furniture and equipment.[14] The number of new outpatients increased by more than 30 percent during the following year (Appendix AC).

The forty-eight-bed Galveston State Psychopathic Hospital opened in August 1931 and Titus Harris, professor of psychiatry, became the hospital's medical director.[15] The number of admissions steadily increased and the state authorized a new addition in 1937 that housed forty-five more beds.[16]

The second Rebecca Sealy Nurses' Home opened in 1932. Adequate care for more patients required more nurses. Soon after the first nurses' home opened in 1915, it could not accommodate the increasing number of student nurses. By 1919 some students were living in four frame cottages opposite the hospital. After John Sealy II died in 1926 the legislature permitted inheritance taxes from the Sealy estate (estimated at $700,000) to be placed in an endowment fund under the joint control of the Sealy & Smith Foundation and the regents. In 1927 the foundation's directors and the regents agreed to use the initial income from this endowment for the second nurses' home. The directors contributed $350,000 and the regents added $50,000. This dormitory contained rooms for 163 nurses and some facilities for teaching.[17]

With Available University Fund income steadily replenished by oil-producing properties, regents could more easily affirm their financial responsibilities to UTMB.
Randall persuaded fellow regents to contribute $421,393 for construction of the east
half of the Keiller Building.[18]

On the last day of May and the first day of June in 1932, UT and UTMB officials
staged a two-day celebratory dedication of the Outpatient Building, the Rebecca Sealy
Nurses' Home, and the Keiller Building. These festivities included the school's forty-
first commencement ceremony and elaborate scientific sessions attended by more than
two hundred physicians. Dignitaries from the state and nation addressed the audiences:
Lewellys Barker from Johns Hopkins, the commencement speaker; Edward H. Cary of
Dallas, the AMA president; J. H. Foster, the TMA president; and Louis B. Wilson, the
AAMC president who offered the congratulations of this chapter's epigraph.[19] J. F. Y.
Paine, UTMB's first dean, would have been ecstatic. Forty-one years after its begin-
nings, UTMB's standards were not trailing in the dust. UTMB was a local, regional,
and national asset.

FEDERAL DOLLARS FOR CAMPUS BUILDINGS

A national asset deserved federal tax dollars. As a result of President Franklin Delano
Roosevelt's New Deal policies, the federal government invested dollars into buildings
at UTMB for the first time during the late 1930s.[20] These dollars supplemented the private and state funds used to construct two replacement buildings: a hospital for blacks
and one for children.

Encouraged by Sealy & Smith Foundation directors, the regents submitted a cost-
sharing proposal to the Public Works Administration (PWA) for a new Negro Hospital
and a separate proposal for a new Children's Hospital. After months of negotiations,
including personal visits to Washington by Edward Randall, the PWA approved these
proposals. For the Negro Hospital, the PWA contributed $128,319, the Sealy & Smith
Foundation $71,478, and the regents $88,750. For the Children's Hospital, the PWA
contributed $90,720, the Sealy & Smith Foundation $14,330, the regents $880, and
the legislature $110,000. The Negro Hospital first accepted patients on August 31,
1937, and the Children's Hospital accepted fifty patients in late October 1937.[21]
Americans everywhere had now invested in health care facilities at UTMB.

The configuration of the campus changed little between 1937 and 1942. The federal government diverted dollars to military uses. Legislators, regents, administrative
executives, and professors coped with the administrative turbulence of the Spies era.
Such turbulence did not inspire confidence and attract "investors." But, after more
than a half-century of sheltering students and teachers, the Medical College Building
stood invincibly, basking in its affectionate regard as the "old red building."[22]

By the end of fiscal year 1942, UTMB's fifty-first year, the estimated value of property was $4,672,447, which included $284,581 for land and improvements; $3,148,083
for eighteen buildings; and $1,239,783 for furniture and equipment.[23] The state had
contributed $905,028 for six academic buildings, $50,000 directly appropriated by the

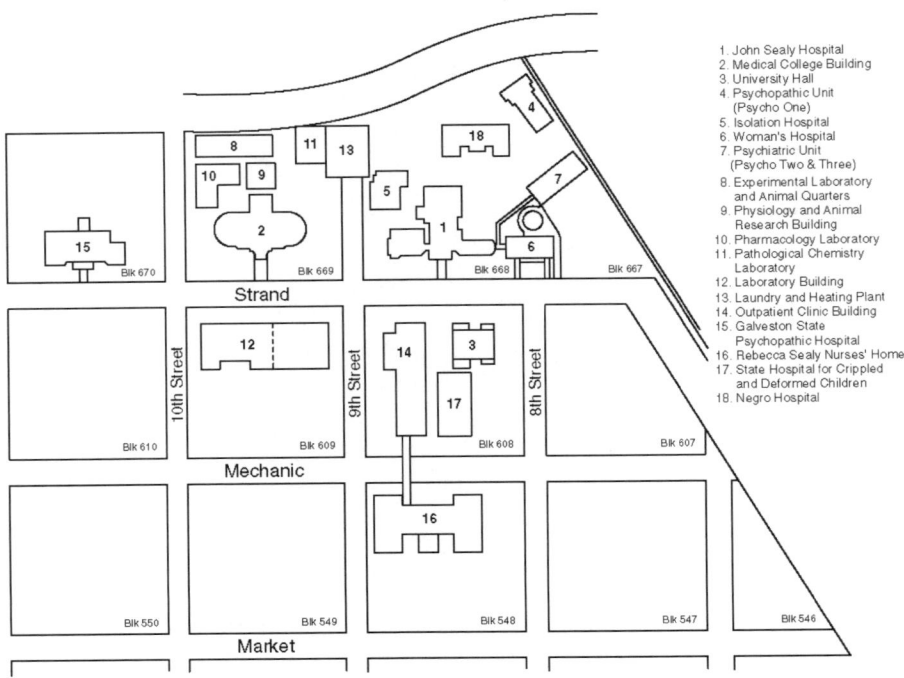

1. John Sealy Hospital
2. Medical College Building
3. University Hall
4. Psychopathic Unit
   (Psycho One)
5. Isolation Hospital
6. Woman's Hospital
7. Psychiatric Unit
   (Psycho Two & Three)
8. Experimental Laboratory
   and Animal Quarters
9. Physiology and Animal
   Research Building
10. Pharmacology Laboratory
11. Pathological Chemistry
    Laboratory
12. Laboratory Building
13. Laundry and Heating Plant
14. Outpatient Clinic Building
15. Galveston State
    Psychopathic Hospital
16. Rebecca Sealy Nurses' Home
17. State Hospital for Crippled
    and Deformed Children
18. Negro Hospital

Schematic of UTMB Campus, 1942

legislature and $855,028 contributed by the regents from Available University Fund income. The Sealy family and the Sealy & Smith Foundation had contributed $1,548,520 to build or remodel eight structures associated with the hospital complex: John Sealy Hospital, Woman's Hospital, Psychiatric Hospital (known as Psycho One, originally the Isolation Pavilion), Negro Hospital, Outpatient Clinic, Rebecca Sealy Nurses' Home, Power Plant and Laundry, and Garbage House. George Brackenridge gave University Hall to the campus, and combined private, state, and federal dollars provided the new Children's Hospital and Negro Hospital. Approximately 51 percent of the funds used for construction during the first half-century came from private sources; 42 percent from appropriations by the legislators and regents, and 7 percent from the federal government.

CHAUNCEY LEAKE'S DREAMS

The second fifty years of campus development began with Chauncey Leake's dreams.[24] He wanted a convalescent home for children, laboratories for the department of pediatrics, better housing for female medical students, and locker and restroom facilities in the hospital. More than anything else, Leake and the faculty wanted a new hospital building that would be large enough to accommodate the patients needed to instruct two hundred medical students (one hundred juniors and one hundred seniors). He also wanted an addition to the Keiller Building, a library building, a large auditorium, an administration building, an addition to the Rebecca Sealy Nurses' Home, a

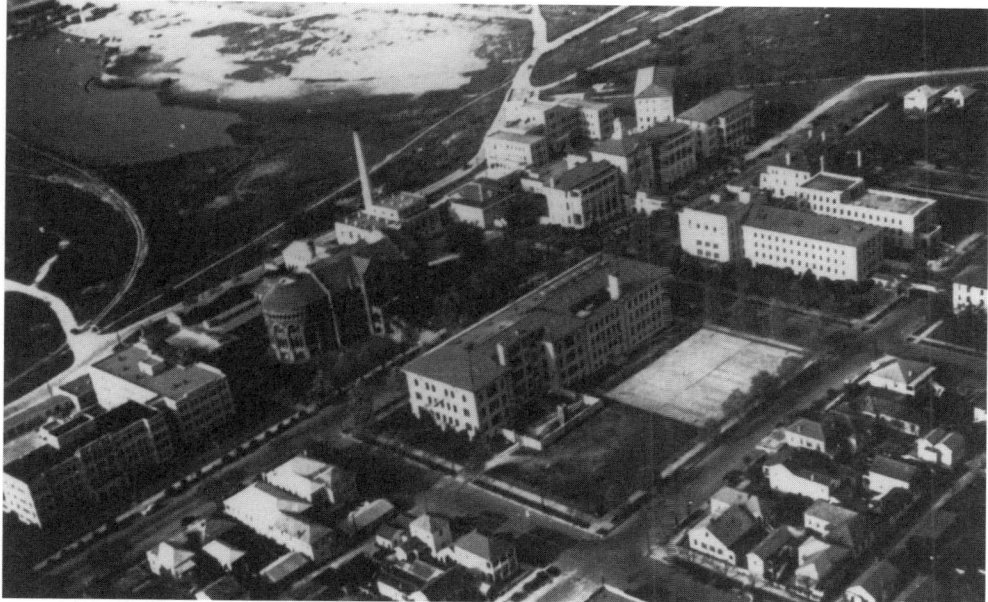

UTMB campus, 1943.

School of Public Health building, and facilities that would provide water and electricity during an emergency. Leake's dreams were Texas-sized.

Wartime conditions, however, slowed progress and only the convalescent home functioned before the end of World War II. In 1944 Maco Stewart and his wife donated their home to UTMB. About ten miles west of the campus, near the Galveston Country Club, the Margie B. Stewart Convalescent Home for Children functioned from February 1946 until February 1949, when the regents closed the home because it was too expensive to operate for the small number of patients usually admitted.[25]

As postwar enthusiasm abounded, Leake envisioned great changes that would require the financial support of just about everybody interested in UTMB. He wanted the Sealy & Smith Foundation to build a new hospital, a separate tuberculosis hospital, an office building for part-time staff, an apartment building, a woman's dormitory, some fraternity houses, and an addition to the power plant. He wanted the regents to issue bonds for a major addition to the Keiller Building and for an administration building that would include library facilities and an auditorium. He wanted the regents to use Available University Fund income for the power plant addition, an expansion of the laundry, a virus laboratory, and some operating expenses. He hoped that legislators would fund additions to the Children's Hospital and the Galveston State Psychopathic Hospital. Finally, he believed that Galvestonians would provide funds for a Students' Union Building. In March 1946 Leake persuaded the regents to develop a comprehensive plan for "further improvement of the Medical Department at Galveston."[26]

Eager to moderate Leake's enthusiasm, Painter and the regents asked the Faculty and Admission Committee to prepare a report on "future building needs." This

111

committee recommended additions to the power plant, John Sealy Hospital, and the Keiller Building, as well as a new Administration Building. Painter supported the power plant and Keiller Building additions, but thought that the other two were "it would be nice" buildings.[27]

None of these dreams had materialized when eight war surplus buildings were transferred from Camp Wallace in Hitchcock to the campus in 1947 and 1948. One of these became a fifty-bed Special Surgical Unit (SSU) for plastic surgery and neurosurgery patients, which opened in the spring of 1948. A 140-seat cafeteria for staff, students, and patients was established in another of these buildings. The other six housed a print shop, general stores, business offices, an animal house, an emergency room, a "time office," a laundry facility, and a gardener's shop.[28]

By the end of 1948 UTMB owned twenty structures plus the war surplus buildings.[29] A house nursing students used was acquired in 1944 and a structure housing a garage and storeroom was acquired in 1945. All of the other buildings had existed before Leake moved to Galveston, though there had been some functional changes. The original Children's Hospital was now an Isolation Building; the original Isolation Pavilion was a Psychopathic Hospital (Psycho One); and the first Rebecca Sealy Nurses' Home was also a psychiatric facility (Psycho Two and Three). The estimated replacement cost of all twenty-eight buildings was $7,462,125.

Leake, however, did not stop dreaming and lobbying. He persistently annoyed Painter about UTMB's failure to receive a fair share of Available University Fund income. Using rather vacuous arguments, Painter made a sharp distinction between the medical school and the hospitals, noting that the former was a "constitutional branch of the University of Texas" and "entitled to share in the Available Fund as much as the Main University," whereas the latter were "statutory appendages" to the medical school and not legally entitled to a share of the fund's income.[30] He believed that the regents were financially responsible for academic buildings and that the legislators were financially responsible for hospital buildings. Painter's hair-splitting appeared to be a desperate attempt to protect the UT Austin campus from losing Available University Fund income that did not work. Leake and others persuaded the regents to be more generous to UTMB and eventually secured support for a new hospital and a new research building.

On May 11, 1949, Painter attended groundbreaking ceremonies for a new John Sealy Hospital, ceremonies made possible after more than ten years of dreaming, drafting, changing, negotiating, redrafting, and replanning. As part of the hoopla about reforming UTMB associated with the hiring of John Spies in the summer of 1938, Edward Randall and other Sealy & Smith Foundation directors began to think about replacing the almost fifty-year-old John Sealy Hospital. Randall hoped that he could obtain PWA money for this project, but fellow regents warned that there would be no Available University Fund income to match a grant from the PWA. Complicating these dreams somewhat was the death of Jennie Sealy Smith in October 1938 and a provision in her will that a portion of her estate be used to build a hospital building in honor of her husband, R. Waverley Smith, a building that would be used by patients who could pay for all or part of their hospital expenses.[31] Planning more or less stopped with the turmoil of the Spies era, the advent of World War II, and Randall's resignation as regent.

When interest in this project reappeared during 1944, the Sealy & Smith Foundation directors offered the regents $2 million for a new six hundred-bed hospital that would include the R. Waverley Smith Pavilion, if they provided furniture and equipment for the new building. Negotiations between these directors and the regents became more stressful as estimated costs of the project escalated to $4 million in 1946, $5 million in 1948, and $6 million in 1949. Many problems appeared during the years of construction as changes in design recurred and as the costs of materials and labor steadily increased. The Texas State Department of Health helped by obtaining $1,500,000 of federal dollars for the project.[32]

The stresses of these years finally gave way to smiles of happiness during the dedication ceremonies for the new hospital held on December 15, 1953, though considerable future income from the Smith bequest and from the university were needed to pay the total costs of about $11 million. Leake's dream became a reality when the completely air-conditioned edifices opened in January 1954.[33]

Leake's hopes for a new research facility had already been fulfilled in 1952. A large increase in the number of basic science faculty during the 1940s generated a need for more laboratory and office space, especially for the departments of physiology, biochemistry, pharmacology, and bacteriology. In May 1950 the regents issued bonds for a new laboratory building. They accepted the completed structure in March 1952 (carrying value of $1,434,385), agreed with Leake's recommendation that the building be named in honor of Gail Borden, and attended dedication ceremonies on June 6, 1952. Members of the departments of biochemistry and physiology moved from Old Red to the Gail Borden Building during the summer of 1952.[34] They had worked in this building for more than a year when the new John Sealy Hospital opened in January 1954.

During the first week of February 1954 patients occupied another new clinical facility, the Ziegler Hospital, a specialized facility UTMB had acquired unexpectedly. During the 1940s the number of adult patients with tuberculosis and other chronic respiratory infections continued to increase. In January 1948 the regents accepted a bequest of more than $300,000 from Rosa M. Ziegler for the construction of a sixty-bed hospital for patients with diseases of the chest. The Texas State Board of Health supplemented this gift with federal grant funds of more than $400,000.[35]

UTMB now had three new patient care facilities and a new basic science research building, all air-conditioned. Living accommodations on the island, however, were inadequate for the dramatic expansion of students and house staff during these years. Using revenue dormitory bonds that were first purchased with a Federal Housing Authority loan and later sold to private interests, the regents authorized the construction of an eight-building dormitory complex on land donated by the Sealy & Smith Foundation.[36] The complex included a dormitory for 36 female medical students, two dormitories for 72 nursing students, three dormitories for 108 interns and residents, one thirty-unit apartment building for married interns and residents, and a building that housed a cafeteria for faculty and apartments for visiting faculty. Occupied in 1955 and 1956, the buildings were named as follows: Bethel Hall, Brackenridge Hall, Clay Hall, League Hall, Morgan Hall, Nolan Hall, Vinsant Hall, and Faculty House (later Unit D).[37]

During Leake's tenure the new John Sealy Hospital and R. Waverley Smith Pavilion crowned campus development. Leake's principal dream had been realized and the Ziegler Hospital was an unexpected bonus. The army barracks came serendipitously and provided housing for clinical and business activities. The number of business personnel expanded so much that a building originally constructed for storage was converted to a business office in 1950. Adjacent to this office, a warehouse for general stores was added in 1951.[38] The Maco Stewart Home became more useful as a residence than it had been as a convalescent home for children. Leake's concern for the care of chronically ill children was partially assuaged with the advent of the Moody State School for Cerebral Palsied Children in 1950.[39] The Gail Borden Building became a major boost for basic science departments and the various dormitories provided low-cost residential space for students and house staff.

During thirteen years, Leake's bombast for more buildings never ceased. He used faculty committees to gather ideas about campus development. He stretched the limits of the regents' tolerance and the Sealy & Smith Foundation's generosity. When he left Galveston toward the end of fiscal year 1955, campus buildings were valued at $18,402,279, a sixfold increase from 1942. Slightly more than 60 percent of this total had come from private gifts, mostly those of the Sealy & Smith Foundation.[40]

JOHN TRUSLOW, DON WALKER, AND COMPREHENSIVE PLANNING

Strongly believing in a philosophy of planned campus development, Don Walker worked carefully with Truslow, who had inherited a report about the physical plant from the faculty's Services, Development, and Space Committee. During discussions in the fall of 1956 Truslow, Walker, Wilson, and others became rather pessimistic about the future of Galveston and UTMB. They did not know if the city would continue to provide funds for the care of indigent patients. Recruitment of new faculty was difficult because of high prices for goods and services in Galveston, an unattractive public school system, and inadequate housing. Doubts lingered about the location of UTMB in Galveston. Instead of recommending new buildings, they decided to renovate certain buildings, use present space more effectively, raze some of the old structures (mostly the war surplus buildings), reduce "the fat" in the current operating budget, upgrade salaries, and use outside consultants to create a plan for campus development.[41]

In 1957 the regents invited the James A. Hamilton Associates of Minneapolis to develop a master plan for the campus. Staff members visited Galveston in July and August 1957 and the consultants submitted a final two hundred-page report in March 1958.[42] The report recommended short-term remodeling projects with an estimated cost of $2,500,000, including rehabilitating the Graves Psychopathic Hospital; transforming the Negro Hospital into a psychopathic hospital to replace Psycho One, Two, and Three; remodeling the outpatient clinics; transforming the Rebecca Sealy Nurses' Home into offices and classrooms for the School of Nursing; and rehabilitating the Keiller Building. They recommended new structures estimated at $8 million: a basic science building, an outpatient building addition, a clinical diagnostic building, a library building, and a building to house central air cooling equipment.

During the next two years Truslow, Wilson, and others explored ways to implement these recommendations. To coordinate these efforts, Truslow appointed Edwin G. Troutman as assistant director for planning. By early 1960 they had decided to raze the original John Sealy Hospital, renovate the renamed Randall Pavilion and other clinical facilities, and make plans for new clinical and basic science buildings.[43]

In September 1960 the regents made tentative decisions about a ten-year development program for the physical plants of the UT System.[44] For UTMB they identified seven projects that would cost an estimated $13,165,000, including an outpatient building, a basic science building, an addition to the central water chilling station and the laundry, remodeling of Keiller and other buildings, and equipment purchases. The regents pledged $3,700,000 in new Permanent University Fund bonds and $1,200,000 in Available University Fund income for these projects.

In January 1962 Ransom reviewed the status of the building program with the regents. Remodeling projects involved Wards 9A and 4C of the John Sealy Hospital, Psycho Two and Three, and the Keiller Building. Bids were about to be opened on a new outpatient building. Plans for two temporary, low-cost (tilt-slab) buildings, to be used for surgical research and the physical plant, were ready for approval, and discussions had begun about an animal care facility and a basic science building. Later that month Truslow pleaded for additional water chilling stations, a large auditorium, modern facilities for the audiovisual department, and an administration building.[45]

As 1962 evolved Truslow became ecstatic about the success of campus planning and the future of UTMB. Campus personnel watched the destruction of the original John Sealy Hospital during the early months of 1962. Construction had started on a centralized cooling plant and the outpatient diagnostic building.[46] The regents approved the remodeling of Keiller, construction of two tilt-slab buildings (the Surgical Research Laboratories and the Physical Plant Storeroom), the transformation of Ward 4-C into a Clinical Research Center, the remodeling of Psycho Two and Three, and the continued construction of the outpatient-clinical diagnostic building. Renovations were in progress or planned for twelve buildings.[47]

In April 1962, the regents authorized the preparation of a five-year building plan for UTMB. To help design this plan, Truslow appointed a faculty building committee that included Willard Verwey (chair), Eric Hall, William Daeschner, John Middleton, Edgar Poth, Don Walker, and Warren Harding. This committee submitted a lengthy report in November 1962. After studying the committee's report, the regents adopted a new master plan in April 1963.[48] They recommended the acquisition of more land and a basic sciences building; remodeling the Gail Borden Laboratory Building, an animal care center, a clinical sciences building, and outpatient facilities; expanding the

Central Water Chilling Station; additions to the warehouse and the laundry; and new parking areas, which would be financed with Permanent University Fund bond proceeds, Available University Fund income, Sealy & Smith Foundation gifts, federal grants, and contributions by other foundations and individuals. The total of Available University Fund income and Permanent University Fund bond proceeds was not to exceed $3,100,000. During the early 1960s the regents pledged about $14 million for campus expansion, an unprecedented affirmation.

Tangible outcomes began appearing in the mid-1960s. Financed by Available University Fund income of $315,000, the Surgical Research Laboratories and the Physical Plant Storeroom were completed by early 1964. The Central Water Chilling Station functioned by then, and the Sealy & Smith Professional Building opened in the spring of 1964. Groundbreaking ceremonies for the new Shriners Burns Institute occurred in late June 1964.[49]

BLOCKER'S BOOM YEARS

A few days after Blocker became CEO the regents accepted his proposal to lease space on the seventh floor of the Sealy & Smith Professional Building for a conference area and faculty lounge that was named the Caduceus Room.[50] With a magnificent view of the Gulf of Mexico, the Houston Ship Channel, and the eastern edge of the campus, the Caduceus Room symbolized Blocker's confident belief that he and the faculty would have much to celebrate as they sustained the campus development momentum initiated during Truslow's tenure.

Blocker was thrilled with the opening of the Shriners Burns Institute in 1966, but disappointed that he could not persuade federal officials to relocate Galveston's U.S. Public Health Service Hospital to the UTMB campus. He focused attention on the McCullough Outpatient Clinic, a Sealy & Smith Foundation proposal for a new hospital, and evolving plans for five buildings that would house some basic science departments, clinical science laboratories, animal care facilities, a centralized library, and physical fitness equipment for students and faculty.[51]

Between 1962 and 1966, the outpatient clinic building was transformed into the six-story John W. McCullough Outpatient Clinic, which opened on October 31, 1966.[52] This building housed clinics for the departments of obstetrics and gynecology, medicine, neurology and psychiatry, radiology, and surgery, and other facilities such as the clinical laboratories, emergency room, pharmacy, blood bank, and medical records.

UTMB had significantly improved its facility for outpatient services, but more inpatient beds were also needed. In early 1964 Ransom asked Don Walker to chair a committee that would review a proposal made by the Sealy & Smith Foundation to build and operate a 150-bed hospital for private patients (100 psychiatric beds and 50 medical beds). More than two years of painful negotiations occurred before construction began in August 1966.[53] University officials dedicated the $5.3 million, six-story, 175-bed hospital on October 29, 1968. Occupied in January 1969, the building was named in honor of Jennie Sealy Smith, the daughter of John Sealy I. The first floor of

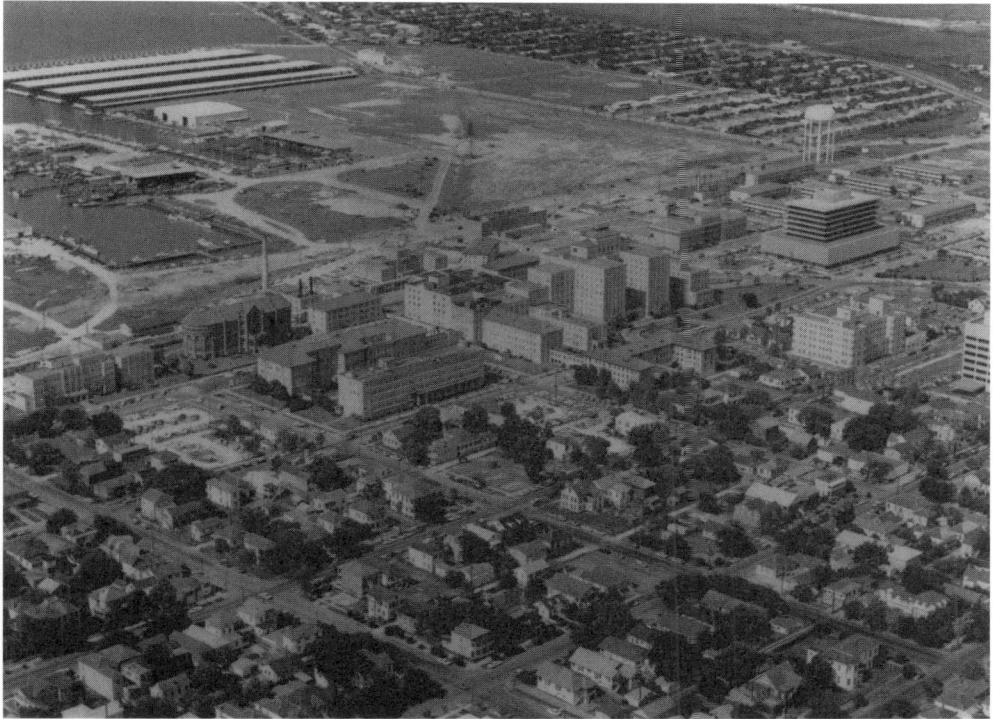

UTMB campus, 1967.

the six-story building housed offices and laboratories, and the second floor housed components of the Department of Radiology. The other floors housed patients, with one hundred beds allocated to psychiatry, fifty to internal medicine, and twenty-five to neurology.[54]

As professors began receiving more federal and private grants for research, more facilities were needed for the personnel and equipment needed to implement the grants. In 1963 and 1964 the building committee provided detailed recommendations for three buildings: an Animal Care Center, a Basic Science Building, and a Clinical Sciences Building. The regents approved final plans for these buildings in the spring of 1967.[55]

The Baxter Construction Company of Houston built the Animal Care Center, which included an operating suite, a dietary kitchen, research labs, administrative offices, and Galveston's animal pound.[56] Opening in 1969, the center cost $943,300. The Baxter Construction Company also built the $4.46 million Libbie Moody Thompson Basic Science Building, which opened in 1971. It was named for Libbie Moody, the daughter of W. L. Moody Jr., who had married Clark Thompson. The five-story building housed the offices and labs of the departments of biochemistry and physiology, and the teaching laboratories for a new interdisciplinary course for sophomore medical students. The building also housed several academic service departments, including student personnel services, medical electronics, medical photography, medical illustrations, audiovisual

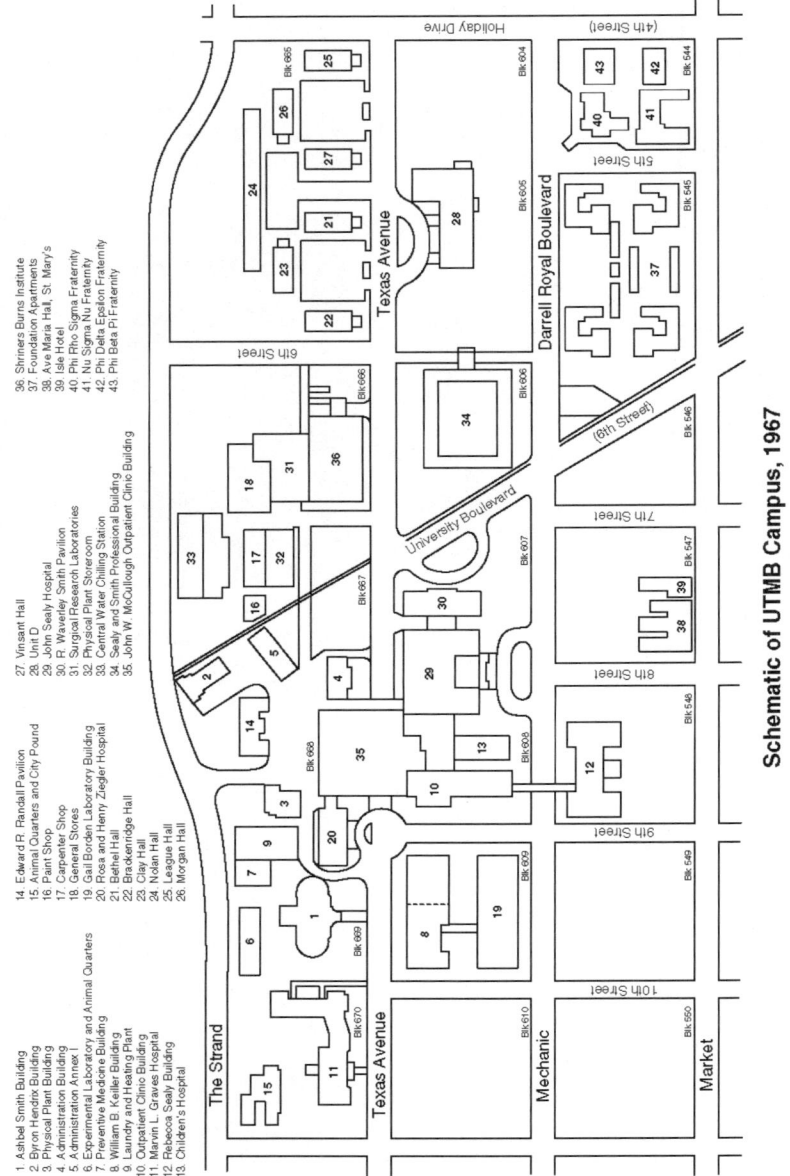

1. Ashbel Smith Building
2. Byron Hendrix Building
3. Physical Plant Building
4. Administration Building
5. Administration Annex I
6. Experimental Laboratory and Animal Quarters
7. Preventive Medicine Building
8. William B. Keiller Building
9. Laundry and Heating Plant
10. Outpatient Clinic Building
11. Marvin L. Graves Hospital
12. Rebecca Sealy Building
13. Children's Hospital

14. Edward R. Randall Pavilion
15. Animal Quarters and City Pound
16. Paint Shop
17. Carpenter Shop
18. General Stores
19. Gail Borden Laboratory Building
20. Rosa and Henry Ziegler Hospital
21. Bethel Hall
22. Brackenridge Hall
23. Clay Hall
24. Nolan Hall
25. League Hall
26. Morgan Hall

27. Vinsant Hall
28. Unit D
29. John Sealy Hospital
30. R. Waverley Smith Pavilion
31. Surgical Research Laboratories
32. Physical Plant Storeroom
33. Central Water Chilling Station
34. Sealy and Smith Professional Building
35. John W. McCullough Outpatient Clinic Building

36. Shriners Burns Institute
37. Foundation Apartments
38. Ave Maria Hall, St. Mary's
39. Isle Hotel
40. Phi Rho Sigma Fraternity
41. Nu Sigma Nu Fraternity
42. Phi Delta Epsilon Fraternity
43. Phi Beta Pi Fraternity

Schematic of UTMB Campus, 1967

118

services, and educational television.[57] The Tellespen Construction Company built the Clinical Sciences Building, which was occupied in 1973. Th s five-story building housed outpatient admitting offices and clinics, laboratories and offices for clinical faculty, and a three hundred-seat auditorium.[58]

With research facilities substantially improved, Blocker turned his attention to expanding and improving clinical facilities. He used idea; from the Lester Gorsline Associates, a hospital consultant firm. After receiving the firm's report in the spring of 1969, Blocker and White appointed Ken Newman as a full-time administrator to coordinate planning. Blocker, White, and Newman solicited ideas from a planning committee that included Bill Daeschner, Bill Deiss, Jack Thompson, David Hoxie, Ed Brandt, Louis Gilliam, and Richard Timmer (chair).[59] After reviewing all proposals, Blocker recommended a new Child Health Center and two additions to the John Sealy Hospital.

In December 1969 the regents selected Pierce, Goodwin and Flanagan of Houston as the project architects for the additions to the John Sealy Hospital, and Goleman and Rolfe of Houston as the architects for a new Child Health Center. After many weeks of working with faculty and staff, Goleman and Rolfe completed their preliminary drawings in October 1971. In March 1972 the regents authorized the sale of construction bonds to raise approximately $32 million of the $40 million required to finance the new Child Health Center and the John Sealy Hospital additions.[60] Other dollars for the Child Health Center came from the Sealy & Smith Foundation ($5,003,686) and from the Bureau of Health Manpower Education of the USPHS ($5,296,314). The regents accepted the $8,299,500 bid of Southwestern Construction Company of Houston, which began work on this six-story building in July 1973.[61]

During 1972 and 1973 Blocker, Thompson, McCullough, Walker, and others met periodically to make decisions about the additions to the John Sealy Hospital. They reviewed detailed reports from architects, engineers, and design consultants. In October 1973 the regents authorized advertisements for bids for the two-story North Addition and the twelve-story South Addition. Early in 1974 the regents awarded the $29.4 million construction contract to Thomas Construction Company of St. Louis, Missouri.[62]

In addition to overseeing these plans for improving patient care facilities, Blocker searched for a way to support the recreational needs of students. In 1967 the revitalized School of Medicine Alumni Association decided to use its accumulated funds, about $162,000, to construct a Field House that would provide recreational facilities for students and faculty. The Sealy & Smith Foundation donated land and offered a loan of $100,000 to meet the estimated cost of the facility. The Field House opened in January 1969 and Blocker happily presided during a dedication ceremony on commencement day, June 11, 1969.[63] UTMB assumed responsibility for operating the Field House after the land and building were given to the university.

Stimulated in part by Leake's interest in libraries and medical history, Truslow's building committee had recommended a library building.[64] After extensive pleading by Ransom and Blocker in 1964, the Moody Foundation pledged $1 million for a new library. In July 1965 the regents authorized the preparation of preliminary plans by the consulting architects. In August 1966 these plans were approved and the regents authorized O'Neil Ford to prepare working drawings and specifications. In 1968 the U.S. Public Health Service awarded UTMB a grant of $1,598,406 for this project and the regents contributed $200,000 from Permanent University Fund bond income.[65] The Tellespen Construction Company began work on the building in March 1969 and the Moody Medical Library was dedicated on June 6, 1972. The five-story concrete-and-steel edifice included storage space for more than 250,000 volumes, a history of medicine and rare book room, individual carrels and group study rooms for students, a book bindery, administrative offices, and an audiovisual resource center.[66]

The new School of Allied Health Sciences needed space for offices and classrooms. In July 1968 the regents approved the rental of space in Ave Maria Hall, a building that formerly housed the St. Mary's Hospital Nursing School. In 1971 the regents purchased this building, now Administration Annex II, which continued to house the School of Allied Health Sciences until it moved to a new building in 1986.[67]

During his last year as CEO Blocker's office was on the sixth floor of the new Administration Building, which was occupied in September 1973. The Sealy & Smith Foundation contributed more than $3 million for this building.[68] The Caduceus Room was moved from the Sealy & Smith Professional Building to the sixth floor of this new building and continued to serve as the site for many meetings, parties, and celebratory dinners.

In 1973 UTMB added four fraternity houses to its property inventory and UTMB's personnel began using Materials Management Warehouses Nos. 1 and 2. A parking garage at Eighth and Market, one of four parking facilities the regents authorized in 1969, began functioning in 1974. During that year, the Gail Borden Building was remodeled, three buildings were under construction (John Sealy Hospital additions, Child Health Center, and another parking facility), and the Eriksson Construction Company added a pre-cast concrete "surge" building for the department of pharmacology. After the department "surged" into this building in September 1974 they did not leave and other "surge" structures never materialized.[69]

Before Blocker retired as CEO the Microbiology Building was authorized and funded, and remodeling of Old Red and the John Sealy Hospital was authorized but not funded. Blocker and Thompson appointed Ed Brandt, Barbara Bowman, Arthur Brown, Bill Deiss, Bill McGanity, David Hoxie, Louis Gilliam, and Ken Newman as a committee to develop the "Long Range Campus Master Plan" for UTMB.[70]

By the end of Blocker's presidency, August 31, 1974, the estimated value of property (land, buildings, equipment, library) was $85,196,085. UTMB owned seventy buildings, with a carrying value of $44,764,624. Thirty buildings were used for patient care, teaching, research, and administration; twenty-six for general services; and fourteen for auxiliary enterprises. Funds used to construct and remodel these buildings came from the following sources: $15,790,678 from private foundations and donors (35.2 percent); $1,211,876 from the state legislature (2.7 percent); $11,502,450 from the sale of Permanent University Fund bonds (25.7 percent); $2,069,728 from Available University Fund income (4.6 percent); $2,296,917 from the sale of revenue bonds for dormitories and power plant addition (5.1 percent); $9,310,627 from federal grants (20.8 percent); and $2,582,344 from Medical Service Research and Development Plan income (5.8 percent).[71]

Levin's Boom Years

Bill Levin carefully shepherded the construction projects initiated during Blocker's tenure: the Child Health Center and the John Sealy Hospital additions. When the Child Health Center was occupied in January 1977, the first floor contained all outpatient clinics, and the fourth, fifth, and sixth floors contained 150 beds for inpatients. The second and third floors housed departmental offices, research labs, and teaching rooms, as well as a "care by parent" unit, which allowed parents to stay with their infants and children. Sick children were admitted to the new rooms in February 1977.[72]

The North Addition to the John Sealy Hospital became functional in December 1976; the South Addition in June 1978.[73] The North Addition included fourteen new surgical operating suites, a central supply, pharmacy, and storage areas. Named the John Sealy Towers, the South Addition of twelve-story twin towers housed individual rooms for 528 beds. The privacy made possible by these rooms was a striking contrast to the multi-patient wards in the previous John Sealy Hospitals.

As the new additions became functional, the twenty-five hospital departments and thirteen academic departments competed for the space released in the old John Sealy Hospital. Charles Tandy coordinated the requests for space from the academic departments and Ray Jarl, director of support services, coordinated those from the hospital departments. Cecil Deming, Tandy, and Jarl correlated these requests, and Jack Thompson and Al LeBlanc made the final assignments. To provide some rationale for these assignments, John Poretto established a space committee, whose members included Alan Ladd (director of ambulatory services), Jarl, and Tim Parker (director of inpatient services). In April 1979 this committee recommended that surge space be "designated separately for the School of Medicine to avoid conflicting priorities."[74] After stormy meetings with this committee and department chairs, George Bryan and others made adjustments that finally permitted all parties to accept the proposed space assignments. The Sealy & Smith Foundation gave $5,650,836 for remodeling space assigned to the departments of internal medicine, pathology, and surgery (approximately forty thousand gross square feet on the fourth, fifth, and sixth floors of the old John Sealy Hospital).[75]

Levin did not neglect the basic science departments that had expanded dramatically during the 1970s. To accommodate the microbiology department, in November 1974 the regents approved a major addition to the Animal Care Center, into which faculty and staff moved in July and August 1978.[76] Levin also supported the auditorium project that the building committee had recommended during the early 1960s. In July 1974 John M. Davis, project architect in the UT System Office of Facilities Planning and Construction, estimated that the structure would cost no less than $3,000 per seat; thus a thousand-seat auditorium would cost $3 million. The solicitation of philanthropic donations began in 1975. Libbie Moody Thompson contributed $500,000 in honor of her husband, Clark Thompson, after whom the auditorium was named. Generous gifts came from the M. D. Anderson Foundation and the Houston Endowment (a total of $3,225,000). Gifts from alumni and faculty amounted to $275,000, as they endowed seats in the auditorium for $2,000 each. The regents assigned $5,373,400 of Permanent University Fund bond proceeds and UTMB contributed $4,491,000 of unexpended plant funds—for a grand total of $13,364,400. Construction began in 1979 and the six-story Learning Center was officially accepted on October 1, 1981.[77] In addition to the Thompson auditorium, the building contained reception areas, offices for biomedical communications, and offices for continuing medical education. Shortly after his arrival in Galveston, Tom James asked the regents to name the Learning Center in Levin's honor. Making an exception to their rule that UT buildings should be named only for deceased persons, the regents renamed the Learning Center as the William C. Levin Hall on October 9, 1987.[78]

Three new clinical facilities opened in 1983: the Mary Moody Northen Pavilion for psychiatric patients, the Texas Department of Criminal Justice Hospital for prisoners, and the Ambulatory Care Center for outpatients.

In December 1977 the regents approved Levin's proposal to renovate 60,000 square feet in the Graves Hospital and add 51,600 square feet at an estimated cost of $4,978,000. The renovated space would house offices and classrooms. The new space would accommodate inpatient beds, an outpatient facility, and a Psychiatric Research Center. The five-story building was completed in December 1982 and named in honor of Mary Moody Northen, chair of the board of directors of the Moody Foundation. Dedication ceremonies occurred on June 7, 1983, and the fifth-floor research center opened in August 1984.[79]

The prison hospital came to UTMB after twenty years of extensive efforts. In the fall of 1963, when seventy-five to one hundred prisoners were taken by bus to UTMB for treatment each week, Truslow appointed Blocker as chair of a committee to study the feasibility of adding a prison hospital to the campus. Further deliberations were not successful then, but the proposal reappeared about ten years later.[80] In December 1973 consultants from the Texas Hospital Association Management Engineering Services evaluated the health care facilities at the prison in Huntsville and concluded that the "TDC must abandon the Huntsville Hospital."[81] In the fall of 1976 the Legislative Budget Board recommended a substantial appropriation for new health care facilities for the Texas Department of Corrections. In the spring of 1977 the Hobby–Clayton Commission recommended that a new prison hospital be constructed on the UTMB campus and the Sixty-fifth Legislature appropriated $40 million for its construction.[82]

During 1977 and 1978 university and prison officials met regularly with architects, engineers, and designers. Details of planning were tedious and taxing; consider housekeeping, for example. Robert Hope, then director of housekeeping services, estimated that it would be necessary to employ two housekeeping supervisors to oversee the work of fifteen trusties. He believed that each of two nursing stations located on four patient care floors needed a cleaning closet large enough to hold supplies and equipment. He estimated that $45,575.05 would be needed for supplies, equipment, and salaries. Establishing functional patterns that would maintain security and provide needed care were also essential. In February 1978 the TDC issued a report that detailed security and other requirements for the new hospital, floor by floor.[83]

The regents approved preliminary plans for the hospital in June 1978. Meeting in an all-day session on August 25, 1978, the TDC Planning Committee made final recommendations to the project's architects. The Texas Health Facilities Commission approved the hospital in May 1979. The regents approved final plans in June and in the fall they selected the J. W. Bateson Company of Dallas to construct the hospital.[84] The Texas Department of Criminal Justice (TDCJ) Hospital opened in June 1983 as the first hospital of its kind in the United States—the only prison hospital situated on the campus of a major academic medical center. The 25,000 square foot, eight-story, $40 million hospital became the state's only centralized facility for tertiary medical care for inmates housed in any of the state's twenty-four correctional institutions.[85]

As hundreds of patients were referred to UTMB for ambulatory care during the 1970s, outpatient facilities became crowded and exasperating for professionals and patients. Levin and Thompson wanted a new Ambulatory Care Center, which would consolidate existing outpatient facilities into a single center that would relieve crowded conditions in existing facilities and accommodate an expanding future population. It would create a model educational environment for the instruction of residents, interns, and students (medical, nursing, and allied health) and create an environment more conducive to clinical research. It would eliminate a two-class system of outpatient health care delivery and promote better efficiency in the use of outpatient support systems such as radiology, clinical laboratories, and medical records. The center would improve the flow of patients to and from specialty clinics and provide each outpatient with better health care at a reasonable cost.[86]

Seven professors and six administrators met with the Page Southerland Page architectural firm on June 15, 1976, to discuss the design of the building's interior. Planning continued during 1976, 1977, and 1978. Jim Donovan, UTMB's planning coordinator, smoothed the interpersonal processes. The regents approved preliminary plans in December 1976 and final plans in June 1978. The J. W. Bateson Construction Company began work in the spring of 1979 and they finished four years later.[87] The center opened in June 1983 and was dedicated on October 13, 1983. The seven-story structure provided 220,400 square feet of space for clinical and laboratory facilities that permitted the consolidation of thirteen major clinics and forty subspecialty clinics.[88]

Two other building projects were dear to Levin's heart: the renovation of Old Red and the construction of a new building for the School of Allied Health Sciences and the School of Nursing.

During the early 1970s Truman Blocker catalyzed widespread interest in preserving and restoring Old Red. With the regents' authorization, Wyatt C. Hedrick Architects and Engineers, Inc. of Houston prepared a feasibility study in 1971. During these years, faculty and alumni staged plays and sold red brick paperweights to secure support and funds for this preservation project. In June 1973 the regents committed $875,000 as matching monies to funds Blocker and others raised.[89] In 1973 and 1974 Wilson, Crain, Anderson, and Reynolds, Inc. in Houston prepared another feasibility study, but no further decisions occurred before Blocker's retirement as CEO.

During the early years of Levin's presidency, numerous Texans joined the "Save Old Red" bandwagon, including "Babe" Schwartz, Truett Latimer, Ray Holbrook, Mrs. Mary Moody Northen, Ed Protz, Emily Whiteside, and Peter Brink. They wrote numerous letters of support and met with the regents more than once to advocate renovation. A national survey revealed that the Ashbel Smith Building was the only extant medical school building of its kind west of the Mississippi River built before 1900 and the only medical school building designated as a state's historical landmark (1969) and listed in the National Register of Historic Places. In 1976 the Galveston County Bicentennial Committee recognized the preservation of Old Red as a state and national bicentennial project, and boosters spread hyperbole in many directions.[90]

In October 1978 the regents decided that the restoration of Old Red was a "necessity." They accepted a Moody Foundation pledge of $500,000, offered to provide a match of $1 million from Permanent University Fund proceeds, and decided to seek $2 million from the legislature for this project. In late February Levin pleaded for money to preserve the building during hearings with the Senate Finance Committee. In April Peter Brink and others lobbied directly with Bill Clayton and staff members in the offices of the lieutenant governor and governor.[91]

A turning point occurred in September 1980, when Levin made an "eloquent" appeal to the regents for additional support. The regents pledged $5 million contingent on the acquisition of another $3 million needed for the total cost of $8 million. During the next three months an Old Red Development Committee evolved into a Task Force for the Preservation and Restoration of Old Red with Ambassador Ed Clark as chair. During 1981 and 1982 this task force displayed extraordinary efforts in the quest for needed funds. With a total of more than $6.5 million secured, the regents approved final plans and authorized advertisements for bids to contractors during their meeting on June 11, 1982. Restoration work began in June 1983 and employees associated with the Department of Anatomy, the Institute for the Medical Humanities, and student personnel offices occupied the building in the summer of 1985. Dedication ceremonies for the restored Ashbel Smith Building were held in Levin Hall on April 10, 1986. Regent Jane Weinert Blumberg viewed the new "Old Red" as a symbol that "renews ties with the past while giving us strength to go forward."[92]

Interest in new facilities for the two baccalaureate schools at UTMB had existed for at least two decades. As early as January 1965 UTMB's building committee had recommended a new building for the School of Nursing. However, the transfer of the administration of the school to Austin in 1967 undermined efforts to secure new quarters in Galveston. The School of Allied Health Sciences had grown steadily since 1968, graduating more than nine hundred students by 1980. The system-wide nursing school was decentralized in 1976 and the political climate about the school's future in Galveston changed favorably during Levin's administration. The School of Nursing was located in Brackenridge Hall, League Hall, and the Port Holiday Mall. The School of Allied Health Sciences was located in Ave Maria Hall. Quarters for these two rapidly expanding schools were quite unsatisfactory by the late 1970s.[93]

In the fall of 1980 the regents approved Levin's proposal for a new building that would house both schools.[94] One year later the regents approved architectural plans and in February 1984 they allocated Permanent University Fund bond proceeds for this building and awarded the construction contract to Robert E. McKee, Inc. of Houston, who had bid $10,686,000.[95]

The schools moved into the four-story building in August 1986 and Levin proudly participated in dedication ceremonies for the $13.75 million building on October 3, 1986. The first floor housed classrooms, a Learning Resources Center, and simulation labs for nursing students. The second floor contained classrooms, basic science labs, and teaching labs for allied health students. The third floor housed offices for faculty and the fourth floor contained offices for faculty and administrators plus the Florence Marie Hall Community Room.[96]

Other events in campus development occurred during Levin's tenure as CEO. Acquired in 1976, the 1700 Strand Building (the former Customs House) housed the book bindery and the print shop by the summer of 1977. Other departments moved into this building as remodeling was completed. Because of the special interests of Edna and Bill Levin and June and Jack Thompson, original paintings and poster art were added to the hallways of John Sealy Hospital and most patient care rooms in early 1980. A redesigned and reconstructed Surgical Research Laboratory was dedicated on November 26, 1980. Located behind the former Shriners Burns Institute building, this expansion and renovation cost $600,000 and included the addition of two sterile operating rooms. In October 1980 a swimming pool was added to the Field House facilities; the 200,000-gallon pool was funded by a donation from the Alumni Association and a bequest from the parents of a former medical student.[97]

The Sealy & Smith Foundation donated a site for the new three-story Physical Plant Building that was completed in the fall of 1982.[98] Four parking garages were added. One included an enclosed floor used by the Moody Medical Library to house a bindery and storage areas for books and journals. An addition to the General Stores Warehouse was constructed in 1985. In 1986 a Visitor's Center was opened at the corner of University Boulevard and Market Street. In 1987 a sculpture titled "Birth" was placed on the campus between the Moody Medical Library and Levin Hall. Arthur Williams, the artist, coated the welded and pressed steel with black lacquer.[99]

By the end of Bill Levin's presidency, August 31, 1987, the estimated value of property (land, buildings, equipment, library holdings) was $368,990,181. UTMB owned seventy-two buildings, with a carrying value of $218,700,361. Thirty buildings were used for patient care, teaching, research, and administration; twenty-four for general services; and eighteen for auxiliary enterprises. The dollars used for constructing and remodeling these buildings came from several sources. They included $36,558,714 from private foundations and donors (16.7 percent), $36,502,982 from the state legislature (16.7 percent), $55,618,693 from the sale of Permanent University Fund bonds (25.4 percent), $1,973,904 from Available University Fund income (0.9 percent), $34,343,865 from the sale of institutional revenue bonds (15.7 percent), $14,289,250 from federal grants (6.5 percent), $7,178,588 from interest earned on construction funds (3.3 percent), and $32,234,366 from other sources such as Medical Service Research and Development Plan income (14.7 percent).[100]

TOM JAMES'S IMPRINTS

Tom James inherited both renovation and new construction projects. In 1989 a $3 million renovation transformed Ave Maria Hall into the Administration Annex II, providing more than 35,000 square feet for administrative and business departments. By 1990 more than $25 million had been invested in other renovation projects: Ewing Hall; the John Sealy Towers and Surgical Suite; and the Waverley Smith Pavilion.[101] Major additions were under construction by early 1990: the Medical Research Building; the Trauma Center; and the new Shriners Burns Institute.

In the fall of 1988 the Texas Higher Education Coordinating Board approved the construction of a $25 million Medical Research Building that would be funded by $20 million from Permanent University Fund bond proceeds and $5 million from the Sealy & Smith Foundation. Groundbreaking ceremonies occurred in March 1989 and dedication ceremonies occurred on April 10, 1991, as one of the centennial year celebrations. The $25 million facility then provided 110,000 square feet of space on the first four floors. Construction of the other three floors was completed in 1995, providing an additional 70,000 square feet for research labs.[102] This building housed the Animal Resources Center, the Sealy Center for Molecular Science, and various offices and laboratories for School of Medicine faculty in basic science and clinical departments.

Groundbreaking ceremonies for the three-story Trauma Center and Emergency Department occurred on September 13, 1989. Made possible by a $38 million gift from the Sealy & Smith Foundation, this 94,000-square-foot structure was dedicated on January 9, 1992. The first floor contained the seven-ton hyperbaric chamber.[103] The second floor included emergency treatment areas that were connected to the ambulance ramp and two helipads. The third floor contained offices and conference rooms, as well as the Southeast Texas Poison Control Center.

Tom and Gleaves James gave special attention to projects that sustained Galveston's architectural legacies and added beauty to the campus, including the renovation of Open Gates, the Louis H. Runge House, and the Henry Rosenberg House, as well as the addition of the Gleaves T. James Centennial Rose Garden.

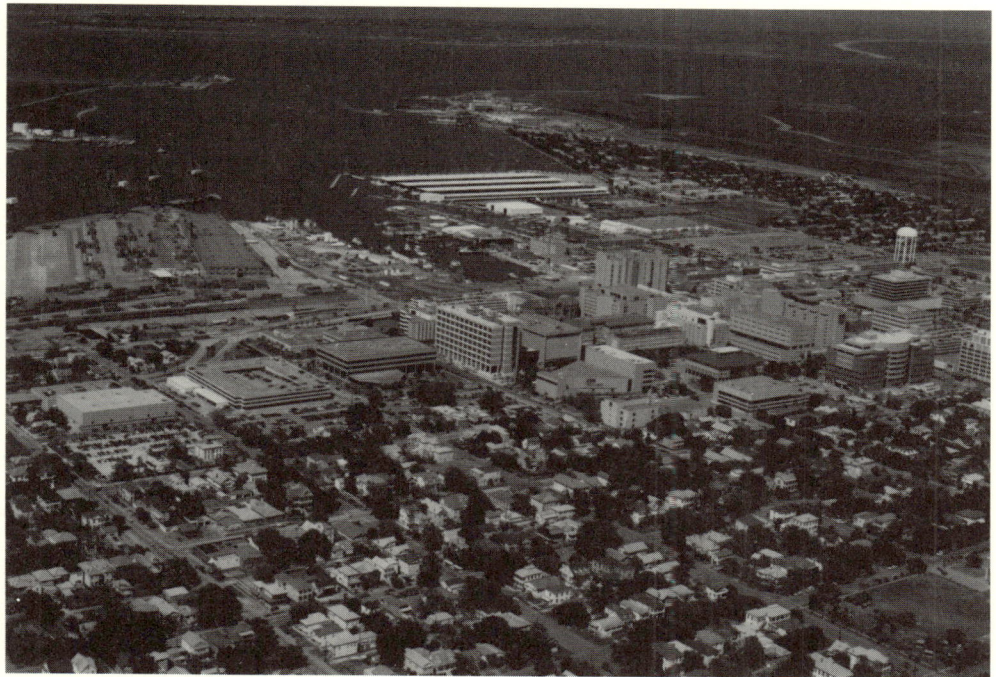

UTMB campus, 1991.

In the late 1880s George Sealy invited New York architect Stanford White to design a family home and Nicholas Clayton to supervise construction of what became known as the "Open Gates" mansion. The massive two-and-a-half-story masonry structure, with encircling galleries and a high-pitched, tiled roof was built between 1889 and 1891. Descendants of George Sealy deeded this Neo-Renaissance mansion to UTMB in 1969. Initial renovations of its roof and outer structures began in the fall of 1982, and restoration of its interior occurred during the 1990s. In 1989 Tom James and others dedicated an oleander garden at Open Gates as a memorial to George Sealy Jr., son of the builder.[104] Open Gates housed the telemedicine program and the George and Magnolia Willis Sealy Conference Center.

Tom and Gleaves James moved into the Louis H. Runge House in the spring of 1990. Located at Market and Thirteenth, the Mediterranean Revival-style house was built in 1916 as the family home for Louis and Anita Runge and their family. Their daughter, Elisabeth, was UTMB's chief librarian for forty-six years. In 1988 the Sealy & Smith Foundation purchased this property and provided funds for its restoration as the residence for UTMB's president.

A gift from Mary John and Ralph Spence of Tyler, the Gleaves T. James Centennial Rose Garden was dedicated on June 14, 1991. Containing thirty-five different varieties of shrubs and roses, this garden was designed by Larry J. Burks, an architect rosarian from Tyler, and Boyce Tankersley, former superintendent of grounds maintenance at UTMB.[105] In 1995 it was named to the All-American Rose Selection, a

127

nationwide network of public gardens that meet strict requirements, including an annual evaluation.

The Sealy & Smith Foundation purchased the Henry Rosenberg House in 1989 and deeded it to UTMB in 1990. Located across Market from the Runge House, this Italianate-style house was first occupied by Henry and Letitia Rosenberg in 1860. After an extensive restoration, this house opened in June 1993 as a conference facility and guest quarters for visiting dignitaries.

By the end of the centennial year, August 31, 1991, the estimated value of UTMB property (land, buildings, equipment, library) was $522,488,463. UTMB owned eighty buildings, with a carrying value of $287,896,654. Thirty-two buildings were used for patient care, teaching, research, and administration; twenty-eight for general services; and twenty for auxiliary enterprises. The sources of funds used for constructing and remodeling these buildings were as follows: $66,361,165 from private foundations and donors (23 percent); $36,500,233 from the state legislature (12.7 percent); $77,718,567 from the sale of Permanent University Fund bonds (27 percent); $1,942,673 from Available University Fund income (0.6 percent); $39,800,562 from the sale of institutional revenue bonds (13.8 percent); $14,043,300 from federal grants (4.9 percent); $8,047,802 from interest earned on construction funds (2.8 percent); and $43,482,352 from other sources such as local practice income (15.1 percent).[106]

CAMPUS CARETAKERS

Employees who took care of the buildings and grounds included janitors and housekeepers, specialized craftsmen, and campus police. In 1900 John Hooper was the janitor and engineer and John Carlson was the assistant janitor. Private contractors did the yard work. In 1903 Provost Johnson employed Michael Little as the engineer and mechanic and Carlson as the janitor. By 1910 there were four janitors who were probably handymen as well as housekeepers. In 1920 Little had an assistant, C. J. McLean, and eight men used the title, "janitor and laboratory attendant." Since a "gasoline lawn mower" was purchased that year and there is no evidence of private contracting, it is likely that some of the janitors also tended the campus grounds. In 1930 Little had two assistants and several "janitors and laboratory attendants."[107] Little and Albert Brautigan did most of the carpentry work, equipment construction, and general maintenance.

Dean Spies appointed Joseph T. Roberts as director of the "shop." A physician and scientist with both M.D. and Ph.D. degrees, Roberts was expected to establish better relationships between the faculty and the shop's craftsmen. Roberts divided functions into three areas: the machine shop, the carpentry shop, and the general maintenance shop. He assigned Brautigan to the machine shop and hired an apprentice for him. He selected Walter Lucas as a carpenter and added another. Harry Lawrence, former night watchman, became supervisor of the general maintenance shop, which included the janitorial staff, the night watchman, a full-time painter, and a plasterer.

Between August 19, 1940, and October 15, 1942, all of the shops handled 710 requisitions. Everyone believed that maintenance of the physical plant and grounds had greatly improved.[108]

When Leake arrived in 1942 Little supervised three assistant mechanics, two carpenters, one painter, and several janitors. By 1954 the Physical Plant Department employed 141 people who exercised more than twenty occupational roles (including architect, welder, plumber, electrician, locksmith, painter, and carpenter). John Moore was foreman of the hothouses and his brother, William, was foreman of the grounds; together they supervised about forty employees. John directed those who cultivated plants and flowers for the hospital, offices, and social events on the campus. William oversaw those who planted and trimmed the hedges, cut the lawns, gathered trash and garbage, and distributed ice.[109]

In October 1955 Reuel S. Purvis became director of the Physical Plant Department. Employees were situated in various locations on the campus: the original John Sealy Hospital, a barracks building behind the Graves hospital, the carpenter's shop, and the business offices facility. These employees provided repairs as needed. They also participated in remodeling and reconstruction projects as the campus expanded.[110]

In 1958 Don Walker appointed Louis Gilliam as the new director of the department. Gilliam and his staff developed an extensive maintenance program for campus buildings. In 1958 this department received more than fifteen hundred requests each month for maintenance and repair items. By 1970 these requests had dropped below eleven hundred, even with significant increases in buildings and services. By 1970 Gilliam supervised a staff of almost two hundred employees and the physical plant's annual budget was more than $1 million. Gilliam served as director for almost twenty-eight years (1958–1986), expertly cooperating with Warren Harding, Vernon E. "Jack" Thompson, and Jere Pederson.[111]

Other caretakers worked at UTMB for many years. Joe McMahan, for example, devoted thirty-four years to the campus. Beginning in 1950 as a painter, he became superintendent of building and grounds maintenance in 1963. Working with him in 1971, Leroy Tolston, landscaper foreman, supervised the work of twenty-seven men, who tended the grass, flowers, shrubbery, and trees on the campus. These caretakers participated in major landscaping projects in 1973, including the construction of pebbled concrete drives and sidewalks, the preparation of elevated grassy plots and flower beds, and the addition of more trees. By 1978 Jim Crow, supervisor of landscaping, coordinated the work of sixteen full-time gardeners and five summer helpers in maintaining the grounds of the eighty-acre campus. McMahan and Crow were especially proud of their landscaping improvements on the campus. 'We can handle that" was McMahan's favorite expression.[112]

By the late 1980s Ed White supervised approximately 250 physical plant employees, who were organized into five functional groups. About twenty were assigned to maintenance of the campus grounds, thirty to administrative tasks including a staff for the physical plant control room at all times, forty each to air-conditioning, electrical, and plumbing tasks, and sixty to other jobs associated with the maintenance of fifty-five buildings.[113]

Housekeeping department employees were responsible for cleaning the buildings. As the number of buildings expanded, the number of housekeepers expanded. By early 1957 Robert G. Lockerman supervised 135 employees in this department. During fiscal year 1961, 157 housekeepers cleaned more than 740,500 square feet of work space, using twenty-eight hundred gallons of liquid cleaner for floors and walls; seventy-five gallons of muriatic acid solution for bathroom plumbing fixtures; and six thousand cans of cleanser for sinks and tubs. In 1968, 181 housekeepers dusted, swept, mopped, and cleaned 1,300,000 square feet of workspace in seventeen campus buildings. In 1976 about three hundred employees worked in this department.[114] By the late 1980s more than five hundred employees were members of the combined housekeeping and transportation department.

Housekeeping tasks involved teams of supervisors, building attendants, and refuse technicians, who were assigned to one of four major areas on the campus. For example, about 128 workers attended 489,000 square feet of floor space in Area Four, which included six facilities: Ambulatory Care Clinic, Clinical Sciences Building, Emergency Room, Keiller Building, Thompson Basic Sciences Building, and the School of Allied Health Sciences Building. Each workday, building attendants emptied wastebaskets, cleaned conference rooms and patient care rooms, cleaned bathrooms (two to four times a day), and cleaned hallways and elevators. They replaced hand towels and toilet paper (672 rolls a month in Area Four alone), wiped walls, dusted furniture and equipment, and mopped, buffed, or waxed floors. Refuse technicians collected contaminated materials in red boxes and red sacks that were incinerated. Two specialized groups of housekeepers cleaned the hospital's operating rooms. Always on "stand by," members of each team had pre-assigned tasks, such as emptying wastebaskets, replacing plastic bags, mopping the floor, cleaning certain kinds of equipment, or washing and drying the overhead lights. The entire team was expected to complete its work in ten minutes, preferably eight.[115]

Night watchmen patrolled the campus during the early decades. In 1950 Paul Leslie became the chief of police. By 1954 he supervised fifteen men, who patrolled the campus, issuing up to ten citations a day for parking violations. By the spring of 1968 Chief Dick Tinney supervised five sergeants and twelve guards, who provided security for about one thousand students and thirty-three hundred employees housed in more than thirty buildings on the sixty-five-acre campus.[116]

Significant expansion occurred after Maurice Harr became director of the twenty-member police force in 1968. In 1973 Barbara Singleton became the first commissioned female police officer at UTMB.[117] By 1978 the sixty-member force included twenty commissioned officers. In fiscal year 1985 the department included sixteen police officers and forty-five police guards, who served a campus population of more than ten thousand people (8,710 faculty and staff and 1,728 students). These police officials investigated 230 incidents involving assaults, theft, criminal trespass, disorderly conduct, and public intoxication. They attended twenty-one traffic collisions and issued 28,490 parking citations. By 1990 the department included more than fifty employees, twenty-eight of them peace officers.[118]

CENTENNIAL YEAR WALK

Persons allotting an hour for a campus walk during the centennial year encountered uniformed police officers, busy housekeepers, and uniformed physical plant employees performing a variety of upkeep and construction tasks in and on the seventy-three major buildings on the eighty-two-acre campus.[119] Beginning their walk between the two concrete pine cones in front of Old Red (1891), they marveled at this red brick and limestone building that mixed "Romanesque arcades with Spanish Baroque parapets, Italian Gothic gables, and vaguely Moorish pinnacles." Carved into each column capital was an image of the state arms: a Lone Star encircled by oak and olive branches—all resting on stylized acanthus leaves borrowed from classical traditions. They probably glanced at the bust of Ashbel Smith, in whose honor the building is named, and they may have read the historical marker erected in 1969.[120]

Walking across the street from Old Red, they carefully inspected the Keiller Building (1925, 1932). They noted its marvelous carvings above the entrances that include rosettes; egg-and-dart motifs associated with goddess temples; lone stars; books; retorts; pans with flames; mortars and pestles; weighing balances; caducei; stylized plants; urns with flames; cornucopiae; skulls and their wings; ribbon swags with tassels probably signifying diplomas; and spiral motifs. These intermingled architectural elements from Greco-Roman, Renaissance, and Modern cultural traditions vividly symbolized the teaching and research activities inside the building.

Walking west, a quick scan of nearby buildings revealed the omnipresence of Galveston buff brick with different hues ("approved equals" from different factories through the years) that provided some color nuances (tawny, brown, yellow, cream) within an overall utilitarian sameness that gave some visual unity and coherence to the campus.

Moving west, walkers saw the Marvin L. Graves Building on their right and the Libbie Moody Thompson Basic Science Building on their left. The Graves Building was originally constructed as the Galveston State Psychopathic Hospital in 1931 and 1937. Though the modified Etruscan and Egyptian motifs evoke some shadows of the past, its sharp, pointed, almost non-ornamented style is "modernistic," like the Shearn Moody Plaza at Twenty-fifth and Strand (the former Santa Fe Railroad Building, built in 1931).[121] Fortress-like, the sides of the Libbie Moody Thompson Basic Science Building (1971) reminded walkers of the need to protect inhabitants from the hot climate and hurricanes.

Continuing west, they encountered the Mary Moody Northen Pavilion (1982) on their right and the Medical Research Building (1991) on their left. They probably liked the windows and curvilinear design of the Northen Pavilion. Though its top

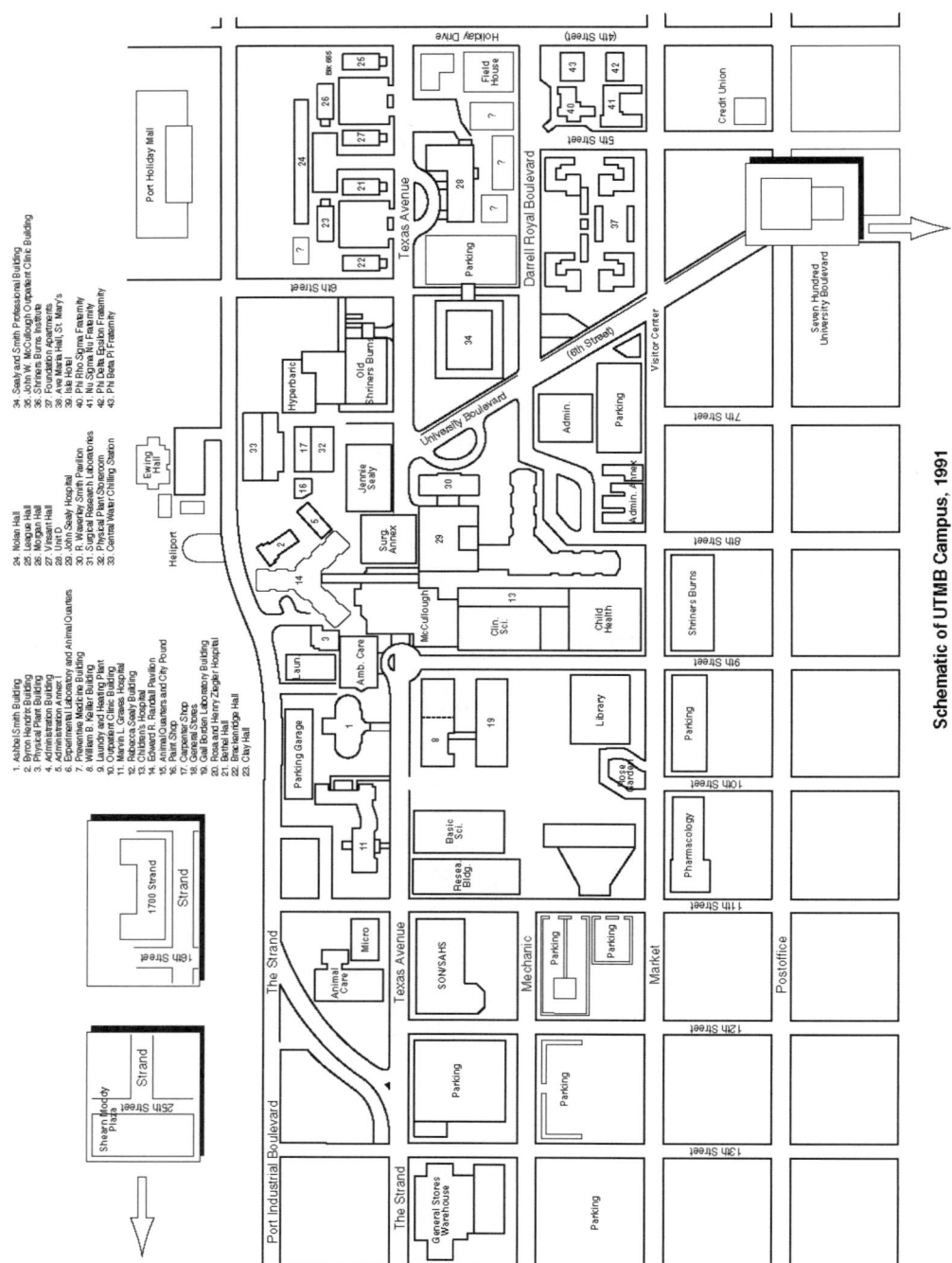

Schematic of UTMB Campus, 1991

1. Ashbel Smith Building
2. Byron Hendrix Building
3. Physical Plant Building
4. Administration Building
5. Experimental Laboratory and Animal Quarters
6. Preventive Medicine Building
7. William B. Keiller Building
8. Laundry and Heating Plant
9. Outpatient Clinic Building
10. Marvin L. Graves Hall
11. Rebecca Sealy Building
12. Children's Hospital
13. Edward R. Randall Pavilion
14. Animal Quarters and City Pound
15. Paint Shop
16. Carpenter Shop
17. General Stores
18. Gail Borden Laboratory Building
19. Rosa and Henry Ziegler Hospital
20. Bethel Hall
21. Brackenridge Hall
22. Clay Hall

24. Nolan Hall
25. League Hall
26. Morgan Hall
27. Vinsant Hall
28. Unit D
29. John Sealy Hospital
30. John Sealy Pavilion
31. R. Waverley Smith Pavilion
32. Surgical Research Laboratories
33. Physical Plant Storeroom
34. Central Water Chilling Station

34. Sealy and Smith Professional Building
35. John W. McCullough Outpatient Clinic Building
36. Shriners Burns Institute
37. Foundation Apartments
38. Ave Maria Hall, St. Mary's
39. Isla Hotel
40. Phi Rho Sigma Fraternity
41. Nu Sigma Nu Fraternity
42. Phi Delta Epsilon Fraternity
43. Phi Beta Pi Fraternity

132

floors were unfinished, the buff brick Medical Research Building was quite imposing with its decorative brick patterns, columns, glass panels, and multi-colored slate tiles. The tiles at the southwest entrance and on the south side added much beauty to the building, suggesting that something imaginative and creative was occurring in its labs. Those venturing inside to the seventh-floor windows enjoyed exquisite views of the island and gulf to the south, and of the harbor and Galveston Bay toward the north.

Leaving the southwest entrance, walkers saw another wonderfully appealing contrast to the "closed-walled" buildings of the campus: the School of Allied Health Sciences/School of Nursing Building (1986) with the openness of its many glass panels. The entranceway was also inviting—welcoming students and faculty for learning and study together. Two magnolia trees had been planted to honor former faculty (John Bruhn and Eugene Kindley). Inside, the strollers saw portraits of previous School of Allied Health Sciences deans and discovered rooms named in honor of four teachers: Ruth Morris (2.216), Sally Mount (2.214), Lisa Leonard (2.228), and Ruby Decker (2.300).

Returning outside and stepping east, walkers viewed Levin Hall (1981) on their right. Inside, they marveled at the huge centennial-year banners streaming down the sides of the auditorium. Depending on the day and time, they might have encountered one of the many celebratory events that year.

Meandering eastward outside, walkers saw the hard, black "Birth" sculpture Arthur Williams created in 1987. Looking south, they quickly moved toward the new Gleaves T. James Centennial Rose Garden, anticipating some moments of pleasurable gazing at its multi-colored, multi-textured flora. While in the rose garden, they probably noticed the rocket-like exhaust pipes atop the gray Pharmacology Building (1974) across Market Street from Levin Hall. Common on campus rooftops (like the communications antennae), these pipes removed noxious gases from the labs inside. Walkers then moved toward the ground-floor columns in the open-air patio, the glass window bays, and the overhanging pitched roofs of the Moody Medical Library just east of the sculpture and rose garden. Those who ventured inside were exposed to exhibits on the ground floor, reference areas on the second floor, portraits of former professors on the walls of the third-floor reading room, and the entrancing designs and contents of the rare books room on the fourth floor that linked UTMB with centuries of Western knowledge and culture.

Returning outside, walkers glanced at the nondescript "modernistic" Gail Borden Laboratory Building, which was UTMB's second freestanding structure for scientific research when it opened in 1953. They probably sat for a moment on a bench or planter to enjoy the most attractive outdoor area on the campus, a tiny university "green" or "mall" that attracted talking, even flirting, students.

Moving east, they encountered the Child Health Center with its "war-on-disease" fortress exterior and its colorful and decorative circus-themed designs for children on the inside. Detouring to the left of the west entrance into a cul-de-sac associated with the service dock area, walkers glimpsed remnants of the original Outpatient

Building (1930), the Children's Hospital (1937), and the second John Sealy Hospital (1954).

Returning to the entrance area, they walked a short distance south on Ninth Street and turned eastward. They noticed the construction of the new Shriners Burns Institute on their right as they walked toward the Administration Annex II and the attractive entrance to the John Sealy Hospital with its award-winning towers. Moving around the east tower, walkers discovered the entrance of the second John Sealy Hospital, clearly visible above the shaded Cafe-on-the-Court(yard).

Retracing steps and moving east on the sidewalk, they saw the gray Administration Building and the Sealy & Smith Professional Building. Climbing the steps to their left, they passed the entrance to the Waverley Smith Pavilion, observed the black entrance to the Jennie Sealy Hospital, and saw the first Shriners Burns Institute building in the near distance. These walkers might have known that portions of the old seawall were dynamited so that proper piling could be placed for the Jennie Sealy Hospital. On the north side of this hospital building, they moved along a sidewalk atop the old seawall as they gazed at the Administration Annex I building, the original Rebecca Sealy Nurses' Home completed in 1915. Though the porches of this home were removed in the 1960s, one of the original mirrors was still perched near the first floor stairway, used by many nursing students to check their uniforms and appearances.

Retracing their steps and entering the east entrance of the John Sealy Hospital, walkers strolled west through the main hallway and encountered a marvelous display of photos of hospital employees engaged in many tasks of patient care, another centennial-year tribute. Passing through the west entrance, walkers turned right and moved under the Clinical Sciences Auditorium and saw the front of the Ambulatory Care Clinic entrance. Moving left, they returned to Old Red, where their campus adventure began.

Depending on the day of the year, they might have talked about the pesky mosquitoes and pigeons, or the sticky humidity, the searing heat, or the blustery norther. Surely they noted the landscaping around and between the buildings. Depending on their location, they could have observed stately palms (Mexican fan, Canary Island date, Texas Sabal); smaller palms (sago, Chinese fan, Mediterranean fan); other trees (ash, live oak, eucalyptus, southern magnolia, crepe myrtle, bald cypress, yaupon holly); broadleaf evergreen shrubs (pittosporum, Indian Hawthorne, wax leaf ligustrum, dwarf holly); sub-tropical shrubs (hibiscus, cape honeysuckle, oleander, bougainvillea); ground covers (widelia, Asian Jasmine, Katie Mexican petunia); annual flowering plants (petunia, penta, pansy, begonia, impatiens, snapdragons); and lawns of St. Augustine and Bermuda grasses.[122]

As the final part of their journey through the heart of the campus, they climbed the front steps of Old Red, noticed the original tablets placed in 1890, and entered the doors of the first floor to discover the John P. McGovern Hall of Medical History.[123] Flanking each side of this entrance floor were statues of outstanding figures in the history of Western medicine sculpted by Doris Appel: Imhotep, Hippocrates, Galen,

Maimonides, Andreas Vesalius, Ambroise Pare, William Harvey, William Morton, Louis Pasteur, Joseph Lister, Wilhelm Roentgen, and Marie Curie. A gift of John P. McGovern, a Houston physician and philanthropist, these figures symbolized centuries of caregiving, teaching, and inquiry, which were sustained in Galveston by the activities described in the next three chapters.

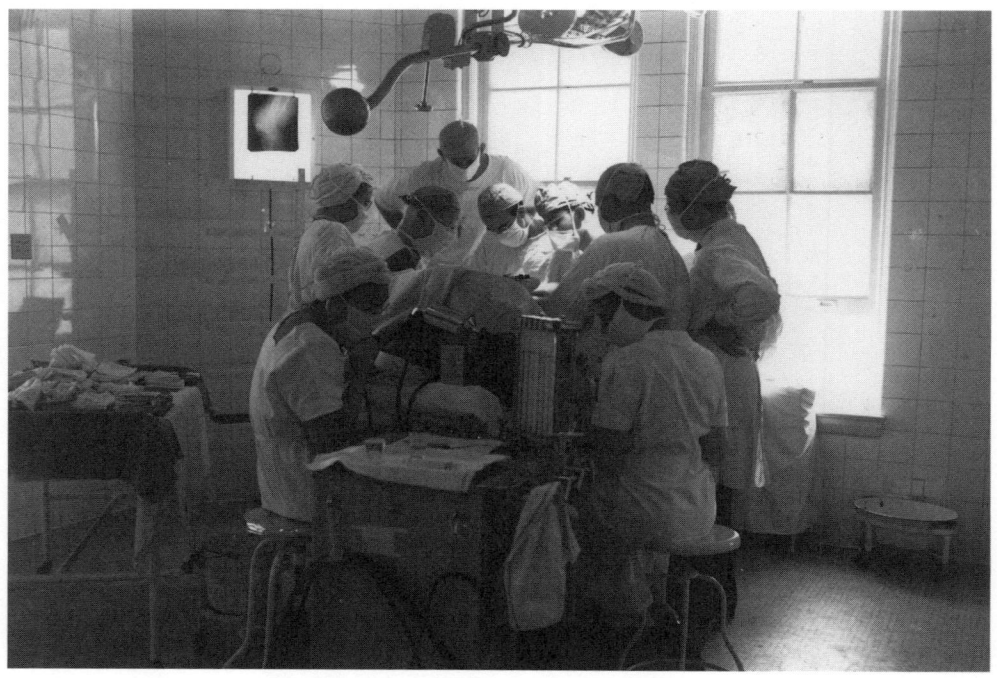

Nurse anesthetist, operating room nurses, and surgeons in the operating room, John Sealy Hospital, 1945.

— 5 —

Caring and Curing

In 1897 Howard Dudgeon Sr. advised an outpatient that he needed a hernia operation. The patient responded: *"Do you remember Mattie Brown? You all operated on her and she died, but I have confidence in you all; and do you remember Brother Jones? You all operated on him too and he died, but I sure have got confidence in you all; and I am going to let you operate on me when I make up my mind."*[1]

Countless conversations between caregivers and patients, like that between Dudgeon and this patient, occurred during UTMB's first hundred years. Sick patients wanted to be healthy. Doctors and others offered ways to restore health. The actual patterns of care at any given time depended on the types of illness or injury, the forms of therapy and the kinds of caregivers available, the physical and technical characteristics of the helping environments, and the power and money contexts that enabled or disabled appropriate care. Divided into three sections, this chapter highlights changes in the components of these patterns. Each section includes information about diseases and injuries, statistical data about patients and caregivers, examples of caregivers and therapies, comments about pertinent buildings and equipment, and a description of certain political and financial events that directly influenced the patterns evolving in that time period.

The transition from acute infectious diseases to more chronic diseases is emphasized in the first section that describes key events between 1901 and 1940. The second section about the years between 1941 and 1968 includes the triumphs of antibiotics and the technical marvels of home dialysis. Intensive care units and transplant surgery are featured among other accomplishments during the years between 1969 and 1991, the focus of the third section. Students are silhouetted in every section because they were struggling to learn a rich assortment of care-giving and cure-giving skills in nearly every clinical venue mentioned in this chapter. Patients and caregivers are the focus of this chapter. Students and teachers are the focus of the next chapter.

Threaded through all of the clinical features of these years is a continuous quest for institutional comprehensiveness. As clinical specialization and sub-specialization evolved, excellence in institutional care required a comprehensive approach to the biological, psychological, social, and spiritual needs of sick and injured humans. For morally adequate clinical care, the conditions of individual patients required different specialists and their assistants. UTMB's executive leaders and professors persistently made choices that honored this comprehensive ideal.

FROM ACUTE TO CHRONIC DISEASES, 1901–1940

UTMB's doctors admitted two thousand inpatients in 1911; three thousand in 1915; five thousand in 1926; and six thousand in 1937 (Appendices AA, AB, and AC). These increases reflected population growth, acceptance of hospital care by more Americans, improved transportation, and more beds in the facilities that appeared on the campus.[2] As described in the previous chapter, these facilities served blacks (1902), patients with contagious diseases (1912), children (1913), women (1915), psychiatric patients (1931), blacks (1937), and children (1937).

More women wanted the care of specialists in obstetrics and gynecology who performed more than thirty-five hundred operations on more than five thousand inpatients between 1901 and 1915. Keiller, for example, treated menorrhagia by performing a hysterectomy on one twenty-seven-year-old patient and two thirty-eight-year-old patients. The annual total increased after the Woman's Hospital opened in 1915. Between 1920 and 1930, doctors admitted 3,880 patients to the obstetrical service. Some pregnant women were quite sick. Between 1930 and 1940, for example, forty-five women presented with ectopic pregnancies; five died.[3] Specialty care did not guarantee survival.

Most parturient women did not experience an infectious disease, though such diseases were still the leading causes of death for all ages. Tuberculosis and typhoid fever were the two leading causes of death in Texas in 1908. Between 1911 and 1915, for example, doctors treated 186 patients with typhoid fever, of whom eleven died. Tuberculosis caused the death of twenty hospitalized patients between January 1, 1911 and January 1, 1913.[4] Many of the children admitted to the Children's Hospital had deformities of the spine and other bones caused by tuberculosis. Some were in the hospital for months, even years.[5] Gradually increasing numbers of children were hospitalized; some required surgery.

By 1906 James Thompson, professor of surgery, had successfully treated a fifteen-year-old girl and a twenty-six-year-old man with congenital cysts of the neck, and two boys with cervical fistulae that developed in their thyroglossal ducts. Many operations to alter congenital anomalies, repair tissues injured by trauma, and remove cancerous lesions occurred in the hospital's operating room. By 1921 in Texas alone, one of eight women and one of twelve men reaching the age of forty-five would die of cancer, with an annual loss of approximately forty-five hundred Texans. By 1922 Thompson had treated fifteen women with cystic carcinoma of the breast.[6]

With each passing year, chronic diseases assumed more importance as causes of morbidity and mortality.[7] The number of deaths from cancer in Texas doubled between 1930 and 1940.The top four causes of death in 231 patients admitted to UTMB's hospitals during fiscal year 1939 were heart disease (55), pneumonia (34), cancer (29)

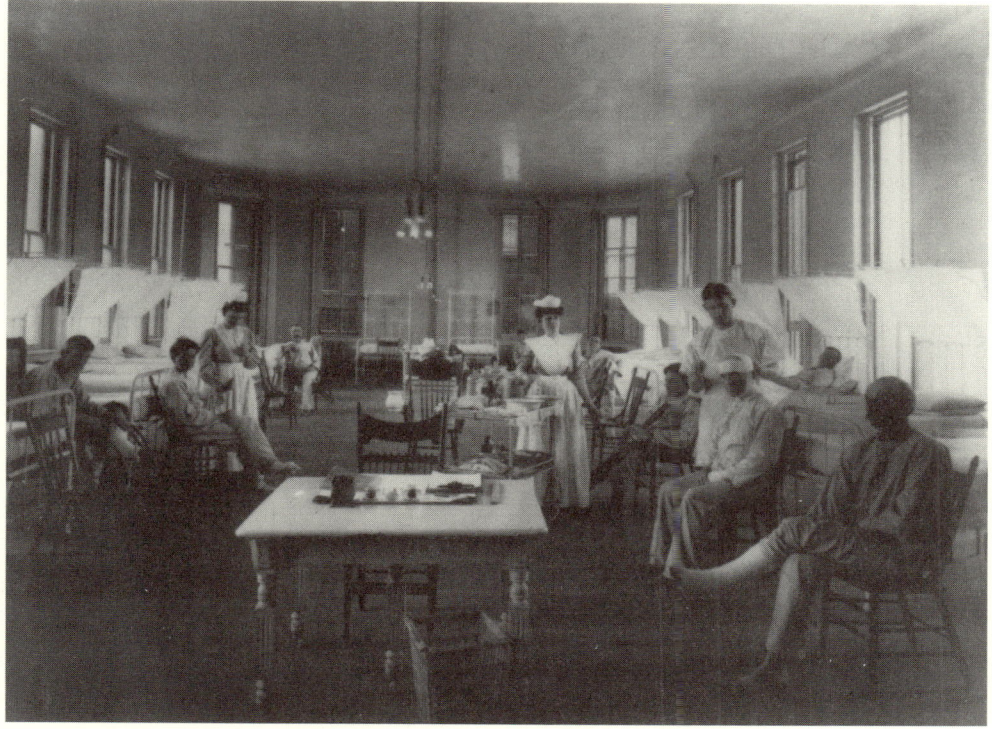

Men's surgical ward, John Sealy Hospital, 1906.

and strokes (29). In 1940 the leading causes of deaths in Galveston were diseases of the circulatory system (259 of 890) and diseases of the respiratory system (148 of 890).[8] The largest number of deaths occurred in people between the ages of forty and eighty years, a striking contrast to the turn of the century when the largest number occurred in infants and children.

Doctors and nurses followed patients with chronic diseases in the outpatient clinics; the total number of new outpatients increased annually from 2,042 in 1901 to 6,799 in 1925 (Appendix AA). The clinics became more crowded as the number of outpatient visits expanded during the 1920s.

The new Outpatient Building opened in October 1930. Patients approaching its registration desk were surrounded with tan and brown faience tile wainscot that covered the walls of the foyer. After registering, whites and blacks walked on inlaid linoleum with terrazo borders to segregated waiting rooms on both the first and second floors. In the first-floor rooms, doctors and students examined children and adults with medical, dermatological, and neurological problems. Most surgical patients went to the second floor. Women needing obstetrical and gynecological care went to the third floor, as did those needing the care of ophthalmologists and otolaryngologists. By the late 1930s doctors and others attended almost twelve thousand new outpatients annually (Appendix AC). By 1941 there were twenty different clinics.[9]

Inpatients and outpatients received care from a remarkable mix of professionals and others, a mix that included more than 150 employees by 1919. There were attending physicians and six interns. Ten nurses exercised supervisory roles: head nurses for the Main, Woman's, Children's, Isolation, and Negro Hospitals; operating nurses for the Main and Woman's Hospital; and a night supervisor. Seventy-five student nurses received $5 each month as well as board, lodging, and laundry services. Others included a superintendent, a pathologist, an X-ray technician, a pharmacist, a dietician, a storekeeper, a housekeeper, a gardener, an anesthetist, a chief engineer, another engineer and two firemen, a head laundress, two laundrymen, twelve female laundry workers, three cooks, three kitchen helpers, two seamstresses, nine orderlies, eleven housemaids, six cleaners, two icemen, eight house helpers, a cashier, a bookkeeper, a clerk, and an office boy. Many of these employees were women, who joined the hundreds of other women entering the national workforce after 1910.[10]

To continue developing comprehensive care for patients, UTMB added professionals who provided different types of services. During the 1920s this included medical record librarians, a social worker, and nurse anesthetists. Margaret McArdle and Miss D. B. Hixon organized the hospital's record room.[11] Between 1923 and 1925, they assembled 11,452 charts, copied 6,100 outpatient histories, inscribed 6,906 follow-up postcards to discharged patients, transmitted 3,371 names to a list for Red Cross nurses who conducted follow-up calls, prepared monthly reports for hospital staff meetings, and prepared reports for UTMB's annual catalogs. With salaries provided by the Junior Welfare League, Agnes Taylor began the hospital's Social Service Department in 1928, assisting 1,132 patients during the first six months. Rosa Lee Arnn was chief anesthetist and instructor in anesthesia between 1920 and 1931; Elvie Shaver between 1932 and 1938.[12]

Graduate and student nurses worked earnestly. UTMB employed twenty-four graduate nurses in 1929; sixty-eight in 1937. In 1929, for example, forty-nine students assisted the graduate nurses in providing daily care to about three hundred inpatients. Twelve students worked ten-hour night shifts. The nurses were stretched to their limits. In June 1940, for instance, one student nurse attended ten gynecologic patients, twelve obstetric patients, a nursery full of babies, and three private patients. She also prepared three or four patients for surgery, and assisted during three deliveries. This situation was far from satisfactory. Obstetrical patients, newborn babies, gynecological patients, and genito-urinary patients were all housed in the same wards in the Woman's Hospital and the Negro Hospital. The same nurses attended these patients, moving from an adult with an infectious disease to a neonate, or vice-versa. Since these arrangements violated "every principle of present day hospital planning," observed Willard Cooke, it was only by the "Grace of God" that there had not been a "serious epidemic."[13]

Finding an adequate number of qualified nurses became a perennial problem for the hospitals because other careers were now possible for women interested in medical work. By the 1930s women could become nurses, medical record librarians, social workers, laboratory technologists, dietitians, physical therapists, or occupational therapists.

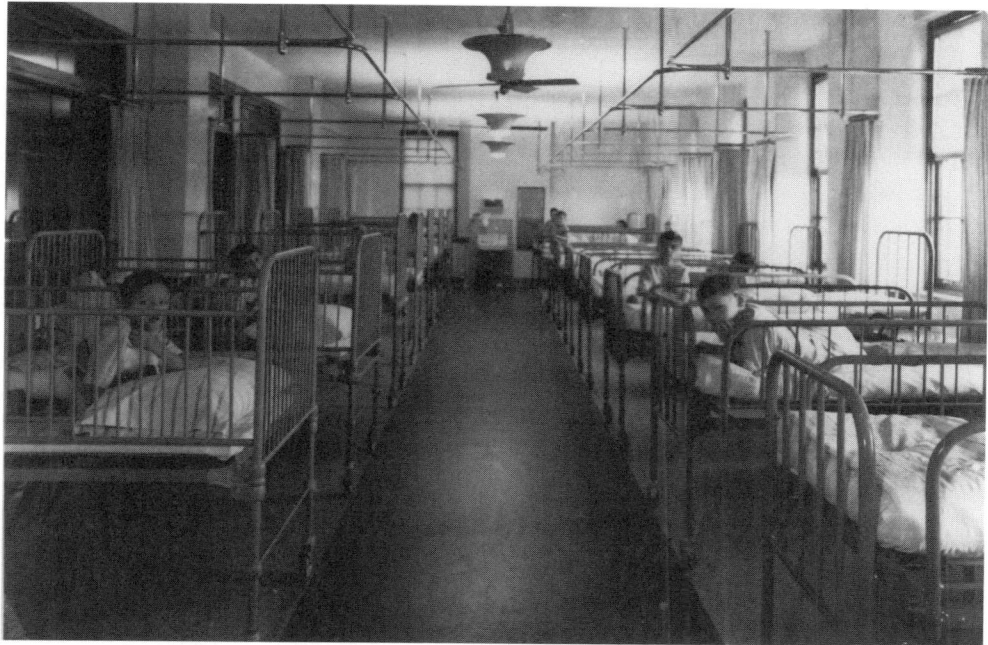

Ward in Children's Hospital, 1938.

Nurses could find employment in general and special hospitals, such as the Galveston State Psychopathic Hospital, which opened on the UTMB campus in August 1931. The first floor contained an admission office, four examination rooms, a hydrotherapy room, a vocational therapy room, recreation rooms, and lecture rooms. The second, third, and fourth floors included private and semi-private rooms that could accommodate forty-eight patients. The staff included a physician-superintendent, a clinical director and an assistant clinical director, three additional physicians, three registered nurses, a business manager, an occupational therapist, a social service worker, a psychologist, and a dietitian. Less than four months after the hospital opened, the medical professionals had treated one hundred patients and discharged forty-eight as improved or cured.[14]

Because the number of mentally ill patients continued to increase, more inpatient rooms were needed. In 1932 the former Nurses' Home was transformed into a unit known as Psycho Two and Three. During the mid-1930s the former Isolation Pavilion was transformed into a thirty-two-bed unit known as Psycho One and a forty-five-bed addition to the Psychopathic Hospital opened in the fall of 1937. These facilities supported a significant increase in the number of psychiatric inpatients between 1934 and 1938 (Appendix AC). In 1936, for example, doctors admitted 265 patients to Psycho One.[15] The staff included attending physicians, a psychiatric resident, rotating interns, a nurse supervisor, three graduate nurses, four student nurses, an occupational therapist, recreational personnel, and ten attendants, who cooperated as needed to provide comprehensive psychiatric care.

Comprehensive care for children also required a sizable group of professionals and assistants. In September 1932, for example, the staff of the Children's Hospital attended thirty-two inpatients. One was a fifteen-month-old infant with a congenital anomaly who had been there since birth and another was a six-year-old girl whose esophagus had been damaged so severely after she swallowed lye that she had been tube fed in the hospital for four years. Others remained in this hospital for long periods of time as they received treatment for burns, broken bones, and polio. A physical therapist exercised post-polio patients in the hospital's pool. The hospital had a schoolteacher whose salary was provided by the Hospital Aid Society until 1930, when state funds became available.[16] These same comprehensive approaches to care guided those who served in the new Children's Hospital, which opened in 1937. During that year, a head teacher and her assistant instructed thirty-five children in grades one through eight (seven hours each weekday for eleven months). By the following year, the hospital's staff included other women: an occupational therapist, a physical therapist, and a social worker.[17]

Women were employed to perform laboratory tests on blood, urine, and other bodily substances from inpatients and outpatients. In 1902 the laboratory of clinical pathology was housed in the Nurses' Home; after 1922 it was in a separate building.[18] Labs for all patients were located in the Outpatient Building: X-ray on the second floor, electrocardiography on the third floor, and a clinical lab on the fourth floor.[19] The hospital housed other labs, such as the electroencephalographic (EEG) lab. In all of these labs, trained women were technologists.[20]

Most of the physicians before 1941 were male. The "visiting staff" usually included those who were employed as professors as well as some practitioners who volunteered as specialists. This group numbered nine in 1900; twenty-seven in 1925; thirty-one in 1937. Those in charge of specialty clinics were designated as the "clinical staff." Some were volunteers and others were part-time or full-time faculty. This group numbered four in 1900; seventeen in 1925; twenty-three in 1937. Their appointments included labels appropriate to a specialty, such as "dermatologist," or "assistant gynecologist," or "chief of the pediatric clinic." Violet Keiller (class of 1914), William Keiller's daughter, was the hospital's surgical pathologist from 1914 to 1927.[21]

Interns were recent graduates who wanted an additional year of hospital training. Before the early 1930s interns were designated as "resident staff" because they received meals, medical care, and laundry services without charge, as well as living quarters while on duty at the hospital. Four interns served the hospitals annually until 1911, when the number increased to six. The total increased to eight in 1922 and twelve in 1937.[22]

First employed during the 1930s, "residents" were graduate doctors who had completed an internship and who desired additional years of training in a specialty. They received a modest stipend plus the same amenities accorded interns. Interns and residents together were classified as house staff. In 1940 the hospital appointed eighteen residents and departmental chairs requested more money from the Sealy & Smith Foundation to pay their salaries.[23]

As recounted in chapter three, dollars from the Sealy family, the Sealy & Smith Foundation, city officials, and fellow citizens who cherished the Sealy legacy provided constant financial support for clinical care during these years. A continuing increase in the number of private patients produced income that offset some of the costs of indigent care in a given year (Appendix U). During fiscal year 1902, for example, paying patients provided slightly more than $4,000; in fiscal year 1905, slightly more than $11,000. The latter amount offset most of the increased expenses between 1901 and 1904. In fiscal year 1919, the hospital received almost $96,000 from pay patients. During fiscal year 1922 the hospital admitted 2,034 charity patients and 2,171 pay patients. To meet all expenses, the hospital collected slightly more than $156,000 from pay patients, $35,000 from the city, and the remainder from the Sealy family and other benefactors.[24]

Though needing the income from pay patients, the boards of managers for UTMB's hospitals did not neglect indigent patients because they were used for the clinical education of students. Fifty-two new charity beds had been added by 1931: twenty at the Children's Hospital; sixteen for patients with tuberculosis; and sixteen for black patients (ten of the sixteen beds were for obstetrical cases).[25]

To help control costs, these boards welcomed the women's groups that provided a variety of volunteer services to patients. In 1916 the Young Ladies' Hospital Aid Society served ice cream to patients during the summer months and fruit during the winter months. During the 1930s volunteer support for hospitalized children came from the Hospital Aid Society and the Galveston Society for Crippled Children.[26] In 1937 the Junior Welfare League established a library of magazines for inpatients; many of the women involved were wives and daughters of professors.

To help balance budgets, the boards kept salaries of hospital employees as low as possible. In 1932 the two highest paid staff members ($300 per month) were the bookkeeper and the director of the clinical laboratories. Jesse P. Johnson, the only radiologist, received $250 each month. Only three employees received $150 a month: the director of the outpatient department; the chief technician in the clinical laboratories; and the hospital's social service worker. About twenty-five employees earned between $100 and $150 a month. This group included the head nurses, dietitians, pharmacists, and the schoolteacher for the Children's Hospital. Earning between $75 and $100 a month were staff nurses, clerks, technicians, painters, anesthetists, a fireman, a night watchman, and an office stenographer.

Hospital employees were quite loyal and often spent their entire working lives at UTMB. In 1932 the iceman, the gardener, and one orderly had worked at the hospital almost as long as the carpenter, who was completing seventeen years of service and earning $105 each month. Such loyalty reinforced the authoritarian style of the boards. These boards controlled the nurses and nursing students, the graduate physicians who provided services to patients, and other hospital personnel. In 1918 a group of doctors organized a "medical staff" to represent their interests in negotiations with the boards (Appendix H).[27] Perhaps some decisions were negotiated more equitably during the

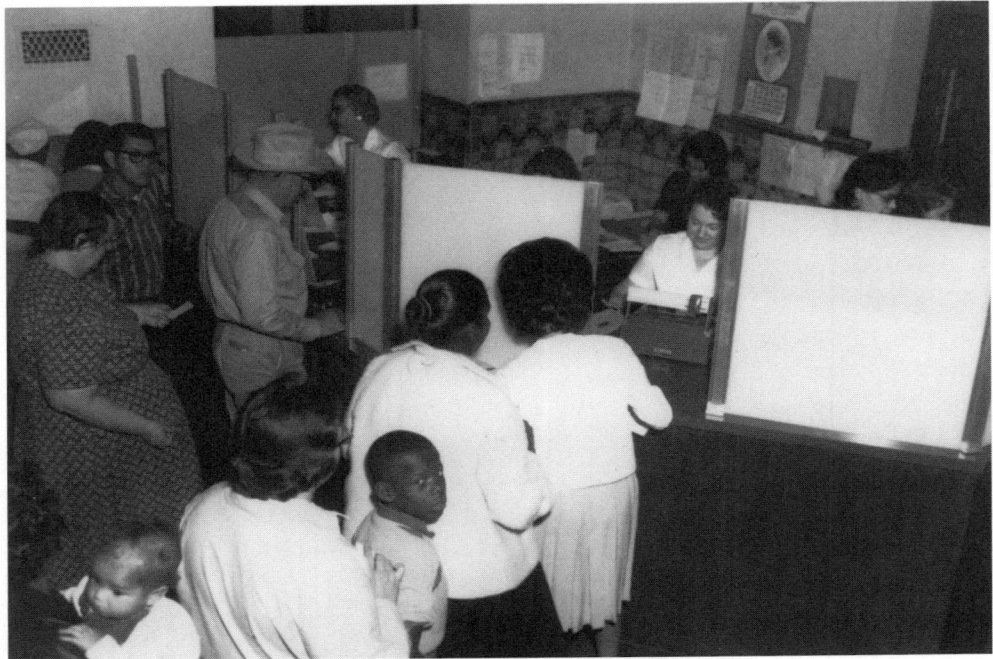

Registration desk, McCullough Outpatient Building, March 1964.

1920s and 1930s. As recounted in chapter two, resistance to the power of these boards was a central feature of the political revolutions that occurred between 1939 and 1942.

FROM PENICILLIN TO HOME DIALYSIS, 1941–1968

Between 1941 and 1968 professionals provided care to inpatients and outpatients that was organized in two ways: (1) according to the specialties and subspecialties of physicians firmly stratified in academic departments (seventeen by 1945) and (2) according to the services provided by other professionals and technicians firmly entrenched in hospital departments.[28]

Doctors in the Department of Obstetrics and Gynecology delivered babies and attended women who needed medical and surgical care associated with their reproductive functions. Doctors in the Department of Pediatrics attended newborns, infants, and children. Some also focused on the care of adolescents, though no rigid boundaries existed between pediatric care and that provided by doctors in the Department of Internal Medicine who focused on the non-surgical diseases of adult men and women. Surgical specialists in the various divisions of the Department of Surgery and in other clinical departments attended infants, children, and adults. Members of the Department of Psychiatry provided mental health care to children and adults. Though patterns of care were segregated according to specialty, consultations among the specialists became more frequent; 4,358 in fiscal year 1949, for example.[29]

Sick and injured patients relentlessly appeared in the clinics. By the 1940s the outpatient clinics were crowded; by the 1950s they were extremely crowded. The

144

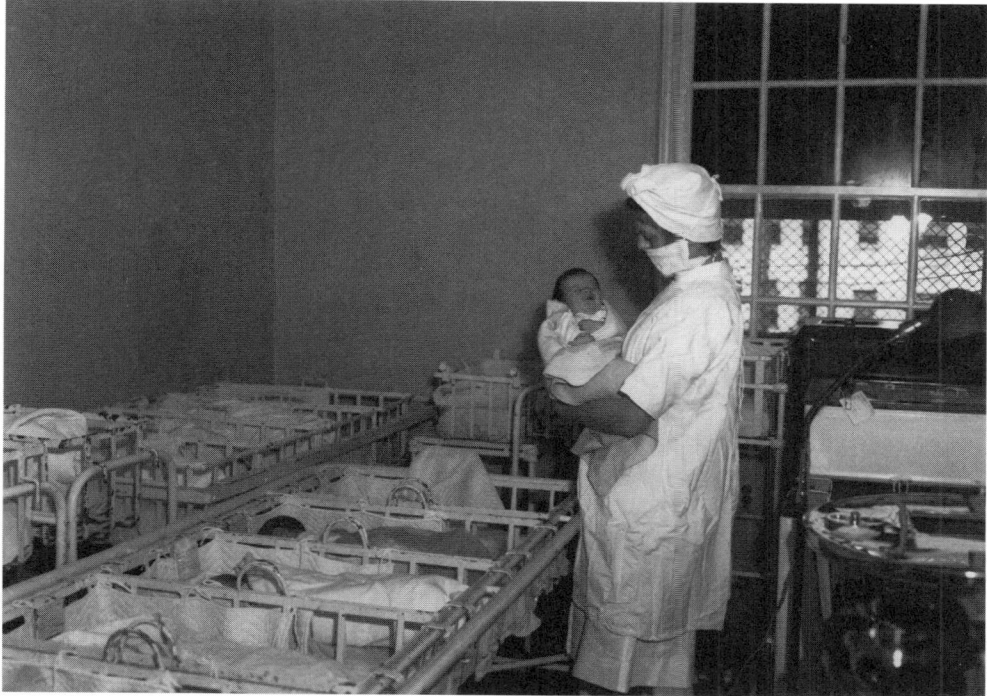

Newborn Nursery, John Sealy Hospital, April 1943.

Outpatient Building had been designed to accommodate a few thousand patients a year. By the summer of 1945 more than six thousand outpatient visits occurred monthly. By 1955 between five and six hundred outpatients daily walked the floors of this building to their appointments in more than thirty specialty clinics. During fiscal year 1960, 12,514 outpatients made 145,068 visits to clinics in the Outpatient Building and the Rebecca Sealy Building (the former Nurses' Home).[30] To handle this increased demand, the Outpatient Clinic Building was transformed into the six-story John W. McCullough Outpatient Clinic Building between 1962 and 1966.[31] The new building included a new emergency room, which opened in October 1962. More than nineteen thousand patients were treated in this emergency room during 1964; during 1968 emergency room personnel handled 25,431 patient visits.[32] The number of inpatients also increased significantly during these years. During fiscal year 1945, doctors admitted 8,323 patients. They admitted 11,825 patients in 1950; 14,222 patients in fiscal year 1957; 16,049 patients in fiscal year 1963; and 17,786 patients in 1968.[33]

Professionals attended these inpatients in fifteen buildings: the original John Sealy Hospital; Woman's Hospital; Isolation Building; Children's Hospital; Negro Hospital (later Randall Pavilion); Margie B. Stewart Convalescent Home for Children; Special Surgical Unit; Moody State School for Cerebral Palsied Children; new John Sealy Hospital and Waverley Smith Pavilion; Ziegler Hospital; Psychopathic Hospital and Psycho One, Two, and Three; and the original Shriners Burns Institute.

Pregnant woman gave birth in the Woman's Hospital, the Negro Hospital, and, later, in the John Sealy Hospital and the Waverley Smith Pavilion. They delivered 908 babies in fiscal year 1944; 1,368 in fiscal year 1956; and 1,891 in fiscal year 1963. Infants born prematurely received special attention. In 1955 a new fifteen-bed premature nursery opened on the fourth floor of the Children's Hospital. Care in this unit reduced the mortality rate of preemies from 50 to 70 percent to 15 to 20 percent.[34]

Infectious diseases still caused deaths and disabilities in children and adults. Infantile paralysis (polio), tuberculosis, and venereal diseases afflicted many families. Only two of the 410 children with polio admitted to the Children's Hospital between 1937 and 1942 died, but most of the others had deformities that were treated with hot packs, massage, warm baths, and other modes of physiotherapy. By September 1945 UTMB's Isolation Hospital could accommodate twenty-five patients with polio. Polio recurred most summers until children nationwide received the Salk polio vaccine, initially in Galveston in 1955.[35]

Tuberculosis was widespread. At UTMB between 1941 and 1944, five teachers, six nursing students, and twenty-eight medical students displayed evidence of pulmonary tuberculosis. Tuberculosis caused the deaths of fourteen infants and children (six months to fourteen years) between July 2, 1948, and September 14, 1952.[36]

To provide care for these patients in a facility that would be separate from other patient care areas, the sixty-bed, four-story Ziegler Hospital opened in early February 1954 with twenty-one patients transferred from the John Sealy Hospital. John Middleton, clinical director of this hospital for fourteen years (1953–1967), witnessed dramatic improvements in the control of tuberculosis as patients received streptomycin, PAS, and isoniazid.[37]

Venereal diseases were widespread. About seventy-five people visited the venereal diseases clinic each day after it opened in the fall of 1938. These diseases became a significant problem among the soldiers stationed at Camp Wallace in Hitchcock and Fort Crockett in Galveston. In 1940, 1,679 cases of venereal diseases were reported in Galveston. An estimated two to five thousand soldiers congregated in Galveston during weekends, eager to associate with an estimated eight hundred prostitutes and "so-called amateurs" who could easily transmit these diseases.[38]

In 1940 Edward Randall Jr. initiated a treatment for venereal diseases known as fever cabinet therapy. Patients were placed inside casket-sized boxes and their body temperatures were increased to approximately 104–106 degrees Fahrenheit. By July 1941, 180 patients had received 1,350 episodes of this treatment. Doctors reported cures of those with gonorrheal arthritis and pelvic inflammatory disease. Fever cabinet therapy disappeared after the advent of penicillin in the mid-1940s. The effects of penicillin on venereal diseases were quite dramatic. In eleven of thirteen neonates treated with penicillin between April 1944 and May 1945, clinical signs of syphilis rapidly disappeared. Of sixty syphilitic pregnant women treated with penicillin during the mid-1940s, only one of their infants was infected with syphilis. Doctors called penicillin "liquid gold."[39]

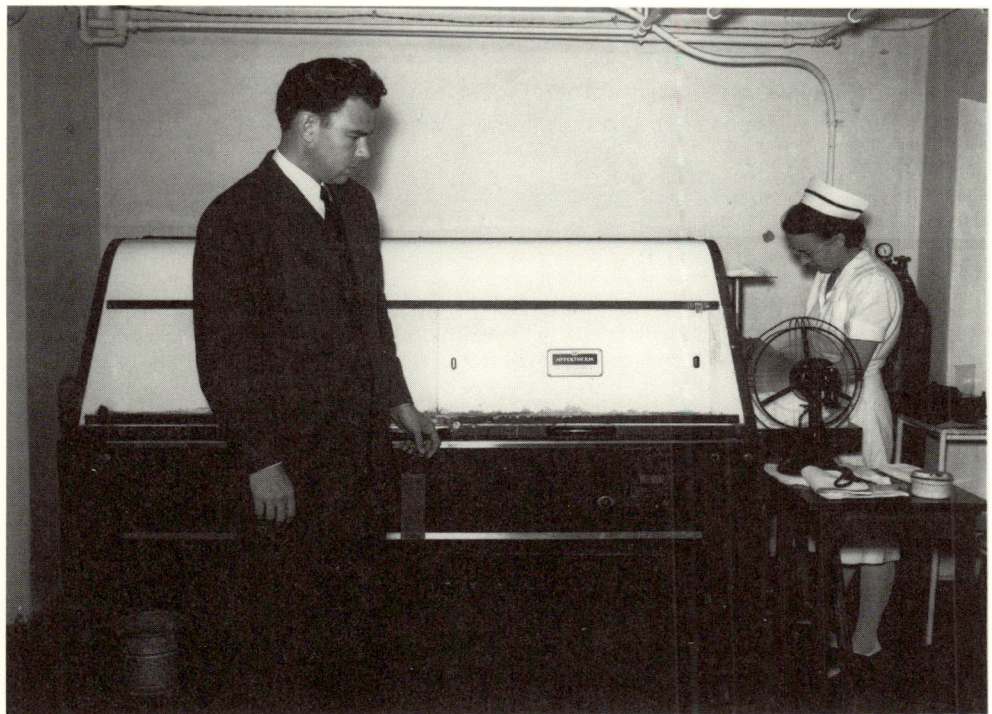

William Bohman, superintendent of the John Sealy Hospital, and nurse with fever therapy cabinet, 1943.

Doctors used sulfa drugs and antibiotics to control other infectious diseases, producing results that seemed liked miracles. By 1941 sulfa drugs had reduced the mortality rate of pneumococcal pneumonia from 30 percent to about 12 percent. In 1943 more than 75 percent of 366 patients with osteomyelitis recovered after treatment with the sulfonamides. During the mid-1950s, doctors attended sixty-eight infants and children from Galveston who presented with fever, diarrhea, abdominal cramps, vomiting, or seizures. Fourteen had sufficient metabolic abnormalities to be in a state of "shock" at the time of admission. Lab studies revealed that each child had bacillary dysentery (shigellosis). All recovered satisfactorily after fluids and electrolytes were replaced and antibiotics given.[40]

Challenges abounded, though, as certain microorganisms began to produce strains that were not inhibited or destroyed by antibiotics. The first outbreak of such pathogenic staphylococci occurred in the nurseries in the fall of 1956, with more episodes in 1957 and 1958. Of 12,458 patients admitted to the hospital, 236 acquired infections with resistant staphylococci and 33 died, mostly older and chronically ill persons.[41]

Severely burned patients became infected with beta hemolytic streptococci, staphylococci, and coliform bacteria. During the 1950s, Blocker and his colleagues discovered that penicillin was useful in preventing blood stream infections from streptococci, but had no effect on the resistant strains of staphylococci and gram-negative flora. Until granulation tissue had formed, mechanical cleansing and frequent changes of dressings often controlled microbial growth better than antibiotics.[42]

Blocker had organized the clinical service for burned patients. As chief of plastic surgery at Wakeman General Hospital in Camp Atterbury, Indiana, between 1942 and 1946, he had performed or supervised more than five thousand operations involving skin grafts, the removal of deforming scars, and the construction of new chins, cheeks, noses, ears, and jaw bones (using cartilage and bone from other areas of the patient's body). After returning to Galveston in 1946, he became director of the new division of plastic and maxillo-facial surgery in the Department of Surgery, a division that received much public attention during the days of the Texas City disaster in 1947.[43]

In the spring of 1948 one of the eight surplus buildings transferred from Camp Wallace became a fifty-bed Special Surgical Unit for plastic surgery and neurosurgery patients. Blocker directed the plastic surgery service and Samuel Snodgrass directed the neurosurgery service. Within a year, they were treating forty to forty-five inpatients daily and performing about ninety operations each month. Blocker's service included all extracranial operations of the head and neck, including congenital defects, cancerous lesions, and traumatic injuries. He and his colleagues developed an open-air treatment for burned patients, used quite successfully on 130 patients by 1952 (including 48 children after June 1950).[44]

Because of this exemplary care, the Shriners of North America established a temporary seven-bed unit for burned children in the John Sealy Hospital in November 1963. The Shriners supported this unit until the new three-story Shriners Burns Institute opened in 1966. The first floor contained an auditorium and some research labs; the second floor housed outpatient treatment rooms, facilities for physical and occupational therapy, and offices for medical records and dietary; and the third floor contained two fifteen-bed inpatient units. Using a comprehensive team approach, Shriners Burns Institute doctors and staff had treated about seven hundred children by July 1968.[45]

Other surgeons attended patients with a variety of tumors, including those of the salivary glands, kidney, and bone. Cancer caused more disabilities and deaths than ever. Golfer Babe Zaharias died at UTMB in 1956 from cancer. Between June 1, 1965, and May 31, 1966, surgeons attended 6,556 inpatients, 24,119 patients in the surgical outpatient clinics and 20,372 patients in the emergency room.[46] Many of these patients received surgical treatment or radiation therapy for cancer. Some forms of cancer were not amenable to surgical treatment. Doctors treated twenty-eight children with leukemia between 1940 and 1950, with no survivors. As antimetabolites, hormones, and irradiation began to be used more systematically during the 1950s, remissions did occur in some children, with an average survival time of forty-one weeks in a group of twenty-five children followed between 1953 and 1957. Some of these children received care in the remodeled Children's Hospital, which was dedicated on February 10, 1956.[47]

Pediatricians treated infants and children with birth defects, infectious diseases, degenerative conditions, and metabolic abnormalities. They established a muscular dystrophy clinic in 1957 and started a summer camp for diabetic children in 1958.[48]

They treated infants with adrenocortical insufficiency or other biochemical dysfunctions, and children with phenylketonuria. Twenty physically abused children received inpatient care between 1966 and 1969. As the department of pediatrics expanded during the 1960s and 1970s, most of the inpatient areas in the Children's Hospital became offices and laboratories. Sick children were housed on the ninth floor of the John Sealy Hospital.[49]

Pediatricians also provided long-term care of children whose brains had been damaged at birth or by trauma. In March 1951 the first brain-injured child was admitted to the Moody State School for Cerebral Palsied Children, located on Teichmann Road adjacent to Offats Bayou. The State Board of Education spent more than $1,500,000 to transform an existing building into an H-shaped structure with classrooms and offices in one arm of the H, and dormitory facilities in the other. Adjacent buildings provided facilities for physical therapy, swimming, occupational therapy, and the construction of braces. Espousing a philosophy of comprehensive care, the staff included physicians, nurses, occupational therapists, physical therapists, speech therapists, teachers, aides, a dietitian, and a psychologist.[50]

Psychiatrists continued providing comprehensive care for those with mental diseases. By 1950 the Galveston State Psychopathic Hospital could accommodate 137 patients. Doctors admitted more than thirteen hundred white patients annually. Approximately 75 percent of these recovered sufficiently to return to their homes, 24 percent were transferred to a state hospital, and 1 percent died in the hospital.[51] Staff psychiatrists, twelve residents, twenty-two graduate nurses, and forty student nurses attended these patients, together with dietitians, occupational therapists, physical therapists, social workers, and others.[52] The number of inpatients began to decline during the late 1950s, as psychiatrists began using tranquilizers (such as Thorazine) and euphoriants (such as Ritalin) in the treatment of manic-depressive disorders. When the Psychopathic Hospital closed for repairs in 1960, patients were transferred to the fifty-seven-bed Randall Pavilion and a sixty-four-bed unit in the former Faculty House (Unit D).[53]

Specialists in internal medicine managed other chronic diseases in adults. In 1942 diseases of the circulatory system caused the deaths of 279 individuals in Galveston, diseases of the respiratory system caused 100 deaths, cancer caused 111 deaths, and 86 died from communicable diseases (35 with pulmonary tuberculosis). Internists attended many patients with these diseases, as well as those affecting the endocrine glands, the blood, and the gastrointestinal system. They treated patients with parathryoid malfunctions, different kinds of anemias, multiple myeloma, and ulcerative colitis—to mention only a few of the diseases in the adults admitted to the new John Sealy Hospital and Waverley Smith Pavilion, which opened in 1954.[54]

The first floor of the John Sealy Hospital included administrative and admission offices, the emergency room, a cafeteria, and some retail shops. The second floor housed a central supply area, offices for doctors, a surgical pavilion with eleven operating rooms, and two patient care areas: Unit 2A and Unit 2B, each with thirty-nine beds. The third floor contained labor and delivery rooms, offices for the department of

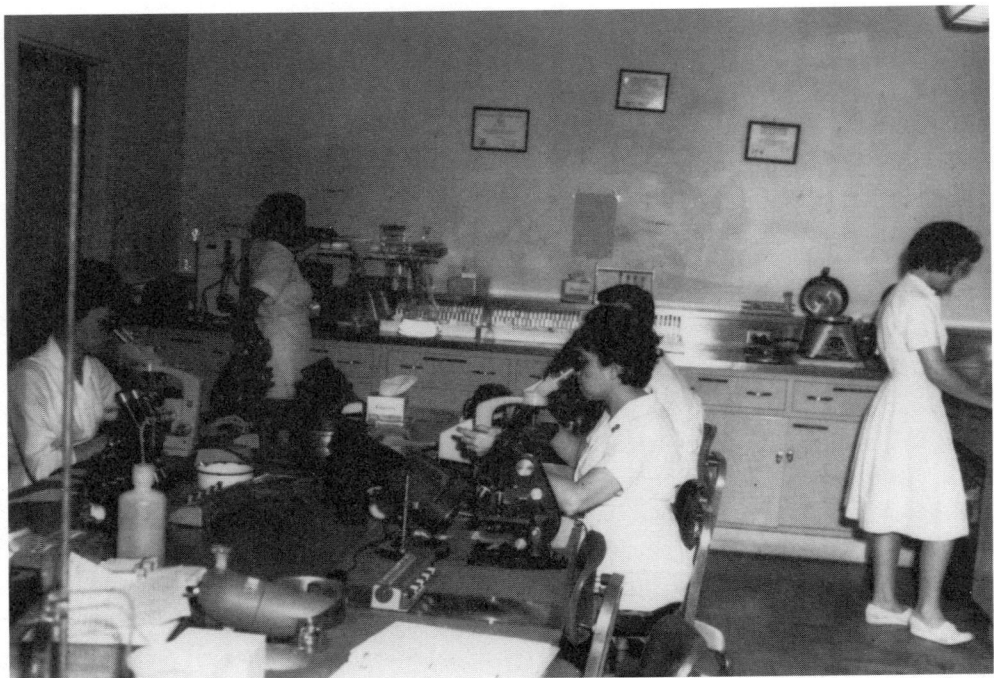

Hematology Lab, c. 1965.

obstetrics and gynecology, and two patient care areas: Unit 3A and Unit 3B. The fourth floor housed the department of internal medicine, the blood bank, a hematology lab, and two patient care areas: Unit 4A (thirty-nine beds for males) and Unit 4B (thirty-nine beds for females). Clinical labs for all patients were located on the fifth floor, as well as more offices for the department of internal medicine and three unfinished patient care areas: Units 5A, 5B, and 5C. The department of surgery occupied the sixth floor together with the Surgical Research Lab and two areas for surgical patients: Unit 6A (twenty-six beds for males) and Unit 6B (twenty-six beds for females). The seventh floor included offices for neurosurgery, ophthalmology, and otorhinolaryngology together with three unfinished patient care areas: Units 7A, 7B, and 7C. Specialists in urology and in plastic surgery had offices and wards for patients on the eighth floor. The ninth floor housed three areas for pediatric patients: Unit 9A and Unit 9B, each with twenty-six beds; and Unit 9C as an isolation ward. Private patients were housed on the third, fourth, fifth, and sixth floors of the Waverley Smith Pavilion; offices and treatment rooms were located on the first two floors.[55]

In 1954 about two thousand hospital employees worked at UTMB, providing direct or indirect services to patients in the institution's 760 beds.[56] As subsequent paragraphs demonstrate, these employees included admitting clerks, nurses, physicians, lab technicians, physical therapists, occupational therapists, respiratory therapists, social workers, medical record librarians, pharmacists, blood bank technicians, dietitians, and workers in the central supply, laundry, and transportation departments.[57]

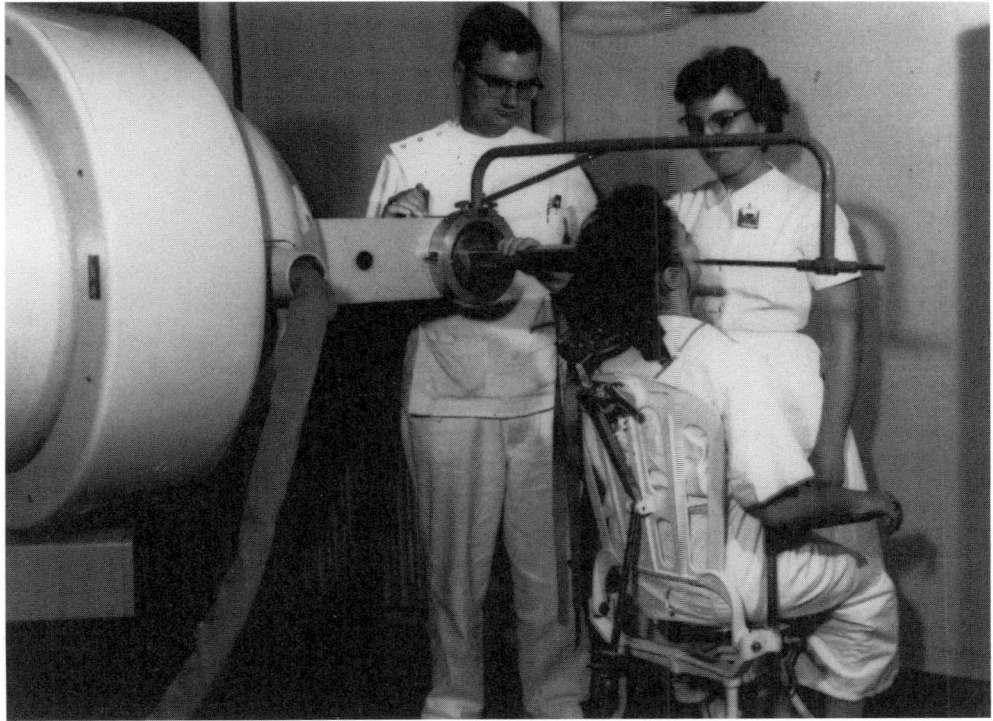

Doctor and nurse using a betatron for treating head and neck cancer, 1955.

Patients admitted to a hospital initially interacted with one of the twenty women who worked in the admitting offices during the mid-1950s. As patients entered wards or rooms, nurses usually extended greetings and provided any clinical services needed at that time. By 1959 a dozen assistants helped the director of nursing services manage an elaborate hierarchy that included assistant directors, supervisors, head nurses, licensed vocational nurses, registered nurses, nurses' aides, ward clerks, and orderlies.[58] In 1961, 126 staff nurses worked in 135 patient care units, attending an average of 750 inpatients and many outpatients each day.[59]

A bevy of physicians and physicians-in-training, including professors, clinical fellows, residents, interns, and medical students, visited with patients after they arrived in their rooms. Each doctor usually asked questions ("taking a history") and performed a physical examination of the patient. In 1962 UTMB employed 34 interns, 50 first-year residents in 16 departments, and 103 second- and third-year residents. These interns and residents worked extremely long and challenging hours in the clinics, wards, and operating rooms.[60]

Physicians and nurses cooperated in providing expert care, especially in the eleven operating rooms. In 1956 twenty staff nurses, two vocational nurses, five orderlies, and twelve aides provided nursing services in these rooms. These persons were responsible for choosing and sterilizing all equipment in autoclaves, preparing all supplies needed for a particular operation, and assisting surgeons during the operations. Nurses and doctors also collaborated in preparing and administering anesthetics to surgical patients. By May 1956 the department of anesthesiology included four professors and fourteen residents. The department established a separate post-operative recovery room during the mid-1950s.[61]

Before these patients went to an operating room, however, students, nurses, or doctors obtained blood, urine, and other bodily substances and sent them to laboratories for analysis. By the mid–1950s these labs processed more than 200,000 tests annually. In 1961 the clinical labs employed about eighty individuals (full- and part-time) who were organized into four sections: bacteriology, hematology, chemistry, and serology. Elwood Baird (director) and William K. Perry (technical director) supervised twenty-nine medical technicians and others who

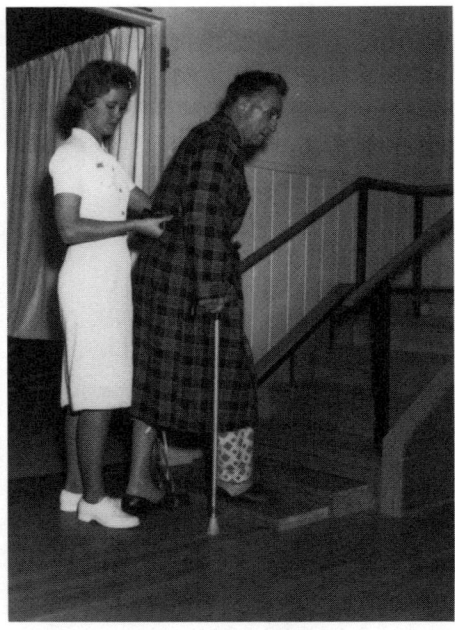

Physical therapist rehabilitating a stroke patient, 1964.

performed more than 1 million diagnostic tests on inpatients and outpatients.[62] Though seldom interacting directly with patients, these lab workers provided essential diagnostic services.

Radiologists and their assistants related directly to patients as they performed diagnostic and therapeutic services. By the mid-1950s, the department of radiology included eight radiologists, five residents, fifteen registered technicians, seventeen technology students, and thirty-three people who were clerks, secretaries, and assistants. In 1955 staff members used fifteen machines in performing about seventy thousand exams; in fiscal year 1961 they conducted 79,716 exams.[63] They also used a new betatron for irradiating cancer.

Other professionals provided specialized therapeutic and social services. Physical therapists worked with patients who experienced neuromuscular malfunctions. In 1960 seven certified therapists, three aides, and two secretaries managed 20,509 visits from 902 inpatients and 752 outpatients, who received 30,085 treatments that included exercises, hot packs, immersion baths, massages, whirlpool treatments, paraffin baths, and applications with a diathermy, infrared, or ultrasound machine. The largest number of patients were those with disabilities from arthritis, traumatic injuries, back pain and "slipped" disc syndrome, and strokes.[64]

Occupational therapists provided assistance to patients adapting to chronic diseases or those undergoing rehabilitation from traumatic injuries. In 1955 Rose Marie Wells directed a group of three certified therapists, one full-time and one part-time occupational therapy assistant, one recreational therapist, and a secretary. By 1961 they offered services to about eighteen hundred patients annually. Their recreational area included punching bags, table tennis, pulleys, shuffleboard, and a practice bowling alley. Patients with spinal cord injuries were taught crafts of working with leather, wood, or metal, and several needlecrafts including weaving. Others were provided with games and puzzles.[65]

During the 1960s trained respiratory therapists begin their association with the anesthesiologists at UTMB. In 1968, for example, fourteen respiratory therapists used sophisticated machines to diagnose, treat, and monitor cardiopulmonary functions that were compromised by a variety of conditions.[66]

Social workers at UTMB's hospitals were formally organized into the Social Service Department in 1942. In 1955 Charles Rosenbloom directed a staff of three case supervisors, four case aides (two were medical students), and four clerical assistants. These personnel helped inpatients and outpatients deal with a variety of social problems. They secured financial aid, located temporary housing, provided emotional support and counseling, helped patients understand their medical care, and coordinated liaison services with state and local agencies. During fiscal year 1961 the department's sixteen members assisted 2,595 patients and 505 relatives.[67]

Medical record librarians, pharmacists, blood bank technicians, and dietitians provided services that were indispensable for efficient and effective care. In 1955 Margaret McArdle supervised about thirty employees of the medical records department, who used typewriters, index cards, and large filing cabinets to organize and manage the clinical records of inpatients and outpatients.[68]

In 1955 the pharmacy department employed seven registered pharmacists, three lab technicians, two delivery persons, and a secretary. Working in rooms on the first floor of the Outpatient Building, the pharmacists and technicians used electric mixers, capsule-filling machines, filtering equipment, and other items to prepare more than six thousand prescriptions each month. Every day, Eddie Green and Elijah Wilson carried these drugs to various hospital areas in about thirty baskets and, three times a week, delivered another twelve baskets to various clinics. In fiscal year 1961 eight registered pharmacists prepared more than 250,000 prescriptions for inpatients and more than 85,000 prescriptions for outpatients.[69]

Many patients needed drugs. Some needed blood or plasma. Galveston's Office of Civilian Defense purchased equipment that was used to establish UTMB's first blood bank in the spring of 1942. Mrs. E. R. "Nonie" Thompson and Mrs. Chauncey Leake co-chaired the American Red Cross Committee that solicited donors. Fifty people volunteered on the first day of the blood drive. By 1955 Bill Levin (medical director) and Jean Stubbins (technical director) supervised a staff of four medical technologists, a vocational nurse, a lab attendant, a secretary, and five night technicians (medical students) who handled requests for about nine hundred transfusions each month.[70]

Most inpatients needed food and drink, and some needed special diets. Dietitians met with patients and their doctors to plan special diets for particular patients. By early

1956 the dietary department (154 employees) prepared and served meals for about eight to nine hundred people each day. During fiscal year 1961 this department (204 employees) prepared and served about 1 million meals. In 1968 the department prepared 2,700,000 meals for inpatients and hospital staff.[71]

Patients seldom encountered other groups of hospital workers whose labors contributed directly to their comfort and safety. In 1956 sixty employees in a new Central Services Department managed central sterile supply, laundry services, transportation, and patient equipment for inpatient rooms. In 1968 forty-two transportation employees responded to 113,353 requests for transferring patients; thirty-four central supply workers cleaned, sterilized, reassembled, and delivered over 2.5 million items; and sixty-two laundry employees poured 120 pounds of soap into washing machines every day.[72]

Patients frequently encountered religious professionals and community volunteers. Local ministers, priests, and rabbis visited members of their congregations who were hospitalized at UTMB. Believing that there was no Episcopalian scarlet fever, Catholic arthritis, or Jewish mumps, Rabbi Henry Cohen, for example, visited many non-Jewish patients. Although these visits by congregational leaders continued after 1942, the largest churches began assigning clergy as part-time or full-time chaplains. In 1954 Weldon Langley became the first hospital chaplain assigned by the Baptist General Convention of Texas. Carl Nighswonger was the Methodist chaplain in 1960; Denton Bassett the Baptist chaplain in 1965; and Bob Wedergren the Lutheran chaplain in 1968. These chaplains provided countless services to appreciative patients and staff.[73]

Inpatients and their families usually rejoiced when approached by the smiling faces and helping hands of those who were volunteer caregivers. The Junior Welfare League, the American Women's Voluntary Services (AWVS), and the American Red Cross organized volunteer programs during the 1940s and 1950s. The Junior League continued the services they had started in 1937. By 1948 twenty Junior League volunteers loaned patients an average of 375 books, 250 paperbacks, and 800 magazines monthly. In 1941 Mrs. Dan Kempner organized an AWVS chapter in Galveston that attracted about seven hundred volunteers by June of that year. AWVS members organized auxiliary nursing groups who told stories and played games with hospitalized children. During the 1950s and 1960s, AWVS members collected clothing for hospitalized infants, purchased layettes for newborns, entertained sick children, rented television sets to patients, and donated other items that enhanced the care of patients. The Galveston chapter of the American Red Cross also provided many volunteers. Their Gray Ladies began serving patients in February 1955. The local chapter trained volunteers and sponsored Christmas parties.[74]

In 1956 AWVS members initiated efforts to organize a hospital auxiliary that could be officially chartered by the American Hospital Association. At their first meeting in March 1960, about 150 women elected Mrs. John B. Truslow as the first president of the UTMB Hospitals Auxiliary. Its members volunteered many hours of service to patients and staff. In 1962 Mrs. Charles T. Stone Sr. received a pin for one thousand hours; in 1963, eight people received thousand-hour pins. During the summer of

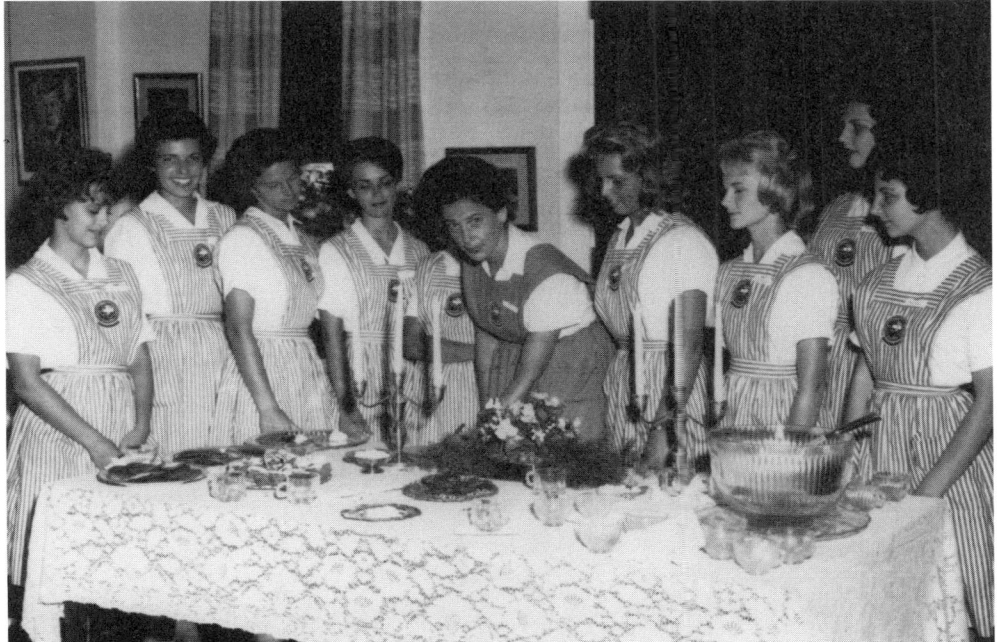

Mrs. Glenn Russell (center) welcoming the first group of candy stripers, August 1962.

1962 the auxiliary enthusiastically supported about fifty high school students who became the first group of candy stripers to do volunteer work in the hospitals. During fiscal year 1966, 347 auxiliary members contributed 22,423 hours of volunteer service. To coordinate all of these services, Blye Green became director of the hospital's volunteer office in March 1956; Pauline Bascom in the fall of 1958; and Mrs. William Hamilton early in 1961.[75]

The services of the aforementioned groups of professionals, employees, and volunteers expanded significantly during the 1960s as the number of patients increased, and as administrators and doctors developed new programs of care. The policy of comprehensive care demanded the addition of new technologies and programs as they emerged nationally.[76] Consider a few examples, beginning with cardiovascular surgery.

In 1960 Leonard Harris directed a new facility for diagnosing and treating patients with congenital heart diseases. By late 1961 doctors had attended 124 patients with 51 requiring medical care only, 40 cardiac catheterization, and 33 surgical procedures. John Derrick directed the surgical cardiovascular team that performed open-heart surgery on adults, implanting cardiac pacemakers in twenty-six patients between 1961 and 1966, for example.[77]

These advances in cardiovascular surgery depended on new types of equipment. In October 1961 the department of radiology began using the first angiograph injector in the Southwest, the seventh in the United States. This instrument monitored physiological functions while injecting radio-opaque substances in the bloodstream for studies of various organ systems. By January 1962 anesthesiologists used three new instruments. A gas chromatograph in the recovery room determined if a patient needed mechanical assistance in obtaining oxygen and eliminating carbon dioxide. An electronic hematocrit in the operating room determined if a patient needed a blood or plasma transfusion. The third was a special FM radio that could transmit an electrocardiogram to an oscilloscope without any direct connections between the patient and the recording device.[78]

The technical marvels of renal dialysis and transplantation came to UTMB in the 1960s. Ray Remmers and Harry Sarles, professors in the department of internal medicine, received a grant of more than $800,000 from the National Center for Chronic Disease Control for establishing a Center for Home Dialysis. In January 1968 the center's staff began teaching patients and their families how to manage the intricate techniques of renal dialysis in their homes. Sheldon Lee was the chief technician in the center's facilities in Clay Hall. Remmers and Sarles also worked closely with Jay Fish in the department of surgery. Fish's team performed the first kidney transplant at UTMB on March 30, 1967.[79]

The expansion and establishment of some programs required more professionals than equipment. In 1960 Nell Boelsche became director of the Child Development Clinic, which provided care for children with cerebral deficits and psychomotor disabilities. By 1967 its professional staff included four pediatricians, three psychologists, two speech and hearing therapists, four social workers, a psychiatrist, and a nurse. In 1961 UTMB employed more speech therapists when the division of otorhinolaryngology in the department of surgery opened a new speech and hearing clinic for children and adults. In 1961 Henry Burks became director of a new division of child psychiatry in the department of neurology and psychiatry. Burks and two residents attended approximately eight hundred outpatients during the summer of 1962. In 1964 Burks established a thirty-bed inpatient unit that was the first of its kind in a public hospital in Texas.[80]

UTMB also reorganized some services in more formal and efficient ways. Pediatricians frequently received calls from mothers about children who had consumed poisonous substances. Spencer Thompson and Armond Goldman acquired federal funds to establish a phone service in the hospital's pharmacy to handle these calls. Harvey Whitney Jr., Joe Nash, and Armond Goldman co-directed the Southwest Regional Poison Control Center, which opened in October 1967. Within five months, they had provided diagnostic and therapeutic advice for more than two hundred patients, usually children, afflicted with toxic substances.[81]

To provide new services, geographically more accessible services, and more efficiently organized services, the department of obstetrics and gynecology established several new clinics. They started a prenatal clinic in Jefferson in 1967 and soon expanded to Beaumont and La Marque. Pap smears enabled doctors to diagnose cervical cancer in an early and usually curable stage and in 1968 this department established a new cervical screening clinic. L. C. Powell Jr., its director, estimated that clinic personnel would perform Pap smears on about eleven thousand women that year. Expecting to provide birth control services to about five thousand indigent women, this department also established three family planning clinics in the spring of 1968; two in Galveston and one in La Marque.[82]

These new and expanded programs of patient care always increased the costs of care because they involved the addition of expensive equipment and salaries for technicians, as well as salaries for additional doctors, nurses, and other professionals. However, the challenging problems associated with increasing costs of care had already begun in the 1940s with the sizable increase in house staff and an administrative decision to attract more indigent patients.[83]

In November 1942 a diagnostic teaching clinic opened under the direction of Raymond Gregory, professor of medicine. This clinic provided care for indigents who could be sent by physicians and county governments from anywhere in the state. In 1942 the clinic's personnel attended 1,277 indigents from 124 counties; in 1943, 1,770 from 143 counties. These services were so appealing that the number of indigent patients from cities other than Galveston exceeded the number of indigent Galvestonians admitted to the hospitals in the spring of 1943.[84]

UTMB's doctors usually treated anyone who needed care. Although valuable for the mission of education, this policy led to financial troubles. Of 11,825 patients from 233 counties admitted in 1950, 3,678 were full-pay; 2,780 part-pay; and 5,367 indigent. During 1955, 9,278 indigent patients were admitted, prompting a significant drain on the hospital's coffers. The costs of operating the John Sealy Hospital, Waverley Smith Pavilion, and Ziegler Hospital led to a deficit of $500,000 by the summer of 1955. Policy changes occurred. After September 1955 indigent inpatients were charged $3 per day and rates for pay patients also increased. Inpatient room charges increased again in 1958 and the Galveston City Commissioners increased their allocation for indigent care from $75,000 to $200,000 per year. The meaning of medical indigency began to change as governing groups assumed more responsibilities for allocating tax dollars to those providing medical care to sick indigents. In May 1956 about 35 percent of UTMB's inpatients were full-pay; about 51 percent part-pay (some with insurance); and about 14 percent indigent. By 1965 almost all (94 percent) inpatients had some form of medical insurance.[85] Patients and their insurance carriers provided about 53 percent of the operating income of the hospitals between 1941 and 1968 (Appendix W).

Receiving more income from insurers helped to balance budgets, as did eliminating duplicate services associated with the patterns of segregation between blacks and whites. By the summer of 1956 the Negro Hospital was so crowded that obstetrical patients lay on beds in the halls. Only two patients could be attended in the extremely hot delivery room, where the noisy fan had to be turned off so the doctor could hear the patient and the baby. Sometimes the elevator would stop working and women in labor could not be taken to the delivery room. Because of these conditions and the shortage of nurses, this hospital closed in June 1957 and black patients were transferred to segregated wards in the John Sealy Hospital.[86]

Integrated services developed between 1959 and 1965. Administrators integrated the newborn nursery in February 1959. Because federal funds were used to create the

Clinical Research Center on 4-C of the John Sealy Hospital, the center became the first integrated adult unit when it opened in June 1963. Sometime in 1964 or early 1965, T. D. Armstrong, a highly respected black Galvestonian, was admitted to the seventh-floor ward for blacks in the John Sealy Hospital. When Sen. Babe Schwartz learned about this situation, he informed Dan Bobbitt and Truman Blocker that Armstrong was a friend of John Connally and Lyndon Johnson and wondered if they really wanted to leave him in the public ward for blacks. Armstrong was soon transferred to a private room in the Waverley Smith Pavilion. At the quarterly meeting of the hospital staff on April 27, 1965, Blocker announced that "a quiet and orderly integration was accomplished last week."[87]

The "quiet and orderly" feature of this change occurred, in part, because of the way physicians had reorganized their governance of hospital activities after the Spies era. The dissolution of the awkward Board of Managers, the departure of an autocratic hospital superintendent, and the resumption of more inclusive self-rule by the doctors produced a new political environment for patient care services. After Leake hired B. I. Burns as director of the hospitals in 1946, the doctors rejuvenated an organized medical staff for the hospitals. By 1953 this staff included active, associate, courtesy, and honorary members, who were subdivided according to the specialized clinical services institutionalized in the academic departments and divisions of the medical school. During monthly meetings they staged scientific programs and adopted policies about education and patient care in the hospitals. By 1960 ten committees did the work of the medical staff: Executive, Medical Records, Tissue Audit, Medical Audit, Liability Insurance, Pharmacy and Therapeutics, Infection, Intern, Program, and Cancer.[88]

These committees and hospital administrators worked diligently to improve working conditions in the hospitals, especially those for house staff. In 1960 they obtained minimum liability insurance coverage for interns and residents at a rate of $20 per year per individual. They also supported salary increases. By 1963 interns earned $275 per month; by 1966, residents earned $424 each month. In 1967 the House Staff Committee, led by Al LeBlanc, successfully lobbied for health insurance coverage for all house staff.[89]

During the 1950s and 1960s UTMB's hospital administrators usually had some formal training in hospital administration (Appendix F). George Currie, a Canadian physician with a master's degree in hospital administration from Columbia, came to UTMB from the University of Colorado Medical Center early in 1954. In 1955 he created five new positions for assistant hospital administrators, naming two at that time: Lyle S. Hartford and Daniel Bobbitt. In 1958 three assistant directors and the director of nursing service reported to Arthur Hennings, Currie's successor.[90]

More patients and more personnel required more managers. After Bobbitt became director in 1959, he used four assistant directors and the director of nursing service to manage the hospital's twenty-eight departments. By 1965 he had four associate administrators and two assistant administrators. Henry Swicegood, Bobbitt's successor, parceled administrative assignments to a total of seven associate and assistant

TABLE 5.1: TOTAL OUTPATIENT VISITS, FY1982–FY 1991

	Clinics	Emergency Room	Total
FY1982	184,352	61,888	246,240
FY1983	209,294	61,808	271,102
FY1984	250,776	58,943	309,719
FY1985	269,442	56,688	326,130
FY1986	290,663	54,845	345,508
FY1987	284,640	61,947	346,587
FY1988	280,633	61,203	341,836
FY1989	288,061	57,636	345,697
FY1990	292,664	56,203	348,867
FY1991	308,135	54,681	362,816

administrators.[91] The delegation of responsibilities to associate and assistant hospital administrators steadily increased managerial bureaucracy as well as the costs of care.[92]

FROM MEDICARE TO AIDS, 1969–1991

Administrative bureaucracy expanded, in part, because federal and state dollars from Medicare and Medicaid catalyzed an unprecedented growth in medical care for thousands of Americans, including those who came to UTMB as outpatients and inpatients during the 1970s and 1980s. To help control the rising costs of hospitalization, there was a shift from less inpatient care to more outpatient (ambulatory) care. During fiscal year 1975, 113,621 patients came to the clinics: 42,238 from the city of Galveston, 70,556 from 226 counties in Texas, 780 from other states, and 47 from Mexico. The totals included 123,120 outpatients and 52,000 emergency room patients in fiscal year 1976; 140,921 outpatients and 57,000 emergency room patients in fiscal year 1978.[93]

As part of the shift to ambulatory care, UTMB gave more support to its emergency room during these years. There was a substantial increase in the total number of emergency room visits during the 1970s. About 4,000 patients visited each month during fiscal year 1973; about 150 to 160 patients each day during fiscal year 1977. Between fiscal years 1982 and 1991, these visits ranged between a low of 54,681 and a high of 61,947 (Table 5.1).[94]

Emergency medical services received considerable public attention when helicopter service began in May 1983. With a staff of four pilots, eleven specially trained flight nurses dressed in bright orange uniforms, and one mechanic, the Life Flight V helicopter began transporting patients to UTMB. These included victims of head injury, multiple trauma, severe burns, and cardiac arrest, as well as premature infants and extremely sick women in labor. During its first two years of service, Life Flight V logged

TABLE 5.2: TOTAL INPATIENT VISITS, FY1982–FY 1991

	Newborn	Adult & Pediatric	Total
FY1982	4,203	25,991	30,194
FY1983	4,873	28,033	32,906
FY1984	5,234	30,259	35,493
FY1985	4,663	31,146	35,809
FY1986	3,726	29,537	33,263
FY1987	3,236	29,161	32,397
FY1988	3,563	27,272	30,835
FY1989	3,374	26,035	29,409
FY1990	3,448	25,194	28,642
FY1991	3,403	23,601	27,004

182,552 miles in 1,172 flights that transported 1,190 patients. In fiscal year 1989, the crew transported 647 patients during 629 flights in a new helicopter with blue, orange, and white colors.[95]

In dealing with the shift to ambulatory care, UTMB expanded its off-campus clinics.[96] The department of obstetrics and gynecology continued its leadership in developing services for patients in other towns. By 1969 about sixty pregnant women visited its prenatal clinic in Beaumont every Tuesday and about forty women visited the one in La Marque every Thursday. By the summer of 1970 personnel in this department attended about two thousand clients at the family planning clinics in Galveston and La Marque, averaging twenty-five new families each week. In February 1982 a satellite clinic was established at the Texas Department of Corrections Women's Unit in Gatesville. By 1988 the department's satellite clinics served pregnant women in twenty-six counties. In 1991 this department cooperated with the Nacogdoches Memorial Hospital in establishing a new Regional Maternal/Child Health Center and the department opened a regional perinatal clinic in Livingston, the department's twenty-third off-campus clinic.[97]

In Galveston, administrators and faculty celebrated the opening of the new seven-story Ambulatory Care Clinic in 1983. By 1989 there were about 250,000 patient visits to all outpatient sites. These included the off-campus clinics; the four major clinics (obstetrics and gynecology, pediatrics, medicine, surgery) and twenty-six subspecialty clinics in the Ambulatory Care Clinic; the teen pregnancy clinic in the 1700 Strand building; the pediatric clinics in the Child Health Center; the day surgery unit in the John Sealy Towers; and the family medicine clinic in Unit D on Texas Avenue.[98]

Every week, some outpatients became inpatients. UTMB's professionals attended 26,500 inpatients in fiscal year 1976; 29,000 in fiscal year 1978.[99] The total number of

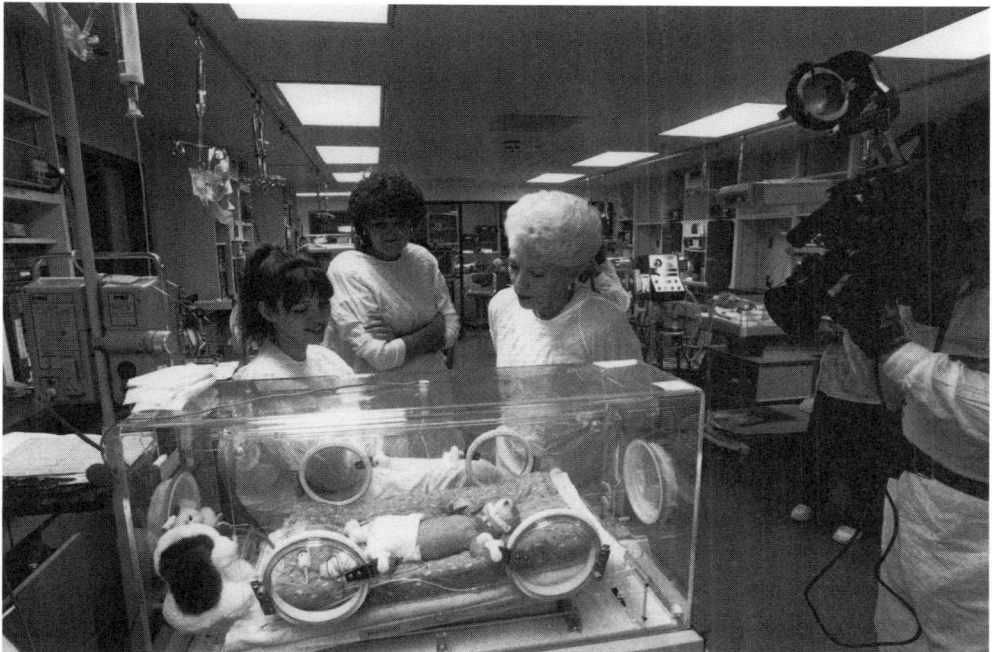

Baby Jessica Barber in Infant Special Care Unit, 1990. Left to right: Jennifer Trahen (mother), Dr. C. Joan Richardson, and Gov. Ann Richards.

inpatients peaked in the mid–1980s, then declined somewhat as less costly ambulatory care expanded (Table 5.2). As these years evolved, personnel attended inpatients in thirteen buildings. These were the Children's Hospital, Randall Pavilion, Moody State School, John Sealy Hospital, Waverley Smith Pavilion, Ziegler Hospital, Marvin L. Graves Hospital, Shriners Burns Institute, Jennie Sealy Hospital, John Sealy Hospital Towers, Child Health Center, Mary Moody Northen Pavilion, and the Texas Department of Criminal Justice Hospital. The number of available beds for inpatients varied from year to year. Between September 1, 1981, and August 31, 1991, it ranged from a high of 1,036 (fiscal year 1984) to a low of 834 (fiscal year 1990). The total number declined as fewer patients were admitted and as multi-bed wards of the John Sealy Hospital were replaced with smaller rooms (single and double occupancy) in the John Sealy Towers.

Inpatient care continued to be organized according to the specialties and subspecialties of physicians. Obstetricians assisted many parturient women. The Sealy & Smith Foundation provided $10,250,000 for a new labor and delivery suite that opened on the third floor of the John Sealy Hospital in November 1986. This unit included four low-risk and eight high-risk labor rooms; a birthing room; an anesthesia induction room; and two major and four minor delivery rooms. About two thousand babies were born in this suite during the next six months. Between September 1, 1981, and August 31, 1991, UTMB's annual total ranged from a low of 3,236 to a high of 5,234 newborns (Table 5.2).[100]

Pediatricians provided care for the newborns. In 1983 UTMB's pediatricians and nurses managed the only neonatal intensive care unit in Texas, attending 450 infants from thirty-seven counties.[101] In the following year, the Department of Pediatrics opened a new sixty-bed newborn nursery and a thirty-two-bed Infant Special Care Unit. ISCU staff attended between four and five hundred babies each year during the mid-1980s. These premature infants needed intensive care because of low birth weight, congenital abnormalities, or addiction (maternal drug abuse). Tiny infants in the ISCU were covered with wires that were connected to a variety of machines that sustained and monitored life functions.[102]

Pediatricians and their colleagues worked as teams in providing care for infants and children with infectious diseases, cancer, degenerative conditions, metabolic abnormalities, physical and sexual abuse, and cerebral dysfunctions. A specialized Extracorporeal Membrane Oxygenation (ECMO) team, for example, attended infants experiencing severe respiratory failure, twenty-one between March 1987 and February 1989. When the lungs of an infant ill with chicken pox were failing, the baby was hooked to the ECMO machine, where the child's blood was oxygenated and medicated. Without the ECMO machine and expert nursing care, the baby would have died.[103]

Teamwork was a distinctive feature of those who provided care to the cerebral palsied children housed at the Moody State School. In 1969, for example, a special helmet and a leather hand splint allowed eight-year-old Sandra Franklin to use wash, line, and dot techniques in her paintings. Nine-year-old Myra Shoemake progressed from watercolor to oil paintings and also did embroidery and leatherwork. After twenty years, the school had "graduated" eight hundred multi-handicapped children; one thousand after twenty-five years (1976).[104]

Other specialized teams emerged during these years. The care of children with renal failure became more technically sophisticated. In 1975 a renal dialysis and transplantation unit opened on the third floor of the Children's Hospital. This unit accommodated children who needed dialysis as well as those who received new kidneys from Jay Fish's transplant team. After eleven years, this team had performed seventy-eight transplants including one for Ryan Bell, a twenty-pound toddler from Midland.[105] During the 1980s Luther Travis directed a team of professionals at the children's diabetes management center that included pediatricians, a clinical nurse specialist, a health educator, a dietitian, a clinical psychologist, and a social worker. This group enthusiastically supported the annual two-week summer camps for diabetic children.[106] David Sapire and his colleagues in pediatric cardiology attended about twenty outpatients a day in 1991.[107]

In addition to the neonatal unit, other intensive care units emerged. On March 24, 1969, UTMB admitted its first patient to the new coronary care unit (CCU) developed by the department of internal medicine.[108] On April 1, 1970, the department of anesthesiology opened a general intensive care unit (GICU) on ward 2B of the John Sealy Hospital. In the GICU personnel attended postoperative patients as well as those admitted from the emergency room and other wards. Death rates were fairly high (Table 5.3). The department of neurology and the division of neurosurgery established a six-bed

TABLE 5.3: DEATHS IN GICU, FY1972–FY 1977

	Patients	Deaths
FY1972	317	57
FY1973	397	64
FY1974	326	50
FY1975	496	56
FY1976	425	58
FY1977	383	69

neurological intensive care unit in October 1975 that expanded to eight beds when it moved to the ninth floor of the John Sealy Towers. After the Children's Hospital was incorporated into the new 150-bed Child Health Center that opened in February 1977, a six-bed pediatric intensive care unit opened on the center's fourth floor.[109]

By 1982 the hospitals at UTMB contained seventy-three intensive care beds. In 1989 internists and colleagues in the eight-bed Medical Intensive Care Unit (MICU) attended patients with pneumonia, cancer, overwhelming infections, renal failure, and cerebrovascular disorders. Though the death rate was high, some patients did respond to the high-tech, high-touch environments of these units. One female patient "died" four times, but eventually recovered and later declared (when visiting the MICU): "My angels, my angels! Look at me! I look great! I look fine! I love you! You are the reason I am alive." An elderly woman living alone on a farm, she had cut herself and contracted tetanus. After several months in the MICU, she recovered completely.[110]

Other patients were alive because of the training and care received by outpatients in the Renal Dialysis Center that had been started by the department of internal medicine. After a training period that usually lasted about two months, these patients dialyzed eight hours a day (three days a week) in their homes, relying on an assistant, usually a spouse, for help in managing the procedure. By the time of its tenth anniversary in the spring of 1978, this center had trained 158 patients.[111] By 1989 the center's staff followed about sixty patients throughout the state and attended about a hundred new patients a year.

Internists and their colleagues also developed a hyperbaric facility that began functioning in 1973. The facility housed one large double-lock decompression chamber about sixteen feet long and three single-lock chambers, one medium and two small. These chambers were used for the treatment of divers with decompression sickness and, more frequently, for patients with gas gangrene, carbon monoxide poisoning, air emboli, and intractable osteomyelitis. In 1980 the facility acquired a larger chamber that could accommodate five patients. Staff members developed techniques for using hyperbaric oxygen to treat severe infections of the face and neck caused by radiation therapy for cancer. In fiscal year 1989, 112 patients received hyperbaric treatment.

Early in 1990 the facility's staff of ten people attended about ten patients a day, with each patient needing an average of fifteen treatments.[112]

During the mid-1970s internists developed a more coordinated approach to the care of patients with cancer.[113] In 1975 William Levin and John Costanzi received two federal grants to develop a Cancer Center that provided immunotherapy for selected patients as well as extensive education programs about cancer. After about two years of operation, Cancer Center personnel had staged more than twenty continuing education programs in sixteen Texas counties; provided research support to some research colleagues such as Thomas Albrecht, Robert Girtanner, and Demitrius Loukas; and stimulated the referral of more cancer patients to UTMB for treatment. These referrals increased from 730 in 1973 to 1,150 in 1985.[114]

As older patients appeared in increasing numbers during the 1980s, internists and their colleagues steadily institutionalized geriatric medicine. In 1983 a geriatric consult team began offering services on the internal medicine floors in the John Sealy Towers and the department of psychiatry opened its first inpatient unit for older patients. In 1986 Derek Prinsley became the first George and Cynthia Mitchell Distinguished Professor in Geriatrics. Between 1986 and 1991 Prinsley, Patsy Koeppe, Barbara Thompson, and their colleagues developed an inpatient geriatric service, a coordinating center on aging, an innovative geriatric day hospital, and an academic division of geriatrics in the department of internal medicine.[115] In November 1989 the geriatric day hospital opened as the first of its kind in the United States. In 1990 the inpatient service (sixteen beds on 3-East of the Jennie Sealy Hospital) admitted 371 patients, and between 15 and 20 patients came to the day hospital each day.[116]

Internists who specialized in infectious diseases treated adults with a host of bacterial, fungal, parasitic, and viral diseases, including the first patient diagnosed with AIDS in 1982. By 1991 Richard Pollard and Michael Borucki had attended more than seven hundred HIV-infected adults, including a substantial number of prisoners receiving outpatient and inpatient care in the TDCJ hospital on the campus.[117]

For many years, prisoners who needed inpatient care were housed with other patients at UTMB, sometimes attended twenty-four hours by a guard, always attended at some time every day by a guard. By the early 1970s between twenty and twenty-five prisoners were inpatients each day. In February 1978 a locked facility with beds for thirty men and five women opened on unit 9-C in the John Sealy Hospital. It moved to units 10-A and 10-B of the John Sealy Towers in the spring of 1980.[118]

After the TDJC Hospital opened three years later, buses transported between 100 and 120 prisoners each day from prison units to the hospital's outpatient clinic. In fiscal year 1986, more than 15,000 prisoners were evaluated in this clinic and 2,914 were admitted as inpatients. Inpatient beds expanded from thirty-six in 1983 to one hundred in 1989.[119] In addition to AIDS and other medical problems, the prisoners developed conditions requiring surgery. Surgeons performed minor surgical procedures in the TDCJ Hospital and major procedures in the operating rooms of the John Sealy Hospital (more than one thousand each year between fiscal years 1985 and 1991).

TABLE 5.4: TOTAL SURGICAL PATIENTS, FY1982–FY 1991

	Patients		Patients
FY1982	9,023	FY1987	11,017
FY1983	9,632	FY1988	9,942
FY1984	11,340	FY1989	9,585
FY1985	11,676	FY1990	9,407
FY1986	11,432	FY1991	8,118

To adapt to the increasing demands for surgical care, these operating rooms were remodeled during 1973 and 1974. During fiscal year 1974, 10,751 surgical cases and 14,781 procedures were completed in the nineteen operating suites, two cystoscopic rooms, and emergency room. After the John Sealy Towers were completed, surgeons used about two dozen operating rooms for performing procedures on an annual number of patients that peaked in fiscal year 1985 and declined thereafter (Table 5.4).[120]

Surgeons continued their legacies of care for infants and children with congenital anomalies, organ failures, cancer, and traumatic injuries. In 1972 Ted Huang (class of 1965) directed a team that treated infants and children with cleft palates and cleft lips. The team usually included a pediatrician, otolaryngologist, plastic surgeon, oral surgeon, audiologist, prosthodontist, speech pathologist, social worker, and special education teacher. Steven Blackwell directed this team during the 1980s.[121]

Blackwell and other plastic surgeons attended drug abusers who had severely damaged the veins of their arms, and they continued their extraordinary work with burned children. In 1978 the Shriners Burns Institute celebrated its twelfth anniversary by discharging three boys: a nine-year-old and a ten-year-old after five months of treatment for each, and a twelve-year-old after four months of care. In 1983 the institute's staff admitted 233 acutely burned children and 394 children needing reconstructive surgery.[122]

Traumatic injuries became "epidemic" during these years. Newspapers carried daily reports of those injured in explosions and fires, as well as those injured in vehicular crashes (bicycle, car, bus, train, boat, and plane). People hurt each other with knives, guns, and other weapons, or hurt themselves during falls from rooftops, ladders, steps, and industrial platforms. Every week, the surgeons treated children and adults with traumatic injuries.

Vehicular accidents challenged the creative skills of the surgeons. In January 1982 they used microvascular techniques during a six-hour procedure to reattach a completely severed arm of a forty-one-year-old shrimp boat crewman. In February 1982 teams of plastic and orthopedic surgeons worked for ten hours to treat a seventeen-year-old Texas City woman who had been injured in a train accident. They transferred her left foot to her right leg after amputating her left leg and they re-attached her partially severed forearm. In December 1989 Martin Robson led the replantation team as they worked nearly ten hours to reattach the arteries, veins, nerves, and bones in a twenty-year-old patient's left arm, which had been severed in an auto accident.[123]

Accidents caused irreversible damage to the brains of some victims, but not to other organs. Surgeons began transplanting these viable organs into patients whose own organs were failing or had failed. Led by Jay Fish, the renal transplant center opened on February 22, 1971. By late 1986 Fish and his colleagues had performed 811 kidney transplants and were following 525 patients with transplants (the second largest renal transplant program in Texas). In April 1988 surgeons performed their first transplant of a kidney and a pancreas into a thirty-two-year-old teacher from Odessa. In 1990 a patient received the one thousandth kidney transplant at UTMB and the state's thirty-eighth dual transplant of a kidney and pancreas.[124]

Other technical advances enabled innovative surgery for babies with severe congenital anomalies. Using new ultrasound equipment, doctors expected the delivery of conjoined (Siamese) twins on July 14, 1976. Six days later, a team of surgeons operated for four hours to separate the conjoined areas, which included the thoracic cage, heart cavity, diaphragm, abdominal cavity, and liver. No complications occurred This was the first case of it kind at UTMB and the eleventh ever recorded. In 1984 surgical teams worked for almost eighteen hours to separate another set of conjoined twins who were less than twenty-four hours old at the time of surgery.[125] In 1985 five-year-old Maria Martinez had no apparent problems after surgeons performed two fourteen-hour operations to correct birth defects.[126]

These extraordinary developments were made possible by the incredible expansion of technical expertise and sophisticated machines that appeared during these years. Because the department of radiology supported the work of every clinical service, it probably acquired more new equipment than any other department. Using a Sealy & Smith Foundation grant, for example, this department obtained a body scanner in 1975. Touted as the "most significant advance in radiology since the discovery of x-rays in 1895," the scanner was a computerized system for diagnosing diseases and injuries of the brain. From July 1975, when it became functional, through June 1976, technicians performed about twenty-two hundred cranial tomographic (CT) scans that helped physicians differentiate between various forms of neurological diseases including trauma, intracranial hemorrhage, aneurysms and arterio-venous malformations, hydrocephalus, cerebral vascular diseases, neoplasms, and inflammatory diseases.[127]

In 1980 radiologists acquired a new million-dollar total body scanner; in 1982, a General Electric 8800 CAT Scanner. In 1984 a $2.35 million Magnetic Resonance Imager (MRI) was installed on the first floor of Jennie Sealy Hospital.[128] Supporting the diagnostic endeavors of most clinicians, radiologists and their assistants annually conducted a large number of examinations during the 1980s, surpassing 200,000 in fiscal year 1991 (Table 5.5).

In 1986 James Belli and his colleagues in the Department of Radiation Therapy acquired a $1.3 million linear accelerator for the treatment of patients with cancer. This

TABLE 5.5: RADIOLOGICAL EXAMS, FY1982–FY 1991

	Exams		Exams
FY1982	135,623	FY1987	171,206
FY1983	139,863	FY1988	169,375
FY1984	143,428	FY1989	171,703
FY1985	136,966	FY1990	182,323
FY1986	135,014	FY1991	200,172

machine could produce two X-ray treatment beams—one of 6 million electron volts, the other of 15 million volts. By 1990 this department used a new orthovoltage machine for irradiating cancerous tissue during surgery. In treating esophageal cancer in 1991, for example, Joseph Zwischenberger and his colleagues combined surgery, chemotherapy, and radiation.[129]

New technologies and new technicians also supported advances in cardiovascular surgery during these years. Vincent Conti, James Arens, and Mark Kuruse led the cardiothoracic surgery team. Kuruse, the chief perfusionist, and his assistants monitored and managed the heart-lung machine during open-heart surgery. UTMB opened a sixteen-bed cardiovascular surgical care unit in the spring of 1984. A surgical team performed the first cardiac transplant at UTMB in May 1985. Using a Sealy & Smith Foundation grant of $8.7 million, a new cardiac catheterization unit was added in 1987. By 1990 Conti and his team were performing more than three hundred open-heart operations a year.[130]

Other departments acquired new diagnostic and therapeutic equipment during these years. In 1984 the department of ophthalmology became the first department in an academic medical center in the United States to acquire a new YAG laser and the division of neurosurgery acquired the Echoflow II Doppler Imaging Unit, a new ultrasound machine. Early in 1987 the Department of Surgery obtained a new KTP/532 Laser that was a significant improvement over the carbon dioxide laser because it could make very small incisions (the least invasive surgical procedures).[131]

In November 1988 the first non-immersion lithotripter in the United States began destroying the kidney stones of patients at UTMB. This lithotripter used electromagnetically generated shock waves to disintegrate kidney stones, thereby avoiding surgery. The smaller particles passed out of the body in the urine. Because patients no longer needed to be anesthetized and immersed in special water baths, this lithotripter could be used with ambulatory patients. It was also used to crush bile stones for the first time at UTMB in late June 1989.[132]

Far less dependent on machines, doctors in the department of psychiatry prescribed a variety of psychotropic drugs during the 1970s and 1980s, and they used various psychotherapeutic programs with families, children, and adolescents. Pat Blakeney, Dan

167

Creson, and others attended patients in a sexual dysfunction clinic. Paul Walker direct-ed a gender identification unit that included counseling programs for sex offenders. A psychiatric adult day program opened in the Mary Moody Northen Pavilion in December 1982. In 1988 this department established an eight-bed unit for patients with eating disorders, especially those with anorexia nervosa.[133]

Most of the clinical and social services that emerged between 1941 and 1968 expanded dramatically between 1969 and 1991. After the Southwest Poison Control Center became part of a national network in 1974, for example, its phone requests rapidly escalated from about four thousand to about eight thousand per year. With Mike Ellis as director, the center's staff handled about four hundred calls each day by the late 1980s.[134]

The evolving panoply of professionals described earlier in this chapter continued to function during these years. Some groups experienced only numerical growth; others experienced structural reformation and further functional differentiation. Consider some examples associated with physicians, nurses, clinical lab technicians, physical therapists, occupational therapists, respiratory therapists, social workers, medical records personnel, pharmacists, blood bank technicians, dietitians, workers in central supply, laundry, and transportation, school teachers, chaplains, and volunteers.

Interns, residents, clinical fellows, attending physicians, and consulting physicians continued to lead clinical care-giving. In 1979, for example, faculty in the ten divisions of the Department of Internal Medicine supervised fifty-three residents and seventeen clinical fellows. A team of residents and students attended fifteen to twenty inpatients daily.[135] The size of these teams varied from department to department.

Graduate and registered nurses worked with doctors and others in providing direct care to patients. Some became supervisors, teachers, and administrators. During the 1980s others became clinical nurse specialists, focusing their attention on one special area such as the care of diabetic children or burned adults.[136]

Usually there was a dearth of nurses for bedside care. To fill this social vacuum, women became licensed vocational nurses and nurse's aides. These groups received less academic training than graduate nurses, but they participated actively in bedside care. In 1969 UTMB organized its first program for training nurse's aides. At the end of June 1972 there were no LVN vacancies, four aide vacancies, and forty-five R.N. vacancies in the hospitals. Between September 1, 1976, and July 11, 1977, 199 nurses began working at UTMB while 138 resigned.[137] Though the problem of an adequate number of bedside nurses continued, more than one bulletin board in the nurses' stations con-tained photos and thank-you notes from patients and families of patients. Mothers sent photos of teenagers who were attended as sick preemies or neonates, reminders that boosted the spirits of nurses, doctors, and others who participated in the daily struggle for life and health.

Nurses assisted students, house staff, and others who obtained samples of blood, urine, and other bodily substances for laboratory analyses. In 1974 the clinical lab added an automated clinical analyzer that could simultaneously perform twenty-five tests on

TABLE 5.6: CLINICAL LAB PROCEDURES, FY1982–FY 1991

	Procedures			Procedures
FY1982	777,221	FY1987		806,637
FY1983	839,210	FY1988		823,814
FY1984	839,313	FY1989		846,028
FY1985	754,501	FY1990		920,345
FY1986	783,938	FY1991		1,057,757

TABLE 5.7: SURGICAL PATHOLOGY TESTS, FY1982–FY 1991

	Tests			Tests
FY1982	19,982	FY1987		24,091
FY1983	21,087	FY1988		26,642
FY1984	24,152	FY1989		26,980
FY1985	24,523	FY1990		29,191
FY1986	24,513	FY1991		27,274

serum and other body fluids. In 1979 the lab employed more than two hundred laboratory professionals (eighty-five technologists) organized in four divisions: microbiology, chemistry, hematology, and blood bank. They performed 658,246 tests during fiscal year 1979; 716,822 tests during fiscal year 1981.[138] The total number of tests surpassed 1 million in fiscal year 1991 (Table 5.6).

In addition to the main clinical lab, technicians operated thirty-two other labs. In 1974 more than three thousand electroencephalograms (EEGs) were performed on patients. Using specialized equipment, technicians could identify and isolate a variety of viruses in the Diagnostic Virology Lab Richard Pollard established in 1978. Technicians in the Surgical Pathology Lab prepared more than sixty-five thousand slides in 1982.[139] The total number of their preparations usually increased each year between fiscal year 1982 and fiscal year 1991 (Table 5.7).

As in previous years, physical therapists, occupational therapists, respiratory therapists, and social workers provided a variety of services to patients. Between fiscal years 1982 and 1991, the annual number of physical therapy treatments ranged between a low of 28,488 treatments in fiscal year 1982 and a high of 47,182 treatments in fiscal year 1988 (Table 5.8). In 1986 John De Santo, then city editor of the *Galveston Daily News*, injured his knee during a volleyball game. After surgical treatment, he received physical therapy, jokingly called p&t (pain and torture). De Santo was "impressed with the whole bunch" of physical therapists: "They're professional, helpful and they work you hard. But they're fair and know their business . . . They care."[140]

TABLE 5.8: PHYSICAL THERAPY TREATMENTS, FY1982–FY 1991

	Treatments		Treatments
FY1982	28,488	FY1987	45,651
FY1983	30,794	FY1988	47,182
FY1984	37,699	FY1989	43,011
FY1985	40,442	FY1990	37,348
FY1986	41,398	FY1991	37,357

TABLE 5.9: OCCUPATIONAL THERAPY HOURS, FY1982–FY 1991

	Hours		Hours
FY1982	47,915	FY1987	60,000
FY1983	41,751	FY1988	73,000
FY1984	50,100	FY1989	69,000
FY1985	55,000	FY1990	54,000
FY1986	60,000	FY1991	48,537

Occupational therapists gave 38,175 hours of therapy in fiscal year 1977, 38,941 in fiscal year 1981. One of the largest in the United States, the occupational therapy department had fifty-six staff members in 1985. During the 1980s the number of hours varied from year to year (Table 5.9). In fiscal year 1988, about sixty staff members provided more than seventy thousand hours of therapy to outpatients and inpatients in twelve locations on the campus.[141] Physical therapists and occupational therapists worked collaboratively, especially in providing rehabilitation services for victims of stroke and spinal cord injuries.

Respiratory therapists gave 501,716 treatments during fiscal year 1977; 931,113 during fiscal year 1981.[142] Between fiscal years 1982 and 1991, these therapists usually administered more than a million treatments each year (Table 5.10).

In early 1969 the social service department included eleven social workers and ten social case assistants, who provided services to between 650 and 750 patients each month. In 1989 this department included fifty social workers and their assistants, and six people with clerical roles.[143] The social workers and their assistants were grouped into teams assigned to specific inpatient and outpatient areas, such as psychiatry, adult services, pediatrics, emergency room, and the intensive care units. Altogether, these teams handled an average of seventy to seventy-five cases a day, or about twenty-two hundred cases each month. Depending on the needs of a patient and the patient's family, they arranged many types of assistance: money, housing, transportation, food,

TABLE 5.10: RESPIRATORY THERAPY TREATMENTS, FY1982–FY 1991

	Treatments		Treatments
FY1982	1,176,091	FY1987	1,002,682
FY1983	1,016,739	FY1988	944,445
FY1984	1,059,526	FY1989	932,948
FY1985	1,134,694	FY1990	1,197,633
FY1986	945,334	FY1991	1,444,991

TABLE 5.11: PHARMACY DISPENSING UNITS, FY1982–FY 1991

	Units		Units
FY1982	19,972,269	FY1987	28,307,188
FY1983	23,255,940	FY1988	30,003,307
FY1984	26,581,548	FY1989	23,208,206
FY1985	25,516,986	FY1990	16,425,678
FY1986	25,739,804	FY1991	14,914,862

clothes, psychotherapy, home health care, hospice care, or placement in a nursing home or foster home.

Also expanding during these years were the more indirect, but essential services medical records personnel, pharmacists, blood bank technicians, and dietitians provided. The Sealy & Smith Foundation provided $2,550,000 in 1979 for an IBM 370/158 Model 3 computer for handling patient records. This system enabled hospital personnel to locate records rapidly and to decode the status of incomplete records more efficiently. By the late 1980s, 157 employees worked in ten different sections of the medical records department.[144]

UTMB's pharmacists filled 13,501,306 prescriptions in fiscal year 1977 and 16,225,351 in fiscal year 1980. Surpassing 30 million in fiscal year 1988, the annual number decreased thereafter (Table 5.11). In 1981 Kathy Horton developed a separate pharmacy for the twenty-two operating rooms. In 1986 the pharmacy issued the thirtieth edition of the formulary, a list of the pharmaceutical substances and formulas used at UTMB.[145]

Blood bank technicians worked tirelessly in responding to a variety of clinical situations. For example, Adam Simon, a father of six from Arcola, became seriously ill in December 1979 with fever, kidney abnormalities, disorientation and other brain dysfunctions, a hemolytic anemia, and a low platelet count. Simon lapsed into a coma on Christmas Day, and doctors exchanged his plasma for six days, believing he had a rare disease known as thrombotic thrombocytopenic purpura. Simon "woke up" on New

TABLE 5.12: DIETARY MEALS SERVED, FY1982–FY 1991

	Meals		Meals
FY1982	690,371	FY1987	590,828
FY1983	677,686	FY1988	559,852
FY1984	700,771	FY1989	534,388
FY1985	654,872	FY1990	524,972
FY1986	611,703	FY1991	496,759

TABLE 5.13: CENTRAL SUPPLIES ISSUED, FY1982–FY 1991

	Supplies		Supplies
FY1982	1,335,887	FY1987	1,611,035
FY1983	1,572,208	FY1988	1,590,878
FY1984	1,679,281	FY1989	1,524,285
FY1985	1,709,343	FY1990	1,433,776
FY1986	1,555,545	FY1991	1,477,147

Year's Day 1980 and recovered completely. The exchange required eighty-four units of plasma and ten units of red cells, provided by ninety-four donors. By the late 1980s donors provided about ten thousand units of the twelve thousand units of blood and blood derivatives used at UTMB each year.[146]

The dietary department expanded considerably. By early 1984 the main kitchen was preparing food each day for about twelve hundred patients and one thousand cafeteria customers. One giant cooking pot could hold about six hundred servings of spaghetti sauce. More than 500,000 meals were served each year between fiscal years 1982 and 1991 (Table 5.12).[147]

Hospital workers in the central supply, laundry, and transportation departments performed tasks that were essential for the safety and comfort of patients and staff. Central supply workers issued 343,612 items in fiscal year 1977 and 1,140,929 items in fiscal year 1981. During the next ten years the annual total continued to surpass 1 million items (Table 5.13). New equipment improved the efficiency of workers in the laundry department until officials decided to outsource these services in the late 1980s. John De Santo also praised the transportation staff: "This often-overlooked group of workers was responsible for wheeling me to and from X-ray, surgery, physical therapy, etc. You can talk to these guys and they'll give you the inside story on what's happening. They do their job well."[148]

The work of schoolteachers, hospital chaplains, and volunteers also expanded during these years. In 1974 the department of school services provided classes for about one thousand students from preschool to high school age. The staff included twenty-seven teachers, four teacher's aides, an educational diagnostician, a speech therapist, an educational material specialist, and a coordinator for the learning resource center. They worked in four sites: audiology and speech pathology for children with hearing losses; the Shriners Burns Institute for burned children; pediatrics for medically disabled children; and the Graves Hospital for emotionally disturbed children. In 1986 these school programs were organized into the Moody Independent School District. By 1991 about twenty-five people taught between thirty and forty students each week.[149]

The expanding work of hospital chaplains became better organized. In 1969 hospital administrators supported the formation of a Council of Hospital Chaplains as a way of encouraging more cooperation among the chaplains.[150] In 1970 this group began hosting annual one-day meetings for physicians and clergy to discuss a variety of issues in pastoral care for patients; the seventeenth annual meeting occurred in January 1987.[151] In 1974 the group transformed itself into the Council on Religious Ministries. In 1975 a department of ministry was established in the hospital administration hierarchy and the chaplains were given an office and a full-time secretary. Eight chaplains provided support for each patient within the framework of the patient's religious orientation or wishes. The chaplains ministered to patients experiencing a variety of diseases and predicaments, including a sizable number of older patients.[152]

In 1969 Antoinette Swinnea became director of the hospital's Department of Volunteer Services. Volunteers performed many services during the 1980s: they sold snacks and soft drinks to patients and staff from their hospitality cart, and distributed reading materials from their library cart (one thousand magazines and one hundred books each month in 1989, for example). They provided new mothers with educational literature about a baby's first year of life, and they comforted anxious and restless infants and children. They enjoyed many play and party activities with hospitalized children. They were escorts for patients and they wrote letters for patients. Volunteers also provided language translation and sign interpretation (350 requests for thirteen languages in fiscal year 1991).[153]

Some volunteers displayed outstanding services. During the annual awards luncheon in November 1984, Frances Moya received an eight thousand-hour bar and Jan Williams a seven thousand-hour bar, and the Junior League of Galveston County received a special award for sponsoring the Pediatric Angels for ten years. During ten years as a volunteer in the Reach to Recovery program, Jean Neal, an administrative assistant who had experienced a mastectomy for breast cancer, logged more than five hundred visits to breast cancer patients. During twenty years, Alice Jenicek contributed 5,199 volunteer hours.[154] B. J. Herz's volunteer experiences with children in the Child Health Center's playroom stimulated her interest in securing the Ronald McDonald House for Galveston that opened in May 1989.[155]

Acquiring dollars from bake sales, snack shops, and other projects, 140 members of the Hospital Auxiliary contributed more than $25,000 for scholarships and other items needed by hospital departments in 1982. Between 1962 and 1982 the auxiliary donated

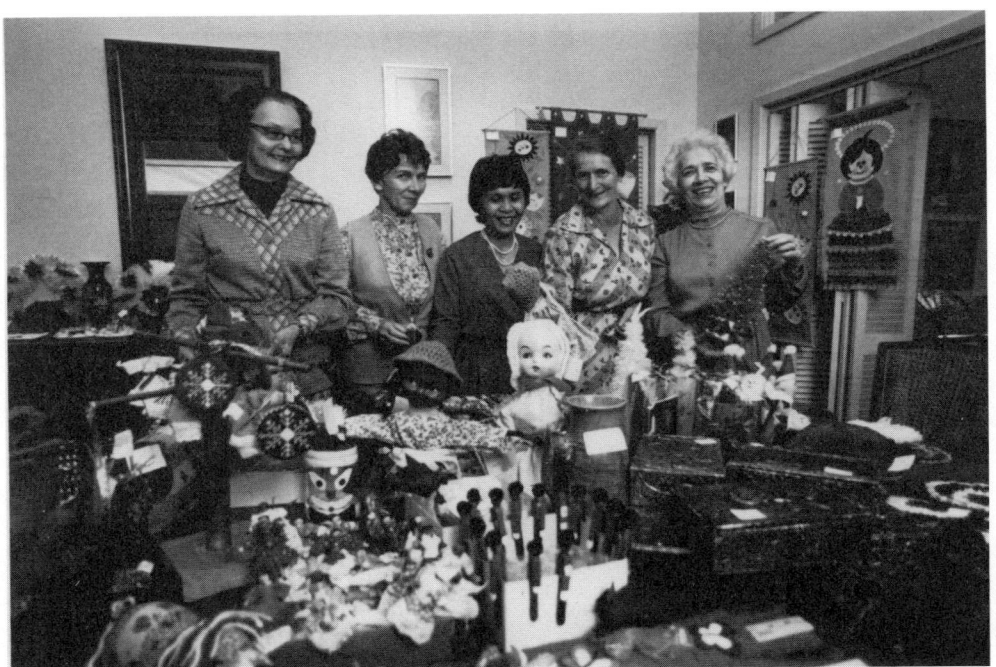

Hospital Auxiliary Arts and Crafts Bazaar Sale, 1980. Left to right: Alice Jenicek, Leni Weidenmeier, Becky Huang, Ursula Hild, and Bonnie Pyle.

almost $165,000 for various scholarship programs and departmental needs. In January 1990 the auxiliary gave $22,585 to various hospital departments and $4,800 for scholarships and loans to medical and nursing students.[156]

As the costs of hospital care continued to escalate between 1969 and 1991, administrators were always happy to receive these gifts. They were a part of the 2 percent of the hospital's operating income received from the Sealy & Smith Foundation and other private sources. As reviewed in chapter three, about 57 percent of this income came from patients and their insurance carriers, and about 41 percent came from county and state tax dollars.

During the 1970s income to the hospitals more than tripled, with substantial increases from state and federal sources (Appendix Y). During fiscal year 1979, for example, 48.32 percent came from state and county funds; 19.52 percent came from Blue Cross and commercial insurance; 15.21 percent from Medicare; 6.81 percent from Medicaid; and 10.14 percent from self-pay and private sources. Income to the hospitals doubled during the 1980s, with a substantial increase of federal dollars between fiscal years 1982 and 1991 (Appendices Y and AD). The percentage contributions from Medicare increased slightly and those from Medicaid increased sevenfold.[157]

As the recession of the early 1980s affected Texans, more patients became "medically indigent," that is, sick but unable to pay for the costs of medical care. In 1983 about 55 percent of UTMB's patients were medically indigent. More than once UTMB officials distinguished between its tradition of accepting many indigent patients and its

TABLE 5.14: HOSPITAL DEPARTMENTS, 1981

Admitting Office	Laundry
Allergy Clinic	Medical Records Library
Anesthesia Service	Moody State School
Autopsy Service	Nuclear Medicine Service
Blood Bank	Nursing Service
Central Supply and Transportation	Occupational Therapy
Chronic Home Dialysis Center	Outpatient Department
Clinical Lab	Pharmacy
Clinical Study Center	Physical Therapy
Cyto-Pathology Lab	Pulmonary Therapy Service
Dental Clinic	Radiology Service
Dietary Service	School Services
Electroencephalography Service	Social Service
Hearing and Speech Clinic	Surgical Operating Suite
Heart Station	Surgical Pathology Lab
Histology Lab	Unit Management
Housekeeping	Vice President for Health Services

legal mandate for education, which required the presence of patients, indigent or non-indigent. For decades the John Sealy Hospital was perceived as the only "general categorical" hospital in the state where indigent patients could receive medical care because the state provided funds for this care. The state legislature had never issued a mandate that required UTMB to care for any indigent Texan, but the state had provided dollars that allowed UTMB to accept a finite number of indigent patients who were referred by licensed physicians in the state. This circumstance encouraged the false perception that UTMB's hospitals had unlimited capacity for patients because it had unlimited funds for their care.[158]

To address the problems of medical indigency, Gov. Mark White authorized a Task Force on Indigent Health Care, which held several meetings between October 1983 and November 1984 before issuing its final report in December 1984.[159] Recommendations from this task force were influential in the decisions of the legislature in 1985 that, in various ways, provided additional funds for the care of medically indigent Texans, including additional dollars for public hospitals that admitted indigents.[160]

In adapting to the financial exigencies of the mid-1980s, administrators and faculty initiated UT-MED in 1985 as a new network for organizing care for both pay and non-pay patients at UTMB. As described in chapter three, they also began contracting for indigent care with other counties in the state as they had done with Galveston County

TABLE 5.15: CLINICAL DEPARTMENTS AND DIVISIONS, 1981

Anesthesiology	Orthopedic Surgery
Dermatology	Otolaryngology
Family Medicine	Patholgy
Hematology/Oncology	Pediatrics
Internal Medicine	Plastic Surgery
Neurology	Psychiatry
Neurosurgery	Radiology
Obstetrics/Gynecology	Surgery
Ophthalmology	Thoracic and Cardiovascular Surgery
Oral Surgery	Urology

since 1969. Attracting more pay patients and contracts with counties for non-pay patients helped somewhat in balancing budgets. But the costs of providing care to an increasing number of non-pay patients continued to escalate. In fiscal year 1990 UTMB expended $110 million in unreimbursed care to indigent patients from 249 of 254 counties in Texas.[161] The challenges of sustaining high quality clinical care during an era of escalating unreimbursed costs become formidable for those managing the hospitals and clinics.

The administrative bureaucracy of hospital management expanded during the 1970s and 1980s. By 1981 these managers coordinated relationships between employees in thirty-eight hospital departments (Table 5.14) and physicians in twenty clinical departments and divisions offering specialized services (Table 5.15).[162]

Reorganization of executive authorities occurred more than once. In 1970 Jack Thompson became vice president for both business affairs and hospital services, David Hoxie became the chief administrator of the hospital, and Bill Levin became chief of the medical staff. Hoxie discussed tasks and problems with the hospital's associate and assistant administrators every Tuesday morning. The hospital's executives provided regular opportunities for mid-level managers to improve their skills, adopted a performance appraisal program for all hospital employees, and began recognizing longtime employees by giving service pins to those who had worked at UTMB for five or more years.[163] These important rituals for development, evaluation, and affirmation continued during the 1980s.

Medical staff committees met regularly to deal with tissue audits, medical records, nosocomial infections, house staff problems, pharmacy matters, use of hospital beds, and the emergency room. Ad hoc committees functioned as needed and the medical staff's executive committee coordinated all activities with Hoxie's executive team and other academic executives.[164]

After Al LeBlanc became medical director of the hospitals in 1977, he used ten "directors" to manage the bureaucracy. He met with these "directors" every Tuesday and with other groups every Wednesday afternoon. Each "director" attended the regular meetings of more than one of twenty-six committees (eleven medical staff, thirteen hospital, and two institutional committees). LeBlanc and the "directors" held periodic retreats to discuss issues that required more time for analysis. When LeBlanc was promoted to associate vice president of university hospitals in 1980, his team included six executive directors and two directors. LeBlanc's team also included some outstanding administrative assistants and secretaries, such as Doris Janek, Kay Cook, Dolores Pena, Barbara Graham, Belinda Rodriquez, and Esther Koleng.[165]

In many important ways, Leblanc's executive team and their assistants transformed interpersonal relationships in the hospitals. This team organized programs that improved communication between hospital employees and clinical professors, programs that improved the skills of managerial personnel and the morale of all hospital employees, and programs that improved the attitudes and skills of hospital personnel as they interacted with patients. Consider some examples.

LeBlanc appointed Ann Smith as the coordinator of a quality assurance program. A quality assurance committee of caregivers from medicine, nursing, and allied health reviewed quarterly reports from all hospital departments. These reports identified three types of problems: intradepartmental, interdepartmental, and those requiring arbitration. This committee provided assistance each department needed to deal with its problems.[166]

In 1981 LeBlanc's team issued a 213–page "House Staff and Clinical Faculty Handbook," which provided everyone with a comprehensive view of hospital operations. In 1986 LeBlanc's team established the Partners in Caring program for all hospital personnel, which featured four-hour training sessions about developing more positive and caring attitudes.[167]

LeBlanc's team also focused on ways to address the daily concerns of patients. Beginning in 1978, the staff of a new patient relations department handled patients' grievances and found solutions to problems patients and their families posed.[168] In 1987 the patient relations department became a six-member office of guest services, whose employees worked to establish patient care systems that were more "guest friendly." During 1989, for example, staff members interviewed 7,027 patients; 426 of these voiced complaints about their care. For example, during a two-month period, seven patients complained about charges for an additional day's stay in the hospital. Staff members discovered that these patients were being charged for an extra day because no one had told them that they had to vacate their rooms by 1 P.M. on the day of discharge. Staff members asked the nursing service to assume responsibility for providing patients with this information.

Guest services employees continued a modified version of the Partners in Caring program by meeting with hospital personnel at the department level to present programs about team building and managing organizational change. Employees in this office also coordinated a group of 386 volunteers who spoke sixty languages and dialects. These persons responded to about 250 requests a year for interpreting and translating communications between patients and caregivers.[169] As the 1980s evolved, these programs generated an extremely high quality of respectful cooperation and regard among hospital employees and patients.

By 1988 an elaborate managerial hierarchy included at least fifteen top-level executives. Expenses for the hospital's general services that included this administrative matrix had grown from slightly more than $13 million in fiscal year 1980 to more than $30 million by fiscal year 1990.[170]

In the spring of 1990 James Arens succeeded LeBlanc as vice president for hospital affairs and Stephen Royal became the chief operating officer of the hospitals (Appendix F). In the fall of 1990 Arens and Royal downsized and streamlined the administrative hierarchy. By the centennial year, the governance and administration of the MSRDP and UT-MED programs had been reorganized in ways that allowed the clinical faculty to coordinate all patient care activities.[171] These events signaled a shift in the quality/quantity seesaw as the tides of unreimbursed indigent care eroded the dreams of those who wanted "the best" for everyone.

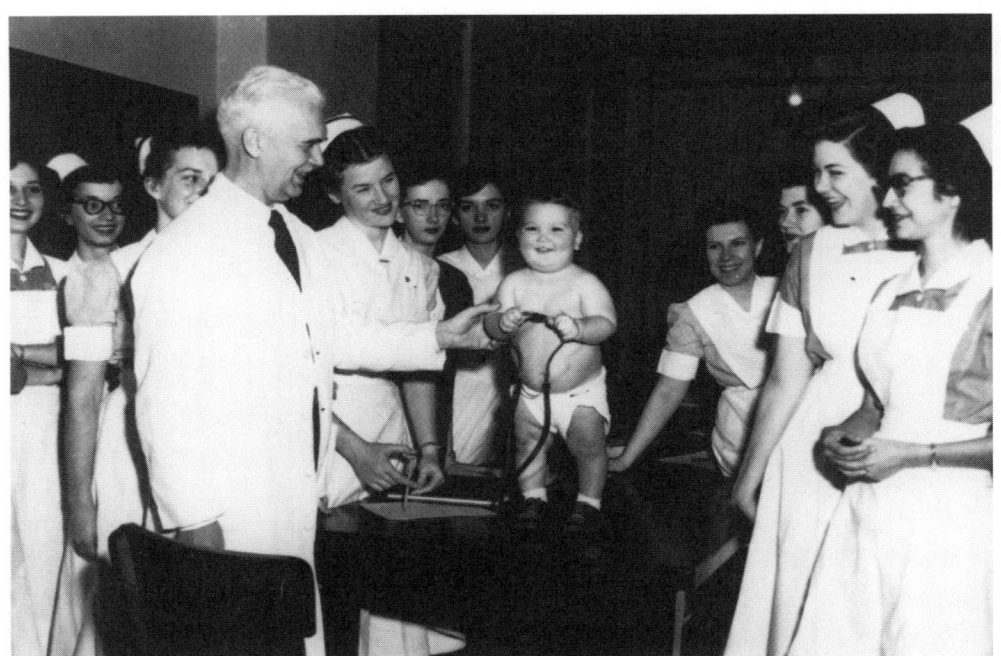

Arild Hansen with student nurses in a well baby clinic, 1952.

— 6 —

Learning and Teaching

"Why," demanded Professor Edward Randall Jr. *"do you look at your watch so often?"* *"I was afraid,"* hastily responded the medical student, *"that you would not have time to finish your interesting lecture."*[1]

During UTMB's first century, hundreds of students wondered if their teachers would ever finish their lectures, interesting or not. Lectures have always symbolized the transfer of knowledge from the more experienced teacher to the less experienced novice. Teachers lectured and students listened on nearly every weekday. By 1900, UTMB was fully recognized as more than a medical school. Though the School of Medicine was dominant, the School of Nursing and School of Pharmacy were distinctive. Each school had separate admission and graduation requirements, and each had a separate curriculum. Although there were important relationships between the schools, distinctive academic territories persisted as each school evolved. Other territories emerged as new schools and institutes were added.

The major teaching units formally appeared in the following sequence: School of Medicine (1891); School of Pharmacy (1893); School of Nursing (1896); School of Allied Health Sciences (1968); Graduate School of the Biomedical Sciences (1969); Marine Biomedical Institute (1969); and Institute for the Medical Humanities (1973). In this chapter, highlights about the development of each unit are presented in the same order. These highlights include an analysis of changes in policies and practices regarding admission and curriculum. Each section also includes information about teachers and students for the relevant years between 1900 and 1991.

THE SCHOOL OF MEDICINE

During the twentieth century administrators and professors changed their curriculum for undergraduate medical students in a variety of ways. They developed new training regimens for graduates who sought additional expertise as interns, residents, and clinical fellows. They also devised a potpourri of "continuing education" programs that allowed graduates to learn new facts and techniques or develop new skills. Changes in each of these patterns are described, together with the vicissitudes in admission practices from decade to decade.

During the early 1900s the School of Medicine faculty struggled with the realities of admitting poorly educated students. Because students seeking admission had such a wide variety of educational backgrounds, the faculty did not require graduation from high school until 1909. During the school's first twenty years, more than half of the students failed and many repeated courses. With each passing year, however, faculty "conditioned" students less frequently. "Conditioned" indicated that the professors required students to meet certain conditions, such as to take another exam or to make a certain grade on the next exam, before being passed to the next sequence. Carter was delighted that those graduating in the spring of 1910 represented a little more than half of the number who had entered four years earlier.[2]

In 1910, when the faculty required one year of college work for admission, the majority of the seventy-two American medical colleges ranked Class A by the AMA's Council on Medical Education required one or more years of college for admission. R. O. Braswell, a member of the Texas State Board of Medical Examiners, resisted this requirement and pledged to battle the faculty until their "standards were lowered" or the school was "driven into the Gulf of Mexico."[3]

Braswell did not succeed. The total number of matriculating first-year students did decrease from seventy-two in the fall of 1909 to thirty-seven in the fall of 1910. But forty-nine students matriculated in the fall of 1911. At the end of that academic year, the faculty conditioned no third-year students on second-year subjects, conditioned only one sophomore on a first-year subject, and required only one student to repeat the entire freshman year. Carter declared ecstatically: "This is the first time that such a thing has happened during the fifteen sessions that I have been connected with this institution."[4]

The faculty continued to honor the higher national standards promulgated by the AMA and the AAMC.[5] By 1914 thirty-two U.S. medical schools required two years of college for admission and twenty-three, including UTMB, required only one year. Because the AMA also required two years of college, UTMB's ranking dropped to the second level of schools designated as Class A. To change this, the faculty decided to require two years of college beginning in the fall of 1917. After that time, no students were admitted who had fewer than ten college courses.[6]

About thirty people (professors and assistants) taught medical students by UTMB's twenty-fourth academic year (1914–1915). Seven of the twelve major departments of instruction each had three teachers.[7] Four of the founding professors still taught (Keiller, Morris, Randall, and Thompson). Whether in a lecture hall or laboratory of Old Red, or a ward or clinic in the John Sealy Hospital, Negro Hospital, Isolation Pavilion, or Children's Hospital, every student could easily interact with the professors, who began revising the curriculum that year.

The professors stopped teaching physics, chemistry, and biology because all students were required to complete courses in these subjects before admission. They "concentrated" basic science subjects into the first two years of the curriculum; clinical subjects

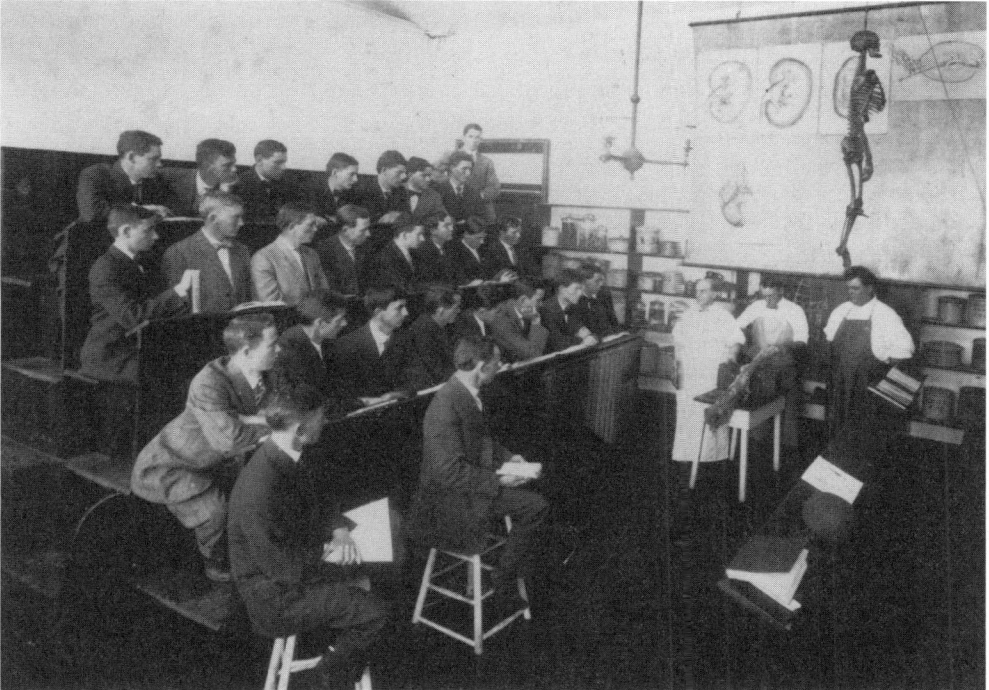

William Keiller, third from right, lecturing to medical students, 1912.

into the last two years. The professors expected students to complete courses in bio-chemistry and pharmacology during the first year; physiology by the end of the first term of the second year; and pathology by the end of the second term of the second year. This encouraged students to learn in a more coherent fashion.[8]

Other changes supported the goal of "concentration." During the 1916–1917 year, the laboratory teaching of pharmacology was extended, and more pathology and bac-teriology were added to the second year. Students assisted with autopsies and they learned more clinical pathology, using a laboratory established in the basement of the Nurses' Home. Teaching expanded in obstetrics and gynecology, pediatrics, medicine, and surgery. Students became more active in the clinics and wards. Both junior and senior students attended outpatients. Expected to be clinical clerks at least two hours each day, seniors were divided into four sections and placed on seven-week rotations in obstetrics and gynecology, medicine, and surgery. By 1920, 884 medical students had successfully survived this rigorous training and graduated.[9]

Even though the attrition rate had decreased, student anxieties remained high. In late November 1922, about eight weeks into the first term, Edith Bonnet wrote in her diary: "Failed in a Materia Medica quiz and am doing very poorly in Anatomy and Chemistry. Its baffling to work hard and get nowhere." The attrition rate remained between 30 percent and 35 percent during the 1920s and 1930s.[10]

Concerned about the increasing numbers of students seeking admission, inadequate lab facilities for the basic science courses, and an insufficient number of patients for clinical teaching, several professors wanted to limit class size. In 1920 they accepted ninety-six men and three women in the first year class. In 1924 they admitted only 60 of 121 applicants. Dean Keiller thought that this was the best group of first-year students ever admitted. The faculty then increased the total to seventy first-year students beginning in the fall of 1926. In 1927 the regents decided to enlarge the teaching laboratories and President Walter Splawn notified Dean Hartman that one hundred students could be admitted to the freshman class.[11]

As the pre-medical education of matriculates continued to improve, UTMB's professors, like those at other schools, searched for criteria that would help them decide about admitting particular students. In 1932 Dean Bethel recommended that the AAMC's Scholastic Aptitude Test for Medical Schools (SATMS) be required of all pre-medical students at UT Austin.[12] Two years later, the admission committee used these SATMS scores for the first time. Assigning an 80 percent value to scholastic achievement and 20 percent to the SATMS score, the committee selected one hundred students from more than two hundred applicants—all from Texas. By 1937 the admissions committee used the following sources of information about each student: scholarship record (together with a rating of the college); SATMS scores; and evaluations of personal qualifications given confidentially by two science teachers with whom the applicant had studied.[13]

With improvements in pre-medical preparation and better screening of applicants, the school's attrition rate decreased considerably by the late 1930s. In the 1937–1938 academic year, for example, there were eighty-one seniors and ninety-one juniors, the largest number ever in a third-year class. One hundred students had entered each class. The attrition rates of 19 percent and 9 percent were far better than the 63 percent of the 1890s.

Students who graduated during the 1920s and 1930s were truly survivors because the medical school curriculum was one of the toughest in the nation. The AMA recommended that the curriculum of a four-year school should not exceed a total of four thousand hours. In 1921 the total at UTMB exceeded five thousand hours. The faculty strongly resisted any changes because they wanted to produce competent general practitioners. By the late 1920s a UTMB graduate had survived a grand total of 5,087 hours of scheduled classes and clinics. In comparison to other schools, the professors taught far more anatomy and substantially more clinical medicine, especially surgery and obstetrics and gynecology.[14]

When Bethel became dean in 1928, about forty professors and another fifteen practitioners shared teaching responsibilities.[15] The professors included Harry "Daddy" Knight, "Crazy" John Sinclair, Byron "Lumpy Jaw" Hendrix, Wilfred Thomas Dawson, Eugene L. Porter, William "Pod" or "Bunny Face" Sharp, "Uncle" Paul Brindley, Charles Stone Sr., George "Pudge" Herrmann, Willard Cooke, A. O. Singleton, Dick Wall, and Seth Morris.

These and other teachers were organized in sixteen departments. Housed in Old Red, the new Laboratory Building (Keiller), and three small laboratory facilities, the seven basic science departments were Anatomy; Bacteriology and Preventive Medicine; Biological Chemistry; Histology and Embryology; Pathology; Pharmacology; and Physiology. Housed in five hospital buildings, the nine clinical departments were Dermatology and Syphilology; Diseases of Children; Neurology and Psychiatry; Obstetrics and Gynecology; Ophthalmology; Otology, Rhinology, and Laryngology; Practice of Medicine; Radiology; and Surgery. The departmental chairs coordinated each department's courses in the curriculum (Appendix G).[16]

Bethel believed that medical students should be thoroughly trained in the fundamentals of medicine, but that training in the specialties should take place after medical school. In June 1931 he appointed a curriculum revision committee, which submitted its report in March 1932.[17] The faculty adopted the recommended changes during the next six years.

Major changes occurred in the "basic science" curriculum in the fall of 1932. The total number of instructional sessions in anatomy was reduced from 741 hours to 522 hours. A course in clinical pathology was added to the second year, but Wednesday afternoons and Saturday afternoons were designated as free time for first- and second-year students. Additional space in the new addition to the Keiller Building permitted the teaching of the entire first-year and second-year classes in most subjects at one time.[18]

By the fall of 1934 Bethel was satisfied with the new curricular arrangements for the first two years. He was distressed, however, that no significant changes had been made for the two clinical years. Junior students learned in outpatient clinics and senior students learned on the wards. He believed that junior students were not prepared to handle outpatients and that the current arrangements needed to be reversed. Charles Stone thought that senior students who had already learned some clinical medicine from work on the wards would be able to perform more acceptably in outpatient clinics. After Carter returned as dean in 1935 he argued strongly for a revision of the clinical curriculum.[19]

Now including Donald Duncan, Wendell "Mickey Mouse" Gingrich, Robert Moore, G. W. N. Eggers, and Titus Harris, among others, the faculty made these changes during the second semester of the 1936–1937 academic year.[20] They eliminated 315 didactic hours from the two clinical years and added two courses to the second year (30 hours of radiology and 15 hours of physical diagnosis). They increased the total time allotted for clinical clerkships and outpatient work by approximately 375 hours, assigning juniors to the hospital wards and seniors to the outpatient clinics. They permitted Wednesday afternoons to remain available for electives. The first full year of the new curriculum was the 1937–1938 academic year.[21]

Nationally, these changes in UTMB's curriculum were similar to those at other schools where an increasing number of part-time clinical faculty in the growing specialties influenced curricular decisions because they attracted paying patients to the teaching hospitals. Even after these revisions at UTMB, the total hours in the school's curriculum (4,565) was still above that recommended by the AAMC. The professors believed that broad-shouldered Texans, like the eighty-five students graduating at the

City Auditorium in 1941, could meet these higher expectations. After fifty commencement ceremonies, the School of Medicine had produced 2,245 doctors.[22]

The advent of World War II prompted certain compromises in both admission and curricular policies. In adapting to the demand for civilian and military physicians, the faculty admitted students after only two years of pre-medical studies. They also shortened the total number of months for the curriculum and they admitted two classes each year. They began a four-quarter system of instruction in June 1941. New students were admitted in the spring and in the fall and they could graduate after three years of study.[23]

Faced with the burdensome administrative details associated with the admissions, courses, and commencements of this accelerated curriculum, Leake appointed D. Bailey Calvin (professor of biochemistry) as UTMB's first associate dean of students in 1942. Calvin was associate dean between 1942 and 1945; then dean of students and curricular affairs between 1945 and 1958.[24]

Leake also wanted more teachers to help with the expanded teaching and he wanted teachers who were experimental scientists. He hired Raymond Blount, George Emerson, Chester Frazier, Arild Hansen, Eric Ogden, and Charles Pomerat—all before the end of 1943.[25]

Some taught in the east lecture room of Old Red, a building that "loomed above the white oleanders at its base, nicely framed in the neat shade trees along the sidewalk in front." Physiology labs were located on its first floor, microbiology on the second floor, and biochemistry on the top floor. The pharmacology lab was still in a separate building, and anatomy and pathology were located in the Keiller Building. Classes were usually "mandatory lectures" in rooms that were not air-conditioned. "Frequently the lecturer was just dripping when the hour was ended, and we'd sometimes have five or six hours of lecture in a row," reported Bill Daeschner, who began his studies in 1942.[26] Junior and senior students learned clinical medicine in the wards and clinics of the John Sealy Hospital, the Woman's Hospital, the Outpatient Building, the Children's Hospital, the Negro Hospital, and the Psychopathic Hospital (until it closed in 1943 because of hurricane damage).

By 1945 the faculty included 126 persons: 35 professors, 28 associate professors, 33 assistant professors, and 30 instructors. They were organized into seventeen departments; the sixteen in place during the 1930s plus the Department of Anesthesiology, which was established in 1942.[27] Department chairs or their designated colleagues coordinated the lecture and lab courses, and the clinical rotations. Every medical student knew all of the major professors.[28] An "extended family" spirit pervaded the learning environment, though it was unlikely that a graduate could name or recognize all of the persons who had been "teachers" at every stage of the curricular process.

The U.S. Navy and Army became part of this "family" as Leake and Calvin negotiated contracts for training navy and army physicians. In the fall of 1944, for example, there were 391 medical students, including 52 civilian students (3 women), 198 army students, and 141 navy students. In early June 1945, 108 students received M.D. degrees, the largest group in the school's history. The last class (twenty-seven navy students, twenty-eight army students, and forty-six civilians) in the accelerated curriculum entered in September 1945.[29] The accelerated curriculum saved a year in preparation, but it was a stressful experience for both students and teachers.

In the fall of 1946 the faculty returned to a four-year curriculum of approximately ten months each year. About 1,223 hours of instruction occurred in each of the two "basic science" years; about 1,200 in each of the two "clinical" years. During the first two years, students learned embryology, histology, gross anatomy, neuroanatomy, biochemistry, physiology, preventive medicine and public health, bacteriology, pathology and clinical pathology, pharmacology, psychobiology and psychopathology, physical diagnosis, and history of medicine. During the last two years, students learned the skills of diagnosis and treatment from the professors, interns, and residents who attended the inpatients and outpatients. More instructional time was allotted to the five major departments (Obstetrics and Gynecology, Pediatrics, Medicine, Surgery, Neuropsychiatry), but all students were introduced to each clinical specialty.[30]

During the 1940s first-year students were told of their failures by public notification. A dismissal notice was delivered to hapless students during the time of the anatomy dissection lab. As an upper classmen stated in 1946, success in medical school was "not a matter of brilliance but a problem of adaptability." A freshman in 1949, Bob Franklin commented that medical school "would work out all right if you didn't have to sleep." The attrition rate did decline during this decade, ranging between 8.6 percent and 19 percent for the years between 1946 and 1949.[31]

After World War II ended, there was a dramatic increase in applicants, many of them war veterans. The total more than doubled between 1940 (325) and 1948 (720). Because there were so many applicants, the faculty encouraged veterans to obtain baccalaureate degrees before applying.[32]

The qualifications of all applicants improved significantly.[33] In 1948 there were 525 applicants with college grade averages of 82.5 percent or higher; 108 were accepted. The remaining 417 had higher averages than the lowest average of a student accepted in 1945. They were qualified to study medicine, but the school had neither the facilities nor the personnel to accommodate such a large number of students. The professors decided that they would usually accept only students with a baccalaureate degree beginning with the class starting in 1952. In 1949 the faculty admitted 162 students (from 740 applicants)—the largest first-year class of any American medical school—and the first class to have a black male student, Herman Barnett.[34]

During the 1950s the number of applicants to American medical schools declined, but the number of applicants with baccalaureate degrees increased. In 1954 Mae Francis McMillan, a graduate of Wiley College in Marshall, became the first black female medical student at UTMB. Although the faculty "required" a baccalaureate degree for admission, they did admit a few students who did not have this degree.[35] During the early 1960s the faculty also admitted more non-residents and some matriculates had post-baccalaureate degrees.[36] Overall, the educational preparation of matriculates was better than ever.

Decisions by state and federal governments affected admissions. The Fifty-sixth Texas Legislature (1959) rejected a request to limit class size to 100 students and the Fifty-seventh Legislature (1961) expected UTMB to admit 160 first-year students. New federal legislation in the early 1960s provided funds to construct buildings in medical schools. To secure funds for these buildings, schools were expected to increase the size of entering classes and develop new facilities for research.[37]

During the 1950s, increased federal support for medical research prompted the professors to place more emphasis on research opportunities in the curriculum. They experimented with small group teaching and individualized laboratory instruction. They decreased the number of lectures, increased the amount of bedside instruction, and began a preceptor program.

In 1952 they inaugurated the preceptor program with the Texas Academy of General Practice. Seventy members of the academy were preceptors for students during ten-week periods. The students resided in the preceptor's home and the preceptor paid the student $25 a month plus the costs of travel, room and board, and laundry. By October 1954, 270 seniors participated; more than 200 with physicians in towns of less than ten thousand people. These experiences were ways for students to learn about the private practice of medicine, the routines of office practice, the importance of personal relationships in a local community, and the types of diseases and injuries experienced by patients outside of Galveston.[38]

The School of Medicine curriculum was still tough. The total number of class hours during the 1950s still exceeded the maximum recommended by the AAMC and the AMA. One student thought that the school was "an efficient mill for gradegrinding quiz passers."[39] Faculty and students struggled with the heavy lecture schedule for juniors, the length of the preceptor periods for seniors, and inconsistencies in the approaches used for grading and evaluating students.

As the attrition rate continued to drop after 1950, student anxieties abated considerably, though not entirely. On the first day of classes in 1951, one teacher told Mary Ellen Haggard's class that a certain number of students in that lecture room would fail, a certain number would commit suicide, and some marriages would end in divorce.[40] The annual attrition rate typically ranged between 10 and 15 percent during the 1950s and early 1960s.

When Truslow became dean and CEO in 1956 there were more than two hundred professors. About 40 percent were full-time teachers; 40 percent were part-time; and 20 percent taught occasionally.[41] To comply with AAMC and AMA recommendations, the School of Medicine needed one hundred additional teachers because of the total number of enrolled students (604 students: 573 men, 31 women). In terms of enrolled students, the School of Medicine had become the third largest medical school in the United States.

In dealing with these circumstances, Truslow made important changes in the political networks. In 1958 he shifted Calvin to a research grants office and appointed two assistant deans: Kenneth Earle for the undergraduate programs and Stephen Lewis for graduate and postgraduate programs.[42] A year later Earle became dean of the School of Medicine and served in that role for three years (Appendix B).

Earle and several professors wanted a new curriculum. They were concerned about a decrease in the number of students applying to medical schools, a decrease in the grade point averages of these applicants, an increase in the number of medical students who left school before graduating, and an increase in the number of married students.

Another concern was the "macho" hangover that had continued from the rugged-individualist, general practitioner legacy of the earlier decades. First-year students in the class entering in 1957, for example, were subjected to three thirty-minute exams in basic science subjects every Saturday morning in the Old Red amphitheater. Every Friday night was a study night.[43] Anatomy and surgery continued to dominate the curriculum. The dissection lab was open every evening except Sunday and many students worked in that lab until late at night. Students would do well in anatomy on the National Board exams, but not well in other basic science subjects. The faculty wanted a new curriculum that would correct such imbalances.[44]

The curriculum committee (chaired by Mason Guest) developed a proposal for a new curriculum. On March 30, 1960, the faculty, by a vote of 66 to 45, adopted this proposal. The new curriculum encompassed nineteen consecutive terms of ten weeks each, arranged into three years of five ten-week terms each year and one year of four ten-week terms. As before, the first two years mostly included the basic science courses taught by faculty in the school's seven basic science departments (Anatomy; Biochemistry and Nutrition; Microbiology; Pathology; Pharmacology and Toxicology; Physiology; and Preventive Medicine and Public Health).[45] The third year involved ward and clinic rotations with professors and house staff in the eight clinical departments (Anesthesiology; Dermatology; Internal Medicine; Neurology and Psychiatry; Obstetrics and Gynecology; Pediatrics; Radiology; and Surgery).[46]

Students in good standing could complete all formal instruction for the degree in fourteen consecutive terms instead of the previous nineteen. Those who preferred a four-year program could design a fourth year of electives that could include departmental courses, clinical clerkships, preceptorships, and sponsored research. The new curriculum was designed to permit qualified students to graduate within three years and to support those who wanted the more traditional four years. Both schedules permitted electives.[47]

First-, second-, and third-year students began the new curriculum in the fall of 1960. In 1961 seniors participated in the new curriculum. By the summer of 1961, 25 students were enrolled in the three-year program; 106 seniors were taking electives; and 80 medical students were doing research.[48]

Many seniors enjoyed the preceptor program. In 1962, for example, 80 percent of the senior class participated. In a West Texas city with two hospitals (one hundred beds and thirty-five beds), Don Gates worked with a general practitioner who was a partner with three other doctors serving the smaller hospital. Gates lived in a room of the hospital near its emergency room. He attended many emergency cases, assisted

TABLE 6.1: TOTAL NUMBER OF APPLICANTS FOR FIRST-YEAR SCHOOL
OF MEDICINE CLASSES, FY1979–FY1991

Years	In State	Out of State	Total
1978–79	1,660	422	2,082
1979–80	1,732	391	2,123
1980–81	1,669	469	2,138
1981–82	1,699	430	2,129
1982–83	1,716	547	2,263
1983–84	1,852	739	2,591
1984–85	1,863	728	2,591
1985–86	1,767	678	2,445
1986–87	1,766	868	2,634
1987–88	1,584	426	2,010
1988–89	NA	NA	NA
1989–90	1,631	357	1,988
1990–91	1,630	442	2,072

with fourteen deliveries and forty-four surgical operations, and participated in the care of children and adults hospitalized with various diseases and injuries. By 1962 the Texas Academy of General Practice had provided preceptors for 1,427 students. By the end of UTMB's seventy-fifth academic year (1965–1966), the School of Medicine had graduated 5,132 doctors.[49]

Pivotal economic and political events set the stage for major changes during Blocker's tenure as CEO. The windfall of more state and federal dollars permitted department chairs to add sixteen new faculty members in the fall of 1964. Two years later the school employed about 190 full-time faculty members.[50] In 1968 Blocker invited Joe White to become UTMB's first vice president for academic affairs and first full-time dean of the medical school. Blocker, White, and department chairs recruited many new teachers, adding fifty-six between April and October 1969, for example.[51]

White and the new teachers wanted another revision of the curriculum. In the fall of 1969 White appointed five committees to design a new curriculum. Barbara Bowman was chair of the Basic Science Core Committee. Other committees included Behavioral Sciences, with Harold Goolishian as chair; Introduction to Clinical Medicine, with Jim Guckian as chair; Clinical Science Core, with Bill McGanity as chair; and the Track Program, with Bill Levin as chair. The faculty accepted many changes these committees proposed.[52]

These changes began in the fall of 1970. Entering students experienced four fifteen-week periods of courses constituting the basic science core. In addition to courses in anatomy, biochemistry, physiology, microbiology, pathology, and pharmacology, students

TABLE 6.2: RESIDENT STATUS, SCHOOL OF MEDICINE STUDENTS,
FY1977–FY1991

Years	All Classes			First-Year Class		
	Texas	Other	Total	Texas	Other	Total
1976–77	747	28	775	189	14	203
1977–78	774	21	795	197	6	203
1978–79	769	28	797	196	7	203
1979–80	757	39	796	184	19	203
1980–81	767	37	804	194	9	203
1981–82	750	51	801	185	18	203
1982–83	742	50	792	183	20	203
1983–84	733	62	795	185	18	203
1984–85	744	45	789	188	15	203
1985–86	757	34	791	195	8	203
1986–87	744	38	782	197	6	203
1987–88	751	35	786	191	12	203
1988–89	724	31	755	180	1	181
1989–90	740	32	772	193	7	200
1990–91	747	21	768	198	2	200

took multidisciplinary courses in cell biology, endocrinology, and neurosciences. They also experienced required courses in medical ethics and medical jurisprudence, and another titled "Introduction to Patient Evaluation," which included the behavioral sciences and techniques for interviewing patients.

A ten-week introduction to clinical medicine course, which included instruction in performing physical examinations, bridged the basic science core and the clinical science core. The latter was a forty-eight-week rotation among the various clinical specialties. During their final year of training, students entered one of three tracks: medical-surgical specialties, family practice, or academic medicine-medical research. Students could include electives within each track, especially if they chose a four-year course. Outstanding students could graduate in three years. With fewer lectures, the new curriculum encouraged integrative learning.[53]

Admission policies and practices also changed during these years. The size of the entering class increased from 160 to 203 because of federal funding policies that connected dollars for construction projects with an increase in the number of students. The number of applicants increased significantly (from 670 in 1965 to 2,378 in 1975, for example).[54] By the late 1970s the annual number of applicants usually exceeded two thousand students (Table 6.1) and at least 90 percent of the matriculates were

TABLE 6.3: ETHNIC ORIGINS, SCHOOL OF MEDICINE STUDENTS, FY1973–FY1991

Years	White		Hispanic		Asian		Black		Other		Total
	M	F	M	F	M	F	M	F	M	F	
1972–73	605	64	13	1	4	3	4	4	1	0	699
1973–74	634	86	10	2	3	2	9	4	2	0	752
1974–75	584	112	14	4	3	2	7	5	1	3	735
1975–76	587	133	13	6	7	4	6	6	3	1	766
1976–77	577	149	16	6	9	4	7	3	3	1	775
1977–78	565	160	18	7	17	6	9	5	7	1	795
1978–79	556	164	21	9	18	5	10	6	5	3	797
1979–80	536	161	36	9	17	2	12	10	7	6	796
1980–81	511	178	41	12	17	3	12	10	16	4	804
1981–82	507	176	40	16	17	4	10	11	15	5	801
1982–83	499	169	50	13	26	4	11	11	6	3	792
1983–84	484	181	39	24	34	9	12	11	3	0	797
1984–85	468	142	37	18	52	8	15	13	2	2	757
1985–86	449	172	44	14	54	17	17	15	3	3	788
1986–87	416	169	50	14	58	24	24	22	1	0	778
1987–88	405	154	50	24	73	33	21	20	2	4	786
1988–89	381	156	43	29	72	28	19	19	3	2	752
1989–90	391	144	41	29	74	30	19	22	1	0	751
1990–91	388	151	37	30	85	34	15	20	5	3	768

Texas residents (Table 6.2). The number of women and ethnic minority applicants markedly increased during the 1970s.[55] Forty-seven women, four Spanish-surnamed students, one black student, and six Asian students were among the 203 students selected for the class entering in 1975, for example. The number of these students significantly increased during the 1980s (Tables 6.3 and 6.4). During the 1970s, most of the applicants had baccalaureate or advanced degrees, though some had completed only three years of college study (Table 6.5). During the 1980s only a few students matriculated without baccalaureate degrees.[56]

Admission committees adopted rigorous procedures for screening, interviewing, and assessing prospective students during the 1980s. Though still not officially required, baccalaureate degrees were strongly recommended as most applicants had acquired these degrees. High grade point averages and good MCAT scores were very important because more qualified students were applying. Two faculty members interviewed most applicants, assessing maturity, motivation, and interpersonal skills. Of the 2,129

TABLE 6.4: SCHOOL OF MEDICINE STUDENTS IN ALL CLASSES,
FY1968–FY1991

Years	Male	Female	Total	Foreign Born
1967–68	556	48	604	6
1968–69	546	45	591	5
1969–70	552	54	606	5
1970–71	569	52	621	4
1971–72	600	54	654	6
1972–73	627	72	699	6
1973–74	658	94	752	2
1974–75	609	126	735	3
1975–76	614	151	765	5
1976–77	612	163	775	10
1977–78	616	179	795	3
1978–79	610	187	797	4
1979–80	608	188	796	0
1980–81	597	207	804	0
1981–82	589	212	801	0
1982–83	592	200	792	0
1983–84	572	225	797	0
1984–85	564	223	787	0
1985–86	570	221	791	0
1986–87	551	231	782	0
1987–88	551	235	786	0
1988–89	525	230	755	0
1989–90	529	227	756	0
1990–91	530	238	768	0

applicants for the class beginning in 1980, 949 (45 percent) were interviewed. By the late 1980s, the faculty found it more difficult to select students with outstanding academic qualifications because the pool of medical school applicants had steadily diminished during the decade.[57]

As the new curriculum evolved during the 1970s and 1980s, opportunities for innovation encouraged the faculty to develop interdisciplinary courses such as the integrated functional laboratory in physiology begun by Sam Kolmen and Dan Traber in 1971. Other innovations involved members of the Marine Biomedical Institute and the Institute for the Medical Humanities. The former led a major reform of the basic science

TABLE 6.5: EARNED DEGREES OF SCHOOL OF MEDICINE FIRST-YEAR CLASSES, FY1968–FY1991

Years	B.A./B.S.	M.A./M.S.	Ph.D.	Other	None	Total
1967–68	147	6	2	2	7	164
1968–69	124	5	4	1	29	163
1969–70	142	5	1	1	14	163
1970–71	147	4	1	0	21	173
1971–72	131	4	4	0	34	173
1972–73	145	14	11	0	32	202
1973–74	160	10	6	0	27	203
1974–75	179	4	2	0	18	203
1975–76	168	8	4	0	23	203
1976–77	169	17	10	0	17	213
1977–78	161	18	7	0	17	203
1978–79	169	13	10	0	11	203
1979–80	162	20	15	0	6	203
1980–81	172	8	14	0	9	203
1981–82	182	10	3	0	8	203
1982–83	175	15	5	1	7	203
1983–84	184	8	4	1	6	203
1984–85	174	20	3	0	6	203
1985–86	170	20	8	0	5	203
1986–87	176	17	4	0	6	203
1987–88	168	29	6	0	0	203
1988–89	167	10	5	0	0	182
1989–90	171	15	11	0	3	200
1990–91	185	6	2	4	0	200

courses and the latter taught new courses in medical history, medical ethics, and medical jurisprudence. During their elective year, seniors could choose training opportunities that were more socially and clinically diverse. Federal dollars from the Area Health Education Center program, for example, permitted some to take clerkships at hospitals in South and Central Texas. The Department of Family Medicine added a family medicine clerkship in the 1989–1990 academic year.[58]

Other noteworthy events affected curricular policies and practices during these years. White established an Office of Research in Medical Education.[59] Bryan and others created an academic reinforcement program. New chairs and new faculty made important

TABLE 6.6: SCHOOL OF MEDICINE STUDENTS WITHDRAWING OR DISMISSED, FY1975–FY1991

Years	1st Year		2nd & 3rd Year		4th Year		Total	
	M	F	M	F	M	F	M	F
1974–75	7	1	6	3	0	0	13	4
1975–76	3	2	3	2	0	0	6	4
1976–77	2	1	7	3	0	0	9	4
1977–78	2	2	2	0	0	0	4	2
1978–79	2	1	0	1	0	0	2	2
1979–80	3	2	4	1	0	0	7	3
1980–81	1	2	5	0	0	0	6	2
1981–82	5	1	1	3	1	0	7	4
1982–83	7	2	2	2	0	1	10	5
1983–84	2	1	4	3	0	0	6	4
1984–85	2	1	8	7	6	3	16	11
1985–86	4	1	7	5	1	1	12	7
1986–87	2	0	7	5	0	0	9	5
1987–88	2	5	1	1	0	0	3	6
1988–89	0	3	0	1	0	0	0	4
1989–90	3	4	1	0	0	0	4	4
1990–91	3	1	3	1	1	0	7	2
Totals	50	30	61	38	9	5	121	73

changes in departmental and interdepartmental courses.[60] The faculty adopted a student competency assessment exercise for seniors. Bryan appointed interdepartmental committees that evaluated students who had failed courses.[61]

In response to the new curriculum and the changes in the administrative services supporting the teaching enterprise, students improved their skills and test scores. In test scores on the National Boards, they moved from the bottom third to the middle third during fiscal year 1974. One year later, the students ranked eighth in the nation among all students who completed part I of these National Board exams.[62] Moreover, the annual attrition rate remained fairly steady, ranging from a low of four in each of two years (1978–1979 and 1988–1989) to a high of twenty-seven in the 1984–1985 year. Between 1966 and 1991, a total of 121 men and 73 women withdrew or were dismissed (Table 6.6).

Bryan and the faculty were generally satisfied with these circumstances. Between 1974 and 1978, the curriculum committee and its subcommittees reviewed and evaluated the

TABLE 6.7: SCHOOL OF MEDICINE GRADUATES, 1967–1991

Years	Total	Male	Female
1966–67	151	143	8
1967–68	139	132	7
1968–69	137	128	9
1969–70	149	137	12
1970–71	133	119	14
1971–72	148	139	9
1972–73	164	148	16
1973–74	193	183	10
1974–75	172	152	20
1975–76	187	160	27
1976–77	180	147	33
1977–78	202	156	46
1978–79	199	155	44
1979–80	193	160	33
1980–81	199	150	49
1981–82	192	133	59
1982–83	183	145	38
1983–84	195	146	49
1984–85	193	135	58
1985–86	190	143	47
1986–87	177	125	52
1987–88	195	139	56
1988–89	183	131	52
1989–90	195	138	57
1990–91	175	120	55
Totals	4,424	3,564	860

new curriculum. In 1978 the faculty adopted some changes that modified the length of certain courses and eliminated late afternoon lecture courses. But, basic patterns and sequences remained the same through the centennial year. During the last twenty-five years of UTMB's first century (1966–1991), the School of Medicine graduated 4,424 physicians: 3,564 men and 860 women (Table 6.7).[63]

To manage the ever-expanding faculty (from 347 full time in fiscal year 1977 to 477 full time in fiscal year 1991), the large number of medical students, changes in admission

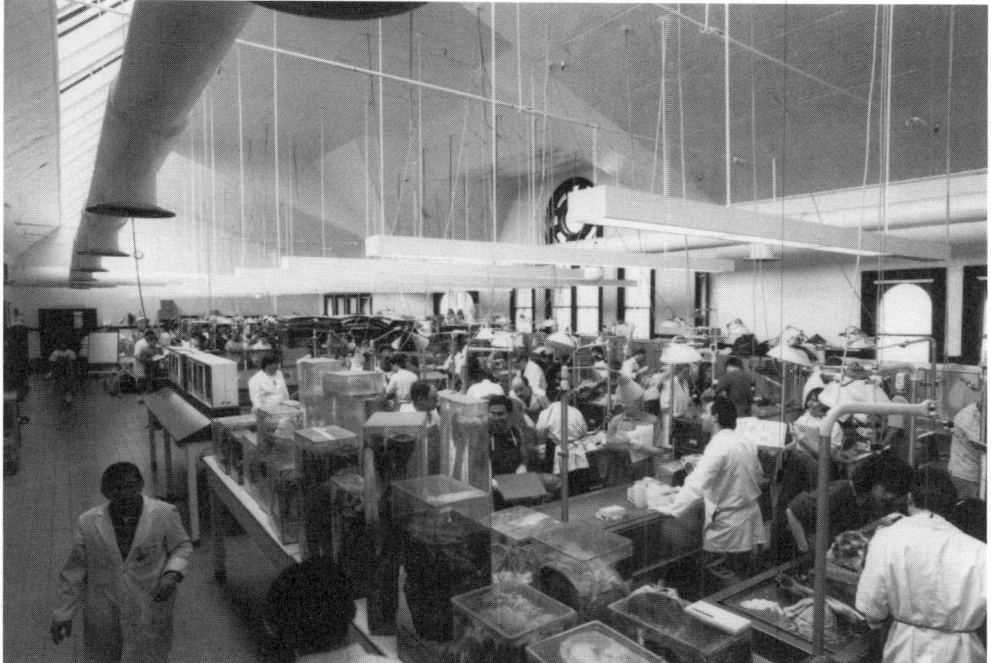

Prof. Gerald Callas, far left, teaching gross anatomy, fall 1990.

and curricular practices, and the new support services for students, an extensive administrative structure emerged for the medical school. Dean Bryan's executive team was fully operational by 1979. David Eiland worked closely with Gene Powell, director of admissions, and Patricia Blakeney, director of a counseling center for students and house staff. Spencer Thompson and Luisa Vaiani managed sponsored research. With their assistants, Julian Kitay managed undergraduate curricular affairs, Al LeBlanc coordinated graduate medical education (house staff training), and Bill Schottstaedt oversaw postgraduate (continuing) medical education. John Bruhn, Phil Rayford, Raymond Lewis, Michael Bowie, and Fernando Trevino gave special attention to recruiting and retaining minority students, as well as other health-related programs in Galveston. Charles Tandy managed the dean's office staff, ably assisted by Dan Oldani (information coordinator), Jean Neal (faculty records), Peggy Brenkus (fiscal services), Bettylu Fitzsimmons (special projects), and Liz Hermann (general administration). As individuals retired or resigned, Bryan appointed others, including Yvonne Russell (1982), Harvey Bunce (1984), Billy Ballard (1988), Judy Carrier (1990), and Walter Meyer (1991). Between 1976 and 1991, Bryan also appointed twenty-four professors as chairs of eighteen departments.[64]

These changes during the 1970s and 1980s caused a dramatic increase in the costs of medical education at UTMB. The expenses for maintaining the school's academic programs were slightly less than $30 million in fiscal year 1976, a sevenfold increase over fiscal year 1966. The expenses of salaries and staff support for maintaining these programs surpassed $60 million in fiscal year 1983, $100 million in fiscal year 1991.[65]

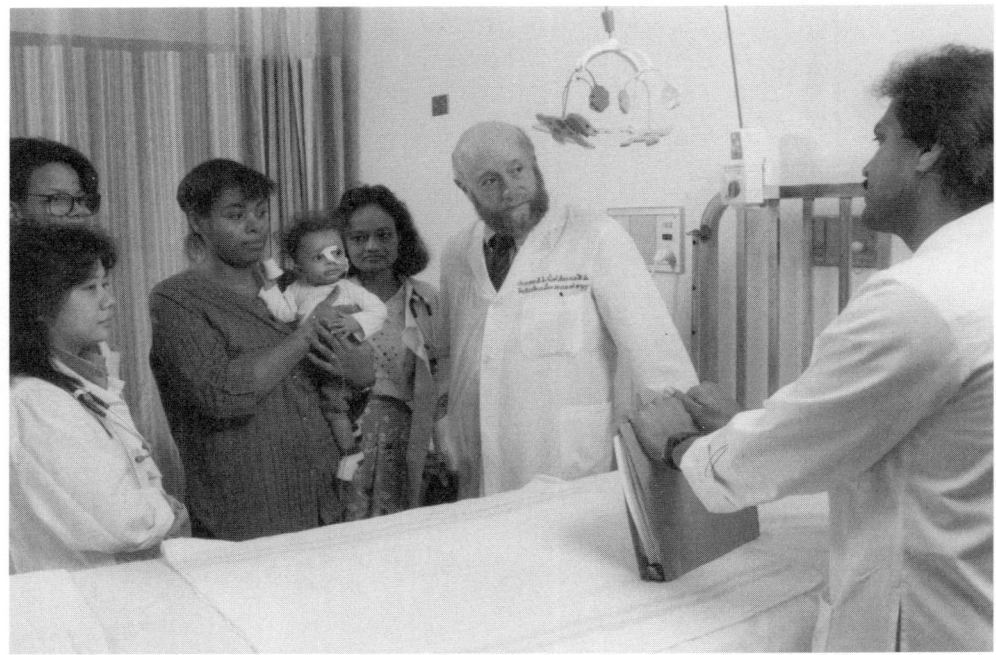

Dr. Armond Goldman during teaching rounds, Department of Pediatrics, 1991.

Some of these dollars were used for the salaries of administrative assistants and secretaries. Like those in the CEO and CBO offices, these personnel were extremely important in managing the daily functions of the offices of the deans and associate deans. Among others, these included Harriet Moody, Marjorie Watson, Joy Hasselmeier, Dorothy Hawkins, Camille King, Ann Kaiser, Pat Perez, Belinda Parker, Betty Ray, Brenda Esther, Bonnie Rhew, Lila Copado, Esther Koleng, Donna Polansky, Sharon Tipton, Patsy Tyler, Cindy Hoover, Shirley Arledge, Mary Jane Rogers, Roxanne Delaney, and Sue Bramel.[66]

Some of these secretaries, especially those in clinical departments, exercised very important roles in supporting the interns, residents, and clinical fellows who received additional training in medical specialties at UTMB. Some School of Medicine graduates became interns, residents, and clinical fellows in UTMB's hospitals. Others sought postgraduate training at other hospitals. Clinical professors selected house staff from among their own students, wrote letters of support for those who wanted to train elsewhere, and selected graduates from other schools who applied for positions at UTMB.

At the turn of the twentieth century, interns were recent graduates who wanted an additional year of clinical experience and training before beginning their private practices. Initially the Sealy Hospital boards awarded internships only to those seniors graduating from UTMB who had the highest general average in their final examinations. In 1900 Ella Devlin and Marie Charlotte Schaefer became the first women graduates who were interns at UTMB. Martha Wood was one of four in 1903–1904; Claudia Potter one of four in 1904–1905. The faculty annually supervised the work of four or

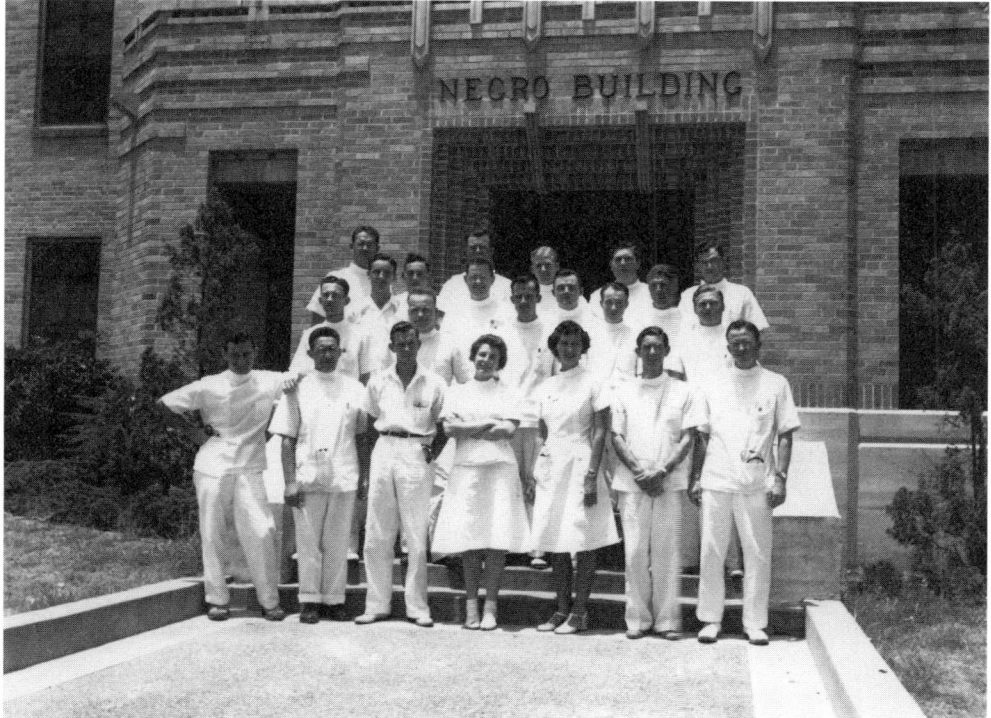

Interns, July 1944.

five interns until 1911, when the number increased to six.[67] As the number of patients increased, the hospital employed more interns: eight beginning in 1922; twelve in 1937. In July 1940, eight (including one woman) were UTMB graduates; the others came from the University of Michigan, the University of Wisconsin, the University of Kansas, and Harvard. The number of non-UTMB graduates continued to increase; for example, only ten of the twenty-five interns in 1950 were UTMB graduates.[68] Between 1891 and 1974, about 1,334 interns continued their training while serving patients in UTMB's hospitals.[69]

Residents were physicians who had completed an internship and who desired additional years of specialty training. Residents also trained interns and medical students, and their help with clinical care allowed the professors to attend a larger number of patients. Surgeons especially appreciated residents because they could handle many pre-operative, operative, and post-operative tasks. Nationally, residency programs steadily expanding during the 1920s and 1930s.[70]

In 1931 the Department of Surgery hired J. Peyton Barnes as the first resident at UTMB. John V. Sessums, another UTMB graduate, became a resident in the Department of Obstetrics and Gynecology that same year. For each year between 1932 and 1935, these two departments appointed a resident. In 1935 Hamilton Ford became an assistant professor in the Department of Neuropsychiatry after completing two years of training as a resident in the Galveston State Psychopathic Hospital. In

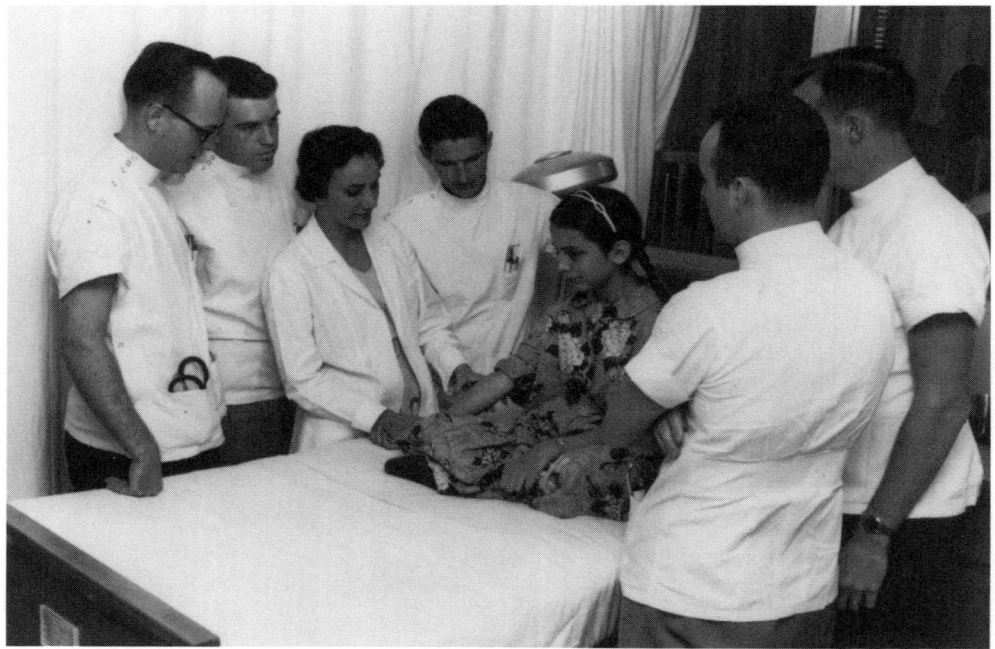

Dr. Nell Boelsche with students and house staff during rounds in the Children's Hospital, 1956.

1936 four clinical departments (Medicine, Neuropsychiatry, Obstetrics and Gynecology, and Surgery) appointed residents. These same departments appointed the following residents in 1937: Charles Mulherin (ob-gyn), Michael Shimkin (medicine), Charley Webb (surgery), and Martin Towler (neuropsychiatry).[71] The number of training programs and residents increased substantially during the 1940s. Eighteen residents were appointed in 1940; sixty-nine in 1946. There were eighty-three residents in fourteen programs by 1949 (Table 6.8).[72]

At mid-century, a shortage of physician graduates from American medical schools prompted hospitals to employ physician graduates from other countries. UTMB's clinical faculty began accepting these doctors for house staff training. Moore J. Yen began a residency in anesthesiology in 1950. In July 1953 the Leakes gave a party for interns and residents from the United States and twenty-two other countries. The house staff in July 1955 included thirty-one interns and fifty-one residents. The interns came from twenty-three states, the territory of Hawaii, Canada, England, Mexico, and Switzerland. Twenty-six residents came from China, Mexico, Japan, Cuba, El Salvador, Chile, Guatemala, Germany, Greece, Honduras, Peru, and Spain. A substantial number of residents at UTMB graduated from medical schools in other countries (Table 6.9).[73]

Similar to national circumstances at other teaching hospitals, the total number of house staff expanded significantly after 1960. As biomedical research expanded triumphantly, clinical specialization and subspecialization accelerated. UTMB's hospitals employed 35 interns and 59 residents in 1960; 37 interns and 214 residents in 1970; 352 residents in 1980; and 451 residents in 1990 (Table 6.9).[74]

TABLE 6.8: RESIDENCY TRAINING PROGRAMS, 1949

Specialty	Year Approved
Surgery	1932
Internal Medicine	1936
Obstetrics and Gynecology	1940
Anesthesiology	1943
Dermatology	1944
Pathology	1944
Pediatrics	1944
Otolaryngology	1945
Radiology	1945
Neuropsychiatry	1946
Urology	1947
Orthopedic Surgery	1947
Ophthalmology	1948
Plastic Surgery	1948

During the 1960s, some departments began hiring "clinical fellows," physicians who had completed their residency training programs and wanted additional years of sub-specialty training. Between 1966 and 1991, for example, the Department of Internal Medicine employed 297 clinical fellows and the Department of Pediatrics hired 102 clinical fellows.[75]

The total number of residents and clinical fellows who trained in the clinical departments varied by department and by year. Fifteen physicians completed training in the Department of Surgery during fiscal year 1961, for example. In 1960 Luther Travis was the first clinical fellow in the Department of Pediatrics. This department trained 320 residents between 1945 and 1991, and 108 fellows between 1962 and 1991. In the fall of 1971 Manon Brenner and David Simons (both UTMB graduates) became the first residents in Family Medicine. In July 1979, the Department of Internal Medicine began a new residency program in general internal medicine with Dan Allensworth as director. Altogether between 1891 and 1991, the clinical departments trained more than ten thousand residents and more than seven hundred clinical fellows (Table 6.9).[76]

Interns, residents, and clinical fellows often established close relationships with their mentors and attending professors. The daily tasks of caring for patients generated countless opportunities for the transfer of information and the practice of skills. At the time of the creation of the Blocker–Lewis Society in 1978, several residents wrote letters of gratitude to Blocker. For example, Tom Baker asserted: "There are not adequate adjectives to describe the gratitude that I have for the hundreds of hours of education

TABLE 6.9: RESIDENTS AND CLINICAL FELLOWS, 1968–1991

Years	Residents			Clinical Fellows
	U.S./Canada	FMG	Total	
1967–68	NA	NA	170	NA
1968–69	NA	NA	182	NA
1969–70	NA	NA	184	11
1970–71	NA	NA	214	16
1971–72	NA	NA	200	23
1972–73	NA	NA	210	32
1973–74	NA	NA	210	NA
1974–75	196	29	225	15
1975–76	232	36	268	20
1976–77	254	48	302	31
1977–78	250	42	292	15
1978–79	265	33	298	28
1979–80	294	29	323	29
1980–81	332	20	352	41
1981–82	324	33	357	34
1982–83	392	4	396	57
1983–84	357	55	412	49
1984–85	359	26	385	53
1985–86	342	35	377	43
1986–87	367	29	396	38
1987–88	346	34	380	38
1988–89	NA	NA	434	45
1989–90	NA	NA	435	46
1990–91	NA	NA	451	41

which you graciously gave to me during my tenure in Galveston. The Sunday morning rounds and conversation with you on a person to person basis gave all of us the stimulus we needed week to week to make our residency profitable." These and similar sentiments exemplified those of many other doctors who were residents in the specialty training programs at UTMB.[77]

Long before these training programs emerged, graduates from the School of Medicine and other schools displayed an intense interest in continuing their medical education. As ways to learn new scientific facts and clinical therapies, physicians read journals, attended meetings of professional societies, and enrolled in postgraduate courses offered by

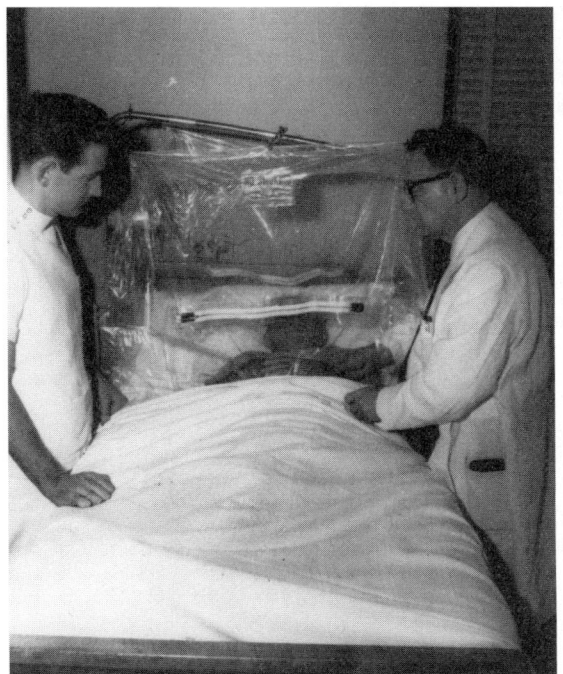

Raymond Gregory and a resident attending a patient in an oxygen tent, c. 1957.

medical school professors. UTMB's first postgraduate course occurred in May and June 1896, when Allen Smith taught a six-week course in clinical microscopy for practitioners. Twenty years later, in May 1916, the faculty staged a two-week course for doctors who served as state, county, and city health officers in Texas.[78]

A systematic approach to the continuing education needs of general practitioners began in the 1920s after Marvin Graves, Moise D. Levy, and William C. Rose recommended that the faculty offer annual postgraduate courses. About fifty physicians attended the first course in June 1922. The professors lengthened the course to two weeks and thirty-one doctors attended in June 1923. Thirty physicians attended in 1926; twenty in 1927. The faculty again taught these courses in 1928, 1929, and 1930, with thirty attending in 1930. None were taught again until June 1940, when twenty-two doctors attended the course in Galveston.[79]

These courses significantly expanded after Leake appointed George Decherd Jr. as director of the "postgraduate medical training program" in 1945. Blocker directed this program between 1946 and 1950. Decherd, Blocker, and faculty committees coordinated the courses offered by various clinical departments each year.[80]

These courses were designed especially for the large number of physicians leaving the armed forces and preparing for specialty board examinations. Expenses were minimal as faculty volunteered their time and attendees paid registration fees to cover the costs of teaching materials. Administrators and faculty also used these courses as opportunities to enhance UTMB's public image by inviting guest speakers from academic medical centers throughout the nation. Between 1945 and 1950 the professors offered several courses in pediatrics, surgery, internal medicine, physical medicine, cancer, obstetrics and gynecology, and psychiatry. Blocker estimated that about 2,500 physicians registered for these courses between 1946 and 1949.[81]

Ivan Bruce Jr. was the program's director between 1950 and 1956; Steve Lewis between 1956 and 1978. The courses in psychiatry, cancer, pediatrics, and ob-gyn continued during the 1950s. New courses in radiology, heart diseases, trauma surgery, electrocardiography, neurology and neurosurgery, dermatology, thoracic surgery, and medical therapy

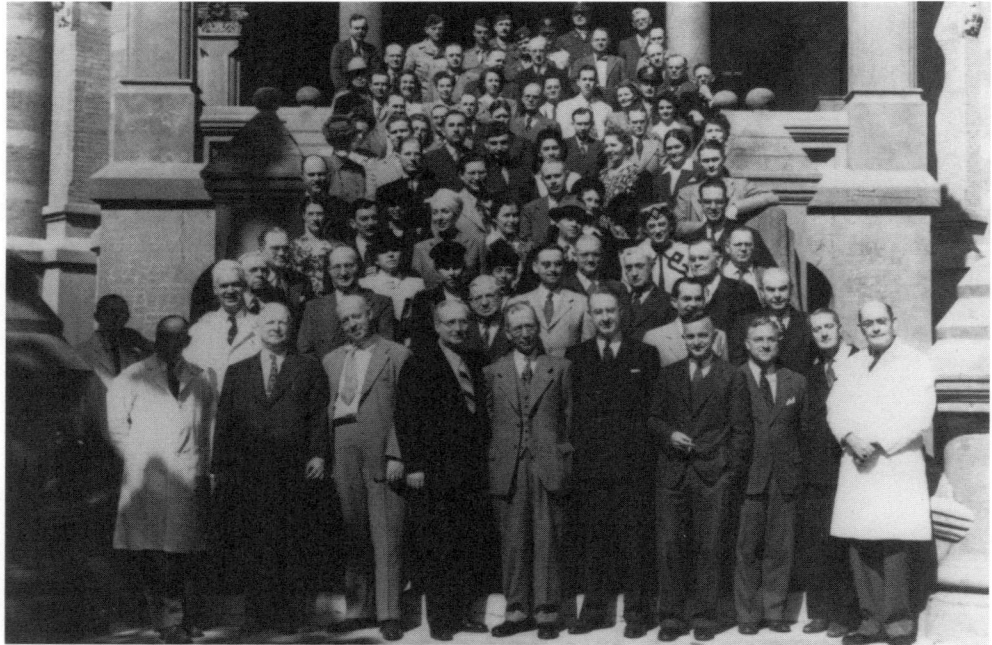

Pediatric postgraduate course, 1945.

appeared during this decade.[82] Some professors also participated in off-campus postgraduate courses.[83]

Continuing education courses in pediatrics and in obstetrics and gynecology continued during the 1960s. During this decade, the faculty also offered courses in neurology, anesthesiology, cardiovascular emergencies, and trauma. During the 1970s UTMB faculty organized between eight and ten continuing medical education (CME) programs each year, including a "Family Physician Review." About sixty of the one hundred participants in the six-day family practice review held in January 1970 planned to take the certification exam of the new American Board of Family Practice. The family practice course and the pediatrics course continued annually. Supported by UTMB's Area Health Education Center, professors participated in numerous CME programs for practitioners in South and Central Texas.[84]

In 1977, Bill Schottstaedt became UTMB's first Associate Dean for Continuing Medical Education, assuming responsibility for coordinating CME programs sponsored by the school's twenty departments as well as those offered by the Cancer Center and the two institutes. After a survey in February of that year, the AMA's Council on Medical Education granted UTMB a full four-year accreditation of its CME programs.[85] These programs expanded during the late 1970s and early 1980s. Between July 1981 and June 1982, for example, 1,727 physicians experienced a total of 337.5 hours of CME in sixty-two courses offered by the faculty. During fiscal year 1983, 2,659 physicians attended sixty-four CME programs.[86] These included conferences and seminars dealing with a wide range of topics in off-campus and on-campus settings, teaching rounds in various hospitals at UTMB and the community, and individualized programs that relied on self-instructional formats as well as direct clinical training. Marty Hotvedt managed UTMB's Academy of Continuing Medical Education, which offered individualized instruction tailored to specific needs. After Schottstaedt retired in 1985, Hotvedt became director of the CME programs. The Department of Ophthalmology held its twenty-third CME meeting in April 1989 and UTMB's twenty-fifth Family Practice Review occurred in April 1991.[87]

THE SCHOOL OF PHARMACY

As the twentieth century began, pharmacy students at UTMB received better pre-professional education. In 1902, for example, twenty of the forty-seven first-year students enrolled after passing exams given by the faculty. Eleven had taken college courses, ten were high school graduates, and six had teacher's certificates. R. R. D. Cline, professor of pharmacy, believed that these students performed better than ever before. Cline was delighted to have John Kemp as demonstrator.[88]

Forty-four juniors and eleven seniors enrolled for the school's fifteenth annual session in October 1908. Cline and John Buckner taught courses in botany and pharmacy; Arthur Austin and Walter Garbade taught chemistry; and Edward Randall taught the course about drugs in clinical practice.[89] These professors attracted more students. Between 1914 and 1919 they admitted 329 students, 280 men and 49 women.

As the School of Medicine faculty elevated admission requirements for medical students, however, educational gaps widened between matriculating pharmacy and medical students. The professors began teaching some separate courses for the pharmacy students. Beginning in 1909 James J. Terrill and Harry Knight taught a course in bacteriology for pharmacy students; William Carter and Oscar Plant taught one in physiology. In 1919 William Rose, Walter Garbade, and Meyer Bodansky began offering separate chemistry courses, which continued in the 1920s.[90]

By the fall of 1922 Henry Henze, Ava McAmis, Harry Little, and DeWitt Neighbors constituted a Department of Pharmaceutical Chemistry. Irma Smith (a one-person Department of Botany) assisted Cline in teaching pharmacy. The faculty required a high school education for admission and the curriculum included laboratory and lecture courses in botany, chemistry, bacteriology, drugs, and pharmacy. Henze and others lobbied for a third year in the pharmacy curriculum that would allow a student to earn the degree of Ph.C. (pharmaceutical chemist).[91]

By 1920, as many as ninety students crowded the unsatisfactory chemistry and pharmacy labs in the basement of Old Red. During that year the regents added a separate building for the chemistry labs, which did improve this situation, and the faculty limited the entering class to sixty students. Knowing that expansion of the school required new faculty and more space, Keiller lobbied for a separate building that would be a memorial to Cline, who died in 1924 after teaching at UTMB for almost thirty years.[92]

W. F. Gidley, Cline's successor, and W. R. Neville, Gidley's associate, wanted to expand the curriculum to three years to meet the standards of the American Conference of Pharmaceutical Faculties [renamed American Association of Colleges of Pharmacy (AAPC) in 1925]. The faculty and regents agreed to this change, with the first year beginning in 1925.[93]

Keiller wanted a faculty representative from the pharmacy school as a member of the Executive Committee and the faculty selected Gidley. In the fall of 1926 the regents named Gidley as dean of the school. He championed high standards and secured membership for the school in the AAPC. As mentioned in chapter two, Gidley and the faculty moved the expanding school to Austin in the summer of 1927. Between 1893 and 1926, the School of Pharmacy awarded Ph.G. degrees to 533 students.[94]

THE SCHOOL OF NURSING

In 1907 the faculty Committee on the Nursing School changed the diploma curriculum from two to three years (Appendices Q and AE). Superintendent Ethel Clay, J. F. Y. Paine, and J. E. Thompson arranged a sequence of lectures, demonstrations, and "ward-work" taught by Clay, sixteen School of Medicine professors, and the graduate nurses who were head nurses and supervisors on the wards.

Because the students were the hospital's nurses, they learned mostly at the bedside. During their first year they attended lectures on anatomy, physiology, drugs, nursing care of "medical cases," and the ethics of nursing. The second year included lectures on dietetics and the nursing care of children and adults (medical and surgical). During the third year students listened to lectures about obstetrics and gynecology; hygiene; nursing care of psychiatric patients and patients with diseases of the eyes, ears, nose, and throat; hospital administration; nursing ethics; and "massage and Swedish Movements." Of the four students who began this curriculum in 1907, Daisy Elizabeth Krebs was the only one who graduated.[95]

The hospital/nursing school environment was militaristic and exhausting. Students worked twelve-hour shifts that included time for lectures and meals. The director of the school dismissed students because they were "unfit for the work" or failed exams or did not follow the rules; a total of fifteen between 1909 and 1914. Others could not endure this environment. Eighteen left in the 1909–1910 year; twenty during the next four years.[96] Those who endured were thrilled with the new Rebecca Sealy Nurses' Home, which opened in 1915.

In 1915 Clay managed the school and worked with Clara Shackford, the hospital's superintendent, to determine staff assignments for the wards in the five buildings that housed about two hundred patients a day (John Sealy, Negro, Isolation Pavilion, Children's, Woman's). Using money donated by the Sealy family, the Board of Managers employed three graduate nurses: one for the "Main Building" and two for the Woman's Hospital (one for the operating room and one head nurse). In 1916 the board added three more graduate nurses: one for the "private operating room" in the Sealy Hospital; one for the Negro Hospital; and one for the Outpatient building.[97] Accountable to both the hospital director and the board, these graduate nurses provided practical instruction to the students.

Administrators experienced conflicts about the dual accountabilities.[98] In 1919 Clay resigned as director of the school and became hospital director for nine years (Appendix F). Martha Eakins and Ella Read, her successors as the school's directors, believed that graduate nurses should be "employed by and under the direction of the Director of Nurses," which would allow them to participate more fully and formally in directing and supervising "the work of the student nurses."[99] Read thought that there was a "distinct disadvantage" in expecting the "graduate charge nurses" to be accountable to the hospital director. "Only by placing them under the direction of the director of nurses can full cooperation be obtained," Read commented. This did not happen. "Charge nurses" continued to experience dual accountabilities—to both the director of the hospital and the director of nurses (who was also the director of the School of Nursing). Eakins and Read, however, were not solo director/teachers like their predecessors. Each had two graduate nurses as instructors/assistants (one full-time and one part-time), and the hospital's dietitian taught dietetics to the nursing students. Moreover, they were the first directors to receive academic titles of instructor in nursing.[100]

Applications for admission remained fairly steady. Between 1910 and 1914, for example, 166 women applied and 144 were accepted. Between 1914 and 1918, 296 students matriculated. In the summer of 1919, sixty-four students enrolled, but the school could have accommodated eighty. Even with a need for more students, the faculty elevated admission standards by requiring a high school diploma beginning with those entering in 1921. This did not reduce the number of matriculates. In the spring of 1923, eighty-five students enrolled. The School of Nursing was competing successfully with the other eighty-four nursing schools that functioned in Texas that year.[101]

As director of the School of Nursing between 1923 and 1926, Grace Grey orchestrated a major transformation in the curriculum. "Active duty" hours for day nurses were reduced from twelve to eight; for night nurses from twelve to ten. Grey added more classroom lectures, recitations, and quizzes. She and her assistants devoted more time to instruction on the wards. She added a lecture course in the history of nursing. She lobbied for more graduate nurse supervisors, who would oversee the care of ward patients and teach students. She told UT President Splawn that the "real crux of the matter is that we are advertising a University School of Nursing and we are not able to carry out our promises." After inspecting the School of Nursing in October 1925, a representative from the New York State Board of Nurse Examiners agreed with Grey. The School of Nursing failed the inspection, thereby losing considerable national prestige.[102]

When Splawn visited Galveston a year later, the school's new director, Sadie Hausmann, and her assistant for education, Zora McAnelly, escorted him on a tour of the hospitals and the Nurses' Home. Afterward Splawn agreed to provide funds for expanding the teaching staff. The school's faculty soon included Hausmann (the first director appointed with the rank of adjunct professor of nursing) and five other graduate nurses; thirteen School of Medicine professors as lecturers, and two Ball High School teachers who gave instruction in chemistry and nutrition.[103]

By 1928 the nursing students were experiencing a rigorous curriculum. It included extensive bedside practice plus 429 hours of classroom instruction during the first year (junior year), 208 during the second year (intermediate year), and 105 during the third year (senior year). By the fall of 1931 UTMB's hospitals employed sixteen graduate nurses, who worked with 134 student nurses.[104]

As a way of maintaining an adequate supply of nurses for these hospitals, the faculty usually admitted two classes each year (February and October). There were not always enough applicants, however, for two classes during the depression years of the 1930s. The school received 125 applications for sixty places in the fall of 1931, but the February 1935 class was not started because only a few students applied. Enrolled students also withdrew or failed; thirty-five in 1931 and thirty-one in 1932.[105]

Nevertheless, the faculty continued to elevate standards for admission. Beginning in 1934, they required a unit of chemistry or physics among the fifteen high school units and, beginning in 1935, they admitted only those who had ranked in the upper half of their graduating high school class. Of seventy-two applicants in October 1937, thirteen withdrew after acceptance and thirty enrolled.[106]

Dorothy Rogers was director between 1931 and 1935. She was the first nurse officially titled professor of nursing and director of the John Sealy College of Nursing. Her assistant, Dora Mathis, was director between 1935 and 1940. Rogers and Mathis were ecstatic about the beautiful Rebecca Sealy Nurses' Residence, which opened in 1932 with its red-tiled roof, red-and-brown-tiled foyer floor, carved walnut chairs and benches with leather backs, and a fireplace with a seal of the University of Texas carved into its stone mantel. In addition to bedrooms and bathrooms, the building contained a living room, library, reception room, auditorium, diet laboratory, classrooms, offices for teachers, a small infirmary, and patio gardens.[107]

By the fall of 1937 the regents provided the salaries of Mathis and six graduate nurses, who were viewed as full-time teachers, and the Hospital Board of Managers and the Sealy & Smith Foundation provided salaries for six other graduate nurses, who were supervisors in the various hospital departments. Because they did a lot of teaching, the regents appointed these supervisors as instructors.[108]

In addition to extensive clinical training in the six hospitals and the outpatient clinics, the students received 570 hours of classroom instruction during their first year in the following subjects: anatomy, physiology, bacteriology, chemistry, dietetics, drugs, ethics, personal hygiene, the principles of nursing, clinical pathology, surgical nursing, and medical nursing. The following subjects were taught in 210 hours of formal courses during the second year: history of nursing, obstetrics, pediatrics, communicable diseases, surgical nursing, psychology, survey of nursing, operating-room technique, and massage. The third year included seventy-five hours of classroom instruction in four courses: psychiatric nursing, public hygiene, professional problems, and sociology. For promotion and graduation, students were expected to pass all of these courses and perform satisfactorily in their practical work with patients. Graduating students received diplomas and they became registered nurses (R.N.) if they passed the state board exam.[109]

No major curricular changes occurred during the late 1930s and early 1940s, when the nursing school was a centerpiece in the dramas involving John Spies. As mentioned in chapter two, Mathis locked horns with Spies.[110] Like her predecessors, Mathis rode the seesaw of dual authorities governing the nurses. She was accountable to Spies for the students as pupils and to the director of the hospital for the students as bedside nurses. But, unlike his predecessors, Spies would not delegate authority and Mathis was accused of usurping his authority. Neither Spies nor Rainey were enthusiastic about Mathis's request that the nursing school participate in the accreditation program of the National League of Nursing Education. However, Spies and Rainey did persuade the regents to declare that the nursing school should be a "university" department and not just a "service agency for the hospital," thereby reinforcing the lines of accountability from Mathis to Spies to Rainey.[111]

Mathis resigned in 1940. Elsa Kibbe, then Anyce Wallace, directed the school through August 1942. At that time, UTMB employed 119 graduate nurses: 15 "instructors," 11 supervisors of hospital departments, 26 head nurses of inpatient units, 16 head nurses of outpatient units, and 51 staff nurses. The faculty formally responsible for teaching the 166 student nurses included everyone except the staff nurses, although this latter group continued to provide bedside instruction.[112]

In September 1942 Marjorie Bartholf assumed the three roles of professor of nursing, director of the School of Nursing, and director of nursing services for the hospitals. Bartholf believed that teaching hospitals associated with university schools of nursing should be able to provide patient care without using student nurses. However, a shortage of graduate nurses, wartime circumstances, inadequate living accommodations for students, and sparse funds made it impossible to employ all of the graduate nurses who were needed.[113]

Bartholf and her colleagues championed higher academic standards. They expected students to possess a better general education, to acquire a more extensive knowledge of the basic medical sciences and nursing theory, and to become proficient in nursing techniques. On the other hand, the increasing numbers of sick patients at UTMB led to a demand for more bedside care and a corresponding demand for more nurses who could provide this care. Many of the vicissitudes of the School of Nursing revolved around these issues of quality versus quantity. Bartholf and her nine colleagues (one associate professor, one assistant professor, and seven instructors) incorporated their ideals into new admission and curricular policies. They admitted only those students who had ranked in the upper third of their high school classes and who had maintained an average grade of C or higher in their college courses. This amounted to twenty-three students in October 1942, eighteen in March 1943, and thirty in June 1943.[114]

Bartholf and Leake transformed the traditional "Committee on Instruction" into a new committee that included two members of the nursing school faculty and two members of the medical school faculty. This committee assumed responsibility for the curriculum of the nursing school between 1943 and 1946. Three educational paths existed then: the diploma program, a B.S. in nursing degree program, and a B.S. in nursing education degree program (Appendix AE). The diploma program included thirty-six months of lecture and lab courses and extensive practice in the various wards (ob/gyn, pediatrics, medicine, surgery, psychiatry). Students who acquired a minimum of sixty-two hours in pre-professional courses taken in the College of Arts and Sciences at UT Austin before coming to Galveston could earn a Bachelor of Science in nursing degree. Designed to prepare graduate nurses for careers in teaching and administration, a Bachelor of Science in nursing education degree program was authorized at UT Austin in 1941.[115] In 1945 the regents transferred this program to the Department of Nursing Education in the School of Nursing at Galveston.

In 1946 the regents sanctioned the School of Nursing as an autonomous unit of the University of Texas and authorized Bartholf to manage all of the school's policies, including the curriculum. School of Medicine faculty no longer participated in the design and implementation of the school's curriculum. Bartholf also relinquished her role as Director of Nursing Services, delegating that job to Ethelyn Peterson (Appendix F). The School of Nursing faculty included Bartholf as the only professor, two associate professors, six assistant professors, and twenty-two instructors. To support the mission to transform the school into a true university school of nursing, the faculty discontinued the diploma program.[116] All students were required to complete two years of college before they could begin their nursing school studies.

With these changes in place, the Association of Collegiate Schools of Nursing admitted the school to membership in May 1948. By that year, 1,114 women had received diplomas from the school; six had received bachelor's degrees in nursing; and six had received bachelor's degrees in nursing education.[117] Bartholf's vision for the school had received national recognition. However, it was not possible to sustain this vision and provide the minimum number of bedside nurses needed at UTMB and elsewhere.

After baccalaureate degree students only were admitted in 1948, Bartholf reluctantly agreed to re-institute the diploma program in the summer of 1949. She was also willing to expand the baccalaureate program to include graduates of diploma programs.[118] Beginning in 1949 diploma graduates could choose a curricular sequence that led either to a B.S. in nursing degree or a B.S. in nursing education degree. UTMB's hospitals also began a six-month (soon twelve-month) training program for women who became "nurse technicians," later named vocational nurses.[119]

By 1955 the School of Nursing included twenty-four full-time teachers, fourteen part-time faculty, and sixteen hospital "supervisors." In various ways, they taught sixteen students in a one-year vocational nurse program, fifty-six diploma students, sixty-five baccalaureate degree students, forty-four master's degree students, and thirty to sixty undergraduate students who affiliated with UTMB for three to six months of training in psychiatric and pediatric nursing.[120] Supported by the Southern Regional Education Board, the W. K. Kellogg Foundation, and the Commonwealth Fund, the master's degree program began in 1952.[121]

To manage all of these programs, Bartholf relied on an assistant dean, four directors, and five departmental chairs by 1955; an assistant dean, one director, and six departmental chairs by 1962 (Appendix B).[122] She presided during weekly meetings of the school's Administrative Council, monthly meetings of the school's Executive Committee, and monthly meetings of the entire faculty. Faculty committees managed academic affairs.[123] By 1958 Brackenridge Hall housed offices for the faculty and dean as well as classrooms.

Bartholf steadfastly adhered to her mission. Between 1958 and 1962 the school ended its bachelor's degree program in nursing education, its diploma program, and its affiliated programs.[124] For the first time in the school's sixty-four-year history, all students in the 1961–1962 academic year were enrolled in the baccalaureate degree program. The number of first-year students in that program increased from thirty-seven in 1960 to seventy-nine in 1962. By the fall of 1962, 209 students had matriculated. Bartholf believed that the quality of the nursing students had improved "markedly." During her last year as dean, thirty-nine students graduated with bachelor's degrees and one student received a master's degree.[125]

Betty Rudnick, a graduate of the school who had served as Bartholf's associate dean, became dean in September 1963 (Appendix B). In 1964 the faculty included Rudnick as the only professor, nine associate professors, nine assistant professors, six instructors, five clinical assistants, and twelve staff nurses from the hospitals.[126]

In the spring of 1964 the baccalaureate students included fifty seniors and forty-four juniors. As a group, the seniors functioned in patient care areas about 840 hours per week; the juniors about 880 hours per week. Supervised by the faculty, the students learned nursing care approaches and techniques as they interacted directly with patients. Hospital supervisors, head nurses, and other staff nurses cooperated with teachers and students as these instructional rituals occurred. [127]

Administrators, physicians, and some nurses were still distressed about the shortage of bedside nurses. In 1964 Blocker asked Rudnick for suggestions about reorganizing the hospital's nursing service. In her twenty-six-page response, Rudnick emphasized that the School of Nursing was not responsible for graduating nurses to staff UTMB's hospitals. Rudnick pleaded for an organizational arrangement that would give the director of nursing political equality with associate or assistant directors of the hospital. She recommended regular meetings between the director of nursing, hospital administrators, and staff physicians; the placement of all registered nurses in patient care areas within networks of accountability to the director of nursing; the assignment of institutional responsibilities about food, drugs, linens, and supplies to persons other than nurses during the 3-to-11 and 11-to-7 shifts; the employment of a full-time director of programs of inservice education for nurses; and the employment of full-time teachers for the vocational nurse training program. She did not expect anyone to pay any attention to her recommendations. Even if they did, she was "pessimistic about the ability of the present General Director of Hospitals [Bobbitt] to effect and maintain effective communication with any qualified director of nursing service."[128]

Rudnick adamantly opposed Bobbitt's efforts to start the diploma program again. She also became embroiled in controversy with Blocker, believing that he was a "firm and consistent enemy of collegiate preparation for nurses." She thought that Bobbitt, Blocker, and others posed a "clear and present threat to the educational integrity of programs in nursing at the University of Texas."[129] To maintain their integrity, Rudnick urged Harry Ransom to consolidate all of the nursing programs on the UT Austin campus. She recommended that the master's degree program be consolidated on the UT Austin campus. Blocker was willing to allow this, though he was quite uncomfortable with the idea of moving both undergraduate and graduate programs to Austin.[130]

Prompted by authentic urges to improve the professional status of the nursing profession, Rudnick's rhetoric portrayed diploma schools as sources of "half-trained, inadequate and incompetent help to a hospital."[131] Her own school, however, had graduated forty-two more diploma nurses than baccalaureate nurses between 1947 and 1957. The number of baccalaureate students had increased after the last diploma student graduated in 1960. In 1965, for example, 270 students were enrolled in the baccalaureate program. However, the university only awarded fifty bachelor's degrees and three master's degrees in 1966, a number insufficient to meet the demand.[132]

By 1966 the school's faculty included twenty-five full-time and two part-time members, as well as seven clinical assistants. Eight of the faculty resided in Austin; the others lived in Galveston. The School of Nursing was the only accredited school in Texas that conducted a bachelor's degree program for high school graduates as well as graduates of diploma and associate degree programs, and a master's degree program.[133]

Intense conflicts persisted. In the summer of 1966 Marie Primm, assistant dean of the Nursing School, told Blocker: "I have yet to hear anyone, except you, on this campus say one good thing about this School of Nursing. It is extremely difficult to function effectively when you are constantly berated, derided, insulted, and criticized." Primm believed that the school was blamed for the shortage of nurses, incompetence among individual nurses, and the organizational inadequacies of the hospital's nursing service. Administrators made arbitrary decisions without consulting the nurses. This lack of mutual regard caused mistrust, conflict, and a demoralization that fed the gossip mills of national associations. Primm blamed those "outside of nursing" for the problems of the school and nursing service. "When will nurses be recognized as responsible individuals who know what they are doing and the direction nursing service and education should be taking?" she asked.[134]

Meanwhile, the nursing service in UTMB's hospitals experienced "crisis" strains during 1966 and 1967 as the new unit management structure spread throughout the wards. For a time, the hospital administration abolished the role of director of nursing services and attempted to decentralize nursing services by connecting them to the unit management system. Problems of communication, authority, responsibility, and accountability appeared everywhere. Some nurses wanted to develop a union that would negotiate with administrators about their grievances. Issues of competence and status triggered many complaints, as the shortage of registered nurses continued. Licensed vocational nurses and nursing students staffed many of the hospital's wards during the 3-to-11 and 11-to-7 shifts.[135]

These realities about nursing education and nursing services catalyzed decisions by the Texas Senate and the coordinating board. Both groups conducted studies of nursing education and the school itself conducted a self-study as part of the system-wide review of the UT health professional schools initiated by Ransom and coordinated by LeMaistre. The Senate committee concluded that UT was not graduating "its share of nurses for the State." In January 1967 the Coordinating Board recommended that the UT System create a unified administrative system for all of its nursing education programs. This system-wide nursing school would be accountable directly to UT's vice chancellor for health affairs, meaning that UTMB's administrators would no longer exercise political control over the local school. The school in Galveston and proposed schools in other cities would offer clinical education only. The graduate program would be moved from Galveston to Austin.[136]

In attempting to adapt to this situation, Blocker persuaded the regents to make the associate deans on local campuses responsible to the dean of nursing education in Austin via the heads of the local institutions. Thus, Rudnick would become accountable to Blocker, who would then report to the dean of nursing education in Austin. This was intolerable for Rudnick and her loyal faculty. During a meeting of the School of Nursing faculty in early February 1967, Blocker's fears led to public humiliation. Rudnick explained to Blocker: "Yesterday, in the presence of my faculty you told me twice that I could do things your way, or resign. Your way is wrong—dead wrong—and neither I nor any self-respecting professional nurse could degrade her professional philosophy by doing things your way." Rudnick, Primm, and ten other faculty members resigned in protest. Rudnick told regent chair Frank Erwin that their resignation was an "emphatic protest of the steadfast refusal of the University of Texas to recognize nursing as a profession or its school as a professional school."[137] The die was cast.

In April 1967 the regents established the UT School of Nursing (system-wide), with a dean accountable to the chancellor via the vice chancellor for health affairs. Marilyn Willman became acting dean and the new school became responsible for both baccalaureate and master's degree programs. Undergraduate students were assigned to Austin or Galveston for their two years of clinical training. Accountable to Willman, associate deans managed the clinical schools. The regents encouraged them to cooperate with the executive officers of each local institution, but no official lines of communication were established.[138] The system-wide school expanded rapidly; twenty-seven new faculty members in fiscal year 1969; twenty-four in fiscal year 1970. By 1972 there were six component schools (Austin, El Paso, Fort Worth, Galveston, Houston, and San Antonio), each with a dean accountable to President Marilyn Willman.[139]

In Galveston Dorothy Damewood was associate dean between 1968 and 1972, then dean between 1972 and 1985.[140] Faculty in Galveston participated in system-wide committees and local committees. They also met monthly as a group and attended quarterly meetings of the entire system-wide faculty.[141]

TABLE 6.10: ETHNIC ORIGINS, SCHOOL OF NURSING UNDERGRADUATES, FY1979–FY1991

Years	White		Black		Hispanic		Asian		Other		Foreign		Total
	M	F	M	F	M	F	M	F	M	F	M	F	
1978–79	15	216	3	15	3	10	0	4	0	2	0	4	272
1979–80	15	219	2	18	2	12	0	2	0	2	0	2	274
1980–81	13	286	1	22	2	16	1	1	0	1	0	1	344
1981–82	8	248	2	22	2	19	1	4	0	2	0	1	309
1982–83	17	265	2	28	2	19	0	1	0	2	0	2	338
1983–84	19	267	1	29	1	17	0	1	0	1	0	0	336
1984–85	22	259	1	24	0	18	0	3	0	1	0	0	328
1985–86	18	233	1	23	1	12	0	3	0	0	0	0	291
1986–87	11	256	2	29	1	17	0	10	1	0	0	0	327
1987–88	15	241	1	27	1	18	0	10	1	1	1	0	316
1988–89	15	198	3	40	2	12	1	14	1	2	0	0	288
1989–90	15	194	4	33	1	8	1	22	0	2	0	0	280
1990–91	20	240	7	39	3	13	0	18	0	1	0	2	343

A new system-wide curriculum for the baccalaureate program began in the fall of 1972. The faculty required sixty semester hours in general education and sixty semester hours in nursing. The curriculum encouraged students to view humans as bio-psycho-social-linguistic beings and to view "nursing process" as a total approach for organizing and providing nursing skills to patients and communities. Curricular experiences in clinical settings became more restricted and staff nurses in the hospitals did little teaching. The system-wide school continued its master's degree program and in 1974 initiated a doctor of philosophy in nursing degree program. Graduate courses were taught in Austin, Galveston, and San Antonio.[142]

In March 1976 the regents dissolved this system-wide arrangement and reorganized the nursing education programs into six separate schools, whose deans were accountable to the CEO of the nearest medical component. The bachelor's degree program was offered in all six schools. The master's degree program was available in all schools except Houston. Doctoral programs were offered in Austin and San Antonio. More than two hundred faculty members taught more than three thousand students then enrolled in these programs.[143]

The school in Galveston realigned itself as one of four schools at UTMB. In 1977 Damewood used three assistant deans, three director/coordinators, and two administrative assistants. Instead of departments and chairs, thirty-five faculty members (one professor, five associate professors, fourteen assistant professors, and fifteen instructors) accomplished their tasks with committees, seven in 1977, ten in 1981, and nine in 1984.[144] Chairs of these standing committees gave reports during monthly meetings of the entire faculty. By 1985 Damewood managed the school with one associate dean, one assistant dean, two directors, two coordinators, and two administrative assistants.[145] Cleo Bryant and others provided excellent administrative assistance.

The demand for graduate nurses was greater than ever during the 1970s and 1980s. Since the late 1960s UTMB alone had expanded its outpatient clinics and added or expanded six inpatient buildings. In adapting to these circumstances, the School of Nursing faculty offered four educational programs: the basic baccalaureate degree program, a flexible option (flex-op) baccalaureate degree program for registered nurses, the master's degree program, and continuing education programs.[146]

Graduation from the baccalaureate program required a minimum of four academic years (120 semester hours). Sixty semester hours of lower-division courses in the sciences and humanities could be completed at any accredited college or university. During two years in Galveston, students completed the program by taking required and elective upper-division courses in nursing. In the fall of 1976, 210 students (121 juniors and 89 seniors) enrolled in this program. Ninety-nine students graduated in 1978. The majority of School of Nursing graduates remained in Texas and practiced as staff nurses in hospitals.[147]

The number of male and ethnic minority students increased significantly during the 1980s. During the decade 1981–1991, 6 percent were male,; 10 percent were black, 5 percent were Hispanic, and 3 percent were Asian (Table 6.10).[148]

TABLE 6.11: RN–BSN FLEXIBLE-OPTION TRACK, SCHOOL OF NURSING, 1978–1991

Years	New Students	Withdrew	Graduated
1977–78	36	7	29
1978–79	44	12	32
1979–80	48	15	33
1980–81	59	30	29
1981–82	57	22	35
1982–83	54	22	32
1983–84	58	17	40
1984–85	54	21	33
1985–86	79	23	56
1986–87	85	22	63
1987–88	75	22	53
1988–89	77	19	58
1989–90	61	10	51
1990–91	66	17	49

In January 1977 the school reestablished a curricular program that allowed registered nurses to earn bachelor's degrees. This "flexible option track" began with nine nurses who were employed in Galveston. Initially directed by Donna Barlow, this program permitted students to design their learning modules and to schedule their written and clinical evaluations by the faculty. Students could maintain a regular work schedule and complete requirements for the baccalaureate degree. By the fall of 1981 ninety-six registered nurses were enrolled in the flex-op program. Aletta Linares became the program's director in 1987. By 1991, 593 students had graduated from this program (Table 6.11).[149]

When the school in Galveston reassumed authority for a Master of Science in Nursing degree program in 1977, there were nine full-time and fourteen part-time graduate students. This program prepared graduates to assume roles as teachers, administrators, clinical nurse specialists (child health or medical-surgical nursing), and nurse practitioners. A master's degree was also a prerequisite for admission to a doctoral program in nursing. Between 1978 and 1991, 1,055 students enrolled in this graduate program (Table 6.12).[150]

Continuing education had become a focus for the system-wide schools, especially after 1969, when Dorothy M. Blume became director of continuing education. In Galveston, Chloe Floyd directed continuing education programs for fourteen years (1971–1985). During the 1976–1977 academic year, for example, eight workshops were organized. During the 1981–1982 academic year, 438 nurses attended fourteen programs.[151]

TABLE 6.12: ETHNIC ORIGINS, SCHOOL OF NURSING GRADUATE STUDENTS, FY1979–FY1991

Years	White		Black		Hispanic		Asian		Other		Foreign		Total
	M	F	M	F	M	F	M	F	M	F	M	F	
1978–79	0	37	0	2	0	2	0	2	0	0	0	2	45
1979–80	0	33	0	1	0	2	0	1	0	0	0	0	37
1980–81	0	37	0	0	0	3	0	0	0	0	0	0	40
1981–82	2	45	1	2	0	1	0	1	0	1	0	0	53
1982–83	1	65	1	4	0	0	0	0	0	1	0	0	72
1983–84	2	72	0	5	0	3	0	0	0	0	0	0	82
1984–85	7	76	0	5	0	3	0	0	0	0	0	0	91
1985–86	8	98	1	4	0	2	0	2	0	0	0	0	115
1986–87	10	108	0	4	0	2	0	2	0	0	0	0	126
1987–88	6	99	0	4	0	3	0	1	0	0	0	0	113
1988–89	4	83	0	5	1	2	0	1	0	0	0	3	99
1989–90	3	64	0	6	0	3	0	2	0	0	0	3	81
1990–91	4	78	0	7	0	5	1	4	0	0	0	2	101

By the fall of 1982 fifty-three people were members of the school's faculty. Thirteen had earned doctoral degrees, forty had master's degrees, and fourteen had received tenure. There were 340 students enrolled in the baccalaureate program and 73 students in the master's program; 6 percent of the students were male and 15 percent were ethnic minority students.[152]

Damewood resigned in 1985 and Mary Fenton became dean *ad interim*, then dean in 1986. Fenton, her colleagues, and their students were thrilled with the new building that housed the School of Nursing and the School of Allied Health Sciences. Many of the 450 students (325 undergraduate; 125 graduate) and faculty (55 full-time; 34 clinical) helped with the move into this building during the summer of 1986. By 1988 the faculty included seven professors, eighteen associate professors, twenty-nine assistant professors, and two instructors. Thirty-nine registered nurses, who were members of the hospital's staff, had clinical or adjunct appointments.[153]

Fenton reshaped the administrative organization of the school, distributing responsibilities among two associate deans, four department chairs, and some coordinator/directors. Other managerial assistants were in place by 1991. Fenton held regular meetings (monthly or bimonthly as needed) with the administrative (later named executive) council. The faculty conducted its tasks with standing committees, task forces, and administrative councils and committees. In 1987–1988, for example, there were nine standing committees, three task forces, three councils, and five administrative committees.[154] Billie Karacostas and others provided outstanding administrative assistance.

During the 1980s the faculty made some minor changes in admission requirements, curricular courses, and graduation requirements for the baccalaureate and master's programs.[155] The faculty made some modest revisions of the curriculum, adding geriatrics, home health care, and health care economics in 1984.

During the late 1980s the school experienced unprecedented growth in international programs. Some nursing students studied in other countries. Terri Paschetag, a graduate nursing student, lived in a tent in Ethiopia for several weeks in 1985 as part of a team dealing with severely malnourished children. In the summer of 1988, thirty-four undergraduate nursing students participated for a week in the International Health Nursing class at the University of Nuevo Leon in Monterrey, Mexico.[156] Contractual agreements for exchanges of students and faculty were made with nursing schools in Bahrain, Barbados, Monterrey, Thailand, Brazil, and Colombia. The school was designated as a World Health Organization Center for Nursing Development, an integral component of the WHO Collaborating Center for International Health at UTMB.

The school conferred one hundred BSN degrees between 1989 and 1990. Enrollment in the generic undergraduate program increased by 45 percent and twenty-seven new students enrolled in the flex-op track. The faculty awarded twenty-three master's degrees. There was a 27 percent increase in graduate student enrollment (from 80 in 1989 to 101 in 1990). The school sponsored twenty-one continuing education programs between December 1, 1989, and November 30, 1990, including one international conference (with twenty-five countries represented) and two national conferences.

To improve collaboration with the hospital's nursing services, Fenton appointed clinical nursing faculty to standing committees of the school and initiated efforts to develop shared continuing education programs. Fenton served on the Hospital Nursing Advisory Committee of Directors of Nursing and the chair of this committee was a member of the school's Executive Council. How to establish and nurture mutually beneficial relationships between the nurses who taught students and the nurses who attended patients had persisted as a recurring challenge throughout the school's history. In recognition of her outstanding leadership, the regents named Fenton as the school's first Rebecca Sealy Centennial Chair in 1990.[157]

THE SCHOOL OF ALLIED HEALTH SCIENCES

The School of Allied Health Sciences began instruction in the fall of 1968, though some of its programs had existed at UTMB for more than twenty years. These programs had emerged nationally in response to technical improvements, clinical needs, occupational opportunities, and social stratifications.[158] By 1955 a variety of training programs existed within the network of hospital services at UTMB. These programs prepared laboratory technologists, physical therapists, radiology technicians, electroencephalographic (EEG) technicians, occupational therapists, medical record librarians, and blood bank technicians.

During the 1930s, Meyer Bodansky taught eight to fourteen student technologists each year in the hospital's clinical laboratory on the fourth floor of the Outpatient Building. These students enrolled in this one-year training program after completing two years of college. After Bodansky's death in 1941, Henry Sweets directed the course, which included 80 hours of lectures and 2,125 hours of lab instruction. Two years of college work were still required for admission. Twenty-four students received certificates in medical technology between 1953 and 1955.[159]

When the new Children's Hospital opened in 1937, G. W. N. Eggers, professor of orthopedic surgery, helped establish a physical therapy (PT) department whose members mostly attended children afflicted by poliomyelitis. Veterans from World War II needing rehabilitation significantly increased the demand for these therapists during the 1940s. Eggers and Billie Louise Crook, director of physical therapy, initiated the first training program for physical therapists in the Southwest in May 1943. Between 1944 and 1954 thirty-two women and twenty-one men received physical therapy certificates.[160]

Ruby Decker directed the physical therapy program between 1945 and 1963. In 1951 the regents approved a baccalaureate program that permitted students with three years of college to earn bachelor's degrees after completing a year of PT studies in Galveston. Thereafter, the hospital's physical therapists taught two groups of students: those seeking certificates and those seeking degrees. In 1954 Alma Alchier became the first student to receive a Bachelor of Science in physical therapy degree.[161]

A one-year training program for radiology technicians began in the 1940s. In 1952 the program was lengthened to two years. In 1953 Nell Recus (chief technician) and eight registered technicians taught eight students in the seven radiographic rooms of the hospitals. Between 1949 and 1955 thirty-eight students earned certificates in radiologic technology.[162]

Juaneva Novak became technical director of the EEG lab in 1943 and continued in that role for more than thirty years. With the support of Martin Towler, who became medical director of this lab in 1949, Novak began a six-month training program for EEG technicians. Five trainees earned certificates between 1952 and 1955.[163]

Occupational therapists (OT) supervised a few students who came to UTMB's hospitals from other training programs seeking "practical experience." In 1952 they submitted a proposal for a bachelor's degree program, but Chancellor James Hart rejected it because the state's appropriation bill prohibited new degree programs.[164]

Wanting to transform these hospital endeavors into more academically sophisticated programs, Chauncey Leake employed George Crosby as the director of a Division of Technical Training Curricula. Crosby began in September 1952, exercising managerial supervision of the following supervisors: Vernie Stembridge for clinical laboratory technology; Nell Redus for radiologic technology; Ruby Decker for physical therapy; Elyda Seeley for occupational therapy; and Mary Catherine Stubbs for medical record librarians. When this division was renamed as the Division of Medical Services Curricula, Stembridge was its assistant director.[165]

Crosby and Stembridge worked diligently to improve these programs. They believed that it was quite peculiar that UT and UTMB could not award bachelor's degrees in medical technology, for example. North Texas State College, Stephen F. Austin State College, and Texas Southern University awarded such degrees after their students completed three years of studies at each main campus and one year of practical training at UTMB. Plans for offering a UT/UTMB degree had been thwarted by a legislative prohibition against new degree programs. After this prohibition was lifted in the spring of 1955, the regents approved bachelor's degree programs in medical laboratory technology and occupational therapy. Leake and Crosby left UTMB, however, and these programs did not materialize under Truslow's aegis. Truslow did support the bachelor's degree program in physical therapy. Between 1955 and 1967 the hospital awarded certificates in physical therapy to twenty-one students and the university granted degrees to ninety-four physical therapy students.[166]

Existing certificate programs continued and new ones were added. Mary Catherine Stubbs established a training program for medical record librarians, beginning with six students who were admitted in 1954 after they had completed two years of college. Twenty-seven women received certificates in medical record library science between 1954 and 1959. In 1955 the hospital's occupational therapists began a certificate training program and three students earned certificates between 1957 and 1959. Between 1957 and 1967 thirty-four people earned certificates in EEG technology. Between 1956 and 1966 UTMB awarded certificates in radiologic technology to ninety-eight students. Between 1956 and 1967 eighty-three people received certificates in medical technology. As technical director of the blood bank, Jean

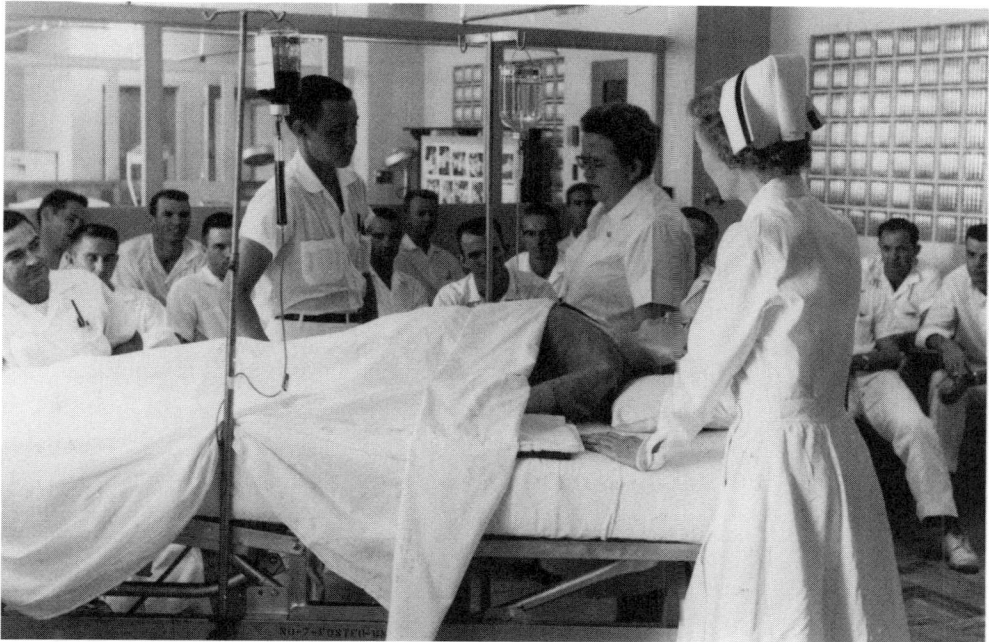

Jean Stubbins (with glasses) giving a demonstration to blood bank technician students, c. 1962.

Stubbins orchestrated a training program for technicians. Between 1962 and 1967 eleven people earned certificates in blood bank technology.[167]

When Blocker became CEO, UTMB supported seven certificate programs and one baccalaureate program (PT). The length of their curricula varied: EEG technology (six months); blood banking technology, medical laboratory technology, medical records library science, and physical therapy (one year); occupational therapy (eighteen months); and radiologic technology (two years). The certificate in physical therapy was the only certificate given to both degree and non-degree students. Blocker and others wanted a more substantial academic umbrella for these programs. In 1967 and 1968 the regents and the Texas Higher Education Coordinating Board approved the establishment of a School of Allied Health Sciences. This school would consolidate existing programs and provide an institutional structure for new programs. Radiologic technology would remain a certificate program. New baccalaureate programs in medical technology, medical records administration, and occupational therapy would join the existing baccalaureate program in physical therapy.[168]

Proud to be associated with the first school of its kind in Texas and the Southwest, the School of Allied Health Sciences faculty began classes with sixty-six students on September 3, 1968. Ave Maria Hall housed offices and classrooms until the new School of Nursing/School of Allied Health Sciences building opened in 1986. Robert Bing, who had directed occupational therapy since 1966 and served as coordinator of planning for the new school, became the first dean and James D. Spitler was assistant dean (Appendix B). Mary Frances Heermans (occupational therapy), Ruth Morris (medical technology), Sally Mount (medical record administration), and Jeanne Schenck (physical therapy) were chairs of the school's four departments (Appendix G). About forty people were faculty members between 1968 and 1971. Bing initially appointed five faculty committees: executive; student affairs; admissions; curricula; and continuing education. By 1983 the faculty used ten committees: admissions; appointment, promotion and tenure; bylaws; continuing education; curricula; faculty affairs; grading and promotion; nominations; research; and student affairs.[169]

The admissions committees devoted much time to the evaluation of applicants. Students who had completed three years of college (ninety semester hours including required courses) could be admitted to the bachelor's degree programs in medical record administration, medical technology, or physical therapy. Those who had completed two years of college (sixty semester hours including required courses) could be admitted to the bachelor's degree program in occupational therapy.[170] Qualified high school graduates were admitted to the two-year certificate program in radiologic technology.

The School of Allied Health Sciences was not an umbrella for all possible allied health careers, but it did add two new departments in 1971 that provided more flexibility and a greater range of choices for prospective students. James Cantwell was chair of the new Department of Associated Health Occupations. In association with Galveston College, this department organized a two-year curriculum that gave high school graduates opportunities to earn associate degrees and certificates as EEG or radiologic technologists, inhalation therapists, OT or PT assistants, hospital management assistants, or community health workers.[171]

Warren Dodge, professor of pediatrics, was chair of the new Department of Health Care Sciences, which developed a two-year curriculum for training physician's assistants. These students completed two years of studies in an accredited college before admission to the physician's assistant program. In 1973 five of the first six graduates of this program joined family practices in Texas and one became a School of Allied Health Sciences faculty member. By 1976 the department had trained sixty-five physician's assistants.[172]

Applications steadily increased. During 1972–1973, the fifth year of the school's existence, 136 students enrolled. By 1973 the School of Allied Health Sciences received about 350 applications and limited its enrollment to fifty new students each year. Between 1975 and 1981, the school's total enrollment ranged from a low of 299 (1977–1978) to 367 (1980–1981).[173]

Curricular committees coordinated the courses that were required for students in each program. Students in the radiologic technology program devoted two years to their studies. The occupational therapy program involved five and a half trimesters of required courses at UTMB and affiliated hospitals. Three trimesters of courses were required for the medical records administration program. The medical technology program involved six months of didactic instruction and six months of rotation through the various clinical laboratories in UTMB's hospitals. Physical therapy students experienced a sequence of three and a half trimesters of required courses and clinical training at UTMB and affiliated hospitals. Between 1972 and 1978 numerous students in SAHS programs

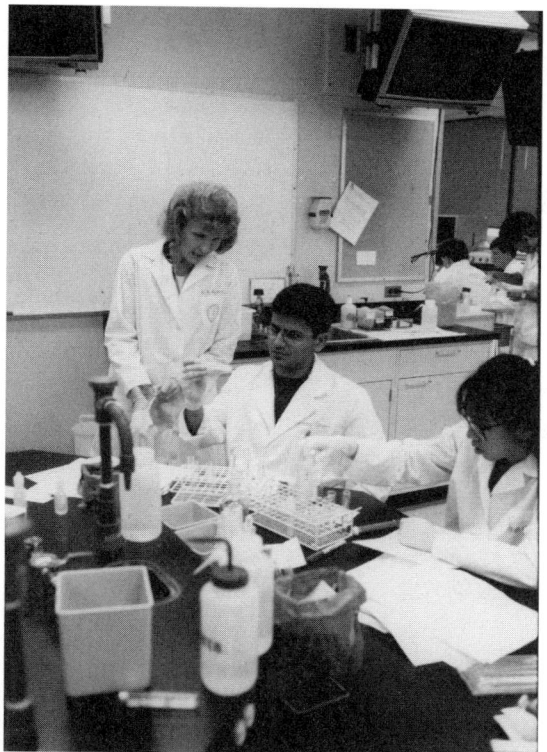

Shirley Richmond, chair, Department of Medical Technology, looking at turbidity reactions with students Anthony Campus and Thuy Vo, 1991.

experienced clinical training at hospitals in South and Central Texas associated with UTMB's Area Health Education Center. Those who successfully completed all courses participated in the school's commencement ceremonies, usually held in August. In 1976 the school graduated 171 students, the largest class to that date. By 1978, the school's tenth anniversary year, 918 students had graduated. Most of these graduates were employed in Texas and between 95 percent and 100 percent had obtained national certification or licensure.[174]

Bing used one associate dean, three assistant deans, one director, and seven departmental chairs in managing the school (Appendix B). Key administrative assistants included Ann Parsons, Pat McGraw, and Lucille Burnworth. After Bing resigned in 1980, John Bruhn was dean between 1980 and 1991. By 1984 Bruhn managed the school with four associate deans, six departmental chairs, one coordinator, and four directors. When Bruhn left in 1991 there were three associate deans, eight departmental chairs, and five directors.[175] Key administrative assistants included Ruth Apolinar, Alice Pineda, and Charles Hayden.

These leaders guided an ever-expanding group of teachers. In 1976 Diane Roberts became chair of the new Department of Allied Health Services, whose members assisted technically prepared students who wished to obtain a bachelor's degree after two additional years of full-time or seven years of part-time studies. In 1978, ten years after its establishment, the School of Allied Health Sciences faculty included fifty-six full-time, thirty-five part-time, and eighty-five adjunct teachers.[176]

By the early 1980s the faculty included about eighty members in Galveston, about one hundred clinical faculty in hospitals in Texas and the Southwest, and about twenty physicians in various Texas cities who were preceptors for the students in the physician's assistant program.[177] During the 1980s the faculty admitted an ethnically diverse group of students who enrolled in a variety of programs (Table 6.13).

The curricula of the departments were fairly standardized during these years. Students in the Department of Allied Health Services could choose to concentrate

TABLE 6.13: ETHNIC ORIGINS, SCHOOL OF ALLIED HEALTH SCIENCES BACCALAUREATE STUDENTS, FY1979–FY1991

Years	White		Black		Hispanic		Asian		Other		Foreign		Total
	M	F	M	F	M	F	M	F	M	F	M	F	
1978–79	44	167	2	8	11	15	0	2	0	1	3	1	254
1979–80	45	185	3	8	5	9	0	3	0	1	3	1	263
1980–81	48	185	4	12	7	13	0	3	0	2	2	1	277
1981–82	53	180	4	13	8	23	0	1	0	0	1	1	284
1982–83	55	174	4	31	7	27	2	5	1	0	0	0	306
1983–84	70	242	4	38	8	27	2	7	1	0	0	0	399
1984–85	69	223	6	18	9	17	1	8	0	0	0	0	351
1985–86	55	181	7	11	9	19	1	6	1	0	0	0	290
1986–87	53	175	3	9	12	23	5	6	1	0	0	0	287
1987–88	54	178	4	13	20	18	8	7	0	0	1	1	304
1988–89	69	192	8	17	31	41	6	14	0	0	2	0	380
1989–90	81	177	8	23	31	35	4	13	0	0	2	1	375
1990–91	81	212	8	24	26	29	4	5	0	0	0	0	389

TABLE 6.14: SCHOOL OF ALLIED HEALTH SCIENCES GRADUATES, 1968–1991

Year	Total Graduates	Year	Total Graduates
1968	23	1980	81
1969	31	1981	86
1970	32	1982	92
1971	48	1983	74
1972	46	1984	86
1973	69	1985	89
1974	82	1986	75
1975	91	1987	95
1976	96	1988	90
1977	90	1989	98
1978	99	1990	112
1979	128	1991	135

their studies in community health education, health care administration, teaching preparation, or research. The Department of Associated Health Occupations coordinated its work with faculty at Galveston College to prepare women and men to become community health workers, EEG technologists, respiratory therapists, occupational therapy assistants, or renal dialysis technologists. After completing the two-year program, students received associate of applied science degrees from Galveston College and certificates of proficiency in an area of specialization from the SAHS. This department also offered certificate programs for those who wanted to prepare for careers as a radiographer, surgical technologist, or unit clerk. In 1982 these two departments merged into a new Department of Health Related Studies led by David Cordova.[178]

The Department of Health Care Sciences offered almost twenty courses for training physician's assistants. These included basic science courses as well as rotations through the clinical specialties of internal medicine, family medicine, obstetrics and gynecology, pediatrics, and surgery.[179] The department was renamed Department of Physician's Assistant Studies when Richard Rahr became chair in 1983.

By the early 1980s the Department of Medical Record Administration trained information specialists. The department offered two educational paths: a five-semester series of courses for those who had completed sixty semester hours of college and a three-semester series of courses for those who already possessed a baccalaureate degree. Students who completed these paths were awarded B.S. degrees and certificates of proficiency in medical record administration.[180] This department was renamed the Department of Health Information Management when John Berkbuegler became chair in 1986.

The Department of Medical Technology offered fifteen courses that included instrumentation, biochemistry, microbiology, immunology, hematology, and clinical chemistry. Six additional courses were available for those who wanted a certificate of proficiency in cytotechnology.[181]

The Department of Occupational Therapy taught a dozen basic courses and the Department of Physical Therapy taught fifteen basic courses.[182]

Courses that addressed topics of common interest to all students, such as anatomy, physiology, and psychology, were organized into a Division of Interdisciplinary Studies in the early 1980s with Jim Spitler as director. Some courses taught in this division became the basis for a "Core Curriculum," which was adopted by the faculty in 1985. The core courses included communication skills, legal and ethical issues in health care, anatomy, physiology, pathology, management skills, and research.[183] This division was renamed the Department of Humanities and Basic Sciences in 1989.

During the late 1980s new courses were added in the Department of Health Information Management and the Department of Health Related Studies. The latter department established a Division of Radiologic Health Sciences that supported the preparation of a variety of radiographic technologists with specialized skills.[184] David Cordova reorganized the department's other programs into a Division of Health Care Administration and a Division of Respiratory Therapy.

In conjunction with the Graduate School of the Biomedical Sciences, the School of Allied Health Sciences began a master's degree program in 1987. By 1988 students could choose two areas of concentration: health education or clinical gerontology. David Chiriboga became chair of a Department of Graduate Studies, which was later renamed the Department of Health Promotion and Gerontology. Initially, seven faculty members offered a variety of required and elective courses.[185]

By UTMB's centennial year, approximately 130 people had faculty appointments in the School of Allied Health Sciences, with slightly more than one-third possessing doctorate degrees. These faculty taught in a variety of degree and certificate programs, which are summarized in Appendix AF. From its first graduation in 1969 thru 1991, 1,948 students had received degrees or certificates or both (Table 6.14).[186]

THE GRADUATE SCHOOL OF THE BIOMEDICAL SCIENCES

In 1913 William Rose became the first professor at UTMB who had earned a Ph.D. degree (Yale) in a biomedical science field. Rose taught biochemistry for seven years before asking UT President Robert Vinson to form a committee that would develop graduate courses in support of a master's degree program.[187] Meyer Bodansky, an instructor in biochemistry, wanted to earn this degree under Rose's tutelage.

Dean Carter supported this proposal because he knew that graduate students who served as assistants to the faculty could ease teaching burdens and increase research productivity. In 1921 the faculty negotiated an agreement with Henry W. Harper, dean of UT's Graduate School.[188] Students who did acceptable work in biomedical science courses taught in the medical school and prepared a thesis on a research problem in anatomy, histology, embryology, biochemistry, bacteriology, or physiology could earn master's degrees from UT Austin. Bodansky acquired his degree in 1922.

The number of faculty with doctoral degrees in the basic science departments increased significantly during the 1920s and 1930s. These teachers were as eager to prepare graduate students for careers in teaching and research as clinical faculty were eager to train new doctors. In 1925 the regents approved master's degrees for supervised work in five basic science departments at UTMB. By 1932 Byron Hendrix was the liaison between the UT Graduate School and the seven departments approved for graduate work (Anatomy, Histology and Embryology, Biochemistry, Pathological Chemistry, Physiology, Pharmacology, and Pathology).[189]

A student could earn a master's degree from UT after completing courses and conducting research in the lab facilities in Old Red, the Laboratory of Experimental Medicine, the Laboratory of Pharmacology and Physiology, the Laboratory of Clinical Pathology, or the Keiller Building. When A. P. Brogan became dean of UT's Graduate School in 1936, he appointed Hendrix, Wilfred Dawson, and George Herrmann as a faculty committee to oversee the work of these students. Fifteen students applied for admission in 1939, for example.[190] By 1941 at least ten had earned master's degrees. In 1942 Joe Dennis became the first student in Galveston to earn a Ph.D. degree after completing courses and conducting original research in biochemistry.[191]

Chauncey Leake enthusiastically supported the faculty who wanted to establish more formal structures for educating graduate students at UTMB. In August 1944 Brogan appointed six professors (Hendrix as chair, Eric Ogden, Charles Pomerat, D. Bailey Calvin, Raymond Gregory, and Arild Hansen) as a committee that would develop recommendations about these graduate degree programs. During the next three years, administrators and faculty developed a set of guidelines and agreed on a list of UTMB's professors who could direct Ph.D. work, but UT's central administration would not authorize formal programs at UTMB.[192]

Conflicts and frustrations impeded progress. Some UT Austin faculty thought that UTMB faculty would admit students who were unacceptable elsewhere just to get their program started and that some students would matriculate in a UTMB graduate program with the hope of eventually gaining entrance to the School of Medicine. President Painter was not convinced that graduate education was a proper function of an academic medical center. He believed that School of Medicine faculty who taught medical students and conducted acceptable research would have little time remaining for the training of Ph.D. scientists. Painter's resistance did not dampen the enthusiasm of UTMB's faculty, who knew that fifty of fifty-seven four-year university medical schools in the United States were offering graduate degree programs in the biomedical sciences by the late 1930s. They also knew that there was a national shortage of trained scientists who wanted to teach in medical schools and they believed that an active graduate program was the best way to recruit and keep good professors.[193]

In 1949 the Departments of Anatomy, Biochemistry, Microbiology, Physiology, and Pharmacology asked the UT central administration to authorize doctoral programs. In 1951 UT's Graduate Council decided to approve individual students who wanted to acquire Ph.D. degrees by studying with faculty in the Departments of Anatomy, Physiology, and Pharmacology. In 1952 this committee permitted these three departments to begin doctoral programs. In 1953 additional programs were authorized for the Departments of Biochemistry, Bacteriology, and Preventive Medicine and Public Health. Donald Duncan became the authorized liaison between the UT Graduate School and UTMB's professors.[194]

Duncan and Mason Guest traveled to Austin many times during the 1950s to represent students and faculty, and to plead for more support of the programs in Galveston. In November 1953 they became members of the Graduate Legislative Council, a group of administrators and elected faculty who determined policies for those in the UT System who taught and supervised graduate students.[195]

UTMB's professors became more aggressive in recruiting graduate students. Though there was not a regent-approved graduate school at UTMB, the catalog for 1953–1954 presented information about graduate studies under the heading, "The Graduate School at the Medical Branch." With professors teaching courses to graduate students and supervising theses and dissertations, a graduate school actually functioned, though without an official name or politically independent status. Nineteen students enrolled in the programs of four departments in the fall of 1954.[196] Between 1942 and 1957, at least thirty-six students earned master's degrees and at least fourteen students earned Ph.D. degrees. The number of graduate students steadily increased. In 1959 forty-nine students, including seven women, enrolled in these programs. By 1964 eighteen "Members" and seventeen "Associates" of the graduate faculty at UTMB supervised fifty matriculates.[197]

In February 1964 the regents adopted new policies for graduate education in the UT System. They designated the UT Graduate School as a system-wide organization of graduate faculty that included members, associates, and special members. Each component institution had a graduate school administrator. Donald Duncan was UTMB's associate dean for graduate studies. Responding to these developments, UTMB's professors adopted bylaws in December 1964, written as if they were policies for a Graduate School at UTMB, though such a school had still not been authorized. These bylaws honored the new system-wide policies. Students in Galveston could earn graduate degrees from six departments: Anatomy, Biochemistry, Physiology, Pharmacology, Microbiology, and Preventive Medicine and Community Health.[198]

Though political perturbations continued, the professors persevered, led fearlessly by Duncan. Two (including Duncan, Mason Guest, Virgil Koenig, and Edwards Rennels, among others) usually trekked to Austin three times a year to represent UTMB during the deliberations of the Graduate Assembly. UTMB's graduate faculty met periodically to adopt changes in courses or programs and to certify students for graduation.[199]

The number of matriculates and graduates continued to increase. The number of matriculates doubled between 1964 and 1968, with a total of seventy-four in the fall of 1968 (fifty-five men and nineteen women). Between 1964 and 1969 forty-seven

TABLE 6.15: GRADUATE SCHOOL OF THE BIOMEDICAL SCIENCES STUDENTS,
FY 1971–FY1991

| Years | M.A. Students | | Ph.D. Students | | Post-doctoral Basic Science Fellows |
	Enrolled	Graduates	Enrolled	Graduates	
1970–71	46	12	56	9	8
1971–72	38	12	50	12	11
1972–73	33	7	62	7	18
1973–74	51	13	55	12	13
1974–75	46	12	48	9	36
1975–76	21	8	79	4	25
1976–77	21	1	101	6	21
1977–78	20	6	103	17	29
1978–79	20	2	115	8	42
1979–80	19	3	121	13	27
1980–81	11	2	116	16	33
1981–82	12	8	102	30	39
1982–83	12	5	101	28	54
1983–84	68	44	102	18	38
1984–85	70	17	93	7	57
1985–86	106	18	111	11	63
1986–87	107	32	138	21	56
1987–88	108	33	153	23	59
1988–89	100	39	143	14	48
1989–90	85	35	155	18	77
1990–91	97	23	158	21	69

students earned master's degrees and forty-six students earned doctoral degrees.[200] These graduates included several who became teachers at UTMB: Earl Adrian Jr., Donald Barnett, Gerald Beathard, Juanita Phipps Bray, Gerald Callas, Jerry Daniels, Jim Dunaway, Richard Fritz, Bryan Holland, Larry Ross, Clifton Smith, Don Stubbs, Dan Traber, Johannes van Lier, Byron Wilkenfeld, and Margaret Broman Young. Beginning in 1965 the University of Texas Medical Branch (not the University of Texas) was designated on the diplomas as the institution authorizing the degrees earned by graduate students at UTMB.

In 1969 the regents permitted each biomedical institution in the UT System to establish a locally independent graduate school. Each school would have a graduate administrator accountable to the president of the local institution. Faculty would be classified as members, special members, and associates.[201] Each academic department offering graduate studies would appoint one of its members as that department's graduate advisor, accountable to both the department's chair and the graduate administrator of the school.

Twenty-eight members of UTMB's graduate faculty met on April 30, 1969, to discuss ways to adapt to these new policies. Duncan presided during a discussion of admission standards and procedures, a need for new bylaws, possible M.D.–Ph.D. programs, recruitment of new students and ways to finance their studies, and a possible graduate program in pathology. The faculty elected Mason Guest as the representative to the system's new Graduate Council.[202]

Ed Brandt became UTMB's first full-time "dean," conducting his initial meeting with the faculty (fifty-eight members present) on February 10, 1970 (Appendix B). Brandt appointed a Student Recruitment Committee and an Admissions Committee. The faculty elected a member from each of the eight existing graduate programs to constitute the Executive Committee: Donald Duncan (anatomy), Gordon Mills (biochemistry), Barbara Bowman (human genetics), Leroy Olson (microbiology), Richard Marshall (pathology), James Hilton (pharmacology), Mason Guest (physiology), and Don Micks (preventive medicine and public health). This committee usually met every month.[203]

In September 1970 the graduate faculty adopted new bylaws. During the early 1970s the faculty taught more than one hundred graduate courses in the nine departments offering graduate degrees.[204] By the fall of 1973 there were 130 graduate faculty members and almost 100 graduate students. Between 1971 and 1974 forty-five graduate students earned master's degrees and forty-four earned doctorates (Table 6.15).[205]

In 1973 the regents eliminated the system's Graduate Council and authorized each UT medical component to title its graduate studies program as the Graduate School of the Biomedical Sciences (GSBS).[206] Brandt automatically became the first dean of the now autonomous GSBS in Galveston, though this was a part-time position for Brandt then, as he had become acting dean of medicine.

In July 1974 Palmer Saunders became the first full-time dean of the fully authorized Graduate School of the Biomedical Sciences at UTMB. Saunders appointed Jim Blankenship as chair of an ad hoc curriculum committee. This committee reviewed and approved all changes in graduate courses, pushed for more uniformity in degree requirements, proposed ways to improve communication between faculty and students, and reviewed proposals for new programs. This committee became a standing committee in December 1977.[207]

Saunders initiated a review of all graduate programs, using faculty committees and outside consultants. Creed Abell chaired the steering committee that included Sam Barranco, Ernie Barratt, Jim Blankenship, John Bruhn, Mason Guest, Alexander Kenny, Elbert Whorton, and Harold Levine. These formal evaluations catalyzed a variety of changes in all programs during the succeeding three years.[208] As the school's first associate dean for curricular affairs, Whorton shepherded many of these changes, including a new set of bylaws adopted in April 1977.[209]

By the 1979–1980 year, 143 faculty supported GSBS programs. These included 40 faculty in physiology and biophysics; 34 in preventive medicine and community health; 24 in human genetics and cell biology; 24 in biochemistry; 17 in pharmacology and toxicology; 14 in anatomy; 14 in microbiology; and 14 in pathology.[210] With substantial growth in the number of faculty, students, and research grants, some departments acquired separate buildings: pharmacology in 1974, microbiology in 1978.

As new faculty, new program directors, and new department chairs appeared during the 1980s, some changes occurred in existing programs and new programs were added. The Department of Preventive Medicine and Community Health divided their courses into three areas of concentration: environmental toxicology, sociomedical sciences, and medical humanities.[211] In 1979 the Graduate School of the Biomedical Sciences became administratively responsible for the master's degree program directed by School of Nursing faculty. In 1980 the coordinating board approved a doctoral program in the neurosciences, the first new doctoral program in the state approved by the board after several years of a moratorium. In 1986 this board approved a master's degree program in allied health sciences with two areas of concentration: clinical gerontology and health education.

In 1981 the Graduate School of the Biomedical Sciences and School of Medicine faculty began a six-year combined M.D.–Ph.D. program. William Willis Jr. chaired the initial faculty committee until Jim Blankenship assumed that role in 1982. After 130 students visited UTMB for interviews, twenty-six formally applied.[212] The faculty accepted nine students. Five matriculated in 1983. In 1990 Mark Cleveland and Shawn David Newlands became the first students to complete this program.

Saunders and the faculty changed the ambience of the Graduate School of the Biomedical Sciences. More rigorous courses were developed for GSBS students, who were also expected to participate in departmental journal clubs, seminars, and professional forums. Saunders expected faculty to give proper credit to students in publications emerging from collaborative research efforts. He held monthly luncheon meetings with students and in the fall of 1975 he initiated an annual welcoming barbecue for students and faculty. In May 1976 Saunders initiated an annual awards dinner for students and faculty. After he established a GSBS minority affairs committee in 1984, more ethnic minority students, especially Asians, enrolled. A separate GSBS commencement ceremony began in 1984.

The number of graduate students grew significantly during these years. In the fall of 1976, 153 students matriculated in the GSBS. These included 101 students in doctoral programs, 22 in master's degree programs, and 30 as special students. In 1986, 300 students enrolled: 152 seeking degrees in the sciences (139 Ph.D. and 11 master's) and 19 as special students; and 101 seeking master's degrees in nursing and 28 as special students. The number of foreign-born students increased dramatically during the late 1980s.[213]

Important political and financial issues surfaced as Saunders neared retirement. He believed that the Graduate School of the Biomedical Sciences was a political stepchild of the School of Medicine. Saunders had little control over the salaries of GSBS faculty because 90 percent of these teachers had their primary appointments in the School of Medicine. He also had no real authority over research programs and resources. The only financial authority vested in the GSBS dean was control over stipends for graduate students. Saunders believed that the GSBS dean should be a vice president for research and graduate studies and should report directly to the president.[214]

In 1987 K. Lemone Yielding succeeded Saunders as GSBS dean and UTMB's first vice president for research.[215] Yielding recognized UTMB's "unrealized potential" as a research institution. He wanted to establish better administrative support for the research activities of the 255 members and 107 special members of the faculty.[216] Yielding held no regular GSBS faculty meetings between March 1988 and August 1991, but he did meet regularly with the four committees (Executive, Curriculum, Program Review, and Recruitment) that managed the school's activities.

Yielding wanted to recruit good students. Distressed that the budget for graduate student stipends permitted only an annual stipend of $7,300 compared to a national norm of almost $12,000, Yielding realigned this budget to provide support to a smaller number of students so that the GSBS would be more competitive in recruiting students. This decision did not produce a decrease in the number of graduate students because the faculty assumed more responsibility for providing student support from research grants.

During commencement ceremonies in May 1991, thirty students received master's degrees and nineteen received doctorates. From 1970 through 1991 at least 332 GSBS students earned master's degrees and 304 students earned Ph.D. degrees (Table 6.15).[217] Resting on contiguous shelves in the Moody Medical Library are 886 theses and dissertations written between 1953 and 1991 by graduate students. They reveal extraordinary efforts to develop and sustain academic programs at UTMB for those who wanted graduate degrees in the biomedical sciences, nursing, and the medical humanities.

In guiding the extraordinary growth of the GSBS between 1974 and 1991, Saunders and Yielding received exceptional administrative assistance from Bob Bennett, Janie Polk, Karen Sevier Thompson, Vera Dobson, and Theresa Copado. With the opening of the Medical Research Building in 1991, their efforts and hopes for the GSBS received tremendous affirmation.

THE INSTITUTES

The Marine Biomedical Institute (MBI) was established in 1969; the Institute for the Medical Humanities (IMH) in 1973. Directors of these institutes held dual accountabilities to the president and the School of Medicine dean until 1983, when they became accountable to the vice president for academic affairs (Appendix B). Teachers affiliated with these institutes were designated as members; their primary appointments were in School of Medicine departments.[218] Their research activities are discussed in the next chapter. The remainder of this chapter describes some of their teaching activities.

The Marine Biomedical Institute's members participated in the basic science courses of the new School of Medicine curriculum that started in 1970, invigorated the graduate programs of most basic science departments, established the graduate program in the neurosciences approved in 1980, and strongly supported the joint M.D.–Ph.D. program initiated in 1981.[219] Initially attracted to the Marine Biomedical Institute's research mission, for example, Bernard Haber (appointed in 1970), Jim Blankenship (1970), Bill Willis (1970), and Richard Coggeshall (1971) were still devoted teachers more than two decades later.

The teaching programs of the Institute for the Medical Humanities during the 1970s and 1980s were built on longstanding legacies in teaching the humanities at UTMB. Medical history, medical ethics, and medical jurisprudence were taught in the medical school during UTMB's first decade. Thomas Ballinger, Robert Street, Allen Smith, and William Gammon gave lectures on law and medicine. Between 1893 and 1897 David Cerna gave a lecture on medical history each week to first-year students. After his retirement as dean, J. F. Y. Paine gave several talks on medical ethics.[220]

Humanities teaching continued in various ways during the first half of the twentieth century. Marvin Graves, professor of medicine, probably gave four to six lectures on medical ethics to senior medical students between 1906 and 1927.[221] Several physicians and lawyers taught medical jurisprudence before 1940: C. K. Peckham, David Lawrence, Dick Wall, Marion Joseph-Levy, L. E. Chapman, Brantley Harris, Russell Markwell, and William Decker. By the mid-1940s, Decker taught a course in legal medicine to seniors and Leake taught a course in medical history to sophomores.[222]

In 1952 Leake wanted to create a Department of Legal and Cultural Medicine whose members would teach medical history, medical ethics, medical jurisprudence, medical economics, medical social service, and health administration. Resisting the establishment of a new department, UT Chancellor Hart believed that faculty with appointments in the existing Department of Preventive Medicine and Public Health should teach these subjects. Accepting Hart's recommendation, Leake employed Patrick Romanell to teach philosophy and ethics. Romanell received his Ph.D. in philosophy from Columbia University in 1937 and taught at two schools before joining UTMB in 1952. After Leake left in 1955, Romanell taught an elective course in the history and philosophy of medicine and public health until his departure in 1962.[223]

Medical ethics received special attention in February 1962 when Joseph Fletcher, then professor of social ethics at the Episcopal Theological School and Harvard University, gave several lectures during a three-day visit sponsored by UTMB's Committee on Religion and Medicine. Though Fletcher's visit sparked considerable interest in medical ethics among students and faculty, there were no formal courses in medical ethics, medical jurisprudence, or medical history when Truman Blocker became CEO in 1964.[224]

Nurtured by Leake and Ransom, Blocker developed an intense interest in rare books and the history of surgery. An area for rare books and history collections was specifically designated in plans for a new library at UTMB. Invited by Blocker, Leake returned to UTMB in October 1965 to give a series of ten lectures on the history and philosophy of medicine. In that same year, responding to Blocker's request, the trustees of the Rockwell Fund in Houston endowed a professorship in medical history in honor of James Wade Rockwell, a former trustee and UT regent.[225]

In August 1969 Blocker and White invited Chester Burns, the first American-born physician to earn a Ph.D. in the history of medicine, to become director of a History of Medicine Division at UTMB. Events associated with the development of this division between 1969 and 1973 led directly to the creation of the Institute for the Medical Humanities. In April 1970, for example, Burns and John P. McGovern hosted a two-day symposium about William Osler and medical humanism, attended by three hundred people from thirty-one states, Canada, and England. George Harrell and Bill Bean were among the speakers. As the first dean of the Pennsylvania State University College of Medicine at Hershey, Harrell had established the first humanities department in an American medical school in 1967. Bill Bean, then professor and chair of the Department of Medicine at the University of Iowa would later become the institute's first director.[226]

To develop some plans for teaching, White appointed Burns as chair of a Medical Humanities Committee, which held twenty-two meetings during the academic year 1971–1972. Composed of six students, fourteen faculty, three hospital employees, and four lay citizens from Galveston, this committee generated more than four hundred pages of minutes that documented a widespread need for humanities teaching at UTMB.[227] Using the committee's final report as a blueprint, Burns, Gammon Jarrell (Episcopal campus chaplain and director of the William Temple House) and H. Tristram Engelhardt Jr. (a physician-philosopher who joined the faculty in 1972) began a teaching program in January 1973. Blocker and White wanted to recognize these teaching activities with a more formal structure, and in April 1973 Blocker asked the regents to establish the Institute for the Medical Humanities, which they did in June.[228]

As the History of Medicine Division became the Institute for the Medical Humanities during the 1973–1974 academic year, some important events occurred. In October 1973 Burns coordinated the Southwest Regional Institute on Human Values in Medicine held at the Holiday Inn in Galveston. For two days fifty teachers and students discussed ways to incorporate the humanities into medical education. In the spring of 1974 *Texas Reports on Biology and Medicine* published a special 368-page issue on "The Humanities and Medicine" edited by Burns and Engelhardt, a volume that generated favorable responses throughout the world.[229] Also in the spring of 1974, Engelhardt organized the first transdisciplinary symposium on philosophy and medicine, a three-day meeting at the Flagship Hotel attended by about two hundred people. In May 1974 the National Endowment for the Humanities (NEH) awarded UTMB a major grant to support the development of the institute. Bean became the first director of the institute in June 1974.[230]

The NEH grant supported the expansion of the institute's teaching program. Four new faculty members were employed between 1974 and 1979. During these years, the

TABLE 6.16: HUMANITIES ELECTIVES FOR SENIOR MEDICAL STUDENTS,
FY 1978–FY1991

Understanding and Caring for Terminally Ill Persons

Medical Lives

Images of Man and Physician in Literature and Film

Philosophy of Medicine

Should Physicians Practice Comprehensive Health Care?

Peer Review for Physicians: How Does It Work?

Medicine in Texas

History of Medicine

The Physician's Role in Judicial Proceedings

The Liability of Physicians for the Acts of Others

Science, Society, and Humanistic Values

---

faculty members developed courses for students in all four schools at UTMB, as well as continuing education courses for medical practitioners and courses for college students attending special programs at UTMB. Institute members taught forty Austin College students during January interterms and 127 college undergraduates attending the Familiarization Program for Minority Students. They taught two courses for 101 School of Nursing and School of Allied Health Sciences students. Institute members taught courses to approximately 1,000 first-year medical students in a required course in medical ethics; 800 second year students in the humanities portion of the required course in preventive medicine and community health; and 950 senior students in the required course in medical jurisprudence. Twenty-five seniors devoted entire four-week periods to electives in the medical humanities (Table 6.16). Institute members also provided humanities instruction to about sixty interns, residents, and clinical fellows in the Departments of Family Medicine, Internal Medicine, and Psychiatry. Some eight hundred doctors attended lectures or courses offered by the institute as continuing education programs. These courses included five extremely demanding four-week seminars.[231]

The IMH faculty also designed eleven humanities courses for Graduate School of the Biomedical Sciences graduate students. Forty-five students took one or more of these courses. Johanna Price completed a Ph.D. program in preventive medicine and community health with an area of concentration in the medical humanities. At the time of her graduation in 1982, Price received the Dean's Award for Academic Excellence.

The NEH grant used to support the growth and development of the Institute for the Medical Humanities was the first grant from a federal agency UTMB received for the purpose of establishing a new academic program with a focus on teaching.[232]

Bill Bean resigned in June 1980. In January 1982 Ronald Carson became the institute's second director. Carson had directed a Division of the Social Sciences and

Humanities in the Department of Community Health and Family Medicine at the University of Florida's School of Medicine in Gainesville. By 1988 the IMH included ten full-time members (Carson, Burns, Harold Vanderpool, Anne Hudson Jones, Tom Cole, Bill Winslade, Sally Gadow, Mary Winkler, Ellen More, and John Douard), who were strongly committed to a multidisciplinary teaching program that was centered in the School of Medicine and the Graduate School of the Biomedical Sciences.[233]

Certain changes occurred in the teaching program during the 1980s. All IMH faculty members participated in the required medical ethics course for first-year medical students, a course Vanderpool directed beginning in 1981. Students met with instructors in small groups for discussions of syllabus readings, readings that included more clinical cases by 1990. In 1984 Winslade assumed responsibility for the medical jurisprudence course required for third-year medical students. Between 1984 and 1990 Winslade met one hour a week with a different group of about twenty-five students every eight weeks; every six weeks beginning in 1990.[234] In 1985 institute faculty began orchestrating four one-hour ethics case conferences for third-year students as they experienced their clerkship rotation in internal medicine. Junior and senior medical students also attended ethics consultations provided by the IMH's ethics consultation service Winslade initiated in 1985. Institute faculty led caregivers in a discussion of specific ethical problems associated with the care of particular inpatients. Finally, senior medical students could take full-time four-week electives with institute members. Between 1985 and 1991 more than three hundred seniors made their selections from fifteen to twenty electives the faculty offered each year.

In 1988 the coordinating board and the regents approved the IMH's request to offer a graduate program for those who wanted to earn master's or Ph.D. degrees in the medical humanities. This was the first graduate program of its kind offered in a university in the United States. By 1991 fifteen students were enrolled in the program and three had earned doctoral degrees.[235]

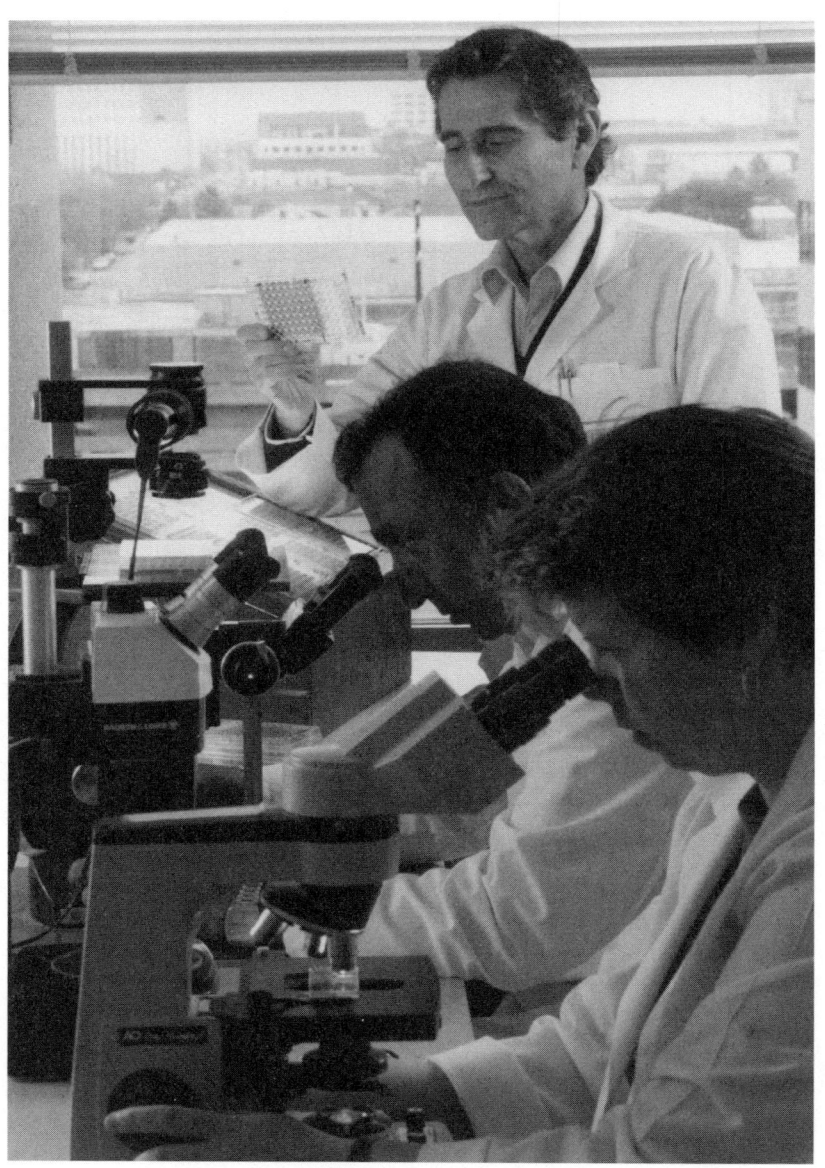

Sam Baron, standing, with I. P. Singh and Joyce Post in the Department of Microbiology's research lab, 1991.

― 7 ―

Inquiry and Research

"While this is primarily a teaching institution, the members of the staff cannot remain efficient in their teaching if they do no research and do not attend meetings of scientific societies where they can report the results of their own investigations and participate in the discussions of presentations by others. Teaching institutions cannot remain static. They must combine original investigation with teaching if they are to progress and keep abreast of the times. If they fail to do so, they are standing still."—Dean William Carter, 1935[1]

UTMB had existed as a university medical center for forty-five years when Carter wrote these words to UT President Benedict in the fall of 1935. Although the care of patients, the teaching of students, and the development of new scientific knowledge had been hallmarks of the top American medical schools during these years, UTMB's faculty members had struggled with some conflicts about their roles as clinicians, teachers, and researchers. The nature and extent of research was at the heart of most conflicts because no one questioned the importance of giving care to patients and teaching students.[2]

Divided into three sections, this chapter highlights three phases of UTMB's evolution as a research university. The first section describes events between 1900 and the arrival of Chauncey Leake in 1942. During these years, most CEOs assigned research a lower priority than teaching and patient care. Nevertheless, they employed enthusiastic and productive researchers as chairs of the School of Medicine's basic science departments. They also selected chairs of School of Medicine clinical departments who hired some clinicians who became highly productive and nationally recognized researchers.[3]

The second section describes the incorporation of research as a primary mission for the School of Medicine and the School of Nursing. Between 1942 and 1964, Leake and John Truslow facilitated this shift in priorities. Leake's achievements in boosting research were stupendous. Truslow made a place for an administrative manager of the research enterprise. Truslow's support of the Student Research Forum and the Clinical Research Center symbolized a new level of commitment by administrators, faculty, and students.

The third section traces the phenomenal expansion of research during the years of leadership by Blocker, Levin, and James (1964–1991). These leaders catalyzed astonishing political and financial support for the research enterprise. Each was a highly regarded researcher who understood the importance of molding a secure and strong infrastructure. Events in molding this infrastructure are described. In response, faculty and students in all four schools substantially increased their productivity as researchers—in the biomedical, behavioral, and social sciences. UTMB also became the site of a special program in the medical humanities.

BEFORE CHAUNCEY LEAKE, 1900–1942

In 1903 Dean Allen Smith asked UT President William Prather to improve conditions for research at UTMB, believing that the school was far behind the best American medical schools. Smith told Prather: "It must be acknowledged no matter how efficient the school is proving itself as an institution for undergraduate instruction, that in one particular it is far behind even less pretentious medical colleges in the country. This refers to the amount and character of original scientific work done by the teaching staff."[4] Smith did not believe that UTMB could maintain its first-class image without more adequate support of research.

Although Smith recognized the need for more scientific investigation, he taught nine subjects and thirteen different courses that year.[5] He always carried a heavy teaching load and it is not surprising that he reported the results of only one set of experiments during his years in Galveston. His colleagues were also busy teaching medical, nursing, and pharmacy students.[6]

Dean Carter believed that UTMB needed "research work more than anything else," but he ceased to be an experimental scientist because of administrative chores.[7] He did hire Oscar Plant (School of Medicine class of 1902) as a demonstrator in physiology and pharmacology. Plant's reports about experimental studies of fat absorption in dogs and the use of nitrates as stimulants appeared between 1908 and 1910.[8] Plant's work earned him an invitation to join the Department of Pharmacology at the University of Pennsylvania, which he accepted in 1910.

In his report about American medical schools published the same year, Abraham Flexner criticized UTMB for its lack of research. Carter told UT President Mezes: "To my mind the most serious criticism of this school made by the [Flexner Report,] although it is eminently just, is its unproductiveness. Of course, this institution ought never to attempt to be a research school primarily, but on the other hand, it is a mistake to make routine teaching the sole function of the school without developing investigation for the expansion of our knowledge."[9]

Between 1900 and 1922, Carter orchestrated major changes in the pre-clinical departments that boded well for experimental science. He hired researchers as full-time chairs for the Departments of Biochemistry, Bacteriology, and Pharmacology. He supported their efforts to attract younger colleagues in these and other basic science departments, and he supported their collective efforts to develop graduate degree programs.

Carter's successors as deans, however, championed teaching. Keiller, a comparative anatomist, believed that teaching was more important than research: "I believe that the

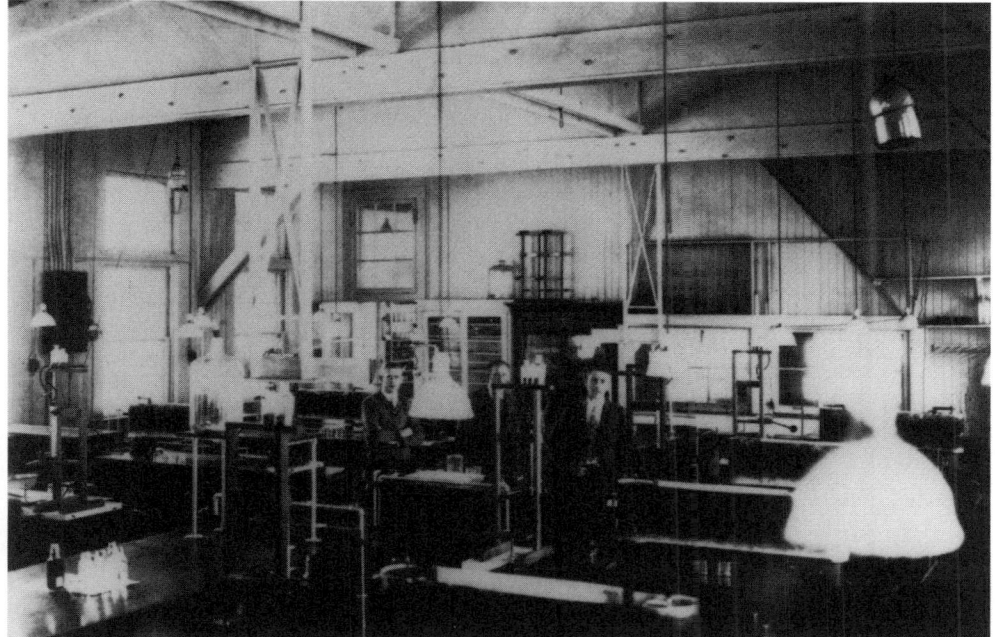

Hans Ash, Oscar Bodansky, and W. T. Dawson in the pharmacology lab, 1927.

first duty of the Medical Branch of the University of Texas is to prepare the largest number of well-equipped general practitioners to serve the people of Texas and while our teaching staff and budget is so limited, and our teaching duties so heavy, only a very small output in research can be expected from those departments whose teaching duties are heaviest." In 1929 Bethel told UT President Benedict that he was glad that research at UTMB ranked third behind teaching and patient care.[10]

Nevertheless, UTMB gradually institutionalized biomedical research during the 1920s and 1930s because of Carter's decisions, the diligence of a small number of devoted experimental scientists, and their support by departmental chairs.

In 1913 Carter selected William C. Rose as professor of biological chemistry. Rose was the first professor at UTMB who had earned a Ph.D. in a basic science field. In Galveston Rose continued the studies of intermediate protein metabolism that he had started with Lafayette Mendel at Yale. Reports about this work appeared in 1916 in the *Journal of Biological Chemistry*, the nation's principal journal for biochemical research. In that same year, Rose told UT President Vinson: "It is our belief that the encouragement of original work should be regarded as an extremely important part of the instruction in every department of the university."[11] As described in the previous chapter, Rose institutionalized such encouragement by initiating successful efforts to develop a master's degree program.

In three other basic science departments, new leaders catalyzed experimental research.[12] In 1921 Carter selected William Sharp as professor and chair of the Department of Bacteriology and Preventive Medicine. In 1922 Carter employed Harry Atkinson as the new chair of the Department of Pharmacology. In 1923 Eugene Porter, who had acquired a Ph.D. at Harvard, became professor and chair of physiology. UTMB now had five basic science faculty with Ph.D. degrees: Hendrix, Sharp, Atkinson, Henry Henze (also in pharmacology), and Porter. Other researchers joined these teachers as their departments expanded.

Sharp (M.D., Rush, 1914; Ph.D., Chicago, 1922), Thurston Johnson (Ph.D., Chicago, 1927), and Wendell Gingrich (Sc.D., Johns Hopkins, 1930) were productive researchers in the Department of Bacteriology and Preventive Medicine during the 1920s and 1930s.[13] Sharp investigated ringworm infections, carriers of pneumococci, and a particular variety of mosquito as a disease vector. Johnson investigated trypanosomal infections, granuloma inguinale, and fungal diseases.[14] Gingrich, trained as a parasitologist, specialized in research about immunity to malaria.[15]

Atkinson was professor and chair of pharmacology for only three years, accomplishing little in terms of research apparently because of the demands of organizing the new department.[16] Wilfred Dawson, Atkinson's successor, studied the regulation of coronary circulation and the pharmacology of cinchona alkaloids. Dawson also collaborated with Porter in studying reflexes as indicators of antagonism between barbiturates and strychnine.[17]

Porter engaged in experimental studies of reflexes and muscle contraction and gave many papers, including one at the historic thirteenth International Congress of Physiology, which met in the United States for the first time in 1929.[18] In that same year, Wilbur Selle became the second Ph.D. employed by the Department of Physiology. Selle studied carbohydrate metabolism and cancer, and he investigated molds and hay fever. Later, Selle used guinea pigs and rabbits in studying asthma, histamine intoxication, and the effects of benadryl and pyribenzamine (antihistamines used in treating hay fever).[19]

The scientific productivity of the Department of Biochemistry did not weaken after Hendrix replaced Rose in 1922. Meyer Bodansky earned a Ph.D. from Cornell in 1923.[20] When Marion Fay arrived in 1925, the department had its second Ph.D. researcher trained at Yale. Hendrix, Fay, and Bodansky also attended the thirteenth International Congress of Physiology in 1929. Hendrix's research involved heavy metal absorption, blood pH, and protein coagulation. Fay's earlier research involved calcium metabolism, but, like Hendrix, she shifted her interest to the intestinal absorption of foodstuffs.[21] Bodansky's research involved liver functions, blood chemistry, the metabolism of creatine, and the metabolism of the sedative paraldehyde.[22]

In 1931 Bodansky left this department to become the "director" of a new academic department titled "Pathological Chemistry" and director of the John Sealy Memorial Laboratory. Bodansky supervised the technicians who performed tests on specimens from patients, trained medical technology students, and used the lab's facilities for research. In 1931, for example, he studied the solubility of fatty acids to obtain more data about hemolysis. He also did collaborative studies with Charles Stone on polycythemia, with William Marr and Paul Brindley on acetylphenylhydrazine used to treat polycythemia, and with Edward Schwab and Titus Harris on certain muscle diseases. More than any other faculty member, Bodansky collaborated with others, even convincing a busy pathologist like Brindley to take on experimental work.[23]

Experimental research in the Department of Anatomy began in 1932 when Harry Knight hired Donald Duncan, a Ph.D. neuroanatomist already recognized as a researcher. As Rose had done for Bodansky and Porter for Selle, Knight supported Duncan's commitment to research. Duncan "was excused from the performance of most other duties in the department," declared Knight, "so that he might reorganize the work in neuro-anatomy and also have the time and opportunity to do library reading and some research work."[24] Duncan initiated several research studies: the relationship of nerve fiber size to function and the formation of myelin, the anatomical paths of certain nerve fibers in the spinal cord, and the effect of amputation on nerve fibers of the opposite limb. Duncan also studied the ratio of nerve fibers to cells in spinal ganglia, and he collaborated with Dawson on the pharmacology of strychnine.[25] John Sinclair, another professor who was employed in 1928 to teach histology and embryology, eventually became an investigator, assisting Bodansky with his project on the functions of the thyroid and parathyroid glands, and initiating an independent study of salivary corpuscles.[26]

Between 1900 and 1942, UTMB's clinical professors continued to report their experiences in treating patients with a variety of diseases and a few did some experimental work. In the Department of Surgery, F. W. Aves knew that patients with prolonged jaundice usually bled extensively when surgeons removed their gallbladders. In 1916 Aves ligated the common biliary ducts of thirteen rabbits to produce obstructive jaundice and then successfully used gelatin to reduce the time needed for coagulation after surgically induced bleeding. He then used the gelatin treatment on two cholecystectomy patients, with excellent results.[27]

In the Department of Medicine, Moise D. Levy studied variations in healthy adults. In 1917 Levy counted the white blood cells of sixty-seven male medical students and forty-seven female nursing students. He claimed that the normal lymphocyte count for a healthy adult between the ages of twenty and thirty was 33–34 percent with variations as high as 50 percent. He concluded that the differential count for asymptomatic humans given in standard textbooks was incorrect.[28]

Earl Crutchfield, William Spiller, and others in the Department of Dermatology and Syphilology investigated the treatment of sexually transmitted diseases, leprosy, and certain fungal conditions. They tested some antimony derivatives used in treating granuloma inguinale and they tested arsenicals used in treating syphilis.

Boyd Reading and others in the Department of Pediatrics assessed the therapeutic value of certain drugs used in the treatment of congenital syphilis and juvenile gonococcus vaginitis.[29]

During the early 1930s experimental research received more support from the chairs of clinical departments. Before becoming chair of the Department of Medicine in 1926, Charles Stone Sr. toured American and European medical schools for fifteen months. Afterward he featured research as a primary mission of this department.[30]

In 1931 Stone hired George Herrmann, an established investigator in cardiology and the first M.D./Ph.D. professor in a clinical department at UTMB.[31] Stone spent about $3,000 to equip a laboratory for Herrmann in the new Outpatient Building. Herrmann did not disappoint Stone. Herrmann initiated numerous research projects and collaborated with several faculty members. He supported Edward Schwab's work on hypertension among blacks and Stone's interest in syphilitic heart disease. He collaborated with Paul Woodard, William Marr, and William Bondurant on their studies of the chemical composition of blood and urine during diuresis. Herrmann and others presented papers at meetings of the Association of American Physicians and the American Society for Clinical Investigation.[32]

While some colleagues adopted some of Herrmann's interest in diuresis and cardiac edema, others developed their own research projects. Schwab continued to study hypertension, Marr developed an interest in anemia, Stone maintained an interest in diabetes and gastrointestinal diseases, and George Decherd studied the role of creatine in cardiovascular functions.[33]

In 1930 A. O. Singleton, chair of the Department of Surgery, hired Robert Moore as an "Associate Professor of Experimental and Research Surgery." Moore wanted to do experimental work and provide surgical care. Moore designed, equipped, and directed a Laboratory of Experimental Surgery, which was housed on the fourth floor of the new wing of the Laboratory Building that opened in 1932. Within a year, professors from the Departments of Surgery, Medicine, Radiology, Anatomy, and Physiology were engaged in more than ten research projects in this lab. Professors from the Departments of Physiology and Radiology studied intestinal absorption, those from Medicine and Surgery studied the effects of pressure on the pericardium and relationships between gastric functions and chemical composition of the blood, and those from Surgery and Physiology investigated the role of the cerebrum in determining thresholds of pain.[34]

Other chairs of clinical departments wanted to support research. Willard Cooke, chair of the Department of Obstetrics and Gynecology, thought that more patients reduced the time and energy needed for research. "As each year increases the number of patients to be handled," Cooke declared, "there is a corresponding increase in the amount of routine work done by each man, and a decrease in the amount of research and other collateral work possible." In 1937 he established a Laboratory for Gynecological and Obstetrical Pathology, hoping that this lab could also be used for research. Clinical tests for patients became so extensive, however, that no time was left for research. Some professors in this department did collaborate with Bodansky in a study of thyroid, parathyroid, and calcium metabolism during pregnancy. By the early 1940s this department evaluated sulfonamides used in treating gonorrhea in women and Jules Lamar investigated aspects of sterility.[35]

Before 1942 deans and departmental chairs made other important decisions that helped institutionalize research at UTMB. They acquired more space for research labs. Before Carter left, three new buildings housed some labs: the Laboratory of Experimental Medicine (1916), the Laboratory of Chemistry for the School of Pharmacy (1920), and the Laboratory of Pharmacology and Physiology (1921). The Laboratory of Experimental Medicine was used mostly for an elective course in experimental surgery that allowed students and faculty to learn and improve surgical techniques. The latter two buildings were used mostly for teaching, though Atkinson undoubtedly conducted some experiments in the Laboratory of Pharmacology and Physiology. Labs in the Keiller Building, which opened in 1925, were used primarily for teaching anatomy and pathology.[36] The Outpatient Clinic building contained the cardiovascular lab Herrmann used and the John Sealy Memorial Laboratory Bodansky directed. In 1932 the Laboratory for Experimental Surgery in the new east wing of the Keiller Building became UTMB's principal site for mammalian research.

Deans and department chairs supported the development of a library with recognized research periodicals. The Keiller Building housed the library in larger quarters, which enabled a fairly rapid growth of the journal collection. From the mid-1920s to the mid-1930s the library's collection of journals quadrupled from about one hundred to about four hundred titles. After Herrmann's arrival, the library began receiving almost two hundred additional titles.[37] As editor of *The American Journal of Syphilis*, he needed access to numerous journals.

Deans and department chairs used research productivity as a criterion for employment, promotion, and salary increases. Carter argued that "the scientific productivity of members of the teaching staff ought to receive consideration in promotions" for both pre-clinical and clinical faculty. In 1924 Keiller recommended salary increases for Hendrix and Bodansky partly because of their research productivity.[38]

Such productivity became even more important during the 1930s. For example, Porter's support of Selle revealed his philosophy about departmental standards. Phillip Gray, with only a master's degree, had returned to UTMB in 1930 after a one-year leave of absence to work on a medical degree. Porter assigned most of the teaching to Gray. In dealing with Gray's distress about this, Porter explained that "to qualify for a position higher than that of instructor a man should have in addition to teaching ability (1) an advanced degree, and (2) a problem of research in experimental physiology underway in which he is actively interested." Gray soon resigned from the department. Felix Butte, who had been a conscientious teacher of anatomy for six years, was distressed about Knight's decision to hire Duncan at the same associate professor level as Butte and at a slightly higher salary.[39] Knight supported Duncan completely and Butte soon left the department.

Revisions in the pre-clinical curriculum of the medical school during the 1930s had a positive effect because eliminating hours of lectures and labs, especially in anatomy, gave basic science faculty more time for research. The presence of graduate students also did much to boost the morale of these professors.

Deans and department chairs encouraged faculty to participate in off-campus meetings with fellow researchers. One problem involved the availability of dollars for reimbursement of travel expenses. Keiller reminded UT President Sutton about the recurring difficulties in attracting basic science faculty. "There is one serious objection which good men have to coming to Texas," asserted Keiller, "viz., that they are so very far away from scientific societies discussing their particular problem and it takes the savings of a year to go to an annual meeting, apart from the fact that they miss the stimulus of discussion of purely scientific problems with men engaged in similar work." Keiller remembered the events of 1920 and 1921, when seven people rejected Carter's invitation to become professor of pharmacology and ten rejected offers to become professor of bacteriology. During Hartman's administration in 1927 the budget included a separate fund for traveling expenses. The total amount ranged from $1,400 to $1,500 until 1933, when it dropped to $650 to $750. In 1939 Spies negotiated an increase from $750 to $1,600.[40]

As the epigraph introducing this chapter indicated, Carter's views about research were even stronger during his second tenure as CEO. He believed that the "advancement of knowledge by promoting research is a responsibility of the University second only to teaching." Carter and others were delighted when Meyer Bodansky received the Award for Outstanding Research from the Texas Pathological Society in 1937.[41]

Rainey and Spies agreed on the need for more administrative support of the research mission. During his commencement address at UTMB in May 1939, Rainey trumpeted a "comprehensive program of research" as his top priority for UTMB's development. Explained Rainey: "A medical school cannot be supported if it only trains rule-of-thumb practitioners."[42]

Spies hired more research-minded faculty, including Joseph Cline, Raymond Gregory, Carl Nau, Ardzroony Packchanian, Luther Terry, and Ludwik Anigstein. Cline came from Bell Labs to support Spies's interest in cancer research. Gregory came from Minnesota to the Department of Pharmacology as UTMB's fourth M.D./Ph.D. researcher.[43] Nau became chair of the Preventive Medicine and Public Health Department, a department that included Packchanian, Terry, and Anigstein. In labs in the Keiller Building, Terry studied undulant fever, Wendell Gingrich and Cline investigated malaria, and Anigstein investigated typhus fever and leprosy.[44]

Spies served on the advisory board for the new *Bulletin of the John Sealy Hospital and the School of Medicine of the University of Texas*, a monthly journal that made its debut in January 1939. Bodansky was editor and Blocker was managing editor. The February issue included an editorial that welcomed Spies and acknowledged his legacy "in both clinical and experimental research" and his authorship of a "large number of scientific publications."[45]

In 1940 Spies established a "Research Council" that included himself, Bodansky, Cline, Terry, and Joseph Roberts.[46] The council informed professors about sources of funding for research, investigated proposed research contracts involving the faculty, mediated political conflicts about research projects, organized an adequate supply of laboratory animals for use by faculty, and recommended ways to improve and expand the animal quarters. Instead of continuing its advisory and booster roles, the council decided to require researchers to submit all manuscripts for publication to the council for its approval. This decision and its reflection of Spies's dictatorial style greatly undermined its effectiveness.[47]

246

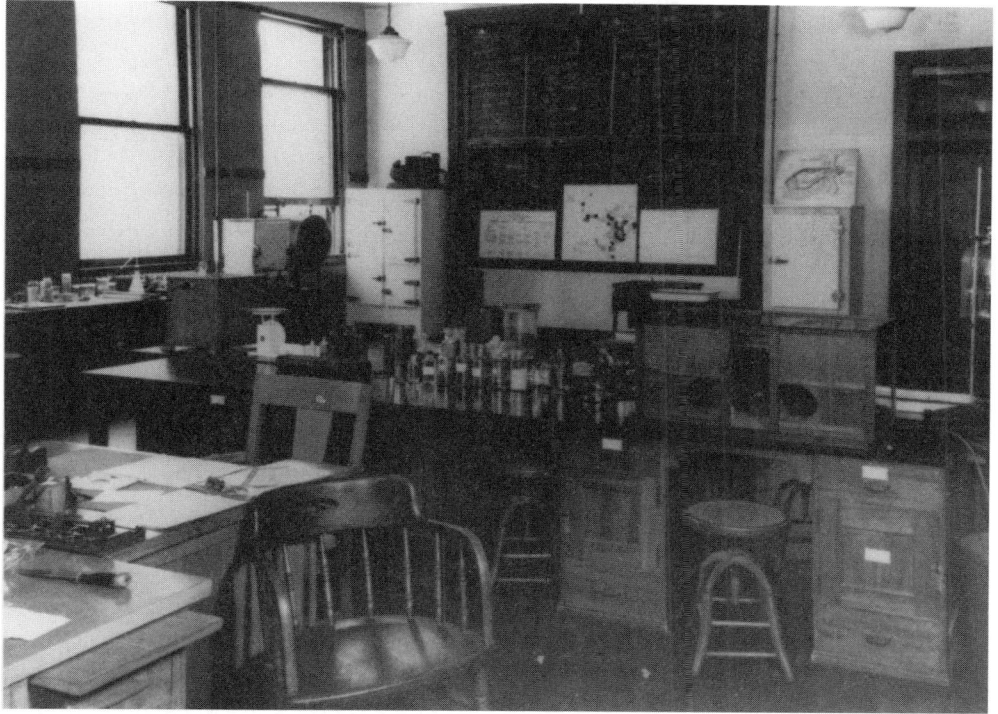

Lab of Ludwik Anigstein and Madero Bader, c. 1941.

Dollars for research expenses were scarce. As described in chapter three, tiny amounts of private money for research came to a few professors before 1942. Spies allocated small amounts of state dollars for research to the School of Medicine departments for fiscal year 1942, about 5 percent of the school's budget. This amount was less than the 8 percent allotted for research by twenty-two four-year public medical schools during 1940–1941; considerably less than the 15 percent allotted by nine private and five public schools with total budgets in the same range as UTMB. The Association of American Medical Colleges team that inspected UTMB early in 1942 concluded that research activities were "underwritten poorly."[48]

In spite of poor financial support and political turmoil, UTMB's professors wrote about sixty articles that were published in national, regional, and state journals during fiscal year 1942. About twenty of these were reports about experimental research.[49]

BETWEEN LEAKE AND BLOCKER, 1942–1964

Because Leake had been a pharmacologist and understood experimental science, he provided more administrative support for research than had ever occurred at UTMB. He recruited talented researchers and supported their specialized laboratories. He established *Texas Reports on Biology and Medicine* and supported successful efforts to develop graduate degree programs. He sponsored conferences and welcomed visiting lecturers, and he expected faculty to give off-campus research presentations. He encouraged faculty to obtain dollars for research from private and federal agencies.[50]

Between 1942 and 1946 Leake employed researchers who became recognized nationally, some internationally. These included Charles Pomerat and Glenn Drager in anatomy, Eric Ogden in physiology, George Emerson in pharmacology, J. A. Scott and Morris Pollard in preventive medicine and bacteriology, Chester Frazier in dermatology, and Arild Hansen in pediatrics.[51]

Pomerat developed a tissue culture laboratory and investigated the effects of drugs and other substances on the growth of different tissues. Numerous scientists from around the world visited Pomerat, and he collaborated with colleagues at UTMB much like Bodansky had done earlier.[52] Pomerat's lab also afforded numerous research opportunities for students. In the early 1950s T. C. Hsu was one of these graduate students. While studying tissue cultures of embryonic human spleen, Hsu accidentally discovered a way to separate chromosomes from other structures in the cells, which became a valuable technique widely used in the development of molecular genetics.[53]

Drager studied the anatomy of the pituitary gland. Ogden came to UTMB from the University of California at Berkeley and continued his research on the role of the kidney in hypertension. Emerson had earned his doctorate in pharmacology while Leake was a professor at the University of California at San Francisco. Emerson investigated a variety of chemotherapeutic agents (including vitamin K derivatives), drugs for leprosy, and central nervous systems stimulants and depressants.[54]

Scott was a senior statistician with the U.S. Census Bureau when he joined the faculty. Before his government service Scott had been a Rockefeller Foundation-sponsored helminthologist in Venezuela and Egypt. Scott studied the epidemiology of filariasis, hookworm, and schistosomiasis.[55] Pollard had been a virologist with the U.S. Department of Agriculture. In Galveston, he established a Virus Research Laboratory that was used for studies of polio, psittacosis, and viral encephalitis.[56]

Frazier and his associates were conducting ten research projects by January 1945; most involved the use of penicillin in the treatment of venereal diseases. Frazier and Wendell Gingrich collaborated in several studies about treating syphilis with penicillin.[57]

Hansen came to UTMB from the University of Minnesota to develop a Child Health Program funded by the William Buchanan Foundation. Hansen's research concerned the relationship between fat metabolism and skin diseases in children. Observing that infants with atopic dermatitis improved after their formulas were supplemented with linoleic acid, Hansen conducted experiments with dogs and infants that proved that linoleic acid was an essential nutrient. In 1957 the American Academy of Pediatrics presented its Gail Borden Award to Hansen for this discovery.[58]

Leake also gave special attention to some of the faculty Spies had hired: Raymond Gregory, Carl Nau, Ludwik Anigstein, and Ardzroony Packchanian. Because Gregory's main interests involved hypertension and kidney disease, Leake moved Gregory into the Department of Medicine and fully supported his research with both dogs and humans.[59] Leake encouraged Nau's interest in the toxic effects of dusts and gases in industrial settings.[60] Anigstein investigated the epidemiology and chemotherapy of rickettsial diseases, and he collaborated with Pomerat in developing an effective intradermal immune serum

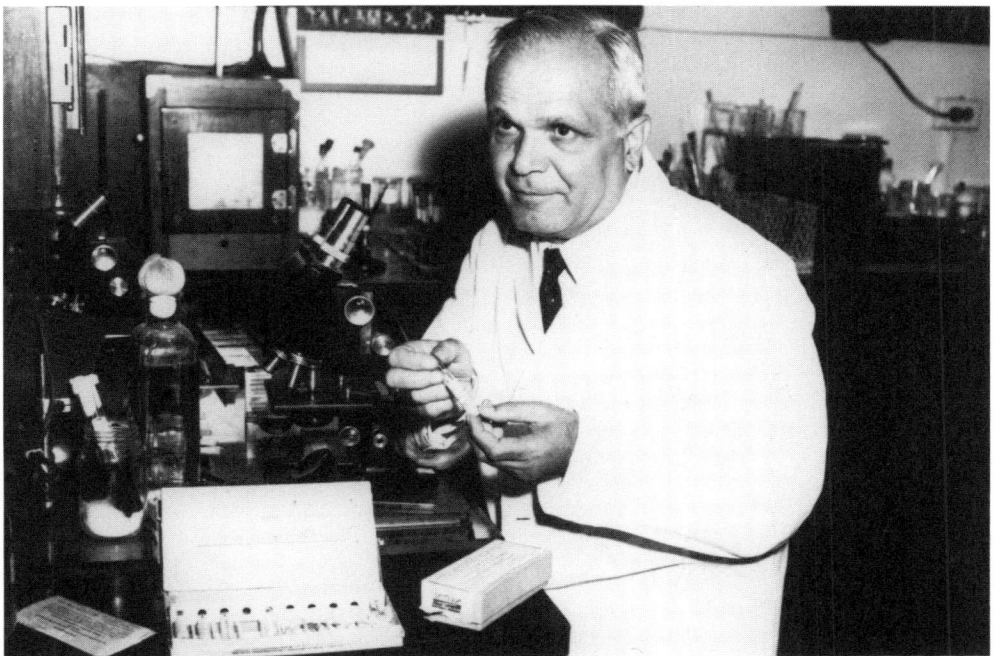

Ardzroony Packchanian in his lab, 1958.

for spotted fever.[61] In the early 1940s Packchanian discovered that the "kissing bug" transmitted Chagas disease, a chronic heart disease. As a researcher at UTMB for more than forty years, Packchanian investigated this disease, African sleeping sickness, and other rickettsial diseases.[62]

As Leake shepherded the new emphasis on research at UTMB during the early 1940s, he wanted a vehicle to publish the faculty's research discoveries. With funding from the Sealy & Smith Foundation, Leake and others prepared the first issue of *Texas Reports on Biology and Medicine*, which was published in 1943. The journal quickly attracted off-campus researchers. By 1950 it published more articles by non-UTMB professionals than those at UTMB. About 4,000 to 4,500 copies were published annually by UT Press and they were distributed without charge to alumni and libraries throughout the world. Many journals in UTMB's library were sent in exchange for *Texas Reports*, about seven hundred by the mid-1950s. As editor of the first thirteen volumes (about eight thousand pages), Leake knew that the journal generated enthusiasm for research among the faculty, gave them some assurance about prompt publication, and garnered prestige for the institution.[63]

Leake encouraged research by attending departmental seminars, inviting visiting lecturers, and supporting conferences in Galveston. Another venue involved meetings of a local affiliate of Sigma Xi, which began as an informal club in 1949 and became an official chapter in 1954.[64] Outstanding scientists and science advocates visited UTMB from a few days to several weeks. These included James Bryant Conant, Linus Pauling, Morris Fishbein, Mary Lasker, Wendell Stanley, and Hans Krebs.[65] Other nationally and internationally recognized scientists worked collaboratively in Galveston for several weeks or even months.[66]

Leake was delighted when the faculty hosted meetings of state, regional, and national scientific societies. In 1944 about seventy-five scientists from Texas, Oklahoma, and Arkansas met on the campus to organize the Southwest Section of the Society for Experimental Biology and Medicine. During annual meetings of the Texas Club of Internists, the faculty presented papers on such topics as the pharmacology of immune responses, the sulfonamides, and the epidemiology of spotted fever on the Gulf Coast. In November 1952 Scott and others hosted the annual meetings of the American Society of Tropical Medicine and Hygiene and the American Academy of Tropical Medicine. The president of the academy that year was R. E. Dyer (School of Medicine class of 1915), who was director of research and professor of medicine at Emory University and had been director of the National Institutes of Health (NIH) between 1942 and 1950. About six hundred members of the American Association of Anatomists attended their annual meeting in Galveston in April 1954.[67]

Leake found the funds to reimburse travel expenses for professors who gave papers during meetings of professional societies. Nineteen professors and colleagues gave research reports at the annual meeting of the American Physiological Society in New Orleans in 1952. In that same year, professors presented reports at the meeting of the American Society for Pharmacology and the Southwest Section meeting of the Society for Experimental Biology.[68]

Leake knew that good research needed adequate funding. In 1942 he revitalized the Research Committee and transformed it into a Research Council three years later. Faculty whose projects exceeded departmental research budgets could apply for some modest support from the council. If it could not provide this support, the council would help the investigator find outside assistance for the project.[69]

During his early years as CEO, Leake hoped that the state government would provide substantial support for research. He was reluctant to tap the federal government. "We do not want Federal support if we can get support from our own people," declared Leake. "We have indicated our firm opposition to bills now in the United States Congress for Federal support of medicine," he added.[70] Like others, Leake feared that public funds for research would obligate scientists to respond to the whims of politicians with special interests.[71]

After a peer-review system was established for federally subsidized biomedical research, Leake and other administrators changed their minds. While Congress was ultimately responsible for the total amount of money appropriated for research and the ways it would be disbursed among different government agencies, the NIH established a system of advisory councils and study sections composed of non-governmental biomedical scientists who evaluated research proposals and made final decisions about which projects to support. After a grant was awarded, the NIH offered no direction, permitted equipment purchased from grant funds to remain in the researcher's institution after the grant

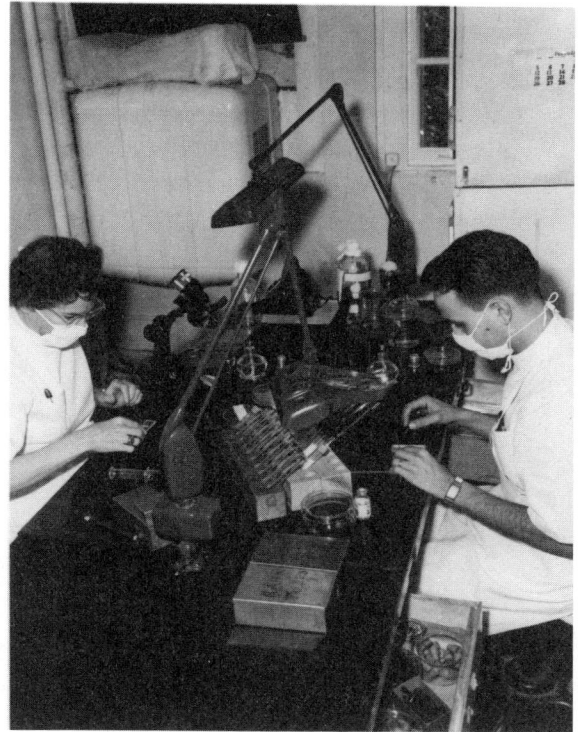

Eva Everett and Ulloa Gregory in the Tissue Culture Lab in the Graves Building during the 1950s.

ended, and monitored the grant only by requiring annual progress reports.[72]

With these guidelines and safeguards in place, Leake encouraged the faculty to apply for federal grants and contracts, and to solicit funds from private companies and foundations. In the summer of 1944 a federal agency, three drug companies, and two private organizations gave grants for research to some professors.[73] In the fall of 1947 seven professors received United States Public Health Service grants that totaled more than $40,000. Between September 1, 1946, and August 31, 1954, researchers received more than $800,000 in support from private sources.[74]

With the impressive changes in infrastructure Leake and departmental chairs fostered, UTMB moved into its second half-century with a new emphasis on inquiry and research. By 1945 nearly every member of each basic science department and some members of each clinical department were involved in a research project.[75] By 1947 eighteen faculty members (thirteen basic science and five clinical) considered themselves qualified to supervise graduate students who wanted to work on Ph.D. degrees in Galveston. Collectively, this group had contributed more than one thousand articles to scientific and clinical journals. Public recognition of this research enterprise reached a new local high in 1951 when the *Galveston Daily News* devoted a full page to a pictorial review of seven faculty working in their labs: Anigstein, Blocker, Gregory, Herrmann, Wiktor Nowinski, Pollard, and Howard Swann.[76]

Leake had enthusiastically supported these and other professors who directed certain research labs at UTMB: the Tissue Culture Laboratory (Pomerat), Tissue Metabolism Laboratory (Nowinski), Rickettsial Research Laboratory (Anigstein), Virus Research Laboratory (Pollard), Laboratory of Industrial Hygiene (Nau), Microbiology Laboratory (Packchanian), Laboratory of Experimental Pathology (Rigdon), Cardiovascular Research Laboratory (Herrmann), Hematology Research Laboratory (Levin), Surgical Research Laboratory (Moore), and the John Sealy Memorial Research Laboratory (Gregory).[77]

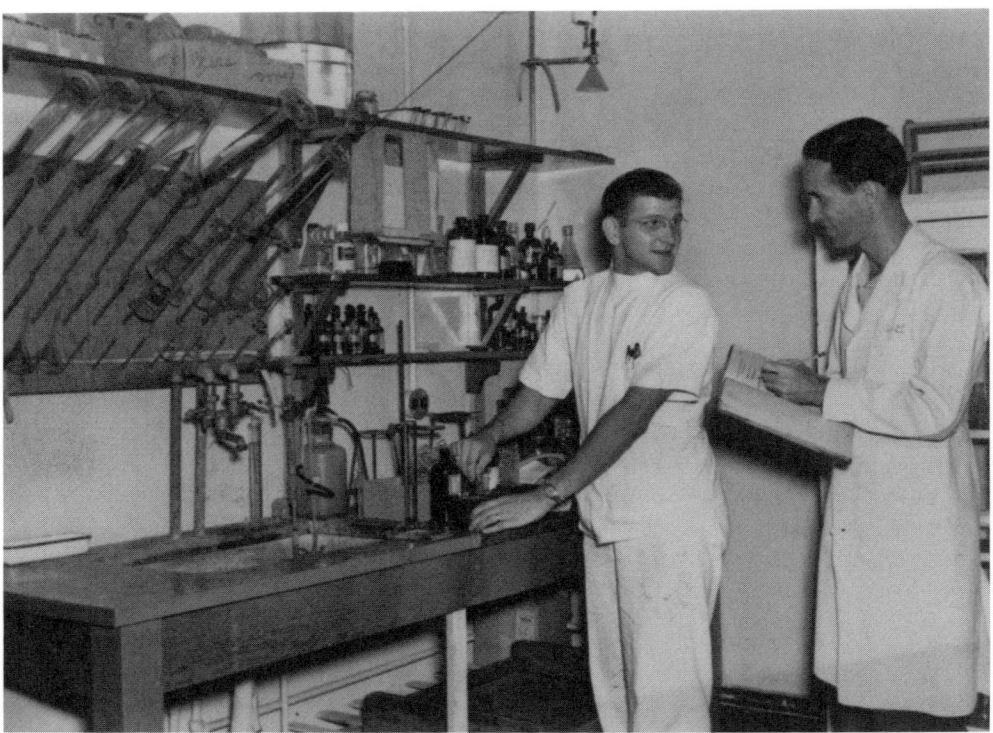

The lab of Wendell Gingrich (far right), 1946.

Nowinski was a European-trained biochemist whom Pomerat hired as a research associate in 1946. In 1951 Nowinski established the Tissue Metabolism Laboratory on the fourth floor of the State Psychopathic Hospital. This lab was moved to the second floor of the Ashbel Smith Building in 1952 and, later, to the Shriners Burns Institute. Nowinski collaborated with numerous faculty on such research projects as metabolic changes in severely burned patients, metabolic requirements during normal growth, hereditary abnormalities of hemoglobin, enzymatic changes in kidneys caused by hypertension, and metabolites excreted in the urine of manic-depressive patients.[78]

Started in 1947 by Raymond H. Rigdon, the Laboratory of Experimental Pathology was located in the basement of the Keiller Building. During the 1950s and 1960s Rigdon studied changes in the blood cells of ducks caused by certain drugs, the effects of certain carcinogens in ducks, and pathological processes in vitamin A-deficient ducks.[79]

Bill Levin directed the research lab in the Division of Hematology for almost thirty years (1946–1975). Levin supported Rose Schneider's work, did collaborative research with other faculty, and obtained a training grant that supported research fellows in hematology.[80]

In addition to support of these specialized labs, Leake and departmental chairs made research a prominent feature of most departments. These features changed as departmental chairs changed, as new faculty began projects, and as more professors secured funds for their research activities.

After Mason Guest became chair of the Physiology Department in 1951, the Carter Physiological Laboratory moved to the second floor of the new Gail Borden Building in 1952. By the mid-1950s Guest, the Halls (Charles and Octavia), Howard Swann, Gerald Seaman, and others investigated the effects of excess potassium on the mammalian heart, functional enlargements of the kidney, cellular changes of acetate and succinate metabolism, neurophysiological reflex actions, diseases in parabiotic rats, and blood clotting and lysing mechanisms.[81]

In 1955 three lab assistants in the Department of Bacteriology and Parasitology assisted faculty in conducting diagnostic tests for inpatients, and they assisted professors and their graduate students with experimental research projects. Mildred Wegner and Etta Mae MacDonald worked in the mycology (fungi) lab. As McLaughlin Fellows, Joe Breckenridge and Warren Stinebring worked with Harriet Felton in the cytology lab. Other faculty included Mary Louise Sigtenhorst in the eye lab, Jim Johnson in the bacterial metabolism lab, Gingrich and Edith Box in the malaria research lab, and Packchanian in the microbiology lab.[82]

The Department of Biochemistry and Nutrition occupied the fourth floor of the Gail Borden Building in the mid-1950s. Lothar Salomon studied the metabolism of ascorbic acid (vitamin C), and Forrest Gish Houston studied trace elements and chelating reactions. Gordon Mills explored the intricacies of red blood cell metabolism, and David Celander studied various aspects of amino acid metabolism.[83]

Professors in clinical departments assessed the efficacy of new drugs in both humans and other mammals. Arthur Ruskin, George Herrmann, Milton Hejtmancik, Raymond Gregory, and John Middleton were among the members of the Department of Internal Medicine who engaged in such studies. Herrmann described the successful use of two drugs: thiomerin in a twenty-three-year-old woman who had thyrotoxic heart disease and aminophyllin in a fifty-year-old man who had rheumatic heart disease and mild congestive failure. Working with Nowinski, for example, Ruskin investigated the effects of mercurial diuretics on the cardiac and renal functions of rats.[84]

G. W. N. Eggers, Truman Blocker, and Edgar Poth were key researchers in the Department of Surgery. Working with Pomerat and others during the 1940s, Eggers demonstrated that pressure splints applied to injured bones increased the rate of healing. Further studies demonstrated that stainless steel splints applied loosely over fracture sites allowed muscle movement and more rapid healing. In 1949 the American Academy of Orthopedic Surgery gave Eggers a gold medal to honor his research. In 1952 the International Society of Surgery gave him another gold medal in recognition of his outstanding discoveries.[85]

Blocker became the "center of gravity" for an enormous amount of clinical and mammalian research about thermal injury. Between 1950 and 1968 he and his colleagues received many federal dollars from contracts with the U.S. Army Medical Research and Development Command and the U.S. Air Force. Blocker also received several United States Public Health Service contracts and grants.[86]

The initial Army contract (DA-49-007-MD-32) funded studies about skin grafting and infection performed by various groups between 1950 and 1953. Other clinical research included studies of burn anemia, antibiotics, biochemical alterations in burns, bone and joint changes in burned patients, microbial growth in burn wounds, debriding agents, drug toxicity, high protein feedings, and lymphodynamics in burned patients. Experimental studies included the effects of hypothermia on burns in rats and dogs, and the effects of certain drugs on burns in rabbits.[87]

Poth directed the Surgical Research Laboratory between 1943 and 1961. A member of the Department of Surgery for more than forty years, he devoted much of his life to research about the best ways to induce intestinal antisepsis before bowel surgery. Someone estimated that the adoption of Poth's recommendations about using sulfa drugs before intestinal surgery had saved an estimated 250,000 lives by 1957.[88]

Even with all of these remarkable accomplishments, the research enterprise still lagged behind the patient care and teaching missions when John Truslow became CEO in 1956. Truslow appointed Don Micks chair of the Research Committee, which included Otto Bessey, Blocker, Duncan, Milton Hejtmancik, Theodore Panos, Pomerat, Poth, and Swann. Truslow wanted this group to oversee animal care facilities, government grants and contracts, the McLaughlin Fellowships, and resources of information about grants. This committee told Truslow that the research budget of approximately $1 million in 1956 reflected "an institutional indifference toward the development of a first-class research center." Without more support for research, UTMB would remain in the "rut of 'back-patting' complacency."[89]

Two surveys in 1958 offered explanations for this alleged indifference. The report of the Committee of 75 highlighted the unsatisfactory conditions for research in the physical plant and the need to add scholars of international reputation to the faculty. The survey of the James A. Hamilton Associates explained the inadequacies as follows:

Reasons advanced for lack of a strong research role were many, but there was general agreement that research has not been encouraged by the university or Branch management in the past; the faculty as a whole has not been research minded; there has been a serious lack of research laboratory facilities; the legislature and state government officials have been unsympathetic toward a research role for the Branch; the level of private practice of full-time faculty has inhibited the development of research and the part-time faculty are generally preoccupied; and the heavy teaching load resulting from the increase in the undergraduate enrollment absorbed the time of faculty which would have been available to pursue research.[90]

Though displaying some rhetorical overkill and distortions, this critique did acknowledge the extensive institutional network required for adequate research and the need for a more systematic development of this network.

Two years earlier Truslow had established a Grants and Contracts Office with a full-time secretary. Don Micks was director until 1958, when D. Bailey Calvin resigned as dean of students and became director of the Office of Research Grants and Contracts. For the first time in its history, a full-time administrator managed the research mission.

When Calvin left in 1964 Truslow assigned the responsibilities of this role to his assistant dean, Spencer Thompson.[91]

With these changes, the administrative infrastructure supporting the research mission improved significantly. Faculty and students steadily engaged in many research projects funded by private and federal dollars during the 1950s and early 1960s.

Private dollars came from the Medical Research Foundation of Texas, the McLaughlin Endowment, and the Harris and Eliza Kempner Fund. In 1955 H. W. Paley announced the creation of the Medical Research Foundation of Texas.[92] The establishment of this foundation reflected a belief that research at UTMB was an enterprise worthy of considerably more support that it had received in the past. In March 1958 this foundation gave grants of $25,000 to researchers in Texas, including $5,000 to support the work of seven professors at UTMB. In 1959 the foundation awarded $5,500 to UTMB researchers; $7,500 in 1960.[93]

The McLaughlin Endowment was far more successful in stimulating research. In 1954 UTMB awarded the first McLaughlin Fellowships for the Investigation of Infection and Immunity.[94] In 1955 the endowment supported thirty-four fellows: eighteen medical student fellows, eleven pre-doctoral fellows, three postdoctoral awards (including fellowships for study at the Institute of Brain Anatomy and the Neurological Polyclinic in Zurich, and the Pasteur Institute in Paris), and two faculty fellowships for study in South America and Italy. Pierre Grabar, chief of the immunochemistry section of the Pasteur Institute in Paris, became the first senior McLaughlin Fellow. He worked with Pomerat and Nowinski for two months in the spring of 1955. For fiscal year 1958, the McLaughlin Fund provided funding for five postdoctoral fellows, one faculty fellow, and twenty-six medical student fellows.[95]

The McLaughlin Fellowships touched almost every part of UTMB's research community. They provided medical students an opportunity to conduct research. They strengthened the graduate program by funding students from around the world who wanted to earn graduate degrees at UTMB. They invigorated faculty by attracting postdoctoral fellows to their research laboratories. They enabled certain faculty to learn new techniques in research centers elsewhere. They brought outstanding researchers to Galveston as lecturers for short visits and as distinguished fellows for long-term visits.[96]

In 1957 the Harris and Eliza Kempner Fund established an endowment to fund Jeane B. Kempner scholarships that provided support for those "pursuing advanced studies in the fields of internal medicine and surgery." Both graduate students and medical students were eligible for these awards. The first Kempner scholar was Samuel Kolmen, a Graduate School of the Biomedical Sciences doctoral graduate who studied in London for a year before returning to UTMB as a professor in the Department of Physiology.[97]

In addition to these private dollars, professors attracted more federal dollars for research and research training. In 1958 Dean Kenneth Earle received a NIH grant of $75,000 to support a training program in neuropathology, and Donald Duncan and

Keith O'Steen received a NIH grant of $125,000 to support a medical student "research training" program.[98] Students received stipends as they worked in faculty research labs, mostly during summer vacations.

These training grants also went to other schools, thereby producing a cadre of young investigators eager to report on their research. In 1959 three professors, James Warren, Glenn Russell, and Willard Verwey, gave special support to three medical students, Ann Cook, J. J. Leonard, and Fred Stegall, who organized a conference for these research-minded students. Between sixty and seventy-five students from schools in Texas, Oklahoma, Arkansas, Louisiana, and Tennessee met at the Galvez Hotel in March 1960. This was UTMB's first Student Research Forum. In March 1962 more than four hundred people attended the third forum, where participants from eleven medical schools presented forty-two papers.[99] The Student Research Forum signaled a new level of extraordinary support from administrators, faculty, and students for the biomedical research enterprise in the United States. UTMB's alleged "indifference" to its research mission had faded in a few short years.

During the early 1960s professors successfully competed for more federal and private dollars for research. Between July 1, 1959, and June 30, 1960, research grants and contracts reached an all-time high of $1,775,900, double the amount received just three years earlier. Four federal agencies and fifty-one private sources provided dollars to seventy-one individuals from each of the medical school's sixteen departments and the nursing school. In 1962 the total was $2,684,603, more than three times the amount received five years earlier. In 1964 the total was more than $3 million. With this rapid increase in dollar support, peers and patrons acknowledged the outstanding quality of research at UTMB.[100]

Research productivity became the dominant missions of the School of Medicine's basic science departments. Like their peers at other American medical schools, these professors used new research tools and techniques to study the physical and chemical laws underlying cellular and molecular dynamics.[101]

Between 1948 and 1958 Donald Duncan, Charles Pomerat, and their colleagues in the Department of Anatomy wrote about three hundred publications describing their research discoveries. Using an electron microscope acquired in 1956, Duncan and others studied the early stages of the chick embryo, the malarial parasite in blood, and carotid bodies. In fiscal year 1961, for example, ten professors in the Department of Anatomy worked on fifteen different research projects and contributed forty articles to the scientific literature.[102]

In 1960 A. W. B. Cunningham, associate professor of pathology, and his team of researchers recorded spontaneous electrical currents from explants of brain tissue for as long as fourteen days. Thought to be the first observations of their kind, the tissue cultures were from the developing brains of birds and mammals. These techniques were used to trace the origin and spread of electrical activity during embryological development. In July 1962 a leased IBM 1620 began processing research data from thousands of punch cards associated with this brain cell research. Truslow appointed Cunningham

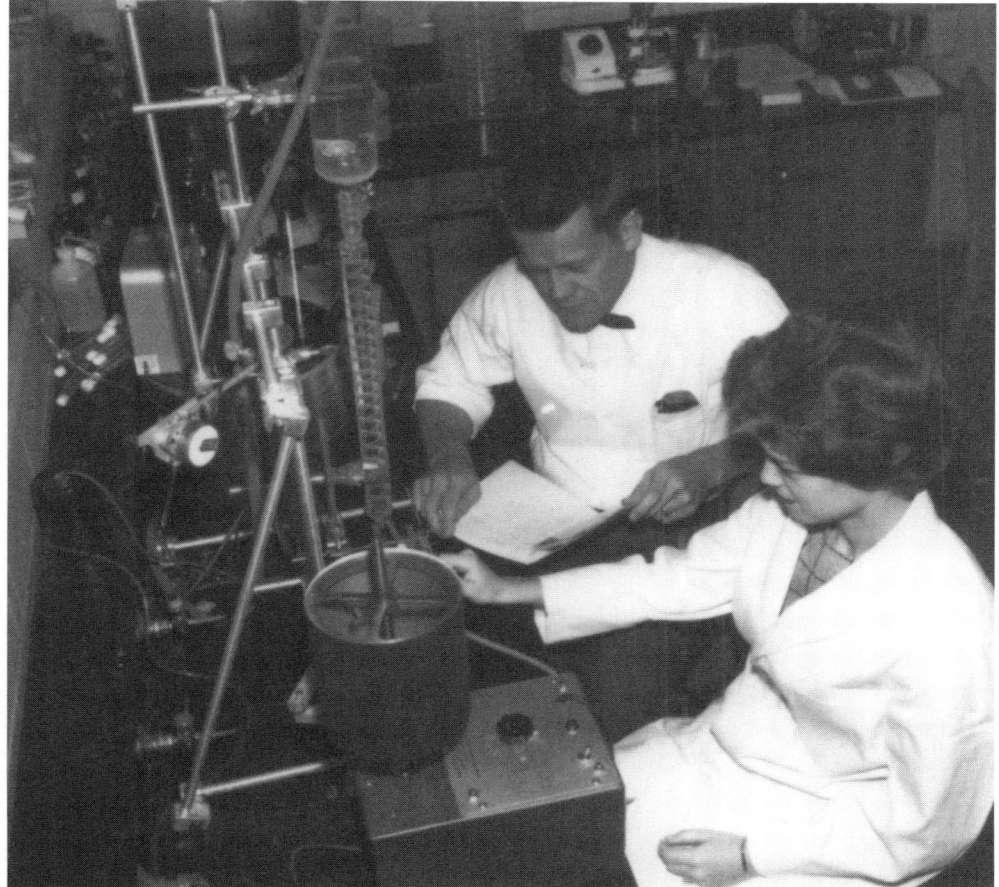

Leroy Olson and Amber Sharp in Microbiology Lab, Gail Border Building, c. 1960.

as director of the Research Computation Center and several researchers began learning "Fortran" so they could use the new equipment.[103]

All forty-one employees in the Department of Microbiology participated in the department's research efforts. These included four animal caretakers, four secretaries, and five research technicians plus seven assistants, six graduate students, two postdoctoral fellows, two research associates, and eleven professors. They worked collaboratively in labs located on the third floor of the Gail Borden Building, the basement of the Keiller Building, and the third floor of the Ashbel Smith Building.[104]

Professors used grant dollars to purchase needed equipment. In 1960, for example, the Department of Pathology acquired an electron microscope, the third at UTMB. Soon thereafter this instrument was used to study renal disease in children, a collaborative project involving Howard Hopps, Robert Turner, Bill Daeschner, and Warren Dodge. In 1961 UTMB acquired a powerful ultracentrifuge that could be used in research projects conducted by Levin (abnormal proteins in blood serum), Gerald Seaman (production of protein by bacteria), Blocker (protein metabolism of burned patients), and Guest (enzymes in blood clotting). Levin directed numerous projects during the 1960s, including studies of protein abnormalities in cancer and drugs used for chemotherapy.[105]

Dollars from grants also permitted researchers to present numerous papers about their discoveries during meetings of national and international societies. Charles Hall and Edward Rennels gave papers during the First International Congress of Endocrinology in Copenhagen in 1960. Hall studied hypertension produced with adrenal hormones in hypophysectomized rats and Rennels studied the effects of burn injuries on cells in the pituitary glands of rats. In 1962 Levin, Bill DeGroot, Guest, Dan Traber, and Don Stubbs were among the faculty who presented research reports at the annual meeting of the Federation of American Societies for Experimental Biology in Atlantic City.[106]

Astonishing improvements in the research enterprise had occurred at UTMB during these years, but more were needed. In fiscal year 1960 UTMB's total expenditures for research and research training was about 25 percent below the average expended by sixteen public medical schools and by fiscal year 1962 the difference was even greater.[107] In 1962 the survey team representing the American Medical Association and the Association of American Medical Colleges commended three departments for achieving a good balance of research, teaching, and service: Anatomy, Pathology, and Obstetrics and Gynecology. But the team thought that the Departments of Biochemistry, Internal Medicine, and Surgery fell far short of honoring the mission of research in a modern medical school.[108]

Later that same year, however, UTMB received a genuine boost to its research mission when the U.S. Public Health Service awarded a grant of $315,000 for establishing a Clinical Research Center (CRC). Bill Levin was the project's director and George Bryan the assistant director. On June 24, 1963, Bryan and Warren Dodge became the first investigators to admit patients to the CRC, a ten-bed unit located on Unit 4C of the John Sealy Hospital.[109]

In that same year, a grant from the National Foundation of Infantile Paralysis to Bill Daeschner and the Department of Pediatrics for the establishment of a birth defects research center prompted a *Galveston Daily News* editor to applaud UTMB's "new achievement—wider recognition as an important research center."[110] There was more pride about research accomplishments at UTMB than ever before.

Inquiry and research at UTMB between 1942 and 1964 also included some projects in the behavioral and social sciences as well as in the humanities.

Behavioral and social sciences research began during the mid-1950s. The Department of Psychiatry hired Gartley Jaco, a sociologist, to conduct research on social variables associated with mental disorders, a project funded by the Russell Sage Foundation. In one project, Jaco studied geographic distribution, age, sex, ethnicity, occupation, marital status, and sources of treatment of all patients in Texas who were diagnosed as psychotic during fiscal year 1952.[111] The Hogg Foundation for Mental Health provided support for the neurobiological and behavioral studies of Jaco, Swann,

Austin Foster, and Glenn Russell.[112] Harold Goolishian, a clinical psychologist in this department, received some USPHS grants in the late 1950s and early 1960s for developing a multiple-impact psychotherapy program. Goolishian also received United States Public Health Service grants for a study of behavioral dynamics in families with children who were considered delinquent. In 1962 Titus Harris hired Ernest S. Barratt as the department's first full-time experimental psychologist.[113]

School of Nursing professors also initiated some behavioral research projects. In the late 1950s and early 1960s Marjorie Bartholf received some USPHS grants to study ways to improve the teaching of maternal and infant care. Betty Beaudry analyzed the hierarchies of nursing service administration and Lucille Moore investigated the psychological needs of nursing students before they began their professional studies. Bartholf also began a longitudinal study of performance variables in nursing education that Betty Rudnick continued.[114]

Inquiry in the humanities was a special feature of research developments at UTMB during these years. During his years as a teacher of philosophy and history between 1953 and 1962, Patrick Romanell wrote four books, twenty articles, and twenty-three book reviews, some in Spanish and Italian.[115] Leake wrote numerous publications involving the history and philosophy of medicine, including four books, thirteen articles, and eighteen book reviews. As editor of *Texas Reports on Biology and Medicine*, Leake's educational visions shaped the only American medical journal that included articles dealing with experimental research, clinical reports, behavioral studies, and humanities topics.[116] At the middle of the twentieth century, no other American medical school had a professional philosopher as a faculty member and a CEO who was a practicing scholar in the medical humanities.

FROM BLOCKER TO JAMES, 1964–1991

UTMB's professors significantly improved their productivity as researchers between 1964 and 1991. During 1968 and 1969 they wrote at least 320 articles for scientific and clinical journals. In 1989 alone they wrote 468 articles that were published in journals or as chapters in books. Many of these publications involved experimental research conducted in basic science labs, hospital wards, and the CRC. Like their peers in other American medical schools, UTMB's experimental scientists investigated significant problems in the neurosciences, cell biology, molecular biology, and immunology. Other publications by UTMB's professors involved behavioral and social studies that relied on statistical analyses, or perspectives from the medical humanities.[117]

Administrators significantly expanded support for the infrastructure researchers needed. The presidents and deans selected full-time administrators to coordinate the research enterprise, expected departmental chairs to hire and support faculty as researchers, and encouraged the research interests of graduate students and medical students, especially by giving enthusiastic support to the National Student Research Forum.[118] The Graduate School of the Biomedical Sciences became a more independent enterprise, long overdue laboratory space became available for several departments, specialized research institutes and centers were established, dollars from federal sources and local foundations expanded significantly, and administrators and faculty established a variety of committees to deal with the growing number of federal regulations. Providing examples of these developments and accomplishments, the following paragraphs are arranged according to the years of Blocker's tenure as CEO, then those of Levin, and finally those of James.

UT System executives, such as LeMaistre and Knisely, strongly supported Blocker, White, and Brandt as they championed the research mission. They worked closely with Spencer Thompson, who managed the funding program for research between 1964 and 1980. By 1965 these leaders understood that UTMB trailed Baylor, UT Southwestern in Dallas,

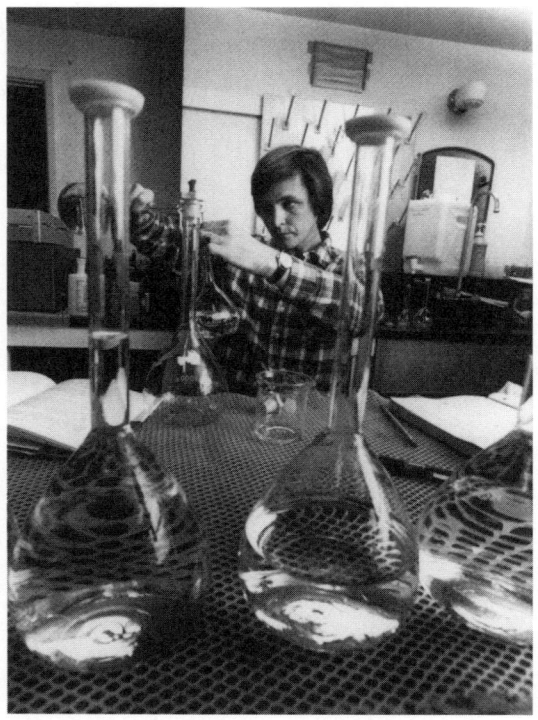

John Forsythe conducting experiments with squids in a Marine Biomedical Institute lab, 1985.

and UT Houston as competitors for federal research grants. They urged professors to become more aggressive in submitting requests for contracts and grants from federal agencies, and for grants from private foundations. Research grant support significantly increased for the schools and institutes (Appendices AG and AH).[119]

Blocker wanted more research-related buildings on the campus. The Surgical Research Laboratory was expanded and incorporated into the Shriners Burns Institute in 1966. Early in that same year, Blocker asked Sen. Ralph Yarborough to lobby for proposals to the Department of Health, Education and Welfare's Division of Research Facilities and Resources requesting federal dollars to help construct an animal care facility, a basic sciences building, and a clinical sciences building.[120] As described in chapter four, these new buildings substantially increased research-related space.

With these improvements in political advocacy, economic support, and more space for labs, departmental chairs added many research-minded professors between 1964 and 1974, sixteen in the Human Biological Chemistry and Human Genetics Department between 1971 and 1973, to give just one example. Pathbreaking discoveries occurred in this department. In 1969 and 1970 Barbara Bowman, Lillian Lockhart, and graduate student Michael McCombs identified a protein in the blood of patients with cystic fibrosis that was believed to be one of the causative factors in this disease. This protein disrupted the rhythmic patterns of cilia in oysters from

Galveston Bay, cilia that functioned similarly to those in the human respiratory tract. In 1973 Bowman and Don Barnett isolated this protein from tissue cultures of skin from cystic fibrosis patients.[121]

Other basic science researchers flourished. In 1967 Rose Schneider received another grant from the NIH to support her seventeenth year of research on genetically variant hemoglobins. By combining fluorescent dyes with antibodies specifically produced against a particular hemoglobin, Schneider studied the location and arrangement of hemoglobins in red blood cells. In 1968 she presented papers at the twelfth International Congress of Genetics in Tokyo and at the twelfth Congress of the International Society of Hematology in New York City. In 1970 she attended meetings in Germany and Czechoslovakia to report on her discoveries of more than ten hemo-globin variants. By that year, Schneider had received more than half a million dollars in research grants.[122]

Some basic scientists wanted specialized research units. Blocker focused much administrative enthusiasm on the creation of a research institute that exploited Galveston's marine environment. In 1968 the UT regents and Texas A&M University directors established the Marine Biomedical Institute for the purpose of advancing "the understanding of the biomedical sciences through research and education associated with the marine environment."[123] Its founders believed that it was the "first marine sci-ence institute devoted specifically to the exploration and solution of problems in bio-medicine and human ecology." In 1969 Stewart Wolf, Regents Professor of Medicine and Psychiatry at the University of Oklahoma, became the first director.[124]

By 1972 the Marine Biomedical Institute's members focused on five areas of research. Wolf directed studies in neurocardiology and William D. Willis Jr. directed studies in comparative neurobiology. James E. Blankenship led those investigating invertebrates. Bernard Haber directed research on the biochemistry of neurotrans-mitters. Edward Beckman led those investigating human adaptation to an underwa-ter environment.[125] In 1973 the Marine Biomedical Institute included sixteen mem-bers with faculty appointments in eight academic departments, five research scien-tists and associates, fifteen graduate students, eleven postdoctoral fellows, and two visiting scientists.[126]

Professors in clinical departments increased their research productivity during Blocker's tenure as CEO. Some published case reports, sustaining the tradition begun by their predecessors in the 1890s. Warren Dodge, Luther Travis, and others traced the long-term effects of post-streptococcal glomerulonephritis in children, discovering that healing usually occurred between two and ten years after the onset of the disease. Marcel Patterson and colleagues reviewed their experiences with seventeen men who were treated for amebic abscesses of the liver between 1956 and 1966.[127]

Some chairs of clinical departments established "basic science" research units in their departments. In 1972 Ron Bailey, chair of the Department of Otolaryngology, hired Manning Correia, an aviation psychologist and vestibular physiologist, as director of a research division in this department.

Other chairs and professors in clinical departments became involved with experimental research involving both humans and other species. In 1964, for example, faculty and students busily worked on a variety of projects in the new Surgical Research Lab. Several studied gastrointestinal problems with Curtis Artz. James Kent investigated a "quick freeze" method for treating ulcers. James Winn studied the use of liquid nitrogen for treating ulcers. Glen Guillet developed ways to use pieces of small intestine to replace a damaged esophagus. Ira Tunnel tested the efficacy of two new drugs used in treating burned patients and John Baker evaluated the benefits of a new high-protein concentrate given orally to seriously ill or injured patients. Some students worked with John Derrick in developing new surgical techniques for treating cardiovascular diseases; others worked with Steve Lewis and John Lynch in devising new cleft palate reconstruction techniques.[128]

Directed by Levin and Bryan between 1963 and 1975, the Clinical Research Center was the principal facility for research using human subjects. In 1968, for example, Harry Sarles, Ray Remmers, Al LeBlanc and others studied sodium excretion patterns in twenty-six pregnant patients hospitalized in the Clinical Research Center. Sarles, Remmers, and Jay Fish discovered ways to reduce the number of blood T-cells in prospective patients by thoracic duct drainage, thereby reducing the likelihood of the rejection of a transplanted kidney. In 1969 Bill DeGroot and Robert Cooley assessed the effectiveness of urokinase in dissolving pulmonary emboli. In 1970 Willard Verwey and Yoshikazu Watanabe tested cholera vaccines in human subjects.[129]

Clinical research was also conducted in other hospital areas. In 1965 fifteen beds in Randall Pavilion were assigned to patients participating in psychiatric research projects. Joe Tupin and colleagues discovered that lithium carbonate administered to four normal subjects and five manic-depressive patients affected the urinary excretion of sodium, calcium, and magnesium.[130]

A few professors received grants for behavioral and social science research from the NIH, the Hogg Foundation, and the Kempner Fund. During the 1960s Ernie Barratt and colleagues received several grants to study impulsive behavior in monkeys, cats, and opossums. In 1967 Barratt received a Hogg Foundation grant to study the effects of school integration on academic performance in high school males. In 1973 Perrie Adams received a NIH grant to study the effects of chronic marijuana use on sleep patterns in primates.[131]

Students participated in these research projects. Administrators and faculty continued to sponsor the National Student Research Forum as an annual opportunity for reports by medical students, house staff, and graduate students. In 1964 ninety-six papers were presented during the fifth forum, which more than four hundred people from twenty-eight schools in nineteen states attended. In 1968 the Student American Medical Association became a co-sponsor of the forum. Almost 140 papers were presented during the 1974 forum.[132]

In addition to this forum, the faculty continued to sponsor a federally funded research training program for medical students. During the summer of 1965, the eighth year of this program, the participants even included twelve students who would matriculate as freshmen later in the fall. In 1970 research fellowships were awarded to twenty-three students.[133]

The expansion of research productivity by faculty and students during these years depended on such support services as the Research Computation Center, the Animal Care Center, and the Biomedical Engineering Shop.[134]

During the 1960s John Overall, then Vernon Benignus, directed the Research Computation Center. During fiscal year 1965, more than fifty people used this center for keypunching services, courses in Fortran and programming, and consultations about the best statistical approaches for specific projects. To provide space for a new IBM 1800 system, Benignus and five staff members moved to new quarters at Mechanic and Tenth Streets in 1968.[135]

In 1963 Abe Levy, a veterinarian, became director of the Animal Care Center. By 1968 this center functioned with twenty-two staff members, who moved to a new building the following year.[136]

In 1965 Norman Welford became director of the Biomedical Engineering Shop. He and his staff repaired, designed, and maintained equipment many researchers used. In 1968 this shop was located in the basement of Psycho One and directed by James A. "Mac" McKay and his assistant, K. T. McClendon. Examples of their work included a stainless steel skull plug used in photo animation, a kidney bath for research, and cat and mice holders for inoculation purposes.[137]

Expanded productivity was also fostered by the continued publication of *Texas Reports on Biology and Medicine*. Between 1964 and 1974, seven professors were editors of *Texas Reports on Biology and Medicine*: John Sinclair (1955–1961), Joe Bass (1962–1964), Samuel Kolmen (1965–1967), Melvyn Schreiber (1968–1970), Robert D. Yates (1971–1972), and James Guckian (1973–1974). Most of the journal's articles involved experimental studies in the biomedical sciences, though a few were behavioral studies.[138] The issue published in June 1966 celebrating UTMB's seventy-fifth anniversary included poems, cartoons, short stories, and art by some employees, and the large issue published in May 1974 was devoted to the humanities and medicine.

UTMB's research enterprise expanded even more during Levin's years as CEO. Levin, Brandt, and Bryan worked closely with Spencer Thompson and David Tabaracci, who coordinated the research enterprise. After Thompson's retirement in 1980, Tabaracci continued to handle the "business office" details while Marjorie Forster and Ray Stinson were the general coordinators.

Levin, Bryan, and Saunders created new cheerleading networks. In 1977 Levin appointed Saunders as chair of a new advisory Research Council, which included the deans of the schools and directors of the institutes.[139] This council's discussions enabled the institution's leaders to make better decisions about improving the infra-structure for research.

In 1983 Bryan appointed a faculty task force to do a critical study of research at UTMB. This eleven-member group, chaired by Bob Rose, concluded that UTMB was only "in the middle ranks" among American medical schools with regard to the quality and quantity of its research. The faculty had "averaged fewer than three new federally funded grants per year involving clinical research for the entire School of Medicine" between 1978 and 1983. During these same years, only 1.5 full-time equivalent faculty in the fourteen clinical departments were supported by research grants. The task force recommended that administrative officers recruit "established research leaders," expect clinical chairs to support more research activities, and secure more funds for research.[140]

Levin and Bryan then harnessed the energies of the previous committees by establishing a Research Advisory Council for the entire institution and they fervently recruited "research leaders" as chairs of medical school departments. New chairs of School of Medicine basic science departments appointed during the 1980s included Cary Cooper (1982), Brad Thompson (1984), Bill Willis (1985), Harold Sandstead (1985), Luis Reuss (1986), and David Walker (1987).[141]

UTMB's research coffers filled steadily during these years. In December 1975 Brandt congratulated the faculty on their outstanding achievements in acquiring more dollars for research. The total for fiscal year 1975 was $9.2 million compared to $6.1 million in fiscal year 1973. Funds awarded to UTMB for research and research training during fiscal year 1979 increased by almost 25 percent over fiscal year 1978. Funding for research and research training surpassed $15,000,000 during each of the three fiscal years: 1980, 1981 and 1982.[142]

In 1981, however, other academic medical centers in Texas surpassed UTMB in attracting federal dollars for biomedical research. Saunders believed that UTMB had a top-heavy faculty of tenured professors who tended "to get lazy" as researchers. Yielding was surprised that grant proposals usually did not include faculty salaries and graduate student support, a phenomenon he labeled "a peculiar form of provincialism." This situation changed as outside funding for research increased 83 percent between 1982 and 1987. In 1987 researchers received 451 grants worth $28.6 million. A significant number of these grants came from private foundations and endowments. The McLaughlin Fund, the Harris and Eliza Kempner Fund, the Moody Foundation, and the Hogg Foundation contributed many dollars for research at UTMB.[143]

A watershed event occurred in 1986 when the Sealy & Smith Foundation established the John Sealy Memorial Endowment Fund for Biomedical Research with a gift of $5 million. "Medical excellence is more dependent than ever on research funding," asserted Ballinger Mills Jr., the foundation's president. The UT regents added a like amount, thereby securing a total endowment of $10 million. Two years later the total increased to $20 million with duplicate gifts from the foundation and the regents.[144]

In addition to substantial increases in federal and private dollars, some institutional funds were used for research support. In 1982 the School of Medicine and the Graduate School of the Biomedical Sciences established an Intramural Research Grants Program. Eight faculty members received grants in 1982. Between 1982 and 1987, 133 professors received more than $1 million.[145]

A few professors hoped to acquire research dollars by forging new commercial links. By 1987 the faculty had made four invention/discoveries that merited license agreements negotiated with four commercial companies. These involved a urinary catheter, a brace for fractured hands, the manufacture of specific DNA sequences in certain recombinant procedures, and the purification and marketing of thymosin.[146]

Administrators and professors focused on other ways to enhance the research enterprise. New and renovated buildings added substantial research space. For basic science departments, these included the Pharmacology Building, the Microbiology Building, and the Maurice Ewing Hall. Labs with specialized equipment evolved, including those for bacterial fermentation, electron microscopy, histopathology, isolation of hybridomas, and tissue cultures. With the opening of its north and south additions in 1977 and 1978, additional space for clinical research became available in the John Sealy Hospital.

Equipment purchased for clinical diagnosis was also used for research. For example, an $850,000 Nuclear Magnetic Resonance Chemical Shift Imaging Unit was acquired in 1986, the first of its kind installed in an American academic medical center. Housed in a building adjacent to the Surgical Research Laboratory, this unit provided information about metabolites in various tissues, including the distribution of compounds composed of phosphorus, sodium, carbon, fluorine, and hydrogen. Radiologists collaborated with other faculty in using this unit for pioneering studies of normal and abnormal development in neonatal brains.[147]

Expansion of certain support offices and faculty committees lubricated the administrative infrastructure for research. In 1979 UTMB established the Office of Environmental Health and Safety, whose members monitored the regulation of biological hazards in research projects involving recombinant DNA and infectious agents; chemical hazards, including carcinogenic, toxic and flammable compounds; and radioactive substances.[148] Two committees were especially important: the Institutional Review Board, which evaluated all research proposals involving human subjects, and the Animal Care and Use Committee, which oversaw all aspects of the use of animals in experimental protocols.[149]

All of these improvements and enhancements created more favorable conditions for research by faculty and students between 1974 and 1987, especially in the Marine Biomedical Institute, the Surgical Research Lab, and the Clinical Research Center.

By 1974 the Marine Biomedical Institute included three divisions. Members in the Division of Comparative Neurobiology investigated neural mechanisms in pain, behavior, and learning; certain problems in neurochemistry; and the physiology of synaptic transmissions. Members of the Marine Medicine Division focused on the use of hyperbaric (high pressure) oxygen treatment for certain anaerobic infections. Members of the Division of Marine Biology and Resources focused on the neurobiology, ecology, and ethology of squids and octopuses. In 1978 Bill Willis, one of America's leading neuroscientists, became director of the Marine Biomedical Institute.[150]

By 1980 the Marine Biomedical Institute included fifteen members, sixteen associate members, and sixteen adjunct members. Working with their graduate students and postdoctoral fellows, they prepared more than three hundred publications between 1972 and 1980. Many members were neuroscientists who used a variety of techniques that included light and electron microscopy, pathways tracing, immuno-cytochemistry, tissue culture, microiontophoresis, gas chromatography and mass spectroscopy, high performance liquid chromatography, computerized models, nuclear magnetic resonance imaging, and behavioral paradigms. In fiscal year 1985, for example, these researchers received thirty-four grants from the National Institute of Neurological and Communicative Disorders and Stroke.[151]

These and other neuroscientists were affiliated with both basic science and clinical departments. J. Regino Perez-Polo, who became a faculty member in 1977, continued his efforts to identify and purify human nerve growth factor protein from placental tissue and measure the amount of this protein in various human tissues. By the late 1980s Perez-Polo, Carol Beck, and Karin Werrbach-Perez, were studying the ways that this protein helped nerve cells adapt to "toxic" molecules produced by aging, disease, and injury.[152]

John Russell, professor of physiology and biophysics, continued his studies of the transport of anions across nerve and muscle cell membranes. Between 1974 and 1988 he received more than $1 million in NIH grants. In 1988 he received the Jacob K. Javits Award for this scientific work.[153]

By 1979 the research section of the Department of Otolaryngology included three neuroscientists: Correia, Avrim Eden, and Ming-Duenn Ni. Each explored certain aspects of the inner ear's vestibular system responsible for balance. Eden studied the anatomical connections of the vestibular apparatus to the brain. Ni studied eye movements (nystagmus) produced by unusual stimulation of the vestibular system. Correia studied eletrical impulses transmitted through the first nerve fibers coming from the vestibular apparatus. These scientists also used data from patients treated in the department's vestibular clinic.[154]

Adrian Perachio became a member of Correia's team in 1979. In 1981 Correia was one of four university scientists invited to participate in a symposium on motion sickness convened in Moscow by the US/USSR Joint Working Group on Space Medicine and Biology. Golda Kevetter joined Correia's group in 1982 and was soon awarded a Research Career Development Grant from the NIH. In 1986 Perachio received a three-year NIH grant to continue studies of primary afferent cells in the vestibular system. By 1987 Correia, Perachio, and Kevetter were engaged in a joint US/USSR project named COSMOS. Members of this project studied the adaptation of animals to microgravity, a collaboration that resulted in two orbital missions over a period of five years. These researchers also received grants from NASA.[155]

Extraordinary work was done in the Surgical Biochemistry Laboratory during the 1970s and 1980s. Jim Thompson's studies in the metabolism of gastrointestinal hormones attracted many students, residents, and clinical fellows. Between 1970 and 1982 the lab's professors worked with more than forty "Research Fellows" and together they wrote more than 150 published articles.[156]

In 1982 Courtney Townsend Jr., one of Thompson's colleagues, received a five-year Research Career Development Award by the National Cancer Institute to support an investigation of the effects of gastrointestinal hormones on the growth of cancer. The overall objective of the research was to discover ways to modify the growth-stimulating effects of the hormones on tumor tissues. By 1986 these researchers had determined the enteric distribution of cholecystokinin, neurotensin, peptide YY, and other gastrointestinal hormones in several animal species. They had studied the metabolism of these hormones, including their roles in expediting and inhibiting the growth of tumors in the gastrointestinal tract. They had identified new relationships between gastrointestinal hormones and the gallbladder in certain patients afflicted with gallstones. They had also conducted long-term studies of thirty-four patients with gastrin-producing tumors.[157]

Several of these studies were conducted in the Clinical Research Center, which was directed by Phillip Poffenbarger between 1975 and 1981, and, afterward, by Walter J. Meyer III and J. Nevin Isenberg.[158] The center attracted more investigators: from nineteen in fiscal year 1964 to seventy-three in 1977 to ninety-five in 1987. Faculty in the Departments of Pediatrics, Medicine, and Surgery extensively used the Clinical Research Center. During the 1970s and 1980s these scientists annually wrote between twenty-five and thirty-five publications that reported the results of this clinical research.[159]

Jim Thompson and colleagues established the importance of serum gastrin measurements in the management of patients with Zollinger-Ellison Sydrome. After a ten-year study, Luther Travis and Warren Dodge demonstrated that the prognosis was excellent for children who developed glomerulonephritis after streptococcal infections. Andy Grant and others studied anaphylactic reactions induced by Polistes wasps, which are common in Texas. Eugene Flewellen and Thomas Nelson developed reliable tests for diagnosing a patient's susceptibility to malignant hyperthermia.

Robert Wolfe conducted extensive metabolic studies. Joseph Jorizzo studied skin diseases and inflammation of joints. Geraldine Powell investigated milk allergies in infants and Nevin Isenberg studied optimal postoperative management of infants with biliary atresia. John Remmers did research on sleep apnea and Bryan Holland investigated aldosterone and hypertension. Frank Gardner studied a drug, etiocholanolone, which stimulated blood cell production by the bone marrow.[160]

In 1983 the Clinical Research Center celebrated its twentieth anniversary with a birthday ceremony and a two-day scientific symposium. In 1989 the center received a five-year renewal grant of $6 million from the NIH. Meyer and Isenberg continued to direct the center as researchers continued their studies of diabetes, viral diseases, hormone regulators of growth, fat and vitamin absorption in chronic liver disease, the effect of cancer on fat metabolism, and the impact of bed rest and exercise on muscle protein metabolism.[161]

Other researchers used different labs located in basic science and clinical departments. Sam Baron, one of the world's leading immunologists, became chair of the

Department of Microbiology in 1975. By 1985 Baron's research group included Robert Fleischmann, Edwin Blalock, John Stanton, and Gary Kimpel.[162] These scientists made important discoveries about interferons. Certain combinations of interferons enhanced their actions against tumors. Gamma interferon, unlike alpha and beta, directly destroyed certain human tumor cells. Combining chemotherapy and hypothermia could protect against experimentally induced cancers. A new substance named "contact-blocking viral inhibitor" prevented infection by some tumor viruses.[163]

Another internationally acclaimed immunologist, Armond Goldman, became director of the Division of Immunology in the Department of Pediatrics in 1959. Goldman and C. Wayne Smith were the first scientists to demonstrate that white blood cells in human milk protected neonates and infants against microbial pathogens. Goldman collaborated with Randy Goldblum, Frank Schmalstieg, and others in determining the components of the chemical systems in human milk that offered this protection and accelerated the maturation of the infant's immune system. Goldman, Goldblum, Schmalstieg, and others also conducted important studies about genetic immunodeficiency diseases. In 1990 they discovered a combined immunodeficiency that led to the elucidation of the central role of the common gamma chain in the immunological system. This was the first discovery of a genetic defect by researchers at UTMB.[164]

Other specialized labs were established in clinical departments. In 1976 John Remmers and William J. DeGroot created a lab for studying sleep disorders, focusing initially on the pathogenesis of upper airway occlusion in certain patients with obstructive sleep apnea. This lab moved to the CRC in 1980. Sam Kuna opened a second one on Towers 5C in 1985. David Rassin and colleagues conducted numerous studies in the Developmental Nutrition and Metabolism Lab established in the Department of Pediatrics in 1980. In their labs on the fourth floor of the Clinical Sciences Building, J. Andrew Grant, Michael Lett-Brown, and David Thueson studied histamine-releasing factors (cytokines) that appeared to function in the pathogenesis of acute allergic diseases.[165]

Under the guidance of Robert Rose, UTMB established a Psychiatric Clinical Research Center (PCRC) that opened in 1984.[166] In 1989 Walter Meyer became director of the PCRC and Eric Smith became director of the PCRC's main lab. During the 1980s Meyer and Smith spearheaded numerous pioneering studies of interactions between the nervous, endocrine, and immune systems in mammals. Smith and J. Edwin Blalock discovered that white blood cells produced adrenocorticotropic hormone (ACTH). With others, they initiated several studies of the production of ACTH in certain stress syndromes such as depression and ways to alter these clinical states by inducing changes in the neuroendocrine and immune systems.[167]

In addition to the neurobehavioral research in the Department of Psychiatry and Behavioral Sciences, other School of Medicine faculty received grants for behavioral and social science research from the Hogg Foundation, Kempner Fund, and Moody Foundation. John Bruhn received three NIH grants that supported a study of ways to reinforce positive health behaviors in preschool children. In fiscal year 1982 Kyriakos Markides received a NIH grant to study the relevance of family relations to health behaviors in three generations of Chicanos. Markides received other NIH grants to conduct studies of aging and health among Mexican Americans. Maradee Davis, Tom Baranowski, Neal Krause, Guy Parcel, Harvey Levin, and David Chiriboga were others who received NIH grants for behavioral and social science studies.[168]

School of Allied Health Sciences and School of Nursing professors engaged in several behavioral research projects during the 1970s and 1980s. In the School of Allied Health Sciences, for example, Bruhn and David Cordova conducted several studies of wellness behavior. During fiscal year 1987, School of Allied Health Sciences faculty received more than $1 million in federal and private grants for research, especially in the areas of health education, health promotion, and gerontology.[169]

By the early 1980s more than twenty School of Nursing faculty were engaged in research about various problems in clinical nursing, nursing education, and nursing services. Harriett Chaney studied the management training needs of health service managers. Sandra Dale investigated the roles of school nurses. Jane DeLoach studied the post-operative consequences of obese patients who had small intestine bypasses. Sara Fuller analyzed the lead content of paper products used by preschool children. Janice Martin evaluated regimens that prepared patients for X-ray studies of the colon.[170]

Leadership and encouragement came from Mary Anne Sweeney after she became assistant dean for research and evaluation in 1985. By the mid-1980s School of Nursing faculty were involved in research projects pertaining to health promotion, geriatric care, the family, clinical practice relationships, nursing education, and nursing management.[171]

Humanities scholars at UTMB were strongly committed to research and inquiry. Between 1974 and 1979, for example, members of the Institute for the Medical Humanities wrote 14 books published as edited volumes or monographs; 130 essays published as articles in journals or chapters in books; and 78 other items published as book reviews, reports, and editorials. During the 1980s sessions were added to the National Student Research Forum for students presenting papers in the behavioral sciences and the humanities. In April 1984, 143 "students" from seventy-nine North American institutions, including twenty from UTMB, attended the silver anniversary meeting of this forum.[172]

Recognizing the vast improvements in research at UTMB and wanting even more accomplishments, the regents employed Thomas N. James as the new CEO in 1987 because they believed that he would catalyze more progress in fulfilling the university's research missions. Between 1987 and 1991 several personnel changes signaled attempts to streamline top-level administrative support for research. Lemone Yielding became UTMB's first vice president for research and Louis Sheppard was appointed as assistant, then associate vice president for research (Appendix B). In 1991 Dorothea Wilson replaced Sheppard.[173]

Within eight months of James's arrival, the permanent endowment for funding bio-medical research established by the Sealy & Smith Foundation had grown to $20 million. UTMB increased its research spending from $26.3 million in fiscal year 1988 (James's first year) to $33.5 million in fiscal year 1989. The faculty attracted about $25.2 million from federal agencies during a time when these agencies were cutting their total grants. In 1991 the Sealy & Smith Foundation gave an additional $5 million to the John Sealy Memorial Endowment Fund for Biomedical Research, making the endowment worth $50 million.[174]

Research activities soared to new heights between 1987 and 1991. In 1988 there were twenty-five fellows and eleven graduate students working on research projects in the Marine Biomedical Institute. The new Sealy Centers progressed in their development, especially in establishing labs with sophisticated equipment, such as the Protein Chemistry Laboratory and the Recombinant DNA Laboratory. Professor-researchers, assistants, and students participated in research adventures in nearly every academic division and department.[175]

In the Department of Human Biological Chemistry and Genetics, Brad Thompson (chair and Kempner Professor), Aubrey Thompson, Paul Weigel, and Darrell Carney steadily pursued their research interests. Thompson and colleagues investigated steroid hormone action. They demonstrated that the DNA binding region of the human glu-cocorticoid receptor is essential for glucocorticoids to lyse leukemic cells and that glu-cocorticoids depress the c-myc oncogene mRNA in leukemic cells. They were the first to determine the structural sequence of the human glucocorticoid receptor, making a clone possible.

Thompson and colleagues studied the mechanisms for the cytostatic actions of Cyclosporin A. They purified the glucocorticoid that regulated transcription initiation factor from RNA polymerase I, a landmark in understanding the antilymphoprolifera-tive effects of glucocorticoid. Weigel and colleagues studied the mechanisms by which liver cells internalized damaged glycoproteins (asialoglycoproteins) from the blood. Carney and colleagues studied the mechanisms by which thrombin initiates cell prolif-eration in wound healing.[176]

In the Division of Environmental Toxicology in the Department of Preventive Medicine and Community Health, Marvin Legator and colleagues made numerous pioneering contributions to the field of genetic toxicology. They exposed the fallacies of using non-mammalian systems for detecting mutagen-carcinogens and they devel-oped multi-endpoint tests for evaluating potential genotoxins in mammals.[177]

The basic research unit of the Department of Otolaryngology flourished. Adrian Perachio and Shawn Newlands conducted studies of vestibular plasticity. In 1991 Manning Correia received a seven-year, $1.7 million Claude Pepper Award from the National Institute on Deafness and Other Communication Disorders for support of his studies about ionic currents in hair cells of the inner ear.[178]

With a grant from the National Cancer Institute, James Belli studied radiation sen-sitivity in hamster cells that were resistant to a chemotherapy drug. Belli and colleagues wanted to discover the mechanisms by which these cells became resistant, hoping that it might be possible to overcome such resistance so that cancer cells would succumb more readily to a combination of chemotherapy and radiation therapy.[179]

Dan Traber, coordinator of research at the Shriners Burns Institute, continued studies of inhalation injuries associated with burns. Inhaling smoke causes increased bronchial blood flow and swelling of the airway, accumulation of water in the pulmonary alveoli, and changes in the pumping abilities of the heart. Traber and colleagues searched for ways to alter these deleterious effects.[180]

Other professors in the School of Medicine, School of Nursing, and School of Allied Health Sciences continued behavioral and social science studies. David Jenkins, Susan Weller, Kyriakos Markides and others were members of the Division of Sociomedical Sciences in the Department of Preventive Medicine and Community Health who received several grants for their research. In 1987 Markides reviewed much of his research in a book titled *Ethnicity and Aging.* In 1989 he became the founding editor of the *Journal of Aging and Health* and in 1990 he became director of this division.[181]

Between 1986 and 1991 the School of Nursing experienced unprecedented growth in research productivity. Ten projects involved geriatric care, maternal/infant care, prenatal care, care of cancer patients, and community health programs for battered women.[182]

Members of the Institute for the Medical Humanities continued their productivity as scholars. Some were involved in off-campus collaborative projects such as the creation of the *New Handbook of Texas* and others participated in six collaborative research conferences held in Galveston between 1983 and 1991: Aging and Meaning (1983), Nursing (1983), Survival (1985), Bioethics (1986), Critical Gerontology (1991), and Good Body (1991).[183] In 1984 Anne Hudson Jones became editor of *Literature and Medicine*, the first scholarly journal devoted to this interdisciplinary field. In 1987 the Institute for the Medical Humanities began publishing a semiannual compilation of reviews of books entitled *Medical Humanities Review* and in 1991 the institute began distributing *Aging and the Human Spirit* as a semiannual newsletter.[184]

The research programs at the Institute for the Medical Humanities received exceptional support in 1990 when the Houston Endowment awarded a grant of $1.5 million to establish the Jesse H. Jones Research Endowment in the Medical Humanities. A $500,000 matching grant from the NEH resulted in a total research endowment worth $2 million.

Between 1987 and 1991, Tom James recognized and supported the research mission in all of its vast breadth and depth. He helped recruit key research-professors such as Robert Hirschfeld as chair of Psychiatry; Stephen Spann as chair of Family Medicine; and Marvin Kronenberg as director of the Cardiology Division in the Internal Medicine Department. He supported the establishment of three new multidisciplinary research centers for environmental toxicology, tropical diseases, and wound healing. Partial funding for these centers came from the $175 million that had been acquired in the Centennial Capital Campaign. In 1991 UTMB received a $500,000 grant from the

Robert J. Kleberg Jr. and Helen C. Kleberg Foundation for the Center for Tropical Diseases and another $500,000 grant from the Amon G. Carter Foundation for the Center for Environmental Toxicology. By 1991 about 450 faculty and staff participated in research projects funded by about 520 grants.[185]

Perhaps James was so successful in leading improvements in the research enterprise because he himself continued to do research every week. From his days as a resident in internal medicine at the Henry Ford Hospital (1950–1953), James displayed an insatiable curiosity about cardiac function in humans and other mammals. To help explain why certain patients would die after air entered their hearts, for example, James and his colleagues studied the effects of air experimentally injected in the hearts of dogs.[186] James developed a perfusion technique that permitted sophisticated studies of certain anatomical, physiological, and pharmacological aspects of the canine heart. This technique was used to study sinus and A-V nodal rhythms, intracardiac reflexes, and the effects of digitalis, quinidine, ATP and related compounds, and acetylcholine.[187] Much of James's experimental work was designed to explain phenomena associated with the structures and functions of human hearts, healthy and diseased.

In addition to experimental studies, James displayed an unequalled interest in the comparative anatomy and pathology of the heart, focusing on the anatomy of coronary arteries and mapping the structures of sinus and A-V nodes as well as other components in the conduction systems of mammalian hearts.[188] Threaded throughout the vistas of James's curiosity is a primary interest in sick human hearts, especially those that manifest arrhythmias that cause sudden death in babies, young athletes, and others.[189]

In New Orleans, Detroit, Birmingham, and Galveston, James never ceased his quest for scientific knowledge. No previous CEO at UTMB had sustained an extensive involvement with research while functioning as the institution's top executive leader. Though some thought this energy misplaced as part of that role, others admired and respected the authenticity of his dedication to the advancement of medical knowledge. Nothing was more symbolic of his legacy and the momentum given to research during the 1980s and the 1990s than the dedication of the new Medical Research Building in April of UTMB's centennial year.[190]

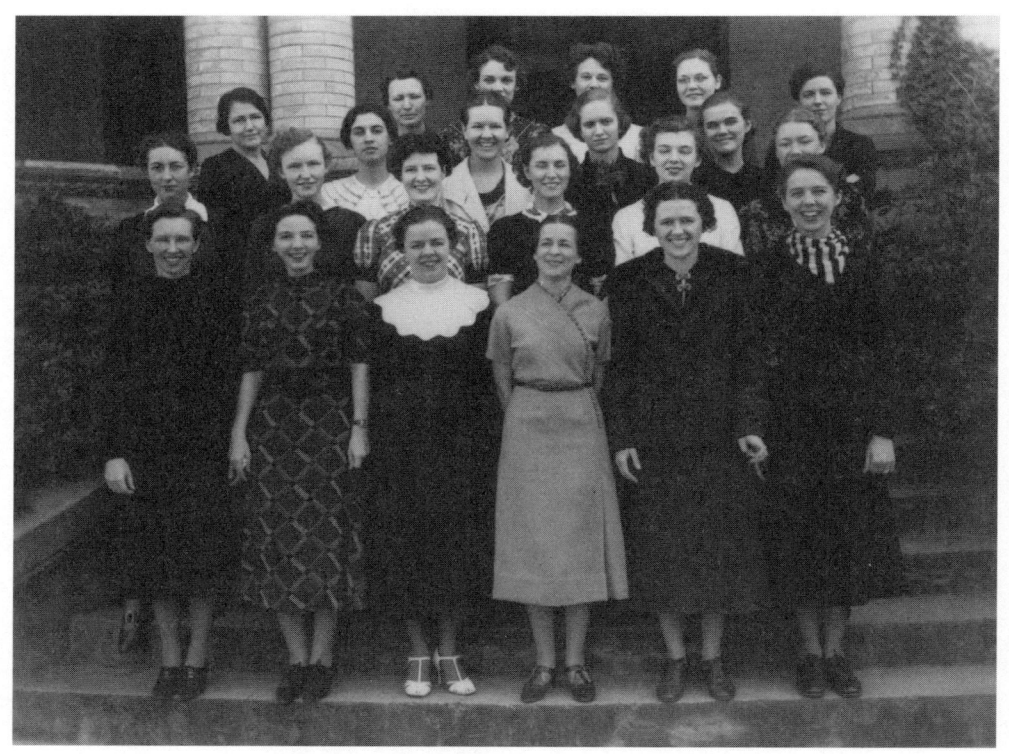

Female medical students, c. 1936–1937. Virginia Irvine is in the third row, second from right.

— 8 —

Identities, Rituals, Images—On Campus

"I had strangers fight with me and for me more than once—to drink a coke at a drugstore counter, to eat in a local restaurant, to have a professor replaced who repeatedly called an old Negro man sitting in a wheelchair in Grand Rounds, a Nigra."—Virginia Stull, School of Medicine class of 1966[1]

As the only black female in her graduating class in the mid-1960s, Virginia Stull experienced many emotional highs and lows during the years of the civil rights movement. Her memory reflects realities that were bound to the cultural and social changes of an era, but they also reflect the ever-recurring emotional predicament of every student who matriculated in a school at UTMB. Each was a stranger, and each wanted acceptance and respect as a person and a budding professional.

The same longing for acceptance and respect affected every other person connected with UTMB during its first century. Each brought specific identities to the institution. Though each wanted relief from suffering, a patient needing surgery for gallstones was not the same as one experiencing chronic depression. A microbiologist was not a neurosurgeon, but each wanted to progress from instructor to professor. A nursing student was not a medical student, though each wanted to become a graduating senior. A secretary was not a lab technician, but each wanted a full complement of job benefits. Patients wanted health; teachers wanted promotions; students wanted degrees; and support staff wanted satisfying jobs. Reaching these goals could occur because each person was a member of particular groups that sustained specific identities and roles. These groups formed distinctive cultures with certain identities, rituals, and images.

Individual patients wanted relief from suffering, relief provided by each other as well as professional caregivers. While sorting their own priorities, corporate officials made decisions that paradoxically fostered institutional stability as well as the more unstable edges of growth and innovation. Whether attending patients, teaching students, or searching for new knowledge, most professors looped together in a variety of committees to handle the rituals and rewards associated with their roles. Students experienced major cultural changes as they forged repetitive patterns of studying, socializing, and playing. The entire institution depended on support staff who made unique contributions to its cultural development. One specialized group created stories and images about UTMB.

This chapter describes certain features of the cultures associated with patients, corporate executives, professors, students, support staff, and storytellers. Some features of each culture were presented in previous chapters. This chapter examines these features from different perspectives and introduces certain themes that deserve special emphasis. Throughout a century of evolving cultures, UTMB's personnel found meaning and purpose in sharing many relationships and experiences. They forged bonds that forever shaped their lives and UTMB's destiny.

PATIENTS: BONDS OF SUFFERING AND RELIEF

UTMB existed because the citizens and political leaders of Texas wanted a trustworthy institution that would provide health care to sick people, educate and train professional caregivers, and discover—by inquiry and research—better ways to provide this care. Suffering humans were always at the center of UTMB's missions.

These humans came to UTMB for diagnosis and treatment of diseases and injuries that had changed their identities. If properly attended, a broken bone would heal and the patient would experience it only as a temporary event. Children often invited visitors to sign casts that protected broken bones. On the other hand, heart attacks, strokes, cancers, and degenerative conditions usually caused irreversible changes in one's identity and life story. Ordinarily, these patients wanted to display their conditions only to their families and to the caregivers previously described. Taboos about diseases and feelings about confidentiality did not encourage socialization among patients and their families, though the latter might share experiences during conversations in waiting rooms, wards, cafeterias, and corridors. Outpatients assembled in "waiting rooms" and some talked to each other about their problems. But nurses and clerks did not summon groups to see a doctor. They called the names of individuals, and special efforts were made to protect the privacy of encounters between a patient and a doctor.

Inpatients admitted to wards also talked about their problems with each other, but doctors and nurses "making rounds" in these wards visited with individuals and not with groups, though it was nearly impossible to establish complete privacy in many ward situations. Teaching caregivers to acknowledge changed identities, taboos, and the feelings of patients was always a formidable challenge in a large bureaucratic institution like UTMB. No single lecture or course or demonstration could inoculate a caregiver with the "human qualities" that constituted the "art" of effective health care. Mel Schreiber believed that these qualities included "the ability to convince, comfort and reassure" as well as "inspire confidence and trust" in a patient. Practicing this art effectively required a "sensitivity to the needs and anxieties of the sick" as well as "benevolence and kindness." In addition to solving diagnostic and therapeutic problems, truly professional caregivers cared about "the patient as a person."[2] Throughout UTMB's first century, this ideal never disappeared.

TABLE 8.1: POEM BY CHARITY PATIENT, JOHN SEALY HOSPITAL, 1903

Though Christmas-tree and holly branch
Are far beyond my reach,
I wish to send my Christmas gift
To the nurses all and each,
Who, when I lay upon my bed,
A pauper patient in a pauper ward,
Did all they could to ease my pain
And looked for pay unto the Lord.

To them I wish to send my thanks—
A small and foolish gift, 'tis true;
But from my heart it issues forth,
It's all that I can do.
I have no mines in which to toil,
For yellow gold to delve,
So all the Christmas gifts I have
Are Christmas thanks from number twelve.

Most patients willingly cooperated with caregivers because they wanted to leave UTMB as soon as possible—to go home. Unlike graduation ceremonies for students, there were seldom any ceremonies when a patient left a clinic or a ward, though nurses and others sometimes shared "happy tears" during goodbye times with some children. Even without ceremonies, professionals and patients often experienced discharge rituals as moments of progress and pride.

Some inpatients could stay for months, such as the children at the Margie Stewart Convalescent Home or those at the Moody State School. In these circumstances, small "communities" of patients did develop. In other circumstances, lay citizens and professionals intentionally developed communities of patients. Pediatricians and their assistants directed summer camps for diabetic children year after year. These children learned that they could manage their conditions while enjoying the fun of summer camps. When the Chronic Home Dialysis Center opened in 1968, families became a vital part of the ongoing care of patients experiencing renal dialysis. Professors Thomas Kirksey and John Derrick founded the Stroke Club in 1968. Its members provided invaluable support and advice to each other. Some patients participated in psychotherapy groups, especially the Family Therapy programs conducted by Harold Goolishian and others during the 1960s and 1970s.[3]

As more cultural openness about diseases appeared during the 1970s and 1980s, employees helped organize other self-help groups. One for cancer patients began in the spring of 1975. The Candlelighters of Galveston, a support group for parents of children with cancer, began in 1983. An Asthma Support Group for adults began in 1986.[4]

Fellowship during the meetings of these and other groups, such as seniors at the Geriatric Day Hospital, revealed the importance of shared support among those experiencing permanent impairments.

Moments of special bonding between patients and caregivers occurred during holiday seasons, especially Christmas and anniversary parties. In December 1903, for example, patients assisted nurses as they decorated certain areas of the John Sealy Hospital with holly, evergreens, and Christmas trees adorned with tinsel, balls, and popcorn. On Christmas Day the nurses walked the wards singing carols, gave each patient "a bag of candy, some fruit, two handkerchiefs, and a cake of soap," and enjoyed the turkey dinner served to all. One charity patient responded with a special poem (Table 8.1). In February 1990 the staff at the Center for Home Dialysis celebrated the center's twenty-second anniversary with William Litchfield, their first patient.[5] Events celebrating survival were special moments of glory for both patients and caregivers.

CORPORATE EXECUTIVES: BONDS OF POWER AND MONEY

Through the decades, CEOs and CBOs managed the distribution of steadily enlarging sums of institutional income. They ultimately controlled many jobs, thereby wielding enormous power. They were responsible for conserving the institution as a whole and guiding its growth and development.

This growth occurred rather slowly during the first half-century, dramatically afterward. In 1901 the academic enterprise included 20 employees, 165 medical students, 59 pharmacy students, and 20 nursing students. In fiscal year 1928, there were 82 employees working for the schools, 8 interns, 248 medical students, and 77 nursing students. Not including employees of the hospitals, about 160 persons received salaries in fiscal year 1941.[6]

After 1942, when the hospital's employees were fully incorporated into the institution and Leake became CEO, expansion was phenomenal. By the fall of 1956 there were almost 2,000 employees and 1,200 students. About 850 people were inpatients and about 600 people visited outpatient clinics each day. Thus, between 4,500 and 5,000 people assembled on the campus each day. The number of employees exceeded 3,000 by the seventy-fifth anniversary year (1965–1966), 6,000 by 1977–1978, and 8,000 by 1982–1983.[7] Including patients and their families, about 10,000 people roamed the campus during workdays by the mid-1980s.

One important example of expansion involved decisions made in the 1970s and 1980s by CEOs, CBOs, deans, and departmental chairs to encourage more women and ethnic minorities to become students, professors, and employees. During 1977 Dan Creson chaired a task force of professors George Bryan appointed to create an affirmative action plan for the School of Medicine and Graduate School of the Biomedical Sciences. Bill Levin appointed an Affirmative Action Advisory Committee that developed an equal opportunity/affirmative action policy for the entire institution by September 1978. Chaired by Philip Rayford and including faculty from all schools, this committee wielded considerable influence in implementing affirmative action policies.

In January 1979 Lucia Guzman, then assistant dean for School of Allied Health Sciences Student Affairs, became UTMB's first affirmative action officer accountable to the president. During the 1980s, she and her successors became outspoken advocates for women and ethnic minorities who wanted to be professors, students, or support staff at UTMB.[8]

These efforts resulted in major demographic changes in the student body, which are described later in this chapter. Demographic changes also occurred among the professors. In 1977 the School of Medicine and Graduate School of the Biomedical Sciences included twenty-eight female faculty members with M.D. degrees and nineteen with Ph.D.s. In 1981 there were thirty-seven with medical degrees and thirty-seven with Ph.D.s. In 1977 there were no blacks. In 1981 there were three. In 1977 there were four Hispanics with medical degrees and one with a Ph.D. In 1981 there were seven with medical degrees and five with doctoral degrees. There were no professors with Asian backgrounds in 1977; there were thirty-seven in 1981. These changes also occurred in the School of Allied Health Sciences and the School of Nursing. In 1977 there were four ethnic minority professors in the School of Allied Health Sciences; in 1981 there were nine. In 1977 there were three Hispanic professors in the School of Nursing. In 1981 there were two Hispanics, two blacks, one American Indian, and one Asian.[9]

Responding to these highly significant demographic changes, Betty Williams, Barbara Bowman, Anne Hudson Jones, Mary Ellen Haggard, Lillian Lockhart, Rose Schneider, and others established the Women Faculty Association of the School of Medicine in 1980. In 1982 the group renamed itself as the UTMB Women's Faculty Association so that professors from other schools could be members. By 1985 sixty women held tenured faculty positions (twenty-nine in the School of Medicine, eighteen in the School of Nursing, and thirteen in the School of Allied Health Sciences) and women occupied 78 of 287 mid-management and senior administrative positions.[10]

While leading expansion, corporate executives also wanted some stability to balance the inevitable instability associated with scientific, technical, social, and cultural changes. As discussed in previous chapters, corporate executives nurtured stability by establishing responsible political networks, by pleading relentlessly for dollars, by involving faculty and others in planning decisions, and by affirming students and employees with special rewards and rituals.

Institutional stability was also dependent on the ways that corporate executives exercised their new roles. Most of UTMB's top executives were not formally trained for their roles.[11] They learned their administrative skills from on-the-job experiences in managing smaller units within the academic bureaucracy. After displaying competence and effectiveness in those roles, they became CEOs or CBOs or deans or department chairs, roles that demanded some adjustments in identity.

One adjustment involved a posture of "distancing" that was needed for maximum effectiveness. To be viewed as fair and judicious to all, executives could not play favorites and give special favors to friends. These were difficult challenges that created troubling feelings of loneliness.[12] Such feelings often surfaced when they appointed new administrators from off-campus instead of applicants from within. Although these appointment decisions perpetuated the important ingredient of "distance" required for effective administration, they were fraught with uncertainty for everyone because no one could predict the outcome and those on the inside were deeply disappointed.

Becoming a CEO, the institution's major powerbroker, demanded additional adjustments. Only fifteen people exercised this role during UTMB's first century. From Paine to James, these CEOs were "professional politicians," continuously adapting within a labyrinth of political networks. The earliest networks were relatively small and streamlined, held together by a self-perpetuating group who seldom shared authority. The battles of the Spies era—with their curtailment of the dominant powers of a few and the dissolution of the John Sealy Hospital Board of Managers—destroyed this relatively closed system.

Though Leake shared authority and responsibility in a more democratic polity, political life became more complex as UTMB expanded and other UT components emerged and expanded. To coordinate and integrate these complex subsystems, the UT System appeared in 1950. UTMB then became the oldest and largest health unit in the system. But it was not the only one; others competed for patients, faculty, students, dollars, and power.

As the UT System evolved, policy decisions were made in different ways at different levels. This plurality and freedom often produced conflicts, perplexities, and inconsistencies, which prompted Leake to resign. Truslow was threatened by these political complexities, displaying a need for more personal control of all decisions. Yet these conditions also provided "a poetry of opportunity," to use Harry Ransom's apt phrase.[13]

Blocker, Levin, and James fully recognized their opportunities. They delegated responsibilities to carefully selected leaders, though each kept pragmatic fingers on the pulses of the entire institution. They changed political structures when they believed that such changes would improve institutional efficiency and quality. They adapted to the most prominent changes in the political networks. These were the absence of regents from Galveston, shifts in the executive powers of the vice chancellor for health affairs, the evolution of four schools and two institutes with their varying styles of leadership and self-governance, and the pleas of students for more institutional power during the 1970s and 1980s.

Another adjustment for a CEO was that of resolving conflicts about previous roles as clinician, teacher, or scientist. Would the incumbent continue to treat patients, give lectures, or work in labs? The daily activities of corporate executives were crucial symbols of their stewardships, symbols that affected personnel throughout the institution. Primarily clinicians and teachers, UTMB's earliest CEOs were not researchers and they gave relatively little "executive" attention to research.[14] Though an experimental pharmacologist, Leake did no lab research at UTMB. He did champion research, unlike any of his predecessors. While CEO, Truslow did not attend patients, give lectures, or do research. He did make important changes in the infrastructure that supported research.

Blocker, Levin, and James were exceptionally skillful as clinicians, teachers, and researchers. Some inner conflicts and public controversies haunted all three as each searched for acceptable balances between previous roles and new roles. While serving as CEO, all three attended patients and gave a few lectures. Only James continued a regular program of scientific research. Their decisions—like those of their predecessors—helped create the social and cultural environments that attracted and motivated teachers, students, and support staff.

TEACHERS: BONDS OF AUTHORITY

Physicians, nurses, allied health professionals, biomedical scientists, and humanities professionals were the cultural authorities at UTMB. Their knowledge and skills gave them influence and power over patients, students, support staff, and each other. Their authorities derived from their identities as knowledge specialists: pediatricians, plastic surgeons, operating room nurses, microbiologists, physical therapists, or medical ethicists, to cite a few examples. Each professor voluntarily chose a particular professional identity and devoted a career to nurturing that identity.

The cultural authorities of the professors were socially organized in specific "departments" in a hospital or school. Each professor found stability and rewards from interactions with other specialists who shared the cultural and social authority of that department. Biochemists worked with biochemists, dermatologists with dermatologists, and occupational therapists with occupational therapists. Professors used their knowledge and skills to treat patients, instruct students, or do research—specialized behaviors and rituals traced in previous chapters.

Faculty cultures emerged for each school and each department. Loyalty to corporate executives was the primary loyalty animating a dean or a departmental chair or a director. Loyalty to a "department" and its chair or director was the primary loyalty animating each professor. These loyalties were sustained or disrupted by the ways that administrators handled the rituals and rewards of the academic culture common to all of the departments. Spouses organized events that added zest to the social routines of academic life. Consider some changes in these communal features during the twentieth century.

Top executives selected departmental chairs and key directors, often using the recommendations of an ad hoc committee. Those being recruited negotiated the perks of their appointments. In terms of status, motivation, and power, for example, a great deal of difference existed between a part-time and a full-time appointment as a professor and chair of a School of Medicine department. Jim Warren was the first full-time chair in the Department of Internal Medicine (1958), Bill McGanity the first in the Department of Obstetrics and Gynecology (1960), and Bill Daeschner the first in Pediatrics (1960).[15] Other full-time clinical chairs were appointed during the 1960s and 1970s, the last in 1978 (Robert Rose). These chairs were expected to devote their entire efforts to managing each department, without any conflicts about the demands of a private practice or a need to seek income elsewhere.

The deans and departmental chairs of each school packaged the power and money variables used to recruit, employ, and reward the teachers and support staff working in a particular department. For the teachers, the variables included salaries; fringe benefits; retirement plans; titles; promotions; tenure; office space, equipment, and furnishings; office and lab assistants; and dollars for research, teaching supplies, and travel to meetings. For many years the chairs controlled these variables exclusively, negotiating terms privately with each teacher and making private decisions about promotions, salaries, and other perks for each member in the department. These prerogatives were viewed as politically sacred.

During the Blocker, Levin, and James eras, the chairs gradually accepted a more corporate approach to management. Decisions about promotions became more equitable as schools and departments adopted written guidelines and faculty committees assumed greater responsibility for recommendations about appointments, promotions, and tenure (APT).

CEOs, CBOs, deans, and chairs devoted countless hours to decisions about salaries, promotions, and the salary increases that ordinarily accompanied promotions. These decisions produced the numbers that were used in developing each year's operating budget and each biennial budget for the legislature. Circumstances, opportunities, and constraints changed from decade to decade, as the following events exemplify.

Carter was concerned about low salaries that prompted teachers like Arthur Austin to resign as professor of chemistry in 1910 and return to private practice.[16] He was also concerned about inequities in salary increases. For example, Keiller served for more than twenty years as professor of anatomy with no change in his annual salary of $3,000. Between 1895 and 1911 Keiller supplemented his income with private practice. In 1913, however, after devoting two years as a professor without private practice, he was distressed that no salary adjustments had been made.[17] As CEOs both Carter and Keiller recognized research productivity and effective teaching as criteria in evaluating recommendations for salary increases, but scarce resources kept salaries low until the late 1950s.[18]

By 1944 all professors in the basic science departments were strictly full time with salaries negotiated annually. About half of the clinical faculty were "geographically fulltime," meaning that they could not engage in private practice, but could still earn extra income from consultations in the hospitals. The other clinical professors were private practitioners who volunteered their teaching services without salary or private practitioners who received part-time appointments with salary. Problems occurred as fulltime members engaged in private practice other than consultation work, and part-time faculty, some with relatively large salaries, neglected their teaching responsibilities.[19]

In 1946 the faculty adopted a new policy about clinical faculty appointments. Parttime appointments were made to qualified specialists who would receive nominal salaries or the privilege of using the hospitals or both. These individuals would retain off-campus private practice offices. Full-time appointments were made to those whose primary responsibilities involved teaching and research. These individuals would have offices at UTMB but they could not attend patients without a specific consultation referral.[20]

Leake championed this consultation approach. The hospitals admitted three classes of patients: those who paid full charges, those who paid only part of the charges, and those who paid nothing. Physicians throughout the state sent their patients to UTMB for consultations. Therefore, none were private patients because no patient could "choose a UTMB physician directly." The regents officially sanctioned this policy in 1954.[21]

Improvements in salaries occurred during Truslow's years. In 1957 the regents adopted a plan for augmenting salaries that Truslow and the clinical faculty had developed. The plan identified three categories of faculty: strictly full-time, geographical full-time, and part-time. Truslow pleaded for an increase in salaries and the regents responded with a 15 percent increase. When the new plan became functional in September 1957, UTMB had forty-two full-time clinical professors. In the summer of 1959 UTMB discontinued payment of salaries to part-time faculty.[22] By 1962 UTMB employed sixty-six full-time clinical faculty, thirty-eight strictly full-time, and twenty-eight geographical full-time.

Truslow and Blocker experienced much stress as changes about salaries and sources of income were negotiated during these years. Some part-time faculty became angry about their loss of salary, and some strictly full-time and geographic full-time faculty were concerned about inequities in their salaries.[23] Disputes also arose about the allocation of practice income.

Under Blocker's leadership, a revised salary plan was adopted in 1967.[24] Income from consultation fees was deposited in a Physicians Referral Service account for each clinical department and the chair of that department could use this income for augmentation of salaries, fringe benefits, professional society memberships, authorized travel, and support of other departmental activities involving teaching, research, and patient care.

The following year the regents changed the name of the Physicians Referral Service Plan to the Medical Service, Research, and Development Plan (MSRDP). An advisory board that included the chairs of all clinical departments and five additional full-time clinical professors administered this plan. By the spring of 1969 ninety faculty members participated in the MSRDP.[25] Administrative leaders and professors amended this plan often during the 1970s and 1980s. To remain nationally competitive, changes were made in base salary rates, maximum augmentation limits, and fringe benefits.[26]

Fringe benefits had become important to faculty during the 1920s and 1930s. In 1924 the regents contracted with the Aetna Life Insurance Company to provide the benefits of group life insurance to qualifying faculty. In 1935 the regents adopted a token form of reimbursement for professors who were required to retire at age seventy. In 1936 Texans amended their constitution to permit the state to make contributions toward a retirement program for teachers in state institutions. This Teachers Retirement System (TRS) was in place by the fall of 1937. Beginning in 1958 a supplementary program allowed those in the TRS program who earned more than $8,400 per year to purchase supplemental annuities with monthly contributions.[27] By the early 1970s faculty could choose the TRS program or programs of private companies offering retirement annuities.

Monthly payroll deductions for hospitalization insurance premiums began in 1947. Group long-term disability income insurance was added in the summer of 1965. By the late 1970s the package of fringe benefits included medical, life, disability, and accidental death insurance; worker's compensation; and retirement programs. Clinical professors were also protected by professional liability insurance.[28] Most of the fringe benefits were also available to professors in the School of Nursing and School of Allied Health Sciences. Salaries in these schools were less than the salaries in the School of Medicine, but nationally competitive with similar schools.

Titles, ranks, and tenure were important features of professional identity. During the 1980s, the School of Allied Health Sciences faculty and School of Nursing faculty adopted policies about appointments, ranks, and tenure in their schools. With their primary appointments in the School of Medicine, members of the Graduate School of the Biomedical Sciences and the institutes were influenced by the evolving vicissitudes of that school.

By the late 1960s most School of Medicine teachers at the associate professor and full professor levels were tenured. Annual contracts of employment were renewed if the teachers continued to exercise their roles competently.[29] Many received appropriate promotions and tenure, though the process for doing this involved ad hoc committees and hours of difficult discussions during Executive Committee meetings. Written guidelines for awarding rank and tenure were first adopted by the School of Medicine faculty in February 1980.[30] Chairs of departments nominated teachers for specified ranks and for appointments with tenure or without tenure. These nominations were reviewed by an Appointments, Promotions, and Tenure (APT) Committee, which included six basic science and six clinical professors (tenured) appointed by the dean of medicine for staggered three-year terms. This committee evaluated candidates and made recommendations to the dean.

Between fiscal years 1982 and 1987, the APT committees approved 80 percent of those proposed for promotion to associate professor (88 of 110) and 83 percent of those proposed for promotion to professor (57 of 69). They also approved 75 percent of those nominated for tenure (80 of 107). By the fall of 1988, 57 percent of the tenure-track faculty in the School of Medicine had received tenure. In 1987 and 1988, the School of Medicine Academic Planning Committee (APC) analyzed the guidelines and rituals involving promotion and tenure. A survey of faculty indicated that a substantial number did not understand the policies about promotion and tenure. Moreover, several departments still had no written guidelines, making it very difficult for faculty to understand departmental expectations and to determine if they were being treated fairly by departmental chairs. During the late 1980s most departments adopted written guidelines that were congruent with those adopted by the school's APT committees. Faculty experienced a historically unprecedented clarity about expectations and procedures involving promotion and tenure.[31]

Special titles were very important for recruiting and keeping professors. To secure needed funds and provide special rewards for outstanding faculty, Blocker sought private dollars to name and endow professorships and chairs. Three were created by the fall of 1965: the Kempner Professorship in Genetics, the Weiss Chair of Otolaryngology, and

TABLE 8.2: ASHBEL SMITH PROFESSORS, 1964–1991

Edgar J. Poth, M.D., Ph.D.	1964
Raymond L. Gregory, M.D., Ph.D.	1966
Donald Duncan, Ph.D.	1968
Maurice Mason Guest, Ph.D.	1973
Hamilton F. Ford, M.D.	1974
George Herrmann, M.D.	1974
Robert N. Cooley, M.D.	1977
William D. Willis Jr., M.D., Ph.D.	1985
William C. Levin, M.D.	1986
William J. McGanity, M.D.	1989
C. William Daeschner Jr., M.D.	1989
Fred J. Wolma Jr., M.D.	1989
E. Burke Evans, M.D.	1991

the Warmoth Professorship of Neurology.[32] Interest from the endowments permitted the named professors to receive appropriate salary supplements, to receive reimbursements for travel to meetings of professional societies, to purchase books and equipment, and to fund other items directly supporting their academic duties.

By 1982 UTMB had seventeen endowed professorships and five endowed chairs. Others were added; in 1984 Bill McGanity became the first professor at UTMB to be awarded the Jennie Sealy Smith Chair in Obstetrics and Gynecology and in 1985 Robert White became the first Marie B. Gale Professor of Psychiatry.[33]

Blocker also began the policy of recognizing outstanding and longstanding School of Medicine professors as Ashbel Smith Professors. During Blocker's tenure, six faculty were named Ashbel Smith Professors: Edgar Poth (1964), George Herrmann (1965), Raymond Gregory (1966), Donald Duncan (1968), Mason Guest (1973), and Hamilton Ford (1974). Thirteen professors had received this honorific title by 1991 (Table 8.2).

Administrative leaders initiated other ways to affirm outstanding performances by faculty. In 1975, for example, Ed Brandt established an annual Teacher of the Year Award for School of Medicine faculty. During the succeeding five years the award was presented to Jim Guckian, Bill Willis Jr., Jay Fish, Betty Williams, and Sally Abston.[34] Several faculty awards were also bestowed during commencement ceremonies.

Evaluating the performance of each individual teacher as a bedside clinician, classroom teacher, or researcher was not an easy task. Patients did not prepare written assessments of clinicians and spoken comments were hearsay. Lack of clinical improvement or death of a patient did not mean that a clinician was incompetent. Written evaluations by students did not begin until the 1970s and even the best teachers received poor evaluations from disgruntled students. Failure to received funding for a grant did not mean that the grant proposal had no merit. Deans, chairs, and APT committees grappled with these realities as they developed their recommendations about particular teachers.

In addition to the daily chores of patient care, teaching, and/or research within a division or department in a school and, for many, with other departments in the hospitals, daily life also involved relentless work as members of various committees. As demonstrated in previous chapters, CEOs, CBOs, deans, and departmental chairs assigned the tasks of institutional maintenance and development to committees of faculty, staff, and students. Effective participation became important measures of a teacher's readiness for promotion and tenure, especially the latter. The specific tasks of these committees also demanded changes in role by faculty as they provided services needed to maintain and develop a department, a school, or the entire institution. As teachers moved from one committee to another, identities changed somewhat and different rituals and interactions were needed to accomplish certain tasks. What was needed for effective work on an Admissions Committee was not necessarily what was needed for effective work on a Curriculum Committee.

During the first fifty years, there were only four faculty committees: Executive Committee, Library Committee, Committee on Entrance Examinations for Admission to the School of Pharmacy, and Committee on the School of Nursing (Appendix H).[35] Others appeared occasionally and a few teachers served on student government committees and the boards of managers for the hospitals.

Nearly thirty committees functioned by the late 1940s. Fourteen School of Medicine committees existed in 1947: Admissions; Animal Quarters; Curriculum and Promotions; Graduate Work; Intern Placement; Library; McLaughlin Fund Advisory; Nominating; Postgraduate Medical Education; Research; Retirement and Group Insurance; Services, Development and Space; Student Affairs; and Student Loan, Fellowship and Scholarship. In 1949 the medical staff of the hospitals functioned with five committees: Executive, Credentials, Intern, Medical Records, and Program. In 1949 Bartholf used eight committees in the School of Nursing: Affiliation, Curriculum–Basic, Graduate Nursing Education, Library, Procedure, Publicity, Scholarship, and Social.[36]

After 1950 the number of committees steadily expanded as leaders, teachers, and tasks changed. In 1956 Truslow used fourteen School of Medicine committees. When Dean Earle and the School of Medicine faculty revised their bylaws in 1958, they named eighteen committees. By the late 1960s the School of Medicine faculty functioned with twenty-one standing committees and several ad hoc committees appointed by the dean or president.[37] In 1991 the School of Medicine faculty organized their work with nine elected committees, thirty-two appointed committees, and nine interdisciplinary course committees.[38]

Faculty in the other schools also accomplished their tasks with committees. In the School of Nursing there were seven committees in 1959, ten in 1981, and twenty in 1987. In the School of Allied Health Sciences there were five committees in 1968 and ten in 1983. In the Graduate School of the Biomedical Sciences there were three committees in 1970 and four in 1991. The institutes also used committees.

Individual professors usually served on one or more committees in any given year. A professor could serve on one or more committees in his/her department, one or more committees for a school or institute, and one or more committees for the institution as a whole. Although committees were necessary for institutional maintenance and growth, some teachers felt that they were sometimes trapped in bureaucratic merry-go-rounds as they regularly interrupted their research, teaching, and clinical duties to attend committee meetings.

Managing these multiple demands was possible because of the assistance of the dedicated secretaries and other support staff mentioned in previous chapters. The care of loyal spouses also enabled more adequate responses to such demands.

Spouses affirmed their partners in some corporate ways that developed during the second half of UTMB's first century. Elizabeth Leake and about seventy-five women (mostly wives) established the Faculty Women's Club in 1946. Usually meeting in homes during the early years, this group hosted monthly luncheons, teas for installation of officers, and seasonal parties, sometimes inviting the Medical Dames or wives of house staff.[39] Picnics, coffees and teas, holiday banquets, luncheons, and dinner-dances occurred during the 1960s and 1970s, as well as meetings of groups interested in bridge, arts and crafts, book reviews, and gourmet food. Betty Hilton produced the Faculty Follies in 1960 and 1965, spectacular evenings of song, dance, and fun. In 1967 and again in 1973 the club sponsored productions of "Sawbones on a Sandbar," a delightful play about UTMB written by Rose Schneider and Eric Hall.[40] In 1977 the club started an annual style show and luncheon, often held during alumni homecoming festivities. In 1979 and 1980 Betty Hilton and other members of the Faculty Women's Club staged a new Faculty Follies. During the 1980s the club continued its style shows and sponsored other events such as the first Faculty Prom at the Moody Civic Center in 1985.[41] Professors and their partners enjoyed the fun and camaraderie of these events.

STUDENTS: BONDS OF METAMORPHOSIS

Students wanted new identities as beginning professionals. Each wanted a metamorphosis. Students searched for ways to remain stable while experiencing the unceasing changes of acquiring professional identities. Students experienced profound changes in these cultures during UTMB's first century. Demographically, there was a major shift from mostly Caucasian men to multiethnic men and women. This resulted in a shift from a rather provincial culture to a diverse, international one. Marriage became more acceptable. In terms of social origins, there was a shift from a mostly rural to a mostly urban heritage. Until 1960 many students had jobs. Afterward, most did not work while attending school. There was a shift in living quarters from boarding and fraternity houses to dorms and apartments.

Students discovered and created a variety of ways to adapt to these changes. They sustained ties with families and some began to form their own families. They found identity and stability as members of particular classes in particular schools. They joined formal political networks by participating in student government entities. They made new

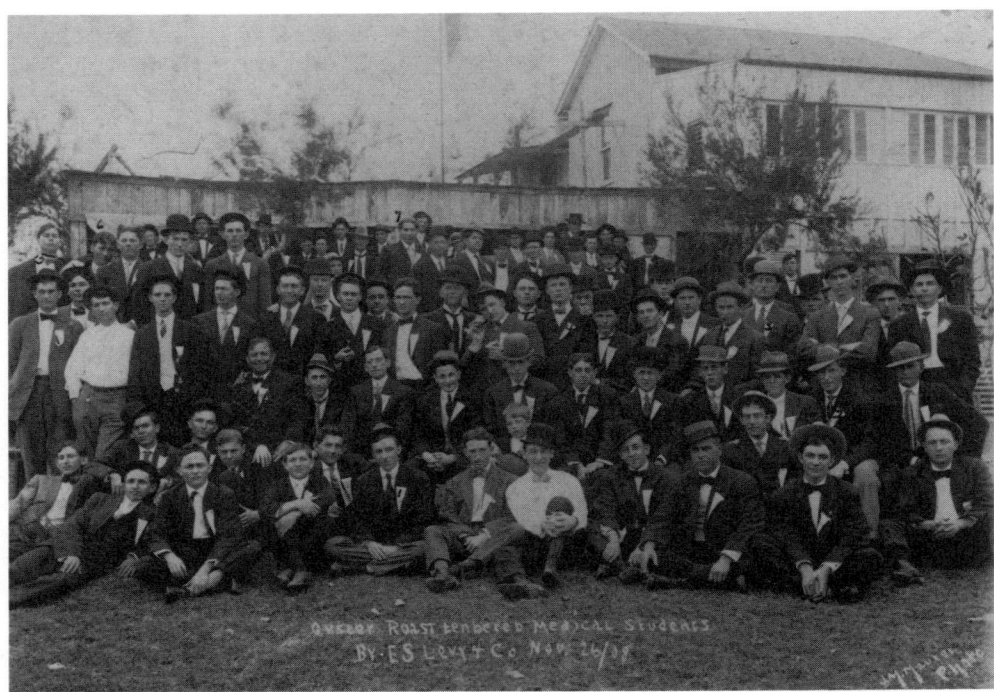

Oyster roast for medical students by E. S. Levy & Co., 1909.

friends as they affiliated with medical fraternities and other recreational and social groups. Outside of clinics, wards, classrooms, and research labs, they established formal and informal relationships with their teachers.

These changes and adaptations are described in the following sequence: demographic changes, living expenses, housing, studies, student government, medical fraternities, other social groups, and student-faculty relationships, including welcoming and graduation rituals.

Demographic changes profoundly influenced all aspects of student culture. The student body as a whole gradually became more heterogeneous as professors admitted more female, married, Hispanic, black, and international students. Consider each change and some of the ensuing responses.

Female School of Medicine matriculates gradually increased during the 1930s and 1940s, representing between 5 and 10 percent of the total. During the 1942–1943 academic year, about a third of the students were female. This included all of the nursing students (149) and 24 of the 397 medical students. During UTMB's last half-century, most School of Nursing students were women, many School of Allied Health Sciences students were women, and the number of female Graduate School of the Biomedical Sciences students expanded. By the 1980s women constituted 25 to 30 percent of the medical students (Table 6.2).[42] Between 1967 and 1991, 20 percent of the medical graduates were women (Table 6.7). Some were married and some were mothers.

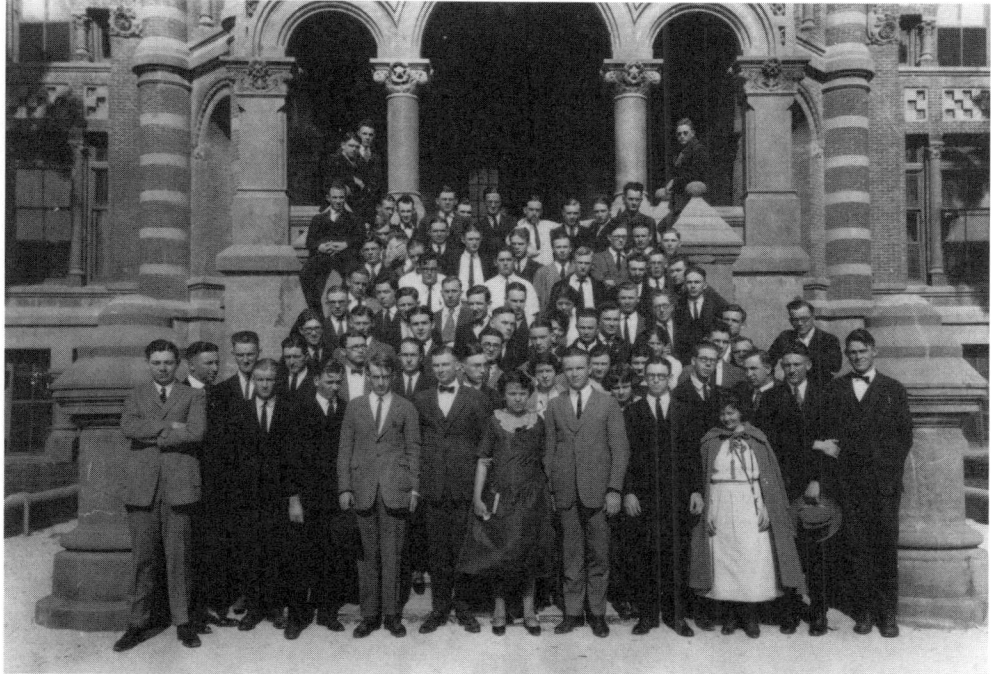

Edith Bonnet (front center) with her class of freshman medical students, 1922.

A few of the female medical students were married when they began school or they married while students. On Lincoln's birthday in 1938, Virginia Irvine, a third-year student, married Truman Blocker Jr. (class of 1933), an assistant professor of surgery. She gave birth to their first son in December, missing only "a week or two of school." Grace Jameson (class of 1949) was married when she entered school in 1945 and she gave birth to her first child during her sophomore year. She missed only ten days of school and continued to nurse her baby after she returned to classes. Like Virginia Blocker, she recalled that her classmates seemed to "cheer her on" through these events.[43]

The number of married students increased significantly during the 1940s and 1950s. Many World War II veterans were married. In 1949 about 190 of the 450 medical students were married (42 percent). This increased to 45 percent in 1955 and 62 percent in 1962. Of 103 medical students graduating in 1961, 76 were married and they were parents of 84 children.[44] These married students altered the cultural life of students in several ways. They lived in apartments with their families, while most single male students lived in fraternity houses. They allotted time to studies, family life, and, for some, part-time jobs. They added maturity to leadership roles in fraternities and other student groups, and, with their wives, they tempered the wildness of some fraternity parties.

Wives of faculty gave special attention to wives of students. In 1937 Mrs. D. Bailey Calvin and Mrs. Willard Cooke revived Medical Dames, a support group for wives of medical students that had been organized in 1924. Elizabeth Leake added much vitality during the 1940s. Members played bingo and card games, staged annual fashion shows, and hosted parties. During the 1950s and 1960s they continued their annual style shows, hosted many festive parties, and cheered during intramural sport competitions among the fraternities. In 1958 Medical Dames became a charter member of the Woman's Auxiliary to the Student American Medical Association (WASAMA) and received the first "Chapter of the Year" award from WASAMA. With 190 members, the Galveston group was named "National Chapter of the Year" in 1961.[45] These wives forged important emotional bonds and shared much practical advice about coping with husbands, dealing with children, and handling multiple frustrations.

By 1972 four of nine female graduates were married and one was the mother of two children. Recognizing these changes, Medical Dames changed its name to Spouses of Students in 1983. This group continued to be very active, sponsoring potluck dinners, brunches, and parties as well as crafts classes, fashion shows, and panel discussions.[46]

There was also much cordiality between these groups and the Resiterns. Initiated by L'Nell Starkey (wife of John Starkey, who was a resident in radiology), spouses of interns and residents organized the Resiterns in July 1959. During the 1960s they produced a cookbook, staged fashion shows, and sponsored numerous parties, including "fun nights" at the Hospitality Room of the local Falstaff Brewery. This group sponsored many events during the 1970s and 1980s.[47]

Other demographic changes occurred. Between 1900 and 1940, a few Hispanic-surnamed students graduated from UTMB. These included Emma Domingo (1900, School of Pharmacy); Alfonso Y. Garcia (1908, School of Pharmacy); Daniel Saenz (1921, School of Medicine); and Simona Lopez (1926, School of Nursing). Manuel Hornedo graduated from El Paso High School in 1925. He began School of Medicine studies in 1927, stopped for two years to earn money, then returned in 1929. After graduating in 1933, he began a career of more than fifty years with the City–County Health Department in El Paso.[48] Hispanic students were named in the *Cactus* between 1942 and 1950, and photographed for the *Syndrome* before 1960.

Professors admitted more Hispanics after 1960. Between 1964 and 1983, 483 of 2,083 (23 percent) Hispanic applicants to the School of Medicine were accepted; 188 enrolled. During the 1980s they constituted between 6 and 10 percent of the medical students; 3 and 7 percent of the nursing students; 7 and 19 percent of the allied health students, and less than 1 to 3 percent of the graduate students (Tables 6.1, 6.13, 6.15, and 6.16). In 1979 about thirty-five students formed the Organization of Hispanic Medical Students, whose members sponsored health fairs at local churches. In 1980 some members participated in the formation of the Texas Association of Mexican-American Medical Students.[49]

The faculty admitted African Americans beginning with Herman Barnett in 1949. A World War II fighter pilot, Barnett was the first black medical student. He was admitted as a "contract student" from the Texas State University for Negroes (TSU). He was registered at TSU and could attend classes at UTMB on a contingency basis until a new medical school for blacks began functioning. In 1950 the Veteran's Administration refused to grant Barnett's GI Bill educational assistance loan because he was not formally enrolled at an accredited medical school. Recognizing the impropriety of this situation, the regents allowed Barnett to enroll officially at UTMB. Although Barnett's presence on the campus generated some apprehension, he was soon recognized as a truly outstanding student who earned considerable respect from classmates and professors.[50]

In 1966 Virginia Stull became the first black woman to receive a medical degree from UTMB. As a junior student on her ob-gyn rotation, Stull was "fired" three times by a nurse supervisor who thought she was a "nurse's aide." Lafayette Williams Jr., a black classmate with Stull, recalled that fraternities were not open to black students and their members would not let blacks use any fraternity quiz files. UTMB's fraternities integrated in 1968.[51]

Between 1949 and 1975 fifty-seven blacks enrolled in the School of Medicine. Of that number, thirty graduated, one transferred, twelve were still enrolled in 1975, and fourteen had failed or quit. Between 1964 and 1983, 151 of 941 black applicants (16 percent) were accepted and 66 enrolled. More were admitted during the 1980s (Table 6.1). In 1980 some students organized a chapter of the Student National Medical Association.[52]

In 1949 Dean Bartholf hoped that black students could be admitted to the School of Nursing. By 1954 eleven women from Prairie View College participated in an "affiliate" program in psychiatry. By 1957 the School of Nursing had accepted black women into its baccalaureate and graduate programs. In 1960 Wilina Iona Gatson became the first black student to earn a bachelor of science in nursing degree from the School of Nursing. Gatson received much support from fellow students, who brought take-out food back to their dormitory from local restaurants that did not serve blacks.[53] During the 1980s blacks constituted between 6 and 15 percent of nursing students, 4 and 11 percent of students in the School of Allied Health Sciences, and less than 1 to 7 percent of students in the Graduate School of the Biomedical Sciences (Tables 6.13, 6.15, and 6.16).

The faculty admitted more students who were natives of other countries. During the first fifty years, a few medical students were born in other countries, eight in 1915–1916; seven in 1936–1937. During the 1980s less than 10 percent of the total number of medical students were natives of other countries (Table 6.5). About fifty foreign-born citizens attended the four schools in 1987; about three hundred in 1991. A Chinese Student Association was established in 1981. When an Asian American Student Association was established in 1985, about eighty students and several faculty members attended its first dinner.[54]

Regardless of birthplace, race, sex, or family background, every student needed adequate dollars for living expenses and school fees. Students obtained money from parents, other relatives, and spouses; worked at various jobs; and received loans and scholarships.

During UTMB's first fifty years, many students came from rural areas in Texas. Less than one-fourth of the medical and pharmacy students entering in the fall of 1916 came from counties with the largest cities. Even in 1941, only 39 percent of the entering medical students came from these counties. The percentage of students from rural areas did decline with each passing decade. In the fall of 1918, 23 percent of the medical and pharmacy students came from rural families; in 1940, only 5 percent of the entering medical students came from these families.[55]

Many students were quite poor. Before 1920, between 40 and 50 percent of the medical and pharmacy students held jobs. The number of those who reported that they were "entirely self-supporting" declined from 32 percent in 1924 to 11 percent in 1940. Yet about 40 percent of the medical students had jobs in 1940.[56]

During summer vacations, students worked in oil fields, on family farms, on the docks in Galveston, or in pharmacies and hospitals. Often the jobs in the hospitals were handed down from upper classmen to lower classmen, from roommate to roommate, or from one fraternity brother to another.[57] Others held part-time jobs during the school year by delivering papers, waiting tables at the school's dining club or in local restaurants, working in the book store, managing a fraternity house, providing teaching or laboratory assistance to faculty, collecting for laundries, soda jerking, or night clerking in a hotel. During 1960–1961, sixty-seven medical students worked at seventy-one weekend and nighttime campus jobs with forty-two of these in hospital areas such as blood bank and clinical labs, Medical Records offices, and food services.[58]

During the first fifty years, a small number of students received financial assistance from scholarship and loan funds. For example, five students received a total of $800 from the Will C. Hogg Loan Fund in 1940. During World War II many medical students received low-interest federal loans by agreeing to serve in the armed services after graduation. The total number of these scholarship and loan funds increased significantly after the war ended. In fiscal year 1960, students received more than $65,000 in loans. In the following year, 167 medical students received $171,421 from loan funds, scholarship funds, and research grants. Eighteen students received part-time support for work as research assistants and ninety-five students received stipends for full-time research work during summer months. By 1966 students could apply for scholarships or fellowships from a dozen programs or for loans from twenty-six different funds.[59]

Wives held a variety of jobs. Several taught in the Galveston public schools and others worked at the Rosenberg Library. Some offered child-care services and some were nurses. The income-earning wives of senior medical students graduating in 1961 included eighteen teachers, ten medical technicians, seven nurses, seven secretaries, one doctor, and one chemist.[60] Spouses of female students also earned needed income.

School of Nursing matriculates were "work-study" students long before that label was invented. They were "employees" of the hospital for many years, learning their skills by directly caring for patients. Sometimes a shortage of students necessitated "double-duty." In 1926, for example, some students were assigned four instead of two months of night duty. After ten hours of patient care, they were expected to attend classes the next day. Moreover, they received no off-duty hours and no half-day on Sunday. The School of Nursing director remarked that "No labor organization would be permitted to treat their people so." In the early 1940s Chloe Floyd could not visit with her Aggie boyfriend one Thanksgiving because she had to work in the diet kitchen.[61]

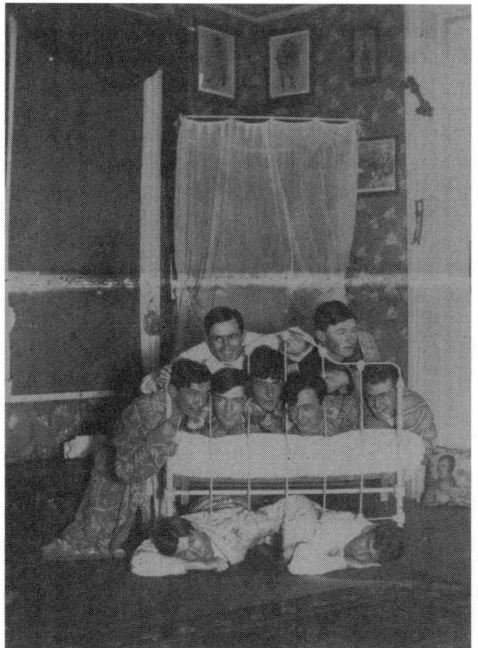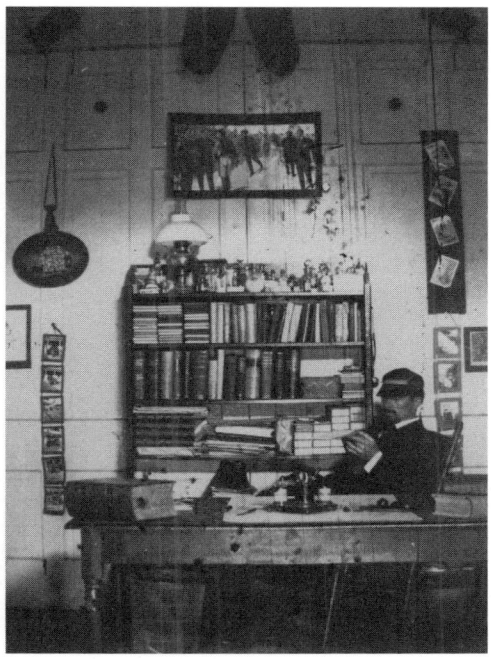

E. C. Northen, right photo, studying in a rooming house at 925 Strand, 1905. Northen's bed, piled with fellow students, is on the left. *Photographs courtesy the Moody Mansion and Museum.*

During the 1970s and 1980s work-study programs emerged in nursing and allied health fields, and loan and scholarship sources expanded greatly. In 1975 the Allied Health Service program in the School of Allied Health Sciences allowed working students to take formal courses for baccalaureate degree credit. In 1980 eleven employees were among the twenty-four students participating in this program. Between 1976 and 1979, $64,340 in scholarships were awarded to minority students. Between fiscal years 1977 and 1981 the total number of scholarships available for all students almost doubled, from 86 to about 160, a total dollar increase from $174,158 to $389,280.[62]

Students used their dollars to pay tuition and other fees, and to secure food, clothing, and housing.

At the turn of the twentieth century, some male students lived at Miss Mary's Boarding House at Ninth and Market and ate at the Old Mess Hall next door. In 1903 the women in University Hall could no longer tolerate the rowdiness of the men who ate in their dining club. The men moved the club to the Old Mess Hall. In 1913, 125 students obtained three meals a day for $12.50 a month in this hall. This dining club closed in 1923.[63]

Until the 1940s, most of the male students lived in one of the fraternity houses, which were east-end Victorian mansions. Between 1941 and 1966 all of the fraternities moved from these mansions into newer houses of contemporary design nearer the campus. Both the old houses and new houses had dining facilities.[64] In the mid-1950s, for example, room and board at the Phi Chi house cost $60 per month.

Before 1943 the female medical and pharmacy students lived in University Hall. In 1914 room and board was less than $15 a month. For many years these students sponsored receptions, dinners, and dances in attractive rooms on the hall's first floor. In the mid-1930s Virginia Irvine (Blocker) and her ten female classmates gathered in someone's room every day to "recite the names of all the boys in the class, making comments (sort of a 1–10 session)."[65] The building closed after it was damaged by a hurricane in 1943. During the 1950s female medical students lived in rooming houses, small apartments near the campus, or the new dormitories.

During UTMB's first fifty years student nurses did not pay for their room and board. They lived in the old City Hospital building, then in the first Rebecca Sealy Nurses' Home from 1915 to 1932, and the second home from 1932 to 1959. In 1943 the former "Isolation Building" housed some nursing students. In 1946 two UTMB-owned frame houses at Tenth and Strand also housed some nursing students. In that year the estimated annual cost of everything for these students (tuition, uniforms, personal items, and pocket money) was less than $500.[66]

The new dorms housed many nursing students when they opened in the mid-1950s. In 1959 the Rebecca Sealy Nurses' Residence closed for repairs and all nursing students moved to the dorms, primarily Morgan and Vinsant Halls. They enjoyed many dorm parties that were labeled "the backbone of dorm social life." By the mid-1960s, they could choose to live on or off campus.[67]

Married students usually lived in apartments, often sections of older houses. In the fall of 1952, for example, 125 of 285 medical students were married and they lived in rooms or apartments in Galveston, Texas City, and La Marque.[68] Until mid-century, nursing students who married while in school were expected to withdraw from the school, but secret marriages were not unknown. Vinsant Hall was named for a nursing student who secretly married while a student. Nolan Hall provided a few apartments for married students.

In 1982 a survey of 468 students from all four schools revealed that 44 percent of the students lived in apartments, 24 percent in a dorm, 19 percent in a single family house, 10 percent in a fraternity house, and 3 percent in a condo or duplex.[69]

Securing income for expenses and finding a place to live enabled every student to focus on the metamorphosis associated with challenging studies. Each student acquired an identity as a member of a particular class in a particular school: a freshman medical student, a senior nursing student, a second-year graduate student. Changing these identities was a common goal. Doing so ushered students into the clinics and wards described in chapter five, the classrooms depicted in chapter six, and the research labs featured in chapter seven. If students performed acceptably in these venues, they were promoted from year to year. If they completed all requirements, they acquired the titles of new professional identities during graduation ceremonies.

Students studied in their rooming and fraternity houses, dorms, apartments, classrooms, and the main library, especially during exam times. The first library was housed in Old Red and attended by Esther Massin, secretary to UTMB's CEO, for more than twenty years. Between 1920 and 1922 it was managed by Kate Feuille, a trained librarian.

In September 1922 Elisabeth D. Runge became caretaker of the library's approximately eleven thousand volumes. "Miss Runge" or "Miss Lillie" managed the library for forty-four years, overseeing moves into the Keiller Building in 1925, then into the Gail Borden Building in 1952. By 1961 she supervised nine full-time and two part-time workers. They prepared catalog cards for new books and bound new journals. They loaned about sixteen thousand books and journals to local patrons each year, and they sent about seven hundred books and journals to off-campus patrons via interlibrary loan. They mailed about three thousand copies of each issue of *Texas Reports on Biology and Medicine*. Miss Runge often worked fourteen to eighteen hours each day, seldom missed a day of work because of sickness, and retired in 1966.[70]

Lee Jones was director when the Moody Medical Library opened in 1972. Succeeding directors included Emil Frey and Brett Kirkpatrick. In the spring of 1984 the library added five personal computers for students and faculty. By 1986 the library's online computerized catalog included all circulating books. When Kirkpatrick became director in 1990, the library employed fifty-six people (fourteen professionals), subscribed to 2,800 journals, and housed more than 230,000 volumes.[71]

In addition to using the library's books and journals, students also purchased the books required for their courses. To obtain these more easily, the Students' Association organized a Students Cooperative Bookstore in 1919, which was housed in a cottage across the street from Old Red. A few students managed this bookstore and their jobs were tightly controlled by the fraternity system. Leake labeled the bookstore "a racketeering enterprise" and in 1950 students and faculty agreed to operate the bookstore as an auxiliary enterprise.[72]

This agreement became more formal in 1959 when UTMB established "The University Medical Branch Cooperative Society" with a board of directors that included administrators, faculty, and students. This board administered the bookstore, which was now operated by a manager, bookkeeper, and clerk. Professors, students, and staff could purchase items from the Cooperative and receive rebates at the end of each year. A new bookstore, which included a student lounge, was opened in the west wing of the first floor of Old Red. In the fall of 1960 this bookstore and lounge moved to the east wing of Old Red, then to Gail Borden in 1972.[73]

Whether using their own books and lecture notes or the library's resources to acquire their knowledge, students pledged to an honor system that proscribed cheating during exams. In 1910 Carter praised the students for their "perfect cooperation" with the faculty in enforcing the system. Formal rules created in 1919 continued for forty years. An Honor Council, composed of an elected representative of each class and chaired by an officer of the student government, investigated allegations of cheating, interviewed witnesses and the accused, determined a verdict, and recommended a penalty to the dean. Most students abided by the rules, but some did cheat.[74]

A new constitution for the honor system was adopted in 1959. Medical and graduate students elected eleven students to serve as an Honor Council. This council reviewed all accusations of cheating and other inappropriate behaviors. A separate Honor Council functioned in the School of Nursing. To reflect changes in UT System policies, a new constitution for the honor system was adopted in 1974, then amended in 1976 to include nursing students after the School of Nursing became an integral part of UTMB again. The Honor Council reviewed all allegations of cheating and misconduct and submitted recommendations to the appropriate administrators. During the late 1970s and 1980s students and faculty expressed some doubts about the effectiveness of the honor system and some amendments were adopted.[75] The Dean's Office established an Honor Education Council in 1990.

The effectiveness of the various honor systems depended on the forms and functions of student government that evolved during UTMB's first century. As noted in chapter one, students wielded corporate power by organizing the Students' Council in 1894, a group that changed its name to Students' Association in 1912 and continued as the center of student government for forty years.[76] During the first half-century, these groups published *University Medical,* supervised the student honor system, coordinated contributions to the *Cactus,* organized recreational events, and established the bookstore.

By the late 1940s, however, the polity of student self-government without faculty involvement had become distasteful to faculty, administrators, and some students. Some professors were unhappy with the excessive drinking and public sexuality at some fraternity parties. During Leake's tenure as CEO, the Students' Association ceased sponsorship of the bookstore, discontinued *University Medical,* and adapted to the desires of the faculty for increased supervision over student affairs. In 1946 Leake appointed some professors to a new Student Affairs Committee.[77] As UTMB's second half-century began, the faculty wanted to withdraw some of the autonomy that had been extended to students during the first fifty years.

Students responded with a new form of self-government. In support of the AMA's successful efforts to establish a Student American Medical Association (SAMA), about eighty-five medical students established a local SAMA chapter in May 1951. In 1952 this chapter became UTMB's "official student government body." The SAMA Council included one representative from each fraternity, one representative from non-fraternity students, and officers elected by the entire student body. In October 1952 the faculty approved SAMA and invited its officers to attend general faculty meetings and those of the Admissions Committee.[78]

The SAMA Council decided to issue a yearbook that was devoted exclusively to UTMB. First published in the spring of 1953, the *Syndrome* featured photographs of all students, fraternities, student organizations, hospital interns and residents, faculty in the departments of the schools, and administrative officers of the schools and hospitals. SAMA also financed the intramural sports program, helped furnish a new student lounge in Old Red, co-sponsored (with Mu Delta) the Gold-Headed Cane award, purchased lockers for junior and senior medical students, and sent delegates to TMA, SAMA, and AMA meetings.[79]

Professors were generally pleased with these developments. Nevertheless, the Student Affairs Committee remained as a supervisory and investigative group.[80] New student organizations were required to submit their bylaws for approval by the faculty, administration, and regents. The faculty would be involved in all matters of discipline for misconduct.

By 1960 the SAMA Council became even more representative as it included officers elected by the student body, presidents from each of the medical school classes, representatives from fraternities, a representative from the Medical Dames, a representative from the Honor Council, and a representative from the *Syndrome*.[81] But it did not include representatives from the graduate students, students in the Medical Services Curricular programs, or nursing students.

Nursing students sustained self-governing groups from the mid-1950s. The group was named "Executive Council" in the late 1950s and "Student Council" in the early 1960s. A separate School of Nursing Honor Council also existed during these years. This Honor Council adjudicated cases about curfew violations in the dorms based on rules that were finally rescinded in 1963. Afterward, separate House Councils monitored dorm life in Morgan and Vinsant Halls, and the Honor Council evaluated "professional and scholastic" infractions.[82]

In 1963 students adopted a constitution for a new University of Texas Student Association at UTMB. This new Student Association included all members of SAMA, all members of the UTMB chapter of the Nursing Student Association, all members of the Graduate Student Organization, and all students in the Medical Services Curricula. Representatives from each student group constituted an Executive Council that elected officers annually. The constitution of this new group stipulated that it would address only those issues that affected the entire student body, and would not in any way usurp the duties and powers of the separate student government organizations in each school.[83]

In 1970 Dennis Whitfield, SAMA's president and vice-president of Region 9 (six states), spearheaded some major changes as he led UTMB's chapter, the largest in the United States with about five hundred students.[84] Students, faculty, and regents approved plans for a Student Government Association (SGA) that included representatives from all four schools.

The SGA included an elected Executive Committee and an elected Student Senate composed of fifteen students, two from each medical school class, two from the Graduate School of the Biomedical Sciences, two from the School of Nursing, and three from the School of Allied Health Sciences. The SGA fully supported the Honor Council, a student group that administered the honor system for all students and conducted hearings on alleged violations. The SGA negotiated an increase in the matriculation fees of students so that a portion would be allocated to SGA projects. In fiscal year 1977, for example, approximately $20,000 of the SGA budget was used for publishing

Synapse (a student newspaper), memberships for all students in the Alumni Field House, a film series, and three all-school parties.[85]

In the early 1980s the SGA changed its constitution. Students in each school elected senators. Students in all schools elected SGA officers. The SGA sponsored surveys about student safety, TGIF (Thank God It's Friday) parties, movies, sports events, lecture series, and volunteer programs. With a contribution of $10,000 from the SGA, mail boxes for students were constructed on a wall of the corridor immediately west of the Clinical Sciences Auditorium.[86] The SGA published a newsletter with information about concerts, parties, and student organizations, including fraternities.

During UTMB's first seventy-five years, fraternities were the most significant agencies of socialization for most medical students and many others. They provided room and board for many of the single male medical students; companionship and psychological support; intramural sports and games; and countless parties attended by students from all schools. They also provided opportunities for students to relate to faculty outside of classes and they provided considerable national publicity for UTMB.[87]

In 1901 the Sigma Ribbon Society, Jolly Bone Jugglers, and Alpha Mu Pi Omega had a combined membership that included 27.5 percent of the medical and pharmacy students. By 1904 the two local groups had faded, but new chapters of two national groups were functioning: Phi Chi and Phi Alpha Sigma. Five more groups appeared during the next dozen years: Phi Delta Chi, Alpha Kappa Kappa, Phi Beta Pi, Theta Nu Epsilon, and Nu Sigma Nu. By 1916 more than half (54.3 percent) of the male medical and pharmacy students belonged to these seven fraternities.[88]

"Rushing" new students was a major ritual of campus life. Cars much fancier than Henry Ford's Model T were the rage during the Jazz Age of the 1920s. In October 1922 Felix Butte, a freshman, wrote to his girlfriend: "The Phi Chis met me at the train Wednesday in a big Pierce Arrow with a chauffeur, then later took me out in a Lincoln. I rode in all kinds of cars till I pledged." Competition during Rush Week increased significantly as three additional groups established local chapters by 1924: Theta Kappa Psi, Tau Phi Gamma, and Beta Phi Sigma. After Rush Week in 1934, eighty students pledged six fraternities.[89]

By the early 1940s Rush Week involved a merry-go-round of meetings, parties, and dinners staged by the fraternities, which competed vigorously for the new students. From the 1920s to the 1960s nearly all male medical students belonged to fraternities: 99 percent in 1924; 98 percent in 1944; 94.9 percent in 1954; and 96.8 percent in 1966.[90]

Phi Chi was the oldest and largest. In 1938 thirty-five of its fifty-eight members lived in its house at 1314 Avenue E. In 1941 this fraternity acquired a new house at 606 Sixth Street, which had two dormitory wings and a central lodge that provided a dance pavilion, kitchen, library, game room, bar, lecture room, and manager's quarters. More than one hundred delegates attended the thirty-first national convention of Phi Chi held in Houston and Galveston in 1949.[91] Phi Chi usually had more than one hundred members each year.

Phi Beta Pi was one of the larger fraternities. The Alpha Kappa chapter was founded in 1910 and its first house was located at 311 Tenth Street. Of seventy active members, thirty-one lived in its house at 1228 Market in 1938.[92] In 1955 the group moved into a new house at Fourth and Mechanic. During the 1950s, a large number of its members were married.

The Alpha Theta chapter of Alpha Kappa Kappa was one of the oldest fraternities. This group relocated its chapter house seven times between 1911 and 1966: 1021 Church Street; 1201 Avenue F (1913); 1521 Avenue E (1914); 1128 Market (1916); 1306 Market (1918); 1426 Avenue E (1925); and 301 Post Office (1966). About 150 delegates and alumni attended the national convention at the Galvez Hotel in 1951. In 1966 the house was a "modern 38-bed building complete with color TV and a swimming pool."[93]

Phi Rho Sigma, Theta Kappa Psi, and Nu Sigma Nu were three other fraternities that acquired new chapter houses on the eastern edge of the campus during the 1950s. The Alpha Nu chapter of Phi Rho Sigma was installed in 1939. This new group accepted members of Phi Alpha Sigma when it disbanded.

The Beta Phi chapter of Theta Kappa Psi was chartered in 1918. In 1938 thirty-eight of its fifty-two members lived in its house at 918 Avenue G. About two hundred delegates attended the national convention of Theta Kappa Psi in Galveston in 1949. Between 1942 and 1966 the local chapter maintained an active membership of about seventy students.[94]

Nu Sigma Nu was one of the smaller fraternities whose legacy featured outstanding scholarship. In 1938 fifteen of its eighteen members lived in its house at 519 Fifteenth Street. In 1954 this chapter hosted the national convention, attended by three hundred members from forty-four chapters.[95]

Phi Delta Epsilon was a national Jewish fraternity. In 1938 ten of its fourteen members lived at its house at 1008 Market.[96]

Alpha Epsilon Iota (AEI) was the only sorority at UTMB. The Rho chapter was organized in 1922. Most female medical students were members of this group. AEI did not have a chapter house. In 1938 most of the twenty-one members lived in University Hall. In 1950 this chapter hosted the AEI national convention, which about fifty women attended.[97] This sorority continued until the women students organized a junior branch of the American Medical Women's Association (AMWA) in fiscal year 1965.

The fraternities and sorority helped their members become successful students. They scheduled study periods, especially before quizzes. Students used files of old quizzes to prepare for new exams. Upper classmen advised lower classmen; they were living proof that a student could survive medical school with a personal identity intact. After the exams, the fraternities helped students play.

Wild partying and excessive drinking did occur in fraternity houses, though increasing numbers of married students tempered the excesses somewhat. During the 1940s some fraternities initiated parties with particular themes that became annual traditions. The Phi Betas became well known for their Hawaiian party. Their house was decorated with palm leaves and coconuts, and everyone wore tropical attire such as grass skirts, floral shirts, or

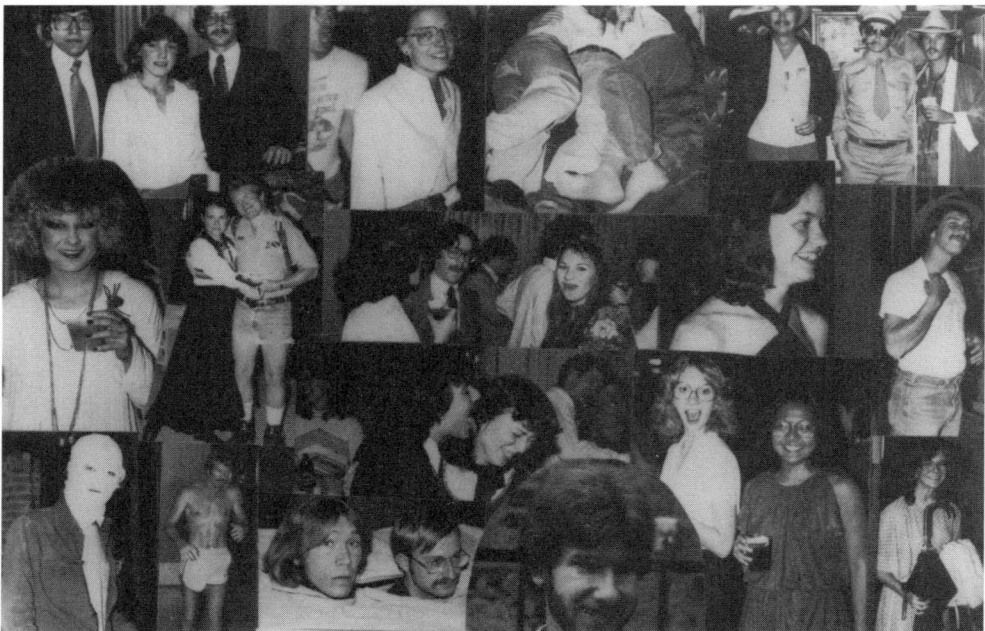

Phi Rho Sigma fraternity montage, 1981.

leis. The Phi Chis initiated Greek toga parties. Some fraternities organized Sunday after-noon lunches attended by members and their families, including alumni.[98]

In addition to parties at the fraternity houses, the Final Ball for seniors became a tra-dition that extended from the early 1900s through the late 1940s. Delegates from the oldest and largest fraternities—Alpha Kappa Kappa, Phi Chi, Phi Beta Pi, and Phi Alpha Sigma (later Phi Rho Sigma)—organized a group named Osteon that coordinated the Final Ball, which was usually held at the Galvez Hotel. Two hundred couples (students and faculty) attended the Final Ball at the Galvez Hotel in 1919. In February 1938 William Seybold Jr. helped decorate the Crystal Palace Ballroom for the Final Ball.[99]

During the 1950s and 1960s the fraternities had increasingly difficult times meeting their financial obligations, especially with the expenses of owning and managing large houses. The Sealy & Smith Foundation provided loans to some fraternities. In 1973 the foundation purchased the properties of four fraternities (Alpha Kappa Kappa; Nu Sigma Nu; Phi Delta Epsilon; Phi Rho Sigma) and gave them to UTMB. UTMB offi-cials assumed responsibility for maintaining the properties, and the fraternities man-aged food and other services for occupants of the houses.[100]

Other changes occurred during the 1970s and 1980s as more women became med-ical students and as more students married before and during medical school. David Eiland helped establish a new Interfraternity Council in 1982. Six fraternity houses still functioned by the late 1980s. Three were university-owned (Alpha Kappa Kappa, Phi Delta Epsilon, and Phi Rho Sigma) and three were privately managed (Theta Kappa Psi, Phi Chi, and Phi Beta Pi).[101]

In addition to the groups and fraternities already mentioned in this chapter, students established other organizations during the twentieth century that nurtured both personal and evolving professional identities.

Students attended local churches and synagogues and participated in various religious groups. About 80 students were members of a YMCA chapter in 1909 and about 120 students enrolled for this chapter's Bible study program in 1910.[102]

After 1950, Baptist, Episcopal, and Methodist chaplains organized numerous activities for students. Earl Rose was director of the Baptist Student Union (BSU) at mid-century. Members of twenty-seven Baptist churches collected about $45,000 as half of the cost of a new brick building constructed at 413 Eighth Street across from St. Mary's Hospital. The Baptist General Convention contributed the other $45,000 needed for this building, which opened in 1951. Doyle Ryan coordinated a variety of programs for students, who congregated for meals, discussions, lectures, and Thanksgiving parties for international students.[103]

In 1955 the Episcopal Church purchased a Victorian structure at 523 Tenth Street and designated it as a Canterbury House that would serve UTMB's students. Mark Boesser, a priest from St. Christopher's Church in League City, and some students furnished one area of the house, known as St. Luke's Chapel. Graham Pulkingham became Episcopal chaplain in 1957, Elmer Arthur "Al" Vastyan in 1960, Gammon Jarrell in 1967, and John Caskey in 1978.[104]

Under Vastyan's leadership the William Temple Foundation incorporated in 1963 and the William Temple Community House opened in 1966. Numerous professors and support staff were trustees of the foundation and boosters for the house.[105] House directors and board members orchestrated a variety of programs for students, patients, and others.

Bill Daeschner chaired the original board of directors for the United Methodist Campus Ministry when Carl Nighswonger became the first Methodist chaplain at UTMB in 1960.[106] Richard Donnenwirth, Hunt Robertson, Nolen Holcomb, and others have served as Methodist chaplains.

Roman Catholics established a Newman Club in 1963, which was located at the Bishop's Palace. It provided a home for a few male students and also hosted religious and social events for UTMB's Catholic students.[107]

Music and dancing have always been a part of student life. In November 1908 students learned songs and cheers for a Texas A&M/UT football game in Houston. In the fall of 1940 more than twenty-five medical students constituted a Glee Club, which made its debut at the First Methodist Church in Galveston and continued performing during the early 1940s. In 1960 Ed Stone, the music director at Ball High School, directed a group of students, house staff, and faculty known as "The Medics." This group made its debut at a Christmas dance hosted by SAMA and Mu Delta. More than six hundred people attended the Cadaver Ball at the Moody Civic Center in 1978; about 550 in 1979. The SGA began sponsoring an annual series of classical music concerts in 1986–1987.[108]

Sports have also been a continuous part of student culture. In 1910 students played tennis on courts in front of Old Red, but there were insufficient funds to construct handball courts or a gym. During the 1950s and 1960s the Athletic Council of the Interfraternity Council organized intramural sports and games for fraternity members, including football, softball, basketball, golf, table tennis, volleyball, and bridge. Truman Blocker encouraged participation in sports. He helped organize a rugby team that won the Sportsmanship Trophy when it participated in a Mardi Gras Rugby Tournament in New Orleans in 1969.[109]

Blocker also catalyzed the creation of the Alumni Field House, which opened in January 1969. By April 1970 members included 350 students, 82 house staff, 41 professors, and 25 support staff. By the early 1980s there were seven tennis courts, two handball courts, two softball fields, an outside basketball court, a swimming pool and sauna, an exercise room, a weight room, and lockers and showers. By 1985 there were fifteen hundred members.[110]

Fraternity intramural athletic contests were popular during the 1980s. Contests in flag football, basketball, volleyball, and softball were organized with the help of Gene Powell, director of campus life. Many students were among the more than seven hundred people who participated in the UT-MED Sesquicentennial Health Run in March 1986.[111]

During the twentieth century, students in each school organized school-based groups that served their needs. For medical students, this included AOA, the Medical Student's Forum, Mu Delta, the William Osler Society, and AMWA. In 1920 the Alpha Omega Alpha Honor Medical Fraternity (AOA) established an Alpha Chapter at UTMB that included five faculty and thirteen senior medical students. Between 1920 and 1991 this chapter inducted 1,430 medical students who had made outstanding grades during their studies.[112]

Mu Delta, an honorary service society of faculty, junior and senior medical students, and alumni, was organized in 1948. Mu Delta members participated in many service roles. During the 1980s, for example, they took prospective students on campus tours, helped teach sophomore students about "taking histories and doing physicals," and helped with various fundraisers, such as those for the Ronald McDonald House.[113]

During the 1940s and 1950s some student groups focused on the cultural traditions of medicine. The Medical Student's Forum offered students an opportunity to discuss the social and cultural aspects of a doctor's life. In 1954 about thirty students organized the Sir William Osler Society, which met periodically for talks and discussions about the history and philosophy of medicine until 1965, when professors organized the Chauncey Leake History of Medicine Society.[114]

Female students organized a junior branch of the American Medical Women's Association (AMWA) in 1964–1965. Lillian Lockhart (class of 1957), a faculty member in the Department of Pediatrics, was the group's first sponsor. In 1966 twenty-seven female medical students were members of AMWA. Members were very active during the 1970s and 1980s. They created files of exams, housed prospective students, organized educational seminars, sponsored weekend orientations for incoming first-year students, and developed a Big-Sib Little-Sib program of support for female students.[115]

As friends of medical students, students in the School of Nursing attended many of the social events sponsored by fraternities during UTMB's first fifty years. But a heavy-handed paternalism sometimes stifled social enthusiasms among the nursing students.[116] This cultural atmosphere changed with the reforms of the Spies era and the arrival of Marjorie Bartholf as dean. During the early 1940s students established an organization that sponsored numerous teas, dinners, and dances. In the late 1940s students staged Halloween carnivals at the Nurses' Residence. In the early 1950s they hosted all-campus dances. This group supported the School of Nursing Honor Council and a local chapter of the Texas Student Nurses Association, whose members chose delegates to attend the annual TSNA meetings. Student groups in the School of Nursing were quite active during the 1970s and 1980s.[117]

In November 1961 thirty-nine graduate students established UTMB's Graduate Student Organization (GSO). Dean Saunders supported a decision by the faculty to give graduate students representation on GSBS governing committees. Beginning in 1977 the GSO elected two students to serve as voting members of the GSBS Executive Committee.[118]

In 1977 faculty and students established a SAHS Student Organization that permitted students to deliberate with the faculty regarding all policy matters affecting the lives of SAHS students. Its Executive Committee included student representatives from all six academic programs in the school.[119]

Students in particular SAHS programs organized groups. In 1980 occupational therapy students organized a Student Occupational Therapy Association. The Student Association of Health Information Managers was organized in 1985. Its members staged annual Christmas parties and banquets for senior students. In 1988 UTMB's student chapter of the American Academy of Physician Assistants (AAPA) was selected as the outstanding student society at the academy's national conference. Toni Deer, a UTMB student, was elected president of the National Student Association of the AAPA. During 1989 about sixty members participated in bake sales, caroling, health fairs, bowling tournaments, blood pressure screening sessions, and the Toys for Tots drive.[120]

About thirty student organizations flourished by UTMB's centennial year. AOA and Alpha Eta were honor societies. Ethnic groups included Baha'i Club, Chinese Student Association, Jewish Student and Faculty Organization, Organization of Hispanic Medical Students, and Student National Medical Association. Specialty groups included American Medical Student Association, Family Practice Student Association, Student Nurses Organization, Student Occupational Therapy Association, and Student Physical Therapy Association. Others included AIDS Education Organization, Graduate Student Organization, and Mu Delta.[121]

Every year some students received extra boosts to their identities as peers selected them for leadership roles in these student organizations. In 1901, for example, some students were elected as officers of each class in the medical, pharmacy, and nursing schools.

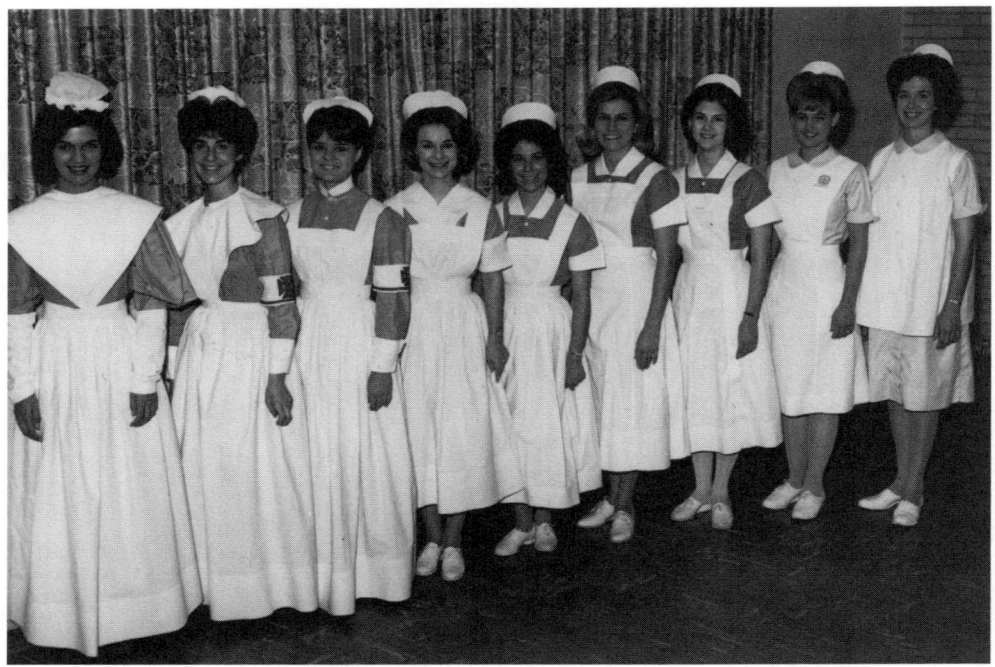

Uniforms of student nurses, 1890–1967.

Others became officers in the Students' Council, University Hall Club, Young Men's Christian Association, and the University of Texas Pharmaceutical Association.[122] These special identities occurred for numerous students throughout UTMB's first century.

Some students received statewide recognition. In 1956 the Texas Nursing Students Association (TNSA) elected Weta Wilson as president, selected Hilda Groner as the Texas Student Nurse of the year, and selected Marion Lemmons as delegate to the National Nursing Students Association meeting in Chicago. In 1958 the TNSA selected Anna Pearl Rains as its Student Nurse of the Year. In 1964 Gene Peterson, the only male nursing student at UTMB, was president of the TNSA. About six hundred students, faculty, and exhibitors attended the four-day annual meeting of the TNSA in Galveston in February 1984 when James Carnes was elected president. In 1988 Deepak Srivastava, a junior medical student, became the first School of Medicine student elected to the Governing Council of the Medical Student Section of the Texas Medical Association.[123]

National recognition also came to some student leaders at UTMB. Dennis Welch, a junior medical student, was elected national president of SAMA in 1961. In 1985 James Carnes became a member of the board of directors of the National Student Nurses' Association and Kathy Howard was elected vice-president of the Student Academy of the American Academy of Physicians' Assistants. The editors of *Who's Who in American Colleges and Universities* began including students from all four UTMB schools in their annual editions. There were twenty-seven students in the 1978 edition; thirty-one in 1981; thirty-five in 1983; thirty-nine in 1986; and forty-five in 1990.[124]

This recognition of outstanding individuals from each school fostered a growing sense of respect for excellence among all students.

A sense of mutual regard between professors and students was expressed in various ways during the first century. Nicknames, suspension of classes for funerals of professors, and a small-town atmosphere were features of student-faculty interactions during the first fifty years. From the days of William "Sam" Carter to "Admiral" D. Bailey Calvin, students enjoyed nicknaming certain faculty.[125] "Wild Bill" Keiller was definitely not wild, just as "Smiley" Edgar Poth never smiled. Byron Hendrix was "Lumpy Jaw" because of a facial nerve paralysis. With jolly red hair, Andrew Ormsby was the "Red Fox." Ever ready to ask questions, Donald "Tennis Shoes" Duncan glided quietly through the anatomy lab. Raymond Gregory was the "Tiger" because of his gruff demeanor. These nicknames usually signified endearment, not lack of respect.

Another feature of the early decades was the suspension of classes that gave medical students the opportunity to attend funerals of professors. When James E. Thompson died in April 1927, some students were active pallbearers and some professors were named as honorary pallbearers. When Charlotte Schaefer died in late May 1927, the prestigious Final Ball was cancelled and considerable sadness permeated the commencement ceremonies. When William Keiller died in February 1931, classes were suspended for two days so that students and faculty could participate in the funeral. In April 1935 classes were suspended for a day so that students and faculty could attend the funeral of Dean George Bethel.[126]

Although these family-like rituals of special regard faded as UTMB expanded during its second half-century, they did not completely disappear. In the mid-1950s, for example, Carl Nau, Don Micks, Rajendra Singh, Patricia Friddel, and others established the International Forum as a venue for welcoming and supporting the increasing number of students and employees from other countries. This forum staged monthly meetings that usually involved programs about the cultures of various countries. About ninety members participated in 1961. In 1966 there were two hundred students and employees from thirty-seven countries at UTMB, with the largest group being fifty-seven exchange visitor nurses from the Philippines. The International Forum sponsored a style show in April 1967 and continued to meet during the early 1970s.[127] Faculty support was essential for the success of this forum.

As demonstrated with other examples in this chapter, professors attended dinners, dances, and other events students sponsored. They were mentors and advisors for many of the groups students organized. They were members of committees appointed by deans to handle issues associated with student conduct.

The deans of each school were the "ultimate" authorities in enforcing policies about student life. During the first fifty years, the deans seldom delegated their authority to a subordinate official. Instead, each dean usually interacted directly with the students, especially with members of the Students' Honor Council. This group reviewed incidents of student misbehavior and made recommendations to the faculty's Executive Council. In 1928, for example, six nursing students had accompanied five medical students to the home of one student after they had been dancing at the Tokio Club one Saturday night. Four of the nursing students returned to University Hall at 4 A.M. on Sunday; the other two did not return until 9 A.M. Although the Honor Council recommended leniency, the Hospital Board expelled one nursing student and suspended the other five for one year. The Executive Council suspended one medical student for six months and the other four for one year (three were not allowed to graduate that year).[128]

During the second half-century, deans appointed subordinate officials who assisted with the management of student affairs. In the School of Medicine, these included D. Bailey Calvin, John Finerty, Warren Harding, Kenneth Walker, Rollin Sininger, Gene Powell, Billy Rankin, David Eiland, Daniel Trevino, Yvonne Russell, and Billy Ballard. Virginia Dryden, Elizabeth Knebel, Shirley Steele, Stephanie Pardue, and Regina Lederman provided this assistance in the School of Nursing. Robert Bennett was the key player for the Graduate School of the Biomedical Sciences, and James Myklebust, Harry Siegel, Lucia Guzman, and Raymond Lewis handled these roles for the School of Allied Health Sciences (Appendix B).

After Eiland became associate dean for student affairs in the School of Medicine in 1974, he pioneered several new approaches. Brandt (later Bryan) and Eiland began regular meetings with small groups of first-year students to discuss issues pertinent to their adaptation to medical school.[129] Faculty who taught small groups in the Introduction to Patient Evaluation course invited students to their homes for dinners. A Student Affairs Committee monitored students with academic or behavioral problems.

In 1975 Eiland established a Student Advisory and Counseling Service Center with Patricia Blakeney as its director. Services were extended to house staff in 1979. By 1980 eight full-time or part-time employees provided counseling about academic difficulties, marital conflicts, psychological problems, legal matters, religious concerns, and financial issues. About one hundred students or house staff visited the center each day.[130]

Eiland gave much support to the Student Government Association, including the allocation of substantial funds from student activities fees beginning in 1976. With the support of Jack Thompson, Eiland established a separate Student Financial Aid office.[131]

Streamlining and centralizing student personnel services continued after Eiland became dean of students and assistant vice president for student affairs for the entire campus in 1984.[132] UTMB's corporate executives supported student life and culture in more effective ways than ever before.

Special moments of interaction between professors and students occurred during welcoming and commencement rituals. During the first half-century, special "capping" ceremonies also occurred in the School of Nursing. During the second half-century, special awards for outstanding students and professors became a part of the graduation ceremonies.

The formal ceremonies that opened academic sessions every fall continued throughout the first half-century. Homer Rainey gave the last "opening" address on October 2,

1941. During the 1940s and 1950s, Leake, Calvin, and others gave more informal welcoming speeches on the days of registration. After moving to the Maco Stewart Home, the Leakes hosted many receptions and parties, including some for incoming students and spouses.[133]

As the years evolved, welcoming receptions and parties varied considerably. In the fall of 1968 Dean White hosted a welcoming party for freshmen medical students. During the late 1970s and early 1980s Dean Bryan hosted annual barbecue receptions that welcomed first-year medical students and their teachers. In 1978 David Eiland initiated a new two-day orientation program for entering medical students that included small group discussions led by senior medical students. By the early 1980s orientation programs for medical students and graduate students occurred together and in 1989 UTMB began a "Quest" orientation program for all students.[134]

Between 1898 and 1967 most students graduated together. These commencements occurred in several places: Old Red, 1894 Grand Opera House, Scottish Rite Cathedral, Martini Theater, City Auditorium, Marine Room at the Municipal Pier, and Moody Civic Center.[135]

In 1910 Regent A. W. Fly gave the address and the senior medical students presented a "Loving Cup" to J. F. Y. Paine, who was retiring. As the commencement address at the City Auditorium in 1927, Rabbi Henry Cohen gave a eulogy on the life of James Thompson, who had died the previous month. The City Auditorium was the location of the fiftieth annual commencement in 1941, when eighty-five medical students and thirty-five nursing students received diplomas.[136]

Two commencement ceremonies occurred in 1942; the first in March for ninety-two medical students and sixty-six nursing students; the second in December for eighty-six medical students. In March 1946 graduation ceremonies occurred at the new Galveston Municipal Recreation Pier, with eighty-eight medical students and twenty-eight nursing students receiving degrees. Two students received certificates in physical therapy. The last accelerated physician class graduated in February 1948.[137]

During the early 1940s, when the School of Medicine staged more than one commencement each year, the School of Nursing held some separate graduations. Special moments affirming the identities of nursing students occurred during capping ceremonies held during some years of the first half-century. Nursing students who had successfully completed their basic studies were honored with special caps that they wore while providing patient care. In April 1931, for example, twenty-five students received caps in a dramatic ceremony held in the amphitheater of the Outpatient Building. Students experienced considerable pride as they accepted the caps and recited the Florence Nightingale pledge.[138]

Special honors and awards became a part of the graduation rituals in 1951 when ten medical students received scholarships or other awards. In 1952 Leake gave special recognition to the fifty-year graduates (class of 1902) and the twenty-five-year graduates (class of 1927). Officials of the Borden Milk Company attended this ceremony, which included the dedication of the new Gail Borden Laboratory Building.

In addition to the medical and nursing students, sixteen laboratory technician students and six radiology technician students received certificates during the sixty-third commencement in 1953. Herman Barnett, the first black medical student, graduated in this class.[139]

As the number of honors and awards increased it became necessary to stage those ceremonies separately from the commencement rituals. The first occurred in June 1955, when 219 students participated in the sixty-fifth commencement, including 100 medical students, 46 nursing students, and 23 students in the medical services curricula. The local chapter of Sigma Xi sponsored these "honors convocations." In 1956 sixty-one students received special awards, including scholarships and summer research fellowships.[140]

In 1957 the graduation ceremonies moved to the Moody Civic Center, where 234 students received diplomas or certificates. During the exercises in 1958, Lois Mendle of La Marque became the first woman to receive a Ph.D. degree in the biomedical sciences during a UTMB commencement. During the seventieth commencement exercises in 1960, Charles T. Stone Sr. (class of 1915) established the Gold-Headed Cane Award honoring the senior medical student selected by the student's class as "the graduate who best exemplifies the qualities of the physician who will put the welfare of his patient first at all times." During the seventy-fifth commencement in 1965, Melvyn Schreiber led the medical students, who recited the Hippocratic Oath, and Betty Beaudry led the nursing graduates, who recited the Nurses' Pledge.[141]

Separate graduation ceremonies for the School of Nursing began when the System-wide School of Nursing existed between 1967 and 1976.[142] Because of curricular schedules, the School of Nursing periodically conducted a graduation ceremony in May and again in December. In December 1976, for example, forty-eight students earned bachelor's degrees and five received master's degrees. Special awards for students and faculty became part of these ceremonies during the 1980s.

The School of Allied Health Sciences held its own commencement ceremonies beginning in 1969, when certificates were given to eleven medical technology students and bachelor's degrees were awarded to six medical technology students and one medical records administration student.[143] Honors awards for students and faculty began in the 1970s. Students and selected faculty recited pledges or oaths pertaining to each professional specialty.

During the 1970s and early 1980s Graduate School of the Biomedical Sciences and School of Medicine students still graduated together. The number of awards for these students significantly increased during these years. Awards and scholarships in twenty-eight categories were given to fifty medical and graduate students during the Honors and Awards Convocation in May 1978, for example. A separate Graduate School of the Biomedical Sciences graduation ceremony began in 1984. Dean Saunders also initiated annual awards dinners for GSBS students and faculty. By 1991 there were sixteen student awards, two faculty awards, and an alumnus award.[144]

Throughout the decades of UTMB's first century, commencement ceremonies affirmed new identities and honored excellence in scholarship and budding professional skills. Graduates, families, spouses, friends, professors, and fellow students typically experienced marvelous moments of joy, unity, and pride.

SUPPORT STAFF: BONDS OF JOBS

Throughout its first century, UTMB employed many people who provided assistance to corporate officials, professors, students, and others who fulfilled the caregiver, educational, and research missions of the institution. Their social origins, educational levels, technical skills, and corporate loyalties varied considerably. Most primarily wanted jobs that provided a living wage and an acceptable work environment. Those who were very dependable and skillful gave extraordinary measures of stability to their departments in the hospitals and schools. Their occupational roles provided opportunities to establish bonds of friendship as well as bonds of loyalty to particular persons and to the institution as a whole.

John Hooper, UTMB's first janitor, was also a "good carpenter, machinist and painter" and attended the cadavers used for dissection. Janitors also functioned as lab technicians in various departments, often for long periods of time. In November 1912, for example, Keiller became quite concerned about the serious illness of Gus Elbert, who had worked in the Department of Anatomy for sixteen years.[145]

Professors repeatedly expressed concern about the low salaries of support staff. In 1918, for example, the black woman who cleaned the anatomical rooms every morning and the pathology rooms every afternoon received $30 each month. The salary situation for these employees became worse during the depression years, when some of the janitor-attendants received as much as a 28 percent salary cut.[146]

The total number of support staff increased steadily. During the 1930s they included housekeepers, lab attendants, technicians, and a photographer, J. E. Beissner. By 1949 there were seven categories of support staff titled laboratory helpers, animal caretakers, technical aides, technicians, general assistants, clerks, and secretaries. In 1950 approximately five hundred people were employed in the hospitals as maids, orderlies, attendants, and ward helpers. The turnover in these occupational roles was extremely high, with as many as thirty-five hundred employees hired in one year.[147]

These roles became more appealing as jobs when certain improvements occurred in the late 1940s and early 1950s. Blue Cross insurance became available in 1947. A workers' compensation plan became effective in 1952. By the summer of 1956 UTMB provided all of its employees with a 20 percent discount on hospital charges and services. The creation of a Personnel Office in 1953 was a key event in supporting numerous efforts to improve salaries, job classifications, and fringe benefits.[148]

With twenty-six hundred employees by 1955, UTMB was Galveston's largest employer. Business officers used approximately 160 "classified salary" categories that also included various levels within certain roles such as secretary, senior secretary, and administrative secretary. Others included accountant, switchboard operator, stores clerk, X-ray technician, ward clerk, social caseworker, speech therapist, laboratory helper, animal caretaker, research technician, electrical engineer, medical illustrator, carpenter, painter, book binder, truck driver, laundry worker, cook, seamstress, and guard.[149] In 1955, after a vote by employees, Social Security coverage was added as a fringe benefit.

During the late 1950s Truslow and others labored successfully to improve the salaries of the support staff. The regents approved salary increases for employees in 57 percent of the 184 job classifications effective September 1, 1957. Even with these increases, distress about low salaries continued. Budget deficiencies, non-competitive salaries, and the absence of a merit plan for salary increases discouraged some employees. In January 1965, 554 hospital employees still received salaries of less than $200 per month. Long-term disability income insurance was added as a fringe benefit that year.[150]

Significant improvements occurred during the Blocker and Levin boom years when the number of classified employees expanded dramatically. Many hands touched the estimated forty thousand purchase orders processed in 1977, for example, and the switchboard operators handled between four and five thousand calls during each twenty-four-hour period in 1978. In the summer of 1979, 6,300 employees worked at more than 560 different jobs.[151]

Improved coverage in the UT System's health insurance plans became effective in September 1980. By the late 1980s the package of benefits available to employees included medical and dental insurance; group term life, accident, and disability insurance; premium sharing; UTFLEX options; annuities and retirement plans; longevity pay; and Social Security and worker's compensation policies.[152]

Other important benefits for all employees emerged at various times during UTMB's first century. Financial self-help became another way to improve economic well being. In the summer of 1949 fifteen people collected $95 to start a Federal Credit Union, which provided low-interest loans to employees. Its charter was changed to the state of Texas in 1952 and its activities expanded considerably under the leadership of John "Pete" Parsons, who became its director in 1957. By 1970, some thirty-eight hundred employees and students were members of the union, which had total assets of $1,750,000.[153]

In addition to sharing money, support staff shared meals together. By 1974 the Dietary Services Department prepared more than five thousand meals every day for UTMB personnel. In August 1987 the hospital opened a new restaurant and food court, which seated almost three hundred people.[154]

Employees sang together. A choral group met regularly in the spring of 1970. Michael Warren organized a "Boys Choir" that sang in 1982. Some employees sang with the Galveston Chorale, a community chorus led by Larry Patton. This chorale sang in the hospital lobby in December 1988 and during the third annual Festival of Carols in Levin Hall in December 1989.[155]

Employees played games together. Officially sanctioned by the American Bowling Congress, a Medical Branch Men's Bowling League was organized in September 1953. Four five-member teams competed for trophies every Friday night at the Bowl Lanes at Twenty-fourth Street and Avenue Q and 1/2. These bowling teams continued during the 1960s and 1970s, sporadically during the early 1980s.[156]

Sports for employees also included softball, rugby, and volleyball. Ten teams from the UTMB employees' softball leagues participated in a World Series tournament in September 1979; thirteen players were named all-tournament stars. A UTMB-Galveston rugby team was one of five teams that formed the Texas Rugby Union in 1967. This team captured the runner-up trophy at the Lone Star Tournament in Houston in 1970. A UTMB volleyball league functioned in the summer of 1981.[157]

Particular groups of employees developed programs that addressed their needs. In September 1956 Bonnie Rickelman (Don Walker's secretary), Sunny Axelsen (James Jannasch's secretary), and thirty other secretaries organized a Secretary's Club. Mary Jane Steding, John Truslow's secretary, was the club's first president. With regular meetings and training programs, the club enhanced the skills of its members while significantly improving communication throughout the campus during the 1960s and 1970s. In 1981 the club staged a "Save Old Red Type-a-Thon" that raised about $3,000 for the Old Red restoration project. By 1986 the club included about three hundred members and many attended its thirteenth annual champagne style show.[158]

During the 1970s and 1980s, decisions by corporate executives and other administrators provided important measures of affirmation, education, and specialized assistance for the support staff.

In 1976 administrative leaders initiated "Employee of the Month" awards for support staff in both academic and hospital areas. Recognizing these employees became a way of affirming outstanding job performances. Committees selected a staff person from the hospital areas and one from the academic areas. In 1979, for example, Lillian Jackson, a custodial worker in housekeeping for twenty years, and Joyce Lunsford, coordinator of the Introduction to Patient Evaluation course in the School of Medicine, received the awards for March. Each received a framed certificate and a $50 U.S. Savings Bond. By the mid-1980s winners received $75 U.S. Savings Bonds.[159]

The Personnel Office sponsored numerous "inservice" education and training classes during the 1970s and 1980s. These included courses in administrative development, defensive driving, management, interviewing techniques, medical terminology, preretirement planning, and typing. In 1980 and 1981 about five hundred department directors and supervisors completed a three-day management training course.[160]

In 1982 a new Employee Assistance Program was organized under the direction of Alan Chesney. This program provided counseling and assistance to any employee who had personal problems that affected job performance. During the first six months, Chesney's office received fifty-six self-referrals and forty-five supervisor referrals. The latter were mostly from 140 supervisors who had received special training in dealing with troubled employees.[161]

In 1982 the regents adopted a new policy about job evaluations in the UT System. Supervisors were required to prepare written performance evaluations of all classified, faculty, and administrative personnel. Appropriate administrators would review these evaluations to determine who qualified for merit pay raises if funds were available in future operating budgets. These policies were implemented at UTMB and other UT components by the mid-1980s.[162]

In September 1988 the Department of Human Resources (formerly the Personnel Office) established a new performance appraisal system for all employees. Administrators periodically assessed employees with criteria that had been carefully reviewed with each employee. This approach permitted them to connect the job performances of each employee to specific goals of the institution, to specify the tasks associated with each job, to measure the competence of each employee, to enhance communication with the employee, and to foster the improvement and development of each employee's skills.[163]

Administrators also developed special awards to recognize longtime service to UTMB. In 1979, for example, 660 employees received these pins, including one given to Charles Allen after thirty-five years of service. Recognizing services ranging from five to forty years of continuous employment, 701 employees received service pins in 1981, 495 in 1982, and 582 in 1985.[164]

Because support staff did find their jobs satisfying, long years of service were not uncommon. John W. Reis, an immigrant from Germany, worked as timekeeper and maintenance man at John Sealy Hospital for twenty-five years before his death in 1941. Seventy-year-old Zelcer Tansey Jr. retired in 1961 after serving fifteen years as an orderly in the emergency room. Six longtime employees retired in August 1966, including John Sullivan (physical plant office, twenty-five years), Rosemary Russell (admitting office, twenty-two years), Jennie Hopson (housekeeping, eighteen years), Madie McMillan (admitting, eighteen years), Rosalie Brick (medical records, fifteen years), and Ruth Ford (EEG office, ten years).[165]

Members of an entire family worked at UTMB. In 1970, for example, Joe Josie Jr. had worked as an incinerator operator for thirteen years and his wife, Earnie, had worked in housekeeping for twelve years. Three of their sons worked for the physical plant department, one son was a hospital orderly, three daughters-in law were nurse's aides, and one nephew was a hospital aide.[166]

Most academic departments also had longtime assistants who provided skills and camaraderie that sustained effective functioning. Thomas "Scotty" MacBeth came to Galveston from Glasgow in 1920 and began working as an orderly at John Sealy Hospital. In 1921 he became a lab assistant in the Department of Anatomy and continued in that job until his retirement in 1963. Highly respected by students and faculty, Scotty charmed all with his magic shows and knowledge of the human skeleton. Born at John Sealy Hospital in 1923, Harry Roberts began working as a lab assistant for Wiktor Nowinski in 1949. He continued in that role for many years until he became a lab supervisor in the HBC&G department in 1973. After thirty-five years of service, Hans Ash retired in 1962. Ash worked as a lab technician in pharmacology for twenty years, animal procurement officer for six years, and director of audiovisual aids for nine years.[167]

In 1977 administrators began conducting annual reception ceremonies for employees who were retiring after ten or more years of service. Thirteen of the sixty-one employees retiring in August 1984 had given thirty or more years of service; twenty-six of ninety-six in 1990. In 1987 an estimated eight hundred retirees organized the UTMB Retirees' Association and elected James Jannasch as president.[168] Loyalty was so intense that even retirees could retain an active UTMB identity.

STORYTELLERS: BONDS OF TIME AND MEANING

Administrators, professors, and students established written records about changes and accomplishments at UT and UTMB. UTMB's students and teachers were included in *Cactus*, the UT yearbook, which began in 1894.[169] Publications that focused exclusively on UTMB during its first fifty years included the annual catalogs, *University Medical* (1895–1946), and the *Bulletin of the John Sealy Hospital and the School of Medicine* (1939–1940).

Students launched *University Medical* in 1895. This journal became a highly regarded monthly record for the UTMB community, on and off campus. Students, teachers, and alumni wrote scientific and professional articles. Other articles reflected the pleasures and pains of student life or acknowledged the accomplishments of alumni. In soliciting and printing advertisements from local businesses, students wielded considerable power over the purchasing of goods in Galveston, and the few who managed the journal acquired some money to help with their living expenses. As this journal degenerated into a mostly advertising medium during the mid-1930s, some professors created the *Bulletin of the John Sealy Hospital and the School of Medicine* as an attempt to provide a more respectable publication that would meet the needs of students, faculty, and alumni. The bulletin, however, was a victim of the turmoil of the Spies era.

Other publications provided new bonds of meaning during the second half-century. Faculty and staff in the School of Nursing edited *Nurses Notes* during the 1940s. To support the community of researchers at UTMB and elsewhere, Chauncey Leake established *Texas Reports on Biology and Medicine* in 1942 and served as its editor for thirteen years. The Personnel Office began issuing *Medi-Texan* in 1953. This monthly publication fostered a strong identity among all employees, especially the support staff. Students created the *Syndrome* in 1953. This photographic yearbook dramatically heightened a new sense of community among students, teachers, and academic support staff. These publications promoted a new level of understanding and respect among the different groups on campus, as well as more regard for UTMB by medical professionals and lay citizens throughout the world.

After Leake's departure, the interim management committee established an Office of Information Services. With funds for this office donated by the Kempner Fund and the Sealy & Smith Foundation, Truslow hired Ralph W. "Bud" Meyer as assistant director of public information in November 1959. Meyer coordinated the preparation of a highly regarded campus newsletter titled *Medical Center News*, first published in the fall of 1960. Meyer resigned on October 31, 1962.[170]

Bobbye Barratt became director of public information in August 1964. Accountable to Blocker, Barratt redesigned and retitled the on-campus publication as *Newsletter*, issuing the first number on November 5, 1964. During her eleven-month tenure, she also initiated the production of a seventy-fifth anniversary history of UTMB, a project completed under the supervision of Patrick J. Conner, who was director of public information between 1965 and 1967.

In October 1967 Myles Knape became director of the Public Information Office. A trained and experienced journalist, Knape managed the expanding office for eighteen years. Two new campus publications included *Faculty News* (1968–1977), initially edited by Lynn Alperin, and *Hospital News* (1968–1976), initially edited by Bill Young.[171] *Faculty News* became a weekly publication in the fall of 1975. Each issue of *Hospital News* usually contained a profile and photo of an employee who represented one of the many occupational roles in UTMB's hospitals.

In 1970 the Public Information Office issued a sparkling new magazine titled *University Medical*, which continued through 1984. This magazine marked a new brand of self-awareness at UTMB. In addition to special features in each issue, there were recurring sections that included alumni news, development news, news about faculty and staff, and a list of publications by the faculty (as reported by ASCA). During the 1980s this quarterly focused on such topics as child abuse, drug abuse, and alcoholism.

In January 1977 the Public Information Office published the first issue of *Impact*. Designed to provide more comprehensive coverage of events at UTMB, *Impact* replaced *Faculty News, Hospital News*, and the *Newsletter/Alumni Bulletin*. As originally configured, this superb newsletter continued until it was reformatted in early August 1986. With photos and text, its pages recognized the full range of employees and activities at UTMB. The roles of housekeepers and gardeners were valued, as well as those of executives and students. By 1985 the Public Information Office distributed about sixteen thousand copies every other week to employees, alumni, benefactors, legislators, and community leaders.[172]

With the incredible growth of UTMB after 1965, however, no single publication could be all things to all people. Various groups at UTMB developed their own publications as ways to secure distinctive identities, foster better communication, and report their "lived experiences" for subsequent generations. In January 1967, for example, students began publishing the *UTMB Student Newspaper*, later titled *Synapse*. Continuing for about a decade, students shared useful information and vented their concerns about life at UTMB.[173]

Other non-Public Information Office publications appeared in the 1970s. The Moody Medical Library published the *Compendium* and the *Bookman*. The Area Health Education Center published *La Salud*, a monthly newsletter. Others included *Now Nursing*, created by the hospital's nursing service; *Child Health*, created by the Pediatric Alumni Foundation; and *School Health*, produced by the School Health Advisory Committee. Some were short-lived; some continued into the 1980s.[174]

In 1979 President Levin created a new Division of Institutional Services, which included the Office of Development and Alumni Affairs, the Office of Personnel Recruitment, and the Public Information Office. Myles Knape became executive director and Linda MacDonald was named director. Gary Merritt became associate director of development and Charles "Chuck" Lawrence was named associate director of personnel recruitment.[175]

The Public Information Office continued producing the acclaimed *Impact* and *University Medical*. Articles from *University Medical* were even reprinted in the monthly Southwest Airlines magazine and other magazines in Texas. In 1983 the Council for the Advancement and Support of Education gave the Public Information Office an Exceptional Achievement Award in recognition of the outstanding quality of *University Medical*.[176]

In 1986 Vicki Saito became director of the Office of Public Affairs, which was renamed the Office of External Affairs. Saito supervised six areas of public interactions: media relations, advertising, marketing, publications, special events, and institutional images.[177] In addition to beginning *Alumni News* and *Newsline* in 1987, and *Biomedical Inquiry* in 1988, Saito and her colleagues were heavily involved in the publicity associated with the centennial year celebrations.

In addition to these centrally administered publications, other departments and programs continued to issue their own publications during the 1980s. The Cancer Center produced *Cancer Perspective* and the clinical labs issued *Clinical Microbiology Update*. The Women's Faculty Association issued a newsletter, as did the Coordinating Center on Aging. The Institute for the Medical Humanities began its *Chronicle* in 1987, and the institute provided support to the students who produced a literary magazine titled *Open Forum* between 1984 and 1989.

The variety and scope of these reports and stories mirrored the diverse identities, rituals, and communities that evolved on the UTMB campus. They recognized and shaped many bonds of times shared, meanings discovered, and missions accomplished.

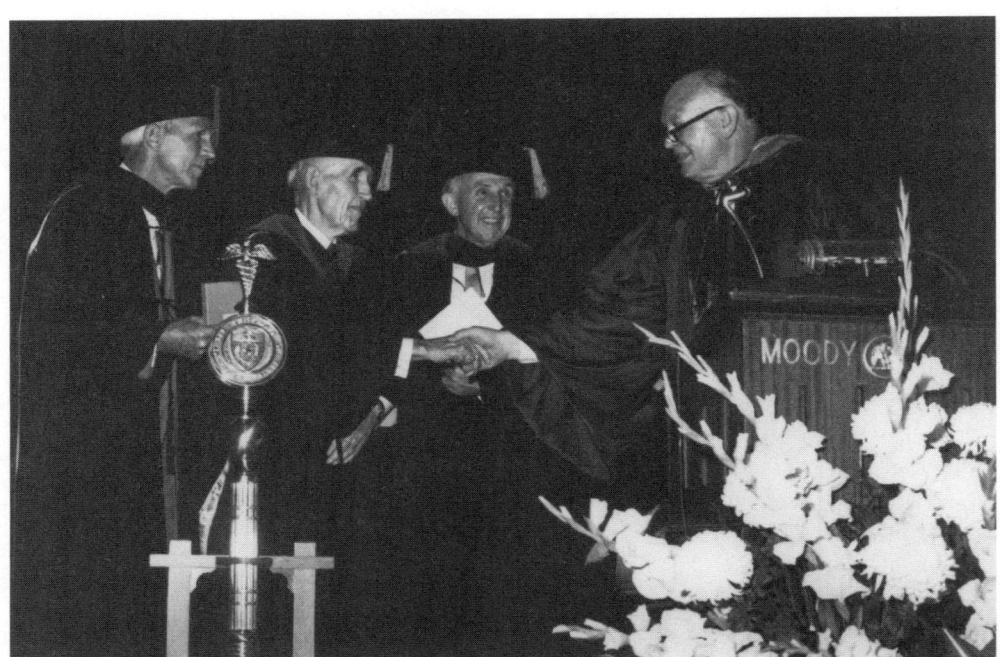

Graduation, 1968. Truman Blocker presents a Distinguished Alumnus Award to Dr. G. V. Brindley (center), who is flanked by his sons, Hanes Brindley, left, and G. V. Brindley Jr., right.

— 9 —

Identities, Rituals, Images—Off Campus

"We are in the dawn of a new era in the history of medical education in this country and our regents imbued with a spirit of patriotism, professional pride and progress, and in the light furnished by the experience of similar institutions, have organized this school upon a plan that is in line with the leading medical colleges of the United States and we here register the solemn edict: its standards shall never trail in the dust."—Dean J. F. Y. Paine, October 5, 1891[1]

Paine concluded his address during UTMB's first opening ceremony with this fervent hope that the new institution would be able to maintain the highest professional standards during its subsequent growth and development. When they became dusty and sandy at times, administrators, faculty, students, and alumni did not permit them to trail for long. Establishing, cleaning, polishing, and reclaiming such standards has been an enduring characteristic of UTMB's commitment to excellence in healing, teaching, research, and service to others. These ideals and values animated alumni, faculty, and students as they influenced the interactive networks and rituals of professionals in Galveston, Texas, the United States, and other nations. Professionals and lay citizens responded with evaluative images of UTMB.

In this chapter, the activities of alumni are considered first because of their central importance to these influences and images. Certain features are considered for each school. The involvement of faculty and others in local, state, regional, national, and international networks are reviewed in the next section of this chapter. To reveal the scope and regularity of this involvement, many examples are given. Peer assessments of standards and behaviors are then described. Their significance in propelling and shaping the institution during its first century must not be underestimated. This chapter concludes with an analysis of some of the ways that storytellers shaped public judgments about UTMB's legacies.

ALUMNI: BONDS OF LOYALTY AND REPUTATION

On commencement days, each graduate became an alumnus or alumna—labels that lasted forever. UTMB's "extended family" spread rapidly throughout Texas, the United

States and other countries.[2] Everywhere a graduate went, he or she carried values, attitudes, and skills from the training received at UTMB. The quality of UTMB as an educational institution was judged by the ways that graduates provided health care to patients, the ways they interacted with other medical professionals, and the ways they served specific groups and communities.

This quality was affirmed, for example, when physicians at other hospitals accepted School of Medicine graduates for postgraduate training. J. S. Jones (class of 1902) attained first place in a competitive exam for internships at Memorial Hospital in New York City. In 1910 twenty-two of thirty-five graduates secured internships, seven at John Sealy or St. Mary's in Galveston, six in other Texas hospitals, and nine in hospitals in other states. Between 1911 and 1920 School of Medicine graduates became more nationally competitive. In 1915 nine became interns in hospitals in Chicago and Milwaukee, five in New York City, three in New England hospitals, and seventeen in Philadelphia.[3]

Most of those graduating between 1920 and 1960 obtained internships. This included thirty-seven of forty-four graduates in 1922, for example, and sixty of sixty-five in 1926. In 1937 about 98 percent of the graduates obtained internships in approved hospitals.[4] Beginning in the 1950s, the majority obtained their first choices. Of 136 students graduating in 1953, for example, 123 received their first choice, 6 their second, 2 their third, and 5 remained unmatched. A match between the hospital and the graduate's first choice usually signified a high regard for the talents of the student. Of 140 graduates in 1960, 135 applied via the National Intern Matching Program and 92 percent of these received their first or second choices.[5]

As training programs for residents expanded in various specialties during the 1940s and 1950s, more graduates chose careers as specialists. In 1961, for example, School of Medicine graduates made the following choices: 41 percent specialty practice (national average 74 percent); 43 percent general or family practice (national average 21 percent); and 16 percent research and teaching (national average 4 percent). By the 1970s "primary care" practitioners were those who practiced obstetrics-gynecology, pediatrics, internal medicine, and family medicine. From 1977 to 1981 between 52 and 58 percent of School of Medicine graduates chose these primary care specialties. From fiscal year 1980 to fiscal year 1991, between 48 percent and 67 percent selected primary care specialties.[6] As interns, residents, and clinical fellows, physician-graduates carried UTMB's values of excellence throughout the state, nation, and world.

During the earliest decades, several alumni entered private practice instead of seeking additional postgraduate training. In 1900 seven of fifteen graduates became general practitioners. Two practiced with their fathers: G. W. Allen Jr. in Flatonia and H. F. Blailock in McGregor. B. S. Brown practiced in Corsicana, F. C. Gregg in Manor, R. S. Jackson in Galveston, J. P. Lokey in McCulloch, and O. H. Radkey in Austin.[7]

A few became faculty members. During fiscal year 1901, Kenneth Aynesworth (class of 1899) was demonstrator of anatomy, replacing Thomas Flavin (class of 1892), who resigned because of illness. As the first female faculty member, Charlotte Schaefer (class of 1900) became demonstrator of general biology, normal histology, and general

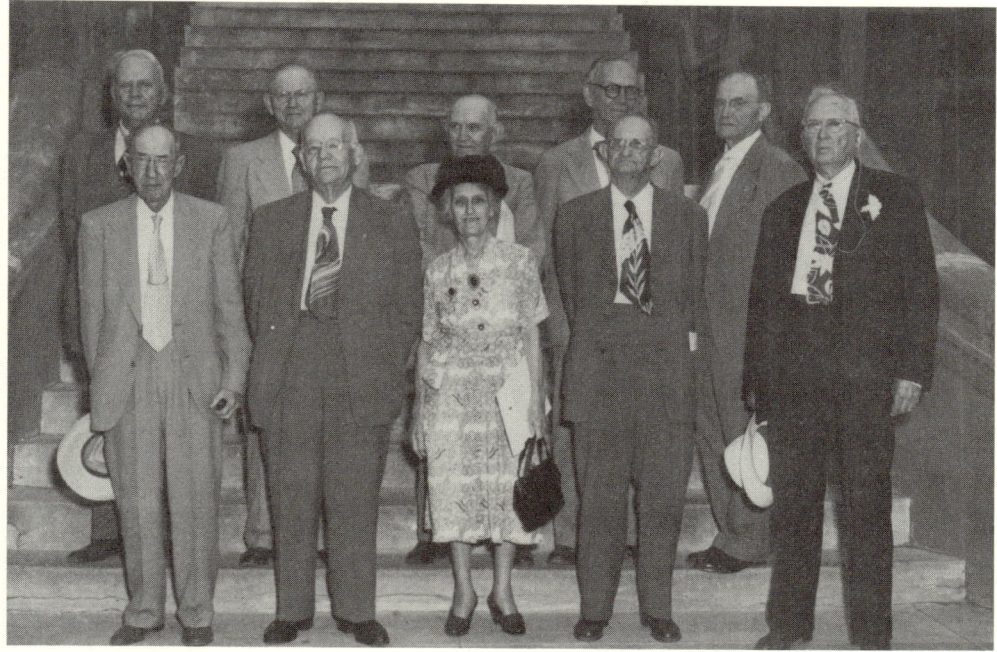

Class of 1902 reunion, 1952.

embryology in 1901, replacing L. E. Magnenat (class of 1895), who became demonstrator of pathology after William Gammon (class of 1893) resigned.

Whether postgraduate trainee, private practitioner, or professor, members of the Alumni Association continued to meet in Galveston in late May or early June to welcome new graduates as members. Beginning in 1905, School of Medicine alumni assembled for festive banquets during the annual meetings of the Texas Medical Association. In May 1909 about 150 male doctors toasted the university, the regents, the faculty, the absent ladies, old-timers, 1900 storm experiences, and West Texas. In 1914 about a hundred people attended the alumni dinner in Houston and about fifty alumni and twenty wives came to Galveston for a luncheon and some clinical presentations. In 1929 Edward Schwab (class of 1928) helped reorganize the Alumni Association and began serving as its secretary for ten years. Annual dinners continued intermittently during the 1930s.[8]

Conversations during these dinners surely involved the exchange of countless stories about their lives as practitioners and public health officials. Thomas T. Jackson (class of 1893) was assistant superintendent at the San Antonio State Asylum. Malone Duggan (class of 1894) was health officer in Eagle Pass, and Charles F. Norton (class of 1899) was a quarantine officer in El Paso and secretary for the state Board of Health. James Jones (class of 1899) was the city physician in Denison and Henry Warner (class of 1899) was the city physician in Thatcher, Arizona. Edwin L. Jones (class of 1903) was an Indian Service physician in New Mexico and Harry K. Speed (class of 1906) was a general practitioner in the Indian Territory (later Oklahoma). Paul Stalnaker (class of

1904) was the quarantine officer in Rockport and Beverly T. Young (class of 1907) was the quarantine officer in Port Lavaca.[9]

Some School of Medicine alumni were general practitioners. Eighty-four-year-old Ella Ware (class of 1899) was honored in the fall of 1954 for her devotion to the citizens of the Stockdale area during more than fifty years of practice. She had delivered more than six thousand babies; about three hundred were named Ella. James Wells Young (class of 1907) was a general practitioner in Roscoe for forty-four years before moving to Sweetwater in 1951 to become a partner with his physician-son. J. Gordon Bryson (class of 1910) was a general practitioner in Bastrop for thirty-seven years, attending many patients at the F. A. Orgain Memorial Hospital.[10]

Some School of Medicine alumni were pioneering specialists. For example, Claudia Potter (class of 1904) was a member of the staff at Scott and White Hospital in Temple for forty-one years, serving as the hospital's chief anesthesiologist for most of those years. Probably the first female physician to practice this specialty in Texas, Potter was president of the Texas Society of Medical Anesthetists in 1947.[11]

Some School of Medicine alumni were remarkable leaders. Two wielded extraordinary influences, one in Houston, the other in Washington. Ernst William Bertner (class of 1911) devoted his career to the development of the Texas Medical Center in Houston. In 1938 he became the seventy-second president of the Texas Medical Association. Rollo Dyer (class of 1915) joined the U.S. Public Health Service in 1916. After five years of field work in New Orleans, he transferred to the Hygienic Laboratory in Washington and became assistant director of the National Institutes of Health in 1922, chief of the Division of Infectious Diseases in 1936, and director of the NIH between 1942 and 1950. He organized the Division of Research Grants and orchestrated the establishment of three new institutes (Heart, Dental Research, and Mental Health).[12]

Alumni served in the armed forces during the 1940s. In 1943 Frances Phillips (class of 1942) received a commission in the Medical Corps of the U.S. Navy. A classmate, Fannie Machles, received her commission as a lieutenant in the U.S. Naval Reserve and was the only female physician at the midshipman's school in Northampton, Massachusetts.[13]

Other alumni and faculty were members of the 30th Surgical Hospital and 127th General Hospital units. The former unit became the 30th Evacuation Hospital and served with distinction in the Pacific. The 127th General Hospital first assembled at Camp Claiborn, Louisiana, in January 1943. This group included Carroll Adriance (class of 1940), William Ainsworth (class of 1940), Norman Duren (class of 1938), and Robert Moore. Capt. Grace Decker (class of 1929) led a group of Army Nurse Corps Officers who joined these doctors in March 1943. In August this fully trained thousand-bed hospital unit, which included five hundred enlisted men and about two hundred professionals (one hundred nurses, thirty-six physicians, five dentists, two chaplains, and others) transferred to southwest England. In buildings located in Sand Hill Park, these personnel attended more than 4,400 patients, performing more than 650 surgical operations. This hospital unit then attended many wounded and

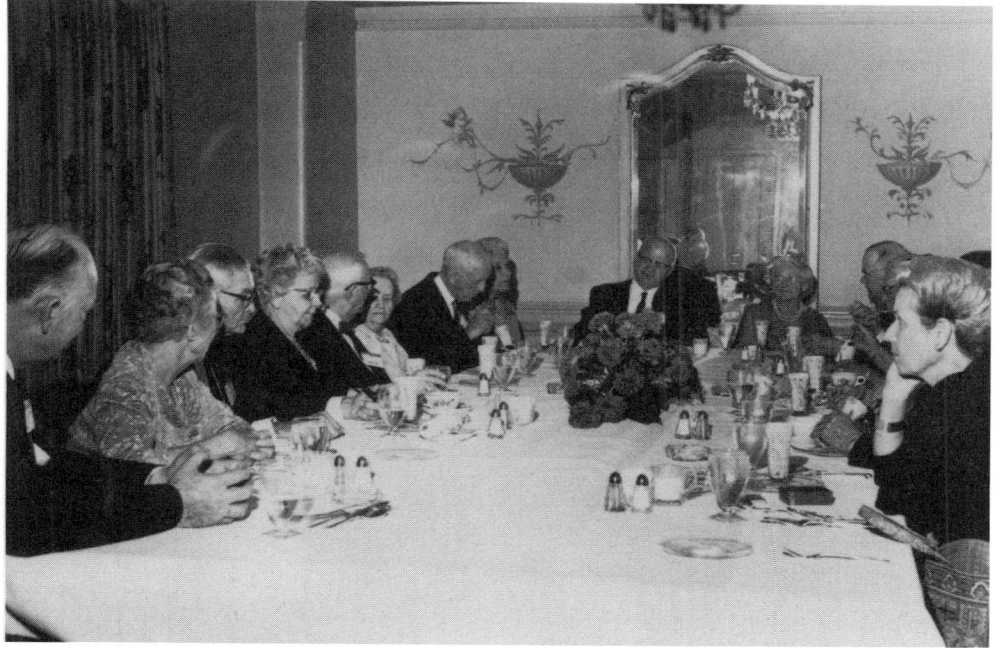

Class of 1915 reunion, 1965. Truman Blocker at front left, Mildred Robertson at front right.

sick soldiers in France, first at Rennes, then at Nancy, before returning to Virginia in October 1945.[14]

In the spring of 1946 Chauncey Leake invited Mildred "Millie" Robertson to become the executive secretary for the School of Medicine Alumni Association (SOMAA), a role she exercised between 1946 and 1978. Millie nurtured alumni with flair, charm, robustness, and constant affection. There were five hundred dues-paying members by June 1947; more than one thousand by December 1952. Millie fostered an extraordinary and enduring spiritual unity among alumni living in Texas, other states, and other countries.[15]

Millie gave special attention to those alumni who were general practitioners.[16] In 1948 Chester Callan (class of 1939) and two partners served more than two thousand citizens living in the thirty-six hundred square miles of Fisher, Stonewall, Kent, and Scurry counties, "the cotton-and-cattle country embraced by the branches of the Brazos River." If necessary, they treated patients in the fifty-bed Callan Memorial Hospital in Rotan, originally built in 1938 in honor of Walter Callan, Chester's father and Rotan's first physician. Together, the three doctors attended between 80 and 120 patients daily. The citizens of Rotan experienced the influences of UTMB every day, as did those in Schulenburg, where Gene Schulze (class of 1936) practiced for many years and those in Iraan where Edwin R. Franks (class of 1949) practiced for twenty-seven years.[17]

Millie continued to organize SOMAA dinners during the 1950s. In April 1951, 430 alumni and guests attended the dinner at the Buccaneer Hotel in Galveston. Ten graduates of the class of 1902 attended the dinner at the Adolphus Hotel in Dallas in 1952.

In April 1953, 363 people attended the dinner at the Shamrock Hotel in Houston. During these dinners, Leake began honoring fifty-year graduates with "Golden T" certificates. From the class of 1904, for example, Claudia Potter, J. Fain Moore, and Paul Stalnaker attended the reunion in 1954. From the class of 1907, Rene Huvelle, J. Guy Jones, and James W. Young attended the dinner in 1957.[18] These certificate ceremonies became a special tradition.

Truman Blocker harnessed the energies and resources of physician alumni unlike any previous CEO. He spurred new life into the SOMAA. Its members adopted a revised constitution and bylaws that designated a fifteen-member Board of Trustees as governing officials. In 1965 this board began selecting School of Medicine graduates to honor during commencement ceremonies with an Ashbel Smith Distinguished Alumnus Award. The first group of awardees included Titus H. Harris (class of 1919), Brittain F. Payne (class of 1927), Leo J. Peters Sr. (class of 1909), and Howard O. Smith (class of 1922). By UTMB's centennial year, ninety-nine alumni had received these awards (Table 9.1).[19]

As mentioned in chapter 3, the regents permitted Blocker to organize a "booster" group of alumni in 1967. This group first named itself the Internal Foundation of UTMB, then the Advisory Council, then the Development Board. Charter members of the Advisory Council included Robert Kimbro (class of 1935), Sam Dunn (class of 1925), McIver Furman (class of 1929), Van Doren Goodall (class of 1933), Harvey Renger (class of 1931), William Seybold (class of 1938), and Courtney Townsend Sr. (class of 1932). This Development Board was an extremely important and influential source of support for UTMB between 1967 and 1991. Blocker, Levin, and James usually gave reports about the institution's development to those alumni who assembled annually as officers and trustees of the School of Medicine Alumni Association, and as officers and members of the Development Board.[20]

School of Medicine alumni exercised other important leadership roles in local, state, regional, and national societies. Between 1950 and 1980 at least forty-three physicians were elected presidents of professional societies.[21]

During the 1950s seventeen alumni were presidents of various societies. These included H. Buford Barr (class of 1926), Jefferson County Medical Society; Herman Weinert Jr (class of 1931), Galveston County Medical Society; Robert E. Leaton (class of 1941), Houston Pediatric Society; William M. Gambrell (class of 1920), Allen T. Stewart (class of 1922), J. Layton Cochran (class of 1924) and C. Denton Kerr (class of 1933), Texas Medical Association; Samuel F. Moore Jr. (class of 1934), Texas Association of Obstetricians and Gynecologists; Dudley Jackson (class of 1917), Texas Surgical Society; L. Bonham Jones (class of 1938), Texas Academy of General Practice; Louis J. Levy (class of 1937), Texas Orthopedic Association; Merton M. Minter (class of 1928), Texas Academy of Internal Medicine; Albert W. Hartman (class of 1934), Southern Society of Clinical Surgery; Rollo Eugene Dyer (class of 1915), American Academy of Tropical Medicine; Ewing S. McLarty (class of 1921) and Holland Jackson (class of 1935), American Academy of General Practice; and Dan E. Jenkins (class of 1940), American College of Chest Physicians.[22]

TABLE 9.1: ASHBEL SMITH DISTINGUISHED ALUMNI, SCHOOL OF MEDICINE, 1965–1991

1965
Titus H. Harris, M.D., '19
Brittain F. Payne, M.D., '27
Leo J. Peters Sr., M.D., '09
Howard O. Smith, M.D., '22

1966
Francis J. L. Blasingame, M.D., '32
Jospeh Kopecky, M.D., '15
Charles C. Sprague, M.D., '43
Charles T. Stone Sr., M.D., '15

1967
H. Frank Connally Jr., M.D., '37
Kenneth M. Lynch, M.D., '10

1968
George Valter Brindley, M.D., '11

1969
James Clarence Cain, M.D., '37
Kenneth Martin Earle, M.D., '45
Edgar Leonard Frazell, M.D., '31
Robert W. Kimbro, M.D., '35
James Roderick Kitchell, M.D., '32
James E. Thompson Jr., M.D., '27
Robert Irby Wise, M.D., '50

1970
Ray K. Daily, M.D., '13
Rolla Eugene Dyer, M.D., '15
Julius Luther Jinkins Sr., M.D., '16
Paul Henry Streit, M.D., '16

1971
Felix P. Ballenger, M.D., '38
Truman G. Blocker Jr., M.D., '33
Leonard Rosoff, M.D., '35
Edward H. Vogel Jr., M.D., '39

1972
Hamilton Ford, M.D., '31
Harvey Renger, M.D., '31

1973
Benjy Brooks, M.D., '48
Frederick Thompson, M.D., '31

1974
Julia M. Baker, M.D., '38
Nicholas Carr Hightower, M.D., '44
M. T. Jenkins, M.D., '40

1975
Alfred Harris Daniell, M.D., '33
James Greenwood Jr., M.D., '31
C. Thorpe Ray, M.D., '31
Courtney M. Townsend Sr., M.D., '32

1976
G. Valter Brindley Jr., M.D., '39
William C. Levin, M.D., '41
C. M. Phillips, M.D., '31

1977
C. William Daeschner Jr., M.D., '45
Jesse B. Heath, M.D., '31
Griff T. Ross, M.D., Ph.D., '45
Raleigh R. Ross, M.D., '35
James M. Vaughn, M.D., '37

1978
Herman A. Barnett, M.D., '53
Julian C. Burton, M.D., '28
Stanley E. Crawford, M.D., '48
Melvyn H. Schreiber, M.D., '55
A. Bryan Spires Jr., M.D., '55

1979
Earl W. Clawater Jr., M.D., '42
William D. Seybold, M.D., '38
James C. Thompson, M.D., '51

1980
Van Doren Goodall, M.D., '33
Ruth Hartgraves, M.D., '32
Edward B. Singleton, M.D., '46

1981
McIver Furman, M.D., '29
Donald R. Lewis, M.D., '44
Herbert M. Seybold, M.D., '51

1982
Jay Collie Fish, M.D., '58
Sam A. Nixon, M.D., '50
Vernie A. Stembridge, M.D., '48
George Willeford Jr., M.D., '46

1983
W. Tom Arnold, M.D., '44
Sterling H. Fly Jr., M.D., '50
Alvin L. LeBlanc, M.D., '55
Wayne V. Ramsey Jr., M.D., '53

1984
C. B. Bruner, M.D., '55
Carlos D. Godinez, M.D., '63
Albert W. Hartman Jr., M.D., '34
Charles E. Putnam, M.D., '67
Fred J. Wolma, M.D., '43

1985
John Childers, M.D., '46
Tracy D. Gage, M.D., '55
James C. Guckian, M.D., '62
Joseph T. Painter, M.D., '49

1986
James A. Allums, M.D., '62
R. Scott Jones, M.D., '61
J. Fred Mullins, M.D., '46
Courtney M. Townsend Jr., M.D., '69
B. Frank Webber, M.D., '60

1987
William S. Hotchkiss, M.D., '39
Mavis P. Kelsey, M.D., '36
Martin L. Pernoll, M.D., '63

1988
W. Kemp Clark, M.D., '48
Sydney M. Finegold, M.D., '49
David C. Miesch, M.D., '51
Richard Ruiz, M.D., '57

1989
Kleberg Eckhardt, M.D., '33
Adolph H. Giesecke, M.D., '57
Ray E. Santos, M.D., '58
Herbert L. Steinbach, M.D., '63

1990
J. Wesley Alexander, M.D., '57
H. Edward Maddox III, M.D., '53
J. Dan Schuhmann, M.D., '35

1991
Harry K. Davis, M.D., '49
Louis J. Girard, M.D., '44
Milton R. Hejtmancik, M.D., '43
Robert L. M. Hilliard, M.D., '56

Eleven presidents during the 1960s included Andrew Magliolo (class of 1938), Galveston County Medical Society; Charles Gillespie (class of 1940), Texas Society of Anesthesiologists; Robert H. Mitchell (class of 1935), Texas Heart Association; Silas W. Grant (class of 1946), Texas Academy of General Practice; Moody C. Bettis (class of 1943), Texas Health Association; George V. Brindley Jr (class of 1939), Texas Medical Association; Glenn Gordon (class of 1947), Oregon Medical Association; W. Grady Morrow Jr. (class of 1942), Southwestern Medical Association; Edward B. Singleton (class of 1946), Society for Pediatric Radiology; Thomas D. Cronin (class of 1932), American Association of Plastic Surgeons; and Bowen Swinney (class of 1926), American College of Allergists.[23]

Fourteen presidents during the 1970s included John Armstrong (class of 1937), Houston Academy of Medicine; Donald M. Gready (class of 1939), Harris County Medical Society and Texas Academy of General Practice; Jack L. Smith (class of 1948), Texas Society of Pathologists; Donald McCready (class of 1939) and Weldon Kolb (class of 1941), Texas Academy of Family Physicians; Henry D. Garrett (class of 1941), Texas Dermatological Society; Robert F. Hyde (class of 1944), Texas Orthopedic Association; Gordon L. Black (class of 1943), Texas Radiological Society; John R. Venable (class of 1953), Texas Occupational Medicine Association; Roger G. Smyth (class of 1941), Texas Public Health Association; William S. Hotchkiss (class of 1939), Medical Society of Virginia; Earl Carter (class of 1955), Aerospace Medical Association; Marion Jenkins (class of 1940), American Society of Anesthesiologists; and Bowen Swinney Jr. (class of 1960), American Association for Clinical Immunology and Allergy.[24]

In 1980 Sam A. Nixon became the thirty-third president of the American Academy of Family Physicians, an organization of 49,000 family physicians in the United States.[25]

Female, black, and Hispanic School of Medicine alumni wielded extraordinary influences in city, state, and national circles. In 1959 Ray Karchmer Daily (class of 1913) was one of eleven physicians selected as Medical Woman of the Year by the American Medical Women's Association (AMWA). An eye, ear, nose, and throat surgeon in Houston, Daily was the first female president of the medical staff at Memorial Hospital and a member of the Houston Independent School District Board of Trustees from 1928 to 1952. In 1956 Ruth Hartgraves (class of 1932), an obstetrician-gynecologist in Houston, organized Houston's chapter of AMWA and in 1962 was president of the national group. In 1974 Hartgraves became the first Texan to receive the AMWA's Elizabeth Blackwell Award in recognition of her outstanding contributions as an advocate for women in medicine. A family practitioner in Austin, Ruth Bain (class of 1942) became the 117th president of the Texas Medical Association in May 1982, the second woman to be honored with that office.[26]

In 1962 Robert Hilliard (class of 1956) became the first black physician selected as chief resident in obstetrics and gynecology at the Robert B. Green Hospital in San Antonio. Hilliard became a private practitioner in San Antonio and a distinguished civic leader and received two special awards from the Texas Legislature for community service. In 1983 he was president of the National Medical Association.[27]

José Antonio García (class of 1934), a general practitioner in Corpus Christi from 1936 to 1971, was the first Hispanic elected as a trustee for the Corpus Christi Independent School District (1940–1951) and the first Hispanic member of the regents of Del Mar Community College (1951–1960). His brother, Hector Perez García (class of 1940), organized the American G.I. Forum in 1948 as a way to improve the status of military veterans. In 1968 Lyndon Johnson selected Hector García as the first Hispanic to serve on the United States Commission on Civil Rights. In 1984 Ronald Reagan awarded him the Presidential Medal of Freedom. Edward Ximenes (class of 1941) practiced internal medicine in San Antonio for more than forty years. In 1967 Ximenes became the first Hispanic to become a UT regent. Ray Santos (class of 1958), an orthopedic surgeon in Lubbock, was a member of the Development Board and a trustee of the SOMAA as well as a member of many civic and professional associations. Carlos Godinez (class of 1963), a McAllen family physician, became the seventieth president of the United States Federation of State Medical Boards in 1984, when he was also president of the Texas State Board of Medical Examiners. During the early 1980s Godinez also chaired UTMB's Alumni Committee on Minority Affairs.[28]

Some School of Medicine alumni were leaders in the AMA. In 1949 F. J. L. "Bing" Blasingame (class of 1932) became a member of the AMA Board of Trustees. A practitioner in Wharton, Blasingame became president of the TMA in 1954. He was the AMA's executive vice president from 1958 to 1969.[29] M. T. "Pepper" Jenkins (class of 1940) and Sam A. Nixon (class of 1950) served on the AMA's Council on Medical Education and Hospitals. Joseph T. Painter (class of 1949), William S. Hotchkiss (class of 1939), and Daniel H. Johnson, Jr. (class of 1963) were AMA trustees and all three served as AMA presidents.

Some School of Medicine alumni had long careers in academic medicine. W. H. Moursund (class of 1906) was dean of the Baylor College of Medicine between 1923 and 1953. Kenneth Lynch (class of 1910) became president of the Medical College of the State of South Carolina in 1949, having served as its professor of pathology since 1926. Charles Sprague (class of 1943) was dean of the medical schools at Tulane and

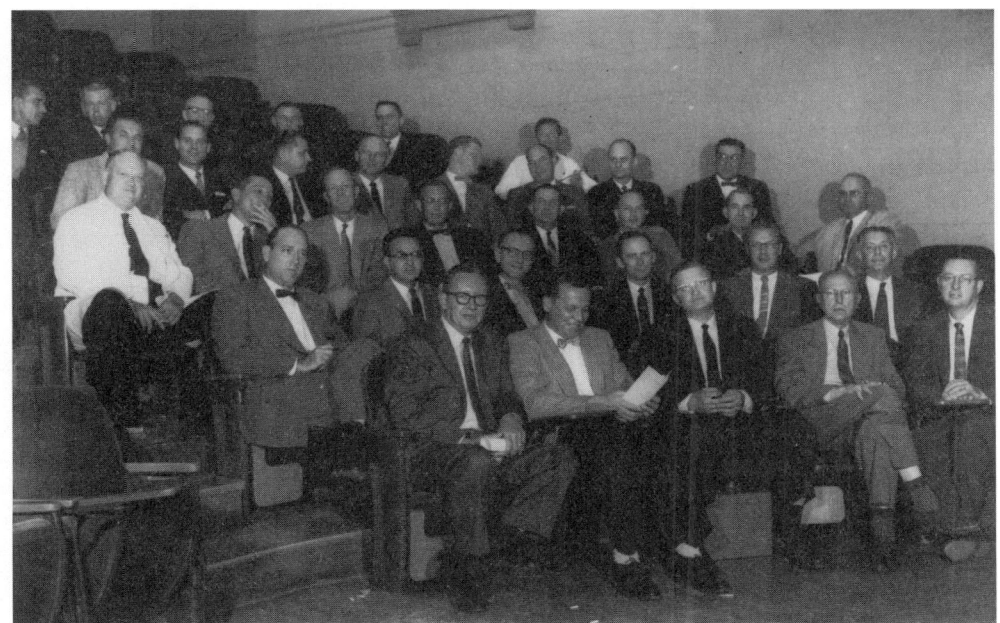

Meeting of Singleton Surgical Society, c. 1954.

UT Southwestern. Bernard Sigel (class of 1953) was dean of two schools: the Women's Medical College of Pennsylvania and the Abraham Lincoln School of Medicine at the University of Illinois. Edward H. Vogel Jr. (class of 1939) became deputy commandant of the U.S. Army Medical Field Service School at the Brooke Army Medical Center in San Antonio in 1970. Stanley Crawford (class of 1948) became dean of the University of Texas Medical School at San Antonio in 1973.[30]

Some School of Medicine alumni created special bonds of tradition and loyalty by establishing societies in honor of five beloved professors. In 1950 alumni and former ob-gyn residents organized the Willard Cooke Club. About thirty-five doctors attended a meeting of this club in Galveston in December 1952 and again in December 1959. Organized in 1953 by about forty-five former students and trainees of A. O. Singleton, the Singleton Surgical Society held its first meeting in Galveston in January 1954. In October 1981 both the Willard R. Cooke Obstetrical and Gynecological Society and the Singleton Surgical Society met in Galveston.[31]

Twenty former residents of the Department of Psychiatry founded the Titus Harris Psychiatric Club in November 1959. About 150 people attended the meeting of the renamed Titus Harris Society at the Galvez Hotel in September 1960. In February 1978 the Singleton Surgical Society held its twenty-fourth annual meeting in Galveston and members of the Titus Harris Society assembled for their eighteenth annual meeting. The Charles T. Stone Society met in Galveston in January 1962. The Robert N. Cooley Radiological Society held its third annual meeting in Galveston in May 1979.[32] By meeting in Galveston periodically, these societies sustained important relationships between alumni and professors in School of Medicine departments.

During Levin's tenure as CEO, the SOMAA organized annual homecoming weekends. More than seven hundred people participated in the first one in March 1978; about five hundred in March 1979. In 1982 the SOMAA sponsored the publication of the first Alumni Directory, which included data for about six thousand School of Medicine graduates. About six hundred alumni and guests from twenty-three states and Canada attended the tenth homecoming in March 1987. Gwen Walker and Jo Lewellyn were executive secretaries of the SOMAA during the 1980s.[33] Forty-five physicians were presidents of the SOMAA between 1946 and 1991 (Table 9.2).

Graduates of the School of Nursing also spread their skills throughout the world and nurtured bonds of loyalty to their school. In November 1919 several graduates working at John Sealy Hospital (JSH) revitalized the School of Nursing Alumnae Association (SONAA). During the 1920s they staged monthly meetings in the Nurses' Home. By 1925 there were 103 members (51 JSH nurses and 52 living outside of Galveston). About 150 people attended the annual homecoming in 1926. Zora McAnelly (class of 1924) was SONAA president in 1927. During the 1930s the SONAA collected funds for scholarships, sponsored teas for honor graduates and visiting dignitaries, and organized "annual boat sails" for seniors.[34]

Graduates were scattered throughout the state and nation. In 1935 Ernestine Schumann Golibart was an instructor at the Medical and Surgical Hospital in San Antonio and Clara Ripperton was an instructor at Breckenridge Hospital in Austin. Lottie Bursey Smith was a school nurse in Fort Worth and Louise Baldwin was a school nurse in Baytown. Anyce Wallace was superintendent of the Elmwood Sanatorium for Tuberculosis in Fort Worth and Xilema Faulkner was superintendent of the Kleburg County Hospital in Kingsville. Mearl Dunham worked at the VA hospital in Biloxi, Mississippi. Hattie Hawkins and Sybil Robertson were private-duty nurses in Fresno, California.[35]

The SONAA organized numerous meetings during the 1940s, 1950s, and 1960s. In June 1940 faculty, students, and alumni assembled to commemorate the school's Golden Jubilee.[36] By 1943 the SONAA had 242 members (92 from Galveston) and the group published an annual *Bulletin of the Alumnae Association of the John Sealy College of Nursing*.

In June 1950 the SONAA sponsored a banquet at the Buccaneer Hotel to celebrate the school's sixtieth anniversary. Elizabeth Bixler, dean of Yale's School of Nursing and president of the Association of Collegiate Schools of Nursing, was the featured speaker. To celebrate the opening of the John Sealy Hospital and the Ziegler Hospital, about two hundred School of Nursing alumni attended homecoming festivities in June 1954. During the reunion dinner, eleven women who had graduated from the school in 1904 or earlier received "Golden T" certificates for their years of service; these included two from the class of 1898 and one from the class of 1899. The SONAA held a homecoming in April 1965 to celebrate the School of Nursing's diamond anniversary. Approximately two hundred nurses celebrated with a picnic, plenary sessions, a Saturday evening banquet featuring folk songs by Alice Anne O'Donell, and a Sunday brunch.[37]

TABLE 9.2: PRESIDENTS, SCHOOL OF MEDICINE ALUMNI ASSOCIATION, 1946–1991

Year	Name
1946–47	George M. Underwood, '17
1947–48	Robert B. Homan Jr., '30
1948–49	George V. Brindley Sr., '11
1949–50	James B. Nail Sr., '19
1950–51	Charles D. Reece, '31
1951–52	Joseph Kopecky, '15
1952–53	Merton M. Minter, '28
1953–54	Thomas M. Oliver, '34
1954–55	Howard O. Smith, '22
1955–56	Kleberg Eckhardt, '33
1956–57	L. Bonham Jones, '38
1957–58	John A. Wall Jr., '34
1958–59	C. M. Phillips, '31
1959–60	James H. Wooten Jr., '38
1960–61	W. Frank McKinley Jr., '40
1961–62	Harvey Renger, '31
1962–63	Howard R. Dudgeon Jr., '35
1963–64	Joe R. Donaldson, '44
1964–65	Travis Smith, '39
1965–66	Jesse B. Heath, '31
1966–67	William L. Marr, '29
1967–68	Ernest E. Anthony Jr., '33
1968–69	John L. Jackson III, '44
1969–70	John L. Otto, '37
1970–71	Courtney M. Townsend, '32
1971–72	Norman E. Halbrooks, '54
1972–73	Van D. Goodall, '33
1973–74	G. Valter Brindley Jr., '39
1974–75	C. Denton Kerr, '33
1975–76	Newton E. Dudney, '49
1976–77	C. Bryan Bruner, '55
1977–78	W. Tom Arnold, '44
1978–79	Earl W. Clawater Jr., '42

1979–80	George M. Willeford Jr., '46
1980–81	Robert B. Crouch, '50
1981–82	John H. Childers, '46
1982–83	Donald R. Lewis, '44
1983–84	Herbert Steinbach, '63
1984–85	James A. Allumns, '62
1985–86	Tracy D. Gage, '55
1986–87	Jack D. Ramsey, '56
1987–88	Jack D. Ramsey, '56
1988–89	David C. Miesch, '51
1989–90	Stephen L. Mark, '74
1990–91	James Len Smith, '55
1991–92	Carlos D. Godinez, '63

TABLE 9.3: DISTINGUISHED ALUMNI, SCHOOL OF NURSING, 1976–1991

Year	Name
1976	Virginia Jarratt, '43
1977	Mary Rose Uher, '59
1978	Elizabeth Knebel, '57
1979	None
1980	None
1981	None
1982	Billye Brown, '53
1983	Beth Jewett, '75
1984	LaVerne Gallman, '49
1985	Lois Mallasanos
1986	Chloe Floyd, '43
1987	Elizabeth Lawhorn, '75
1988	Clair Jordan, '68
1989	Wilina Iona Gatson, '60
1990	Mary Alice Beaver Collerain, '38
1991	Bonnie Rickelman, '63

TABLE 9.4: DISTINGUISHED ALUMNI, SCHOOL OF ALLIED HEALTH SCIENCES, 1982–1991

Year	Name
1982	Jeanette Winfree, '61, Physical Therapy
1983	Arene Gustafson, '53, Medical Technology
1984	Ruby Decker, '61, Physical Therapy
1985	Herbert J. Sauer, '57, Physical Therapy
1986	John W. Young Jr., '73, Physician's Assistant
1987	J. D. Wendeborn, '59, Physical Therapy
1988	Susan McPhail, '74, Physical Therapy
1989	Richard Rahr, '75, Physician's Assistant
1990	Dorit Haenosh Aaron, '77, Occupational Therapy
1991	Mary Rapp Daulong, '70, Physical Therapy

TABLE 9.5: DISTINGUISHED ALUMNI, GRADUATE SCHOOL OF THE BIOMEDICAL SCIENCES, 1976–1986 AND 1990–1991

Year	Name
1976	Joe Wood, Ph.D.
1977	Melvin Hess, Ph.D.
1978	Leroy Olson, Ph.D.
1979	Gilbert Castro, Ph.D.
1980	William B. Stavinoha, Ph.D.
1981	Sam Kolmen, Ph.D.
1982	Cantel Adrian, Ph.D.
1983	Johannes Van Lier, Ph.D.
1984	Matthew La Vail, Ph.D.
1985	Daniel Traber, Ph.D.
1986	Martin Wasserman, Ph.D.
1990	Jerry Daniels, M.D., Ph.D.
1991	J. Arly Nelson, Ph.D.

Nurse alumni reorganized the SONAA in 1978. By 1982 more than fifteen hundred graduates were members. During the 1980s they staged luncheon and dinner meetings, style shows, teas for graduating students, tours and receptions for incoming students, and fund-raising events for various School of Nursing projects. The SONAA began two important events in 1982: coordinating the program of Distinguished Alumni Awards given during commencement ceremonies (Table 9.3) and organizing annual homecomings for graduates. Members also played key roles in staging the school's centennial celebration in 1990.[38]

During the 1970s and 1980s, School of Allied Health Sciences graduates organized alumni groups. Established in 1970, the Physical Therapy Alumni Association held its first reunion in Galveston in August 1978. In 1982 graduates from several programs established a SAHS Alumni Association that included approximately two hundred members by October 1986, when the group held its first homecoming.[39] Beginning in 1982 a Distinguished SAHS Alumnus was honored annually during the SAHS commencement ceremony (Table 9.4).

Beginning in 1984, a Distinguished GSBS Alumnus was recognized periodically during Graduate School of the Biomedical Sciences commencement ceremonies. Thirteen graduates had received this honor by the centennial year (Table 9.5).

A separate book could be written about the accomplishments of the alumni selected for "distinguished" awards. By the time of UTMB's centennial era, these particular graduates and many others had manifested extraordinary bonds of loyalty to their schools, and their reputation for competence and excellence was a core ingredient of UTMB's distinctive legacies.

PROFESSIONAL NETWORKS: BONDS OF LEADERSHIP AND REPUTATION

Throughout the twentieth century, alumni, teachers, students, and support staff attended meetings of other professional societies, hosted meetings of these groups in Galveston, and served as officers of these societies. Like those in alumni groups, member and leader roles in these societies were voluntary, usually requiring tremendous amounts of time and effort with no monetary rewards.

Each meeting mentioned in this chapter required months of planning. Officers and host committees attended to details about advertising, hotel accommodations, transportation, and schedules for business, scientific, and recreational sessions. Social events for the forty-first annual TMA meeting in Galveston in May 1909, for example, included boat rides, auto tours of the beach and city, a "bathing party," and a "fish supper, music and dancing" at the Surf Club.[40] Like residents of other cities, Galvestonians wanted to showcase their tourist attractions.

Officers and committee members especially wanted to develop scientific programs that would honor the cultural purposes of their professional societies. They knew that each meeting provided fellow members with information that could be used in the care of patients, the teaching of students, and the search for new knowledge. The presidents mentioned in this chapter endured countless rituals of handling phone calls, writing letters, appointing committees, developing agendas and priorities, and orchestrating meetings. They relied on secretaries, clerks, audiovisual technicians, photographers, printers, and other support staff at UTMB. Alumni, professors, and staff understood that staging excellent meetings and exercising leadership roles effectively could generate an astonishing number of positive images about UTMB's reputation. Consider some examples for local, state, regional, national, and international organizations, in that order. Notice that numerous individuals participated in one or more societies within each of the geographical subdivisions.

In Galveston, alumni and faculty continued as members of the medical staff at St. Mary's Hospital.[41] They were staunch supporters of the Galveston County Medical Society (GCMS). Abiding by the new reorganization schemes of the AMA and the TMA, the GCMS reorganized in July 1903. In 1905 forty-five of its forty-eight members were from Galveston. Throughout the twentieth century alumni and professors continued to support the GCMS by attending regular meetings, giving presentations about clinical and professional topics, and serving as officers and members of committees.[42]

Alumni and professors supported a variety of other health-related organizations and initiatives in Galveston. Edward Randall Sr. chaired the Sanitary Committee, which was responsible for cleaning the streets and alleys of Galveston after the 1900 hurricane. During the early 1900s the faculty cooperated with the Women's Health Protective Association, whose members lobbied for improved living conditions in Galveston. In 1913 J. P. Simonds, chair of UTMB's new Department of Preventive Medicine, coordinated a sanitary survey whose results officials used to improve sanitary conditions in the city.[43] Doctors assisted the Public Health Nursing Service during the late 1930s and early 1940s. In 1944 Chauncey Leake was chair of the Galveston Health Council, which coordinated the public health efforts of twenty-five local organizations.[44]

During the 1970s and 1980s local initiatives involved emergency services, the health of school children, and cardiac surgery for children from other countries. In 1974 Sally Abston, John Bruhn, Jim Baird, and Jim Williams conducted an extensive study of Emergency Medical Services (EMS) in Galveston County. Funded by a planning grant from the Texas Regional Medical Program, this study became the blueprint for establishing an effective EMS program for Galveston. Ron Bailey chaired a Citizens Committee that helped persuade the City Council to begin a 911 EMS service late in 1974. During the 1970s Phil Nader, Guy Parcel, Nathalie Vanderpool, and others participated in a collaborative project with the Galveston Independent School District to improve the health of students attending schools in that district. Cooperating with local Rotary clubs, UTMB's cardiovascular surgery team voluntarily performed open-heart surgery on twenty children from Korea and four from Panama.[45]

Alumni, teachers, students, and support staff attended meetings of state societies, hosted meetings of these groups in Galveston, and served as officers of these societies. Teachers and alumni exerted major influences in the development of the state's medical organizations.[46]

Graduates of the pharmacy school regularly supported the Texas Pharmaceutical Association. During the years that UTMB had a pharmacy school (1893–1927), this association held three annual meetings (1908, 1913, and 1923) in Galveston.[47]

Professional nurses organized the Graduate Nurses' Association of Texas, later renamed the Texas Nurses Association (TNA). About thirty-five nurses attended the first meeting in Houston in 1907. Three years later they met in Galveston and elected

Ethel Clay (the School of Nursing director) as their first vice-president and Clara Shackford (the superintendent of John Sealy Hospital) as their delegate to the national association of nursing school alumni that met later that year in New York City. More than one hundred nurses attended the fourteenth annual TNA meeting at the Galvez Hotel in 1921. During the twenty-seventh annual convention in Galveston in 1934, public health nurses organized the Texas Organization of Public Health Nursing. The TNA, the Texas League of Nursing Education, and the Texas Organization for Public Health Nursing held their annual meetings in Galveston in 1948.[48]

After 1950 School of Nursing alumni, faculty, and students continued to participate in state organizations by attending annual meetings, serving as officers, and hosting meetings in Galveston. Marjorie Bartholf was president of the Texas League of Nursing Education in 1952 and president of the Texas League of Nursing when that group held its third annual meeting at the Galvez Hotel in 1955. Billye Brown was president of TNA's District 6 when more than three hundred people attended the fifty-first annual TNA meeting in 1959. Catherine Bane was elected TNA treasurer in 1963 and reelected in 1965. Anna Pearl Rains served two two-year terms as TNA president (1985–1989).[49]

School of Medicine alumni and faculty provided extraordinary support to scientific, clinical, and public health societies in Texas. When the Texas Academy of Science (TAS) was revived during the 1930s, for example, UTMB's basic science professors and graduate students actively participated. Several hundred scientists attended a TAS regional meeting at UTMB in 1936. John Sinclair was vice-president; Dean Carter and other professors gave talks. The TAS met again in Galveston in 1944 and Sinclair became president in December 1946.[50]

UTMB faculty continued to participate in the TAS until the mid-1960s. Charles Pomerat was president in 1950. More than seven hundred people attended the annual meeting in Galveston in 1953, when D. Bailey Calvin was president. John Finerty was president when six professors gave papers at the annual meeting in 1955. The sixty-fifth annual TAS meeting convened in Galveston in December 1961. About twenty-five students and professors from UTMB gave papers at the sixty-sixth annual meeting in Austin in 1962, when Donald Duncan was president. Six professors, a research associate, and two medical students participated in the sixty-ninth annual meeting in Dallas in 1965.[51] Participation of UTMB's personnel dropped dramatically after this, as teachers and students became more active in national and international scientific societies.

School of Medicine alumni and teachers continued their extraordinary support of the Texas Medical Association. They hosted annual TMA meetings in Galveston during nine years: 1901, 1909, 1916, 1928, 1938, 1946, 1951, 1956, and 1961. More than two thousand people attended the meeting in May 1938; about eighteen hundred in 1946; more than two thousand in 1951; and about twenty-six hundred in 1956.[52]

Hamilton West was the TMA secretary from 1891 until his death in 1904. John T. Moore of Galveston (class of 1896) became the new secretary, then president in 1911 and chair of the Board of Trustees for twenty-nine years. In 1913 Marvin Graves became president and Holman Taylor of Fort Worth (class of 1899) became secretary-treasurer. In 1926 Keiller was president, Graves was a trustee, and Harry Knight and Henry Hartman were members of committees. Throughout the century, many alumni practicing in various areas of the state were delegates or alternate delegates to the House of Delegates; 157 in 1986, for example. Professors or alumni gave many presentations at annual meetings and served on various committees or as officers of various sections.[53] In 1964 George Herrmann received the TMA's first Distinguished Service Award.

School of Medicine alumni and teachers were leaders in the state's clinical specialty societies that emerged after 1910. During the TMA meeting in 1914 small groups of specialists began discussing the formation of statewide specialty organizations. Later that year radiologists organized the Texas Radiological Society and surgeons organized the Texas Surgical Society.[54]

During the ninth annual meeting of the Medical Association of the Southwest at the Galvez Hotel in 1914, James E. Thompson spearheaded the organization of the Texas Surgical Society (TSS). Thompson was president when about thirty doctors attended the group's first formal meeting in San Antonio in 1915. The TSS decided to meet twice a year. About fifteen members assembled in Galveston in 1916; about fifty in 1932; about one hundred in 1935. The TSS met in Galveston in 1941, 1944, 1947, 1951, and 1954. Altogether, the group held twenty meetings in Galveston between 1916 and 1990. In 1991 James C. Thompson became president-elect.[55]

Beginning in the 1930s other specialty groups met in Galveston, or elected alumni and professors as presidents. The Texas Neurological Society held its fifth semi-annual meeting in 1930. The Texas Association of Obstetricians and Gynecologists held its fifth annual meeting in 1934. This group met in Galveston again in 1941, 1946, 1958, and 1974. John J. Delaney (class of 1932) was president in 1955; Hiram P. Arnold (class of 1940) in 1967; Julius Jinkins (class of 1947) in 1972; and Harry Little Jr. (class of 1957) in 1991. The Texas Radiological Society met in 1936 and again in 1951. Melvyn Schreiber (class of 1955) was president in 1987.[56]

The Texas Neuropsychiatric Association met in 1942. In 1954, when Edgar Ezell (class of 1942) was president, this association held a joint meeting with the Mexican Neuropsychiatric Association and the Western Institute on Epilepsy.[57] Titus Harris (class of 1915), Hamilton Ford (class of 1931), John Otto (class of 1937) and Ivan Bruce (class of 1942) served as presidents.

Members of the Department of Medicine regularly participated in the Texas Club of Internists and the Texas Academy of Internal Medicine. George Herrmann was re-elected secretary-treasurer of the club in 1940 and became president in 1941. Forty internists attended the club's meeting in Galveston in 1943; about fifty in 1949; about two hundred in 1954. The Texas Academy of Internal Medicine held annual meetings in Galveston in 1952, 1954, and 1958. About 150 members attended the meeting in 1954 when William W. Bondurant (class of 1929) was president. By the end of that year, the academy had 264 members in Texas who had been certified by the American Board of Internal Medicine. George Herrmann was president in 1962.[58]

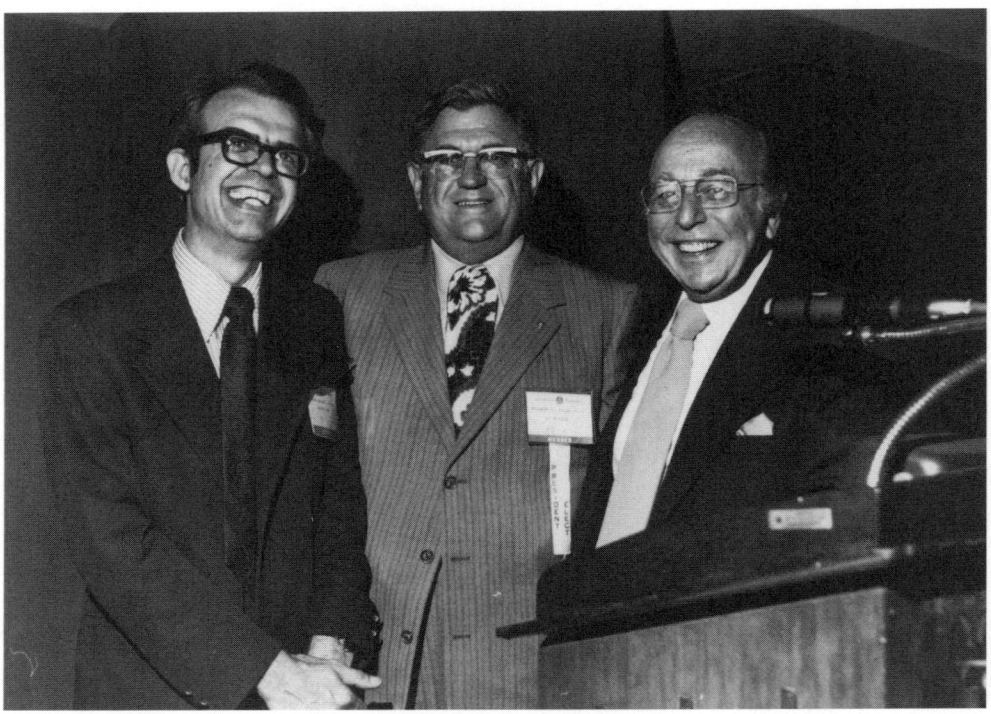

Texas Academy of Family Physicians, twenty-fifth annual scientific assembly, 1974. Edward N. Brandt, left, new president Weldon G. Kolb, center, and luncheon speaker Phil Thorek.

The Texas Academy of General Practice held its fifth annual meeting in Galveston in 1954 and its tenth in 1959. About fourteen hundred doctors attended the fifth; more than one thousand participated in the tenth. Alumni who served as presidents included Chester U. Callan (class of 1929), Van D. Goodall (class of 1933), Holland T. Jackson (class of 1935), and Frank Beall (class of 1934). Renamed the Texas Academy of Family Physicians, three hundred members celebrated its twenty-fifth anniversary during a four-day meeting in Galveston in 1974.[59]

Alumni and faculty organized meetings in Galveston for their colleagues in other specialty societies and served as presidents of these groups. The Texas Pediatric Society met in 1940 and 1955. Francis Garbade (class of 1931) was president in 1964. Robert E. Cone (class of 1919) was president of the Texas Urological Society in 1953. This society held its annual meeting at the Jack Tar Hotel in 1958.[60]

Eight professors were presidents of the Texas Society of Pathologists: Moise D. Levy (1921); John F. Pilcher (1937); Paul Brindley (1945); John Childers (1958); Raymond Rigdon (1961); Elwood Baird (1972); Lamont Jennings (1975); and P. Ridgeway Gilmer (1987). This society held annual meetings in Galveston in 1948, 1957, 1962, 1980, and 1988.[61] In 1937 this society gave its Award for Outstanding Research to Meyer Bodansky.

G. W. N. Eggers (class of 1923) was president of the Texas Orthopedic Association in 1951. Thomas J. Vanzant (class of 1933) was president of the Texas Ophthalmological

Association in 1956. M. T. Pepper Jenkins (class of 1940) was president of the Texas Society of Anesthesiologists in 1962; Steve Lewis was president of the Texas Society of Plastic Surgeons in 1964; and Ben T. Withers (class of 1940) was president of the Texas Otolaryngological Association in 1966.[62]

Alumni and professors also supported groups of volunteers who organized public advocacy groups against specific diseases and they supported the state's public health institutions and organizations. For example, Dean Carter was a member of the delegation from Texas that attended the International Congress on Tuberculosis held in Washington, D.C., in 1908. During the train ride to Washington, this group organized the Texas Anti-Tuberculosis Association, which became the Texas Public Health Association (TPHA) in 1917. The TPHA staged six annual meetings in Galveston between 1950 and 1955. Henry A. Holle (class of 1927) became the director of the Texas Department of Health in 1954.[63]

Titus Harris (class of 1919) spearheaded the organization of the Texas Society for Mental Hygiene at a meeting in Austin in 1934. Harris became president in 1943 and the society met in Galveston in 1946. Renamed the Texas Society for Mental Health, the group held its sixteenth annual meeting in Galveston in 1951, when Hamilton Ford (class of 1931) was president. Renamed the Texas Mental Health Association, M. Lake Fowler (class of 1947) was president in 1967.[64]

Charles Stone Sr. was president of the Texas Heart Association in 1941, George Herrmann in 1953, and John Derrick in 1970. William D. Seybold (class of 1938) was president of the Texas Division of the American Cancer Society in 1964. In 1973 Truman Blocker was president of the Texas Division of the American Trauma Society.[65]

Some professors received special honors from these advocacy groups. In 1990 the Texas Cancer Council gave its Public Education Achievement Award to Billy Philips Jr. and in 1991 Courtney Townsend Jr. received the council's Gibson D. Lewis Physician Achievement Award.[66]

Alumni, professors, and other employees participated in statewide networks of allied health, hospital, and paramedical personnel. With about thirty-five members, the Texas Association of Occupational Therapists (TOTA) organized in 1935. In 1937 about twenty-five members convened in Galveston for a two-day conference. In 1990 about five hundred members and guests attended the fifty-sixth annual TOTA meeting in Galveston.[67]

The Executive Council of the Texas Hospital Association (THA) met for two days at the Galvez Hotel in 1945, and the THA held three annual meetings in Galveston (1949, 1950, and 1953).[68]

About two hundred people attended the nineteenth annual convention of the Texas Society of Medical Technicians at the Galvez in 1951. The society met in Galveston again in 1961. In 1967 Arene Gustafson became president of the renamed Texas Society of Medical Technologists during its thirty-fifth annual meeting in Galveston in April. This society returned to Galveston in 1975 and in 1979 named Mary Jane Webb, supervisor of UTMB's Hematology Laboratory, as its Member of the Year.[69]

Other groups met in Galveston. In 1952 the Texas Association of Blood Banks held its third annual meeting at the Galvez Hotel. The Texas Society of X-Ray Technicians met in 1953. Approximately 120 scientists attended the first meeting of the Texas Society for Electron Microscopy at the Flagship Hotel in 1966. The society met at the Jack Tar Hotel in 1973 and again in 1982. The Texas Speech and Hearing Association held its annual meeting in 1975. The Texas Society for Gastrointestinal Endoscopy came to Galveston in 1978.[70]

Members of allied health professional societies elected professors as presidents. After five years as a member of the SAHS faculty, Juanita Caskey became president of the Texas Medical Record Association in 1981. Susan McPhail was president of the Texas Physical Therapy Association in 1984 and two SAHS faculty were presidents of their societies in 1985: Camellia St. John (Texas Society for Medical Technology) and Donald Davidson (Texas Occupational Therapy Association).[71]

Alumni and faculty also participated in meetings of regional organizations, some multi-county within the state, others multi-state within the country. The South District Medical Association staged meetings in Galveston during the following years: 1903, 1905, 1909, 1913, 1914, 1919, 1921, 1924, 1928, and 1941. Presidents included John Moore (1905), William Keiller (1910), and James E. Thompson (1918). To coordinate continuing education for its members, the South District Medical Association established the Post Graduate Assembly in 1932. Professors from UTMB, Baylor, and other schools gave presentations during meetings of this assembly that attracted large number of doctors. Some professors at UTMB were directors and officers of this assembly.[72]

Members of other regional groups elected professors as officers. James E. Thompson was president of the Southern Surgical Association in 1919, A. O. Singleton in 1939, and Robert Moore in 1962. In 1941 John Spies was secretary of the Medical Education and Hospital Training Section of the Southern Medical Association. In 1943 R. E. Cone was president of the South Central Region Section of the American Urological Association. In 1960 Austin Foster was president of the Southwestern Association of Medical Psychologists and Patrick Romanell was president of the Southwest Philosophy Society. Charles L. Hooks (class of 1935) was president of the South Central Urological Association in 1963. Curtis Artz was president of the Southeast Surgical Congress in 1966 and William L. Marr (class of 1929) was president of the Southwest Allergy Forum in 1967. Hamilton Ford (class of 1931) was president of the Southern Psychiatric Association in 1970 and George V. Brindley Jr. (class of 1939) was president of the Southern Surgical Association in 1973.[73]

Regional multistate medical associations held annual meetings in Galveston. About two hundred neurologists and psychiatrists attended the twenty-third annual meeting of the Central Neuropsychiatric Association in 1947. The Southwestern Psychological Association held its thirty-ninth annual meeting at the Jack Tar Hotel in 1960. When Titus Harris was president, the Southern Psychiatric Association held a three-day convention at the Galvez Hotel in 1962. Approximately three hundred

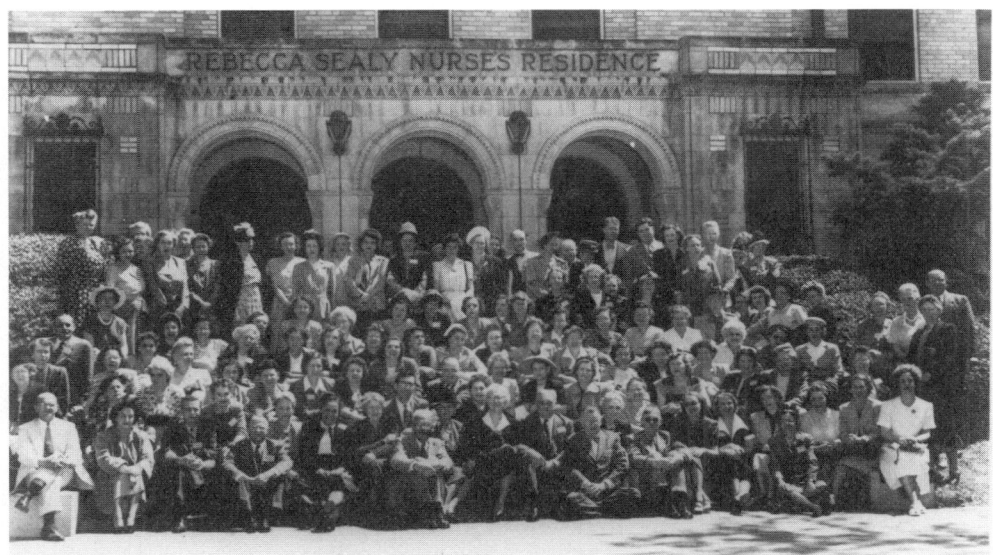

Medical Library Association, 1949.

doctors from thirty-nine states and Canada attended the seventy-first annual meeting of the Western Surgical Association in 1963.[74]

Ed Brandt, then chair of the Southern Region Council of Deans, hosted the Southern Group on Medical Education in 1976. In 1977 about sixty toxicologists met at UTMB for the fall meeting of the Southwestern Association of Toxicologists. George Bryan hosted another meeting of the Southern Group on Medical Education in 1987.[75]

Teachers, alumni, students, and support staff attended meetings of national societies, hosted meetings of these groups in Galveston, and served as officers of these societies.

Dean Carter and Allen Smith presented papers at the AMA meeting in New Orleans in 1903. Keiller attended the AMA's annual Congress on Medical Education in 1922. Some students accompanied faculty members to the AMA meeting in Dallas in 1926. Lucius Wilson, A. O. Singleton, George Herrmann, Meyer Bodansky, W. F. Spiller, James Bennett, Hamilton Ford, Samuel Snodgrass, and William Marr attended the AMA meeting in St. Louis in 1939.[76]

Charles Stone Sr. served ten years (1952–1961) as a member of the AMA's Council on Medical Education and Hospitals, as did M. T. Pepper Jenkins (1976–1985). In 1971 George Herrmann became the thirty-fourth American physician and the first UTMB professor to receive the Distinguished Service Award of the American Medical Association, the AMA's highest honor. When Dean Joseph M. White was a member, the AMA's Council on Medical Education and Hospitals met at the Flagship Hotel in 1973.[77]

Professors gave presentations during meetings of other national societies. Fourteen professors gave talks at the annual meeting of the American Association for the Advancement of Science in Dallas in 1941. Willard Cooke, George Herrmann, and Titus Harris were frequent speakers at meetings of national groups during the late

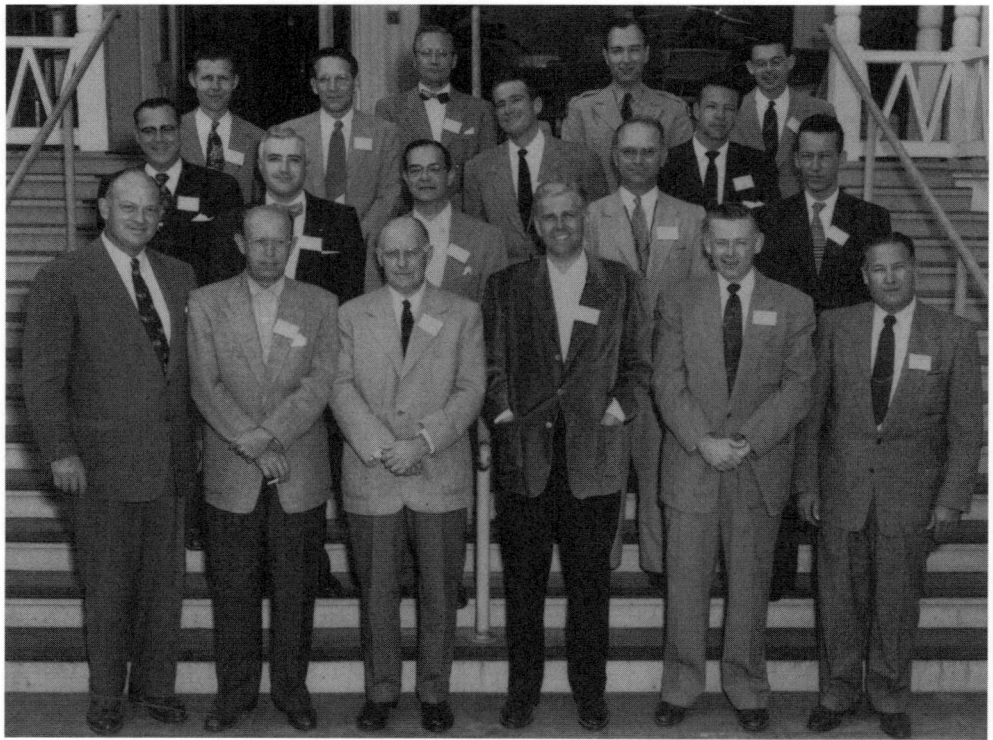

Annual meeting, Texas Society of Plastic Surgeons, 1953. Truman Blocker is on the front row, first from left, and Steve Lewis is on the front row, second from right.

1930s and early 1940s. About twenty professors gave talks during the meeting of the Federation of American Societies for Experimental Biology in Chicago in 1953. In January 1966 twenty-three members of the Department of Internal Medicine attended meetings of the Southern Society for Clinical Investigation and the American Federation for Clinical Research. In February 1985 the Department of Pediatrics rented a bus to take twenty-eight people (faculty, staff, and students) to New Orleans for the annual meeting of the Southern Society for Pediatric Research.[78]

In Galveston, faculty and staff hosted meetings of national societies. The Society of American Bacteriologists held its annual meeting in 1942. About three hundred people attended the meeting of the American Society of Anesthetists in 1944. More than two hundred people attended the annual meeting of the Medical Library Association in 1949. During the 1950s, six national societies met in Galveston: the American Society of X-Ray Technicians (1951), the American Academy of Tropical Medicine and the American Society of Tropical Medicine and Hygiene (1952), the American Association of Anatomists (1954), the American Society of Plastic Surgeons (1954), and the American Psychiatric Association (1955).[79]

By the 1960s and 1970s, many national organizations were too large to be accommodated by the hotel and meeting facilities in Galveston. Nevertheless, a few groups did meet in the Oleander City. The Department of Microbiology hosted a meeting of the American Society of Microbiology at the Jack Tar Hotel in 1964 and the Institute for the Medical Humanities hosted the American Association for the History of Medicine at the Flagship Hotel in 1976. In 1991 the Department of Surgery hosted the fifty-second annual meeting of the Society of University Surgeons.[80]

UTMB's professors and staff also hosted meetings of regional sections of national societies. About one hundred urologists and guests attended the twenty-first annual meeting of the South Central Section of the American Urological Association at the Galvez Hotel in 1941. Chauncey Leake was chair of the Southwestern Section of the Society of Experimental Biology and Medicine when the section met in 1946. Five regional groups met during the 1950s. These included the Society of Experimental Biologists (1951), the Texas branch of the Society of American Bacteriologists (1952), the southern district of the state chapter of the American Physical Therapy Association (1953), the Southern Section of the American College of Surgeons (1955), and the Southern Regional Group of the Medical Library Association (1959).[81]

A regional meeting of the American College of Physicians was held at the Galvez Hotel in 1962. More than twelve hundred people attended a regional meeting of the American Ortho-Psychiatric Association in 1972. The Texas Branch of the American Society for Microbiology met in 1974 and 1979. Jay Fish was president of the South Texas Chapter of the American College of Surgeons when this chapter met at the Holiday Inn in 1975. The Southwest Section of the Society for Experimental Biology and Medicine met in 1980. The Texas Academy Chapter of the American College of Physicians and the Texas Society of Internal Medicine held a combined meeting in 1982.[82]

Peers throughout the country honored some professors with special awards and honored others by electing them as members or officers of national associations. In 1913 James Thompson was a founding member and first vice president of the American College of Surgeons. In 1917 Dean Carter was president of the Association of American Medical Colleges and in 1919 he was elected to the National Board of Medical Examiners. In 1914 William Gammon, Henry Haden, George Lee, and Seth Morris became fellows of the American College of Surgeons (ACS) and in 1928 George Bethel, Boyd Reading, and Raymond Reitzel became fellows of the American College of Physicians (ACP). A. O. Singleton became second vice president of the ACS in 1939 and a trustee in 1942. Charles Stone Sr. became a regent of the ACP in 1942.[83]

During the 1940s some professors received other honors from their national peers. Robert Moore became the third Texan admitted to membership in the prestigious American Surgical Association, which was limited to two hundred surgeons in North America. Moore was also appointed to the American Board of Surgery (1947) and elected second vice president of the American College of Surgeons (1948). In 1942 Truman Blocker became a member of the American Board of Plastic Surgery and Willard Cooke was president-elect of the American Association of Obstetrics, Gynecology, and Abdominal Surgery. A. O. Singleton was vice-president of the American Surgical Society

(1944); Jack Ewalt was elected a fellow of the American Psychiatric Association (1944); and Wendell Gingrich was vice president of the National Malaria Society (1946).[84]

Such honors continued during the 1950s. George Herrmann was elected a director of the American Heart Association (1954) and president of the American College of Chest Physicians (1956). Robert Moore became a vice president of the American Surgical Association in 1954. Chauncey Leake was elected to the board of directors of the AAAS (1955). Truman Blocker was president of the American Association of Plastic Surgeons (1955) and the American Association for the Surgery of Trauma (1958).[85]

Peers in national associations presented special awards to two professors. In 1949 the American Academy of Orthopedic Surgery gave G. W. N. Eggers a gold medal in honor of his outstanding discoveries about the healing of burn wounds. In 1957 the American Academy of Pediatrics presented its Gail Borden Award to Arild Hansen for his discoveries about linoleic acid.

During the 1960s some School of Medicine professors were presidents of national societies or of state or regional sections of national groups. These included Samuel Snodgrass, American Academy of Neurological Surgery (1960); G. W. N. Eggers Sr., American Board of Orthopedic Surgery (1960), American Academy of Cerebral Palsy (1961), and American Orthopedic Association (1962); John Middleton, Texas Chapter, American College of Chest Physicians (1962); C. A. Hooks, South Central Section of the American Urological Association (1964); J. M. Robison, American Society of Ophthalmologic and Otolaryngologic Allergy (1965); and Donald Duncan, American Association of Anatomists (1966).[86]

Some professors exercised other leadership roles assigned by their national peers. During the early 1960s Elwood Baird chaired the board of directors of the National Board of Schools of Medical Technology, the national accrediting board for more than eight hundred schools of medical technology and eighty-three schools of cytotechnology in 1965. In 1966 Stephen Lewis was elected to the American Board of Plastic Surgery and in 1968 Fred Mullins began a nine-year term as a member of the American Board of Dermatology. In 1968 Roy Wilson was appointed to the Board of Medical Advisors of the American Association of Inhalation Therapy.[87]

Some non-physician staff and faculty were officers of national associations during the 1960s. Robert Weilacher was president of the South Texas Chapter of the American Association of Inhalation Therapy in 1964. In 1968 Sally Mount was president of the Texas Association of Medical Record Librarians and she was elected to the executive board of the American Association of Medical Record Librarians.[88]

During the 1970s their national peers continued to elect UTMB's professors as presidents of professional societies. School of Medicine faculty included: Bill Daeschner, American Association of Pediatric Department Chairmen (1970); Martin Towler, American Medical EEG Society (1970); Stephen Lewis, American Society of Plastic Surgery (1971); Robert Cooley, American Board of Radiology (1974); Chester R. Burns, Society for Health and Human Values (1975); Fred Mullins, American Board of Dermatology (1976); Byron Bailey, Society of University Otolaryngologists (1976);

William P. Deiss, American Board of Internal Medicine (1977); James Arens, Society of Academic Anesthesia Chairmen (1979); and Philip Nader, American School Health Association (1979).[89]

School of Allied Health Sciences faculty included Sally Mount, who was president of the American Medical Record Association in 1972, and Ruth Morris, who was elected in 1973 to a five-year term as a member of the Board of Registry for the American Society of Clinical Pathologists.[90]

After 1980 members of national associations continued to elect faculty and staff as presidents or directors. These included Barbara Bowman, American Society of Human Genetics (1981); Bill Daeschner, American Board of Pediatrics (1982); Ronald A. Carson, Society for Health and Human Values (1982); Phil Nader, Ambulatory Pediatric Association (1982); Melvyn Schreiber, Society of Chairmen of Academic Radiology Departments (1985); Byron J. Bailey, American Academy of Otolaryngology—Head and Neck Surgery (1988); James Arens, American Society of Anesthesiologists (1988); Ben Smith, American Academy of Dermatology (1989); and James C. Thompson, American Surgical Association (1991).[91]

In 1985 P. Ridgeway Gilmer Jr. began a three-year term as governor of the College of American Pathologists, an organization of about ten thousand members. Anne Hudson Jones was president of the Southwest Chapter of the American Medical Writers Association in 1987. In that same year Julian Kitay was chair of the AAMC's Group on Medical Education. In 1991 members of the Radiation Research Society selected James Belli as their president-elect.[92]

In 1986 three School of Allied Health Sciences faculty were elected as directors of the Texas Society of Allied Health Professions: David Cordova, Richard Rahr, and Lynn Verret. In 1988 Billy Philips Jr. began a two-year term as a director of the American Society of Allied Health Professions. In 1990 Regina Lederman (School of Nursing professor) was elected president of the American Society for Psychosomatic Obstetrics and Gynecology.[93]

Throughout the century, other faculty and alumni also served as directors or trustees, vice presidents, secretaries, treasurers, and committee members and chairs in other local, state, regional, national, and international societies. In 1979, for example, Richard Stream was elected vice president for administration of the American Speech-Language-Hearing Association and in 1990 Linda Phillips became vice president of the Association of Women Surgeons.[94]

During the 1980s national groups gave special honors to some School of Medicine faculty. Luther Travis received the National Award for Outstanding Contributions to Youth with Diabetes from the American Diabetes Association and Phil Nader received the American School Health Association's Distinguished Service Award. In 1981 the March of Dimes Birth Defects Foundation presented its Agnes Higgins Award for Outstanding Achievement in the field of Maternal and Fetal Nutrition to Bill McGanity. In 1982 the AMA gave its Abraham Jacobi Award to Bill Daeschner for outstanding contributions to American pediatrics. In 1990 the Society for Surgery of the

Alimentary Tract awarded its Founder's Medal to James C. Thompson in recognition of his outstanding research on peptide hormones.[95]

Throughout the century professors visited colleagues in other countries, attended meetings of international societies, hosted meetings of these groups in Galveston, served as officers of these societies, and received special awards from their peers in these groups.

Grace Grey, director of nursing, attended an International Congress for Nurses at Helsingfors, Finland, in 1925. Joseph Kopecky, professor of clinical pathology, was a visiting professor at the University of Mexico in 1929.[96]

Paul Brindley and George Herrmann visited Guatemala in 1944. J. Allen Scott studied parasitic diseases in Brazil during two months in 1944. In 1946 Ludwik Anigstein gave several lectures on tropical medicine and taught physicians during a three-month visit to Poland. Ardzroony Packchanian was one of nine American delegates attending the first Inter-American Congress of Medicine in Rio de Janeiro, Brazil, in 1946. Between 1942 and 1948 George Herrmann, Charles Pomerat, A. Packchanian, and Edgar Poth made more than one visit to schools and labs in Mexico City and Monterrey. For his research studies on bone healing, G. W. N. Eggers received an award from the International Surgical Society in 1949.[97]

Travel by faculty in other countries expanded during the 1950s and 1960s. In 1950 George Herrmann gave papers at the First International Congress of Internal Medicine and the First Cardiological Congress in Paris. Arild Hansen, Hilda Wiese, Edward Randall, and Elisabeth Runge attended the Sixth International Pediatric Congress in Zurich in 1950. In 1953 Truman Blocker was a consultant for the U.S. Army during six weeks in Japan and Korea. He taught plastic surgery techniques to Japanese surgeons who were attending survivors from the atomic bomb explosions in 1945. In 1954 Charles Pomerat and John Finerty gave papers during the International Congress of Hematology in Paris, and John Bieri spoke during the third International Congress on Nutrition in Amsterdam.[98]

In 1955 Blocker participated in the first International Congress of Plastic Surgery in Stockholm. During this congress, Blocker became a member of the executive committee of a newly organized International Society of Plastic Surgeons. In 1956 Hansen and Wiese gave papers during the eighth International Congress of Pediatrics in Copenhagen. Wiktor Nowinski was a visiting professor at the National University of Buenos Aires for four months beginning in November 1958.[99]

After John Truslow's visit to the University of Hamburg in 1960, a few exchange visits occurred between members of their faculty and some professors at UTMB, including Ludwik Anigstein, Harry Levine, and Al LeBlanc. George Herrmann attended the fourth International Congress of Cardiology in Mexico City in 1962. Eight professors attended the third International Congress on Plastic Surgery in Washington, D.C., in 1963. During the mid-1960s some exchanges of faculty and students occurred between UTMB and the University of Nuevo Leon Medical School in Monterrey, Mexico. In 1968 Blocker visited medical schools in Mexico City, Lima, Buenos Aires, and Santiago to consult with their chiefs of plastic surgery. All four had trained as residents at UTMB.[100]

During the 1970s and 1980s some professors hosted international meetings in Galveston. In 1970 about three hundred people from Canada, England, and the United States attended a conference honoring the legacies of William Osler. In 1980 about fifty people attended an international symposium on Fundamental Mechanisms in Human Cancer Immunology. Funded by the Moody Foundation, the International Center for Health at Galveston staged a three-day Conference on the Control and Prevention of Injury in May 1982. Sally Abston, Truman Blocker, Michael Warren, and others participated in this conference.[101]

Designed to promote international collaboration among nurses, the School of Nursing hosted a two-day conference in 1988 entitled "Global Nursing: Education, Research and Practice." UTMB hosted the 1988 International Conference on Nutrition and Aging, co-sponsored by the World Health Organization, the American Board of Family Practice, the American College of Nutrition, and the American Society on Aging. In 1974 and again in 1989 the Department of Surgery sponsored two international symposia on gastrointestinal hormones.[102]

Peers in other countries honored some professors by selecting them as officers in international societies. In 1977 Luther Travis began a six-year term as a counsillor for the International Pediatric Nephrology Association. Between 1981 and 1983 James C. Thompson was president of the Society for Surgery of the Alimentary Tract, an international organization of seven hundred gastrointestinal surgeons. In 1989 Ernest S. Barratt was president of the International Society for the Study of Individual Differences. In 1991 Janet Gottschalk became co-chair of the National Council for International Health, and Chester Burns became a treasurer for the International Society for the History of Medicine.[103]

School of Allied Health Sciences faculty made special overtures to China during the 1980s. In 1985 Ruth Morris lived in China for four months as a visiting teacher. At the Zhejiang Medical University in Hangzhou, one hundred miles southwest of Shanghai, she helped teachers develop a Learning Resource Center and taught technicians how to use videocassette recorders. Morris and other School of Allied Health Sciences faculty later hosted six educators from China who studied the SAHS's Learning Resource Center.[104]

The World Health Organization (WHO) affirmed UTMB's expanding international roles in several ways. In 1985 the Pan American Health Organization, WHO's regional office, designated UTMB as the site for a World Health Organization Collaborating Center for Research and Training in Psychosocial Factors in Health. During a four-year period, some professors taught health care professionals about the social and cultural factors pertinent to the delivery of primary health care in developing nations.[105]

Administrators and professors established a Center for International Health in 1988 and added a Division of International Health to the Department of Preventive Medicine and Community Health. Abdul Sajid was named center director and division chief. The new center incorporated the WHO Collaborating Center for Psychosocial Factors and Health and the WHO Collaborating Center for International Health

Manpower Research and Allied Health Science Education. In 1991, for example, School of Allied Health Sciences faculty taught courses in medical laboratory technology, physical therapy, and radiography to students in the College of Arts, Science and Technology in Kingston, Jamaica.[106]

Throughout UTMB's first century, alumni, faculty, students, and support staff exercised many leadership roles in numerous local, state, regional, national, and international networks of professionals. Their extraordinary commitment to these voluntary roles signaled a quality of caring and generosity that produced admiration and respect throughout the world. These behaviors significantly shaped UTMB's reputation for excellence.

Peer Reviews: Bonds of Accountability and Reputation

Throughout UTMB's history, professors, students, and staff prompted each other to discover better ways of treating patients, instructing students, conducting research, and managing institutional tasks. The standards for UTMB's reputation as an academic institution were defined and sustained by intramural peer reviews and by formal extramural assessments rendered by those who voluntarily participated in challenging exercises of professional accountability. Bonds of accountability were shared and nurtured.

More systematic intramural evaluations occurred after the UT System was established in 1950. System officers initiated institutional self-studies as ways to assess schools and make plans for future developments. As noted in chapter two, these included the Committee of 75 report in 1958, the studies initiated by LeMaistre in 1966, and the UT System reviews in 1976.

These assessment rituals were standardized in the UT System's planning policies adopted in the early 1980s. George Bryan began orchestrating thorough reviews of the policies and practices of each School of Medicine department. These reviews included a self-study, a site visit by a review panel that included professors from other departments at UTMB and professors from non-UT institutions, and a final report of recommendations that Bryan and other administrators used to assess departmental progress and evaluate biennial budget requests.[107]

As mentioned in chapter one, the more formal extramural patterns of accountability began during the 1890s with the establishment of the Association of Southern Medical Colleges and the Association of American Medical Colleges. UT President Prather attended a meeting of representatives of southern colleges and preparatory schools in Charlottesville, Virginia, in November 1900 and reveled in their high regard for UTMB. By adopting the four-year course of study, UTMB had become "the best of the South," Prather declared. For UTMB's professors, though, national standards were more important than regional ones. At the beginning of the twentieth century, they shifted their allegiance to the AAMC and the AMA as these organizations championed higher standards.[108]

With the support of the AMA's Council on Medical Education, the Carnegie Foundation for the Advancement of Teaching sponsored Abraham Flexner's site visits to 155 North American medical schools in 1908, 1909, and 1910. Flexner visited Galveston in November 1909 and his report was published in June 1910. He thought that UTMB was the only medical school in Texas "fit to continue in the work of training physicians."[109]

Using Flexner's data, an unnamed editor of *Collier's*, a weekly magazine, named five schools in "different sections of the country which are doing their work well. The Johns Hopkins at Baltimore, the University of Pennsylvania at Philadelphia, Western Reserve at Cleveland, the University of Michigan at Ann Arbor, and the University of Texas at Galveston, all appreciate what good medical teaching requires, and go far to provide it in all its essential features."[110] Twenty years after UTMB began, its reputation was dust-free and sparkling.

Dean Carter was also pleased that the AMA's Council placed UTMB among the top thirty-five American medical schools in its report issued in the *Journal of the American Medical Association* in 1910. Viewing Flexner's evaluation as "justly gratifying to State pride," the UT regents were thrilled with UTMB's high rank because the medical school was the first UT school that had been evaluated by an outside educator who used nationally superlative criteria.[111]

In terms of national reputation, the decade after 1910 was a high point for UTMB. In April 1913 nearly one hundred physicians attended the thirty-third semi-annual meeting of the South Texas District Medical Association in Galveston. Attendees included N. P. Colwell and F. C. Waite, who were then inspecting UTMB. Colwell was secretary of the AMA's council and Waite was a member of the AAMC's executive council. After Colwell's evaluation the AMA gave UTMB an A-plus rating, one of only four in the South; twenty-seven in the nation.[112]

John Witherspoon, then dean at Vanderbilt, inspected UTMB as an official AAMC representative. After recommendations by Waite and Witherspoon, UTMB was accepted as a member of the AAMC.[113] In 1914 Dean Carter began attending AAMC meetings regularly. He became a member of the Committee on Education and Pedagogics (1914–1916) and the Auditing Committee (1915). Fellow deans elected him vice president in 1916, president in 1917. These honors were truly symbolic of their high regard for Carter and UTMB.[114]

During the 1920s and most of the 1930s UTMB maintained a high national reputation and UTMB's deans maintained acceptable relationships with the AMA's Council and the AAMC. Dean Keiller attended five AAMC meetings, actively reading papers and participating in discussions. Dean Hartman attended the annual meetings in 1926 and 1927. Dean Bethel attended four AAMC meetings. During his second tenure as dean, Carter attended AAMC meetings in 1936, 1936, and 1937.[115]

As recounted in chapter two, Carter was dean when AMA representatives visited UTMB in January 1936 as part of the Survey of Medical Education the AMA's council conducted.[116] The results of this visit eventually prompted the employment of John Spies in 1938, probationary status assigned to UTMB by both the AAMC and the AMA in 1942, the replacement of Spies by Chauncey Leake, and the reinstatement of

UTMB as an acceptable AAMC member and an AMA-approved institution in 1943. The evaluations of a few physicians (deans of medical schools outside Texas and officers of professional organizations) propelled these extremely significant events between 1936 and 1943.[117] Bonds of national accountability were extremely powerful.

Leake, other administrators, professors, students, and support staff reclaimed UTMB's reputation. After each of three site visits to the School of Medicine between 1947 and 1950, representatives of the Liaison Committee on Medical Education (LCME) praised UTMB as an outstanding educational institution.[118]

The School of Nursing reached new levels of national status during the 1940s. In 1942 the School of Nursing met the minimum requirements of the Texas State Board of Nurse Examiners, though no nursing school in Texas was yet accredited by the National League of Nursing Education. Under Marjorie Bartholf's leadership, the School of Nursing became a member of the Association of Collegiate Schools of Nursing in 1948. In 1949 the National League of Nursing Education accredited the School of Nursing and the National Committee for the Improvement of Nursing Services ranked the school among the top twenty-five nursing schools in the United States. The National Nursing Accrediting Service accredited the School of Nursing in 1950.[119]

After 1950 accountability and accreditation became more complex as additional agencies and protocols began functioning. As the following examples demonstrate, separate groups evaluated the hospitals and their training programs as well as the four schools.

Hospital facilities were always considered during the accreditation inspections of the School of Medicine and School of Nursing. The adequacy of hospital care at UTMB, though, was primarily determined by another set of standards initially developed by the American College of Surgeons (ACS) in 1918. The John Sealy Hospital received a Class A ranking by the ACS from the onset of what was labeled the "Hospital Standardization Movement." Symbolic of the faculty's regard for the highest standards of hospital care, A. O. Singleton represented UTMB during the twenty-fourth annual Hospital Standardization Conference in 1941. These ACS approvals of John Sealy Hospital continued every year until the JCAH was established in 1952.[120]

During the 1940s some evaluative intersections occurred between hospital care and the allied health training programs in John Sealy Hospital. The training programs for laboratory technicians, X-ray technicians, and physical therapists were approved initially by the AMA's Council in 1944. In 1949 Dr. Edgar Hull (a member of the council) and a representative of the various specialty boards inspected the fourteen residency training programs at UTMB and recommended that all be fully approved.[121]

In December 1952 the ACS conveyed its Hospital Standardization Program to the newly established Joint Commission on Accreditation of Hospitals (JCAH) that was composed of representatives from the ACS, the American College of Physicians, the American Hospital Association, the American Medical Association, and the Canadian Medical Association. JCAH committees visited UTMB hospitals in 1954, 1957, 1958, 1961, and 1964.

The first visit occurred during the same month that the new John Sealy Hospital opened in 1954. The visiting team submitted thirteen recommendations for improvements, such as rehearsals of a fire disaster plan, monthly cultures of autoclaves, better attendance at medical staff meetings, and more active participation by the staff in clinico-pathological conferences. The JCAH accredited UTMB for the maximum three years. The JCAH team noted several problems during its visit in January 1957 and UTMB was re-accredited for only one year. Administrators and hospital personnel responded satisfactorily because UTMB was re-accredited for three years after another inspection in January 1958. Only minor deficiencies were cited in 1961 and 1964. In each year, UTMB was re-accredited for three years.[122]

Representatives from the member organizations of the JCAH visited UTMB's hospitals again in 1967, 1970, 1973, 1974, 1976, 1977, 1979, 1980, 1982, 1985, 1988, and 1991. These representatives reviewed written reports, met with administrators and hospital personnel, and inspected hospital facilities. The teams assessed every activity in the hospitals in terms of the highest standards that had been adopted for the practices and policies of all North American hospitals that wished to receive accreditation by the JCAH. After each of the visits, the teams made recommendations about specific improvements and decided how many years could elapse before another inspection or report was necessary.[123]

The flurry of activities associated with these visits should not be underestimated. Believing that a satisfactory national reputation was always at stake, UTMB's personnel displayed continuous and intense vigilance as they sought and secured JCAH approval. Enormous levels of energy were expended in correcting deficiencies and in responding to JCAH recommendations. Failure to receive JCAH accreditation of its psychiatric facilities in 1976, for example, prompted the regents to spend more than $2 million to renovate the Graves Hospital so that it would conform to new JCAH fire and safety standards.[124]

To improve efficiency in handling accreditation policies, Ann Smith became the full-time coordinator of quality assurance and accreditation for the hospitals in 1979. She organized visits by accreditation teams, established a risk management training program, and coordinated the development of UTMB's quality assurance program.[125]

Other programs in the hospitals were accredited by different agencies, including the College of American Pathologists; the American Association of Blood Banks; the Houston-Galveston Area Council Health Systems Agency; the Department of Health, Education and Welfare; and the American Society of Hospital Pharmacists. In 1980, for example, an eighteen-member team of pathologists, clinical chemists, microbiologists, and certified medical technologists from four medical centers (Baylor, UT Houston, M. D. Anderson, and UT San Antonio) inspected twenty-five clinical laboratories at UTMB. Afterward, the CAP accredited UTMB for two years.[126]

Some patterns of extramural policing for UTMB's schools remained similar after 1950 while others changed considerably.

The School of Medicine continued its accreditation program with the Liaison Committee on Medical Education. LCME teams visited in 1962, 1970, 1977, 1984, and 1991. UTMB's administrators always attended to specific problems identified by these teams of peers from other academic medical centers.

In 1962 the team believed that the activities of the faculty were efficiently organized in departments, but that Dean Truslow's executive network was "not clearly defined as to its lines of responsibility." Although the educational efforts of most School of Medicine departments were "of high caliber," the team urged improvement by "a more vigorous program of research." The team commended the school for its new student admission policies and curriculum. The team believed that UTMB's physical facilities were inadequate and urged implementation of existing plans to expand them. The team concluded that UTMB had made "considerable strides in the past decade" and that there was "every indication of its potentiality to become a leading medical center."[127]

In 1970 the LCME team congratulated UTMB for its progress and commended Truman Blocker and Joe White for their "splendid leadership."[128] The team encouraged UTMB to improve its long-range planning process and Joe White responded by hiring Ken Newman to coordinate this planning.

When the team members visited UTMB in January 1977, they praised the School of Medicine's self-evaluation efforts that John Bruhn had coordinated during a six-month period. They recognized a major problem that involved "frustrations with hospital administration" and "lack of medical expertise in hospital administration." To deal with this, Bill Levin appointed Al LeBlanc as the coordinator of all hospital affairs. In 1977 the LCME gave the School of Medicine a maximum accreditation of seven years, with the following comments: "the school seven years ago and the school now bear little relationships to one another except for geographic location and . . . facilities."[129]

In 1984 the LCME team noted that the "momentum of positive change has not slackened" since 1977.[130] The comments in 1977 and 1984 were extraordinary testaments to the progressive evolution of programs of excellence in the School of Medicine during the Blocker and Levin eras.

After its visit in October 1991 the LCME team submitted a 150-page report that included commendations for several accomplishments. These included the employment of new basic science and clinical chairs; the sense of "community" among faculty, students, and administrators; innovative approaches to student evaluation; the high autopsy rate and its educational value; the addition of the TDJC hospital; good academic support services for students; the John Sealy Memorial Endowment Fund; the Moody Medical Library; and the reorganization of UT-MED. The team also commended UTMB for its well-managed budget: "The institution has managed to balance decreasing state revenues with other sources of funding, permitting the maintenance or expansion of existing programs and the introduction of new initiatives." The LCME granted UTMB an unconditional seven-year accreditation.[131]

After each visit between 1962 and 1991, the LCME re-accredited the School of Medicine for the maximum period of seven years. This continuing affirmation was extremely important for maintaining the school's national reputation.

The postgraduate training programs of the School of Medicine were reviewed by board-certified specialists accountable to the Liaison Committee on Graduate Medical Education. In 1981, for example, nineteen residency training programs had been accredited for specified periods of time that ranged from two to five years.[132] By 1991 thirty-seven postgraduate training programs were accredited by appropriate boards.[133]

Off-campus educators also evaluated the educational programs of the School of Nursing, School of Allied Health Sciences, and the Graduate School of the Biomedical Sciences during the 1960s, 1970s, and 1980s. The School of Nursing met state board requirements every year and the National League for Nursing re-accredited this school after survey teams visited in 1961, 1977, 1980, and 1989. In 1989 the team strongly commended Dean Fenton and the nursing school faculty. Between 1976 and 1980 the educational programs in six School of Allied Health Sciences departments were re-accredited by the American Medical Association Council on Allied Health Education and Accreditation in conjunction with nine other national agencies.[134] Between 1977 and 1981 all graduate programs in the Graduate School of the Biomedical Sciences were evaluated with internal and external reviews.

Another feature of Blocker's leadership was his desire to have UTMB evaluated as a total institution. In November 1970 Gordon Sweet, executive secretary of the Commission on Colleges of the Southern Association of Colleges and Schools (SACS), met with various UT and UTMB administrators. In the spring of 1972 Blocker and White invited Sweet to initiate an accreditation process for UTMB. In November 1973 a SACS team of eleven professors (three from medical schools) inspected UTMB. This was the first accreditation effort that involved an evaluation of all four schools and both institutes. The team praised UTMB as "one of the finest medical centers in the southern United States" and UTMB received full accreditation.[135]

The team made twelve specific recommendations. For example, the team thought that counseling programs for students and policies for handling student grievances should be included in a more streamlined and efficient Office of Student Affairs. In response, Dave Eiland established the counseling program in that office. Again, the stimulus for improvement came from evaluations of professors from other universities who were willing to participate in voluntary accreditation programs.

To prepare for the next SACS visit in 1978, committees of faculty, students, and staff met regularly throughout 1977 and early 1978. Ed Brandt and, later, Palmer Saunders chaired the sixteen-member steering committee. Other employees were members of subcommittees that reviewed such items as financial resources, the Moody Medical Library, and student development services. Separate self-study committees were organized for each of the four schools and two institutes. John Bruhn chaired the eleven-member editorial committee that integrated several self-study reports into a final report of more than six hundred pages. George Bryan believed that everyone participated in this self-study process "with more openness, fairness, and understanding than ever before." Levin and Saunders acknowledged an emergent "unity of purpose" throughout the various components of the complex institution. During its visit in March 1978 the twenty-four-member SACS team complimented UTMB for its thorough and compre-hensive self-study. During a week in Galveston, the SACS team reviewed all reports, inspected facilities, observed programs, met with numerous administrators and faculty, and discussed their findings and recommendations.[136] In March 1978 UTMB administrators received the forty-nine-page final report, which included twenty-four recommendations.

During the next four years administrators and professors responded in specific ways to these recommendations. Each school developed faculty handbooks, for example, and an affirmative action plan was established for the entire campus. In December 1983 Bill Levin sent a one hundred-page report to the SACS describing the changes that had occurred at UTMB between 1978 and 1983 in response to SACS recommendations and in recognition of SACS standards. That report was accepted and no further reports were required until the next inspection scheduled for 1988.[137]

Early in 1986 Levin appointed Julian Kitay as the director of the new self-study required for the SACS site visit in 1988. Karyl Norcross chaired a steering committee, whose members included Joel Gallagher, Alice Hill, Jim Spitler, Betty McAshan, Jim Swinnea Jr., Rose Marie Philips, and Judy Carrier. The four schools constituted thirty-one committees, which reviewed all policies and programs. Judy Carrier edited the 175-page final self-study report the eleven-member SACS team used during the April 1988 visit.[138] Their seventy-eight-page report acknowledged the high quality of education at UTMB. The institution was re-accredited for ten years.

Peer review by colleagues from other institutions was an ongoing and prominent feature of life at UTMB throughout the century. By the late 1970s and early 1980s faculty and staff responded regularly to about forty accrediting agencies. Nearly all of these accountability exercises were voluntary, established and maintained by profes-sionals who chose to have their competence evaluated by off-campus peers who used the highest national standards established for specific programs of patient care, edu-cation, and research.[139]

STORYTELLERS: BONDS OF TIME AND MEANING

In the section about storytellers in the preceding chapter, the bilateral function of reporters employed in UTMB's public information offices was emphasized. On the one hand, their publications nurtured a sense of community and purpose on-cam-pus. These publications provided faculty, staff employees, and students with a broadened sense of value and understanding about what individuals and groups were doing to fulfill the missions of the university. They provided some integrated views of the roles and contributions of individuals who functioned in the varied and multiple communities in the institution. They provided a sense of order in the ever-changing complexity.

On the other hand, the same publications were sent to alumni and others off-campus. They provided information about the continued growth and progress of UTMB. They nurtured loyalty among alumni and they secured trust and goodwill from the various public groups that supported the institution as well as those served by the institution.

During the earliest decades corporate leaders at UT and UTMB appreciated the importance of issuing publications that addressed the interests of alumni. Articles by and about UTMB alumni appeared in the original *University Medical* and in two publications produced by officials in Austin for UT alumni: the *University of Texas Record* (1898–1913) and the *Alcalde* (1913 to present).[140]

Beginning in the 1940s two publications from UTMB fostered loyalty among School of Medicine and School of Nursing alumni. Marjorie Bartholf enthusiastically supported those nursing school graduates who intermittently edited a bulletin for the School of Nursing's Alumnae Association between 1944 and 1960. After becoming executive secretary of the SOMAA in 1946, Mildred Robertson transformed her Overseas Letters into an Alumni Bulletin that she edited for twenty-three years.

In addressing the needs of alumni, some important changes occurred after Myles Knape became Public Information Office director. Robertson's *Alumni Bulletin* was integrated into the campus *Newsletter* for four months in the fall of 1969. Between 1970 and 1984 the Public Information Office sent *University Medical* to employees and alumni. Alumni also enjoyed receiving issues of *Impact* beginning in 1977.[141] In 1987 the Office of External Affairs began publishing *Alumni News*. All of these publications included news items about the bonds of leadership reviewed in this chapter.

UTMB's CEOs also understood the importance of providing information to newspaper reporters and other media professionals who told stories about UTMB to the general public. During UTMB's first seventy years its CEOs provided these reporters with official publications and they interacted with them directly. Leake, for example, established excellent relationships with reporters for the *Galveston Daily News*. In turn, they wrote many reports about activities at UTMB, including some about its research mission.[142] These journalists and their stories were important links of accountability between UTMB and the publics served by the institution.

During these seventy years journalists obtained information from the offices of the deans and hospital directors and they interviewed faculty and students. Eager for drama, they lost no time in chronicling conflicts such as those associated with the issues of relocation, financing, and governance recounted in chapter two. But they also wrote many articles of praise for progressive accomplishments, especially those that resulted from the astonishing political and financial support of Galveston's citizens and foundations. These newspaper reports forged images about UTMB's reputation for lay citizens in Galveston and Houston, other parts of the state, the nation, and the rest of the world.[143]

In addition to creating the *Medical Center News* in 1960, Ralph Meyer used a Houston newspaper as a forum for aggressive publicity about UTMB. With Meyer's support, Jean Walsh wrote eight carefully researched articles that appeared in the *Houston Post* between January 8 and January 15, 1961. Walsh depicted serious problems caused by inadequate funds from antagonistic legislators, insufficient salaries for faculty and staff, too many indigent patients, and too many new medical students. She concluded the series by wondering "when the day will arrive when the Medical Branch will be properly evaluated and given credit which seems to be long past due."[144]

Reprinted in booklet form and distributed to legislators and physicians throughout the state, this series surely shaped the more positive attitudes toward UTMB that emerged during the early 1960s.

During and after the 1960s, employees in UTMB's Public Information Office prepared more in-house publications and assumed more responsibilities for direct communications with off-campus journalists. Their bilateral roles continued, prompting difficult decisions about the best ways to nurture on-campus communities and the best ways to provide information about UTMB to off-campus communities. Between 1977 and 1984 *Impact* and *University Medical* successfully honored the Public Information Office's bilateral responsibilities.

The incredible expansion of UTMB presented challenges for on-campus and off-campus journalists. Off-campus journalists interviewed UTMB's personnel much less frequently than before. Off-campus reporters typically reprinted or rewrote the stories that first appeared in the in-house publications prepared by Public Information Office writers. Because of the expanding panorama of events associated with an ever-enlarging and complex institution, bonds of time and meaning—on and off campus—became more highly circumscribed.

Coverage in off-campus media became even more selective. Before 1960, for example, local newspapers regularly reported the extremely important events involving peer evaluation and accreditation. After 1960, these events seldom appeared in newspaper, radio, or television reports. The daily routines and rituals of patient care, teaching, and research were typically offered in small and focused glimpses when sensational events occurred, like conflicts between executives, or the surgical reattachment of a severed hand. Off-campus news reporters typically avoided complexities and nuances. They presented what they heralded as "defining moments," both negative and positive.

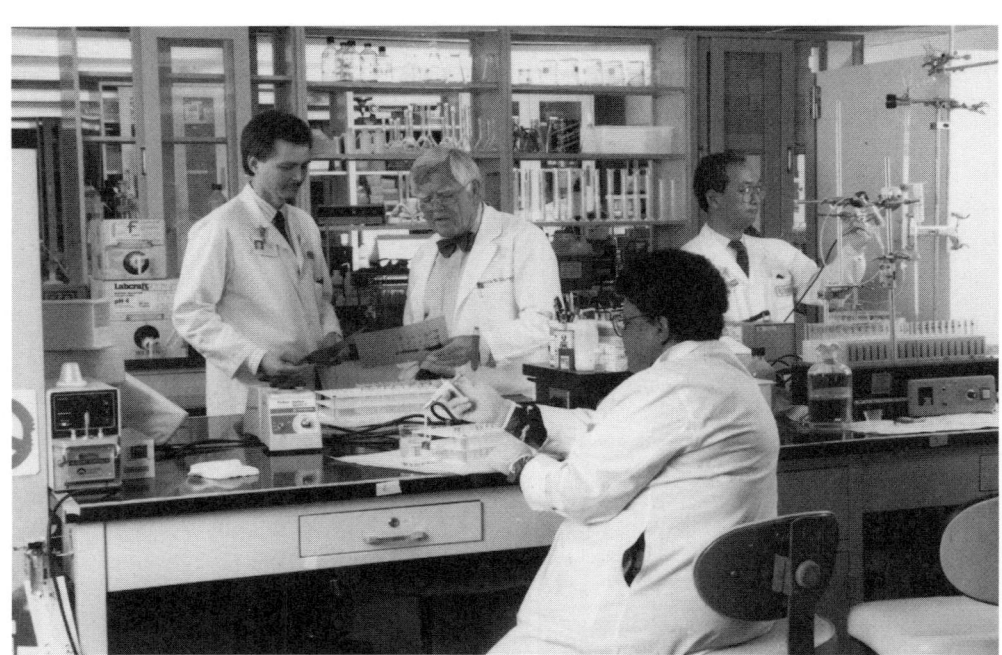

Surgical Biochemistry Lab, 1992. Left to right, Robert "Dan" Beauchamp, James C. Thompson, Freddie Hill, and Jin Ishizeka.

— 10 —

A Centennial Perspective

"What the future has in store for the school cannot now be known, it largely rests with the votes of the present Legislature. To believe that body of representative citizens capable of deserting an institution built up from nothing in ten years to take place with the first medical and pharmaceutical schools of the land, steadily maintaining the highest type of curriculum in the face of the most eager competition by schools all over the South and West offering short courses, brief terms of study and easy graduation, is to believe that the old Texan spirit, which made men die before surrender, has lost its force and changed its type. When that happens the heart will have gone from the Texan's boast, and the proud distinction of Texan citizenship will indeed be but a bluff."—Dean Allen Smith, after the 1900 storm[1]

The "old Texan spirit" did not desert UTMB. As depicted many times in the previous chapters, that spirit propelled the institution during more than one hundred years of countless events. Powerbrokers and moneytenders made momentous decisions. Construction workers and caretakers built, remodeled, and maintained campus buildings. Doctors, nurses, and others attended sick people. Teachers interviewed, lectured, and nurtured students. Scientists and other scholars embarked on journeys of discovery in labs, libraries, and offices. Support staff scheduled appointments and typed letters, lectures, reports, and minutes of committee meetings. Students and faculty busily worked and played. Faculty, alumni, students, and support staff led peers during meetings of committees and societies, on and off campus. Faculty permitted peers to evaluate their professional competence periodically. Individuals and groups prepared stories about UTMB that were presented in a variety of media formats for on-campus and off-campus audiences.

Some storytellers crafted "histories" about the institution's past. Reminiscence urges, deaths, developmental landmarks, "birthday" years, and major changes motivated the preparation of these historical accounts. Though many of the "historians" were insiders, so to speak, their experiences, perceptions, and interpretations provided a variety of differing views. More than one type of "history" appeared. One was the autobiographical report of "lived experiences." These informal, firsthand accounts were indisputable as testimonies, though their authors might have altered, intentionally or unintentionally, certain details about the "lived" events. With their details, these reminiscences and autobiographical reports provided some depth and vivid imagery. Biographical accounts of cherished professors were a second type of history. Professors identified strongly with their departments and some wrote histories of these departments, a third type. These departmental histories could be quite comprehensive. A few storytellers wrote more formal reports about continuities and changes in UTMB's overall development. They relied on evidence and claims that could be disputed by those who provided more reliable evidence and arguments. These histories provided some breadth and more "objective" analyses, sometimes pointing to timeless values within time-dependent decisions and behaviors.

The "centennial perspective" of this chapter includes three components. The first section includes contextual summaries of each twenty-five-year period in UTMB's first century together with an analysis of some "histories" about UTMB created during those years. Histories about UTMB have been an important feature of UTMB's legacies. It is instructive to juxtapose today's views of the events in each quarter-century with the previous histories written about them. This juxtaposition is not intended to be overly critical of previous storytellers, but to remind us that histories of an evolving institution can be revised with the passage of time and different interpretive frameworks. The next section is a chronicle of activities during UTMB's two centennial years and the last section offers a third "centennial perspective" by using glimpses of the institution's continuing development during the 1990s to highlight recurring moral values in UTMB's legacies and destiny. These glimpses are organized with the same conceptual frameworks used in chapters two through nine.

QUARTER-CENTURY LANDMARKS

During the first decade of the twentieth century, "progress" was a key cultural theme in Texas and the other United States.[2] With its new commission form of government; its construction projects involving grade-raising, the seawall, and new bridges; and its worldwide reputation for commercial shipping, Galveston was viewed as a very "progressive" city. "Other cities have made progress and improvements with a rapid growth and increase of population, but it is doubtful if any other city has ever accomplished so much in such a short time, in spite of a decrease in population," proclaimed the anonymous author of an advertisement for the TSMA annual meeting scheduled for Galveston in May 1909. Almost eight hundred people attended this meeting.[3]

UTMB enjoyed an outstanding reputation during its first twenty-five years (fiscal years 1892–1916). As a teaching enterprise, its School of Medicine was viewed as one of the best medical schools in the United States. In 1913 James Thompson was a founding member and first vice president of the American College of Surgeons. Two years later he was the founder and first president of the Texas Surgical Society. In 1916 Dean Carter was president-elect of the AAMC, only three years after UTMB became a member of this national group of medical school deans. This was "high cotton" for the first entry into American academic medicine from the University of Texas.

How did "historians" report the events of these years? As noted in chapter one, William Gammon, the fourth student to graduate from the School of Medicine and the founder of the Alumni Association, wrote the earliest historical account of UTMB in 1895. Three deans (Smith, Paine, and Carter) prepared the next histories.

In 1901 Allen Smith opened the institution's eleventh session with a review of its first decade. He focused on struggles of the founders and improvements after the hurricane in 1900. UTMB began its second decade, he declared, "better and more fully equipped in a material sense and full of the strength of the past decade's growth, calm in the reliance which triumph over difficulties and danger ever brings, a fixed part of the great educational scheme of Texas—to stay while Texas stands." He believed that the School of Medicine was a leading institution among American medical schools, especially in the South. In 1906 J. F. Y. Paine opened the sixteenth annual session with a lecture on the history of medical education in Texas. He traced the story of the Galveston Medical College and the Texas Medical College and Hospital. He gratefully acknowledged the trust of those Texans who voted to locate UTMB in Galveston and the financial contributions of the Sealy family, the city, and the legislature. Still CEO in 1914, William Carter described the progressive changes that occurred during his first ten years as dean (1903–1913). He acknowledged the new facilities that enabled better medical care for blacks, those with infectious diseases, and children; and he eagerly awaited construction of the Woman's Hospital and the Nurses' Home. The increasing number of inpatients and outpatients had enhanced practical instruction. He celebrated improvements in the educational preparation of entering medical students and improvements in the School of Medicine curriculum. He was delighted that every medical school graduate who wanted an internship had been able to obtain one. Carter was thrilled about Flexner's evaluation and about UTMB's ranking among medical schools evaluated by the AMA's Council on Medical Education in 1907, 1910, and 1913. "Each time," declared Carter, "the University of Texas has been in the first-class, and in the last classification of 1913, there are only twenty-one other colleges in Class A plus. May it always maintain this standing and may it continue to progress in the future as it has in the past."[4] Carter celebrated progress based on honorable regard for high standards.

The advent of the twenty-fifth year invited the creation of more stories. The July 1915 issue of *Alcalde* included several items. Willard Cooke contributed a biographical sketch of Paine, who had died in 1912, and a brief history of UTMB. Allen Smith, R. L. Wilson, James T. Downs, Howard R. Dudgeon Sr., W. D. Jones, and James J. Terrill contributed reminiscences. Cooke praised the majestic Paine, who was six feet, four inches tall, as a "real Southern gentleman" with "true dignity." Terrill praised Keiller as the "little sandy-haired . . . Scotchman" with "the nerve of a giant, a heart as big as the world, a brain of first quality" as "the greatest teacher of anatomy" in the United States. Dudgeon recalled the influences of Clopton, Keiller, Flavin, and Carter; his days as a surgical intern assisting Paine; the 1900 hurricane; and some of his patients. Smith described his first days in a city whose "streets were deep with sand" and alleys "disgraceful and menacing." Citizens collected drinking water from "dirty roofs," rode "little street cars pulled each by a single tiny mule," and traveled to the mainland by a "single railroad bridge across the bay." He gave splendid depictions of the first faculty, the "chips and shavings on the floors" of Old Red, the students and their courses, and the pride that appeared when "Galveston graduates proved their worth by the highest grades" on the Texas licensure exams during the early 1900s.[5]

Cooke's "brief history" was a portrait of conditions in 1915, including the "gloomy, wet-floored cave" of Old Red's ground floor that housed the pharmacy and chemistry labs; the obsolete plumbing and light fixtures in this building; the pitiful condition of the Nurses' Home that made it necessary for "nurses on the north side of the building to sleep under mackintoshes during every wet norther"; and the poverty of an institution "hopelessly handicapped" by its dependency on legislators who believed that "money appropriated for the support of an institution of learning is totally wasted." Cooke listed faculty appointments between 1891 and 1914, commented on improvements in the quality of students, traced the growth of inpatients and outpatients, listed current needs of the schools and hospitals, championed the School of Medicine as one of the "best in the United States," and labeled the future of the institution as "problematic" unless more income was provided for both teaching and research.[6] Smith was awestruck with the institutional support received after the hurricane. Carter was ecstatic about progressive changes. Dudgeon embellished portraits of the faculty. Cooke's passionate rhetoric reflected high hopes and deep fears. Each story revealed the interests and interpretations of its author. Each story had its own timeless integrity that cannot be fully captured with a few quotes or paraphrases. Each evinced justifiable pride and devotion. Quite realistic, Cooke's fears reflected the sentiments of UT's executives who wanted UTMB in Austin, the constraints on legislators who were obligated to parcel scarce resources to multiple state agencies, the frustrations of Galveston's city officials who did not want to spend more tax money for the medical care of indigents, and prevalent anxieties about survival in a city located on a sandbar in the northern Gulf of Mexico.

On August 17, 1915, a hurricane similar to the one in 1900 tested the city's stamina again. Though there were damages and injuries, only eight residents died.[7] The seawall and grade-raising had protected the city's inhabitants. These protective measures had also stopped the exodus after the 1900 storm and had encouraged people to settle in Galveston. More than thirty-five thousand citizens lived in the city by 1910; forty-five thousand by 1920. Their courage and persistence were not unlike that displayed by Dean Carter, the regents from Galveston, members of the Sealy family, I. H. (Ike) Kempner, Thomas Nolan, and Edward Randall as they battled fervently and successfully for UTMB during its first quarter-century. The Woman's Hospital and the Rebecca Sealy Nurses' Home that opened in 1915 were more than mere survival. They represented a special blend of the same power and money that had created and sustained the institution. Like University Hall, they also symbolized genuine improvement in the social and cultural status of women at UTMB.

But none of the institution's "historians" then acknowledged this cultural progress. Even though they taught pharmacy and nursing students, they also gave little attention to the pharmacy and nursing schools. They said nothing about the historic "firsts" of the School of Nursing. They reported nothing about staff support, faculty committees and research, the Students' Council, *University Medical*, the Alumni Association, and the incredible involvement of faculty and alumni in local, state, regional, national, and international organizations. In considering the panorama of people and events during UTMB's first quarter century, these histories were limited in scope. Their major themes were survival, growth, and robust leaders.

From a centennial perspective, however, UTMB had originated and developed as a product of the national reform movement in medical education. UTMB had also been a corporate leader for further reform. In his survey of American medical schools in 1910, Abraham Flexner identified forty-six proprietary and university-affiliated medical schools in twelve states in the South and Southwest. Because they did not have connections to a teaching hospital, he used the term "half-school" when describing the University of North Carolina (1890) and the University of Oklahoma (1898). Although the University of Virginia had initiated progressive changes in 1907, UTMB's School of Medicine was the only school embedded in a state university that had adopted and enforced Flexner's high ideals for two decades.[8] It was a bellwether institution among American medical schools, especially in the South and Southwest.

The second twenty-five years (fiscal years 1917–1941) began on these high notes of state and national repute. In 1917 Carter was the national leader of all medical school deans and in 1918 the John Sealy Hospital received full approval by the American College of Surgeons when this group began its efforts to standardize practices in American hospitals. In 1920 Abraham Flexner visited the two medical schools in Texas.[9] Baylor University College of Medicine in Dallas received some Rockefeller money; UTMB did not. What UTMB received was even better: the Sealy & Smith Foundation, established in 1922. The two professors (Keiller and Thompson) and one UT executive (Splawn) who crafted "histories" of UTMB during the 1920s acknowledged this Sealy legacy.

During commencement ceremonies in June 1923, UT President Robert Vinson announced Keiller's selection as UTMB's next CEO. A state and national leader, Keiller used his graduation address as an opportunity to review thirty-two years of changes at UTMB. He noted the growth in faculty and operating budget, and the addition of important hospital facilities. He championed the teaching mission: "A small school, but the best teaching institution for general practitioners in the United States, aye, in the world—this and nothing short of this must be our aim." He happily announced that construction would soon start on a new Laboratory Building, a structure that would ensure superior teaching in the basic sciences.[10] Keiller also knew that this building was made possible by the largest amount of Available University Fund income the regents had yet given to UTMB.

Some professors hoped that this building would encourage more research. Surely those graduating during the thirty-fourth annual ceremony in May 1925 listened attentively to the autobiographical remarks of Thompson, who had been professor of surgery during those thirty-four years. Thompson believed that the idealism, enthusiasm, and loyalty of the faculty balanced the institution's relative poverty during its first nine years when the legislature "in its most generous moods . . . never gave us more than a bare sustenance." He acknowledged the extraordinary improvements after the 1900 hurricane, the addition of eight buildings between 1910 and 1925, and the beneficence of the Sealy family that enabled so many campus improvements. A state and national leader, Thompson was proud of UTMB's reputation: "The glory of our school in the past has been its teaching." But he knew that a university school should also be advancing scientific knowledge. He hoped that the new Laboratory Building would encourage research as well as improve teaching facilities. "We cannot hide the fact that few members of our faculty have contributed much to the advancement of medicine and its ancillary sciences," Thompson asserted. Using stories about John Hunter, Louis Pasteur, and Claude Bernard, Thompson encouraged students and faculty to become industrious scholars and scientists.[11]

When he became UT's CEO in 1924, Walter Splawn used historical perspectives to secure public trust. He wrote a series of fifteen historical articles about UT, which appeared in the *Galveston Daily News* during 1924 and 1925. The fourteenth and fifteenth articles described the evolution of UTMB, particularly campus development.[12]

When the Sealy & Smith Foundation began its grants to UTMB in 1926, Splawn spoke to the Rotary Club of Galveston about the magnificence of the Sealy bequest: "A great fortune made by a genius for business, has been turned over to all the people of Texas to further the interest of medicine and insure better protection against disease. As long as men and women live in Texas the name of John Sealy will be honored."[13] Splawn celebrated the Sealy legacy, fully understanding its promise for shaping UTMB's destiny. Gifts from the Sealy & Smith Foundation, allocations from regents and legislators, and some federal dollars enabled the addition of eleven new structures to the campus during this second quarter-century. These included the Galveston State Psychopathic Hospital, the state's first tax-supported hospital for the mentally ill located on the campus of an academic medical center. New and improved clinical facilities attracted more inpatients and outpatients. Dollars from these patients, the Sealy family, and the Sealy & Smith Foundation were used to pay the salaries of new types of professionals who appeared in the caregiving networks of the hospitals during these years. Managers added these professionals to maintain UTMB's identity as a nationally respectable institution that provided comprehensive care to each patient.

Nearly all of the dollars from private sources had been assigned to the care of patients, not teaching or research. Tax-based dollars financed the major changes that occurred in the educational programs of the three schools during these years. The School of

Nursing directors and faculty periodically elevated admission standards, and they made the curriculum more rigorous for an increasing number of students. They were thrilled with the beautiful Rebecca Sealy Nurses' Residence, but they were not satisfied with their school's national reputation. The School of Pharmacy moved to Austin in 1927 because its dean, faculty, and alumni wanted an expanded school that would receive full national accreditation.

The School of Medicine faculty acknowledged the steady expansion of scientific knowledge and clinical specialization among America's physicians. They adapted to these changes by revising the undergraduate curriculum, initiating specialty-training programs for graduates, and offering postgraduate courses for practitioners. They also remained steadfast in their determination to train doctors who could be general practitioners at the time of graduation or upon completion of an internship. The medical school professors fully understood that their undergraduate curriculum was one of the toughest in the nation.[14]

UTMB was enthusiastically celebrated in the images about Galveston crafted during the "Roaring Twenties." "Galveston: Where the World Comes to Play" was the title of the article advertising Galveston as the site of the TSMA annual meeting in 1928. E. S. Holliday, the assistant secretary for Galveston's Chamber of Commerce, touted Galveston as an "all-season, resort city" of sixty thousand inhabitants who are "proud" to host this meeting. "It can safely be said that no institution has had such a large part in the molding of medical affairs in Texas as the Medical Department of the University of Texas," added Holliday. In his opening address welcoming new students in the fall of that same year, Meyer Bodansky included a few laudatory comments about UTMB, specifically paying tribute to the School of Nursing as the first school of its kind in the South.[15]

Except for some paragraphs in the annual university catalogs, the only historical overview of UTMB that appeared in print during the 1930s was a three-page entry in Samuel Griffin's *History of Galveston, Texas* (1931). A businessman with managerial roles in Sugarland Industries, Griffin emphasized UTMB's clinical and educational missions: "There are few hospitals in which the patients can be utilized so fully for bedside and clinical instruction as in the John Sealy Hospital."[16] Griffin hailed progressive developments in Galveston, noting growth at UTMB as a major example. However, he did not mention research at UTMB as an example of progress.

During this second quarter-century UTMB's executives struggled with decisions about developing an infrastructure for research. Most individuals or groups who donated or allocated dollars to UTMB wanted these funds used for the care of patients and teaching. Accordingly, most professors were very busy with teaching and patient care, leaving little time for research. Executives did increase space for laboratories, expand the library, use research productivity as a criterion for promotion and increased salaries, and provide released time for researchers to present reports during off-campus meetings of professional societies. Scientists with Ph.D. degrees were chairs and members of basic science departments, and some clinical departments included a few experimental scientists. Some professors (Bodansky, Duncan, Herrmann, and Moore) were highly productive researchers.

Although countless articles about UTMB and its development had appeared in local newspapers, research was seldom mentioned before the early 1930s. Though not a historical analysis, a summary of some research projects appeared in the *Galveston Daily News* in the fall of 1933.[17] More than forty years after UTMB began, one local newspaper finally acknowledged research as one of the institution's primary missions. Perhaps the "hope" attached to scientific research motivated recognition at this time, as social conditions worsened during the years of the Great Depression.

Though unemployment, business failures, and impoverishment occurred in Galveston during these years, the city's economy remained relatively strong because of tourism, commercial shipping, insurance companies, and UTMB. Galveston did not have a bank failure and the American National Insurance Company was the fifth largest in the United States by 1932. Although UTMB's faculty and employees experienced salary cuts, a new Outpatient Clinic Building, the Galveston State Psychopathic Hospital, and a new Rebecca Sealy Nurses' Home were constructed on the campus during the early 1930s. In 1931 someone estimated that UTMB's students spent approximately $500,000 a year in the city.[18]

Students graduating in 1936 were surely mesmerized by Seth Morris's reminiscences. At the age of sixteen he enrolled in the first class admitted to UT Austin in 1883. With firsthand stories, the "Old Test Tube" (nickname given by students) provided colorful portraits of Smith, Clopton, West, McLaughlin, Graves, Carter, Paine, Lee, Randall, and Keiller. Venerable and beloved, Morris was a symbol of steadfast loyalty to an institution that had attracted federal dollars for a new Negro Hospital and a new Children's Hospital that were being constructed as he spoke. New Deal optimism infused the spirits of UTMB's personnel, who showed these structures to President Franklin Delano Roosevelt when he visited the campus in May 1937.[19]

This same optimism also animated Adah Grant, who wrote the article advertising Galveston as the site of the seventy-second TSMA annual meeting in the spring of 1938. "No matter what you seek, whether it be beauty for the nourishment of the soul, pleasure for the relaxation of the mind, or rest and recuperation for the body, it awaits you in Galveston," she declared. More than two thousand people attended this meeting.[20]

Two years later this optimism had faded, as Galvestonians—like other Americans—were frightened by the war in Europe and UTMB's fiftieth year (1940–1941) was lost in the turmoil associated with John Spies. Spies himself displayed little interest in history. Bob Nesbitt, a reporter for the *Galveston Daily News*, interviewed seventy-three-year-old Seth Morris and C. W. Sanders (School of Medicine class of 1926) wrote a brief chronological overview for the *Phi Chi Quarterly*.[21] The political revolution associated with Spies clouded everyone's perception of the institution. It was difficult then to believe that there was any legacy at UTMB worth celebrating. That there were no historians writing about UTMB at its fifty-year mark signaled a tragic loss in trust and credibility.

UTMB's first century of roller coaster rhythms reached a low point when the third quarter-century (fiscal years 1942–1966) began. The AAMC representatives who visited the campus in January 1942 recommended probation. In a short article about UTMB in the 192-page supplement published in April 1942 celebrating the one hundredth anniversary of the *Galveston Daily News*, there was no recognition of the institution's fiftieth-year milestone.[22]

The arrival of Chauncey Leake in the fall of that year was a good omen for those who believed that this milestone had not been celebrated properly. Leake named John Sinclair as chair of a Fiftieth Anniversary Committee. In November 1942 Sinclair invited the chairs of each department to prepare a brief history of their departments. With typescripts ranging from seven to thirty-three pages, nine of these men wrote remarkable summaries that varied considerably in style but generally focused on the location of the department, changes in personnel, evolution of courses, and research activities. With Leake's strong interest in history, it is somewhat surprising that these were not published. With the political sensibilities of a new CEO, though, Leake was probably fearful that someone would be offended by the rhetoric and contents of one essay that characterized Paine as a "master" of profanity and a "holy terror" in the operating suite.[23]

In recognition of the fiftieth anniversary of the first graduation in 1892, Leake focused historical energies on the graduation exercises held on December 18, 1942. During daylight hours, six nationally prominent speakers gave talks on various topics associated with military medicine. Fraternities hosted luncheons in honor of alumni. Historical exhibits were displayed and a "Founder's Room" was opened in the library. An early evening reception honored the two surviving members of the original faculty, Randall and Morris.

Judson Taylor, the TMA president and commencement speaker, declared: "The school is now, on its fiftieth anniversary, on the threshold of a great medical history, and the state is all set for a marvelous expansion of medicine here." Leake's first graduation program, as a newspaper editorial noted, was an "occasion singularly filled with memories of a great past and promise of an even greater future."[24] As UTMB's second half-century gathered some momentum, Leake used the values of historical perspective to encourage alumni, faculty, students, and boosters to adopt a positive attitude about UTMB's destiny.

Early in 1943 the Sealy & Smith Foundation Board, with Edward Randall Sr. still president, published a forty-nine-page brochure on the history of UTMB, its hospitals, and the foundation. This brochure included legal documents about the establishment of UTMB and the John Sealy Hospital and a summary description (with photos) of hospital expansion between 1890 and 1943. It also included the wills of John Sealy II and Jennie Sealy Smith, documents that enabled the creation of the foundation, which had secured and propelled UTMB for more than two decades.[25] This historical account reminded everyone of the one light that had remained bright throughout all the cloudy storms of the Spies era.

Extraordinary changes occurred at UTMB after Leake arrived. The model of the "rugged-individualist, all-powerful, can-do-no-wrong" political hero gradually receded in the dynamics of UTMB's political networks. It was replaced by the model of a leader who could share responsibility with many people who worked together to accomplish corporate goals. Chauncey Leake was one of these leaders.

Leake and the faculty worked diligently to establish a better balance between hospital care and academic programs. B. I. Burns, the hospital's director between 1946 and 1954, and the organized medical staff made so many improvements that the new John Sealy Hospital received full accreditation after its first Joint Commission on the Accreditation of Hospital review in 1954. Much pride infused the atmosphere when executives walked Vice President Richard Nixon through the hospital's corridors on Sunday morning, June 12, 1955.[26]

Leake's influence on teaching was profound. He supported the School of Medicine's clinical faculty as they significantly expanded postgraduate training programs for interns, residents, and community practitioners. With his enthusiastic endorsement, Marjorie Bartholf and her colleagues assumed full responsibility for the School of Nursing's educational programs. The School of Nursing became fully accredited and ranked among the top twenty-five nursing schools in the nation by mid-century. Leake wholeheartedly supported the expansion and improvement of degree programs in the biomedical sciences, as well as the expansion and formalization of certificate and degree programs in the allied health sciences, including the first training program in physical therapy for the Southwest. Teaching a popular history of medicine elective and employing a professional philosopher as a faculty member, Leake also championed the addition of humanities perspectives to medical curricula.

During his tenure as CEO, research became a primary corporate mission at UTMB. Leake was the principal cheerleader for expanding research. Because he had been an experimental pharmacologist, he could "talk the talk" with those who chose careers as scientists. He understood their need for an effective infrastructure. He worked tirelessly to secure political support, dollars, space, and publicity for research-minded faculty. He was thrilled when the research contributions of a professor at UTMB (G. W. N. Eggers) were recognized with a gold medal from the American Academy of Orthopedic Surgery and a gold medal from the International Surgical Society.

Leake was also a sophisticated storyteller. For the centennial issue of the *Texas State Journal of Medicine*, published in May 1953, he traced the historical development of internal medicine in Texas.[27] He described the research and clinical contributions of several professors at UTMB, as well as the advent of residency training in internal medicine at six hospitals in the state. Leake clearly understood the progressive changes that had occurred in medical science, education, and practice in Texas since his arrival in 1942.

Only two short histories about UTMB appeared in the early 1950s. Emmett N. Wilson, a sophomore medical student, wrote a chronological overview for fellow members of the Alpha Kappa Kappa fraternity meeting in Galveston. In 1952 the Texas State Historical Association published a two-volume *Handbook of Texas* that was hailed as the "best systematic work of reference on any of the fifty United States." This *Handbook* included a very short (but not error-free) entry about UTMB written by a former UT president.[28]

In telling stories about UTMB at mid-century, biography was the principal approach. The Alumni Association published Mildred Robertson's collection of biographical sketches of twenty-five professors. The *Handbook of Texas* contained biographical entries about twelve deceased professors. In 1953 Anne Brindley wrote a short unpublished history of the Department of Pathology chaired by her husband, Paul Brindley.[29] Like Robertson, Brindley focused on the careers of individual teachers. Neither the overview essayists nor the biographers addressed the dynamics of interactive groups and institutional changes.

These dynamics became more pronounced at mid-century as both Galveston and UTMB struggled with competing cultural and social values used to define credibility and progress. On the one hand, there was a view of Galveston as "one of the most romantic and colorful cities in the South." "Galveston today is a rather carefree resort and port town concerned over the growth of the municipality to no more than 71,000 in 1950 and busily absorbed in ways of attracting more tourists and residents to the only large Texas city girdled by the Gulf of Mexico," added the anonymous author of the article advertising the eighty-fourth annual TSMA meeting planned for Galveston in the spring of 1951.[30]

On the other hand, Galveston was "America's liveliest, naughtiest, least-inhibited city." Between the 1920s and the 1950s Galveston had become a major "sin city" on the Gulf Coast as prostitution, gambling, and illegal consumption of alcohol flourished. These activities were a way of recouping some of the city's economic losses associated with the expansion of the petrochemical industries and commercial shipping in Houston and other parts of Galveston County.[31] Would Galveston continue to function outside the state's legal network?

During the late 1950s and early 1960s, Galvestonians reformed their city's reputation. In 1954, the Negro Chamber of Commerce and the Galveston Chamber of Commerce merged. Beginning in June 1957 Will Wilson and the Texas Rangers closed many gambling clubs, bingo parlors, and brothels. In 1960 Galvestonians changed their commissioner form of government to a city-council, city-manager structure, and elected a woman (Ruth Kempner) and a black (T. D. Armstrong) to the new city council. In 1962 the National Municipal League selected Galveston as one of eleven "All-American cities."[32] As the last half of the twentieth century gained momentum, Galvestonians chose more progressive values for their city's destiny.

Though a major player in the city's economy by mid-century, UTMB was still plagued by a lingering provincialism. School of Medicine department chairs and other managers justified their paternalistic attitudes as a necessary protection against competitors in Houston and Dallas, as well as those in Austin who still thought that UTMB had been a strange tail wagging the UT dog from its very beginning. UTMB was the oldest, but not the only medical unit in the UT System. Among other components,

UT's Southwestern Medical School in Dallas, the M. D. Anderson Cancer Hospital in Houston, and UT's School of Dentistry in Houston competed for power, money, and prestige.[33] Would UTMB be eclipsed or swallowed by other institutions evolving in the larger, expanding, and wealthier cities of rapidly industrializing Texas?

During the late 1950s and early 1960s UT's corporate executives reformed their attitudes about UTMB's status in unprecedented ways. Major turning points occurred between 1958 and 1963 as these executives took a long look at their entire system (Committee of 75 Report) and as UTMB's executives asked disinterested, outside consultants for guidance with long-range planning (Hamilton Report). Ransom and the regents publicly affirmed UTMB's future in Galveston with strong rhetoric and lots of money. They enthusiastically chose more progressive values for UTMB's destiny.

Corporate executives supported progressive changes in all three of UTMB's missions. Racially segregated clinical services ended and cardiovascular surgery began. The first inpatient unit for emotionally disturbed children in a public hospital in Texas opened at UTMB. School of Medicine faculty adopted a drastically revised curriculum and School of Nursing faculty streamlined their educational mission by eliminating the diploma program and enrolling all new students in one baccalaureate degree program. More administrative coordination of hospital training programs for allied health workers occurred and a bachelor's degree program in physical therapy was added.

A dramatic increase in private and federal dollars enabled unprecedented growth of research endeavors and many contributions to medical science. Three professors received national awards for their research discoveries (Hansen, Pomerat, and Herrmann). The first Student Research Forum in 1960 signaled a profound enthusiasm among professors and students for corporate leadership in American medical research. The Clinical Research Center that opened in 1963 signaled a strong measure of peer approval by fellow scientists. Like other academic medical centers in the United States, UTMB was rapidly progressing as a multi-specialty, multi-school, multi-disciplinary institution that fully embraced its interrelated academic missions of patient care, education, and research. Its first comprehensive self-study in 1966 revealed this new image, as it refreshed and renewed the spirits of all connected with the institution.

As UTMB became larger, more specialized, and more bureaucratized during this third quarter-century, it became more and more difficult to comprehend the entire institution historically. Historically minded School of Medicine professors focused on the development of their departments. In 1957 Mary Ellen Haggard and Arild Hansen offered a history of the Department of Pediatrics. In 1960 Benedict Abreu wrote an unpublished history of the Department of Pharmacology, which he chaired between 1961 and 1965. After serving thirty-six years as chair of the Department of Microbiology, William Sharp retired in 1957 and began working on a history of this department. At the time of his death in 1961 the 182-page typescript included sixteen chapters and outlines for two more.[34]

These histories reflected the growing importance of scientific and clinical specialization, and the more substantial professional identities associated with specific departments.

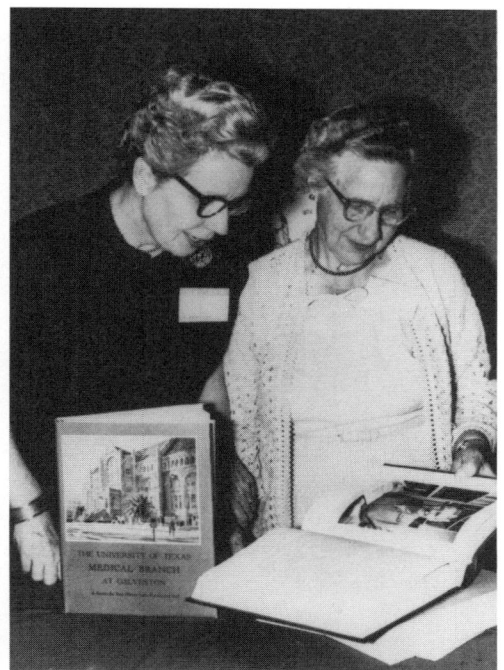

Mildred Robertson and Lillie Runge, 1968.

As UTMB expanded and the era of training for "general practice" faded, professional identities mostly involved relating to colleagues in a distinctive department in a specific school. Truman Blocker displayed this focus with an obituary of A. O. Singleton (1948), an unpublished history of the Department of Surgery (1956), and an obituary of G. W. N. Eggers (1963). The centennial annual session issue of *Texas Medicine* in March 1967 included nineteen historical articles about clinical specialties in Texas, including Charles T. Stone's review of the development of internal medicine.[35] Specialization encouraged a more limited historical identity, though some still wanted a broader perspective.

Orchestrating major changes for UTMB in the mid-1960s, Harry Ransom and Truman Blocker were keenly aware of the School of Medicine's upcoming seventy-fifth birthday year (1965–1966). Learning the value of historical perspective from both Leake and Ransom, Blocker wanted a comprehensive history of the institution with which he had been associated for thirty-five years. As director of the Public Information Office, Bobbye Barratt initiated a systematic approach to the collection of materials needed for writing this history. Using questionnaires completed by department chairs in the fall of 1964, Gay Eddy and Nancy Brown interviewed these chairs and other employees in the spring of 1965. Eddy, Brown, and Darlene (Dodie) Messer continued research and writing during 1965 and 1966. After several months of editing, the University of Texas Press printed the book, *The University of Texas Medical Branch at Galveston: A Seventy-five Year History by the Faculty and Staff*, late in 1967.[36]

Alumni, administrators, professors, students and support staff entered UTMB's fourth quarter-century (fiscal years 1967–1991) with a richer historical perspective than any that existed previously. Available for sale in the Public Information Office by January 1968, the 435-page book included six chapters of text, twenty-five appendices, a bibliography and index, and more than one hundred marvelous photos. Five of the chapters were organized chronologically and the sixth focused on student life richly embellished with anecdotes from alumni. Recognizing features of geographic location, survival after hurricanes and political controversies, scientific development in the service of human welfare, and recipient of the philanthropies of a "great foundation," Ransom's foreword noted that "few centers of medical education" had "combined such distinctive elements of growth" as UTMB.[37]

John Duffy, Tulane's eminent professor of medical history, described the book as "a remarkable production job, an excellent piece of public relations, and a detailed reference work" that should "warm the cockles of the heart of every alumnus of the University of Texas Medical Branch." Duffy noted the book's focus on individual personalities, mostly chairs of School of Medicine departments. "The medical profession, more than any other group, tends to see its history in terms of individuals," Duffy asserted.[38] Many alumni purchased and enjoyed the book. They realized that its authors, conditioned by the circumstances of its origins, focused on the powers and skills of department leaders and key professors as the principal catalysts for progress during UTMB's first seventy-five years. Although important features of those years were absent from the book, its stories and images generated a new historical awareness for alumni, students, employees, and boosters. This awareness also heralded a profound faith in the possibility of a new and even better future for the institution.

This future became a reality. The extraordinary boom years of the late 1960s, 1970s, and 1980s were "a magic time."[39] The magic was everywhere. Gov. John Connally catalyzed improvements in education for the entire state. As the senator orchestrating the allotments of state dollars, Aaron "Babe" Schwartz helped UTMB acquire more public dollars than ever before. A spectacularly forceful regent, Frank Erwin won many battles for the university he loved. Chancellor LeMaistre, a physician, guided the UT System for most of the 1970s, then was replaced by Don Walker, a former UTMB official, who selected Ed Brandt, a former UTMB dean, as UT's vice chancellor for health affairs. Blocker and Levin were insiders who developed mutually productive relationships with these power and money "magicians."

As described in previous chapters, Blocker, Levin, and their colleagues guided previously unimagined expansion in administrative hierarchies, budgets, buildings, and programs of patient care, teaching, and research.[40] There was an enormous increase in dollars from private, state, county, and federal sources. The operating budgets for the schools expanded from a little more than $9 million in 1964 to more than $135 million in 1987; for the hospitals from a little more than $9.5 million to more than $185 million. Blocker and Levin oversaw the addition of twenty-six buildings to the campus.

Unprecedented advancements occurred in patient care services during the fourth quarter-century. These included renal transplants and home dialysis, plus new services for those with speech and hearing disorders. Various intensive care units were created, as well as a day surgery unit. Other advances included new cardiovascular and transplant surgeries, laser therapies, lithotriptic treatments for kidney and bile stones, laparoscopic surgeries, and spectacular changes in diagnostic radiology and imaging. Emergency care services, rehabilitation services, ambulatory care services, and home health services expanded in dramatic ways. New services for cancer patients, patients with diabetes, and geriatric patients were created. A center for managing responses to accidental poisonings became a regional and national asset, as did a facility for hyperbaric therapy. When it opened in 1983, the Texas Department of Criminal Justice Hospital was the only prison hospital in the world directly affiliated with an academic medical center. UTMB's international reputation for the care of burned patients continued as the Shriners of North America chose to expand their services in a new building on the campus.

Unprecedented advancements occurred in educational programs. The School of Medicine expanded dramatically, reforming some departments and adding new ones. The medical school faculty revised their curriculum for medical students, initiated new programs for training clinical residents and fellows, and expanded continued education programs.

The School of Nursing faculty experienced major political reformations, becoming part of a centralized UT System in 1967. After decentralization and administrative reincorporation into UTMB in 1976, the nursing faculty continued their basic baccalaureate degree program, master's degree program, and continuing education programs. They initiated a new program that allowed registered nurses to earn bachelor's degrees.

In 1969 the UT regents formally authorized autonomy for each graduate school affiliated with the system's medical units. The graduate programs at UTMB that had evolved over many years were now officially designated as the University of Texas Graduate School of the Biomedical Sciences at Galveston. New leaders and professors revitalized its destiny. Five new graduate degree programs emerged during the 1980s. GSBS faculty attracted more graduate students because of their reputation as scientists and scholars.

During these years, UTMB established one school and two institutes. In 1968 UTMB formally incorporated several hospital-based training programs into the first School of Allied Health Sciences in the Southwest. In 1969 UTMB established its Marine Biomedical Institute as the first organized research program of its kind in an academic medical center in the United States. In 1973 UTMB established its Institute for the Medical Humanities. Fifteen years later, this institute initiated a graduate program that was the first of its kind in the United States.

Executives and faculty reformed the infrastructure for UTMB's research mission during the fourth quarter-century. Nationally and internationally recognized researchers became directors and chairs of divisions and departments. The research productivity of faculty in the schools and institutes expanded in previously unimagined ways. Research contributions flowed from the Marine Biomedical Institute, the Institute for the Medical Humanities, General Clinical Research Center, research labs in the Department of Surgery, a new Psychiatric Clinical Research Center, and labs in the School of Medicine's other basic science and clinical departments. Research became more prominent in the School of Nursing and the School of Allied Health Sciences.

Although the enormous increase in state and federal dollars during the 1960s and 1970s propelled fantastic growth, certain events of the 1980s chastened executives and reined excessive enthusiasm. The oil and gas setbacks of the national and state economies of the mid-1980s influenced all institutions of higher education in Texas. Financial crunches were severe and some institutions "lost" their "savings" as officials adapted to the setbacks. The regents, for example, reallocated about $11 million of UTMB's budget to bail out other UT institutions. In 1986 cutbacks on state income caused UTMB's business executives to "freeze" positions, stop merit increases, curtail promotions, reduce maintenance programs, and postpone capital outlay expenditures. Moreover, competition for state dollars became fiercer as existing institutions slowly expanded and new ones began.[41]

As the centennial year approached James and Pederson exerted valiant efforts to alter myths about the economic impact of UTMB's "tax-exempt" status. In 1987 they commissioned economic impact studies of UTMB by the Bureau of Research in the School of Business and Public Administration at the University of Houston at Clear Lake. The bureau's first report in 1988 revealed that UTMB had become the "dominant force" in Galveston's economy. UTMB's annual payroll of $179 million exceeded the combined payrolls of twenty of the city's next largest employers. Either directly or indirectly, UTMB supported 39 percent of the civilian jobs in Galveston. Moreover, UTMB—from utility charges, franchise fees, and permits—contributed more than $4 million in tax revenues to city government. A newspaper reporter proclaimed: "It's time Galvestonians put UTMB in perspective. The branch is the number one positive component of the city."[42]

James captured the upbeat tone of the late 1980s in an editorial in the *Galveston Daily News* on February 26, 1989. "From almost any perspective, there's much to be said for Galveston County," James declared. "Restful seascapes and balmy breezes. Active cultural and civic groups. Established businesses. Local performing arts. Proximity to a bustling metropolis, with minimal traffic jams of our own. Good fishing. They add up in any quality-of-life tally, and chief among them is my own vocation, that of health care." "We in Galveston County have access to health resources simply unavailable in most other communities of this size," James added. UTMB's century of roller coaster rhythms in Galveston had reached another high mark.[43]

A variety of historical accounts appeared during this quarter-century of extraordinary expansion. Two alumni wrote biographical essays about two professors of surgery. Walter B. King Jr. (School of Medicine class of 1940) discussed the career of James E. Thompson and Joseph P. McNeill (School of Medicine class of 1942) reviewed the contributions of A. O. Singleton Sr.[44]

Though dealing with specific components only, some histories were quite detailed. As her doctoral dissertation, completed in 1975, Billye Brown wrote the first comprehensive history of the School of Nursing. Henry Burlage, professor emeritus of pharmacy and former dean, and Margot Beutler, a professional historian, wrote the first comprehensive survey of the School of Pharmacy as part of their history of UT's College of Pharmacy, which was published in 1978.[45]

A lab technician and four former chairs prepared histories of their School of Medicine departments. In 1969 Hans Ash, a longtime technician in the Department of Pharmacology, completed an illustrated overview of that department. Donald Duncan's story of the development of the Anatomy Department between 1891 and 1932 was published in 1974. Robert Cooley wrote a detailed, unpublished history of the Department of Radiology in 1985, Don Micks prepared a short, published history of the Department of Preventive Medicine and Community Health in 1986, and Charles Allen wrote a detailed, unpublished history of the Department of Anesthesiology in 1991.[46]

Some histories appearing during these years reflected the more analytic styles of professional historiographers. In 1976 the Texas State Historical Association published a supplementary volume to its *Handbook of Texas*, which updated previous entries and added new ones. The concise update about UTMB noted the changes involving research and signaled expansion plans for the future. In his general history of Galveston published in 1986, David McComb devoted a few pages to UTMB, noting that the medical center became "the most important industry on the island" after World War II. In commemoration of the 150th anniversary of the establishment of the Republic of Texas in 1836, *Texas Medicine* published a monthly medical heritage series during 1986. A few of UTMB's legacies were examined in four of these articles.[47]

The institution expanded and changed in many ways as the fourth quarter-century evolved. The kaleidoscopic whirlwind of events was daunting for anyone who wanted a more comprehensive historical perspective. CEOs, as previously exemplified, were usually interested in such histories because they were the administrative caretakers of the entire institution. In the summer of 1985 Bill Levin authorized the preparation of this centennial history.

THE CENTENNIAL YEARS

UTMB celebrated two centennials: the birth of the John Sealy Hospital and the School of Nursing, and the birth of the School of Medicine. Formal planning for these celebrations began in the fall of 1989 when Tom James established a UTMB Centennial Commission of more than two hundred people. Chaired by Ann Brinkerhoff, this commission included faculty, students, staff, alumni, foundation representatives, and others willing to plan centennial celebrations. Nine subcommittees were appointed to shepherd special events, scientific symposia, artistic endeavors, alumni activities, professional meetings, community events, a centennial history, hospitality, and publicity. Some celebrations would focus on the hospital, some on component schools, and others on the institution as a whole. These celebrations were planned for 1990 and 1991.[48]

The John Sealy Hospital celebrated its centennial during a dinner at the San Luis Hotel on January 10, 1990, exactly one hundred years after the hospital opened its doors on January 10, 1890. As master of ceremonies, Ballinger Mills introduced the featured speakers, who included Jack Blanton, Charles Mullins, Tom James, Al LeBlanc, Preston Shirley, and George Sealy. Tom James appropriately conveyed the evening's spirit: "Without the Sealy & Smith Foundation, which has been a source of absolute inspirational confidence in this institution, there would certainly be no present form of the University of Texas Medical Branch." Robert Nichols, a writer in the Office of External Affairs, prepared a 126-page book about this legacy that chronicled the contributions of the Sealy family and the Sealy & Smith Foundation to UTMB.[49]

The School of Nursing celebrated its centennial anniversary during three major events in 1990. A homecoming weekend for alumni in early March featured lectures, a tea, a Victorian fashion show, and special dinners. In April the School of Nursing faculty staged the 1990 Global Nursing Conference, which was the third annual meeting of the World Health Organization Network of Collaborating Centers for Nursing Development. In September the American Association for the History of Nursing held its annual meeting at the Tremont Hotel. Poldi Tschirch prepared an excellent brochure titled "A Century of Excellence, A Vision for the Future: School of Nursing, 1890–1990" and a splendid exhibit about Edward Randall, the John Sealy Hospital, and the School of Nursing, which was displayed in the Galveston County Historical Museum.[50]

The Centennial Opening Ceremony occurred on January 25, 1991. After a luncheon for the commission featuring Sir Peter Froggatt from Belfast, dignitaries and guests assembled in the courtyard in front of John Sealy Hospital. Larry Patton directed the Centennial Chorus and Sister Anastasia Enright from St. Mary's Hospital gave the invocation. Tom James gave welcoming and closing remarks. Regent Louis A. Beecherl Jr., Charles B. Mullins, Ballinger Mills, and Mayor Barbara Crews offered comments. Ball High's Junior ROTC Color Guard assisted with the raising of three flags (United States, Texas, and UTMB Centennial) while the chorus sang "America the Beautiful." Afterward, guests attended a reception and viewed the Centennial Quilt hung in the lobby of the hospital.[51] That evening, UTMB's President Club staged a gala dinner at the San Luis Hotel.

Leslie Watts and her colleagues in the Office of External Affairs prepared a thirty-eight-page color brochure entitled "A Century of Service," which was distributed to all dinner guests. The text and photos of this brochure highlighted various facets of UTMB's century of service. In its foreword, James emphasized the future: "There is much here to be proud of, but our pride must go beyond applauding yesterday's achievements and acknowledging today's successes. Tomorrow's dreams are also a part of this significant anniversary." With the Capital Campaign, James had begun building for this future soon after his arrival in 1987. By the time of this dinner, this campaign had already generated gifts of $178 million.[52]

The centennial logo featured a profile of the front of Old Red that symbolized strength and endurance. This logo was placed on a huge Centennial flag, which flew throughout 1991 on the pole adjacent to the John Sealy Towers. Mementos and artifacts with this logo could be purchased. These included centennial medallions, posters of a painting of Old Red by Pam Heidt, centennial stationery, calendars, mailers (with an Old Red cancellation stamp), ties for men and scarves for women, Old Red T-shirts, coffee mugs, watches, lapel pins, and keepsake replicas of the 1891 School of Medicine catalog.[53] Issues of *Impact* included a Centennial Calendar of Events and Centennial "spotlights" on various celebrations and memorabilia.

More than seven hundred School of Medicine alumni and guests attended the week-long Centennial Homecoming festivities in March. This group included thirty-four

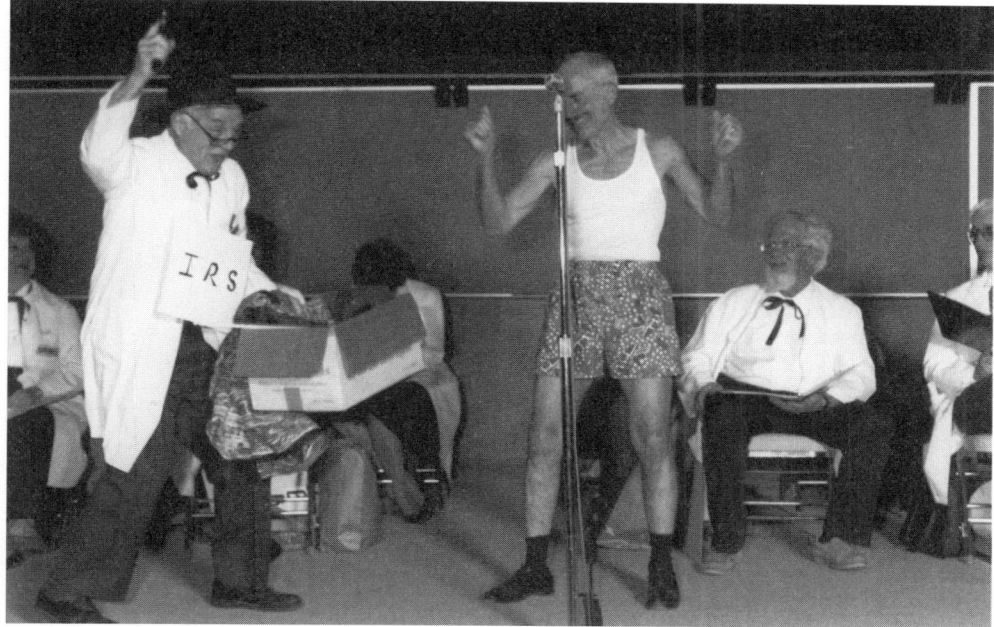

"Sawbones on a Sandbar," 1991. Left to right, Rene Kempen, Myron Nichols, and Charlie Powell.

graduates from the class of 1941, several from the class of 1936, and two from the class of 1926. John Tupper, AMA president, and Gov. Ann Richards gave keynote addresses. Volunteer faculty again presented Rose Schneider's play "Sawbones on a Sandbar."[54]

A Centennial Convocation Week occurred in June 1991. Several distinguished educators gave lectures. The Jubilee Banjo Band played a concert for faculty and guests. The U.S. Postal Service conducted first-day-of-issue ceremonies for the dedication of the latest addition to their Historic Preservation Series: a postcard featuring Old Red. Faculty representatives marched from the Moody Medical Library to the Clark W. Thompson Auditorium in Levin Hall for a Convocation Ceremony featuring a concert by the Centennial Chorus and a speech by Elspeth Rostow, Stiles Professor Emerita in American Studies at UT Austin. The Gleaves T. James Centennial Rose Garden was dedicated on the esplanade between the library and Levin Hall.[55]

In honor of the centennial, the editors of the *Journal of the American Medical Association* devoted its September 11, 1991, issue to UTMB. With a painting of Old Red on the cover, the 150-page issue included eight articles, ten abstracts, and two editorial-commentaries written by professors. One of the articles focused on UTMB's early years. Ron Bailey, Wiess Professor and chair of otolaryngology and longtime member of the journal's editorial board, coordinated the preparation of this issue. George Lundberg, *Journal of the American Medical Association* editor, believed that UTMB enjoyed "a tremendous reputation as a great school, particularly in terms of education, where it has placed graduates virtually everywhere. . . . You will find UTMB medical graduates at the top of the heap everywhere you look."[56]

Thousands of employees and their families participated in special festivities in early October, including a family picnic, a fajita cook-off, a fun run, a dunking booth, bingo, face painting, and children's games. An Employee Appreciation Ceremony occurred and the U.S. Postal Service issued a limited-edition commemorative postal "cachet" together with a "Century of Service" cancellation design.[57]

During 1991 several professional societies held special or annual meetings in Galveston. These included the Society of University Surgeons, the South Texas Chapter of the American College of Surgeons, the AMA's Council on Medical Education, the Texas Society for Medical Technology, the Southern Regional Group of the AAMC/GSA, the American Society for Rickettsiology and Rickettsial Diseases, the Texas Society for Histotechnology, the Texas Society of Anesthesiologists, the Texas Society for Gastrointestinal Endoscopy, the Texas Dermatological Society, the Texas Chapter of American College of Physicians with the Texas Society of Internal Medicine, the American Board of Internal Medicine, and the American Board of Otolaryngology. The willingness of these groups to meet in Galveston was a glowing testimonial to the professors and alumni who sustained UTMB's longstanding legacy of extensive involvement with state, regional, and national societies.

In honor of the centennial, the editors of *Texas Medicine* devoted "The Journal" section of its December issue to UTMB. Ron Bailey edited the eight articles contributed by seventeen members of UTMB's faculty. Bailey and Tom James declared that "UTMB takes great pride in the completion of its first century of service to Texans."[58]

On the plaza in front of John Sealy Towers on December 11, James and Ann Brinkerhoff presided during the UTMB Centennial Closing Ceremony, which featured songs by the Centennial Chorus and the lowering of the Centennial flag from the pole adjacent to the towers.[59]

FACING THE TWENTY-FIRST CENTURY

Securing regard and respect from many, the celebrations of the centennial years spurred its executives, faculty, students, and staff employees to move steadily toward the twenty-first century. Expansion and further development characterized many programs during the 1990s. Using the same conceptual frameworks presented in the previous chapters, a few representative changes are now described. These examples remind us of the moral values that animated UTMB's personnel as they faced the new century.

The networks of political power and authority remained relatively stable. There were a few structural changes. The Division of Orthopedic Surgery became a new School of Medicine department with Jason Calhoun as chair. The School of Allied Health Sciences added a new Department of Respiratory Care with Jon Nilsestuen as chair. There were numerous personnel changes that generated transitional adjustments for the affected groups. In the early 1990s, for example, William Cunningham became chancellor of the UT System; Gary Rounding became vice president for university relations; George Bernier Jr. became dean of medicine and vice president for academic affairs; Donald Prough became chair of anesthesiology and Courtney Townsend Jr.

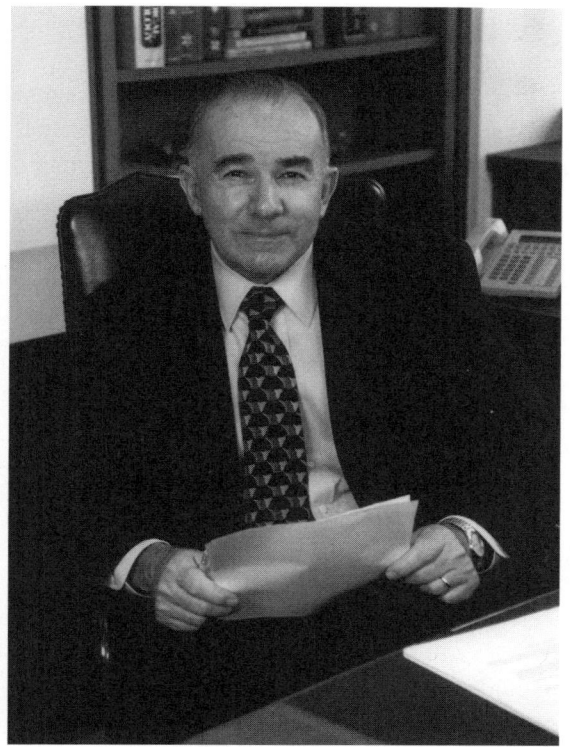

John D. Stobo, 1997.

became chair of surgery in the School of Medicine; Charles Christiansen became the School of Allied Health Sciences dean; and Cary Cooper became the Graduate School of the Biomedical Sciences dean.[60]

The regents and UT System executives adopted an elaborate strategic plan for the entire university during the 1990s. In the spring of 1995 UTMB's corporate leaders announced four strategic initiatives: training more primary care physicians; a more focused research agenda; networks for competing effectively in a managed health care environment; and a Texas Department of Criminal Justice managed care system.[61] These initiatives guided priorities in making policy and budgetary choices.

During 1996 and 1997 Charles Mullins coordinated a search for a new UTMB president as Tom James wanted to retire as CEO. In October 1997 John Stobo became UTMB's fifteenth CEO and fourth president. Stobo came to Galveston from Baltimore, where he had served for fifteen years in various roles at the Johns Hopkins University Medical Institutions. Energetic and personable, Stobo visited every building on the campus during his first day at work and, during subsequent months, met with many individuals and groups to become acquainted with faculty, students, and staff.[62]

Signaling his desire to relate the management of UTMB to success stories in the corporate world, Stobo asked UTMB's executives to read two books: *Built to Last: Successful Habits of Visionary Companies* by James C. Collins and Jerry I. Porras, and *Leading Change: The Argument for Values-Based Leadership* by James O'Toole. Stobo also employed Susan H. Coulter as UTMB's vice president for university relations. Coulter changed the title of her office from external affairs to university advancement.[63]

Symbolizing a new management style, Stobo also staged regular town meetings for the entire campus beginning on January 22, 1998. During the first part of each meeting, he addressed particular issues, such as overall missions, structural changes in administration, financial challenges, and topics involving patient care, teaching, and research. He fielded questions from the audience during the second part of each meeting. These were historically innovative sessions as no previous CEO had made systematic efforts to communicate openly and directly with all employees who wanted the opportunity to see their president "on the firing line," so to speak.[64]

A centennial perspective about UTMB reminds us that the decisions and behaviors of CEOs were the most important factors that propelled the institution's progress during its first century. Their integrity and professional competence were crucial in determining the institution's destiny. Their central role in harnessing or deflecting the moral energies of the entire institution must never be underestimated.

A centennial perspective reminds us that UTMB has always depended on multiple sources of income for its operations and growth. Soliciting dollars from private and governmental agencies continued during the 1990s. The Centennial Campaign raised more than $275 million. Galveston's local foundations continued their fantastic generosity during the 1990s. The Kempner Fund established an endowment for scholarships for minority students. The Moody Foundation contributed $4 million to the library's endowment fund. The Sealy & Smith Foundation gave about $70 million for construction projects, $50 million for the John Sealy Biomedical Endowment, and $2 million to the Institute for the Medical Humanities in support of its visiting faculty program.[65]

A centennial perspective reminds us that the decisions and behaviors of CBOs and their colleagues were essential to UTMB's progress. In 1992 John Sharp, the state's comptroller, praised UTMB as one of the "most efficiently run institutions in the state." In implementing new purchasing guidelines, business officials reduced costs that saved approximately $17.5 million for Texas taxpayers. In recognition of this accomplishment, Sharp gave a special award to UTMB in 1996.[66]

As the 1990s evolved, everyone reeled from the changes associated with the expansion of health maintenance organizations. Some decisions involved cutbacks. For example, continued financial losses prompted officials to close the Life Flight base in 1997 and return all responsibilities for helicopter transportation to Hermann Hospital in Houston. Decisions at UTMB about the purchase of physician practices and the expansion of primary care clinics provoked controversies among the state's physicians and fiscal agencies.[67]

Stobo and his executive team encountered major economic challenges. At the end of fiscal year 1998, UTMB had an operating deficit of about $80 million caused by shortfalls in reimbursement for indigent care from counties, reductions in Medicare and Medicaid reimbursements, inflation in the costs of supplies, and increases in wages to maintain a competitive edge. These circumstances made it necessary to close about 120 of 915 hospital beds, decisions that were largely responsible for the loss of jobs by more than three hundred employees early in 1999. Though the economic circumstances affected all teaching hospitals nationwide, the events in Galveston produced some clouds of stressful anxiety throughout UTMB as the end of the millennium approached. The Seventy-sixth Texas Legislature relieved some of this anxiety with a 13.1 percent increase in its biennial appropriations to UTMB.[68]

During the 1990s UTMB's CBOs initiated several changes. The Department of Human Resources completed a new compensation program that correlated salary ranges with specific jobs. Business-related support services underwent a major transformation from a hierarchical management structure to a team-oriented, process-centered organizational structure. About 270 employees—many cross-trained or retrained—became part of the "Logistics" segment of Support Services, which was designated as Acquisition, Creative, Lease/Rent/Reserve, Mail, and Warehouse/Store. Designed to improve efficiency by streamlining and coordinating roles, these changes offered many opportunities for adaptation by those working in the buildings of a still expanding campus.[69]

Certain changes occurred on the campus. The old John Sealy Hospital was renamed the John Sealy Annex and the John Sealy Towers were renamed the John Sealy Hospital. Renovations and/or additions occurred in the R. Waverley Smith Pavilion, the Keiller Building, the Medical Research Building, the Rebecca Sealy Hospital (former St. Mary's Hospital, purchased early in 1996), the Alumni Field House, the West End Chilled Water Plant, Open Gates, the 1902 Harborside Drive and 1700 Strand Buildings, and the John W. McCullough Building. The U.S. Department of Commerce gave UTMB $1 million to transform Open Gates into a telecommunications center.[70]

In 1992 officials dedicated the new Emergency Room and the Children's Hospital (renamed Child Health Center). The Rosenberg House opened in 1993 and the plaza between the Administration Building and the John Sealy Hospital was named the E. Burke Evans Plaza in honor of the physician-professor who served as chief of the Division of Orthopedic Surgery between 1965 and 1992. The Port Holiday Mall building was transformed into the Primary Care Pavilion, which opened in October 1996. The Lee Hage Jamail Student Center was dedicated in 1997.[71]

By 1998 about 1,250 plants representing forty species of roses were arranged in thirty-five beds of the Gleaves T. James Centennial Rose Garden, a site of beauty and tranquility employees and visitors enjoyed throughout the year.[72] A centennial perspective reminds us that the campus changes continuously as executives and others search for ways to improve and adorn the university's physical environment.

A centennial perspective reminds us that the care of sick patients has always been a primary mission at UTMB. As patients came for this care during the 1990s (36,000 inpatients and 654,000 outpatient visits by residents of 226 counties in 1996, for example), physicians, nurses, and others continued previously established services and discovered new approaches that led to improvements in patient-satisfaction ratings during the mid-1990s.[73]

The Extracorporeal Membrane Oxygenation (ECMO) team treated its one hundredth infant in the summer of 1993. By the summer of 1995 the Department of Obstetrics and Gynecology had established thirty-seven maternal/child health satellite clinics in Texas. The first satellite family medicine clinic was established in West Columbia. A new newborn nursery opened in the Waverley Smith Pavilion and the Children's Hospital established the first pediatric hospice program in the Houston–Galveston area, directed by Marcia Levetown.[74]

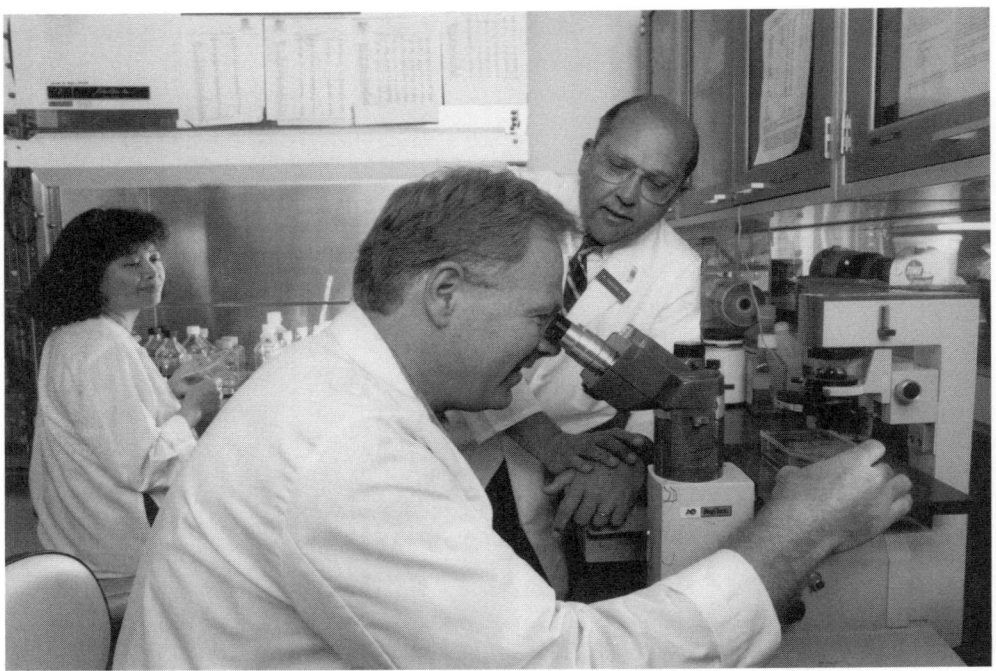

Tissue Culture Lab of the Surgery Department, 1992. Left to right, Jell H. Shieh, Kirk Ives, and Courtney M. Townsend Jr.

UTMB was selected as the only regional site in the Southwest to participate in the AIDS Clinical Trial Group, a research project involving thirty-seven institutions. To support this effort, UTMB received a multi-million dollar grant from the National Institute of Allergy and Infectious Disease to establish an AIDS Research Center. By 1994 about six hundred HIV-infected patients participated in this project. By 1996 Pediatric HIV Clinic personnel were treating about thirty children.[75]

Open Gates housed telemedicine equipment that was used for both patient care and new educational ventures in "distance learning."[76] Using a two-way interactive video system between doctors in Galveston and patients in off-campus TDCJ units and other clinical sites, UTMB initiated an extensive program of telemedicine care. By 1995, for example, doctors representing seventeen specialties examined and treated forty to sixty-five prisoners each week.

Transplant surgery expanded and improved radiographic equipment was purchased. In April 1992 more than one thousand people attended a reunion celebrating twenty-five years of kidney transplantation. Since 1966 the transplant team had performed 1,164 renal transplants on 1,101 patients; since 1988, the team had performed 34 dual kidney-pancreas transplants. The first heart-lung transplant occurred in October 1994. The Department of Radiology added a new CT Scanner and a new MRI Breast Scanning Unit.[77] A centennial perspective reminds us that UTMB's health care professionals are adamant about acquiring new machines and providing new services that honor a moral commitment to comprehensive care for individual patients.

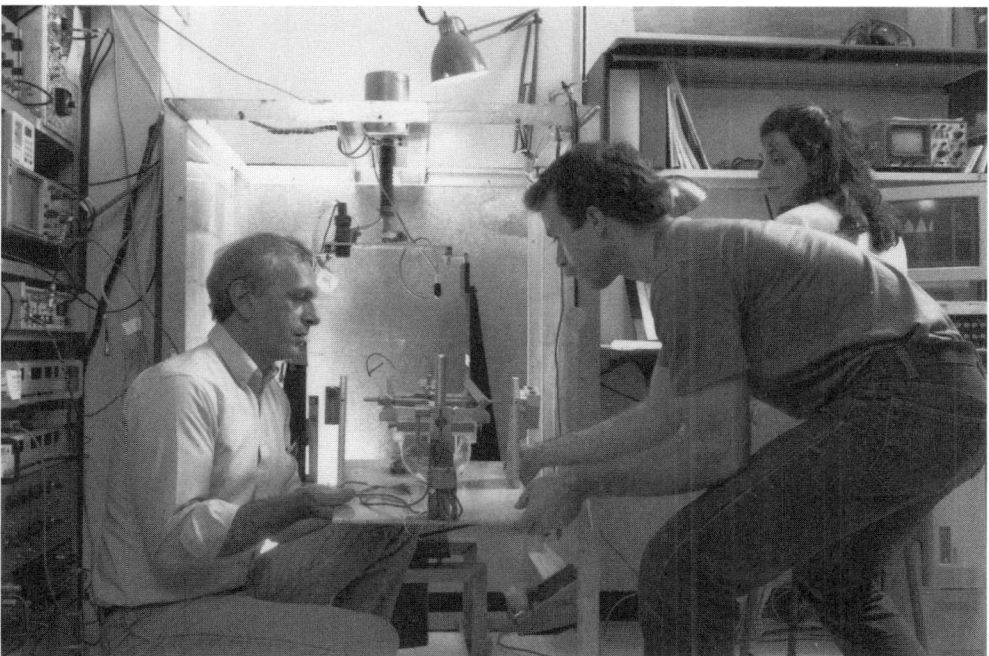

Research Lab, Department of Otolaryngology, 1992. Left to right, Adrian Perachio, Ian Purcell, and Heather McMullen.

A centennial perspective reminds us that volunteers have always provided extremely important caregiving services to patients and their families. In 1996 alone, nearly three hundred volunteers donated forty-seven thousand hours. Some volunteers addressed special needs. Over a ten-year period, Lana Meunier, a UTMB secretary, made 150 pairs of booties for premature infants and 350 stuffed animals for hospitalized children. By 1997 Judy Bahr and Betty Langer, two members of the Busy Bees Club, had brought handcrafted gifts to inpatients in the Children's Hospital every other month for six years.[78]

A centennial perspective reminds us that the education of students has always been a primary mission at UTMB. Discovering ways to improve teaching programs has been a central moral value for UTMB's teachers. Expansion of existing programs and some innovations occurred in the curricula of each school during the 1990s.

To improve communication between major committees, and between the faculty and administrators, the School of Medicine established a Faculty Coordinating Council in 1991. In 1994 the School of Medicine received a three-year, $1.5 million grant from the Robert Wood Johnson Foundation to support a collaborative project involving the Departments of Family Medicine, Internal Medicine, and Pediatrics that increased the number of primary-care physicians trained at UTMB. UTMB was the only school in Texas and one of fourteen nationwide to receive such a grant. In a survey of 125 accredited medical schools in the United States in 1996, UTMB ranked twenty-first with respect to the number of graduates choosing careers in primary care. The Department of Family Medicine also developed a new program that educated students and residents about rural practice in Texas.[79]

In the fall of 1995 twenty-four of two hundred first-year medical students voluntarily enrolled in a new four-year, problem-based curriculum named the Interactive Learning Tract. These students were introduced to clinical situations early, met in small groups to discuss case-based patient situations, assumed more personal initiative in obtaining information needed for analyzing and understanding the clinical cases, and, like their fellow students in the traditional curriculum, were expected to pass the required USMLE exams. A new Integrated Medical Curriculum for all other medical students began functioning in the fall of 1998.[80]

In 1998 the Department of Preventive Medicine and Community Health became the only academic medical center in the United States to have approved residency training programs in all three preventive medicine areas: general preventive medicine; aerospace medicine; and occupational medicine.[81]

Major improvements also occurred in the other three schools at UTMB. To provide off-campus educational opportunities for students (especially those in the School of Allied Health Sciences), Steve Shelton and colleagues established a Coastal Area Health Education Center in La Marque in 1992, followed by the Piney Woods AHEC and the Greater Houston AHEC. The School of Nursing restructured its governance polity and admitted its first Ph.D. students in the fall of 1997. Cary Cooper provided superb leadership for the Graduate School of the Biomedical Sciences. Cooper developed a new alumni organization for the GSBS that enabled the school to expand its scholarships and awards for students. The GSBS enrolled 442 students from twenty states and twenty-two countries in 1996, for example. To evaluate programs and make plans for the new century, GSBS faculty participated in an extensive internal assessment of policies and programs.[82]

Another event signaled a new era as faculty faced the twenty-first century. To provide an opportunity for faculty representatives to communicate their concerns about policies and directions, the faculty of all four schools established a Faculty Senate in 1998 and 1999. This innovative approach to shared governance symbolized a hope that more mutual respect, active collaboration, and direct communication among all faculty would occur during the new century.[83]

A centennial perspective reminds us that research became more of a primary mission at UTMB after 1942. During the 1990s, Dorothea Wilson, assistant vice president for research, reorganized research support services and George Bryan sponsored two faculty retreats organized by the Research Advisory Council. Wilson, Rosemary Simpson, and their assistants generated catalogs and reports that gave everyone a comprehensive view of the breadth and depth of research activities at UTMB.[84] A new corporate understanding of research emerged as faculty faced the twenty-first century. This understanding revitalized a moral commitment to this primary mission.

During the 1990s previously established research centers and departments continued their work, as numerous investigators received grants. In the Department of Physiology and Biophysics, for example, Harvey Fishman received a four-year, $1.1 million grant from the National Institute of Neurological Disorders and Stroke to discover the ways that nerve cells in earthworms and squid repair themselves after injury. In the Department of Pediatrics, Armond Goldman and Frank Schmalstieg located the abnormal gene on the "X" chromosome of a large family in East Texas whose members have an inherited immuno-deficiency disease. In the Department of Preventive Medicine and Community Health, Kyriakos Markides and colleagues received a five-year, $3.5 million grant from the U.S. Department of Health and Human Services to conduct field research on the health care needs of Mexican Americans in the southwestern United States. About twenty professors conducted studies in the General Clinical Research Center, attracting more than $7 million in research funding by 1996.[85]

New research centers and laboratories emerged during these years. Thomas G. Wood directed a new Recombinant DNA Laboratory in the 1700 Strand Building in 1992. The John Sealy Memorial Endowment Fund provided partial support for five research centers. Samuel Wilson directed the Sealy Center for Molecular Science; Marshall Runge directed the Sealy Center for Molecular Cardiology; Stratford May Jr. directed the Sealy Center for Oncology and Hematology; David Gorenstein directed the Sealy Center for Structural Biology; and James Goodwin and Mary Fenton directed the Sealy Center on Aging.[86]

Chrysalis BioTechnology, UTMB's first biotechnology company, was founded in 1995. UTMB received royalties from the sale of Chrysalin products that enhanced tissue repair during the treatment of wounds and injuries. Darrell Carney, professor of human biological chemistry and genetics, developed Chrysalis, a synthetic peptide with the same properties as a portion of the naturally occurring enzyme thrombin, which plays a key role in blood clotting and tissue repair.[87]

A centennial perspective reminds us that the energies and dreams of UTMB's students have propelled the institution during its first century and beyond. In forging bonds of metamorphosis, their moral courage and incessant struggles have been extraordinary. Guided by Rebecca Saavedra, director of the Office of Campus Life, students achieved more cohesiveness and camaraderie as a multi-school student body during the 1990s. This spirit was facilitated and symbolized by *Omni*, a regular publication of the Student Government Association and Office of Campus Life that began early in 1991. This newsletter addressed student government elections, sports activities, concerts, student health services, student organizations, community service projects, Quest orientation programs for new students, counseling and peer support programs, and dances and parties. Both the Student Government Association and the Office of Campus Life nurtured mutual respect among all students. Symbolizing and facilitating this respect, UTMB orchestrated its first all-schools orientation program for entering students in August 1998.

A centennial perspective reminds us of the tenacious moral commitment of "service to others" that animated UTMB during its first century and beyond. Without any expectation of personal monetary gain, alumni, faculty, staff, and students continued to generate positive images about UTMB locally and throughout the world. Leslie Charles Powell Jr., professor of obstetrics and gynecology, received the 1999 Rabbi Henry Cohen Humanitarian Award for his work as a volunteer physician on Indian reservations in the United States and at hospitals in Africa and Bosnia.[88]

School of Medicine alumni continued their leadership roles in professional societies. Joe Painter (class of 1949) was president of the AMA in 1994; Daniel Johnson Jr. (class of 1963) in 1996.[89] Between 1991 and 1999 five alumni were presidents of the Texas Medical Association: Sam Nixon (class of 1950), William Gamel (class of 1963), Robert Tenery Jr. (class of 1968), Mark Kubala (class of 1958), and Alan Baum (class of 1968).

Some professors became presidents of state, regional, and national associations during the 1990s. These included David Herndon, Society of University Surgeons; James Belli, Radiation Research Society; Byron Bailey, American Board of Otolaryngology and American Laryngological Association; James Blankenship, Association of Neurosciences Departments and Programs; Linda Phillips, Association of Women Surgeons; Martin L. Nusynowitz, American College of Nuclear Physicians; Billy Philips, Texas Society of Allied Health Professions; and Richard Rahr, Association of Physician Assistant Programs.[90]

During the 1990s James C. Thompson received more recognition and honors than any other professor. Thompson was president of the American Surgical Association, the Society for Surgical Chairmen, and the Southern Surgical Association. Recognizing his extraordinary leadership, Mayor Barbara Crews proclaimed January 29, 1992, as Dr. James C. Thompson Day. Earlier that month, Thompson had hosted the American Surgical Association's midwinter council meeting at the Tremont House. In 1999 Thompson was president of the American College of Surgeons.[91]

UTMB's Center for International Health, led by Harold Drayton and Ulysses Panisset, celebrated its tenth anniversary in 1997. This center coordinated communication between the WHO Collaborating Centers at UTMB and staff members at Pan American Health Organization headquarters (Washington, D.C.) and WHO headquarters (Geneva). Professors participated in an extraordinary array of research, teaching, and patient care activities that interfaced directly with health care professionals in many parts of the world. Tom James directed the WHO Collaborating Center for Cardiovascular Diseases; Elizabeth Anderson directed the WHO Collaborating Center for Nursing Development in Primary Health Care; and David Walker directed the WHO Collaborating Center for Tropical Diseases. Numerous professors and students from several departments participated in programs in Latin America, the United Arab Emirates, Nigeria, India, Vietnam, Russia, China, Mexico, and several European countries.[92]

A centennial perspective reminds us that UTMB's professors were morally committed to the "highest standards" in patient care, teaching, and research during the institution's first century and beyond. They invited peers from outside UTMB to provide a critical evaluation of all programs as a systematic way of maintaining their commitment to these high standards. This voluntary commitment was a crucial component of UTMB's reputation extended by peers and lay publics. Peer assessments continued during the 1990s.

In 1998, for example, the Joint Commission on Healthcare Organizations accredited UTMB's hospital and clinics for three years.[93]

A centennial perspective reminds us that telling stories about UTMB has been a prominent feature of the first century and beyond. During the 1990s UTMB's journalists produced a variety of publications for on-campus and off-campus groups. Employees of the Office of External Affairs and its successor, the Office of University Advancement, also embraced the challenges of the Internet age by developing a remarkable home page, www.utmb.edu, which opened unprecedented vistas of communication for the approaching new century.

Spurred by Tom James, the Office of External Affairs worked diligently to establish good relationships with the public media. Reporters for the *Galveston Daily News* wrote several stories about events during UTMB's centennial year. Bob Whitby captured a "defining moment" of the year with his article about research.[94] Whitby highlighted six areas: neurophysiology and hyperbaric studies at the Marine Biomedical Institute; studies in the Center for Environmental Toxicology about the effects of chemicals on fetal and adult development; studies of yellow fever, malaria, African sleeping sickness, Chagas' disease, and Rickettsiae japonica in the Center for Tropical Diseases; studies of ethical, legal, and philosophical problems in patient care by members of the Institute for the Medical Humanities; studies at the Shriners Burns Institute about wound healing and other bodily responses in severely burned patients; and studies of genetic and molecular mechanisms conducted by faculty in most School of Medicine departments. As UTMB celebrated its first century and faced a new century, no citizen could deny the central role of its research mission.

Among the stories about UTMB published during the 1990s, some histories appeared. Andy Grant analyzed the work of three outstanding professors, Meyer Bodansky, Charles Marc Pomerat, and George Herrmann. Harold Levine wrote a superb history of the Department of Pediatrics, which was published in 1992. Chester Burns discussed UTMB's hospitals in an overview of Galveston's hospitals published in 1993, and he wrote a history of the Graduate School of the Biomedical Sciences for its twenty-fifth anniversary in 1994.[95]

UTMB was a sponsor of the six-volume *New Handbook of Texas* the Texas State Historical Association published in 1996. The "Health and Medicine" entries included about 375 biographical sketches of deceased professionals (including several UTMB alumni and twenty-six professors) and about 145 entries on organizations, institutions, and special topics (including John Sealy Hospital, Moody Medical Library, Sealy & Smith Foundation, Shriners Burns Institute, and UTMB). In 1997 Heather Campbell assessed the historical significance of the School of Nursing.[96]

In 1999 Campbell and Burns depicted the influences of William Keiller and James E. Thompson on medical education and practice in Texas and the United States. Vernie Stembridge (class of 1949) included UTMB in his story of medical schools in Texas and Mavis Kelsey (class of 1936) contributed an extraordinary autobiography to the state's medico-historical literature. Harry Davis (class of 1949) edited a unique and

The Path I Choose

What is this freedom which men boast they own?
My barque seems free upon the waters,
Yet no matter what the course I set
I only partly guide.
You, like a lodestar, turn my compass north
Across the trackless miles
A feeble force but constant
And a source directive in my better hours.

For life is unknown ocean,
And winds may blow destructive rancor to my soul,
Or anchor it becalmed on surface of a liquid glass
To shrivel 'neath the blazing sun.
At other times I race before a cooling draft
And speak of progress toward a port
The tide may raise my song to buoyant tone
Or wring a minor wail at its recess,
And under all, the oceans move in vaster whirls.

Men speak of final ports. This craft was ocean born
And knows no rest.
If port there be, it yet has sighted none.
But this is life, not yonder, and the best we have
Lies in this frame and not in distant scene.
Let me speak fair to all of those who pass,
Hail and farewell or traveling abreast.
May I no wreckage cause nor halt the travelers fast
Who know where they are bound.

Yet wandering to touch at many strands,
The known and loved, the new uncharted isles,
I seek the gems of each and hope to land
Upon your restful shore before the end.

extraordinary set of recollections prepared by the School of Medicine class of 1949 for its fiftieth anniversary reunion.[97]

As the twentieth century receded and the twenty-first century beckoned, alumni, professors, and others crafted histories and images about a remarkable institution still expanding and evolving on an island in the Gulf of Mexico more than one hundred years after its establishment. Their stories and images focused on the paths chosen by many people who established, sustained, and renewed UTMB during its first century and beyond (Table 10). A centennial perspective reminds us that UTMB has been and is an institution composed of many different kinds of caregivers. Countless moments of caring sustained and propelled UTMB. Memories forged in the bonds of many caregiving relationships and experiences became the stories about UTMB's past. One way to be a caregiver to the entire institution is to tell stories about the institution as a whole.

A centennial perspective about UTMB reminds us that historical inquiry can be a path of affirmation and empowerment. Historical inquiry can be a tool for recognizing, understanding, and interpreting the multiple factors that influence the choices and lives of individuals and groups. Historical inquiry can be a tool for sorting moral values as professionals and citizens. Moral values and daily choices determine legacies and destinies. A centennial perspective reminds us that humans created and recreated UTMB by choice, not by chance. Every day and night offered new beginnings and new endings. Today, others make their choices and walk their paths along "the new uncharted isles" of UTMB's second century. Tomorrow, others will follow in their footsteps.

Appendices

LIST OF APPENDICES

A. UTMB Chief Executive Officers, 1891–1991   391

B. Administrative Officers, UTMB Schools and Institutes, 1891–1991   392

C. Committees on Medical Institutions, UT Board of Regents, 1891–1991   399

D. UT Chief Executive Officers, 1891–1991   405

E. John Sealy Hospital Boards of Managers, 1891–1941   406

F. Chief Administrative Officers, John Sealy and UTMB Hospitals, 1890–1991   412

G. Department Chairs, Schools, 1891–1991   415

H. Power Centers and Administrative Organization, UTMB, 1891–1939   424

I. Executive Committees, Faculty, 1898–1943   425

J. UTMB Chief Business Officers, 1891–1991   426

K. Income, Schools and John Sealy Hospital, 1888–1900   427

L. Budgets, John Sealy Hospital, 1890–1900   428

M. Expenses, Schools, 1891–1900   429

N. Major Buildings Associated with UTMB, 1890–1991   430

O. Patient Care Statistics, John Sealy Hospital, 1891–1900   438

P. The Fate of New Matriculates, 1891–1900   439

Q. Medical Faculty Who Served on the Committees on Instruction
for the School of Nursing, 1896–1939   441

R. General Administrative Organization, UTMB, September 1954   443

S. General Administrative Organization, UTMB, November 1984   445

T. Directors of the Sealy & Smith Foundation for the John Sealy
Hospital, 1922–1991   446

U. Budgets, Hospitals, 1901–1940   447

V. Budgets, Schools, 1901–1940   449

W. Income, Hospitals, 1941–1968   451

X. Income, Schools, 1941–1968   453

Y. Income, Hospitals, 1969–1991   455

Z. Income, Schools, 1969–1991   457

AA. Patient Care Statistics, Hospitals, 1901–1912   459

AB. Patient Care Statistics, Hospitals, 1913–1924   460

AC. Patient Care Statistics, Hospitals, 1925–1938   461

AD. Total Collections, Patient Services Revenue, Fiscal Years 1982–1991   462

AE. Major Educational Programs in Nursing, 1890–1991   463

AF. School of Allied Health Sciences Degree and Certificate Programs, 1991   464

AG: Grants for Research and Research Training by Source, 1976–1990   468

AH: Grants for Research and Research Training by Department, School,
or Institute, 1967–1991   469

Appendix A

UTMB Chief Executive Officers, 1891–1991

1891–97	John Fannin Young Paine
1897–98	Allen John Smith
1898–1901	Henry Pendleton Cooke
1901–03	Allen John Smith
1903–22	William Spencer Carter
1922–26	William Keiller
1926–28	Henry C. Hartman*
1928–35	George Emmett Bethel*
1935–38	William Spencer Carter
1938	Byron M. Hendrix (A)
1938–42	John William Spies
1942–55	Chauncey D. Leake
1955–56	Truman G. Blocker Jr.*
1956–64	John B. Truslow
1964–74	Truman G. Blocker Jr.*
1974–87	William C. Levin*
1987–	Thomas N. James

Assistant Executive Director
1958–59	H. Frank Connally Jr.*

Associate Director
1964–65	E. Don Walker

Vice President for Administration
1965–70	Warren G. Harding

NOTE: An asterisk signifies a graduate of UTMB's School of Medicine. During the 1955–1956 year, Truman G. Blocker Jr. was chairman of an Interim Executive Committee that included G. A. W. Currie, Donald Duncan, Raymond Gregory, Titus H. Harris, Robert M. Moore, and Charles T. Stone. The (A) signifies an interim role as the acting administrator.

APPENDIX B

ADMINISTRATIVE OFFICERS, UTMB SCHOOLS AND INSTITUTES, 1891–1991

ADMINISTRATIVE OFFICERS, SCHOOL OF MEDICINE

VICE PRESIDENTS

1968–73	Joseph M. White (Academic Affairs)
1983–	George T. Bryan (Academic Affairs)
1985–88	James C. Guckian* (Medical Professional Affairs)
1987–	K. Lemone Yielding (Research)
1989–91	Fred Wichlep (External Affairs)
1990–	James F. Arens (Clinical Affairs)

ASSOCIATE VICE PRESIDENT

1990–	Louis C. Sheppard (Research)

ASSISTANT VICE PRESIDENTS

1984–	Alvin L. LeBlanc* (Clinical Affairs)
1984–	Julian I. Kitay (Academic Affairs)
1984–88	David Eiland* (Students)
1985–87	Charles Tandy (Planning and Public Affairs)
1986–	Harvey Bunce III (Academic Administration)
1988–	A. Yvonne Russell (Student Affairs)
1988–90	Louis C. Sheppard (Research)
1991–	Clifford W. Houston (Multicultural Affairs)
1991–	Dorothea C. Wilson (Research)

EXECUTIVE DEAN

1976–77	Edward N. Brandt Jr.

DEANS

1891–97	John Fannin Young Paine
1897–98	Allen John Smith
1898–1901	Henry Pendleton Cooke
1901–03	Allen John Smith

DEANS

1903–22	William Spencer Carter
1922–26	William Keiller
1926–28	Henry C. Hartman*
1928–35	George Emmett Bethel*
1935–38	William Spencer Carter
1938–42	John William Spies
1942–53	Chauncey D. Leake Jr.
1945–58	D. Bailey Calvin (Students and Curricular Affairs)
1953–55	Truman G. Blocker Jr.*
1955–56	Truman G. Blocker Jr.* (A)
1956–59	John B. Truslow
1959–62	Kenneth M. Earle*
1962–64	John B. Truslow
1964–67	Warren G. Harding (Student Affairs)
1964–65	William J. McGanity
1965–66	Warren G. Harding
1967–68	Kenneth P. Walker (Student Affairs)
1968–73	Joseph M. White
1973–74	Edward N. Brandt Jr. (A)
1974–76	Edward N. Brandt Jr.
1976–	George T. Bryan
1984–88	David Eiland* (Students)
1988–	Yvonne Russell (Students)

VICE DEAN

1991–	Walter J. Meyer III

ASSOCIATE DEANS

1941–42	Jarrett E. Williams
1942–45	D. Bailey Calvin (Student Affairs)
1963–64	Warren G. Harding
1968–80	Spencer G. Thompson* (Sponsored Programs)
1969–73	Richard F. Timmers (Curriculum Affairs)
1972–73	Edward N. Brandt Jr. (Clinical Affairs)
1972–81	John Bruhn (Community Affairs)
1973–75	James Guckian* (Clinical Affairs)

ASSOCIATE DEANS

1974–83	David Eiland* (Student Affairs)
1974–77	George T. Bryan (Curricular Affairs)
1977–84	Al LeBlanc* (Graduate Medical Education)
1978–84	Julian I. Kitay (Curricular Affairs)
1978–85	William W. Schottstaedt (Continuing Education)
1982–88	A. Yvonne Russell (Community Affairs)
1984–	Julian I. Kitay (Academic Affairs)
1986–	Harvey Bunce III (Administration)

ASSISTANT DEANS

1939–41	Jarrett E. Williams
1941–42	William S. Wallace
1954–56	John C. Finerty (Students and Curricular Affairs)
1958–59	Kenneth M. Earle* (Undergraduate)
1958–62	Stephen R. Lewis (Graduate and Postgraduate)
1959–63	Warren G. Harding (Admissions)
1964–65	Rollin A. Sininger (Student Affairs)
1964–66	Spencer G. Thompson* (Grants and Contracts)
1966–68	E. Gene Powell (Student Affairs)
1967–69	Joe Tupin*
1968–69	Billy B. Rankin (Student Affairs)
1978–80	Philip L. Rayford
1981–87	Daniel Trevino (Student Affairs)
1984–86	Charles Tandy (Administration)
1984–86	Harvey Bunce III
1987–88	Billy B. Rankin (Admissions)
1988–	Billy R. Ballard (Student Affairs)
1990–	Judy Carrier (Faculty Affairs)

ADMINSTRATIVE OFFICERS, SCHOOL OF NURSING

DIRECTORS/DEANS

1890–92	Dorothea Fick
1892–93	Anna L. Locke
1893	F. Edith Howard*
1893–96	Josephine Durkee
1896	Augusta Gilminot
1896–1900	Hanna Kindbom
1900	Minnie Ferguson*
1900–01	Emma L. Cartmell*
1901–02	Marie Overton*
1902–03	Margaret G. Fay
1903–05	Marjorie M. Taylor
1905–19	Ethel D'Arcy Clay
1919–20	Martha St. John Eakins
1920–23	Ella E. Read
1923–26	Grace Gertrude Grey
1926–28	Saidee Nolan Hausmann
1928–31	Xilema Faulkner*
1931–36	Dorothy Rogers
1936–40	Dora Mathis
1940–41	Anyce Wallace*
1941	Elsa Maurer Kibbe
1942	Anyce Wallace*
1942–63	Marjorie Bartholf
1963–67	Betty Rudnick*
1967	Chloe Floyd* (A)
1967–68	Virginia Walker (A)
1968–85	Dorothy Damewood
1985–86	Mary Fenton* (A)
1978–	Mary Fenton*

Associate Deans

1978–85	Elizabeth Knebel* (Administration)
1979–86	Helen Ptak (Research and Evaluation)
1979–83	Shirley Steele (Graduate Studies)
1985–90	Stephanie Pardue (Academic Affairs)
1986–90	Mary Anne Sweeney (Research)
1989–	Regina P. Lederman (Academic Affairs)
1990–	Jerry Lester (A) (Research)

Assistant Deans

1956–62	Virginia Dryden
1962–63	Betty R. Rudnick*
1964–68	Marie C. Primm
1978–79	Helen Ptak (Research and Evaluation)
1978–79	Shirley Steele (Graduate Studies)
1985–86	Mary Anne Sweeney (Research)
1990–	Michael Manheimer (Business Affairs)

Adminstrative Officers, School of Pharmacy

Dean

1926–27	William F. Gidley

Adminstrative Officers, Graduate School of the Biomedical Sciences

Deans

1970–74	Edward N. Brandt Jr.
1974–87	J. Palmer Saunders
1987–	K. Lemone Yielding

Associate Deans

1952–70	Donald Duncan
1975–80	Elbert B. Whorton Jr. (Curriculum)
1980–	James E. Blankenship (Curriculum)

Assistant Dean

1981–	Robert C. Bennett

ADMINSTRATIVE OFFICERS,
SCHOOL OF ALLIED HEALTH SCIENCES

DEANS

1968–80	Robert K. Bing
1980–91	John G. Bruhn
1991–	Billy U. Phillips (A)

ASSOCIATE DEANS

1978–79	James D. Spitler
1982–	Patrick McGraw (Administration)
1982–91	Billy U. Phillips
1982–	D. Lisa Leonard (Curricular Affairs)
1982–86	Harry Siegel (Student Affairs)
1986–	Raymond Lewis (Student Affairs)

ASSISTANT DEANS

1971–76	Robert Plunkett
1978–80	Lucia Guzman
1978–80	Roger A. Lamer (Academic Affairs)
1978–82	Patrick McGraw (Administration)
1980–82	D. Lisa Leonard (A) (Academic Affairs)
1981–82	James Myklebust (A) (Student Affairs)
1981–82	Billy U. Phillips

ADMINSTRATIVE OFFICERS, MARINE BIOMEDICAL INSTITUTE
DIRECTORS

1969–77	Stewart Wolf
1977–78	William D. Willis (A)
1978–	William D. Willis

ADMINSTRATIVE OFFICERS,
INSTITUTE FOR THE MEDICAL HUMANITIES

DIRECTORS

1974–80	William B. Bean
1980–81	Chester R. Burns (A)
1981–82	William W. Schottstaedt (A)
1982–	Ronald A. Carson

ASSOCIATE DIRECTOR

1975–80	Chester R. Burns

NOTE: An asterisk signifies a UTMB graduate. The (A) signifies an interim role as the acting administrator.

APPENDIX C

UT BOARD OF REGENTS
COMMITTEES ON MEDICAL INSTITUTIONS, 1891–1991

1891–94	T. M. Harwood
	T. C. Thompson
	T. D. Wooten
1894–98	Beauregard Bryan
	T. C. Thompson
	T. D. Wooten
1898–99	Beauregard Bryan
	Frank M. Spencer
	T. D. Wooten
1899–1903	George W. Brackenridge
	Beauregard Bryan
	Frank M. Spencer
1903–05	George W. Brackenridge
	Beauregard Bryan
	R. Waverley Smith
1905–06	George W. Brackenridge
	Beauregard Bryan
	Marcellus E. Kleberg
1906–08	George W. Brackenridge
	M. Marx
	J. W. McLaughlin
1908–09	George W. Brackenridge
	A. W. Fly
	J. W. McLaughlin

1909–10	George W. Brackenridge
	A. W. Fly
	Hampson Gary
1910–13	Joseph Faust
	Alex. Sanger
	W. H. Stark
1913–14	A. W. Fly
	Will C. Hogg
	W. H. Stark
1914–17	A. W. Fly
	Will C. Hogg
	G. S. McReynolds
1917–19	George W. Brackenridge
	Frederick W. Cook
	John Sealy II
1919–20	Henry J. L. Stark
	Ralph Steiner
	Louis J. Wortham
1920–23	Frederick W. Cook
	Frank C. Jones
	Mrs. H. J. O'Hair
1923–24	Frederick W. Cook
	Frank C. Jones
	Tucker Royall
	Joe S. Wooten
1924–27	Marcellus E. Foster
	Mart H. Royston
	George W. Tyler

1927–29   None appointed

1929–31   W. M. Odell
               Edward Randall
               H. J. Lutcher Stark

1931–32   Beauford Jester
               W. M. Odell
               Edward Randall

1932–33   Charles I. Francis
               Beauford Jester
               Edward Randall

1933–35   K. H. Aynesworth
               Edward Randall
               M. Frank Yount

1935–40   K. H. Aynesworth
               Edward Randall
               J. R. Parten

1940–41   K. H. Aynesworth
               Fred C. Branson
               J. R. Parten

1941–42   K. H. Aynesworth
               Fred C. Branson
               H. H. Weinert

1942–43   K. H. Aynesworth
               W. Scott Schreiner
               H. H. Weinert

1943–44	Orville Bullington
	D. F. Strickland
	H. H. Weinert

1944–46	Orville Bullington
	W. H. Scherer
	C. O. Terrell

1946–47	James W. Rockwell
	W. Scott Schreiner
	C. O. Terrell

1947–50	James W. Rockwell
	A. M. G. Swenson
	C. O. Terrell

1950–53	L. S. Gates
	James W. Rockwell
	Mrs. Margaret B. Tobin

1953–55	L. S. Gates
	Leroy Jeffers
	Dudley K. Woodward Jr.

1955–57	Leroy Jeffers
	Merton M. Minter
	L. S. Oaten
	J. R. Sorrell

1957–59	J. P. Bryan
	Merton M. Minter
	J. R. Sorrell
	Joe C. Thompson

1959–61   J. P. Bryan
                 Mrs. Charles Devall
                 J. Lee Johnson III
                 Wales H. Madden Jr.

1961–63   J. P. Bryan
                 H. Frank Connally Jr.
                 Wales H. Madden Jr.
                 A. G. McNeese Jr.

1963–65   H. Frank Connally Jr.
                 Frank C. Erwin Jr.
                 Wales Madden Jr.
                 Levi A. Olan

1965–67   H. Frank Connally Jr.
                 Frank N. Ikard
                 Jack S. Josey
                 Levi A. Olan

1967–81   See note

1981–83   Janey Briscoe
                 Sterling H. Fly Jr.
                 Jon P. Newton

1983–85   Janey Briscoe
                 Jess Hay
                 Mario Yzaguirre

1985–87   Jack S. Blanton
                 Janey Briscoe
                 Mario Yzaguirre

1987–89   Sam Barshop
               Jack S. Blanton
               W. A. "Tex" Moncrief Jr.
               Mario Yzaguirre

1989–91   Jack S. Blanton
               W. A. "Tex" Moncrief Jr.
               Mario Yzaguirre

NOTE: These names, arranged alphabetically, were taken from annual catalogs and the Minutes of the Meetings of the University of Texas System Board of Regents. Because of changes in the composition of the board (due to death, resignation, or new members) and because of changes in the composition of committees of the board, there may be errors in this list. After 1946 the committee was named the Committee on the Medical and Dental Branches; after 1955, the Committee on Medical Affairs; after 1979, the Health Affairs Committee. A Medical Branch Committee was not appointed between 1927 and 1929. All members of the board served on each committee established by the board between 1967 and 1981. Janey Briscoe, Sterling H. Fly Jr., Jon P. Newton, Howard N. Richards, and Walter G. Sterling served on special Subcommittees on Hospitals between 1979 and 1981.

Appendix D

UT Chief Executive Officers, 1891–1991

1895–96	Leslie Waggener
1896–99	George T. Winston
1899–1905	William L. Prather
1905–08	David F. Houston
1908–14	Sidney E. Mezes
1914–16	William J. Battle
1916–23	Robert E. Vinson
1923–24	William S. Sutton
1924–27	Walter M. W. Splawn
1927–37	Harry Y. Benedict
1937–39	John W. Calhoun
1939–44	Homer P. Rainey
1944–50	Theophilus S. Painter
1950–54	James P. Hart
1954–61	Logan Wilson
1961–71	Harry H. Ransom
1971–78	Charles A. LeMaistre
1978–84	E. Don Walker
1984–	Hans M. Mark

Appendix E

John Sealy Hospital Boards of Managers, 1891–1941

1891–92	T. C. Thompson
	C. Campbell
	George Sealy
	John Reymershoffer
	C. J. Allen
1892–95	T. C. Thompson
	C. Campbell
	George Sealy
	D. B. Henderson
	Ben Levy
1895–97	T. C. Thompson
	C. Campbell
	George Sealy
	A. Ferrier
	H. A. West
1897–98	T. C. Thompson
	C. Campbell
	George Sealy
	J. D. Skinner
	D. S. Davison
1898–99	J. D. Skinner
	W. C. Fisher
	Henry P. Cooke
	George Sealy
	D. S. Davison

1899–1900   Henry P. Cooke
F. M. Gilbough
George Sealy
C. H. Hughes
J. D. Skinner

1900–01   Henry P. Cooke
F. M. Gilbough
George Sealy
Ben Levy
J. D. Skinner

1901–02   James E. Thompson
V. E. Austin
John Sealy II
I. H. Kempner
C. W. Trueheart

1902–06   James E. Thompson
V. E. Austin
John Sealy II
I. H. Kempner
Edward Randall

1906–09   James E. Thompson
Edward Randall
John Sealy II
V. E. Austin
I. H. Kempner

1909–11   Edward Randall
James E. Thompson
John Sealy II
V. E. Austin
Lewis Fisher

1911–13	Edward Randall
	M. L. Graves
	John Sealy II
	V. E. Austin
	I. H. Kempner
1913–16	Edward Randall
	M. L. Graves
	John Sealy II
	A. P. Norman
	H. O. Sappington
1916–17	Edward Randall
	M. L. Graves
	John Sealy II
	A. P. Norman
	H. O. Sappington
	Mr. and Mrs. R. Waverley Smith (Hon.)
1917–19	Edward Randall
	M. L. Graves
	John Sealy II
	Charles Suderman
	E. D. Cavin
	Mr. and Mrs. R. Waverley Smith (Hon.)
1919–23	Edward Randall
	M. L. Graves
	John Sealy II
	A. P. Norman
	George E. Robinson
	Mr. and Mrs. R. Waverley Smith (Hon.)

1923–24
Edward Randall
M. L. Graves
John Sealy II
A. P. Norman
R. P. Williamson
Mr. and Mrs. R. Waverley Smith (Hon.)

1924–25
Edward Randall
M. L. Graves
John Sealy II
R. P. Williamson
I. E. Pearce
Mr. and Mrs. R. Waverley Smith (Hon.)

1925–26
Edward Randall
A. O. Singleton
John Sealy II
R. P. Williamson
Alvin T. Lang
Mr. and Mrs. R. Waverley Smith (Hon.)

1926–27
Edward Randall
A. O. Singleton
R. P. Williamson
Alvin T. Lang
Mr. and Mrs. R. Waverley Smith (Hon.)

1927–29
Edward Randall
A. O. Singleton
E. H. Ivey
Frank H. Mellina
Mr. and Mrs. R. Waverley Smith (Hon.)

1929–30
Edward Randall
A. O. Singleton
R. P. Williamson
O. E. Casey
Mr. and Mrs. R. Waverley Smith (Hon.)

1930–32
Edward Randall
A. O. Singleton
Mrs. R. Waverley Smith
R. P. Williamson
O. E. Casey

1932–33
Edward Randall
A. O. Singleton
Mrs. R. Waverley Smith
R. P. Williamson
Arthur J. Peterson

1933–35
Edward Randall
A. O. Singleton
Mrs. R. Waverley Smith
R. P. Williamson
P. H. Wilson

1935–38
Edward Randall
A. O. Singleton
Mrs. R. Waverley Smith
Raymond Stewart
Adolph Suderman

1938–39
Edward Randall
A. O. Singleton
Mart H. Royston
Raymond Stewart
Adolph Suderman

1939–40

Edward Randall

A. O. Singleton

Mart H. Royston

Raymond Stewart

George H. Gymer

1940–41

L. E. Dowd

George H. Gymer

Arthur J. Peterson

George Sealy Jr.

Raymond Stewart

NOTE: These names were obtained from various sources, including annual catalogs; Minutes of the UT Board of Regents, June 18, 1891; an unpublished list in box VF 9/C, UT President's Records; and A. L. Singleton to Homer P. Rainey, June 3, 1940, letter, box VF 9/P, UT President's Records.

Appendix F

Chief Administrative Officers, John Sealy and UTMB Hospitals, 1890–1991

Year	Directors, Hospitals	Directors, Nurses
1890–91	J. H. Wysong	Dorothea Fick
1891–94	J. P. Hendrick	M. E. Wygant
		F. Edith Howard
		Anna L. Locke
1894–95	William Gammon	C. Josephine Durkee
1895–96	W. F. Starley Jr.	C. Josephine Durkee
1896–98	W. F. Starley Jr.	Augusta Gilminot
		Hanna Kindbom
1898–99	Edward L. Batts	Hanna Kindbom
1899–1900	Hanna Kindbom	Hanna Kindbom
	Kenneth H. Aynesworth	
1900–01	Kenneth H. Aynesworth	Emma Lee Cartmell
1901–02	H. O. Sappington	Emma Lee Cartmell
		Marie Overton
1902–03	H. O. Sappington	Margaret G. Fay
	James J. Terrill	
1903–04	Margaret G. Fay	Margaret G. Fay
1904–05	Marjorie M. Taylor	Marjorie M. Taylor
1905–06	Marjorie M. Taylor	Ethel D'A. Clay
1906–17	Clara L. Shackford	Ethel D'A. Clay
1917–18	John E. Fay	Ethel D'A. Clay
1918–19	Tamar Milne	Ethel D'A. Clay
1919–20	Ethel D'A. Clay	Martha St.J. Eakins
1920–23	Ethel D'A. Clay	Ella E. Read
1923–26	Ethel D'A. Clay	Grace G. Grey
1926–28	Ethel D'A. Clay	Saidee N. Hausmann
1928–31	Lucius R. Wilson	Xilema D. Faulkner
1931–35	Lucius R. Wilson	Dorothy Rogers
1935–40	Lucius R. Wilson	Dora Mathis
1940–41	Jarrett E. Williams	Elsa M. Kibbe
		Anyce J. Wallace

Year	Directors, Hospitals	Directors, Nurses
1941–42	Jarrett E. Williams	Anyce J. Wallace
1942–43	Jarrett E. Williams	Marjorie Bartholf
	Chauncey D. Leake	
	William O. Bohman	
1943–46	Chauncey D. Leake	Marjorie Bartholf
	William O. Bohman	
1946–47	Beryl I. Burns	Ethelyn Peterson
1947–48	Beryl I. Burns	Aurelia C. Willers
1948–49	Beryl I. Burns	Aurelia C. Willers
	Jack R. Ewalt	
1949–50	Jack R. Ewalt	Aurelia C. Willers
1950–51	Jack R. Ewalt	Aurelia C. Willers
	Truman G. Blocker Jr.	
1951–53	Truman G. Blocker Jr.	Aurelia C. Willers
1953–54	G. A. W. Currie	Aurelia C. Willers
1954–55	G. A. W. Currie	Catherine Bane
1955–56	G. A. W. Currie	Isabella Tremor
1956–57	Daniel J. Bobbitt	Isabella Tremor
1957–59	Arthur G. Hennings	Catherine Bane
1959–67	Daniel J. Bobbitt	Catherine Bane
1967–68	Henry A. Swicegood	Patricia M. Bosworth
1968–70	Warren G. Harding	Dorothy C. Felis
1970–72	David E. Hoxie	Dorothy C. Felis
1972–78	David E. Hoxie	Anna P. Rains
1978–80	John P. Porretto	Anna P. Rains
1980–90	Alvin L. LeBlanc	"Decentralized"
1990–	James F. Arens	"Decentralized"
1991–		Jana Stonestreet

NOTE: These names were obtained from various sources, including Minutes of the UT Board of Regents, annual catalogs, annual budgets, and the Human Resource Information Systems Office of the Human Resources Department. Some names may have been missed because the sources were confusing and incomplete at times. In the 1899–1900 year, for example, Hanna Kindbom was superintendent and Kenneth H. Aynesworth was house surgeon. In the following year Aynesworth served as both superintendent and house surgeon. In addition to such shifts in roles, there were sometimes temporary appointees. For example, James J. Terrill acted as interim superintendent during the summer months of 1903. During his first three years as executive director and dean, Chauncey Leake was also the principal administrator of the hospitals, although William O. Bohman handled most of the daily administrative tasks. When two names are given for a particular year, it usually means that the individual named second succeeded the first person, who had resigned or died. For example, Jack R. Ewalt assumed the role of director of the hospitals after B. I. Burns resigned on March 1, 1949. Truman G. Blocker Jr. became director of the hospitals after Ewalt resigned on September 30, 1950. Warren G. Harding administered the hospital with the title of vice president for health services. John P. Porretto was named assistant vice president for hospital affairs and Alvin L. LeBlanc succeeded Porretto with the title of associate vice president for university hospitals. LeBlanc "decentralized" control of nursing services by assigning nursing care areas to different executive directors. In 1985 LeBlanc became vice president for university hospitals. In 1990 James F. Arens became chief executive officer for the UTMB hospitals and Stephen L. Royal became associate vice president for hospital operations and chief operating officer.

Appendix G

Department Chairs, UTMB Schools, 1891–1991

Department Chairs, School of Medicine

Anatomy

1891–1931	William Keiller
1931–39	Harry O. Knight
1939–42	Donald Duncan
1942–46	John Sinclair
1946–68	Donald Duncan
1968–85	Walther J. Hild
1985–86	William D. Willis Jr.

Anatomy and Neurosciences

1986–	William D. Willis Jr.

Anesthesiology

1942–53	Harvey Slocum
1953–77	Charles R. Allen
1977–90	James F. Arens
1990–	Harry K. Wallfisch (A)

Bacteriology and Preventive Medicine

1917–21	Mark F. Boyd
1921–40	William B. Sharp

Bacteriology

1941–57	William B. Sharp

Biochemistry

1891–1908	Seth M. Morris
1908–10	Arthur E. Austin
1910–13	George F. Gracey
1913–22	William C. Rose
1922–48	Byron M. Hendrix
1948–51	Wendell Griffith

1952–56	Otto A. Bessey
1956–63	Andrew A. Ormsby
1963–71	Virgil K. Koenig

DERMATOLOGY

1923–27	Earl Crutchfield
1927–42	William Spiller
1942–49	Chester Frazier
1949–53	Clarence S. Livingood
1953–77	J. Fred Mullins
1977–78	William B. Bean (A)
1978–	Edgar Ben Smith

FAMILY MEDICINE

1973–79	M. Lamar Ross
1979–80	William Schottstaedt (A)
1980–88	Paul Young
1988–90	Alice Anne O'Donell (A)
1990–	Stephen J. Spann

HISTOLOGY AND EMBRYOLOGY

1912–27	Charlotte Schaefer
1928–40	John G. Sinclair

HUMAN GENETICS

1967–71	Barbara Bowman

HUMAN BIOLOGICAL CHEMISTRY AND GENETICS

1971–81	Barbara Bowman
1981–84	Creed Abell (A)
1984–	E. Brad Thompson

INTERNAL MEDICINE

1891–97	Hamilton A. West
1897–1905	James McLaughlin
1905–26	Marvin Graves
1926–58	Charles T. Stone Sr.
1958–61	James V. Warren
1961–66	Raymond Gregory

1966–68	Raymond Gregory (A)
1968–84	William P. Deiss
1984–85	James Guckian (A)
1985–90	Walter G. Johanson Jr.
1990–	Donald W. Powell

MICROBIOLOGY

1957–74	Willard F. Verwey
1974–75	Leroy J. Olson (A)
1975–	Samuel Baron

NEUROLOGY

| 1973– | John Calverly |

NEUROLOGY AND PSYCHIATRY

| 1926–63 | Titus H. Harris |
| 1963–73 | Hamilton Ford |

OBSTETRICS AND GYNECOLOGY

1891–1910	John F. Y. Paine
1910–24	George H. Lee
1924–54	Willard R. Cooke
1954–60	Garth L. Jarvis
1960–89	William McGanity
1989–	Garland Anderson

OPHTHALMOLOGY

1907–37	Seth M. Morris
1937–54	Clarence Sykes
1954–60	Gaynelle Robertson
1960–62	Wendell Gingrich
1962–63	Gaynelle Robertson
1963–64	David Haney (A)
1964–81	Edward Ferguson
1981–82	John C. Barber (A)
1982–90	John C. Barber
1990–91	Byron J. Bailey (A)
1991–	Wayne March

OTOLARYNGOLOGY

1924–39	Dick Wall
1939–61	Jehu M. Robison
1961–68	George McReynolds
1968–	Byron J. Bailey

PATHOLOGY

1891–1903	Allen J. Smith
1903–07	Alfred E. Thayer
1907–13	James J. Terrill
1913–29	Henry C. Hartman
1929–54	Paul Brindley
1954–56	Elwood E. Baird
1956–63	Howard C. Hopps
1963–76	F. Lamont Jennings
1976–85	Edward G. Reynolds Jr.
1985–87	Peachy R. Gilmer (A)
1987–	David H. Walker

PEDIATRICS

1924–43	William Boyd Reading
1943–58	Arild E. Hansen
1958–60	Harry Stoeckle and Mary E. Haggard (A)
1960–89	Charles William Daeschner Jr.
1989–91	C. Joan Richardson (A)
1991–	Pearay Ogra

PHARMACOLOGY

1922–27	Harry V. Atkinson
1927–40	Wilfred T. Dawson
1940–44	Raymond Gregory
1944–61	George A. Emerson
1961–65	Benedict E. Abreu
1965	James G. Hilton
1966–67	Charles R. Allen (A)
1967–77	Sydney Ellis
1977–79	J. Palmer Saunders (A)
1979–82	James G. Hilton (A)
1982–	Cary W. Cooper

Physiology

1891–98	A. G. Clopton
1898–1922	William S. Carter
1922–24	Charles C. Gault
1924–41	Eugene L. Porter
1941–43	Carl A. Nau (A)
1943–49	Eric Ogden
1949–51	Howard G. Swann (A)
1951–71	M. Mason Guest
1971–73	M. Mason Guest (A)

Physiology and Biophysics

1973–85	Arthur M. Brown
1985–86	John Russell (A)
1986–	Luis Reuss

Preventive Medicine

1912–14	James Person Simonds
1914–16	Burdett Loomis Arms

Preventive Medicine and Public Health

1940–41	John W. Spies
1941–61	Carl A. Nau
1961–66	Don W. Micks (A)

Preventive Medicine and Community Health

1966–85	Don W. Micks
1985–90	Harold Sandstead
1990–91	John Bruhn (A)
1991–	Harvey Bunce (A)

Psychiatry

1973–74	Hamilton Ford
1974–77	Ivan Bruce (A)
1977–78	Dan Creson (A)

Psychiatry and Behavioral Sciences

1978–89	Robert M. Rose
1989–90	John Calverly (A)
1990–	Robert M. A. Hirschfeld

RADIATION THERAPY

1982–	James A. Belli

RADIOLOGY

1931–39	Jesse B. Johnson
1939–40	William Wallace
1940–46	Jesse B. Johnson
1946–49	Martin Schneider
1949–53	Joe C. Rude
1953–76	Robert N. Cooley
1976–91	Melvyn Schreiber
1991–	Leonard Swischuk (A)

SURGERY

1891–1927	James E. Thompson
1927–47	Albert O. Singleton
1947–60	Robert M. Moore
1960–65	Truman G. Blocker Jr.
1965–68	Roger Williams
1968–70	Samuel Snodgrass
1970–	James C. Thompson

MATERIA MEDICA AND THERAPEUTICS

1891–1944	Edward Randall

DEPARTMENT CHAIRS, SCHOOL OF NURSING

ADMINISTRATION AND CURRICULUM

1965–67	Virginia Dryden

ADULT HEALTH

1989–90	Bernadette McKay (A)
1990–	Mary Lou Shannon

COMMUNITY HEALTH/GERONTOLOGY

1989–	Elizabeth Anderson

Fundamentals of Nursing

1960–61	Marie Arganbright
1961–63	Edith M. Samartino

Maternal/Child Health

1957–60	Virginia Lane
1960–61	Lucille Moore (A)
1961–64	Gwen Roberts
1964–69	C. Grace Schexnayder
1989–90	Eloise Boortz (A)
1990–	Mary L. Moore

Medical-Surgical

1956–58	Virginia Brantl
1958–67	Chloe Floyd

Mental Health/Management

1989–90	Ernestina Forman (A)
1990–	Helen K. Kee (A)

Psychiatric

1956–62	Beatrice Carruth
1962–68	Betty Beaudry

Public Health Nursing

1958–60	Mary E. Beikert
1960–64	Loretta Roberts
1964–66	Eleanor Danysh (A)

Department Chairs, School of Allied Health Sciences

Allied Health Services

1976–78	M. Diane Roberts
1978–79	Evelyn Scott
1979–80	F. David Cordova (A)
1980–81	F. David Cordova

Associated Health Occupations

1971–80	James L. Cantwell

HEALTH CARE SCIENCES

1971–73	Warren F. Dodge
1973–77	Robert C. Greaser
1977–78	Byron Williams (A)
1978–82	Byron Williams
1982–83	Richard R. Rahr

HEALTH INFORMATION MANAGEMENT

1986–89	John W. Berkbuegler
1989–	Beth H. Anderson

HEALTH PROMOTION AND GERONTOLOGY

1988–	David Chiriboga

HEALTH RELATED STUDIES

1981–91	F. David Cordova

HUMANITIES AND BASIC SCIENCES

1989–90	Salah Ayachi
1990–	Kyungsoon Chang Chung (A)

MEDICAL RECORDS ADMINISTRATION

1968–76	Sally A. Mount
1976–79	Beverly A. Ripple
1979–84	Kathryn Howard
1984–85	Billy U. Phillips (A)
1985–86	John W. Berkbuegler

MEDICAL TECHNOLOGY

1968–86	Ruth E. Morris
1986–	Shirley A. Richmond

OCCUPATIONAL THERAPY

1968–77	Mary Frances Heermans
1977–78	Gretchen Schmalz (A)
1978–79	Robert Bing (A)
1979–83	Charles Christiansen
1983–84	Gretchen Schmalz (A)
1984–	Donald A. Davidson

PHYSICIAN'S ASSISTANT STUDIES

1983–	Richard R. Rahr

PHYSICAL THERAPY

1968–76	Jeanne M. Schenck
1976–84	Eugene C. Rembe
1984–89	Betty R. Landen
1989–	Claire Peel

NOTE: The (A) signifies an interim role as the acting chair.

APPENDIX H

POWER CENTERS AND ADMINISTRATIVE ORGANIZATION, UTMB, 1891–1939

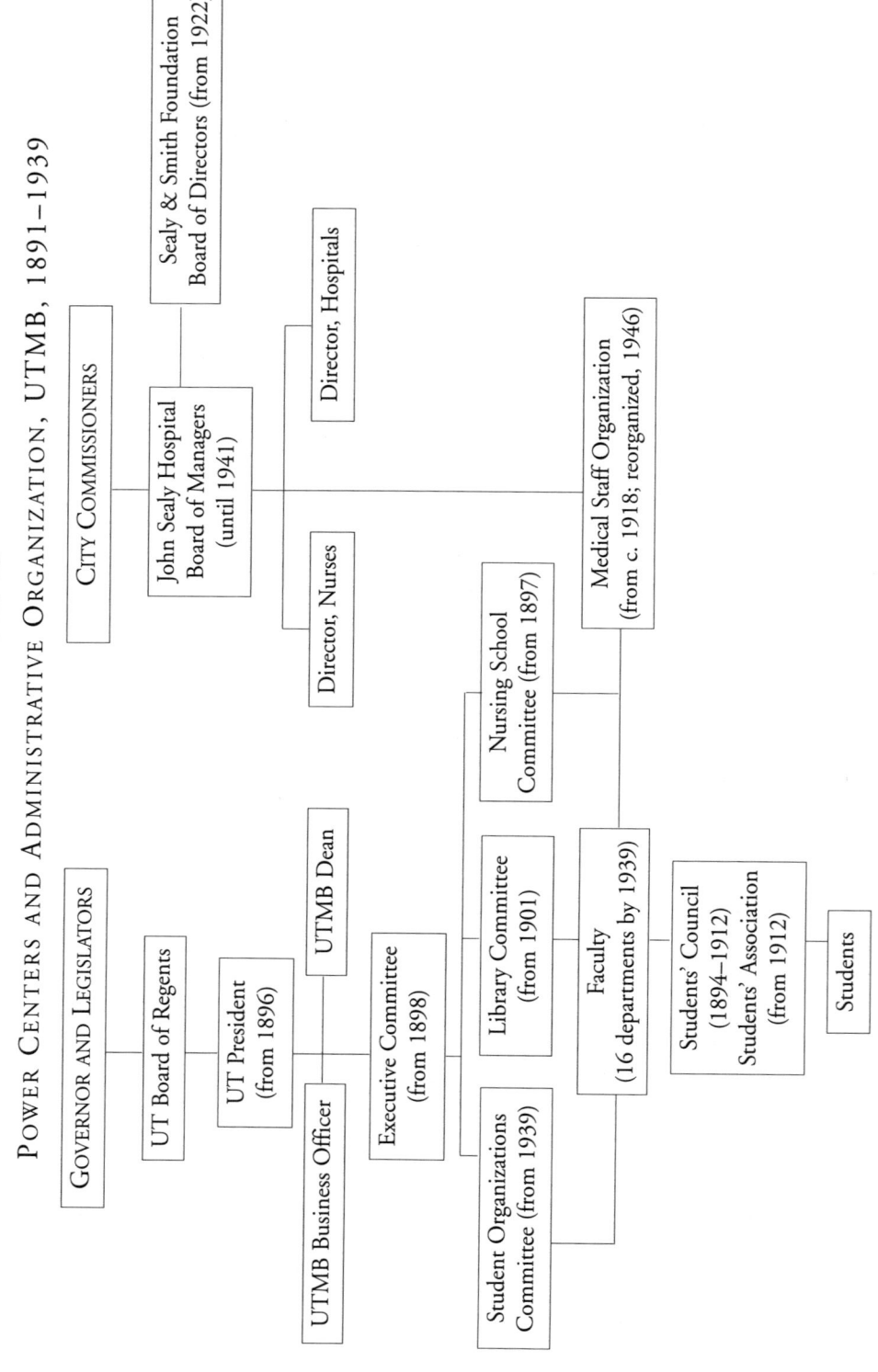

424

Appendix I

Executive Committees, UTMB Faculty, 1898–1943

1898–99	Seth Morris, Edward Randall
1899–1900	R. R. D. Cline, William Keiller
1900–02	William Carter, James Thompson
1902–03	Not known
1903–04	Edward Randall, James Thompson
1904–05	Edward Randall, James Thompson
1905–06	William Thayer, James Thompson
1906–14	Marvin Graves, Edward Randall
1914–19	Marvin Graves, William Keiller, Edward Randall Jr., James Thompson
1919–22	Marvin Graves, Edward Randall Jr., William Rose, James Thompson
1922–25	Marvin Graves, Henry Hartman, Edward Randall, James Thompson
1925–27	W. F. Gidley, Henry Hartman, Byron Hendrix, Edward Randall, James Thompson
1927–28	Byron Hendrix, Harry Knight, Edward Randall, A. O. Singleton
1928–39	Byron Hendrix, Harry Knight, A. O. Singleton, Charles T. Stone Sr.
1939–40	Paul Brindley, Willard Cooke, William Boyd Reading, William Sharp
1940–41	Paul Brindley, Willard Cooke, Raymond Gregory, Clarence Sykes
1941–42	Paul Brindley, Raymond Gregory, Jehu Robison, Clarence Sykes
1942–43	D. Bailey Calvin, Donald Duncan, George Decherd Sr., Titus Harris, William Sharp, Samuel Snodgrass

NOTE: These names were obtained from various sources including annual catalogs, Minutes, UTMB Faculty Meetings, Minutes, UTMB Executive Council, and an unpublished list in box VF 9/C, UT President's Records. Over the years, this committee experienced some changes of titles and responsibilities. Between 1898 and 1914, it was called the Advisory and Executive Committee. The word "Advisory" was dropped in 1924 when the Executive Committee, together with the dean, assumed executive authority for the entire faculty. This committee and its power continued until Dean John Spies obtained a change in the rules of the regents that transformed the role of the committee into one that was only "advisory" to the dean (1940). Renamed Faculty and Admissions Committee in 1943, this committee continued only as an advisory committee during Chauncey Leake's tenure as CEO.

Appendix J
UTMB Chief Business Officers, 1891–1991
Chief Business Officers

1891–1903	James P. Johnson
1903–21	Thomas H. Nolan
1921–45	John C. Nolan
1945–55	Edgar N. Capplemann
1955–64	E. Don Walker
1964–67	Warren G. Harding
1967–86	Vernon E. Thompson Jr.
1986–	E. J. "Jere" Pederson

Vice President for Business Affairs

1989–	Richard M. Moore

APPENDIX K

INCOME, SCHOOLS AND JOHN SEALY HOSPITAL, 1888–1900

Year	Schools		Hospital			
	Student Fees	State	City	Private Patients	Sealy	Other
1887			$62,500			
1888		$50,000			$50,000	
1889		25,000←	25,000		35,000	
1890–91			10,500	NA		
1891–92	$2,520	52,000	12,500	NA		
1892–93	2,790	22,000	15,980	$3,290	201	
1893–94	5,400	33,700	15,555	2,820	3,025	
1894–95	6,125	31,200	NA	2,448	NA	
1895–96	7,545	38,500	18,000	4,089	NA	
1896–97	8,555	38,500	15,272	4,433	3,105	
1897–98	6,175	38,500	16,270	4,037	3,146	$41,000
Sept. 98		38,500				
1898–99	5,322	35,500	17,613	2,532	2,964	
1899–1900	6,660	41,500	18,940	3,654	5,241	
					40,000	

NOTE: T. C. Thompson, "Brief Review," 1897; Minutes, UT Board of Regents; *Report of the UT Board of Regents* (1881–1901); unpublished typescript showing Medical College income, 1891–1917, box 4Q22, UT President's Records; *Galveston Daily News*, Aug. 30, 1902; and Edward Randall to R. E. Vinson, Jan. 10, 1917, box 4Q21, UT President's Records. In 1887 the city donated Block 668 and the City Hospital building. In 1897 Thompson estimated their worth at $62,500. The Sealy family donated $85,000 for construction of the John Sealy Hospital and improvements of Block 668. The Medical College Building and the lots on Block 669 cost $100,000 ($25,000 from the city and $75,000 from the state). In 1891 the legislature granted $30,000 for equipment and furnishings for the Medical College Building and $22,000 per year for salaries and operating expenses during the 1891–1893 biennium. In fiscal year 1894 the professor of pharmacy received $2,500 for equipment and supplies. After matriculation fees were reduced in 1893, the number of students dramatically increased, resulting in more income from student fees. In 1897 George Brackenridge gave $47,000 to build University Hall. City dollars and deficit balances are taken from Appendix L without any changes. However, there would be unknown differences in these totals because of different fiscal year sequences used by the state and by the city. The Sealy family presumably absorbed the hospital's deficits. Between 1898 and 1900 the Sealy family spent at least $40,000 for a horse-drawn ambulance and renovations of the hospital. Totals, which should be viewed as approximate, are rounded to the nearest dollar. NA means not available from cited sources.

Appendix L

Budgets, John Sealy Hospital, 1890–1900

Year	Income		Expenses	Balance (Deficit)
	City Dollars	Pay Patients		
1890–91	$10,500	NA	NA	NA
1891–92	12,600	NA	NA	NA
1892–93	15,980	$3,290	$19,471	$(201)
1893–94	15,555	2,820	22,400	(3,025)
1894–95	NA	2,448	17,917	NA
1895–96	28,000	4,089	19,160	2,929
1896–97	25,272	4,433	22,810	(3,205)
1897–98	15,270	4,037	23,453	(3,146)
1898–99	27,623	2,532	23,109	(2,954)
1899–1900	18,940	3,654	27,835	(5,242)

NOTE: Account books of the John Sealy Hospital Board of Managers and the City of Galveston are not extant for these years. Data for the Expenses and Pay Patients columns are taken from *Galveston Daily News*, Aug. 30, 1902, and May 26, 1920. City Dollars are calculated from estimates given in the unpublished minutes of meetings of the Galveston City Council. Balances (deficits) are calculated by subtracting Pay Patients and City Dollars from Total Expenses. These deficits were presumably absorbed by the Sealy family and they are shown as Sealy contributions in Appendix K. Operating expenses of the hospital included salaries for those employed as superintendent, steward, engineer, druggist, nurse, cook, and laundry woman, and expenses for furnishings, food, drugs, clothing, coal, ice, gas, telephone, printing, and insurance. See *Galveston Daily News*, Feb. 11, 1890, and Mar. 1, 1894. NA means not available from cited sources. The totals, rounded to the nearest dollar, were for each fiscal year, March 1 to March 1.

Appendix M

Expenses, UTMB Schools, 1891–1900

Year	Salaries	M&O	Total
1891–92	$22,425	$1,352	$23,777
1892–93	23,900	8,144	32,044
1893–94	25,700	12,885	39,585
1894–95	25,700	11,123	37,823
1895–96	33,633	15,131	48,765
1896–97	37,236	9,907	47,144
1897–98	34,428	11,458	45,886
Sept. 1898	17,098	3,225	20,322
1898–99	37,257	5,597	42,854
1899–1900	37,155	5,733	43,887

NOTE: The data came from an unpublished typescript of Medical College expenditures, 1891–1917, box 4Q22, UT President's Records; and Minutes, UT Board of Regents and *Report of the UT Board of Regents* (1891–1901). Salaries included those for professors, demonstrators, provost, janitors, and physical plant personnel. Maintenance and Operating Expenses (M&O) included purchases for the library, equipment and supplies for teaching laboratories, and overhead expenses (fuel, gas, water, stamps, stationery, printing catalogs, painting and repairs, care of grounds, etc.). The sources show a separate appropriation for September 1898 and a separate total of expenditures for that same month. The reason for this is not known. It may be a reporting error and these separate items may be a part of the 1897–1898 or 1898–1899 totals. Not included is the $41,000 gift from George Brackenridge that was expended in constructing University Hall. Figures are rounded to the nearest dollar and should be considered approximate.

Appendix N

Major Buildings Associated with UTMB, 1890–1991

In the following list, particular buildings and building clusters are separated by asterisks. Years given in the left column are those in which they opened for use or were renamed or significantly restructured for continuing use. Years given in the right column are those in which they were demolished. Buildings in brackets are situated on the campus, but are not owned by UTMB. UTMB owns other buildings that are not included in this list. The Office of the Director of UTMB's Physical Plant has a computerized master file of all buildings.

***

1875	Galveston City Hospital	
1890	Nurses' Home and Negro Hospital	
1902	Laboratory of Clinical Pathology	1915

***

1890	John Sealy Hospital	1962

***

1891	Medical College Building (Old Red)	
1950	Ashbel Smith Building	
1985	Ashbel Smith Building	In use

***

1898	University Hall	1945

***

1902	Negro Hospital	1937

***

1912	Isolation Pavilion	
1936	Psycho One	
1962	Byron Hendrix Building	1989

***

1913	Walter Colquitt Memorial Children's Hospital	
1915	State Hospital for Crippled and Deformed Children	
1937	Isolation Building	
1950	Physical Plant Building	1988

***

| 1915 | Woman's Hospital | |
| 1954 | Administration Building | 1973 |

***

1915	Rebecca Sealy Nurses' Home	
1932	Psycho Two and Three/House Staff Quarters	
1962	Administration Annex I	In use

***

1916	Laboratory of Experimental Medicine	
1942	Animal Building	After
1950	Experimental Laboratory and Animal Quarters	1967

***

| 1920 | Laboratory of Chemistry (Pharmacy) | Before 1942 |

***

| 1921 | Laboratory of Pharmacology and Physiology | 1961 |

***

| 1922 | Laboratory of Clinical Pathology/ Pathology Chemistry Laboratory | After |
| 1942 | Preventive Medicine Building | 1962 |

***

1925	Laboratory Building/West half	
1932	Laboratory Building/East half	
1951	William B. Keiller Building	In use

***

1929	Power Plant and Laundry	
1949	Annex added	
1963	Power Plant and Laundry	1989

***

| 1930 | Outpatient Clinic Building | |
| 1966 | Integrated with John W. McCullough Outpatient Clinic Building | |

| 1973 | Integrated with Clinical Sciences Building | |
| 1983 | Integrated with Ambulatory Care Center | In use |

***

1931	Galveston State Psychopathic Hospital	
1937	A 45-bed addition opens	
1943	Closed for repairs	
1946	Reopened as Galveston State Psychopathic Hospital	
1958	Marvin L. Graves Hospital	
1960	Closed for repairs	
1962	Marvin L. Graves Hospital	
1979	Marvin L. Graves Hospital	In use

***

| 1932 | Rebecca Sealy Nurses' Home | |
| 1960 | Rebecca Sealy Building | 1973 |

***

1937	State Hospital for Crippled and Deformed Children	
1954	Children's Hospital of new John Sealy Hospital	
1956	Children's Hospital	
1977	Integrated with Child Health Center	In use

***

1937	Negro Hospital	
1957	Closed for repairs	
1960	Edward R. Randall Pavilion	1979

***

1944	Margie B. Stewart Convalescent Home for Children	
1949	Home of Dr. and Mrs. Chauncey Leake	
1958	Home of Dr. and Mrs. John Truslow	
	Sold	1967

***

1947	Eight Surplus Army Barracks transformed into	
1948	Special Surgical Unit, Cafeteria, Print Shop,	
	General Stores, Business Offices, Laundry,	After
	Gardener's Shop, Emergency Room	1955

432

***

| 1950 | Storage Building No. 1 | |
| 1954 | Carpenter Shop | In use |

***

1951	Storage Building No. 2	
1954	General Stores/Surgical Research Annex	
1973	MBI's Hyperbaric Facility	In use

***

| 1953 | Gail Borden Laboratory Building | In use |

***

| 1954 | Rosa and Henry Ziegler Hospital | |
| 1969 | Department of Internal Medicine | 1979 |

***

[ALL OF THE FOLLOWING BUILDINGS ARE IN USE]

***

| 1954 | New John Sealy Hospital |
| 1954 | R. Waverley Smith Pavilion |

***

| 1955 | Bethel Hall, Brackenridge Hall, Clay Hall, Nolan Hall |
| 1956 | League Hall, Morgan Hall Vinsant Hall, Unit D |

***

| 1962 | Central Water Chilling Station |

***

| 1963 | Physical Plant/General Stores |

***

1964	Surgical Research Laboratories
1966	Integrated with new SBI
1980	Expanded and renovated

***

1964	[Sealy and Smith Professional Building]

***

1966	John W. McCullough Outpatient Clinic Building
1973	Integrated with Clinical Sciences Building
1983	Integrated with Ambulatory Care Center

***

1966	[Shriners Burns Institute]
1992	SBI moved to new building on Market Street
	Old building used for UTMB offices and labs
1969	Jennie Sealy Hospital

***

1969	Animal Care Center

***

1969	Alumni Field House
1980	Swimming pool added

***

1971	Libbie Moody Thompson Basic Science Building
1979	Extensive renovations

***

1972	Ave Maria Hall for School of Allied Health Sciences
1989	Renovated and renamed Administration Annex II

***

1972	Moody Medical Library

***

1973   Clinical Sciences Building   ·

***

1973   Administration Building

***

1973   Materials Management Warehouses

***

1974   Pharmacology Building
1983   Additional floors added
1985   Containment Laboratory added

***

1975   1700 Strand Building (former Customs House) deeded to UTMB

***

1976   North Addition, John Sealy Hospital
1978   South Addition (Towers), John Sealy Hospital

***

1977   Child Health Center

***

1978   Microbiology Building
1984   Ground floor enclosed

***

1979   Heliport

***

1979   Strand Street Parking Garage (Tenth and Strand)

***

1980   Open Gates (Sealy Mansion, Twenty-fifth and Broadway)
                Given to UTMB to become the George and Magnolia Willis Sealy
                Conference Center

***

| 1981 | Learning Center |
| 1987 | Named William C. Levin Hall |

***

| 1981 | Space leased in Shearn Moody Plaza |

***

| 1982 | Mary Moody Northen Pavilion |

***

| 1982 | Physical Plant Building |

***

| 1982 | Texas Department of Criminal Justice Housing |
| 1987 | Additional units |

***

| 1983 | Ambulatory Care Center |

***

| 1983 | Texas Department of Criminal Justice Hospital |

***

| 1985 | Physical Plant Construction Storage Facility |

***

| 1986 | School of Nursing/School of Allied Health Sciences Building |

***

| 1986 | Parking Garage (Twelfth and Texas Avenue) |

***

| 1986 | Parking Garage/Library Storage and Bindery (Tenth and Market Street) |

***

| 1987 | Maurice Ewing Hall |

***

1987   Construction Warehouse

***

1988   Parking Garage (University and Market)

***

1989   Pumping Station for Vehicle Maintenance Facility

***

1989   Rosenberg House acquired

***

1990   Runge House

***

1991   Medical Research Building

***

1991   Trauma Center/Emergency Room

Appendix O

Patient Care Statistics, John Sealy Hospital, 1891–1900

		INPATIENTS										OPERATIONS	
Year	Outpatients	Total	Med	Surg.	Ob-Gyn	Pedi	Cured	Improved	Deaths			Surg	Gyn
1891	600	1,039	533	412	94	NA	615	303	78			216	62
1892	610	1,078	NA	NA	NA	NA	NA	NA	NA			NA	NA
1893	1,217	1,057	491	462	104	NA	502	433	75			177	67
1894	1,831	1,061	500	431	130	NA	614	286	62			219	99
1895	2,247	1,080	526	409	145	NA	657	288	68			324	132
1896	2,734	1,073	460	393	156	64	676	273	76			366	163
1897	2,801	1,329	638	459	179	53	810	312	102			326	129
1898	3,560	1,326	603	484	192	47	865	260	110			376	124
1899	3,729	1,645	818	493	276	58	886	462	95			207	160
1900	3,216	1,738	842	568	241	87	1,080	313	148			381	120
Totals:	22,545	12,426	5,411	4,111	1,517	309	6,705	2,930	814			2,592	1,056

NOTE: Most of the totals came from reports in the annual catalogs of the Medical Department. However, these reports are confusing. Data for 1891 are included in a preliminary catalog issued in 1893 and data for 1893 are included in a later catalog for the 1893–1894 year. Two catalogs (1894–1895 and 1895–1896) state that 1894 data are presented, but the data are different. The 1896–1897 catalog states that 1895 data are included. Subsequent catalogs stipulate that data of the first year are included, 1897 data in the 1897–1898 catalog, 1898 data in the 1898–1899 catalog, etc. The only other extant sources of comparable information are three articles in the *Galveston Daily News*, Mar. 1, 1894 (a report for 1893–1894), May 10, 1899 (a report for 1898–1899), and Aug. 30, 1901 (a ten-year summary). Because of the confusing reports and unexplained differences in the totals, these data must be viewed as approximate. Medical inpatients include those with neuropsychiatric and skin diseases. Surgical inpatients include those with eye, ear, nose, and throat diseases. NA means not available from cited sources.

Appendix P

The Fate of New Matriculates, 1891–1900

School of Medicine

Year	1st Yr. Mat.		2nd Yr. Mat.		Total Mat.		Total Grad.		% Grad.		
	M	F	M	F	M	F	M	F	M	F	T
1891	14/7	0	5/2	0	22	0	12	0	55	0	55
1892	14/4	0	2/2	0	16	0	6	0	38	0	38
1893	98/37	0	2/1	0	100	0	38	0	38	0	38
1894	81/35	2/1	0	0	81	2	35	1	43	50	43
1895	102/36	7/2	1/0	0	103	7	36	2	35	29	35
1896	125/47	0	4/2	0	129	0	49	0	38	0	38
1897	53/5	2/0	5/5	0	58	2	10	0	17	0	17
1898	51/12	2/0	3/2	1/1	54	3	14	1	26	33	26
1899	86/35	3/1	1/1	0	87	3	36	1	41	33	41
1900	53/21	1/1	2/2	0	55	1	23	1	42	100	43
Total	677/239	17/5	25/17	1/1	705	18	259	6	37	33	37

School of Pharmacy

Year	1st Yr. Mat.		2nd Yr. Mat.		Total Mat.		Total Grad.		% Grad.		
	M	F	M	F	M	F	M	F	M	F	T
1893	11/2	0	0	0	11	0	2	0	18	0	18
1894	26/7	0	3/2	0	29	0	9	0	31	0	31
1895	20/8	4/4	2/2	0	22	4	10	4	45	100	54
1896	23/8	0	0	0	23	0	8	0	35	0	35
1897	32/8	0	1/1	0	33	0	9	0	27	0	27
1898	24/12	2/1	0	0	24	2	12	1	50	50	50
1899	32/13	2/1	0	0	32	2	13	1	41	50	41
1900	34/13	0	0	0	34	0	13	0	38	0	38
Total	202/71	8/6	6/5	0	208	8	76	6	37	75	38

School of Nursing

Year	1st Yr. Mat.		2nd Yr. Mat.		Total Mat.		Total Grad.		% Grad.		
	M	F	M	F	M	F	M	F	M	F	T
1896	0	11/9	0	7/7	0	18	0	16	0	89	89
1897	0	12/12	0	0	0	12	0	12	0	100	100
1898	0	6/5	0	0	0	6	0	5	0	83	83
1899	0	12/12	0	0	0	12	0	12	0	100	100
1900	0	9/9	0	0	0	9	0	9	0	100	100
Total	0	50/47	0	7/7	0	57	0	54	0	95	95

NOTE: Data for the School of Nursing and the School of Pharmacy were taken from the annual catalogs. Data for the School of Medicine were obtained by correlating specific names included in the annual catalogs with those in the unpublished register of Matriculates and Graduates, 1891–1938 (Blocker Collections). Because first names like Shirley can be male or female, readers should view these figures as highly probable but not error-free. These figures are much closer to the truth than those provided in the annual reports of the UT Board of Regents. In the first column, the figure to the left of the slash represents the number of male students admitted to the first-year class for that academic year; the number to the right is the number of those matriculates who eventually graduated. This same format is used for the next columns, which show female students initially admitted to the first-year classes and males and females intitially admitted to the second-year classes. The total number of medical school matriculates in the first academic year includes three men initially admitted as third-year students (all three graduated). For the remainder of the decade, no other medical students were admitted initially to either the third-year classes or the fourth-year classes. In the next columns, totals are given for matriculates and graduates. The last column is the percentage of matriculates actually graduating. These figures do not represent total enrollment in a given year. Those totals depended on the number of those promoted, those repeating, and those admitted for the first time.

Appendix Q

Medical Faculty Who Served on the Committees on Instruction for the School of Nursing, 1896–1939

1896–97	H. A. West
	Allen J. Smith
1897–98	J. W. McLaughlin
	Allen J. Smith
1898–99	H. P. Cooke
	J. W. McLaughlin
1899–1900	H. P. Cooke
	J. W. McLaughlin
1900–03	J. W. McLaughlin
	J. E. Thompson
1903–05	W. Keiller
	J. W. McLaughlin
1905–06	M. L. Graves
	J. F. Y. Paine
1906–07	J. F. Y. Paine
	J. E. Thompson
1907–08	M. L. Graves
	J. E. Thompson
1908–23	M. L. Graves
	J. E. Thompson
1923–24	M. L. Graves
	A. O. Singleton
1924–25	W. R. Cooke
	J. Kopecky
1925–29	W. R. Cooke
	J. Kopecky
1929–30	W. R. Cooke
	R. J. Reitzel
1930–31	M. Bodansky
	W. R. Cooke
	T. H. Harris

1931–32	M. Bodansky
	W. R. Cooke
1932–34	W. R. Cooke
	W. B. Reading
1934–38	W. R. Cooke
	W. T. Dawson
	W. B. Reading
1938–39	W. T. Dawson
	J. L. Jinkins
	W. B. Reading
	D. P. Wall

```
                    ┌─────────────────────┐
                    │ EXECUTIVE DIRECTOR  │
                    └─────────────────────┘
```

Librarian	Dean Students & Curriculum	Dean Faculty of Medicine	Associate Dean Grad. Studies

Book Binding
Cataloging
Exchanges
Periodicals
Reading Room
Reference Service
Stacks

Admissions
Alumni Relations
Announcements &
Catalogs
A-V Aids
Class Schedules
Collegiate Relations
Degrees Certificates
& Records
Scholarships &
Loans
Student Activities
Student Health

Anatomy
Anesthesiology
Bacteriology &
Parasitology
Biochemistry &
Nutrition
Dermatology
Internal Med.
Neurology &
Psychiatry
Ob-Gyn
Ophthalmology
ENT
Pathology
Pediatrics
Pharmacology
Physiology
PM&PH
Radiology
Surgery
Co-ordinated Cancer
Training Program
Mental Health
Training Program
Post-Graduate
Training

Graduate Studies

Organized Research

Grants & Contracts
Interdepartmental
Research
Special Research
Laboratories

Saving Lives, Training Caregivers, Making Discoveries

```
                    ┌─────────────────────────┐
                    │   EXECUTIVE DIRECTOR    │
                    └─────────────────────────┘
```

Dean School of Nursing	Director Medical Services Curricula	Medical Administrator of Hospitals	Business Manager
Affiliate Nurse Prog.	Clinical Lab.	Admissions	<u>Bus. Office</u>
Degree Course	Technology	Clinics	Accounting
Diploma Course	Clinical Psychology	Med. Records	Financial &
Graduate Nurse	Medical Case Work	Medical Case	Statistical Reports
Prog.	Med. Records	Service	Payroll
Nursing Education	Librarians	Nursing Serv.	Personnel
& Admin.	Occupational	Operating Rooms	Purchasing &
Vocational	Therapy	Wards & Services	Receiving
Curriculum	Physical Therapy	Dietary Serv.	Vouchering
	Radiation	Housekeeping	
	Technology	Laundry	<u>Gen. Serv.</u>
	Extension	Interns & Residents	Animal Hosp.
	Preceptor Program	Hospital Admin.	Auxiliary
			Enterprises
		Professional	Gen. Stores
		Division	Mail & Tele.
		Anesthesia &	Med. Illus. &
		Resuscitation	Photo.
		Blood Bank	Print Shop
		Clinical Lab.	Tech. Appar. Shop
		Dental Serv.	Workers' Comp.
		Heart Station	
		Pharmacy	<u>Phys. Plant</u>
		Radiology Service	Grounds & Buildings
		Rehabilitation	Pest Control
			Police & Fire
			Shops & Maintenance
			Utilities

444

APPENDIX S

GENERAL ADMINISTRATIVE ORGANIZATION, UTMB, NOVEMBER 1984

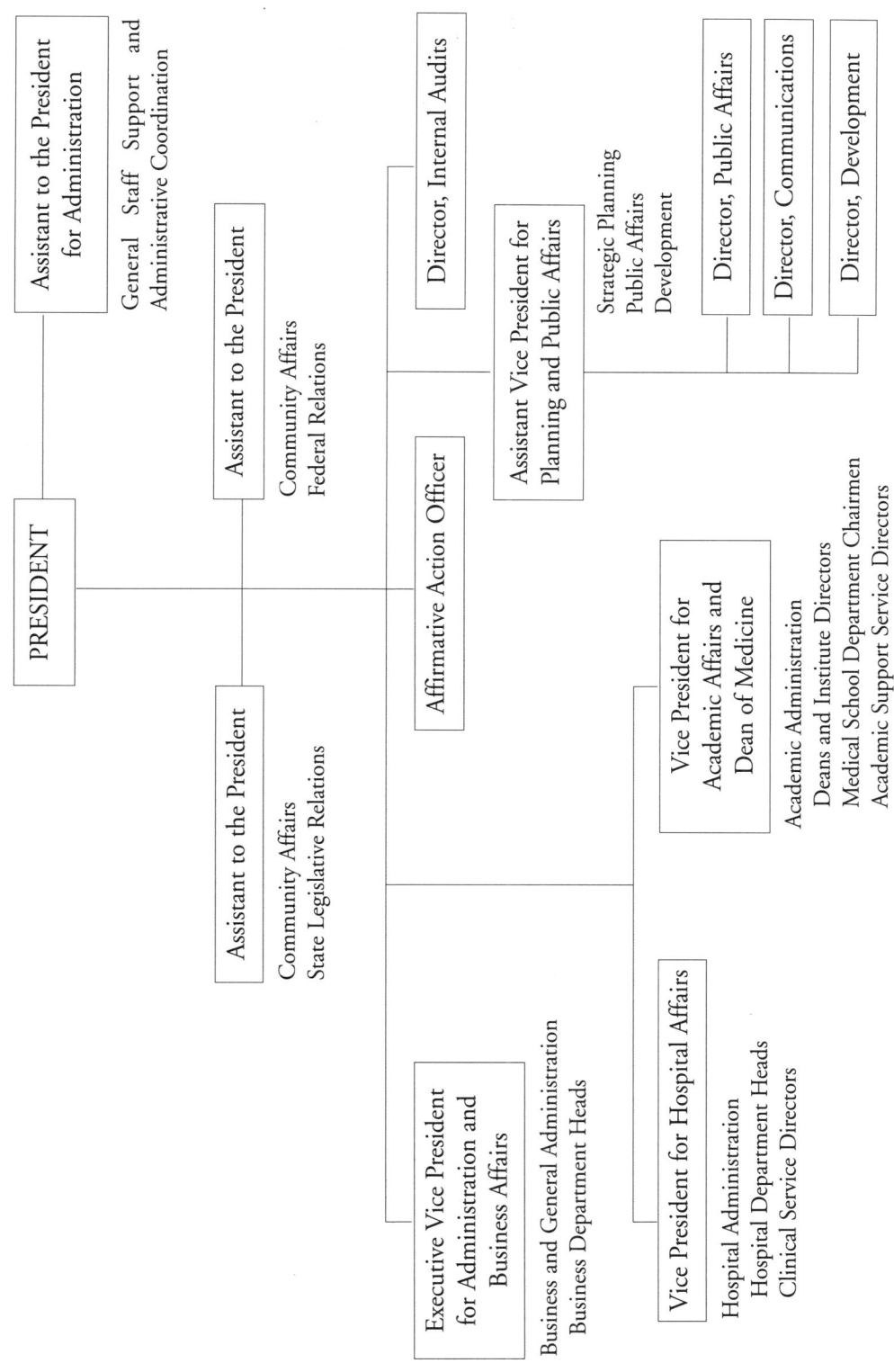

PRESIDENT

Assistant to the President for Administration

General Staff Support and Administrative Coordination

Assistant to the President

Community Affairs
Federal Relations

Assistant to the President

Community Affairs
State Legislative Relations

Director, Internal Audits

Affirmative Action Officer

Assistant Vice President for Planning and Public Affairs

Strategic Planning
Public Affairs
Development

Director, Public Affairs

Director, Communications

Director, Development

Vice President for Academic Affairs and Dean of Medicine

Academic Administration
Deans and Institute Directors
Medical School Department Chairmen
Academic Support Service Directors

Executive Vice President for Administration and Business Affairs

Business and General Administration
Business Department Heads

Vice President for Hospital Affairs

Hospital Administration
Hospital Department Heads
Clinical Service Directors

Appendix T

Directors of the Sealy & Smith Foundation for the John Sealy Hospital, 1922–1991

1922–26	John Sealy II
1922–38	Jennie Sealy Smith
1922–30	R. Waverley Smith
1922–32	Charles S. Peek
1922–44	Edward Randall Sr.
1922–30	Edward O. Cone
1922–57	Fred W. Catterall
1922–32	Mart H. Royston
1930–47	Ballinger Mills
1930–36	J. W. Terry
1932–44	George Sealy Jr.
1936–86	John W. McCullough
1938–85	John W. Harris
1944–71	Edward Randall Jr.
1945–51	Leland S. Dennis
1947–	Ballinger Mills Jr.
1949–57	William M. Morgan
1952–77	V. W. McLeod
1957–70	Alvin N. Kelso
1958–87	Homer F. Sanderford
1970–90	Preston Shirley
1972–80	Bryan F. Williams Jr.
1977–	Charles A. Worthen
1980–	George Sealy III
1985–	John W. Kelso
1986–	Joe C. Blackshear
1987–	J. Fellman Seinsheimer III
1991–	John Eckel

Appendix U
Budgets, John Sealy Hospital, 1901–1940

FISCAL YEAR	INCOME			EXPENSES
	CITY DOLLARS	PAY PATIENTS	SEALY/ S&S FOUN./ OTHERS	TOTAL
1901	$16,316	$3,697	NA	$23,410
1902	20,785	4,012	NA	24,797
1903	24,631	5,659	NA	30,289
1904	23,878	8,170	NA	32,048
1905	22,413	11,108	NA	33,520
1906	21,188	11,812	NA	39,612
1907	25,959	13,005	NA	38,964
1908	29,262	14,578	NA	43,840
1909	29,386	13,682	NA	43,068
1910	30,788	11,955	NA	42,743
1911	29,364	15,954	NA	45,318
1912	32,009	17,276	NA	49,286
1913	32,504	19,316	NA	51,820
1914	39,261	24,766	NA	64,026
1915	45,310	29,587	NA	74,896
1916	47,302	34,477	NA	81,779
1917	39,975	56,085	$18,290	114,350
1918	39,993	80,015	25,547	145,555
1919	27,335	95,920	21,455	144,710
1920	30,000	128,637	16,385	175,022
1921	29,989	177,432	23,091	230,512
1922	34,995	→ $158,686 ←		193,681
1923	34,999	→ 169,245 ←		204,244
1924	35,000	→ 165,982 ←		200,982
1925	39,000	→ 176,619 ←		215,619
1926	39,000	142,361	36,442	217,803
1927	39,000	123,058	50,569	212,627
1928	40,000	105,570	101,199	246,769
1929	40,000	141,453	101,190	282,643
1930	40,000	131,118	90,253	261,371
1931	NA	NA	119,690	NA
1932	40,000	122,879	125,191	288,070

447

FISCAL YEAR	INCOME			EXPENSES
	CITY DOLLARS	PAY PATIENTS	SEALY/ S&S FOUN./ OTHERS	TOTAL
1933	NA	NA	$90,028	NA
1934	NA	NA	87,117	NA
1935	$40,000	$116,820	97,642	$254,462
1936	40,000	183,955	76,375	300,330
1937	45,000	233,568	84,214	362,782
1938	46,411	251,428	107,007	404,846
1939	41,255	294,741	112,654	448,650
1940	NA	NA	120,964	NA

NOTE: The data are from an untitled two-page typescript in box 4Q18, UT President's Records; *Galveston Daily News*, Aug. 30, 1902; May 26, 1920; and Aug. 1,1921; extant published budgets of the city of Galveston for some of the years; and the annual financial reports of the Sealy & Smith Foundation. In comparing these sources there are unexplained differences in some of the totals. The total costs for each year before 1916 were usually met by income from the city and paying patients. There are puzzles, though. In 1906, for example, the total costs were $6,000 higher than the sum of the income from the city and the patients. John Sealy II presumably absorbed this deficit. In 1910 the Advisory Board of Lady Managers of the John Sealy Hospital raised $3,000 for the hospital from the churches of Galveston (see Carter's Annual Report, May 2, 1910, box 4885, UT President's Records). However, that amount is not included in any reported totals and how it was incorporated into the operating expenses for that year is not known. Before 1922, operating deficits were met mostly by the Sealy family; after 1922, mostly by the Sealy & Smith Foundation plus the Hospital Aid Society and a few private donors. The extant published budgets of the city of Galveston list only John Sealy Hospital income. For the years 1922–1925, records do not indicate how much of the totals represented contributions by the foundation and how much came from paying patients. From 1926, the totals in the Pay Patients column were calculated by subtracting the contributions of the foundation and the city's contributions from the total expenses given in the city's published budgets. These Pay Patients totals included miscellaneous donations from other private sources, but these amounts are not known because the hospital's financial records are not extant. Therefore, the actual income from paying patients must be viewed as approximate. Five thousand dollars of the city's contribution for fiscal year 1937 were for furniture and equipment for the Negro Hospital. The figures for fiscal years 1938 and 1939 are taken from Lucius Wilson's annual report to the John Sealy Hospital Board of Managers dated August 22, 1939, box VF 9B, UT President's Records. Between 1901 and 1920, the city's fiscal year began on March 1 and ended on the last day of February. Between 1920 and 1941, the city's fiscal year began on July 1 and ended on June 30. Figures are rounded to the nearest dollar. NA means not available from cited sources.

Appendix V

Budgets, UTMB Schools, 1901–1940

FISCAL YEAR	INCOME				EXPENSES			
	State	St. Fee	Other	TOTAL	Salaries	M&O	Other	TOTAL
1901	$75,563	$5,145	$5	$80,713	$36,783	$25,812	$19,916	$82,511
1902	40,000	6,490	3,145	49,635	39,257	23,296	249	2,802
1903	40,000	6,225	13	46,238	40,178	8,264	200	48,642
1904	48,007	6,640	5,013	59,660	42,399	15,070	1,733	59,202
1905	48,007	7,289	415	55,711	42,984	10,236	2,300	55,520
1906	49,000	8,867	361	58,225	46,014	11,448	1,077	58,539
1907	49,000	7,556	250	56,806	46,206	9,858	210	56,274
1908	50,000	7,881	250	58,131	48,062	11,579	0	59,641
1909	50,000	9,204	250	59,454	50,112	8,603	240	58,955
1910	55,000	8,897	250	64,237	50,459	12,878	0	63,337
1911	55,000	6,638	250	61,888	50,642	11,903	240	62,785
1912	65,000	6,642	844	72,486	52,691	13,174	2,234	68,099
1913	67,000	7,586	15,912	90,498	56,802	13,286	20,440	90,528
1914	71,000	9,005	750	80,755	59,561	14,876	2,196	76,633
1915	70,000	8,382	794	79,176	62,356	13,847	2,244	78,447
1916	82,755	8,635	1,230	92,620	66,346	18,544	2,063	86,955
1917	75,205	10,315	1,183	86,703	70,462	22,144	1,626	94,232
1918	98,755	8,212	1,032	107,999	77,445	26,897	2,091	106,433
1919	98,755	6,203	2,255	107,213	89,212	23,899	3,221	116,332
1920	114,066	9,992	3,223	127,282	94,840	25,761	3,802	124,043
1921	136,316	11,253	3,020	150,588	112,583	35,180	4,483	152,246

FISCAL YEAR	INCOME				EXPENSES			
	State	St. Fee	Other	TOTAL	Salaries	M&O	Other	TOTAL
1922	$135,775	$14,072	$25,490	$175,337	$109,630	$36,594	$4,332	$150,558
1923	135,775	14,234	7,240	157,250	126,289	28,202	18,854	173,345
1924	157,883	13,178	6,300	177,361	133,881	25,594	14,278	173,753
1925	160,500	35,879	(2,903)	193,476	148,478	29,215	10,582	188,275
1926	202,375	34,397	5,893	242,665	170,968	33,254	25,979	230,201
1927	216,895	34,172	7,892	258,959	184,303	34,383	20,634	239,320
1928	237,506	12,422	744	250,672	179,072	50,674	24,125	253,871
1929	232,085	14,350	11,758	258,193	191,163	31,888	31,684	254,735
1930	250,260	16,504	604	267,368	206,049	41,419	18,670	266,618
1931	250,260	17,476	9,475	277,211	203,137	34,616	26,809	264,562
1932	238,580	16,950	10,845	266,375	207,810	29,482	22,815	260,107
1933	238,580	17,079	9,905	265,564	214,176	44,134	19,010	277,320
1934	172,662	25,597	12,518	210,777	161,654	33,274	15,917	210,845
1935	172,154	26,499	16,934	215,587	162,083	40,187	17,166	219,436
1936	207,500	26,798	11,675	245,973	196,518	32,532	18,186	247,236
1937	207,500	27,791	11,176	246,467	197,939	31,959	14,670	244,568
1938	264,175	27,608	9,247	301,030	225,639	32,116	17,161	274,916
1939	264,175	28,122	10,490	302,787	241,761	39,582	22,858	304,201
1940	408,909	28,978	8,664	446,551	272,555	126,576	28,085	427,216

NOTE: Data for this table were taken from appendices in the biennial reports published by the Board of Regents between 1900 and 1928, and from the Auditor's Reports published between 1928 and 1940. These bound reports are located in the office of the University of Texas Board of Regents, Ashbel Smith Hall, Austin, Texas. Other (income) included miscellaneous gifts and scholarships, rental fees for rooms at University Hall, and interest on bank deposits. For reasons unknown, UTMB transferred $10,894 to UT Austin in fiscal year 1925, resulting in a negative balance. Other (expenses) included equipment, furniture, supplies for University Hall, scholarship aid to students, and transfers to other funds. Expenses may exceed income because of a balance carried forward from previous years. Figures are rounded to the nearest dollar. This table does not include funds for construction of new buildings.

Appendix W

Income, Hospitals, 1941–1968

Fiscal Year	State	City	Sealy & Smith	Gifts & Grants	Patient Services	Other Services	Professional Fees	Total
1941	$123,171	$40,000	$115,055		$282,320			$560,546
1942	376,700	40,000	60,000	$95	274,371			751,166
1943	440,130	40,000	114,002	17,442	325,959			937,533
1944	405,213	40,000	74,478	103,047	362,769			985,507
1945	417,260	40,000	77,496	93,755	414,086			1,042,597
1946	644,691	40,000	101,261	32,564	536,634			1,355,150
1947	865,737	80,833	30,000	47,790	774,498			1,798,858
1948	961,075	75,000	129,802	29,104	902,544			2,097,525
1949	970,171	75,000	212,449	43,284	1,096,162			2,397,066
1950	1,771,322	81,250	86,304	37,746	1,141,119			3,117,740
1951	1,811,047	75,000	61,565	52,208	1,152,449			3,152,269
1952	52,136	75,000	70,268	42,256	1,312,752			1,552,412
1953	72,697	75,000	68,000	50,771	1,328,182			1,594,650
1954	2,857,551	75,000	65,201	39,226	1,588,362			4,625,340
1955	2,948,220	75,000	104,500	38,933	2,020,829			5,187,482
1956	2,371,754	75,000	76,125	50,434	2,721,196			5,294,509
1957	2,371,504	50,000	80,168	46,729	2,852,080	$17,373		5,417,854
1958	2,586,418	218,750	33,500	49,931	2,713,118	21,237	$99,903	5,722,857
1959	2,586,418	200,000	↑	374,956	3,047,223	12,020	95,170	6,315,787
1960	2,776,663	200,000	↑	102,121	3,155,073	12,572	110,841	6,357,270
1961	2,778,103	200,000	↑	85,769	3,559,876	14,032	141,381	6,779,161

Fiscal Year	State	City	Sealy & Smith	Gifts & Grants	Patient Services	Other Services	Professional Fees	Total
1962	$2,691,985	$200,000	↑	$83,298	$3,609,073	$14,767	$138,288	$6,737,411
1963	2,889,758	200,000	↑	89,456	4,904,961	11,572	120,535	8,216,282
1964	3,149,431	200,000	↑	209,017	5,866,492	7,413	183,452	9,615,805
1965	3,267,244	200,000	↑	263,934	6,402,935	5,340	228,608	10,368,061
1966	5,194,616	200,000	↑	279,432	7,435,914	7,206	293,319	13,410,487
1967	5,339,180	200,000	↑	145,504	8,263,172	13,169	101,221	14,062,246
1968	7,236,446	200,000	↑	236,786	6,857,462	16,055	121,583	14,668,332

NOTE: The State column refers to monies received by legislative appropriation or from other state agencies. All of the appropriations listed between fiscal years 1941 and 1951 were specifically earmarked for the hospitals. For fiscal years 1952 and 1953, legislative appropriations for schools and hospitals were included in those designated for the schools. Legislative appropriations for schools and hospitals were again separated between fiscal years 1954 and 1968. However, hospital appropriations do not include coverage of the indirect costs (electricity, water, etc.) that were shared between the hospitals and schools. Income to cover those costs were included in the appropriations for UTMB schools. During these years, modest funds were received from other state agencies for specific programs such as vocational rehabilitation or the care of crippled children. City refers to appropriations from the city government of Galveston for the care of indigent patients. The Sealy & Smith column does not include monies given for construction of buildings nor interest income from the endowed fund jointly held by the UT Board of Regents and the Sealy & Smith Foundation. The Gifts & Grants column includes this interest income and income from other private sources, although the hospitals did receive some federal income between fiscal years 1944 and 1947 for military training programs. Beginning in fiscal year 1959, the Annual Financial Reports do not report Sealy & Smith income separately from other Gifts & Grants. The Patient Services column includes all service charges for inpatient and outpatient care. The Other Services column is first used in fiscal year 1957 and includes revenue received from cot and equipment rental, fees for technical courses, telephone and telegraph services, and other miscellaneous services. After the Faculty Augmentation Plan was adopted in 1957, Professional Fees were listed separately.

Appendix X
Income, Schools, 1941–1968

Fiscal Year	State	Federal	Private	Student Fees	Sales/Services	Other	Total
1941	$305,000		$647	$49,805	$10,661	$622	$366,735
1942	644,781		1,396	49,300	8,707	824	705,008
1943	614,059	$21,044	2,848	46,966	9,627	1,612	696,156
1944	613,520	220,491	66,774	15,804	416	1,459	918,464
1945	628,512	192,573	36,012	9,070	459	3,014	869,640
1946	713,605	82,857	102,877	33,156	542	4,197	937,234
1947	821,835	207,186	111,057	45,681	61	23,269	1,209,088
1948	1,195,724	167,202	104,018	35,867	18,728	9,403	1,530,942
1949	1,258,293	185,032	74,185	42,718	93,341	14,286	1,667,855
1950	1,925,623	184,198	69,341	37,539	128,488	22,246	2,367,435
1951	1,655,500	218,496	146,469	45,373	229,322	15,695	2,310,855
1952	3,890,000	273,841	151,347	51,292	260,891	14,798	4,642,169
1953	4,599,750	261,854	165,056	67,332	273,717	19,766	5,387,475
1954	2,100,800	294,193	238,929	73,711	314,403	89,029	3,111,066
1955	2,178,490	331,685	338,571	81,920	465,734	507,489	3,966,889
1956	3,090,828	405,092	527,627	78,025	636,874	25,072	4,763,518
1957	2,955,228	533,573	625,446	80,777	691,691	20,477	4,907,192
1958	3,601,559	646,864	681,161	171,982	721,992	35,359	5,858,917
1959	3,533,633	904,069	780,382	199,801	671,053	47,224	6,136,162
1960	3,801,499	1,108,472	785,752	179,327	606,607	54,239	6,535,896
1961	3,754,664	1,345,279	812,212	174,399	613,277	62,232	6,762,063

Fiscal Year	State	Federal	Private	Student Fees	Sales/Services	Other	Total
1962	$4,136,586	$1,601,979	$975,567	$189,495	$517,580	$86,352	$7,507,559
1963	4,064,280	2,025,922	942,332	208,463	583,213	89,337	7,913,548
1964	4,598,937	2,475,196	1,131,119	215,865	516,292	121,477	9,058,859
1965	4,635,843	2,735,071	1,648,023	230,092	446,904	142,967	9,838,900
1966	3,787,608	2,839,675	1,801,897	241,413	431,947	100,434	9,202,975
1967	4,292,281	3,331,917	2,426,091	257,382	389,712	252,849	10,950,232
1968	5,306,316	5,123,816	3,051,989	250,895	407,722	333,054	14,473,792

NOTE: Not listed in this table were $12,850 received from the city of Galveston for bacteriological examinations between fiscal years 1946 and 1957. The State column includes appropriations earmarked for the "Educational Units" between fiscal years 1941 and 1951. In fiscal years 1952 and 1953, these figures also include legislatively appropriated monies for the hospitals. Appropriations for fiscal years 1954 through 1968 included dollars for the indirect costs shared between the hospitals and the schools. Also included in this column are state monies received for specific health programs or research activities. The Federal column includes revenues from both training and research grants and contracts from the U.S. Public Health Service, the Children's Bureau, Food and Drug Administration, Vocational Rehabilitation, Department of Defense, and National Aeronautic and Space Administration. The Private column includes gifts, grants, contracts, and endowments received from private sources (individuals, foundations, corporations) for research, health programs, scholarships, fellowships, endowed chairs, library expenses, and capital expenditures. Student Fees include registration, laboratory, and graduation fees. Most of the revenue listed under Sales/Services was derived from sales, rentals, and fees associated with teaching manuals, parking stickers, health services, dormitories and apartments, snack shops, hospitality shops, and the John Sealy Hospital Cafeteria. The Other column includes such items as microscope rentals, income from journals and publications, sale of assets, transfer of funds, interest on time deposits, room rentals, and vending machine commissions. The fiscal year 1955 total included a transfer of $500,000 from the Available University Fund to UTMB.

Appendix Y

Income, Hospitals, 1969–1991

Fiscal Year	State	Sealy & Smith	Gifts & Grants	Patient Services	Other Services	Professional Fees	Total
1969	$7,608,398	$45,942	$214,465	$9,376,067	$465,758	$3,474,682	$21,185,312
1970	9,554,996	35,548	125,362	13,573,326	536,225	3,428,718	27,254,175
1971	9,908,373	22,960	52,552	16,235,257	760,793	4,382,080	31,362,015
1972	11,511,375	34,866	161,790	17,002,598	928,667	4,506,937	34,146,233
1973	11,997,543	40,531	147,832	16,830,630	1,131,998	4,502,655	34,651,189
1974	16,025,630	48,757	207,006	18,705,367	1,092,918	5,064,265	40,936,937
1975	18,657,846	26,980	201,888	22,538,722	1,187,024	6,775,453	49,387,913
1976	24,653,304	42,418	151,059	26,747,340	1,366,122	7,667,958	60,628,201
1977	28,027,309	3,699,971	199,855	29,684,742	1,502,998	8,792,779	71,907,654
1978	31,761,083	1,437,843	203,459	33,765,878	2,047,393	8,997,020	78,212,676
1979	32,622,675	536,447	101,873	37,806,529	3,014,688	10,257,508	84,389,721
1980	40,290,955	1,085,861	379,948	41,502,643	89,020	11,903,999	95,252,426
1981	43,272,119	1,366,822	508,600	46,742,216	284,035	13,483,286	105,657,078
1982	60,509,349	2,533,496	468,943	58,463,716	333,857	15,523,247	137,832,508
1983	78,262,832	3,611,615	506,696	59,844,274	650,067	18,304,576	161,180,060
1984	74,485,634	3,627,532	298,447	60,431,507	471,327	17,728,915	157,043,362
1985	89,190,741	3,193,707	443,042	68,964,591	607,479	17,776,707	180,176,267
1986	87,724,437	2,512,324	327,360	71,330,191	1,004,650	22,134,081	185,033,043
1987	78,542,762	649,519	368,027	78,680,985	544,734	26,798,137	185,584,164

Fiscal Year	State	Sealy & Smith	Gifts & Grants	Patient Services	Other Services	Professional Fees	Total
1988	$69,671,667	$1,454,903	$322,045	$75,358,600	$444,517	$27,640,432	$174,892,164
1989	70,632,783	4,471,764	348,740	84,326,774	530,832	34,212,056	194,522,949
1990	80,252,851	6,750,100	747,455	101,459,809	500,684	50,761,312	240,472,210
1991	78,583,007	6,021,717	779,093	136,954,809	562,497	25,688,598	248,589,720

NOTE: The State column includes funds for inpatient, outpatient, and emergency services in the hospitals, and research and teaching programs such as the Educational Cancer Center, Interferon Research Program, and Chronic Home Dialysis Center. Though most of the income listed in the Sealy & Smith column was used for equipment, some was designated for the nurse recruitment program, repair and maintenance of buildings, and work-scholarship programs. Funds in the Gifts & Grants column include all private gifts and endowments specifically designated for hospital-based activities, except for those shown in the Sealy & Smith column. The Patient Services column includes dollars received for room charges, nursing services, and other hospital services from patients, private and federal insurance carriers, and city and county governments. Patient Services income in fiscal year 1991 includes $28,638,634 received as part of Medicaid's Disproportionate Share Programs. The Other Services column includes hospital-based programs not associated directly with patient care, such as barber shop services and telephone and telegraph services. The significant decrease in 1980 resulted from the discontinuation of contract service agreements with the Sealy & Smith Foundation after UTMB assumed full management of hospitals previously provided under contract with the foundation. Professional Fees means fees for physician services.

456

Appendix Z
Income, Schools, 1969–1991

Fiscal Year	State/Local	Federal	Cost Recovery	Private	Student Fees	Sales/Services	Other	Total
1969	$5,467,489	$4,539,822	$717,382	$668,678	$244,282	$570,785	$403,523	$12,611,961
1970	7,393,754	4,935,151	748,605	947,223	235,938	440,927	664,772	15,366,370
1971	7,938,833	5,427,313	734,837	1,507,909	264,303	324,119	659,167	16,856,481
1972	10,307,053	5,712,390	805,267	1,180,378	295,448	352,213	1,260,876	19,913,625
1973	11,761,773	6,955,064	1,037,303	1,529,194	348,160	419,251	1,011,655	23,062,400
1974	18,272,395	6,995,3344	1,128,008	1,994,828	393,605	462,927	1,300,440	30,547,537
1975	21,374,102	8,844,213	1,527,695	2,556,921	382,464	576,221	1,561,365	36,822,981
1976	30,337,176	8,235,903	1,719,068	2,979,576	474,677	1,131,074	1,229,541	46,107,015
1977	32,977,011	10,240,238	2,025,203	3,334,553	509,589	1,265,324	1,711,878	52,063,796
1978	42,742,793	9,465,233	2,050,705	2,862,358	533,855	1,343,506	1,888,450	60,886,900
1979	48,261,142	9,857,755	2,404,187	3,072,667	565,232	1,564,098	2,629,583	68,354,664
1980	62,584,016	10,887,109	2,558,993	3,429,512	609,793	1,847,949	2,846,112	84,763,484
1981	69,523,878	11,526,885	2,699,384	3,976,350	596,981	2,053,603	4,140,446	94,517,527
1982	96,375,645	10,805,026	2,566,347	4,106,287	604,248	2,484,314	5,520,779	122,462,646
1983	106,401,528	9,787,299	2,633,459	4,998,321	770,769	2,492,772	5,287,522	132,371,670
1984	110,529,466	10,828,963	2,908,566	4,778,293	795,885	2,773,246	8,093,855	140,708,274
1985	106,126,955	12,303,699	3,599,770	5,379,886	713,555	2,736,254	9,270,257	140,130,376
1986	102,895,139	14,081,231	4,367,436	6,158,401	1,814,023	3,243,331	7,992,737	140,552,298
1987	94,519,226	15,148,613	4,694,401	6,560,894	2,822,317	3,572,085	8,441,303	135,758,839
1988	124,907,314	17,089,038	5,727,196	7,615,291	3,818,676	5,819,776	11,345,819	176,323,110
1989	138,001,916	19,533,395	6,643,344	8,802,909	4,673,437	4,234,598	11,653,256	193,542,855
1990	134,737,526	19,391,537	6,342,802	9,225,817	5,240,765	4,614,251	13,545,367	193,098,065
1991	138,696,774	19,019,326	6,126,052	10,882,787	5,355,695	5,149,342	15,953,373	201,183,349

NOTE: The State/Local column includes legislative appropriations for educational activities, repair and maintenance of the Physical Plant, administrative and library services shared by schools and hospitals, and staff benefits for employees. This column also includes monies from state agencies for specific programs and funds for contracted or shared services with county health departments or county governments. The Federal column includes funds awarded by several agencies: Department of Health and Human Services, U.S. Public Health Service, Environmental Protection Agency, Department of Defense, National Science Foundation, National Aeronautics and Space Administration, National Research Foundation Aging, and National Endowment for the Humanities. Cost Recovery includes funds associated with federal and private grants and contracts that reimbursed the schools for indirect (overhead) costs. The Private column includes gifts, grants, contracts, and endowments received from private sources (individuals, foundations, corporations) for research, health programs, scholarships, fellowships, endowed chairs, library expenses, capital expenditures, and travel expenses for professional meetings. Student Fees include tuition, activity fees (e.g. student government), laboratory fees, break fines and forfeits, and graduation fees. The rapid increase after 1985 reflected a substantial increase in tuition for medical students (350 percent increase distributed over a few years). Sales/Services includes revenue derived from the operation of the Auxiliary Enterprises, including the John Sealy Hospital Cafeteria, dormitories and housing facilities, the Alumni Field House, parking facilities, television rentals, and student government projects. This category also includes income generated by affiliation agreements with other institutions, especially after 1976. The Other column includes funds from vending machine commissions, interests on time deposits and other investments, as well as miscellaneous fees, rentals, and charges.

Appendix AA

Patient Care Statistics, John Sealy and Other UTMB Hospitals, 1901–1912

Year	Outpatients New	Outpatients Old	Medical Total	Medical Gen	Medical NP	Medical Derm	Surgical Total	Surgical Gen	Surgical EENT	Ob/Gyn Total	Pedi Total	Grand Total	Total Deaths	Operations Surg	Operations Gyn
1901	2,042	NA	507	460	43	4	418	385	33	174	16	1,115	85	373	88
1902	1,368	NA	458	368	45	13	333	308	25	216	32	1,007	90	319	80
1903	1,494	NA	530	431	68	NA	434	381	53	264	31	1,228	127	264	218
1904	889	4,375	644	577	67	NA	541	449	92	286	NA	1,471	150	245	197
1905	1,063	4,142	544	497	46	NA	596	564	32	295	NA	1,435	119	273	174
1906	2,245	4,321	552	493	59	NA	635	612	23	306	NA	1,493	97	325	169
1907	2,985	5,353	746	673	73	NA	771	727	44	362	NA	1,879	157	380	187
1908	5,031	7,458	720	645	75	NA	749	719	30	335	NA	1,804	151	445	208
1909	5,414	7,102	553	465	88	NA	796	719	77	413	NA	1,762	139	437	238
1910	5,886	6,333	564	480	84	NA	792	693	99	423	NA	1,779	138	494	275
1911	6,627	9,440	725	633	92	NA	926	808	118	519	NA	2,170	169	614	301
1912	7,136	10,303	806	676	130	NA	870	754	116	605	NA	2,281	194	580	343
Totals:	42,180	58,827	7,349	6,398	870	17	7,861	7,119	742	4,198	79	19,424	1,616	4,749	2,478

NOTE: The data are taken from reports included in the annual catalogs of UTMB. The peculiarities of these reports determined the categories of this table. For example, the totals in the Medical and Surgical columns do not always equal the sums of the numbers in the other categories. NP means neuro-psychiatric. Derm means diseases of the skin. EENT means diseases of the eye, ear, nose, and throat. NA means not available from these reports.

APPENDIX AB

PATIENT CARE STATISTICS, JOHN SEALY AND OTHER UTMB HOSPITALS, 1913–1924

	OUTPATIENTS		INPATIENTS										OPERATIONS			
Year	New	Old	Med	NP	Derm	Surg	EENT	Gyn	Ob	Pedi	Total	Deaths	Surg	Gyn	EENT	Ob Del
1913	6,911	9,052	654	100	NA	780	103	NA	NA	NA	2,049	166	613	564	100	NA
1914	7,438	9,234	842	110	NA	812	79	332	135	155	2,465	197	559	237	112	114
1915	7,048	8,841	1,030	101	NA	1,028	49	333	205	200	3,085	264	525	312	109	139
1916	6,849	8,939	1,002	118	NA	1,045	161	437	206	200	3,621	232	638	458	163	133
1917	6,065	12,018	959	144	NA	1,102	311	424	236	114	3,877	268	915	447	245	136
1918	4,870	11,065	1,404	112	NA	1,048	328	402	266	173	4,961	320	717	365	202	157
1919	5,240	11,861	798	155	NA	995	392	406	158	106	3,963	221	952	357	369	105
1920	4,331	11,416	814	189	NA	1,146	381	387	178	112	4,148	243	1,018	367	395	137
1921	6,371	19,163	700	215	63	1,138	412	422	217	158	4,171	226	1,054	390	432	150
1922	5,042	19,550	759	269	20	1,066	250	415	216	147	3,871	225	953	424	242	153
1923	5,434	21,316	677	257	16	985	234	451	238	161	3,812	236	906	442	248	188
1924	6,734	23,909	783	253	51	1,134	331	542	253	272	4,539	276	1,141	478	339	221
Totals:	72,393	166,364	10,422	2,023	150	12,279	3,031	4,551	2,308	1,798	44,562	2,874	9,991	4,841	2,956	1,633

NOTE: The data are taken from reports included in the annual catalogs of UTMB. The peculiarities of these reports determined the categories of this table. Ob Del means obstetrical deliveries. NA means not available from these reports.

APPENDIX AC

PATIENT CARE STATISTICS, JOHN SEALY AND OTHER UTMB HOSPITALS, 1925–1938

Year	OUTPATIENTS		INPATIENTS										OPERATIONS			
	New	Old	Med	NP	Derm	Surg	EENT	Gyn	Ob	Pedi	Total	Deaths	Surg	Gyn	EENT	Ob Del
1925	6,799	26,048	842	269	57	1,316	366	580	322	371	4,982	294	1,074	498	353	268
1926	5,767	26,508	1,132	219	39	1,336	287	604	356	226	5,219	319	992	509	265	298
1927	6,265	31,583	982	142	36	1,362	338	556	474	216	5,168	295	1,042	547	313	369
1928	5,359	34,031	977	220	38	1,288	366	547	444	342	5,305	325	1,136	493	372	367
1929	4,317	36,090	840	263	37	1,405	356	516	421	277	5,442	343	1,312	433	387	415
1930	8,692	45,830	938	230	21	1,486	303	579	655	382	5,675	358	1,325	543	347	444
1931	11,434	50,472	964	237	31	1,551	269	570	660	375	5,452	310	1,317	549	265	487
1932	12,904	58,327	1,108	213	42	1,458	293	534	686	395	5,242	311	1,122	521	283	507
1933	12,210	61,462	1,077	279	38	1,733	321	649	691	416	5,744	325	1,300	586	302	536
1934	11,215	60,281	1,177	400	25	1,751	284	587	637	420	5,817	366	1,298	531	283	532
1935	11,055	57,303	1,230	429	24	1,878	250	546	668	371	5,915	385	1,569	482	241	511
1936	10,688	55,998	1,228	578	41	1,771	323	532	636	316	5,938	372	1,518	496	298	508
1937	11,587	61,818	1,167	595	28	1,198	341	597	746	328	6,377	355	940	463	315	615
1938	12,595	75,122	1,109	737	52	1,300	342	533	689	367	6,644	331	1,006	477	326	610
Totals:	130,887	680,873	14,771	4,811	509	20,833	4,439	7,930	8,085	4,802	78,920	4,689	16,951	7,128	4,350	6,467

NOTE: Most of the data are taken from reports included in UTMB's annual catalogs. Data from 1938–1939 are taken from Lucius Wilson's annual report, which is in box VF 9/B, UT President's Records. In the 1929 report, the time designated by the cited year changed from a calendar-year to a July 1–July 1 pattern. Thus, 1928 and the preceding years signified twelve calendar months. The year 1929 signifed July 1, 1929, to July 1, 1930. This new pattern was followed during subsequent years.

Appendix AD

Total Collections, Patient Services Revenue, Fiscal Years 1982–1991

Fiscal Year	Medicare	Medicaid	Blue Cross	Commerical-Insurance	Private Patient	Other	Total
1982	$22,562,856	$5,447,750	$6,650,281	$16,119,522	$2,231,676	$2,919,635	$55,931,720
1983	21,045,930	5,613,013	5,096,478	20,207,995	2,324,408	3,104,949	57,392,773
1984	21,550,228	6,120,958	3,843,392	24,378,618	2,395,157	3,602,020	61,890,373
1985	25,841,332	5,509,252	3,383,108	26,182,317	2,567,418	3,376,423	66,859,850
1986	28,543,433	8,730,682	3,431,179	24,948,864	2,557,400	2,827,349	71,038,907
1987	28,104,272	10,254,888	3,503,367	29,272,061	2,436,116	3,766,313	77,337,017
1988	24,685,294	13,811,115	2,480,499	27,433,829	2,541,021	3,493,678	74,445,436
1989	26,353,033	17,706,038	2,458,846	25,745,110	2,734,922	5,045,357	80,043,306
1990	34,802,158	25,811,451	2,270,697	28,311,947	2,743,301	6,240,092	100,179,646
1991	29,838,310	37,355,425	2,726,873	27,375,564	2,485,577	6,247,957	106,029,706
Total:	263,326,846	136,360,572	35,844,720	249,975,827	25,016,996	40,623,773	751,148,734

Appendix AE

Major Educational Programs in Nursing, 1890–1991

1890–1960	Diploma program (no degree). Changed from two-year to three-year program in 1907. No students in 1948. Last students admitted in 1957.
1923–40	Bachelor of Science in Nursing degree. First graduate, 1933; last in 1940.
1937–61	Bachelor of Science in Nursing Education degree program for diploma graduates. Began in School of Education at UT Austin. Administrative control transferred to Galveston in 1945.
1944–71	Bachelor of Science in Nursing degree. First graduates in 1947.
1949–68	Bachelor of Science in Nursing for diploma graduates.
1952–67	Master of Science in Nursing program with degrees granted by the UT Graduate School at Austin.
1967–76	UT System-wide Graduate Nursing School at Austin with master's degree (1967) and doctoral degree (1974) programs.
1972–76	Integrated Bachelor of Science in Nursing degree program for all campuses in the system-wide school.
1976–	The UT School of Nursing at Galveston reassumes degree-granting authority for bachelor's degree program.
1977–	Flexible Option program begins for registered nurses who want to earn a bachelor's degree.
1977–79	The UT School of Nursing at Galveston reassumes degree-granting authority for master's degree program.
1979–	The master's degree program now authorized via the UT Graduate School of the Biomedical Sciences at Galveston.

Appendix AF

School of Allied Health Sciences Degree and Certificate Programs, 1991

Graduate Level

Program: Graduate Studies

Basic Entrance Requirements: Baccalaureate degree with overall 3.0 GPA; appropriate score on Graduate Record Examination

Length of Program: 1.5–2.5 years

Beginning Term: Fall, Spring, or Summer

Applications Accepted: September 1–August 1

Type of Diploma/Certificate: M.S. and Certificate in either Health Education or Clinical Gerontology

Baccalaureate Level

Program: Health Information Management (formerly Medical Record Administration (Baccalaureate)

Basic Entrance Requirements: 60 hours of prescribed college coursework; overall 2.0 GPA with minimum GPA of 2.0 in English language, statistics, and computer sciences; competitive admissions

Length of Program: 2 years

Beginning Term: Fall

Applications Accepted: September 1–July 1

Type of Diploma/Certificate: B.S. in Health Information Management

Program: Health Information Management (Baccalaureate—Accredited Record Technician Progression)

Basic Entrance Requirements: Same as baccalaureate program listed above plus certification as an A.R.T.

Length of Program: 2 years

Beginning Term: Fall, Spring, or Summer

Applications Accepted: September 1–July 1

Type of Diploma/Certificate: B.S. in Health Information Management

Program: Health Information Management (Postbaccalaureate)

Basic Entrance Requirements: Same as baccalaureate program listed above plus a baccalaureate degree in a related field.

Length of Program: 1 year

Beginning Term: Fall

Applications Accepted: September 1–July 1

Type of Diploma/Certificate: B.S. in Health Information Management

Programs: Health Care Administration, Long Term Health Care Administration, Substance Abuse Counseling and Therapy Program Administration, and Radiologic Health Services Administration

Basic Entrance Requirements: 60 hours of prescribed college coursework; overall 2.5 GPA; competitive admissions

Length of Program: 2 years

Beginning Term: Fall, Spring, or Summer

Applications Accepted: 2 weeks prior to matriculation

Type of Diploma/Certificate: B.S. in Health Care Sciences and Certificate in Health Care Administration, Long Term Health Care Administration; Substance Abuse Counseling and Therapy Program Administration; or Radiologic Health Services Administration

Program: Medical Technology

Basic Entrance Requirments: 60 hours of prescribed college coursework; overall 2.0 GPA with a minimum 2.0 GPA in science courses

Length of Program: 24 months

Beginning Term: Second Summer Term

Applications Accepted: Open

Type of Diploma/Certificate: B.S. in Medical Technology

Program: Medical Technology

Basic Entrance Requirments: 79 hours of prescribed college coursework; overall 2.5 GPA with a minimum 2.5 GPA in science courses

Length of Program: 18 months

Beginning Term: Second Summer Term

Applications Accepted: Open

Type of Diploma/Certificate: B.S. in Medical Technology

Program: Occupational Therapy

Basic Entrance Requirements: 60 hours of prescribed college coursework; overall 2.5 GPA with a minimum 2.0 GPA in biological sciences

Length of Program: 26 months

Beginning Term: Second Summer Term

Applications Accepted: August 1–January 1 of year proceeding matriculation

Type of Diploma/Certificate: B.S. in Occupational Therapy

Program: Physical Therapy

Basic Entrance Requirements: 65 hours of prescribed college coursework; overall 2.8 GPA with a minimum 2.0 ("C") in each course and 2.8 or above in science and mathematics. 150 clock hours of paid or volunteer work in physical therapy

Length of Program: 2 years

Beginning Term: Fall

Applications Accepted: September 1–January 1 of year preceeding matriculation

Type of Diploma/Certificate: B.S. in Physical Therapy

Program: Physician's Assistant Studies

Basic Entrance Requirements: 60 hours of prescribed college coursework; overall 2.5 GPA on all previous coursework

Length of Program: 2 years

Beginning Term: Second Summer Term

Applications Accepted: May 1–January 15

Type of Diploma/Certificate: B.S. in Physician's Assistant Studies and Certificate as Assistant to the Primary Care Physician

CERTIFICATE/ASSOCIATE LEVEL

Programs: Radiographic Technology, Radiation Therapy Technology, and Nuclear Medicine Technology

Basic Entrance Requirements (Cooperative Program with Galveston College): Liberal arts courses completed at Galveston College or other college. Professional courses completed at University of Texas Medical Branch.

Length of Program: 2 years

Beginning Term: Fall

Applications Accepted: Early application encouraged. No later than two weeks prior to matriculation. Limited space.

Type of Diploma/Certificate: Certificate of Completion from School of Allied Health Sciences at Galveston and Associate in Applied Science Degree from Galveston College

Program: Respiratory Care

Basic Entrance Requirements (Cooperative Program with Galveston College): Liberal arts courses completed at Galveston College or other college. Professional courses completed at University of Texas Medical Branch.

Length of Program: Self-paced (2 year equivalent)

Beginning Term: Enrollment may occur at any time

Applications Accepted: Open

Type of Diploma/Certificate: Certificate of Completion from School of Allied Health Sciences at Galveston and Associate in Applied Science Degree from Galveston College

Programs: Computerized Tomography Technology, Magnetic Resonance Imaging Technology, and Radiation Therapy Dosimetry Technology

Basic Entrace Requirements: Graduate of an accredited radiologic health science program with a 2.5 GPA and certified, or licensed for same

Length of Program: 1 semester

Beginning Term: Fall and Spring

Applications Accepted: June 1–Fall, October 1–Spring

Type of Diploma/Certificate: Advanced Certificates from School of Allied Health Sciences at Galveston and Galveston College

Program: Special Procedure Technology

Basic Entrace Requirements: Graduate of an accredited radiologic health science program with a 2.5 GPA and certified, or licensed for same; competitive admissions

Length of Program: 2 semesters

Beginning Term: Fall and Spring

Applications Accepted: June 1–Fall, October 1–Spring

Type of Diploma/Certificate: Advanced Certificates from School of Allied Health Sciences at Galveston and Galveston College

APPENDIX AG

GRANTS FOR RESEARCH AND TRAINING BY SOURCE, 1976–1990

Fiscal Year	Project Grants		Training Grants		Fellowships		Career		Other		Total
	Federal	Non-Federal	Federal	Non-Federal	Federal	Non-Federal	Federal	Non-Federal	Federal	Non-Federal	
1976	$6,627,034	1,467,822	670,699	135,400		88,992		45,500		864,765	$9,900,212
1977	6,819,126	1,536,330	718,179	54,350		215,000		138,283		741,390	10,222,658
1978	7,433,618	1,339,510	613,736	48,496		300,425		182,940		838,512	10,757,237
1979	9,728,248	1,651,510	607,681	28,720		345,385		240,990		796,278	13,398,812
1980	11,544,124	1,892,697	682,096	88,338		400,281		157,655		1,104,695	15,869,886
1981	10,324,464	2,514,342	720,508	45,000		452,015		273,139		1,276,241	15,605,709
1982	9,908,087	3,059,162	617,470	97,000		313,505		325,432		768,274	15,088,930
1983	11,162,923	2,763,025	394,953	52,000	129,800	73,197	291,042	38,010	713,514	604,174	16,222,638
1984	12,363,737	2,563,241	428,522	69,000	176,378	312,504	328,408	0	770,896	71,394	17,084,080
1985	13,934,995	5,412,190	193,116	88,000	148,436	495,916	534,459	0	726,403	36,733	21,570,248
1986	16,859,444	5,027,694	156,043	66,000	80,617	410,544	484,728	29,000	861,809	1,050,555	25,026,434
1987	19,689,409	5,867,872	308,810	78,315	112,423	322,823	674,381	151,820	262,912	36,975	27,505,740
1988	22,144,038	9,948,719	421,371	137,700	36,996	387,242	607,728	151,820	243,048	127,842	34,206,504
1989	24,786,077	10,504,202	535,849	72,700	662,056	587,913	431,897	109,540	214,767	304,528	38,209,529
1990	22,908,357	12,177,814	1,082,424	272,909	717,967	467,431	648,056	72,795	589,087	106,255	39,043,095

NOTE: These totals were taken from the annual reports prepared by the Office of Sponsored Programs–Academic entitled "Awards for Support of Research and Research Training." A set of these reports is in the office of the assistant vice president for research. Because of a change in the format for these reports, comparable data are not available for fiscal year 1991.

Appendix AH

Grants for Research and Research Training by Department, School, or Institute, Fiscal Years 1967–1991

SOM: Human Biological Chemistry and Genetics	48,405,338
SOM: Surgery	42,667,811
SOM: Internal Medicine	40,346,523
SOM: Physiology and Biophysics	36,479,641
SOM: Microbiology and Immunology	26,639,402
SOM: Pediatrics	23,192,690
SOM: Preventive Medicine and Community Health	15,897,315
SOM: Pharmacology and Toxicology	14,728,732
SOM: Psychiatry and Behavioral Sciences	11,923,171
SOM: Pathology	10,094,091
SOM: Anesthesiology	8,789,745
SOM: Otolaryngology	7,166,712
SOM: Obstetrics and Gynecology	6,306,439
SOM: Radiation Therapy	5,185,186
SOM: Anatomy and Neurosciences	4,778,650
SOM: Neurology	3,642,497
SOM: Dermatology	2,203,892
SOM: Ophthalmology	1,529,182
SOM: Family Medicine	954,894
SOM: Radiology	917,823
Administration	41,135,240
School of Nursing	4,307,228
School of Allied Health Sciences	6,006,973
Marine Biomedical Institute	37,842,424
Institute for the Medical Humanities	2,558,425
Office of Educational Development	179,289
Cancer Center	343,210
Clinical Research Center	1,140,459
Grand Total, UTMB	$405,362,982

NOTE: Department totals for fiscal years 1972–1974 were taken from the Minutes, UT Board of Regents. Totals for the other years (except fiscal year 1991) were taken from the annual report prepared by the Office of Sponsored Programs–Academic entitled "Awards for Support of Research and Research Training." The totals for fiscal year 1991 were provided by the office of the assistant vice president for research.

Notes

INTRODUCTION

1. Rupert Norval Richardson, Ernest Wallace, and Adrian N. Anderson, *Texas: The Lone Star State* (4th ed.; Englewood Cliffs, N.J.: Prentice-Hall, 1981), 181–183; Charles W. Hayes, *Galveston: History of the Island and the City* (2 vols.; Austin: Jenkins Garrett Press, 1974), I, 366; David McComb, *Galveston: A History* (Austin: University of Texas Press, 1986), 66. Also see Earl Wesley Fornell, *The Galveston Era: The Texas Crescent on the Eve of Secession* (Austin: University of Texas Press, 1961), and Kenneth W. Wheeler, *To Wear a City's Crown: The Beginnings of Urban Growth in Texas, 1836–1865* (Cambridge: Harvard University Press, 1968). "Public Sanitation," *Scientific American*, 39 (1878), 241 (quotation). Originating from the efforts of a sanitary committee established in December 1873 and authorized by a new charter for Galveston approved by the state legislature on August 2, 1876, Galvestonians had organized a board of health in March 1877. For details about the sanitary improvements initiated by this board, see Chester R. Burns and Heather G. Campbell, "Sanitizing Galveston: Politics, Policies, and Practices Before 1915," *Houston Review*, 19, no. 1 (1997), 5–26. The image of Galveston as a clean and healthy city was generally acknowledged. See Maggie Abercrombie, "Sketch of Galveston County," *American Sketch Book*, 6, no. 5 (1881). She thought that Galveston's sanitary laws were "the best on earth" (p. 332) and that Galveston was "one of the healthiest cities on the face of the globe" (p. 340).

2. For general features of Texas during these years, see Robert Calvert and Arnoldo De Leon, *The History of Texas* (Arlington Heights, Ill.: Harlan Davidson, Inc., 1990), 127–152; and Alwyn Barr, "Reconstruction," in Roy R. Barkley and Mark F. Odintz (eds.), *The Portable Handbook of Texas* (Austin: Texas State Historical Association, 2000), 51–63. Before 1881 Galveston was the only city in Texas with a medical college and doctors who edited medical journals. Other cities supported professional societies, hospitals, and boards of health or licensure. Short-lived societies appeared in Houston (1868) and Dallas (1870), with more enduring societies organized in Austin (1870) and San Antonio (1876). Private hospitals opened in Houston (1867), San Antonio (1869), and Austin (1873). A city hospital existed in Dallas (1872). In 1873 several counties organized boards of medical examiners. Boards of health appeared in Austin (1871), San Antonio (1873) and Dallas (1873). For details, see Walter H. Moursund Sr., "Medicine in Greater Houston 1836–1956," unpublished manuscript, Texas Medical Center archives (Houston Academy of Medicine Library, Houston), 36, 281; Marie Louise Giles, "The Early History of Medicine in Dallas, 1841–1900," (M.A. thesis, University of Texas, 1951), 86, 90, 97, 156; James M. Coleman, *Aesculapius on the Colorado* (Austin: Encino Press, 1971), 46, 49–51; and Pat Ireland Nixon, *A Century of Medicine in San Antonio* (San Antonio: Privately published, 1936), 98, 113, 164–166.

3. *Galveston Daily News*, Dec. 23, 1894. The number of steamers loading or unloading at Galveston increased from 177 in 1891 to 372 in 1898; see *Galveston Daily News*, Nov. 27, 1898.

4. Association of American Medical Colleges, *AAMC Directory of American Medical Education 1990–91* (Washington, D.C.: Association of American Medical Colleges, 1990). For the estimated total of sixteen thousand and a list of the most important schools, see John Shaw Billings, "Literature and Institutions," in Edward H. Clarke, Henry J. Bigelow, Samuel D. Gross, T. Gaillard Thomas, and J. S. Billings (eds.), *A Century of American Medicine, 1776–1876* (Brinklow, Md.: Old Hickory Book Shop, 1962), 355–359. For the names of physicians practicing in Texas before the Civil War, see Chester R. Burns, "Medicine in Texas: The Historical Literature," *Texas Medicine*, 82 (Jan., 1986), 61. At least seventeen Texans graduated from medical schools outside their home state before 1869; see *Galveston Medical Journal*, 4 (Aug., 1869), 353. See P. I. Nixon, "Greensville S. Dowell," in Walter Prescott Webb and H. Bailey Carroll (eds.), *The Handbook of Texas* (2 vols; Austin: Texas State Historical Association, 1952), I, 517, and Inci A. Bowman, "Greensville S. Dowell," in Ron Tyler, Douglas E. Barnett, Roy R. Barkley, Penelope C.

Anderson, and Mark F. Odintz (eds.), *The New Handbook of Texas* (6 vols.; Austin: Texas State Historical Association, 1996), II, 691–692.

5. Kenneth M. Ludmerer, *Learning to Heal: The Development of American Medical Education* (New York: Basic Books, 1985), 29–46; Thomas Neville Bonner, *American Doctors and German Universities* (Lincoln: University of Nebraska Press, 1963), and Thomas Neville Bonner, *Becoming a Physician: Medical Education in Great Britain, France, Germany, and the United States, 1750–1945* (New York: Oxford University Press, 1995), 231–308; Martin Kaufman, Stuart Galishoff, and Todd L. Savitt (eds), *Dictionary of American Medical Biography* (2 vols.; Westport, Conn.: Greenwood Press, 1984), I, 206. Dock remained in Galveston for three years before moving to the medical school at the University of Michigan, where he developed an extraordinary teaching program. See Horace W. Davenport, *George Dock: Teaching and Learning Medicine at the Turn of the Century* (New Brunswick, N.J: Rutgers University Press, 1987).

6. Patricia Bellis Bixel and Elizabeth Hayes Turner, *Galveston and the 1900 Storm: Catastrophe and Catalyst* (Austin: University of Texas Press, 2000), 41 (quotation), 61–62, 74–77.

7. *The University of Texas Medical Branch at Galveston: A Seventy-five Year History by the Faculty and Staff* (Austin: University of Texas Press, 1967; cited hereafter as *UTMB: Seventy-five Year History*), 62 (quotation). For photos of damaged buildings, see pages 56–63. To assist with the medical care of survivors, several out-of-state physicians and nurses immediately came to Galveston. For details, see R. H. Harrison, "The Great Storm at Galveston—From a Medical Standpoint," *Texas Medical Journal*, 16 (Oct., 1900), 164–169; "The Great Storm at Galveston," *Texas Medical News*, 9 (Oct., 1900), 699–716; Isadore Dyer, "A Note on the Medical Relief Work Done in Galveston After the Storm," *New Orleans Medical and Surgical Journal*, 53 (Nov., 1900), 261–265; Allen J. Smith, "The Medical Department and the Galveston Storm," *University Record*, 3 (Mar., 1901), 53–67; H. A. West, "Medical and Sociological Aspects of the Galveston Storm," *Transactions, Texas State Medical Association* (1901), 118–127; and H. A. West, "Further Observations on the Medical Aspects of the Galveston Storm," *Transactions, Texas State Medical Association* (1901), 128–136.

8. Bradley Robert Rice, *Progressive Cities: The Commission Government Movement in America, 1901–1920* (Austin: University of Texas Press, 1977), 1–18; Bixel and Turner, *Galveston and the 1900 Storm*, 89–126, 130.

9. Ludmerer, *Learning to Heal*, 143.

10. Chester R. Burns, "Traditions and Transformations: How Texas Medicine Changed in the 20th Century," *Texas Medicine*, 96 (Jan., 2000), 45–47.

11. William G. Rothstein, *American Medical Schools and the Practice of Medicine: A History* (New York: Oxford University Press, 1987), 225; Chester R. Burns, "Health and Medicine," in Tyler, et al. (eds.), *The New Handbook of Texas*, III, 531; Edward N. Brandt Jr., "Medical Education: The Past 80 Years," *Texas Medicine*, 76 (May, 1980), 4–5.

12. Paul Starr, *The Social Transformation of American Medicine* (New York: Basic Books, 1982), 290–378; David E. Rogers, *American Medicine Challenge for the 1980s* (Cambridge, Mass.: Ballinger Publishing Company, 1978); Steven A. Schroeder, Jane S. Zones, and Jonathan A. Showstack, "Academic Medicine as a Public Trust," *Journal of the American Medical Association*, 262 (Aug. 11, 1989), 803–812; and Kenneth M. Ludmerer, *Time to Heal: American Medical Education from the Turn of the Century to the Era of Managed Care* (Oxford: Oxford University Press, 1999), 260–348.

13. Jack Lait and Lee Mortimer, *U.S.A. Confidential* (New York: Crown Publishers, 1952), 213. "Around Galveston," the muckrakers added with exaggeration, "the breeze wafts gently and the breakers woosh softly. No one works very hard. There is little labor trouble. There is no unemployment. There are no Communists. Gaiety echoes in the balmy air even during droughts. The good life pervades this island of iconoclastic isolation, as it always has under six flags— not including the skull and crossbones" (p. 218–219). See also David G. McComb, *Galveston: A History and a Guide* (Austin: Texas State Historical Association, 2000), 41–52; *Galveston County Daily News*, Dec. 19 and 26, 1999; and "The Best Places to Live Now," *Money*, 20 (Sept., 1991), 134.

14. Geoffrey Leavenworth, "Glorious Galveston: Forward-Looking Footprints on the Sea-Washed Sands of Time," *Texas Business*, 8 (Jan., 1984), 49–64 (quotation on 53).

15. Chester R. Burns, "The University of Texas Medical Branch at Galveston: Origins and Beginnings," *Journal of the American Medical Association*, 266 (Sept. 11, 1991), 1400–1403. Six state universities west of the Mississippi River established schools of medicine before 1891: University of Iowa (1870), University of California, San Francisco (1873), University of Colorado (1883), University of Southern California (1885), University of Oregon (1887), and University of Minnesota (1888). See John H. Rauch, *Illinois State Board of Health Report on Medical Education, Medical Colleges and the Regulation of the Practice of Medicine in the United States and Canada* (Springfield, Ill.: Roker Pub. Co., 1890), 5–7, 21, 50–51, 76–77, 127–128. Three state universities west of the Mississippi established schools of pharmacy before 1893: University of Iowa (1885), University of Kansas (1885), and University of Minnesota (1892). See Glenn

Sonnedecker (ed.), *Kremers and Urdang's History of Pharmacy* (4th ed.; Philadelphia: J. B. Lippincott, 1976), 383–385. Before 1890, private, hospital-based nursing schools had started in San Francisco, Minneapolis, St. Louis, and Denver. See Heather G. Campbell, "A Note on the First Nursing School in Texas and its Role in the Nineteenth Century Experience," *Houston Review*, 19, no. 1 (1997), 49–58.

CHAPTER 1

1. General Laws of the State of Texas (1881), Texas State Archives (Texas State Library, Austin), 79.

2. Texans used the words "Medical Department," "Medical Branch," "Medical College," and "Medical School" more or less interchangeably during the early years of the institution's development. The original tablet, situated to the right of the first floor entrance to today's Ashbel Smith Building, is inscribed: "School of Medicine, Medical Department of the University of Texas." This did not please Regent T. C. Thompson, who preferred Medical College. See T. C. Thompson to T. D. Wooten, Dec. 24, 1889; Jan. 14, 1890; and Oct. 4, 1890, letters, box 2H407, Thomas D. Wooten Papers (Center for American History, University of Texas at Austin). F. James MacKie kindly provided copies of these and other letters by Thompson; see RF226, Centennial History Project Archives, Blocker Collections; hereafter cited as CHP Archives, with the research folders designated RF and the writing folders designated WF. In a referendum on November 4, 1919, Texans approved a legislative amendment to the Texas constitution that designated the Medical Department a "branch" of the University of Texas. See General Laws of the State of Texas (1919), 350–354. Since that time the institution's official name has been the University of Texas Medical Branch at Galveston, commonly shortened to UTMB, the label that will be used throughout this book. See also A. P. Wooldridge, "A History of the Location of the University of Texas at Austin, Texas," *Alcalde*, 2 (Nov., 1913), 26–41. Article VII, Sections 10–14 of the Texas constitution of 1876 included specific stipulations about "The University of Texas." Since the legislative bill of March 30, 1881, authorizing the establishment of the university involved amendments to these sections of the constitution, a plebiscite was necessary.

3. Chester R. Burns, "The Development of Hospitals in Galveston During the Nineteenth Century," *Southwestern Historical Quarterly*, 97 (Oct., 1993), 238–263. Physicians, pharmacists, and dentists were named in the city directories for Galveston. Twenty doctors were named in the *Galveston City Directory* for 1868–1869; thirty-one in 1874–1875; fifty-two in 1875–1876; thirty-four in 1876–1877; and thirty-eight in 1877–1878; see *Galveston City Directory for 1868–9* (Galveston: Shaw and Blaylock, Publishers and Job Printing, 1868–1869); *Haller's Galveston City Directory, 1874* (Galveston: Strickland & Clarke, Stationers, Printers, and Lithographers, 1874); *Fayman & Reilly's Galveston City Directory for 1875–6* (Galveston: Strickland & Clarke, Stationers, Printers, and Lithographers, 1875–76); *Haller's Galveston City Directory 1876–7* (Galveston: John H. Haller, 1876–1877); and *Galveston General and Business Directory for 1877–8* (Galveston: Shaw & Blaylock, Publishers & Printers). See also *Galveston Daily News*, Oct. 2–3, 1875; and Sister Mary Loyola Hegarty, *Serving with Gladness: The Origin and History of the Congregation of the Sisters of Charity of the Incarnate Word Houston, Texas* (Houston: Bruce Publishing Co., 1967), 233–236, 246–247.

4. Fourteen doctors had organized the Galveston Medical Society in July 1865; see *Galveston Medical Journal*, 1 (Nov., 1866), 5–13. In June 1869 three members (T. J. Heard, Greensville Dowell, and John Webb) attended the reorganizational meeting of the TSMA in Houston. Heard was elected president. For details, see *Transactions, Texas State Medical Association*, 1 (1869), 8; and Pat Ireland Nixon, *A History of the Texas Medical Association, 1853–1953* (Austin: University of Texas Press, 1953), 31–40. In 1876 the Galveston Medical Society reorganized as the Galveston County Medical Society. For details, see *Galveston Daily News*, Dec. 28, 1875; Jan. 13, 1876; Mar. 22, 1876; Apr. 12, 1876; and May 14, 1876. See also *Transactions, Texas State Medical Association*, 9 (1877), 1–4 (quotation on 2). Only two American cities exported more cotton than Galveston. See McComb, *Galveston: A History*, 47–50. Between 1870 and 1881 Galveston almost doubled its total value of exports, from over $14.8 million to more than $26.6 million; see Alwyn Barr, *Reconstruction to Reform: Texas Politics, 1876–1906* (Austin: University of Texas Press, 1971), 13. See also *Galveston Daily News*, Apr. 4–7, 1877. A graduate of the University of Pennsylvania School of Medicine and a former Confederate army surgeon, Kelley had moved to Galveston in 1865. See William Wallace McCullough Jr., *Doctor William Dennis Kelley, 1825–1888: Texas Physician and Surgeon* (Galveston: Privately printed, 1961).

5. Other places of origin included Nova Scotia, New York, Virginia, Tennessee, North and South Carolina, and Mexico; see *Galveston Medical Journal*, 4 (Aug., 1869), 343–351. Graduation totals were calculated from data provided by a "Tabulated History of Galveston Medical College," in *Texas Medical Journal*, 5 (Apr., 1876), 41–50, and from the Texas Medical College and Hospital Register of Matriculates and Graduates, 1873–1891, unpublished register, Truman G. Blocker Jr. History of Medicine Collections (Moody Medical Library, University of Texas Medical Branch at Galveston; hereafter cited as Blocker Collections). The main building of Soule University was in Chappell Hill, but medical teaching occurred in Galveston. The relationship of the Galveston Medical College to Soule University was substantial.

The university's board of trustees signed diplomas, approved catalogs, and provided money for a new building. See Ralph W. Jones, "The First Roots of the University of Texas Medical Branch at Galveston," *Southwestern Historical Quarterly*, 65 (Apr., 1962), 465–474; Galveston Medical College Register of Students and Minutes of Faculty Meetings, 60, 78, 93–94, 126–127, 128–137, Blocker Collections; cited hereafter as Galveston Medical College Register.

6. After the 1866–1867 session, for example, each teacher received $255.43; after the 1870–1871 session, $96.42, see Galveston Medical College Register, 69, 129. For a roster of the teachers during the seventh and final session of the Galveston Medical College, see the advertisements in *Transactions, Texas State Medical Association*, 3 (1871), 60–61.

7. Galveston Medical College Register, 117–118.

8. Galveston Medical College faculty had graduated from Jefferson, University of Pennsylvania, University of New York, and Augusta Medical College. Dowell traveled to New Orleans, Baltimore, Philadelphia, and New York City to visit medical schools and attend annual meetings of the American Medical Association (AMA). Dowell also attended special conferences of medical professors convened during the AMA's annual meetings in 1866 and 1870; see *Galveston Medical Journal*, 1 (July, 1866), 261–267, 283–290; 2 (June, 1867), 736–742; 2 (July, 1867), 774–793; and 5 (Apr., 1870), 183–186.

9. Special Laws of the State of Texas (1871), Texas State Archives (Texas State Library, Austin), 499–501; supplement to *Galveston Daily News*, Jan. 19, 1873.

10. Donald W. Whisenhunt, *The Encyclopedia of Texas Colleges and Universities: An Historical Profile* (Austin: Eakin Press, 1986), 122, 133–134; Special Laws of the State of Texas (1873), 170–175.

11. *Journal of the House of Representatives of the State of Texas: Being the Session of the Thirteenth Legislature Begun and Held at the City of Austin, January 14, 1873*, 461 (Texas State Library, Austin). By the middle of the nineteenth century, legislators in Massachusetts, New York, Pennsylvania, Illinois, and Louisiana provided state funds to hospitals in Boston, New York City, Philadelphia, Chicago, and New Orleans. See Charles E. Rosenberg, *The Care of Strangers: The Rise of America's Hospital System* (New York: Basic Books, 1987), 106.

12. Special Laws of the State of Texas (1873), 174. A local newspaper reporter mistakenly claimed that Galveston would now save five thousand dollars per year because of this law. He either missed the political charade of "not otherwise appropriated" or did not recognize the steady growth of indigent patients who were dependent on public funds from city, county, or state governments. See *Galveston Daily News*, Mar. 30, 1873.

13. In 1856 legislators authorized the establishment of asylums for Texans who were insane, blind, or deaf. The asylum for blind persons and the one for deaf persons began functioning in 1857; the insane asylum in 1861. Between 1856 and 1873 the legislators allocated at least $600,000 for the maintenance of these three institutions. This total was calculated from amounts budgeted by successive state legislatures. See General Laws of the State of Texas (1856), 39–40, 58–59, 60–61; (1858), 120–121, 153–154, 251; (1860), 79–80, 106; (1862), 49; (1863), 31; (1864), 42–44; (1866), 115, 216; (1870), 296; (1871), 104, 137; (1873), 214, 216. Also see Elizabeth Borst White, "Patterns of Development in Texas Hospitals, 1836–1935: Preliminary Survey," *Texas Medicine*, 82 (Dec., 1986), 55–60.

14. *Galveston Daily News*, Jan. 9, 1876. A native of Hartford, Connecticut, Ashbel Smith completed undergraduate and medical studies at Yale University. After additional medical studies in France and practice as a physician in North Carolina, Smith came to Texas in 1837 to serve as surgeon general for the army of the Republic of Texas. He later served as the republic's ambassador to France and England, as an elected representative in the Texas legislature in 1855, 1866, and 1878, as a surgeon in the Confederate army, and as a leader for higher education in Texas. See Elizabeth Silverthorne, *Ashbel Smith of Texas: Pioneer, Patriot, Statesman, 1805–1886* (College Station: Texas A&M University Press, 1982) and an assessment by J. J. Lane in *History of Education in Texas* (Washington, D.C.: Government Printing Office, 1903), 313–316. For the faculty, see *Transactions, Texas State Medical Association*, 7 (1875), n.p.; *Galveston Daily News*, Feb. 23 and Mar. 26, 1876, and Sept. 16, 1877.

15. *Galveston Daily News*, Mar. 16, 1876. One of these graduates was John A. O'Brien. Gratitude is extended to his granddaughter, Elaine F. O'Brien of Ventura, California, who provided a photograph of her grandfather's diploma, which is in WF232, CHP Archives.

16. *Galveston Daily News*, Mar. 7, 1878. Reacting to an influx of pretenders, Texans were among the earliest post–Civil War legislators to adopt a medical licensure law. The same legislature that established the TMCH in 1873 also passed "An Act to Regulate the Practice of Medicine" in the entire state. See General Laws of the State of Texas (1873), 74–76. A physician could not practice legally in Texas without evidence of graduation from a "regularly established and well accredited medical college" or without a certificate attesting that the physician had passed an examination given by a board of medical examiners established by the district judge of the county in which the physician

resided. Physicians were expected to register their diploma or certificate with the clerk of the district court in the county. Galvestonians responded promptly. Edward Randall, Greensville Dowell, J. M. Callaway, Edwin H. Watts, and W. S. Rogers constituted the first Board of Medical Examiners for Galveston County; Galveston County Board of Medical Examiners, notice, 1873, Blocker Collections. Between November 25, 1873, and January 3, 1877, fifty physicians registered in Galveston County; Register of Physicians, Galveston County, 3–15, district clerk's office (Galveston County Courthouse, Galveston, Texas). Texas legislators revised this licensure act on August 21, 1876; see *Galveston Daily News*, Dec. 7, 1876. Diplomas alone were no longer accepted as sufficient evidence of qualification. A board could certify only on the basis of its own exam, which was offered semi-annually. In November, William H. Stewart, judge of the Twenty-sixth Judicial District of Texas, appointed a new board for Galveston County consisting of Edwin H. Watts, Edward Randall, William D. Kelley, Charles W. Trueheart, MacKenzie Johnston, Greensville Dowell, and Clarke Campbell. By September 1881 another twenty physicians had registered in Galveston County; Register of Physicians, Galveston County, 15–21.

17. Information about the Association of American Medical Colleges was obtained from the annual meeting reports that are bound as *AAMC Proc., 1876–1879 and AMCA Proc., 1880–1882*, box 1, AAMC Proceedings (AAMC Archives, Washington, D.C.). For Dowell's letter, see *AAMC Proc., 1877*, 12. For other meetings see *AAMC Proc., 1878*, 4; *AAMC Proc., 1879*, 4; and *AAMC Proc., 1880*, 2.

18. *Texas Medical Journal*, 6 (Jan., 1877), 20–31. At the New York meeting in 1880, AMCA delegates were so optimistic about reform standards that they agreed to extend the required curriculum to three years. Within two years, however, thirteen member schools had resigned because they could not support this requirement. Only twelve delegates came to Cincinnati in 1882, and the group did not meet again until fifty-five schools sent representatives to a reorganizational meeting held in Nashville on May 21, 1890. These delegates adopted the original name of Association of American Medical Colleges (AAMC).

19. When Dr. Percival Butler McCutchon visited the school on its opening day in November 1879, only "six or eight students" were present. Percival Butler McCutchon, "Diary and reminiscences of the Medical Officer of Morgan's iron steamship, *City of Norfolk*, during the voyage from New Orleans to Indianola via Galveston and from Indianola back to Galveston thence by steamship *Josephine* of the same line to Morgan City and from there to New Orleans by railroad," unpublished. McCutchon's visit to the TMCH occurred on the morning of November 3, 1879. Dr. McCutchon had graduated from Tulane earlier that year. He became a prominent physician in New Orleans. I am grateful to his grandson, Dr. F. James McCutchon of Corpus Christi, for permission to use this diary. The assertion about state funds may be incorrect, but there is no evidence that state funds were ever transferred to the TMCH. This claim is based on an examination of selected ledger pages in the Register of Warrants Paid by the Treasurer's Office of the State of Texas 1871–1877 and the General Warrant Register, vol. IV, 1871–1874, Archives Division (Texas State Library, Austin).

20. *Galveston Daily News*, Mar. 4, 1880.

21. *Journal of the Senate of Texas* (1881), 100–101 (Texas State Archives, Texas State Library, Austin). A few weeks earlier, in anticipation of the legislative authorization, the Galveston City Council had offered to lease the former City Hospital buildings and grounds to the state for temporary use by the new medical school. The councilmen also offered to purchase and donate nearby land as a site for a new building; see Galveston Medical College Register, Feb. 21, 1881. James B. Stubbs (1850–1925) and Charles J. Stubbs (1867–1948) were brothers and partners in a busy law office in Galveston. Some of their papers are deposited in the Galveston and Texas History Center of the Rosenberg Library in Galveston. For a list of those members of Texas legislatures who represented the citizens of Galveston between 1846 and 1991, see Appendix A-1, WF441, CHP Archives. See also Inci Bowman, "Beginnings of Medical Journalism in Texas," *Texas Medicine*, 82 (Feb., 1986), 51–55.

22. "Proceedings of the Texas State Medical Association, Thirteenth Annual Session," *Texas Medical and Surgical Record*, 1 (June, 1881), 213. Members of the TSMA began the successive numbering of their annual sessions with the re-organizational meeting of 1869. Nixon, *History of the Texas Medical Association*, 93–94.

23. "Record of Minutes Locating University of Texas," 3–54, 200–217, unpublished record, Office of the Board of Regents of the University of Texas (Ashbel Smith Hall, Austin; hereafter cited as "Record of Minutes"); Wooldridge, "A History of the Location of the University of Texas," 30.

24. "To the People of Texas," *Dallas Weekly Herald*, June 30, 1881. Cary Wilkinson reiterated these arguments in two lengthy editorials that appeared in the *Texas Medical and Surgical Record*, 1 (July, 1881), 291–298; and 1 (Aug., 1881), 336–341.

25. "Record of Minutes," 22; Alwyn Barr, *Reconstruction to Reform: Texas Politics, 1876–1906* (Austin: University of Texas Press, 1971), 63, 77–79. For examples of ads these cities placed in newspapers, see the *Dallas Weekly Herald*, July

21, 1881, and Aug. 18, 1881, and the *San Antonio Daily Express*, Aug. 20, 1881. For sentiments in Galveston, see *Galveston Daily News*, Sept. 3–4, 1881.

26. Stubbs's prediction about voter preference in Galveston County came true: 1,359 county residents were for separation; 250 against. Tyler received 1,041 votes for the main university; Austin received only 363. See election return, September 1881, Galveston County, Secretary of State records, RG307, Archives Division (Texas State Library, Austin). In the election, 1,735 Galveston County residents chose Galveston, 3 chose Houston, 1 Austin. Some Houstonians were not happy with the outcome. In the October 19, 1881, issue of the *Houston Post*, an editor argued that those who voted for Austin as the site of the entire university were voting against any other place as the site of the medical school. Therefore, the 14,607 votes for Austin for the entire university, as well as the votes for the other cities named for the entire university should have been added to those cast for Houston for the medical department, which would have resulted in 35,565 votes against Galveston, thereby defeating it as the location for the medical school. For the legal citation to these events, see *Vernon's Annotated Constitution of the State of Texas* (1993), vol. 2, Article VII, Sec. 10, pp. 432–434.

27. Minutes, UT Board of Regents, Nov. 16–17, 1881, Office of the UT Board of Regents (Ashbel Smith Hall, University of Texas at Austin). Other details about these early months can be found in the *Report of the Board of Regents of the University of Texas* (1883), 1, 3–12, and several newspaper articles included in the "Record of Minutes Locating University of Texas," 254–262. Details can be found in J. J. Lane, *History of the University of Texas* (Austin: Hutchings, 1891), 75–137 and Lane, *History of Education in Texas*, 135–145, 194–208. Roger A. Griffin, "To Establish a University of the First Class," *Southwestern Historical Quarterly*, 86 (Oct., 1982), 135–160.

28. Minute, UT Board of Regents, Sept. 14, 1883. For information about the allegations, see *Galveston Daily News*, June 29 and 30, 1883, and Sept. 12 and 20, 1883. Minutes of the UT Board of Regents, May 16, 1884; *Report of the UT Board of Regents* (Dec. 18, 1884), 12. The regents published their reports somewhat irregularly before 1900. The *Third Biennial Report* was issued in 1886; the seventh and eighth in 1897 and 1899. Beginning with the *Ninth Biennial Report* of 1900 the reports were published regularly in even-numbered years through 1930.

29. The best source for understanding the early history of these two funds is Berte R. Haigh, *Land, Oil, and Education* (El Paso: Texas Western Press, 1986), 1–78.

30. During these early years, there is no evidence that the regents considered any city other than Galveston. In a letter to Dr. J. E. Burke, secretary of the Galveston County Medical Society, dated January 10, 1885, Ashbel Smith reaffirmed his commitment to Galveston: "The Medical Department when properly organized as it needs must be, will by force of circumstances be the leading, paramount School of Medical Instruction of the great South Western region of the American Union. That Galveston is the preeminently suitable location for the Institution for Medical Instruction in the wide region I have adverted to, does not admit of reasonable doubt." See Ashbel Smith to J. E. Burke, Jan. 10, 1885, letter, box 2G229, Ashbel Smith Papers (Center for American History, University of Texas at Austin); *Report of the UT Board of Regents* (1886), 13–14, 65–66.

31. Minutes, Galveston City Council/Commissioners, Jan. 22, 1887, 114–115; *Galveston Daily News*, Jan. 23, 1887; Minutes, Galveston City Council/Commissioners, Feb. 11, 1887, 121; and *Galveston Daily News*, Feb. 15, 1887. A shrewd businessman who matured at the beginning of the postbellum commercial and industrial revolutions, John Sealy amassed his fortune first by merchandising, then by banking, and finally by active participation in railway, shipping, and natural gas companies. For more on Sealy, see Robert B. Nichols, *A Bridge to a Better World* (Galveston: The Sealy & Smith Foundation for the John Sealy Hospital, 1989), 9–25. For the ordinance accepting his gift, see City of Galveston, Ordinances 1871 to 1891, 618–619, and J. D. Kelley, *An Appendix Containing Special Ordinances, Contracts and Other Acts Affecting the Rights and Interests of the City of Galveston* (Galveston: Oscar Springer Print, 1916), 660–661.

32. Minutes, Galveston City Council/Commissioners, Feb. 21, 1887, 121–128. For the ordinance, see City of Galveston, Ordinances 1871 to 1891, 658–659. Dr. C. W. Trueheart played an extremely important role in persuading the Sealys to construct a hospital and in lobbying throughout the state for Galveston as the best site for the new medical school; C. W. Trueheart to J. W. McLaughlin, May 18, 1909, box 4R19, UT President's Records, Office of the University of Texas Board of Regents (Ashbel Smith Hall, University of Texas at Austin). For a biographical sketch of Trueheart, see Chester R. Burns, "Charles William Trueheart," in Tyler, et al. (eds.) *The New Handbook of Texas*, VI, 577–578.

33. For more about Thompson, see L. E. Daniell, *Personnel of the Texas State Government, with Sketches of Representative Men of Texas* (San Antonio: Maverick Pub. Co., 1892), 558–559; *University Record*, 1 (Dec., 1898), 62–64; *University Medical*, 4 (Oct., 1898), 9; Minutes, UT Board of Regents, May 16, 1898; and Chester R. Burns, "Thomas C. Thompson," in Tyler, et al. (eds.), *The New Handbook of Texas*, VI, 475. For Wooten, see "The Father of The University," *Alcalde*, 2 (Nov., 1913), 1–12; a biographical sketch in *Daniel's Texas Medical Journal*, 3 (Nov., 1887), 175–179; and "Thomas Dudley Wooten," in Tyler, et al. (eds.), *The New Handbook of Texas*, VI, 1075. Ashbel Smith died on January 21, 1886.

34. Thomas D. Wooten, "The University of Texas," 1887, p. 6, biographical files, Office of the University of Texas Board of Regents (Ashbel Smith Hall, University of Texas at Austin). Wooten was infuriated by the legislators' willingness to give scarce funds to Texas A&M and Prairie View, monies that would have enabled the regents to build the medical college building. Wooten was also angry about an alleged alliance between supporters of Texas A&M and a group of Galvestonians, including Walter Gresham. This alliance had attempted unsuccessfully to get the legislature to pay a debt of $87,000 due to the university, specifically designating $50,000 of that payment for a medical school building in Galveston, and the remainder to A&M. These maneuvers had occurred behind the backs of the UT regents. See Lane, *History of the University of Texas*, 156–159, and Lane, *History of Education in Texas*, 219–221.

35. Minute Book, Board of Trustees, Texas Medical College and Hospital, 1887–1888, Blocker Collections; and *Galveston Daily News*, Oct. 30, 1887. Physicians in Fort Worth and Austin celebrated the revival of the Texas Medical College and Hospital; see *Texas Courier–Record of Medicine*, 5 (June, 1888), 381; 6 (Sept., 1888), 23; and *Daniel's Texas Medical Journal*, 3 (July, 1887), 17–19; 3 (June, 1888), 530–532; 4 (Sept., 1888), 123–127, 133. For the city's ordinance leasing the City Hospital building to the Texas Medical College and Hospital, see City of Galveston, Ordinances 1871–1891, 652–653.

36. Minutes, UT Board of Regents, Apr. 16, 1888; General Laws of the State of Texas (1888), 19–20. "Loaned" was the term used in the law. However, Michael Green, reference archivist at the Texas State Library, was unable to find mention of a "loan" or of repayment in the treasurer's and comptroller's annual and biennial reports. The legislators probably used the word "loan" to circumvent the provision in the state's constitution that prohibited the use of general revenue funds for the construction of university buildings. Minutes, UT Board of Regents, June 19, 1888, Sept. 3. 1888.

37. General Laws of the State of Texas (1889), 74 and Minutes, Galveston City Council/Commissioners, May 9, 1889. For the city ordinance, see Kelley, *An Appendix Containing Special Ordinances, Contracts and Other Acts Affecting the Rights and Interests of the City of Galveston*, 662–663. Minutes, UT Board of Regents, Sept. 17, 1889. To obtain new ideas about designing Old Red's interior, Clayton visited several medical colleges in the northeastern part of the United States. For his report, see Lane, *History of the University of Texas*, 168–171. Some of Clayton's drawings are in the Blocker Collections and a few are in the Texas and Galveston History Center at the Rosenberg Library (accessions no. 1033).

38. Both T. C. Thompson and C. W. Trueheart worked extensively with Wooten to determine the exact wording of this lease. See C. W. Trueheart to T. D. Wooten, Oct. 4, 1889, letter, box VF 11/E, UT President's Records and T. C. Thompson to T. D. Wooten, Sept. 27, 1889; T. D. Wooten to T. C. Thompson, Sept. 28, 1889; T. C. Thompson to T. D. Wooten, Sept. 29, 1889; and T. C. Thompson to T. D. Wooten, Oct. 6, 1889, letters, Wooten Papers. A copy of the lease is included in the Minutes, UT Board of Regents, Sept. 17, 1889. There is also a copy in box 24 of the UTMB Dean's Office Records, Blocker Collections. For discussion of the lease, see Lane, *History of the University of Texas*, 162–165. The professional staff of the hospital would include a house surgeon who would be selected by the board of managers and compensated by the city, visiting physicians and surgeons who would be members of the faculty and receive no compensation from the city, and two or more interns who would be selected by the regents or their authorized agents and receive only board and lodging for their services.

39. McComb, *Galveston: A History*, 118–120. The quickest way to appreciate this situation is to examine photographs of homes and buildings constructed in Galveston during the late 1880s and early 1890s. For two collections, see *Galveston Tribune, A Souvenir of Galveston* (Galveston: *Galveston Evening Tribune*, 1893), and *Art Work of Galveston* (Chicago: W. R. Parish Pub. Co., 1894). Any one who doubts the dominant cultural power of Galveston at this time should read the speeches H. A. West and Sam Burroughs gave to welcome the TSMA members who assembled in Galveston in late April 1888 for their twentieth annual meeting. Attendees elected J. F. Y. Paine, the former TMCH dean, as their new president; see *Transactions, Texas State Medical Association* (1888), 9–13.

40. T. C. Thompson to T. D. Wooten, Nov. 12, 1889, letter, Wooten Papers.

41. During these three weeks, the hospital incurred expenses of $373.82 for food, drugs, coal, wood, and ice, and $249.00 for salaries paid to the house surgeon and superintendent, a cook and an assistant cook, a steward, a druggist, a matron, a laundry woman, an engineer, and a fireman; *Galveston Daily News*, Feb. 11, 1890; *Galveston Daily News*, Mar. 16, 1890 and *UTMB: Seventy-five Year History*, 88–93. The Lady Board of Managers selected Dorothea Fick, a graduate of Mount Sinai Hospital's School of Nursing in New York City, as the first superintendent. Fick had come to Galveston to care for an injured child who was a member of the Sealy family. See Ella Sealy Newell to Chauncey Leake, July 22, 1944, letter, Chauncey D. Leake Papers, History of Medicine Division (National Library of Medicine, Bethesda, Md.; cited hereafter as NLM); Lane, *History of the University of Texas*, 171.

42. *Report of the UT Board of Regents* (1890), 9–10, 44.

43. On October 24, 1889, Galveston's City Council authorized this arrangement with the TMCH faculty and students. On September 7, 1889, the council had authorized the creation of a John Sealy Hospital Board of Managers, but the charter amendment legitimizing that board was not approved by the state legislature until March 25, 1891; Special Laws of the State of Texas, Regular Session, Twenty-second Legislature (1891), 68–70. Presumably the original board drafted the first set of rules governing the hospital, since they were published in 1890; see *General Rules for the Management of the John Sealy Hospital, Galveston, Texas* (Galveston: J. C. & W. E. Strickland, 1890); a copy is in the Blocker Collections. The new board was functioning by mid-July, 1891; *Galveston Daily News*, July 12, 1891, Mar. 21, 1891. Thirty-eight students matriculated at the TMCH during the three years of its reincarnation (1888–1891). Four graduated, two in 1890 and two in 1891. The faculty's standards were high, the three-year curriculum was tough, and total fees amounted to $435. The faculty included J. F. Y. Paine as dean, H. P. Cooke, George Dock, A. W. Fly, B. E. Hadra, G. P. Hall, G. H. Lee, Edward Randall, H. A. West, and J. H. Wysong. Wysong became the first superintendent of the John Sealy Hospital. Some TMCH matriculates continued their studies at UTMB. For details, see TMCH Register of Matriculates and Graduates, 1873–1891, Blocker Collections; Announcement of Re-opening Sessions of 1888–1889 in folder 6, box 1, University of Texas Medical Branch Materials (Galveston and Texas History Center, Rosenberg Library, Galveston); *Galveston Daily News*, Apr. 25, 1888; May 20, 1888; Aug. 29, 1888; Nov. 11, 1888; Mar. 17, 1889; Mar. 21, 1891; and Rauch, *Illinois State Board of Health Report on Medical Education, Medical Colleges and the Regulation of the Practice of Medicine in the United States and Canada*, 143–144. This latter listing was the first time that Texas appeared in a national catalog of medical colleges. For a report of instruction at the TMCH during its last year (1890–1891), see "Reminiscences of an Alumnus of '93" in *University Medical*, 5, no. 4 (1900), 132–135.

44. T. C. Thompson to T. D. Wooten, Apr. 13, 1891, letter, Wooten Papers; General Laws of the State of Texas (1891), 124. See comments in *University of Texas Faculty Report* (1890–1891), 7–9. This report, included in a volume bound as *Annual Faculty Reports 1883–1903*, is in the Office of the University of Texas Board of Regents (Ashbel Smith Hall, University of Texas at Austin). By the early 1890s annual income from the university's investments approximated $50,000, though this was not enough to meet the expenses of the main campus; see *Report of the UT Board of Regents* (1890), 3–4; (1892), 5–6; (1894), 12–14.

45. T. C. Thompson to T. D. Wooten, Apr. 22, 1891, letter, Wooten Papers.

46. Minutes, UT Board of Regents, June 17, 1891; *UTMB: Seventy-five Year History*, 27–28; Minutes, UT Board of Regents, Aug. 25–26, 1891; and *Galveston Daily News*, Sept. 10, 1891.

47. T. C. Thompson to T. D. Wooten, Apr. 13 and 22, 1891, letters, Wooten Papers; and *Galveston Daily News*, Aug. 28, 1891.

48. *Galveston Daily News*, Oct. 2, 1891.

49. *UTMB: Seventy-five Year History*, 51. For a biographical sketch, see Chester R. Burns, "John Fannin Young Paine," in Tyler, et al. (eds.), *The New Handbook of Texas*, V, 12–13.

50. Additional biographical details and photos of these teachers are found in *UTMB: Seventy-five Year History*, 25–49 and in *Daniel's Texas Medical Journal*, 7, no. 3 (1891), 101–103; 8, no. 1 (1892), 27–38; 8, no. 4 (1892), 136–138.

51. Minutes, UTMB Faculty Meetings, Sept. 29, 1891, UTMB Archives, Blocker Collections. Although some lecturers taught during the first academic year, the regents did not extend official appointments to the six lecturers until April 1892; Minutes, UTMB Faculty Meetings, Apr. 22, 1892. The regents selected private practitioners for three lectureships: R. C. Hodges as lecturer on diseases of the eye, ear, nose, and throat; R. W. Knox as lecturer on diseases of the skin; and H. P. Cooke as lecturer on diseases of children. The regents named T. J. Ballinger, a Galveston lawyer, as lecturer on medical jurisprudence. The regents named two incumbent faculty as lecturers: Randall as lecturer on diseases of the chest and Smith as lecturer on nervous and mental diseases. Four of these six had been nominated by the faculty.

52. William Keiller to Board of Regents, Mar. 31, 1892, and George Lee to Board of Regents, Apr. 18, 1892, letters, box 4R85, UT President's Records.

53. For a discussion of this veto power, see Fred Gantt Jr., *The Chief Executive in Texas: A Study in Gubernatorial Leadership* (Austin: University of Texas Press, 1964), 169–191. Between 1891 and 1991, twenty-four people served as governors of Texas. For a list of names and years, see Appendix A-2, WF441, CHP Archives.

54. Eight appointees constituted the early UT Boards of Regents, nine after 1913. See *Rules and Regulations, UT Board of Regents* (1912), 27; (1925), 28. In 1991 the *Rules and Regulations* were recorded on approximately 280 typescript pages kept in two loose leaf binders in the office of the Executive Secretary of the Board of Regents. The *Rules* adopted in 1891, 1904, and 1912 were quite general, allowing much freedom to line authorities, as long as exercises of that freedom did not circumvent the policies of the regents and their appointed executive officers. The lengthy *Rules*

adopted in 1936 and amended several times through 1943 were much more detailed than preceding ones. In this book, *Rules and Regulations* is used for citations, together with the appropriate year and pages. Approximately two hundred people, including nine women, were UT regents between 1881 and 1991. Margaret Berry named 190 regents who served through January 1979. See Margaret C. Berry, *The University of Texas: A Pictorial Account of Its First Century* (Austin: University of Texas Press, 1980), 413–415. In the university bureaucracy, executives moved in political seesaws with those immediately "above" and those immediately "below" in the hierarchies. On the one hand, they honored the desires of the person or group immediately superior. On the other, they led and guided those immediately inferior. Corporate "superiors" established this hierarchy to motivate "inferiors" to implement policies, to protect subordinates from arbitrary manipulations by competitors or enemies, and to provide a lattice of accountability that presumably assured everyone that the university accomplished its social missions satisfactorily.

55. Before 1991 the regents issued major revisions of their rules about a dozen times (1904, 1912, 1920, 1925, 1936, 1950, 1953, 1960, 1967, 1977, 1979, and 1988). See "Rules and Regulations for the Conduct of Business by the Board of Regents of the University of Texas. Adopted August 25, 1891"; "Regulations for the Government of the University of Texas. Adopted by the Board of Regents, September 16, 1904," *University of Texas Bulletin*, no. 87 (Jan. 15, 1907); "By-laws of the Board of Regents and Rules and Regulations for the Government of University of Texas. Adopted by the Board of Regents, November 11, 1912," *University of Texas Bulletin*, no. 270 (Mar. 8, 1913); "Revised Section of the Rules and Regulations of the Board of Regents," 1920; "Bylaws of the Board of Regents and Rules and Regulations for the Government of the University of Texas adopted by the Board of Regents, December 8, 1925," *University of Texas Bulletin*, no. 2548 (Dec. 22, 1925); "Rules and Regulations of the Board of Regents for the Government of the University of Texas," 6th ed., Mar. 14, 1936, *University of Texas Bulletin*, no. 3631 (Aug. 15, 1936); "Rules and Regulations of the Board of Regents for the Government of the University of Texas," 6th ed., with amendments to Aug. 1, 1943, part I, *University of Texas Bulletin*, no. 4331 (Aug. 15, 1943); "Rules and Regulations of the Board of Regents for the Government of the University of Texas," 6th ed., with amendments to Aug. 1, 1943, part II, *University of Texas Bulletin*, no. 4332 (Aug. 22, 1943); "The Rules and Regulations of the Board of Regents for the Government of the University of Texas," 1960, copy no. 1202 in folder 3, box 3U380, Ransom Papers, University of Texas Chancellor's Records (University of Texas at Austin); "Rules and Regulations of the Board of Regents for the Government of the University of Texas," 1967, Material Supporting the Agenda for Meetings of the UT Board of Regents, vol. XIV b; "Rules and Regulations of the Board of Regents of the University of Texas System for the Government of the University of Texas System," Sept. 16, 1977, Material Supporting the Agenda for Meetings of the UT Board of Regents, vol. XXV a; "Regents' Rules and Regulations," Feb. 7–9, 1979, Material Supporting the Agenda for Meetings of the UT Board of Regents, vol. XXVI d; "Rules and Regulations of the Board of Regents of the University of Texas System for the Government of the University of Texas System," June 1, 1988, with amendments to Oct. 7, 1988, Material Supporting the Agenda for Meetings of the UT Board of Regents, vol. I–1.

56. Born in Maryland and educated in Washington, D.C., Frank Spencer (1835–1907) moved to Galveston in 1866. He was a district attorney for fourteen years, a district judge for three years, and a regent for six years. For more details, see "Frank Maury Spencer," in *Biographical Encyclopedia of Texas* (New York: Southern Publishing Co., 1880), 71–72, and *Galveston Daily News*, July 15, 1907.

57. How decisions were made about the distribution of fees received from private patients is not known. Presumably the attending faculty member pocketed the fees received for services, and the hospital received those charged for food, medicines, technical procedures, and nursing care. This aspect of health care economics irritated some of the legislators who parceled state funds, leading some professors to defend their rights to private practice; see *Galveston Daily News*, May 1, 1893.

58. Minutes, UT Board of Regents, June 21, 1893. The faculty of the pharmacy school also included two faculty members from the School of Medicine: the professor of materia medica and the professor of chemistry. Paradoxically, the elimination of tuition fees led to a total increase in revenue. A much larger number of students were required to pay laboratory fees; see Minutes, UT Board of Regents, May 15–16, 1895. See Paine's report for the 1893–1894 year in box 4R85, UT President's Records.

59. From 1883 until 1895 the faculty of UT Austin elected one of the professors as chairman of the faculty, a *de facto* chief executive officer. In 1895 the regents invited Leslie Waggener, a former chairman, to serve as *ad interim* president until a full-time president could be employed. See *UTMB: Seventy-five Year History*, 312, and *Galveston Daily News*, Mar. 5, 1893; May 1, 1894; and Oct. 2, 1895. For biographical information about Winston, see *University Medical*, 2, no. 1 (1896), 8–13 and *Galveston Daily News*, July 12 and 19, 1896. *Rules and Regulations* (1897), 11, 16. For reports about his week-long visits to UTMB in 1897, see *Galveston Daily News*, July 17, 1897 and Dec. 14, 1897. *University*

Medical, 2 (Feb., 1897), 195; Minutes, UT Board of Regents, July 27, 29–30, 1897. Winston probably reassured everyone that the budget reduction was not as frightening as it could have been. Six weeks earlier, he told regent Thompson that he had expected only $30,000 from the legislature; George Winston to T. C. Thompson, June 2, 1897, letter, T. C. Thompson Papers (Rosenberg Library, Galveston).

60. These decisions involved issues of political patronage since Clopton and West had been ardent supporters of Paine. The old guard of Paine, Clopton, Randall, and West were challenged by the "foreigners," Keiller and Thompson. When Randall was absent at a meeting in November 1892 the faculty elected Thompson to represent them at a meeting of the Association of Southern Medical Colleges. Clopton was distressed that neither he nor Paine was selected; see A. G. Clopton to T. D. Wooten, Jan. 22, 1893, letter, Wooten Papers. Moreover, Clopton's wife did not like Galveston; see A. G. Clopton to T. D. Wooten, Feb. 22, 1896, letter, Wooten Papers. David Cerna also resigned; see *Texas Medical News,* 6, no. 10 (1897), 434. Minutes, UT Board of Regents, Sept. 18, 1897. For a biographical sketch, see Chester R. Burns, "Allen John Smith," in Tyler, et al. (eds.), *The New Handbook of Texas,* V, 1088–1089.

61. For information on Carter and McLaughlin, see *UTMB: Seventy-five Year History,* 74–80, and Inci Bowman, "James Wharton McLaughlin (1840–1909)," *The Bookman,* 7, no. 5 and no. 6 (1980), no. 5, 3–8, no. 6, 3–8. For details about the search for new faculty, see *Galveston Daily News,* July 31, 1897. The regents selected Adolph Bernhard of the Johns Hopkins University School of Medicine to replace Cerna. Bernhard fled when yellow fever appeared to exist in Galveston during the fall of 1897; see *Texas Medical News,* 6, no. 10 (1897), 473; 7, no. 2 (1897), 81.

62. Minutes, UT Board of Regents, Jan. 18–19, 1898. The faculty had adopted a constitution and bylaws in October 1891. Neither a copy of the original nor the proposed revision has been found. For an anecdote about Prather's view of Smith's "Constitution," see page 5 of Anne Brindley's biographical sketch of Smith in the Pathology Department's scrapbook for 1891–1942 in the Blocker Collections. Smith was also unhappy about the stinginess of the legislators and the "old, rotten, dirty" former city hospital building; see "Some of the Needs of the Medical Department," *University Record,* 1, no. 1 (1898), 42–49. In 1914 Dean Carter expressed distress about the absence of any bylaws written by the professors; see W. S. Carter to A. W. Fly, Mar. 5, 1914, letter, box VF 2/B, UT President's Records. In October 1916 Carter and the faculty created a set of "Regulations for the Guidance of the Faculty of the Medical Department"; a copy is in box 4Q24, UT President's Records. Presumably eager to preserve their ultimate political authority, the regents had not approved them by 1925; see William Keiller to W. M. W. Splawn, June 2, 1925, letter, box 4Q24, UT President's Records.

63. Minutes, UT Board of Regents, May 14, 1898; Dec. 10, 1897. After resigning as demonstrator of anatomy, George Lee became a lecturer in dermatology and, after Paine retired, professor of obstetrics and gynecology. See *UTMB: Seventy-five Year History,* 84.

64. In 1890 the first board authorized salaries for a superintendent, steward, druggist, matron, cook, assistant cook, laundry woman, engineer, and fireman; see *Galveston Daily News,* Feb. 11, 1890, and *By-Laws and Rules of the John Sealy Hospital Medical Department of the University of Texas, Galveston, Texas* (Galveston: Clarke & Courts, Stationers and Printers, 1891). They expected the nurses and nursing students to monitor just about everything associated with patient care and they adopted rules governing social functions in the hospital, including smoking, gifts of food, and visitors; *Galveston Daily News,* June 8, 1898. The original rules for nurses, patients, and their families are reprinted in *The Bookman,* 9 (Oct., 1982), 8–11. In 1896 the board appointed Hanna Kindbom as director of the nursing school. Kindbom had trained in Sweden and acquired much practical experience from working in several hospitals in Europe and New York City. In 1899 the board appointed Kindbom as director of the hospital, much to the distress of male interns, who feared supervision by a woman who was not a physician. See *Galveston Daily News,* Mar. 8–9, 1899; May 10, 1899.

65. *Rules and Regulations* (1936), II, 13–14. During the early years, adjunct professor was the label used for today's assistant professor. These arrangements were codified in the *Rules and Regulations* adopted during the 1920s. Preparing Appendix G was not a simple matter. When UTMB began, the regents appointed eight "professors" with specific titles: Anatomy; Physiology and Hygiene; Chemistry and Toxicology; Pathology, Histology and Bacteriology; Materia Medica and Therapeutics; Obstetrics and Gynecology; Theory and Practice of Medicine and Diseases of Children; and Surgery. As these professors added other faculty, departments emerged and the original professors usually served as chairs. As the years evolved, incumbent chairs delegated some departmental interests to teachers who wanted political independence and the regents appointed professors who organized new departments. At which point in time does the designation "department" become appropriate in referring to the political status of these individuals? Atmar Steele Holley became an instructor in radiology in 1917, but no one referred to Holley as a "department." William Boyd Reading became an instructor in pediatrics in 1919 and was promoted stepwise during the next five years, subsequently serving as professor of pediatrics from 1924 to 1943. In Appendix G, Reading is designated as a chair, but not Holley. Chairs or acting

chairs were individuals who had been given administrative authority to self-direct and guide others committed to a career in a particular academic or clinical discipline.

66. T. L. Kennedy, "The Students' Council—Its Origin and Growth," *University Medical*, 1, no. 3 (1895), 111–115. The first comparable effort at UT Austin occurred in 1901; see *Cactus*, 8 (1901), 45, and 9 (1902), 25. See also *University Medical*, 1, no. 3 (1895), 132; 2, no. 7 (1897), 269–270. Smith did return to the University of Pennsylvania as professor of pathology in 1903. For a description of a Friday evening soirée in the west lecture room that included music and readings, see *University Medical*, 1, no. 6 (1896), 255–256, and *Galveston Daily News*, Feb. 22, 1896. Students did cheat and were suspended. For examples during the 1897–1898 year, see the Dean's Office Record Book, 1897–1929, Blocker Collections.

67. *University Medical*, 5, no. 1 (1899), 13–14; W. F. Starley Jr., "The Duty of Our Alumni to State and Alma Mater," *University Medical*, 1, no. 1 (1895), 21–28; F. R. Karback, "Business Managers' Department," *University Medical*, 1, no. 2 (1895), 71–73; and "The Deficiency of the Appropriations for the Medical Department," *University Medical*, 5, no. 4 (1900), 121–126.

68. *Galveston Daily News*, Jan. 6, 1899; *Rules and Regulations* (1897), 13–14; (1899), 6–8.

69. In 1898 pay patients were charged $7 per week for a ward bed, and $15 to $36 for a private room. Before admission, pay patients were expected to make arrangements for reimbursing their physicians; *Galveston Daily News*, June 8, 1898. Burke claimed that "the hospitals of Galveston are well patronized by people from the interior, but they are mostly pay patients who have been attracted here by the superior advantages offered," *Galveston Daily News*, Mar. 22, 1896, Jan 14, 1895 (quotation). Some of these patients were poor immigrants, though how many is not known. Between July 1, 1897, and June 30, 1898, for example, twelve hundred immigrants arrived in Galveston; *Galveston Daily News*, Sept. 1, 1898. According to the U.S. Census for 1890 (p. 509), 20 percent of the population of Galveston County was foreign-born.

70. Minutes, UT Board of Regents, June 15, 1899, and Jan. 25, 1900; *Galveston Daily News*, June 19, 1899. A passionate editorial, "The Deficiency of the Appropriations for the Medical Department," appeared in *University Medical*, 5, no. 4 (1900), 121–126. *Galveston Daily News*, May 2, 1899 (quotation). Competitors in Texas during the 1890s included the University of Texas, Texas A&M, Sam Houston Normal, and Prairie View Normal. In May 1899, for example, the senate discussed appropriations for the University of Texas during three night sessions and one morning session. Afterward, a proposal to appropriate $75,000 was defeated by a vote of 66 to 41, and another for $40,000 was defeated by a vote of 56 to 51; *Galveston Daily News*, May 2, 1899.

71. *Galveston Daily News*, May 26, 1899.

72. For a photo, see *UTMB: Seventy-five Year History*, 99. During the early years, the western half of the building housed blacks (women on the first floor, children on the second, men on the third) and the eastern half housed the nursing students (all three floors). Ordinarily up to thirty patients could be accommodated, though that number could change as circumstances warranted. The faculty voiced concerns about the unsanitary conditions of the rooms for blacks, the attitudes of the nursing students toward black patients, and the difficulties of admitting black patients. See Minutes, UTMB Faculty Meetings, 1891–1893; Minutes, Galveston City Council/Commissioners, Oct. 16, 1893; and William Gammon, "A Brief Sketch of the John Sealy Hospital and the Medical Department of the University of Texas," *University Medical*, 1, no. 3 (1895), 79–80. The nursing students moved to a new house some time in the late 1890s. For photographs, see *Cactus*, 6 (1899), 86, and 7 (1900), 116. Another photo of a "View from Nurses' Home," *Cactus*, 7 (1900), 126, suggests that this house was located just east of University Hall. After the nurses moved to this house, black patients and white children were housed in the original building; *Galveston Daily News*, May 15, 1898.

73. "University Hall, Galveston," *University Record*, 1 (Dec., 1901), 36–39 and *Cactus* (1898), 8. The quotation is from Regent T. S. Henderson's remarks during the dedication of this building in May 1898; see *University Record*, 1 (Dec., 1901), 41. Nursing students were excluded from this residential hall. Early in 1898 the regents named a twelve-member Lady Board of Managers for University Hall. This board gave a formal evening reception in the new building on commencement day, May 14, 1898; see *Galveston Daily News*, May 15, 1898. Breakfast was first served in the dining hall on Sept. 29, 1898; see *Galveston Daily News*, Sept. 29, 1898. Brackenridge was disappointed that the building did not attract more female students, but he continued to provide personal funds to offset the differences between income and the cost of maintaining the building; see Marilyn Sibley, *George Brackenridge: Maverick Philanthropist* (Austin: University of Texas Press, 1973), 178. Honoring his generosity, some referred to the dormitory as Brackenridge Hall; *Galveston Daily News*, May 15, 1910.

74. *Galveston Daily News*, Sept. 9, 1890. Chauncey Leake recalled his view of Old Red for the first time in the fall of 1942. "I was amazed at its unusual construction: curved brick walls at both ends; indented brick work that took master

masons to lay; large and lofty arched windows; graceful towers, and a red tile roof. Clearly this was the work of a great architect." See "A Message from Dr. Chauncey D. Leake," *University Medical*, 4 (Sept., 1972), 17. Gammon, "A Brief Sketch," 86–89.

75. For an explanation of the pavilion design Clayton chose, see Larry Wygant, "The John Sealy Hospital: A Study of Late 19th Century Hospital Design," *Texas Architect*, 30 (Sept./Oct., 1980), 52–55. The 1891–1892 catalog stated that the total capacity was 180 beds; *UTMB Annual Catalog* (1892), 138. This larger number reflected what was possible if maximum capacity was reached in both buildings that housed patients. Regent Thompson reported that the John Sealy Hospital could accommodate ninety-six beds in the general wards and twelve beds in private rooms, and that the city hospital building could expand from thirty to seventy beds if needed. See Lane, *History of the University of Texas*, 171. Also see *Galveston Daily News*, Oct. 2, 1891.

76. For a concise analysis of the emergence of specialization and training hierarchies in American hospitals, see Rosenberg, *The Care of Strangers*, 166–189.

77. The hospital reported its patient care statistics in UTMB's annual catalogs published between 1893–1894 and 1937–1938. Data for the first year were included in the 1893–1894 catalog (pp. 17–21). Until the 1914–1915 year, these catalogs provided diagnostic labels for the diseases or injuries experienced by the patients. None of the reports included demographic data about patients, such as age, race, sex, or occupation.

78. *Galveston Daily News*, Apr. 8, 1894.

79. J. F. Y. Paine, "Report of the Obstetrical Service of the John Sealy Hospital for the Ten Years Ending with 1900," *Transactions, Texas State Medical Association* (1901), 210–216.

80. Officials established a separate ward for white children in the John Sealy Hospital during the 1898–1899 year; see *University Record*, 1, no. 4 (1899), 367.

81. Hospitalized patients from Louisiana, Galveston, and the interior of Texas did acquire malaria, though it is highly probable that some non-malarious febrile illnesses were included in the group labeled "malaria." In evaluating seventy-six patients thought to have malaria, George Dock observed the plasmodium parasite in the blood specimens of only forty-one patients. Dock had examined these patients in Galveston while a member of the Texas Medical College and Hospital faculty between 1888 and 1891; see "Further Studies in Malarial Disease," *Medical News*, 58 (May 30, 1891), 602–606, and (June 6, 1891), 628–634. The most comprehensive source of information about the diseases mentioned in this book is Kenneth F. Kiple (ed), *The Cambridge World History of Human Disease* (Cambridge: Cambridge University Press, 1993).

82. There were fifty-six cases of endometritis between 1891 and 1893; *Transactions, Texas State Medical Association* (1893), 329–330.

83. James Thompson wrote all of these reports: "Operative Procedures in Glandular Tumors of the Neck," *Texas Medical Journal*, 10, no. 7 (1895), 331–338; "Tumors of the Upper Jaw and Naso-Pharynx," *University Medical*, 3, no. 1 (1897), 4–16; "The Technique of Early Operations for Cleft Palate," *Transactions, Texas State Medical Association* (1900), 279–291; and "Treatment of Hare-lip," *Transactions, Texas State Medical Association* (1901), 232–244. See also John T. Moore, "Empyema," *University Medical*, 2, no. 5 (1897), 159–167; John T. Moore, "Report of Case of Strangulated Umbilical Hernia," *University Medical*, 1, no. 2 (1895), 57–60; James Thompson, "When to Operate in Appendicitis," *University Medical*, 3, no. 6 (1898), 208–212; James Thompson, "The Surgical Treatment of Hepatic Neoplasms," *Transactions, Texas State Medical Association* (1899), 216–229; J. Gilbert, "Misplacement of the Kidney, with Report of a Case Operated upon by Dr. J. E. Thompson," *University Medical*, 2, no. 1 (1896), 13–20; J. E. Thompson, "Faecal Fistulae and Artificial Anus," *Texas Medical Journal*, 11, no. 1 (1895), 1–8; and Julius H. Ruhl, "Popliteal Aneurism," *University Medical*, 3, no. 1 (1897), 16–20.

84. Henry P. Cooke, "Cases of Chloroform Anesthesia," *Transactions, Texas State Medical Association* (1896), 248–255; T. D. Berry, "Suggestions on Anaesthesia," *University Medical*, 5, no. 1 (1899), 47–53; J. C. Ralston, "Local Anaesthesia by Infiltration," *University Medical*, 2, no. 8 (1897), 284–286. Via lumbar puncture, William Keiller injected cocaine to numb a patient's gluteal region so that he could investigate infected muscles; see William Keiller, "Cocaine Anesthesia by Lumbar Puncture," *Texas Medical News*, 10, no. 3 (1901), 141–144. Keiller reported: "An attack of vomiting prevented our patient from feeling festive, making jokes, or smoking a cigar, but he had no pain and was able to answer questions which suggested themselves to me during the operation" (p. 141). Thompson removed a sebaceous cyst from the face of a student who was hypnotized by Allen Smith; see "Local and Personal," *University Medical*, 2, no. 5 (1897), 195.

85. "Local and Personal," *University Medical*, 2, no. 5 (1897), 194. Witnessed by other professors and several students, Seth Morris and William Keiller conducted "x-ray experiments" in a small utility room in the basement of Old Red in September 1896; see *Galveston Daily News*, Sept. 12, 1896. Using a Crookes tube, radiographs were made of

fractured or injured limbs of three patients, the arm of a young female visitor, and several tools and coins. During this gathering Morris also demonstrated a fluoroscope. See Seth M. Morris, "Sciagraphy," *University Medical,* 2, no. 6 (1897), 215–219. Before the hospital acquired proper equipment, Morris took X-rays of patients at his office on Twenty-third and Market; *UTMB: Seventy-five Year History,* 158–160; *Galveston Daily News,* May 30, 1937.

86. H. A. West, "Report of Eighteen Cases of Typhoid Fever," *Daniel's Texas Medical Journal,* 8, no. 7 (1893), 249–260; James Thompson, "A Study of Some Surgical Diseases of the Kidney," *Texas Courier–Record of Medicine,* 14, no. 5 (1897), 131–137; and William Gammon, "The Antitoxine of Diphtheria in Practice," *Transactions, Texas State Medical Association* (1895), 325–334.

87. These teachers recommended textbooks. The first list for medical students is in the *UTMB Annual Catalog* (1891–1892), 150–151 (also in *UTMB: Seventy-five Year History,* 395–396). The first list for pharmacy students is in the *UTMB Annual Catalog* (1893–1894), 67–68, and the first one for the nursing students is in the *UTMB Annual Catalog* (1896–1897), 84. Some wrote "texts" for students. David Cerna wrote *Notes on the Newer Remedies, Their Therapeutic Application and Modes of Administration* (Philadephia: W. B. Saunders, 1893). Seth Morris wrote "Laboratory Exercises in Inorganic Chemistry" and "Laboratory Exercises in Physiological and Medical Chemistry," *University Medical,* 1, no. 6 (1896), 260, which were later combined in a single volume titled *Laboratory Exercises in Medical and Pharmaceutical Chemistry* (3rd ed.; n.p., 1902). Allen Smith wrote *Lessons and Laboratory Exercises in Bacteriology* (Philadelphia: P. Blakiston's Son and Co., 1902). Students also used journals and books housed in a small reading room in Old Red. Within a few years, this library contained five hundred volumes and regularly received about one hundred journals; see *UTMB: Seventy-five Year History,* 122. The library circulated 226 items between November 2, 1894, and August 19, 1901; see UTMB Library Circulation Record, 1894–1902, Blocker Collections.

88. Even those who taught basic science subjects, such as Keiller and Morris, continued practicing medicine. Those who taught the basic science subjects had not earned Ph.D. degrees studying those subjects. Those who taught the clinical specialties had not experienced any residency training programs. Graduate degree programs in the basic medical sciences and organized residency training programs were yet to be developed.

89. The following could be admitted to the first year: graduates of recognized colleges, graduates of recognized high schools, those who had a certificate indicating satisfactory performance on an examination given by a county medical society, or those who had passed an entrance exam given by UTMB's professors. The following could be admitted to the second year: graduates in good standing from colleges of pharmacy who had passed the entrance examination and exams in anatomy, histology, and pathology given by the professors; and students who had attended one year of courses in a regular medical school (not homeopathic or eclectic) and had passed exams in anatomy, chemistry, pathology, and materia medica (drugs) given by the professors. The following could be admitted to the third year: graduates of regular medical schools or those who had attended two years of courses in a regular medical school and passed exams in anatomy, chemistry, physiology, pathology, and materia medica given by the faculty.

90. These were the dominant basic science subjects in American medical schools at the turn of the twentieth century. Concise histories of their teaching are in Ronald L. Numbers (ed.), *The Education of American Physicians* (Berkeley: University of California Press, 1980). John B. Blake reviews anatomy (pp. 29–47); John Harley Warner, physiology (pp. 48–71); James Whorton, chemistry (pp. 72–94), David L. Cowen, pharmacology (pp. 95–121), and Russell Maulitz, pathology (pp. 122–142). Keiller shifted dissection to daylight hours for the second term. In April 1892, after six months of classes, the faculty decided that six of the nine students had to complete "make up" work in anatomy and histology, and another had to repeat examinations in three subjects. These students performed satisfactorily and were promoted to the second year. What happened to them after that? One died during his second year. One could not pass the second year courses. Seven completed all three years, with five graduating on schedule in 1894, one in 1896, and the other in 1897. Data about these students were found in the Register of Matriculants and Graduates (1891–1938), and the Register of Grades (1892–1910), Blocker Collections. For the schedules of the classes during 1891–1892, see *UTMB: Seventy-five Year History,* 397–399.

91. Internal medicine, surgery, and obstetrics and gynecology were the dominant clinical subjects in American medical schools at the turn of the twentieth century. Concise histories of their teaching are in Numbers (ed.), *The Education of American Physicians.* Edward C. Atwater reviews internal medicine (pp. 143–174); Gert H. Brieger, surgery (pp. 175–204), and Lawrence D. Longo, obstetrics and gynecology (pp. 205–225). Both Gammon and Jackson were interns during their third year and they were the only graduates in the spring of 1893. For details about Jackson's career, see the Thomas Terrell Jackson Papers, Blocker Collections.

92. J. F. Y. Paine, "Status of Medical Education in the United States, Being the Annual Report of the Dean to the Board of Regents at the Commencement Exercises of the First Session of the Medical Department of the University of

Texas," *Transactions, Texas State Medical Association* (1892), 235–244. Paine re-read this address at the twenty-fourth annual meeting of the Texas State Medical Association held in Tyler a few days after the commencement in Galveston. Privately, Paine's colorful rhetoric did not glow as brightly. The labs for the basic sciences were poorly equipped. Clopton had no animals for vivisection and no equipment for the physiology laboratory. Morris needed equipment for the chemistry laboratory. Smith needed better microscopes and improved facilities for autopsies. Paine had no manikins, models, or charts for teaching obstetrics and gynecology, and Keiller, Randall, and Thompson needed funds to purchase teaching instruments. In spite of these deficiencies, Paine praised the versatility of the faculty as Keiller and Smith had taught chemistry during Morris's six-week-long illness, and Keiller had substituted for Thompson during his prolonged illness. Paine's comments were based on reports submitted by the professors, which are in box 4R85, UT President's Records. For Thompson's first impressions of UTMB, see *Galveston Tribune*, June 5, 1925, and for Smith's negative comments about Old Red, see "Some Memories of the Medical Department in its Beginning," *Alcalde*, 3, no. 8 (1915), 746.

93. Minutes, UT Board of Regents, Apr. 22, 1892. The Medical College building was officially completed on February 23, 1892, fifteen months after the contractor promised to have it ready. Shortly thereafter, Thompson became embroiled in controversies. The attorney general's office helped to resolve those involving payments to the contractor, subcontractors, and suppliers. For details, see letters between Thompson and Charles Culberson (the attorney general), Apr. 11 and 12, 1892, and Thompson's report to Wooten on Apr. 22, 1892, box 4R85, UT President's Records. Other problems involved the provosts and available balances in UTMB's accounts. For details, see letters of T. C. Thompson in UTMB Provost's Office Letterpress Book, Blocker Collections. As provost of the university, James P. Clark thought that his duties were too extensive, and he wanted to transfer fiscal responsibility for UTMB to its provost, J. P. Johnson. Clark was surely correct, if one can judge from the huge ledger of itemized operating expenses for the main university and UTMB between 1888 and 1892, box 4L470, UT President's Records. The regents agreed with Clark, who made no transactions for UTMB after February 9, 1892. On May 24, 1892, there was a balance of $5,116.71 in UTMB's account. See Minutes, UT Board of Regents, Jan. 21, 1892, and *Rules and Regulations* (1892), 27–32 and 23–24 (quotation).

94. *UTMB Annual Catalog* (1900–1901), 17–28. Four demonstrators in the basic sciences (anatomy, pathology, biology, and chemistry) and three in the clinical specialties (gynecology, obstetrics, and surgery) were appointed for the 1900–1901 year. Funds were appropriated for those in the basic sciences, but none were specified for the others. They probably received salaries from the hospital's budget. Such political and financial accountabilities were not inconsequential, as the demonstrator in gynecology, T. L. Kennedy, formally charged J. F. Y. Paine in April 1901 with improper conduct as a clinician and teacher. After an investigation the regents exonerated Paine of all charges and gave him the only salary increase awarded to any of the original professors during the first eleven academic years; Minutes, UT Board of Regents, July 1, 1901.

95. For examples of exams, see the *UTMB Annual Catalog* (1894–1895), 11–12. Of seventy-five students applying for the second-year class in 1897, only three passed the entrance exams; *Galveston Daily News*, Sept. 5, 1897. See Paine's report to the regents, Apr. 30, 1894, box 4R85, UT President's Records, and *Galveston Daily News*, Nov. 13, 1893. By 1897, 60 of the 468 tax-supported public high schools in Texas prepared students for university studies; see George Winston, "Education in the South," *Galveston Daily News*, July 18, 1897. During 1897 and 1898, President Winston visited nearly every high school in Texas; *Galveston Daily News*, Dec. 14, 1897. All of these schools had developed since 1881, when none existed in the state. By 1898 UT allowed graduates of eighty-four of these schools, including Ball High School in Galveston, to enroll without further exams; see C. E. Evans, *The Story of Texas Schools* (Austin: Steck Co., 1955), 122–123, 149–150; and *UTMB Annual Catalog* (1898–1899), 258–263. Though its curriculum prepared them for college studies, only a few Ball High graduates actually attended UT. Not everyone thought that it was a first-class institution. O. H. Cooper, former superintendent of public instruction for the state, harshly criticized UT during his days as superintendent of public schools in Galveston. For information about Ball High, see *Galveston Daily News*, June 26, 1894; Aug. 18, 1894; and Sept. 28, 1894. For the controversies surrounding Cooper's criticisms, see *Galveston Daily News*, Feb. 26, 1893; Mar. 5, 1893; Mar. 19, 1893; and Apr. 3, 1893. Information is available about the educational preparation of 187 physician graduates during UTMB's first ten years. Only eleven from that group received bachelor's degrees from UT; "Department of Medicine, School of Medicine," *University Record*, 4, nos. 1 and 2 (1902), 136–160.

96. See Morris's annual report in box 4R85, UT President's Records; *Galveston Daily News*, Oct. 2, 1895.

97. Minutes, UT Board of Regents, Jan. 15, 1896. The faculty actually initiated the four-year course in the fall of 1896, though they did not require it of all students until the fall of 1897. Strangely, the regents decided that any UT arts and sciences graduate should be allowed to graduate in three years. This rule caused considerable perplexity until it was repealed on January 25, 1900.

98. Catalogs from 1893 to 1896 included questions from some exams: see *UTMB Annual Catalog* (1893–1894), 14–31; (1894–1895), 15–32; and (1895–1896), 16–32. The requirements for promotion and graduation were usually included in the catalogs under the section entitled "Requirements for Admission." For example, see *UTMB Annual Catalog* (1900–1901), 15–17. Special rules for reexamination applied to some students who had failed exams.

99. "Faculty Reports of the Medical Department," *University Record*, 1 (Aug., 1899), 303–315; and "Medical Department Notes," *University Record*, 1 (Oct., 1899), 366–368. For the names of graduates, see *UTMB: Seventy-five Year History*, 327.

100. A list of the names of matriculates between 1893 and 1926 is in a bound volume 17, Blocker Collections. Students eligible for admission to the School of Pharmacy were those who had college degrees or had passed entrance examinations of recognized colleges, or possessed diplomas from recognized high schools, or held a first-grade teacher's certificate, or passed exams in arithmetic and writing given by UTMB professors. Matriculates could not be younger than seventeen years old. Students who had attended another pharmacy school for one year and passed exams given by UTMB teachers could be admitted to the second year. Henry M. Burlage and Margot E. Beutler, *Pharmacy's Foundation in Texas* (Austin: Pharmaceutical Foundation of the College of Pharmacy of the University of Texas at Austin, 1978), 40.

101. The first complete description of the school (including a schedule of courses) is in the *UTMB Annual Catalog* (1895–1996), 69–78. Beginning in the *UTMB Annual Catalog* (1896–1897), 75–76, names of the matriculates were listed for each year.

102. For their names, see *UTMB: Seventy-five Year History*, 352.

103. Using several sources, Cheryl Vaiani prepared the list of names in Table 1. Even before the medical school opened, these politically adroit women sponsored a luncheon reception for the regents when they met in Galveston in August 1891. Regent E. J. Simpkins admitted that the outstanding work of the nursing students had caused a change in his attitude about the overall value of UTMB; *Galveston Daily News*, Aug. 27, 1891. For a glimpse of the esteem accorded the nursing school, see reports in *Galveston Daily News*, Jan. 14, 1894; Apr. 8, 1894; and Apr. 11, 1895. Some of the women managers were also involved in other charitable organizations in Galveston; see Elizabeth Hayes Turner, *Women, Culture, and Community: Religion and Reform in Galveston, 1880–1920* (New York: Oxford University Press, 1997), 121–150. The best source of detailed information about the School of Nursing is Billye J. Brown, "The Historical Development of the University of Texas System School of Nursing, 1890–1973" (Ed.D. diss., Baylor University, 1975). Also see Inci Bowman, "John Sealy Hospital Training School for Nurses," *The Bookman*, 9 (Oct., 1982), 3–5, and the excellent brochure titled "A Century of Excellence, A Vision for the Future School of Nursing 1890–1990." Poldi Tschirch wrote this brochure for the school's centennial celebration; a copy is in WF338, CHP Archives. For more on the history of nursing and nursing education in Texas, see Poldi Tschirch and Eleanor L. M. Crowder, "Nursing," in Tyler, et al. (eds.), *The New Handbook of Texas*, IV, 1079–1082, and Eleanor L. M. Crowder, "Nursing Education," in Tyler, et al. (eds.), *The New Handbook of Texas*, IV, 1082–1083. For the history of nursing in the United States, see Philip A. Kalisch and Beatrice J. Kalisch, *The Advance of American Nursing* (Boston: Little, Brown and Company, 1986) and Susan M. Reverby, *Ordered to Care: The Dilemma of American Nursing, 1850–1945* (Cambridge: Cambridge University Press, 1987).

104. Mrs. J. G. Goldthwaite to Board of Regents, Dec. 19, 1894, letter, box VF 11/E, UT President's Records; Minutes, UT Board of Regents, Jan. 16, 1895, and June 20, 1895. Durkee, for unknown reasons, resigned a few months later; see Minutes, UT Board of Regents, Jan. 15, 1896. In T. C. Thompson to T. D. Wooten, Mar. 3, 1896, letter, Wooten Papers, Thompson reported that the Sealy Hospital Board would pay the balance of the expenses of the Training School if the regents would continue to give between $1,200 and $1,500 each year. *Galveston Daily News*, Mar. 22, 1896. The nursing students received room, board, and seven dollars each month. Paine was also delighted that the ratio of nurses to Sealy hospital inpatients (one to six) was better than anywhere else. For a concise summary of the emergence of professional nurses in American hospitals, see Rosenberg, *The Care of Strangers*, 212–236.

105. Eight members of the former Lady Board became an Auxiliary Board of Lady Managers, serving as an advisory group to the Hospital Board. The names in Appendix Q were obtained from annual catalogs and a list John Spies gave to Homer Rainey, Aug. 5, 1939, box VF 9/C, UT President's Records. Between 1934 and 1939, Edward H. Schwab Jr., physician to the nursing school, also served as a member. *UTMB Annual Catalog* (1896–1897), 77–79; *Galveston Daily News*, Mar. 22, 1897.

106. The student nurses could matriculate any time between May and October. No academic requirements were specified. Caucasian women between the ages of nineteen and thirty-five were expected to bring two letters of reference about their moral character and one from a physician regarding their "sound health." By 1898 the minimum age had increased to twenty-three years, and a UTMB physician evaluated the health of prospective students in the presence of the superintendent of nurses. For photos of uniforms, see *UTMB: Seventy-five Year History*, 90, 92, and 192. For a photo

of the nurses on the surgical ward of the hospital in 1900, see Eleanor Crowder, *Nursing in Texas: A Pictorial History* (Waco: Texian Press, 1980), 8.

107. For interesting examples of Kindbom's approach to the management of inflammation, to techniques of administering enemas, and to the preparation of operating room supplies, see Hanna Kindbom, "Inflammation: Its Cause, Symptoms and Treatment," *University Medical*, 2 (Dec., 1896), 96–98; 2 (Jan., 1897), 142–143; 2 (Feb., 1897), 180–182; 2 (Apr., 1897), 251–253; and 2 (May, 1897), 294–295; "Enemas—Enemata—Clyster," *University Medical*, 3 (Nov., 1897), 35–40; and "Preparation of Op. Room Supplies," *University Medical*, 3 (Dec., 1897), 77–78; 3 (Jan., 1898), 117–118; 3 (Feb., 1898), 153–155; 3 (Mar., 1898), 195–197; and 3 (Apr., 1898), 236–237. Kindbom also urged nurses to use silver dishes or china for serving meals to patients, with the dishes arranged "like a beautifully painted picture, each dish a piece of art in itself." See Hanna Kindbom, "The Serving of Food to Invalids," *University Medical*, 4 (Jan., 1899), 151–155 (quotations on 152).

108. *Galveston Daily News*, Jan. 11, 1897. Ninety-year-old Fanny Durst Putegnat vividly remembered her hard work as a student nurse who graduated in the class of 1893; *Galveston Daily News*, Aug. 2, 1963. Eighteen students enrolled in the 1896–1897 year (eleven first years and seven second years), twenty-one in 1897–1898 (twelve first years, nine second years), nineteen in 1898–99 (ten first years, nine second years), twenty-one in 1899–1900 (twelve first years, nine second years) and twenty-one in 1900–1901 (nine first years, twelve second years). See *UTMB Annual Catalog* (1896–1897), 83; (1897–1898), 85; (1898–1899), 253; (1899–1900), 85; and (1900–1901), 85. Four of the women named as first-year students in 1897 were named again as first-year students in 1898. Perhaps they were asked to repeat the year, or perhaps there was an error in listing. These four were not included in the total number of matriculates designated for 1898 in Appendix P. Also, in every year, two or three of the nursing students were listed as "Mrs." Whether single, divorced, or married, they were expected to live on campus. After the March graduation, *Galveston Daily News*, Mar. 22, 1897, fifty women applied for the seven vacancies created by the new graduates. While the school was privately operated between 1890 and 1896, eighty-two students had survived the first month's probation. Of those, thirty-two graduated, eighteen withdrew voluntarily, twenty-two were dismissed, and ten were still enrolled. For the names of some early graduates, see *UTMB: Seventy-five Year History*, 344. *Galveston Daily News*, Jan. 11, 1897 (quotation).

109. Articles by H. A. West included "Address by H. A. West, M.D.," *Transactions, Texas State Medical Association* (1891), 63–75; "The Diagnosis of Miliary Tuberculosis," *Transactions, Texas State Medical Association* (1892), 96–106; "The Association of Diseases and Morbid Processes," *Transactions, Texas State Medical Association* (1893), 84–96; and "Bacteriological Aspects of Croupous Pneumonia," *Transactions, Texas State Medical Association* (1894), 75–93. Reports by James E. Thompson included "Operative Treatment in Typhoid Perforation of the Intestine," *Transactions, Texas State Medical Association* (1893), 266–275; "The Operative Treatment of Neglected Cases of Hip Joint Disease," *Transactions, Texas State Medical Association* (1894), 177–183; and "Cysts of the Spermatic Cord and Testicle," *Texas Medical Journal*, 9, no. 9 (1894), 433–437. By the summer of 1901 Thompson had written twenty-nine publications. See a complete bibliography in folder 3, James E. Thompson Papers, Blocker Collections. J. F. Y. Paine's essays included "Some Practical Observations on the Management of Albuminuria in Pregnancy," *Transactions, Texas State Medical Association* (1891), 151–166; "Report of Chairman, J. F. Y. Paine, M.D.," *Transactions, Texas State Medical Association* (1893), 313–330; "The Present Status of Symphyseotomy and its Relation to Other Obstetric Operations," *Transactions, Texas State Medical Association* (1894), 324–331; and "Some Remarks on the Essential Etiology of Eclampsia," *Transactions, Texas State Medical Association* (1898), 146–151. Reports by Cooke included "The Relation of Chorea to Rheumatism," *Transactions, Texas State Medical Association* (1892), 146–153; "Protracted Varicella," *American Journal of Obstetrics*, 33, no. 4 (1896), 497–501; and "Progress in Treatment of Typhoid Fever," *Transactions, Texas State Medical Association* (1900), 135–151. Articles by George Lee were "Report and Address of the Chairman," *Transactions, Texas State Medical Association* (1892), 267–273; "Diagnosis in Diseases of the Skin," *University Medical*, 1, no. 3 (1895), 93–100; "Report of Chairman Geo. H. Lee, M.D.," *Transactions, Texas State Medical Association* (1896), 425–431; and "The Diagnosis of Eczema," *University Medical*, 3, no. 5 (1898), 159–164. Reports by R. C. Hodges included "Clinical Notes," *Daniel's Texas Medical Journal*, 6, no. 12 (1891), 493–497, and "Polypi of Middle Ear and Auditory Canal as a Cause of Suppurative Otitis," *Daniel's Texas Medical Journal*, 7, no. 5 (1891), 199–204. George Hall wrote "A Contribution to the Study of the Insufficiencies of the Ocular Muscles, with Measures Directed to Their Relief," *Transactions, Texas State Medical Association* (1893), 373–378, and "Some of the Toxic Effects of Tobacco on the General Organism, with Especial Reference to Its Effects on the Eye," *International Medical Magazine*, 3, no. 3 (1895), 178–181.

110. Robert P. Hudson, *Disease and Its Control: The Shaping of Modern Thought* (New York: Praeger, 1983), 121–139.

111. A. G. Clopton to T. D. Wooten, Aug. 29, 1891, July 7, 1892, and Sept. 13, 1892, letters, Wooten Papers. For a biographical sketch of Cerna, see "Biographical. Dr. David Cerna," *Daniel's Texas Medical Journal*, 8, no. 7 (1893),

286–287. At the University of Pennsylvania, Cerna had studied the physiological actions of anesthetics and certain alkaloids; see "The Antagonism between Opium and Belladonna," *Daniel's Texas Medical Journal*, 8, no. 6 (1892), 205–215. Cerna's mentor was Horatio C. Woods, one of America's first experimental physiologists and pharmacologists. See Horatio C. Wood, "Reminiscences of an American Pioneer in Experimental Medicine," *Transactions of the College of Physicians of Philadelphia*, 42, 3rd ser. (1920), 195–234. See Edward Randall and David Cerna, "A Contribution to the Study of the Action of Chloroform," *Transactions, Texas State Medical Association* (1894), 201–216. Though Randall had learned about experimental medicine during postgraduate studies in Europe, the stimulus for this research came from Cerna, who had an interest in this drug before coming to Galveston. This paper is the only example of Randall's participation in experimental research during his long career at UTMB.

112. David Cerna, "Phenacetin as a Toxic Agent," *Transactions, Texas State Medical Association* (1895), 126–132 and "A Note on the Action of Apolysin," *Transactions, Texas State Medical Association* (1896), 176–186. William S. Carter, "Preliminary Communication on the Relation of the Parathyroids to the Thyroid Gland," *Transactions, Texas State Medical Association* (1901), 387–398.

113. Minutes, UT Board of Regents, Apr. 30, 1894. After his appointment in 1891 Morris had journeyed to Europe twice for postgraduate studies in chemistry. His promotion to professor at the age of twenty-seven was probably the fastest in the annals of UTMB. See T. C. Thompson to T. D. Wooten, Feb. 18, 1895, letter, Wooten Papers, and *Daniel's Texas Medical Journal*, 8, no. 4 (1892), 153. A devoted assistant and popular teacher, Flavin agreed with Keiller that the only way to learn anatomy was by dissecting a cadaver; see B. T. Flavin, "Teaching Anatomy in Medical Schools," *Texas Medical Journal*, 9, no. 4 (1893), 155–159. Unexplained differences in salaries among the professors occurred from their first appointments. Why one should earn $500 more or $250 less than another was never specified. Such inequities persisted with no apparent rationale. Regent Thompson was distressed that the salaries paid to UTMB's professors were $2,000 to $3,000 lower than those at the better medical schools in the United States; see T. C. Thompson, "Brief Review of the Medical Department, University of Texas," 1897. This pamphlet was published as an unnumbered *University of Texas Bulletin* (Center for American History, University of Texas at Austin). Though specific amounts are not known, most of these professors earned income from providing clinical services to private patients, presumably enough to offset the smaller salaries of the region as well as the salary differentials between individual professors.

114. Since published statistics for these years do not indicate race, conclusions about race are based on class photos in the *Cactus*, the yearbook for University of Texas students that began publication in 1896. Hometowns are given in the annual catalogs.

115. *University Medical*, 1, no. 1 (1895), 40. In 1898 Keiller unequivocally declared that doctoring was man's work and nursing was woman's work; see William Keiller, "Address Delivered to the Class of '98 at the Regular Commencement Exercises," *University Medical*, 4, no. 1 (1898), 1–10. Also see Larry J. Wygant, "A Note on the Early Medical Education of Women at UTMB," *The Bookman*, 7 (Mar., 1980), 3–5, and *University Medical*, 2, no. 6 (1897), 236; 3, no. 3 (1898), 147; and 5, no. 5 (1900), 163.

116. These numbers were derived from the student directory for 1899–1900 published in *University Record*, 1, no. 4 (1899), 392–396. There were four rooming houses that sheltered eight or more students and eleven with six or more. E. C. Northen lived at 925 Strand. Matriculating in 1904 at the age of thirty-one, he withdrew in 1907 after developing an eye disease. He became an insurance broker in 1913 and married Mary Elizabeth Moody on December 1, 1915. For other details about living arrangements for students, see the "Student Housing" folder, WF383, CHP Archives. Information about the dining hall is in *University Medical*, 5, no. 1 (1899), 22; 5, no. 3 (1899), 99–100; 5, no. 6 (1900), 196; 7, no. 2 (1902), 42–45; and *Cactus*, 7 (1900), 126, 201.

117. The poem is from "History," *Cactus*, 5 (1898), 72–73. Other examples of class spirit are depicted in *Cactus*, 5 (1898), 66–67, and 8 (1901), 82–83. For examples of bonding, see *University Medical*, 1, no. 8 (1896), 335; 3, no. 3 (1898), 113–114; 3, no.4 (1898), 148; 4, no. 2 (1898), 81; 5, no. 2 (1899), 63; and 5, no. 5 (1900), 159.

118. "History of Class of 1902," *Cactus*, 7 (1900), 97 (1st quotation); "History of the Class of '97," *Cactus*, 4 (1897), 66 (2nd quotation). Also see "Medicine '98," *Cactus*, 4 (1897), 68; and "History," *Cactus*, 5 (1898), 66–68, 78.

119. *Cactus*, 4 (1897), 131, 134–135; 5 (1898), 124, 127–128; and 6 (1899), 121, 123, and 119; *University Medical*, 1, no. 6 (1896), 260; 2, no. 4 (1897), 157; 2, no. 5 (1897), 199–200; 3, no. 1 (1897), 33; 3, no. 4 (1898), 144; 4, no. 2 (1898), 73; and 5, no. 3 (1899), 106; *Cactus*, 5 (1898), 115; 7 (1900), 199. For the YMCA, see *Galveston Daily News*, Oct. 7, 1899. Medical students and pharmacy students organized pre-professional associations. For example, in December 1895 a group of senior medical students organized a Senior Class Medical Society, whose members met monthly to read and discuss scientific papers, some of which were published in *University Medical*; see *University Medical*, 1, no. 3 (1895), 129; 1, no. 4 (1896), 180; 1, no. 8 (1896), 341–342. In 1896 pharmacy students organized

the Pharmaceutical Association of the University of Texas, which maintained a membership of thirty to forty through-out the 1890s; see *University Medical*, 2, no. 1 (1896), 35–36; 2, no. 6 (1897), 231; 2, no. 8 (1897), 300; 5, no. 1 (1899), 23; 5, no. 4 (1900), 129; 5, no. 5 (1900), 159; and *Cactus*, 5 (1898), 81.

120. *University Medical*, 1, no. 6 (1896), 255–256; 1, no. 7 (1896), 288–291; 3, no. 4 (1898), 146; 5, no. 1 (1899), 15; *Cactus*, 4 (1897), 78; and *Galveston Daily News*, Oct. 20, 1899. See also Howard R. Dudgeon Sr. "My Recollections of the Medical Department of the University of Texas at Galveston," 11, typescript prepared in the early 1950s by Howard R. Dudgeon Jr., Blocker Collections. Theft of microscope lenses from the histology lab, mutilation of speci-mens in the anatomy museum, and other incidents of vandalism occurred; see *University Medical*, 2, no. 6 (1897), 234; 3, no. 2 (1897), 64; 4, no. 5 (1899), 205; and *Cactus*, 4 (1897), 76. Minutes, UTMB Faculty Meetings (1891–1893), Sept. 30, 1892 (quotation).

121. For descriptions of some opening ceremonies, see *Galveston Daily News*, Oct. 3, 1893; Oct. 2, 1894; Oct. 2, 1895; Oct. 2, 1896; Oct. 2, 1897; Sept. 29, 1898; and Oct. 3, 1899. Graduation ceremonies for nursing students were held separately between 1892 and 1897. For examples of ceremonies, see *Galveston Daily News*, May 3, 1893; May 2, 1894; May 16, 1895; May 16, 1896; May 16, 1897; May 15, 1898; and May 14, 1899. Medical students who attained the highest grades on certain exams or in all their courses received medals, books, or cash prizes. For undisclosed rea-sons, these prizes were discontinued in 1898. See *UTMB Annual Catalog* (1897–1898), 61.

122. See *University Record*, 4, nos. 1 and 2 (1902), 136–167, for information about the graduates' careers. For more information about particular graduates, see the regular sections of *University Medical* variously entitled Alumni Notes, Personals, Locals, or Alumni Department. For nursing graduates, see *University Medical*, 4, no. 3 (1898), 102–103. Between 1892 and 1896, twenty-six nurses graduated from the privately operated John Sealy Hospital Training School; see Paine's comments in *Galveston Daily News*, Mar. 22, 1896. Unfortunately, little is known about the careers of those graduating from the School of Nursing before 1900. Seventy-eight pharmacy students had graduated by 1902 and most were practicing pharmacists in Texas. Six lived in other states and six had entered medical school. See *University Medical*, 7, no. 3 (1902), 89; and *University Record*, 1, no. 2 (1899), 139–143.

123. *Galveston Daily News*, May 2, 1894. A member of UTMB's first graduating class, Gammon was a distinguished practitioner in Galveston until his death in 1937; see *Texas State Journal of Medicine*, 32 (May, 1937), 67. *University Medical*, 1, no. 8 (1896), 337–338; 2, no. 8 (1897), 308; *Galveston Daily News*, May 16, 1897; *University Medical*, 4, no. 1 (1898), 16; *Texas Medical News*, 7, no. 7 (1898), 306; *Galveston Daily News*, May 14, 1898, and May 13, 1899; *University Record*, 2, no. 2 (1900), 201–202. The loyalty of Medical Department graduates even preceded that of alum-ni from the main campus. UT graduates residing in Galveston organized a short-lived alumni association that was super-seded by a statewide alumni association, which held its first banquet in Dallas on October 21, 1899; see *Galveston Daily News*, July 28, 1897, and July 29, 1898; and *University Record*, 2, no. 1 (1900), 44–45.

124. *Galveston Daily News*, Jan. 24, 1897; Register of Patients of St. Mary's Infirmary from 1899 to 1903, 7–10 (Villa de Matel archives, Houston).

125. "Galveston County Medical Society," *Texas Medical Journal*, 9, no. 6 (1893), 290. Jacob Sampson, a senior med-ical student, was first vice-president. Twelve members, three physician guests, and five medical students listened to Keiller's paper on "Uterine Hemorrhages" given during their meeting in December 1893; see *Texas Medical Journal*, 9, no. 7 (1894), 313–320. Active participation in civic organizations was also characteristic of faculty and alumni. Citizens elected Hamilton West as alderman in 1895 and again in 1897; see Minutes, Galveston City Council/Commissioners, June 8 and 17, 1895, June 11 and 21, 1897; and *Galveston Daily News*, June 8, 15, and 22, 1897. In both years he was appointed to the aldermen's Health and Hospital Committee. Allen Smith and David Cerna were members of the Texas Historical Society, and Cerna was appointed Mexican Consul in Galveston; see *Galveston Daily News*, Mar. 17, 1896, and Oct. 13, 1896; and *Texas Medical Journal*, 12, no. 8 (1897), 463. Cerna left Galveston in 1897 to return to his eighty thousand-acre family hacienda in the state of Coahuila; see *Galveston Daily News*, Sept. 22, 1898.

126. TSMA members in Galveston included Charles C. Barrell, David Cerna, W. I. Ducie, Thomas Flavin, J. M. Gary, John B. Haden, J. P. Hendrick, William Keiller, W. A. McAlpine, Allen J. Smith, and James E. Thompson. See *Transactions, Texas State Medical Association* (1893), 19. This list is incomplete as Clopton and Paine were not named even though they were the official UTMB delegates; Minutes, UTMB Faculty Meetings, Apr. 29, 1893. West reported that only half of the fifty-four scheduled papers were read, but each prompted vigorous discussion. At this meeting the doctors decided to allow women to become members; see *Daniel's Texas Medical Journal*, 8, no. 12 (1893), 515–517. See also *Transactions, Texas State Medical Association* (1893), 9–11. New graduates and professors readily joined the TSMA: William Gammon and Seth Morris in 1894, Isaac Cline in 1895, Thomas L. Kennedy and W. F. Starley Jr in 1896, William S. Carter in 1899, James W. McLaughlin in 1900, and John T. Moore in 1901.

127. All of the information about the academy is taken from the Academy's Minute Book, box 2H27, Texas Academy of Science Collection (Center for American History, University of Texas at Austin), and from volume 1 of the *Transactions of the Texas Academy of Science.*

128. *Galveston Daily News,* Dec. 28, 1895 (quotation); "South Texas Medical Association," *University Medical,* 2, no. 3 (1896), 109–114; "South Texas Medical Association—Second Annual Meeting—Galveston," *Texas Medical Journal,* 12, no. 12 (1897), 682–684; "South Texas Medical Association," *University Medical,* 4, no. 3 (1898), 112–114.

129. "Foreign Correspondence Letter from Prof. J. E. Thompson, M.D.," *Daniel's Texas Medical Journal,* 8, no. 2 (1892), 67–68; "Medical News and Miscellany," *Daniel's Texas Medical Journal,* 8, no. 11 (1893), 482; and "Axis Traction Forceps. Letter from Prof. Wm. Keiller, M.D. of Edinburg, Professor of Anatomy, University of Texas Medical College," *Daniel's Texas Medical Journal,* 8, no. 12 (1893), 512–515; "The Professors," *Texas Medical Journal,* 10, no. 1 (1894), 32. Thompson attended the meeting of the British Medical Association in July 1892, whose attendees decided to permit women to become members. "Medical News and Miscellany," *Daniel's Texas Medical Journal,* 8, no. 12 (1893), 525. T. C. Thompson to T. D. Wooten, Feb. 18, 1895, letter, Wooten Papers, and "Medical News and Miscellany," *Daniel's Texas Medical Journal,* 8, no. 4 (1892), 153. T. J. Bennett, M.D., and J. W. M'Laughlin, M.D., "Society Proceedings. The First Pan-American Medical Congress. Notes of the Meeting," *Texas Sanitarian,* 2, no. 11 (1893), 457–466. Cerna, Smith, and West presented papers at the Pan-American Medical Congress. For Gammon, see "Personal," *Texas Courier–Record of Medicine,* 13, no. 7 (1896), 180, and "Medical News and Miscellany," *Texas Medical Journal,* 11, no. 10 (1896), 583. For Cerna, see David Cerna, "Random Notes on the Second Pan-American Medical Congress held at the City of Mexico, November 16, 17, 18, 19, 1896," *University Medical,* 2, no. 3 (1896), 88–96; and *Galveston Daily News,* Nov. 28, 1896. See also Hanna Kindbom, "Impressions by the Way," *University Medical,* 4, no. 1 (1898), 21–24; 4, no. 2 (1898), 67–70; and 4, no. 3 (1898), 105–106.

130. "The Alleged Medical College of Texas," *Texas Health Journal,* 5, no. 11 (1893), 289 (1st quotation); "The Medical Department of the University of Texas," *Texas Sanitarian,* 4, no. 9 (1895), 396 (2nd quotation).

131. Using data from John Rauch's report of the Illinois State Board of Health about American medical schools published in 1891, Paine noted that the admission and graduation requirements of many schools had improved significantly. In 1882, only 29 schools specified any admission requirements, whereas 129 did in 1891. In 1891, 85 schools required attendance at three annual courses of lectures, whereas only 22 had that requirement in 1882. In 1882, 42 schools had annual sessions of six months or longer; in 1891, 111 schools had such sessions. In the better schools, students were required to do practical work in laboratories of histology, chemistry, physiology, pathology, bacteriology, and pharmacology. Paine used this data to claim that UTMB had been established according to the higher standards of the better schools. During the 1890s, there were numerous controversies about proper standards for those judged as worthy members of the AAMC and the ASMC. In the fall of 1894, a professor (unnamed) praised the thorough clinical training at UTMB, claiming that its standards were much higher than those championed by the AAMC; *Galveston Daily News,* Oct. 1, 1894. Even former presidents of the AAMC were distressed about that organization's reputation at the turn of the century. In E. Fletcher Ingals of Rush Medical College (president of the AAMC in 1894–95) to William Howells of Johns Hopkins University, Dec. 18, 1899, letter, box 1, Miscellaneous Historical Documents (AAMC Archives, Washington, D.C.), Ingals remarked that it was a "disgrace" to belong to the AAMC because too many "poor colleges" had become members and lowered the standards of the association.

132. "An Epoch in Medical History," *Daniel's Texas Medical Journal,* 8, no. 6 (1892), 230–235, 243–244. The faculty had elected Allen Smith as their representative in 1892, but Smith's wife died and Thompson replaced Smith. "Association of Southern Medical Colleges," *Texas Sanitarian,* 2, no. 2 (1892), 88–89 (quotation). For matriculation at member colleges, students were required to have college or high school diplomas or certificates attesting educational qualifications equivalent to those required for second-grade teachers. For graduation, students were required to attend three years of not less than six months of formal courses annually that included dissection, laboratory work, and clinical training. At the meeting in 1898, representatives agreed to a four-year medical school curriculum for all students matriculating after January 1, 1899; see "Southern Medical Colleges," *Texas Medical News,* 8, no. 2 (1898), 92, and "Meeting of the Southern Medical College Association, Memphis, December 5, 1899," *New Orleans Medical and Surgical Journal,* 51, no. 7 (1899), 400. Nine schools sent representatives to the meeting in New Orleans in December 1899. The medical college in Fort Worth was represented, but no one attended from UTMB; see "Meeting of the Southern Medical College Association, Memphis, December 5, 1899," *New Orleans Medical and Surgical Journal,* 52, no. 7 (1900), 404.

133. *Galveston Daily News,* Oct. 2, 1895. See the letter by T. C. Thompson dated Feb. 23, 1895, in Lane, *History of Education in Texas,* 222. In 1892, twenty Texans were among the ninety-six physician graduates from Tulane; see "Editorial Notes and Miscellany," *Texas Sanitarian,* 1, no. 8 (1892), 439. Between 1834 and 1890 Tulane graduated

2,500 physicians and 199 pharmacists; see "Annual Report of Professor S. E. Chaille Dean of the Medical Department of Tulane University of Louisiana," *New Orleans Medical and Surgical Journal*, 17, no.11 (1890), 825. Thirty-seven of the 122 graduates from the Memphis Hospital Medical College in 1894 were from Texas, 15 in 1895, 11 in 1897; see *Texas Medical Journal*, 9, no. 12 (1894), 646; 10, no. 10 (1895), 546–547; and 12, no. 12 (1897), 692. Vanderbilt had 43 matriculates from Texas in 1893, 15 in 1897; see "Publishers' Notes," *Texas Medical Journal*, 10, no. 1 (1894), 41; and "Publishers' Notes," *Texas Medical News*, 6, no. 9 (1897), 394. In 1895–1896, there were 25 students from Texas at the University of Louisville and 18 at the University of Tennessee; see *Texas Medical News*, 5, no. 10 (1896), 472–473.

134. Gammon, "A Brief Sketch," *University Medical*, 77–89.

CHAPTER 2

1. Chauncey D. Leake to Chauncey Jr., Wilson, and Dorothy, Feb. 13, 1952, letter, box 1, Leake Papers, NLM.

2. These included Smith (1903–1905), Marcellus E. Kleberg (1905–1907), M. Marx (1907–1909), A. W. Fly (1909–1911; 1913–1917), John Sealy II (1917–1919), Mart H. Royston (1925–1927), Edward Randall Sr. (1929–1940), and Fred C. Branson (1940–1942).

3. For a biographical sketch of Carter, see Chester R. Burns, "William Spencer Carter," in Tyler, et al. (eds.), *The New Handbook of Texas*, I, 1002.

4. After President Houston's visit to Galveston in October 1907, for example, he and Regent George Brackenridge discussed the possibility of teaching the first two years of the medical school's courses in Austin. See *Galveston Daily News*, Oct. 10, 1907, and David Houston to George Brackenridge, Dec. 23, 1907, letter, box 4R19, UT President's Records.

5. Abraham Flexner, *Medical Education in the United States and Canada* (New York: The Carnegie Foundation for the Advancement of Teaching, 1910), 312 (quotation). The Carnegie Foundation had invited Flexner to visit and evaluate all North American medical schools. W. S. Carter to S. A. Mezes, n.d. [c. April 1910], letter, box 4R82, UT President's Records.

6. S. E. Mezes to G. W. Brackenridge, June 16, 1911, letter, box VF 2/B, UT President's Records. When visiting Galveston, however, Mezes publicly praised UTMB and declared its location in the port city as ideal; *Galveston Daily News*, Oct. 11, 1908; Apr. 11, 1909; Jan. 22, 1910; Jan. 23, 1910; and May 30, 1911.

7. S. E. Mezes to Clarence Ousley, Apr. 26, 1911, letter, box VF 2/B, UT President's Records; W. S. Carter to S. E. Mezes, May 3, 1911, letter, box 4R82, and May 17, 1911, letter, box 4Q18, UT President's Records.

8. W. S. Carter, M. L. Graves, and Edward Randall to the UT Board of Regents, Oct. 13, 1911, letter, box 4Q18, UT President's Records; W. S. Carter to S. E. Mezes, Jan. 27, 1913, Jan. 31, 1913, May 2, 1913, letters, box 4Q19, UT President's Records. The new lease contained provisions that directly addressed the relocation issue: title to Block 668 would revert to the City of Galveston if UTMB closed, and lots in Block 667, which John Sealy II had given to the hospital, would revert to him if the property was not used for hospital facilities. See B. F. Looney to O. B. Colquitt, Nov. 19, 1914, letter, box VF 11/E, UT President's Records.

9. *Rules and Regulations* (1918), 4–7, and Minutes, UT Board of Regents, June 9, 1919, and June 7, 1920. City and state politicos resisted demands for more "charity" dollars. W. S. Carter to R. E. Vinson, Jan. 26, 1919, letter, box 4Q22, UT President's Records.

10. Ludmerer, *Learning to Heal*, 191–206; W. S. Carter to Abraham Flexner, Oct. 18, 1919, letter, box 4Q22, UT President's Records.

11. *Galveston Daily News*, Jan. 6, 1920; W. S. Carter to R. E. Vinson, c. Jan. 10, 1920, letter, box 4Q22, UT President's Records.

12. The $30,000 figure was about twice that expended by the city of Houston for its indigent sick and about two and one half times that expended by the city of San Antonio for the same purpose, even though both of these cities had populations that were more than twice as large as Galveston. Such comparisons appeared to justify the decisions of the city commissioners, but power politics may have played a more crucial role. In March 1920, Mayor H. O. Sappington told a John Sealy Hospital intern that the commissioners intended "to close the institution up as the hospital was run by Drs. Randall, Thompson, and Graves." See W. S. Carter to R. E. Vinson, Nov. 29, 1920, letter, box 4R81, UT President's Records; Minutes, UT Board of Regents, Apr. 27, 1920 (1st quotation); W. S. Carter to R. E. Vinson, Mar. 27, 1920, letter, box 4Q22, UT President's Records (2nd quotation); *Galveston Daily News*, May 25, 1920 (3rd quotation).

13. W. R. Brents to R. E. Vinson, Apr. 1, 1920, letter, box VF 2/A, UT President's Records (1st quotation). Carter told Vinson that the trustees of the Hermann estate were developing a plan to move UTMB to Houston; see W. S.

Carter to R. E. Vinson, May 9, 1920, letter, box 4Q22, UT President's Records. W. H. Dougherty to R. E. Vinson, May 20, 1920, letter, box VF 2/A, UT President's Records (2nd quotation).

14. *Galveston Daily News*, June 14, 1920. For a list of the governors of Texas between 1846 and 1991, see Appendix A-2, WF441, CHP Archives. "The people of Galveston should wake up to the fact that the Medical College is a valuable asset to the City, and make some effort to provide for it," proclaimed T. J. Crow, secretary of the Texas State Board of Medical Examiners, which met in Galveston during the latter part of June; *Galveston Daily News*, June 25, 1920. The board applauded Hobby for establishing a committee to investigate the fate of UTMB. The board correctly believed that UTMB ranked with the "best medical colleges in the country," but that it would not be able to maintain this high standing if its facilities were not improved; see T. J. Crow to W. P. Hobby, June 30, 1920, letter, box 4R84, UT President's Records. *Galveston Tribune*, June 26, 1920; *Galveston Daily News*, July 1 and 4, 1920; T. J. Manton to R. E. Vinson, July 14, 1920, and W. S. Carter to R. E. Vinson, July 19, 1920, letters, box 4Q22, UT President's Records; and *Galveston Daily News*, July 30 and 31, 1920. The protesting groups included the Galveston Commercial Association, the Young Men's Progressive League, the Retail Merchants' Association, the Cotton Exchange and Board of Trade, the Galveston Ministerial Association, the Rotary Club of Galveston, and the Longshoremen's Association.

15. *Galveston Daily News*, Oct. 1, 1920. Also see T. E. Jackson and Mabry Seay to Members Special Legislative Committee on State Medical School, Nov. 1, 1920; Frank W. Rozengraft to R. E. Vinson, Nov. 2, 1920; and N. P. Colwell to W. S. Carter, Oct. 29, 1920, letters, box 4R81, UT President's Records.

16. W. S. Carter to R. E. Vinson, Oct. 21, 1920, letter, box 4R84, UT President's Records. This committee included Reps. Leonard Tillotson of Sealy and C. T. Bass of San Marcos, Sen. W. H. Bledsoe of Lubbock, Dr. A. C. Scott of Temple, Dr. Everett Jones of Wichita Falls, T. S. Reed Sr. of Beaumont, and W. H. Fuqua of Amarillo. All except Fuqua came to the first meeting. *Galveston Daily News*, Nov. 5 and 6, 1920.

17. "Report of the Committee on Inquiry on the Location and Organization of the Medical Branch of the University of Texas," Dec. 3, 1920, box 4R85, UT President's Records. For more information about the main campus controversies, see "Facts Relating to Removal of the University," n.d., box 4R81, UT President's Records.

18. W. S. Carter to R. E. Vinson, Jan. 17, 1922, letter, box 4R84, UT President's Records; and *Galveston Daily News*, Feb. 6, 1922. To accept a permanent role with the Rockefeller Foundation, Carter officially resigned as professor of physiology and dean in February, 1923; see W. S. Carter to R. E. Vinson, Feb. 10, 1923, letter, box 4R80, UT President's Records. Carter died in 1944; for an obituary, see *Galveston Daily News*, May 13, 1944. William Keiller to W. S. Sutton, Dec. 15, 1923, letter, box 4Q23, UT President's Records (quotation); William Keiller to W. M. W. Splawn, Aug. 4, 1924, letter, box VF 1/A, UT President's Records; W. Keiller to W. M. W. Splawn, Mar. 11, 1926, letter, box 4Q24, UT President's Records. Keiller recovered satisfactorily and continued to teach until his death on February 22, 1931. See *UTMB: Seventy-five Year History*, 39, and *Galveston Daily News*, Feb. 23, 1931. Also see Chester R. Burns, "William Keiller," in Tyler, et al. (eds.) *The New Handbook of Texas*, III, 1047.

19. W. F. Gidley, UTMB's professor of pharmacy, had danced some important political moves. In 1925 he successfully lobbied for membership on UTMB's Executive Committee; Minutes, UTMB Faculty Meetings, Feb. 26, 1925. In 1926 the regents appointed Gidley as dean of the pharmacy school, actions that permitted the school to become a member of the American Association of Colleges of Pharmacy (AACP). Until these decisions, the UT School of Pharmacy had been the only university school of pharmacy in the United States that was not a member of the national association; *Galveston Daily News*, Oct. 27, 1926; Jan. 1, 1927; and Feb. 27, 1927. With a steady increase in students, the school needed more space for classrooms and laboratories; *Galveston Daily News*, Feb. 25, 1927. When a chemistry building burned on the campus in Austin, influential pharmacists began lobbying for a new building that would house the pharmacy school and the chemistry department; *Galveston Daily News*, Oct. 20, 1926, and Dec. 7, 1926. In July 1927 the regents and Harry Y. Benedict, UT's new president, decided to move the school from Galveston to Austin. The Texas Pharmaceutical Association recommended this transfer because the location in Galveston was "isolated, unsuited, and detrimental to the best interest of the college"; *Galveston Daily News*, June 23, 1927, and July 19, 1927. Benedict and the regents believed that the school could be operated more economically in Austin and that the pharmacy students would receive better training in chemistry, botany, and business. For details, see letters in the College of Pharmacy folder, box VF 1/A, UT President's Records, and Burlage and Beutler, *Pharmacy's Foundation in Texas*, 146–175. *Galveston Daily News*, July 21, 1927; Aug. 6, 1927; May 20, 1928; Aug. 7, 1928; and Aug. 16, 1928. For tributes about Bethel at the time of his death in April 1935, see *Galveston Daily News*, Apr. 18, 1935; Apr. 19, 1935; Apr. 20, 1935; and May 2, 1935; and Minutes, UTMB Faculty Meetings, May 27, 1935.

20. Bethel lobbied unsuccessfully for a dental school in Galveston. See *Galveston Daily News*, Feb. 11, 1927; Feb. 25, 1927; Apr. 19, 1927; Oct. 1, 1927; May 23, 1930; June 4, 1930; Mar. 29, 1931; and May 14 and 15, 1931. See also

George E. Bethel to H. Y. Benedict, Aug. 16, 1928, letter, box 4Q24, UT President's Records (1st quotation); George E. Bethel to H. Y. Benedict, Sept. 16, 1933, letter, box VF 9/C, UT President's Records (2nd quotation).

21. For samples of public regard for Randall, see *Galveston Daily News*, June 11, 1933; Nov. 16, 1934; Feb. 17, 1935; Mar. 31, 1935; and Mar. 2, 1937. Also see the obituary in *Galveston Daily News*, Aug. 13, 1944; *UTMB: Seventy-five Year History*, 32–36, and Chester R. Burns, "Edward Randall Sr.," in Tyler, et al. (eds.), *The New Handbook of Texas*, V, 437. For additional insights into Randall's personality, see the typescripts of interviews with Edward Randall Jr. and Willard Richardson Cooke conducted in 1965, folder 35, box 1, 75th Anniversary History Papers, Blocker Collections.

22. Edward Randall to H. Y. Benedict, Apr. 13, 1935, letter, box VF 9/C, UT President's Records; *Galveston Daily News*, Aug. 8 and 31, 1935; *Rules and Regulations* (1936), 30.

23. *Rules and Regulations* (1936), 60; *Rules and Regulations* (1936), part II, 54–56, 66. Still in the throes of the depression, students failed to pay their debts, especially to fraternities. Carter hoped that a faculty committee could improve this situation, since many of the professors were also members of these fraternities. See W. S. Carter to H. Y. Benedict, Feb. 13, 1936, and John C. Nolan to H. Y. Benedict, Feb. 13, 1936, letters, box VF 9/C, UT President's Records.

24. W. S. Carter to H. Y. Benedict, Jan. 29, 1936, letter, box VF 9/C, UT President's Records; H. G. Weiskotten and J. N. Baker, "University of Texas School of Medicine, Galveston, Texas, January 27, 28, 29, 1936." The original report is in the Office of the Liaison Committee on Medical Education, Association of American Medical Colleges, Washington, D.C. Only rank orders and graphs are included in the published report that is in the Blocker Collections. See American Medical Association Council on Medical Education and Hospitals, *Survey of Medical Schools, 1934–1937* (Chicago: American Medical Association, 1937). For UTMB's ranks, see pp. 1000–1001.

25. For details about standardization, see Ludmerer, *Learning to Heal*, 256–260, and Rothstein, *American Medical Schools and the Practice of Medicine*, 140–178.

26. Byron M. Hendrix, professor of biochemistry, was appointed acting dean; *Galveston Daily News*, July 7 and 28, 1938. See J. R. Parten to K. H. Aynesworth, Mar. 9, 1938 (quotation); J. R. Parten to Edward Randall, Mar. 9, 1938; and K. H. Aynesworth to J. R. Parten, Mar. 15, 1938, letters, all in the J. R. Parten Papers (Center for American History, University of Texas at Austin). This subcommittee had visited UTMB in the spring of 1938 to develop "a plan for the future for the Medical Department." See K. H. Aynesworth to J. R. Parten, Apr. 5, 1938, letter, J. R. Parten Papers.

27. K. H. Aynesworth to J. R. Parten, Sept. 13, 1938, letter, J. R. Parten Papers (quotation). For additional details about Aynesworth's criticisms of UTMB, see K. H. Aynesworth to Edward Randall, Aug. 25, 1937, letter, series 3, box 11, "Letters, Documents, Discussions, etc.," pp. 18–22, Kenneth Hazen Aynesworth Papers, Blocker Collections. Aynesworth was also disturbed about the "relatively low rating of the John Sealy Hospital in many departments," as revealed in the report evaluating various hospitals in the country that appeared in the August 27, 1938, issue of *Journal of the American Medical Association*. See K. H. Aynesworth to John W. Spies, Aug. 14, 1939, letter, series 3, box 11, p. 440, Aynesworth Papers. For biographical details about Aynesworth, see the obituary in *Galveston Daily News*, Oct. 31, 1944, and Larry J. Wygant, "Kenneth Hazen Aynesworth," in Tyler, et al. (eds.), *The New Handbook of Texas*, I, 324. K. H. Aynesworth to J. R. Parten, Mar. 15, 1938, letter, J. R. Parten Papers.

28. Edward Randall to J. W. Calhoun, May 18, 1938, letter, box VF 4/E, UT President's Records; and the following letters: Edward Randall to J. R. Parten, May 31, 1938; J. R. Parten to Edward Randall, June 2, 1938; Edward Randall to J. R. Parten, June 3, 1938, all in J. R. Parten Papers. For biographical details about John Spies, see *Galveston Daily News*, Nov. 11, 1938; UTMB Dean's Office Records, Inactive (1938–1939); and box VF 9/C, UT President's Records. For biographical details about Tom Spies, see "Editorial," *Southern Medical Journal*, 53, no. 2 (Feb., 1960), 219–220. There are numerous articles about his career in the Tom Spies Papers in the Jefferson County Medical Society/University of Alabama at Birmingham Health Sciences Archives in Birmingham, Alabama. As early as the summer of 1934, both brothers told UT President Benedict that they were interested in becoming professors at UTMB; see George Bethel to H. Y. Benedict, July 21, 1934, letter, box VF 9/C, UT President's Records.

29. Edward Randall to J. W. Calhoun, July 26, 1938, letter, box VF 4/E, UT President's Records; Tom D. Spies to Edward Randall, Aug. 22, 1938, J. R. Parten Papers; Edward Randall to J. R. Parten, Sept. 1, 1938, letter, J. R. Parten Papers; J. W. Calhoun to Edward Randall, July 27, 1938, letter, box VF 4/E, UT President's Records; Tom D. Spies to Edward Randall, Aug. 4, 1938, J. R. Parten Papers; Tom D. Spies to J. R. Parten, Aug. 19, 1938, letter, J. R. Parten Papers. Maybe Aynesworth hoped the regents would employ both John and Tom Spies; K. H. Aynesworth to J. R. Parten, Sept. 13, 1938, letter, J. R. Parten Papers.

30. Edward Randall to J. R. Parten, Aug. 17, 1938, letter, J. R. Parten Papers; J. R. Parten to Don E. Carleton, July 1983, interviews, J. R. Parten Papers; K. H. Aynesworth to J. R. Parten, Nov. 1, 1938; J. W. Calhoun to J. R. Parten, Nov.

8, 1938; J. R. Parten to Edward Randall, Nov. 11, 1938, letters, all in J. R. Parten Papers. Also see J. W. Calhoun to Edward Randall, Nov. 22, 1938, and Edward Randall to J. W. Calhoun, Nov. 23, 1938, letters, box VF 9/C, UT President's Records. Spies especially nurtured a cordial relationship with Aynesworth; for evidence, see the letters exchanged between Aynesworth and Spies between Nov. 8, 1938 and Nov. 14, 1939 in series 3, box 11, "Letters, Documents, Discussions, etc.," pp. 414–473, Aynesworth Papers. Minutes, UT Board of Regents, Nov. 10, 1938; J. W. Calhoun to B. M. Hendrix, Jan. 5, 1939, letter, box VF 9/C, UT President's Records. Tom Spies never accepted this professorship.

31. *Galveston Daily News*, Jan. 20, 1939. On Rainey's support, see John W. Spies to Homer P. Rainey, Feb. 9, 1939, and John W. Spies to Homer P. Rainey, May 26, 1939, letters, box VF 9/C, UT President's Records; and Minutes, UT Board of Regents, July 15, 1939. Regarding the promotions, see K. H. Aynesworth to J. R. Parten, Mar. 15, 1938, letter, J. R. Parten Papers; and Edward Randall to Homer Rainey, Aug. 3, 1939, and Homer Rainey to Edward Randall, Aug. 4, 1939, letters, box VF 4/E, UT President's Records. On the fight with Lucius Wilson, see John W. Spies to J. R. Parten, Mar. 10, 1939; Edward Randall to J. R. Parten, June 2, 1939; J. R. Parten to Edward Randall, June 3, 1939; letters, all in the J. R. Parten Papers. On the recommendations for dismissal, see John W. Spies to Homer P. Rainey, July 31, 1939, letter, box VF 9/C, UT President's Records. On the report to Rainey, see John W. Spies to Homer P. Rainey, Oct. 5, 1939, report, box VF 9/B, UT President's Records. In this report, Spies claimed that his decisions had nothing to do with the suicides of two faculty members, Harry Knight and Wilfred Thomas Dawson. For an excellent summary of events before the October hearing, see Don E. Carleton, *A Breed So Rare: The Life of J. R. Parten, Liberal Texas Oil Man, 1896–1992* (Austin: Texas State Historical Association, 1998), 221–222. University of Texas Board of Regents, Special Session in Galveston, Oct. 7–9, 1939, Blocker Collections (cited hereafter as Special Session, UT Board of Regents).

32. "Memorandum Regarding Meeting of Executive Committee Medical Branch July 21, 1939," box VF 9/C, UT President's Records (1st quotation); Special Session, UT Board of Regents, 53–54 (2nd and 3rd quotations).

33. Special Session, UT Board of Regents, 80–82.

34. Special Session, UT Board of Regents, 76 (quotation), 91. What Spies meant by federal approval of cancer research facilities is not clear. By 1934 the American College of Surgeons had approved 181 hospitals in North America as suitable sites for proper cancer treatment; see James T. Patterson, *The Dread Disease: Cancer and Modern American Culture* (Cambridge, Mass.: Harvard University Press, 1987), 94.

35. Special Session, UT Board of Regents, 266 (1st quotation), 275–276 (Singleton and Parten quotations). For comments about Singleton, see Edward B. Singleton to Greg Diamond, Jan. 18, 1987, interview, and W. W. Stephen to Greg Diamond, Dec. 19, 1986, interview, Blocker Collections.

36. Special Session, UT Board of Regents, 301–307.

37. Carleton, *A Breed So Rare*, 226–228; Special Session, UT Board of Regents, 828–829 (quotation).

38. [John W. Spies], "Confidential Report to President Rainey on the Medical Branch," Jan. 1, 1940, box VF 9/B, UT President's Records; Minutes, UT Board of Regents, Jan. 13, 1940. For a diagram of this proposed administrative arrangement, see Appendix A-14, WF441, CHP Archives. It was never adopted. Minutes, UT Board of Regents, Mar. 9, 1940. Aynesworth correctly interpreted Stark's motion as a signal that full-scale war had begun. "Every method of attack upon him personally and professionally, both fair and unfair, both gossip and rumor, based on hatred, jealousy, and the fear of losing prestige, has been used to vilify, traduce, and destroy the Dean personally and professionally, all of which is a veiled and covert attack upon the authority of the Board of Regents," Aynesworth proclaimed. "The battle has been launched; the forces have been organized, and nothing will be left undone to destroy completely the authority of the Board of Regents to control the Medical School. Among these weapons which are being used are the Sealy and Smith Foundation, the City Council of Galveston, and every friend of the small but willful group who have had control of the Medical School since they seized control in 1914. It is my opinion that they will eventually go to the press and make attacks upon the members of the Board of Regents, the President, and the Dean of the Medical School, with the sole purpose of retaining their strangle hold on the Medical School." See K. H. Aynesworth to J. R. Parten, Mar. 12, 1940, letter, J. R. Parten Papers.

39. Edward Randall to Gov. Lee O'Daniel, Jan. 24, 1940, letter, box VF 4/E, UT President's Records; Minutes, UT Board of Regents, Apr. 27, 1940. Thus, Randall and Royston no longer had dual roles as directors of the Sealy & Smith Foundation and directors of the hospital's board. Royston's distress is demonstrated in a lengthy statement published on May 3, 1940, in both the *Galveston Daily News* and the *Galveston Tribune*. For a passionate defense of the proposal to dissolve the hospital's board and assign full control of hospital affairs to the UT regents, see George Sealy's letter dated Feb. 28, 1940 that accompanies Minutes, Sealy & Smith Foundation Board of Directors, Apr. 3, 1940, Sealy & Smith Foundation (Suite 500, Bank of America Building, Galveston). Between January and May 1940, Randall and

his supporters mounted vicious public attacks on Spies, and they did all that they could to obstruct efforts to dissolve the hospital's board; see Carleton, *A Breed So Rare*, 231–237.

40. A. O. Singleton to Homer P. Rainey, June 3, 1940, letter, J. R. Parten Papers; *Galveston Daily News*, Oct. 23, 1940. Wilson declared that service to patients had been impaired by the administrative controversies at UTMB. George Sealy Jr., who replaced Singleton as a member of the hospital's board and who was treasurer of the Sealy & Smith Foundation Board, strongly denied Wilson's claims; *Galveston Daily News*, Oct. 24, 1940. Randall defended Wilson and announced that Sealy was not authorized to speak for the foundation; *Galveston Daily News*, Oct. 29, 1940, and Nov. 4, 1940.

41. John W. Spies to W. Lee O'Daniel, Nov. 5, 1940, and Dec. 2, 1940, letters, box VF 9/B, UT President's Records; Minutes, UT Board of Regents, Dec. 7, 1940; Feb. 22, 1941; and Mar. 22, 1941; and *Galveston Daily News*, Jan. 7, 15, and 31; Feb. 11 and 22; and Mar. 7 and 14, 1941.

42. *Galveston Daily News*, July 12, 1941, and drafts of Rainey's announcement in box VF 18/A, UT President's Records. This cancer research program eventually became the M. D. Anderson Hospital in Houston. Had Spies accepted Rainey's offer, the program would probably have developed in Galveston, and Spies's credibility as an academic leader would have been salvaged. For negotiations with the Anderson Foundation board, see Carleton, *A Breed So Rare*, 247–248. Forty-three faculty members signed a petition in support of Spies (see petition in box VF 9/B, UT President's Records) and 229 of 382 medical students cast secret ballots in favor of Spies (see *Galveston Daily News*, July 15, 1941). For alumni, see *Galveston Daily News*, July 18, 1941, and E. W. Bertner to Homer Rainey, July 21, 1941, letter, box VF 9/B, UT President's Records. For the Galveston County Medical Society, see the petition of members in box VF 9/B, UT President's Records; for the TSMA, see *Galveston Daily News*, July 16 and 17, 1941; and for the state board, see a resolution adopted by the board on July 20, 1941, in box VF 9/B, UT President's Records and *Galveston Daily News*, July 22, 1941. For the legislators, see *Houston Chronicle*, July 20, 1941; *Galveston Daily News*, July 20, 1941; and the *Summer Texan*, July 20, 1941. For Sealy and Kempner, see George Sealy to Board of Regents, c. July 23, 1941, letter, box VF 18/A, UT President's Records, and Daniel W. Kempner to Homer P. Rainey, July 13, 1941, letter, box VF 9/B, UT President's Records. Ella Sealy Newell believed that her father supported Spies because he had acquired more state dollars for UTMB than anyone ever before; see Ella Sealy Newell to Chauncey Leake Jr., July 22, 1944, letter, box 53, Leake Papers, NLM. Minutes, UT Board of Regents, July 26, 1941.

43. Minutes, UTMB Faculty Meeting, Aug. 27, 1941 (quotation); Minutes, UT Board of Regents, Sept. 29, 1941. For details about the actions of the faculty, see *Galveston Daily News*, Aug. 23–24, 28–30, and Sept. 3, 1941. Minutes, UT Board of Regents, Oct. 25, 1941; *Galveston Daily News*, Oct 23–24, 26, and 30, 1941.

44. A copy of this undated, anonymously authored document is in box VF 9/B, UT President's Records (quotation). Also see *Galveston Daily News*, Nov. 17, 1941, and Minutes, UT Board of Regents, Nov. 22, 1941.

45. Minutes, UT Board of Regents, Dec. 22, 1941. Even with these developments, Rainey continued to support Spies and to believe that the problems at UTMB could be solved with simple changes in the power structures. For evidence of this assertion, see Homer P. Rainey to Samuel Shelburne, Dec. 4, 1941, letter, box VF 9/B, UT President's Records. For Rainey's retrospective view of these events, see Homer P. Rainey, *The Tower and the Dome: A Free University versus Political Control* (Boulder, Colo.: Pruett Publishing Co., 1971), 50–51.

46. Occurring during the early months of American involvement in World War II, the "un-American" label was also used because doctors had told the legislators that the turmoil at UTMB was designed to limit the output of doctors as a way of protesting the war efforts; *Galveston Daily News*, Feb. 14 and 15, 1942. The committee included Jack Love (Fort Worth), Jimmy Phillips (Angleton), Marvin Simpson Jr. (Fort Worth), Arthur Cato (Weatherford), and Pat Dwyer (San Antonio). For details about the imposter, David Walton Fell, see "Meeting of the Board of Regents of the University of Texas, Medical School, Galveston, Texas," vol. 1, pp. 513–588, box 14, Aynesworth Papers. For more on Fell and comments about a student prank on "Comrade" Cato, see Robert B. White to Chester R. Burns, Dec. 10 and 20, 1991, interview, Blocker Collections.

47. For details, see *Galveston Daily News*, Feb. 21–23, 1942. More than one student was discouraged by these events. In the fall of 1942 Denton Cooley applied to four other schools for acceptance to their third-year classes. In February 1943 he transferred to Johns Hopkins. See Denton A. Cooley to Chester R. Burns, Sept. 4, 1987, letter, WF358, CHP Archives, Blocker Collections.

48. Though a search was conducted, I did not find a copy of this transcript. For some details, see *Galveston Daily News*, Feb. 27, 1942, and Minutes, UT Board of Regents, Feb. 28, 1942. For other comments about this investigation, see Carleton, *A Breed So Rare*, 249–250.

49. Minutes, UT Board of Regents, Feb. 28, 1942 (quotations). For details, see *Galveston Daily News*, Feb. 21, 1942, and Mar, 11, 1942; John W. Spies to Homer P. Rainey, Apr. 15, 1942, and John W. Spies to J. K. Kline, Apr, 15, 1942,

letters, both in box VF 9/A, UT President's Records. Remember that Rainey had offered Spies the directorship of a cancer program at UTMB in July 1941 when the regents first decided that Spies should not be reappointed as dean. Spies had refused that offer.

50. *Galveston Daily News*, May 9, 1942. The quote is from a "To Whom It May Concern" letter Spies wrote on May 13, 1942; a copy is in box VF 9/A, UT President's Records. The exact distribution of the letter is not known, but its contents were used for an article that appeared in the *Dallas Morning News* on May 16, 1942.

51. *Galveston Daily News*, June 6, 1942. The regents officially terminated Spies in August; Minutes, UT Board of Regents, Aug. 1, 1942. A six hundred-page transcript of testimonies given during three days of the regents' meeting (May 22–24) is in box 14, Aynesworth Papers. Published comments about these meetings can be found in *Galveston Daily News*, May 23–26, 28–29, and 31, 1942, and June 3–5, 1942.

52. For a public statement of Spies's beliefs, see *Galveston Daily News*, Mar. 19, 1941. J. R. Parten believed that Spies should be given full credit for creating the M. D. Anderson Hospital in Houston. See Carleton, *A Breed So Rare*, 250.

53. Leake had to pay his own moving expenses because one regent believed that if he had been unable to accumulate enough savings in San Francisco, he was "a poor business man." See D. F. Strickland to Homer P. Rainey, Aug. 15, 1942, letter, box VF 10/B, UT President's Records.

54. Mrs. I. D. Fairchild, the only female regent, expressed alarm over the absence of a plan. "If some definite decision as to a future program could be reached before a Dean or Vice-President is secured," she observed, "I have a feeling that we would be in better shape to state definitely what is expected of him in developing such a program." With extraordinary accuracy, she added: "I have always felt in Dean Spies case that the blame was as much ours as his. As I see it, he came to us with meager knowledge of the background of the School and was told that the former Deans were as rubber stamps and that the school needed reorganizing without really outlining in what respect the reorganization was needed. He set about to reorganize. We see what followed." See Mrs. I. D. Fairchild to Homer P. Rainey, Aug. 17, 1942, letter, box VF 10/B, UT President's Records. In the letter offering the job to Leake, Rainey explained that "as Executive Vice-President it is our purpose to give you the responsibility for developing and carrying through the University's medical program in the State." See Homer P. Rainey to Chauncey Leake, Aug. 10, 1942, letter, box VF 10/B, UT President's Records.

55. Chauncey D. Leake to dear all, Sept. 23, 1942, letter, box 2, Leake Papers, Blocker Collections; Chauncey D. Leake to J. C. Geiger, Sept. 19, 1942, letter, box 2, Leake Papers (Medical School Library, University of California at San Francisco; cited hereafter as UCSF); Chauncey D. Leake to Robert Gordon Sproul, Oct. 20, 1942, letter, box 2, Leake Papers, UCSF. Leake's correspondence is extraordinary. There are seventy-nine cartons of letters and papers at the National Library of Medicine in Bethesda, Maryland; seven in the library of the Medical School at the University of California in San Francisco; and five in the Blocker Collections at UTMB. Mary Jane Rogers (then Steding) began secretarial work for Leake in 1945; see Mary Jane Rogers to Megan Seaholm, July 21, 1989, interview, Blocker Collections.

56. Chauncey Leake to Judson Taylor, et al., Nov. 3, 1942, letter, box 3, Leake Papers, Blocker Collections; Minutes, UTMB Faculty Meeting, Nov. 4, 1942; *Houston Post*, Feb. 14 and 21, 1943. In 1944 Marjorie Bartholf became the first chief administrative officer of the School of Nursing to receive the title of dean in the official budgets adopted by the UT Board of Regents; *Report of the UT Board of Regents* (July 15, 1944), 391. Minutes, UT Board of Regents, May 21, 1943.

57. For the AAMC inspectors, see *Galveston Daily News*, May 16, 1943. For the AMA inspectors, see *Galveston Daily News*, Sept. 23, 1943. For AAMC and AMA data, see reports and correspondence in box VF 18/C, UT President's Records. For confirmation of accredited status, see Minutes, UTMB Faculty Meeting, Nov. 5, 1943, and Victor J. Johnson to Chauncey D. Leake, Nov. 9, 1943, letter, box 3, Leake Papers, Blocker Collections. For publicity about the removal of probation, see *Galveston Daily News*, Oct. 14, 24, and 28, 1943.

58. The complete text was published in *Texas Reports on Biology and Medicine*, 1, no. 1 (1943), 79–86; *Dallas Morning News*, Jan. 1, 1943 (quotation). "We are very friendly with Baylor and the Southwestern Medical Foundation. We've been helping both to get men and material. We've given duplicates from our Library to help both institutions build up their libraries. I've gotten Baylor their physiologist and pharmacologist. We're lending equipment to Southwestern. We probably will cooperate with Baylor in Houston with organization"; see Chauncey D. Leake to Dean Langley Porter, Sept 8, 1943, letter, box 57, Leake Papers, NLM. Leake cooperated with F. C. Elliott (dean of the UT Dental School), W. H. Moursund (dean of the Baylor Medical School), and E. W. Bertner (a UTMB graduate who was acting director of the M. D. Anderson Cancer Hospital) in preparing a memo about the development of the Texas Medical Center. See "Memorandum on Proposed Houston Medical Center," Sept. 23, 1943, box VF 10/B, UT President's Records.

59. Minutes, UT Board of Regents, Nov. 25, 1943.

60. Homer P. Rainey, "The Future Development of the University of Texas, a Report to the Board of Regents by the President of the University, July 15, 1944," Minutes, UT Board of Regents, July 15, 1944. In his report, Rainey used the same data from the AMA survey of 1937 that had been used to justify the reforms associated with Spies. Moreover, he placed that data within a context of false generalizations about the "glaring deficiencies" at UTMB that had been demonstrated "in report after report for twenty-five years by the American Medical Association and the Association of American Medical Colleges."

61. "Remarks by Chauncey D. Leake at meeting of the Board of Regents, Saturday, July 15, 1944," box VF 10/B, UT President's Records. In preparation for this meeting, Leake had prepared two reports: "Needs of the University of Texas Medical Branch, Galveston," July 12, 1944, box 2, Leake Papers, Blocker Collections, and "Statement Regarding Clinical Material at the University of Texas Medical Branch, Galveston," July 14, 1944, box VF 9/D, UT President's Records.

62. Minutes, UT Board of Regents, Feb. 25, 1944; Chauncey D. Leake to Alan Gregg, July 28, 1944, letter, box 36, Leake Papers, NLM.

63. Chauncey D. Leake to M. F. Ashley Montagu, Aug. 31, 1944, letter, box 50, Leake Papers, NLM.

64. See copies of various resolutions in box VF 10/C, UT President's Records; E. H. Klatt and George S. McReynolds to Board of Regents, Aug. 7, 1944, letter, box VF 10/C, UT President's Records (quotation); R. E. Bowen and A. D. Simpson to John H. Bickett Jr., July 25, 1944, box 1, Leake Papers, Blocker Collections. See the letters and other documents in file folders 2, 3, and 5 in box 28, H. Kempner Records (Rosenberg Library, Galveston). Also see Harold M. Hyman, *Oleander Odyssey: The Kempners of Galveston, Texas, 1854–1980s* (College Station: Texas A&M University Press, 1990), 432–433.

65. Medical Committee report, Sept. 29, 1944, box VF 9/A, UT President's Records (1st quotation); *Galveston Daily News*, Sept. 30, 1944; and Chauncey D. Leake to all, Sept. 30, 1944, letter, box 2, Leake Papers, Blocker Collections (2nd quotation).

66. Minutes, UT Board of Regents, Nov. 1, 1944; Chauncey D. Leake to A. J. Carlson, Oct. 16, 1944, letter, box 24, Leake Papers, NLM (quotation). Leake was correct. Rainey placed second in a field of thirteen candidates for governor of Texas in 1946.

67. The transcriptions of these hearings were compiled in four volumes, which are deposited in the Legislative Reference Library in Austin. These volumes will be cited as "Proceedings (1944), I, II, III, or IV." A printed summary of these hearings was issued with the title: "An Educational Crisis . . . A Summary of Testimony Before a Senate Committee Investigating the University of Texas Controversy, November 15–28, 1944." A copy of this summary is in box 3L382, Rainey Controversy Scrap Book, UT President's Records.

68. Proceedings (1944), II, 491–493 (1st quotation on 492), 663 (2nd quotation), 731 (3rd, 4th, and 5th quotations). Charles Stone Sr. and Raymond Gregory, two professors of medicine at UTMB, retold many of the stories associated with the Spies saga. Stone and Gregory's testimonies and documents about UTMB constituted more than two hundred pages of the third volume of the proceedings; see Proceedings (1944), III, 115–250, 332–438. "The University of Texas Controversy," statement by J. R. Parten, Nov. 28, 1944, box 3L382, Rainey Controversy Scrap Book (Center for American History, University of Texas at Austin) (6th quotation).

69. Minutes, UT Board of Regents, Jan. 26, 1945. For details about these controversies, see Alice Carol Cox, "The Rainey Affair: The History of the Academic Freedom Controversy at the University of Texas, 1938–1946," (Ph.D. diss., University of Denver, 1970); Henry Nash Smith, *The Controversy at the University of Texas, 1939–1945: A Documentary History* (Austin: Students' Association of the University of Texas, 1945); and Rainey, *The Tower and the Dome.* Because of these controversies, the American Association of University Professors censured the UT Board of Regents for seven years (1946–1953). Theophilus Painter to C. D. Leake, Aug. 3, 1945, letter, box VF 18/B, UT President's Records (quotation) and *Galveston Daily News*, Aug. 11, 1945.

70. In 1943 the Texas Medical Association published photos of sixty-five representatives and fourteen senators in the Texas legislature who had been especially supportive of efforts to improve medical care in the state. Galveston's William E. Stone was one of these senators; *Texas State Journal of Medicine*, 39 (Aug., 1943), 224. For examples of Stone's exhortations in support of UTMB, see *Galveston Daily News*, June 9–10, 1945; July 25 and 29, 1945; and Aug. 22, 1945. For Kempner and the chamber's committee, see the letters in folders 6–8, box 28, H. Kempner Records; *Galveston Daily News*, Jan. 12 and 14 and Feb. 16–18, 1945; Mar. 6, 8, 9, 20, 23, and 25, 1945; and Apr. 11–12, 1945; and "University of Texas," *Texas State Journal of Medicine*, 41 (Feb., 1946), 543. For Stone, see June 9 and 14, 1945; July 25 and 29, 1945; and Aug. 22, 1945. For Kempner, see *Galveston Daily News*, Aug. 26 and 30, 1945, and Sept. 2, 1945.

71. Theophilus Painter to UT Regents, Feb. 14, 1946, letter, box VF 9/D, UT President's Records.

72. Chauncey Leake to John Fulton, July 16, 1946, letter, box 2, Leake Papers, UCSF (1st quotation); Chauncey Leake to Ella Sealy Newell, July 25, 1946, letter, box 53, Leake Papers, NLM (2nd quotation). Ella was the sister of George Sealy Jr., who had died in 1944; see the obituary in *Galveston Daily News*, Nov. 5, 1944. To cope with the budget cut, Leake and the faculty recommended the closing of five charity wards in the hospitals; see *Galveston Daily News*, Sept. 18, 1946.

73. Chester R. Burns, "The Health Sciences," in Leo J. Klosterman, Loyd S. Swenson Jr., and Sylvia Rose (eds.), *100 Years of Science and Technology in Texas* (Houston: Rice University Press, 1986), 286–287. The scientists began their work in the main residence of the Baker Estate in Houston. For photos, see *Cactus*, 51 (1944), 450. Minutes, UT Board of Regents, Mar. 24, 1945; *Galveston Daily News*, Mar. 25, 1945; and Minutes, UT Board of Regents, July 12, 1947 (quotation).

74. Minutes, UT Board of Regents, Apr. 28, 1950; *Galveston Daily News*, Jan. 22, Feb. 22, and Mar. 26, 1950; "Report of Committee of Administrative Reorganization," March 1950, box 5, UTMB Alumni Association, Blocker Collections. The other four components included the University of Texas Main University (Austin), Texas Western College of the University of Texas (El Paso), the University of Texas McDonald Observatory (Fort Davis), and the University of Texas Institute of Marine Science (Port Aransas).

75. T. S. Painter, "Talk Before the AAUP on April 19, 1950," box VF 18/B, UT President's Records; *Galveston Daily News*, July 28, 1950. Hart was the father of Sherman Little, wife of Harry Little, former professor of obstetrics and gynecology at UTMB.

76. For details about Currie, see Chauncey D. Leake to James P. Hart, Sept. 19, 1953; Tom Sealy to all members of the Board of Regents, Sept. 19, 1953; James P. Hart to the members of the Board of Regents, Nov. 16, 1953; G. A. W. Currie to J. P. Hart, Nov. 23, 1953; letters, all in box VF C/1, UT Chancellor's Records; see also *Galveston Daily News*, Dec. 11, 1953. A Canadian-trained physician, Currie came to UTMB from the University of Colorado, where he was director of the university's hospitals. For details, see *Medi-Texan*, 1 (Feb., 1954), 1, 3.

77. Chauncey D. Leake to F. J. L. Blasingame, Oct. 1, 1954, letter, box 12, Leake Papers, NLM.

78. Chartered in 1952, the Texas Research League was a private, non-profit, educational corporation governed by a seventy-two-member Board of Directors (mostly bankers) who employed a staff of a dozen or so professionals. These professionals were expected to apply the techniques of business management research in studying governmental operations and programs. The chair of the league's board believed that the league's recommendations from the University of Texas survey, if implemented, would significantly improve "the administration of the University's several branches, and achieve savings of more than $900,000 annually in the non-academic operations of the system"; see Hines H. Baker, *Business Management in Texas Government* (Austin: Texas Research League, 1955). For a list of the "top administrative problems" at UTMB, see the nineteen-page excerpt from the league's survey in box VF I/4, UT Chancellor's Records. See also Minutes, UT Board of Regents, Sept. 18, 1954. Wilson had become president of UT Austin in February 1953; see *Galveston Daily News*, Oct. 29, 1953. When Hart resigned in the spring of 1954, the regents appointed Wilson as acting chancellor; see *Galveston Daily News*, Apr. 10, 1954. For a brief obituary of Wilson, see *Galveston Daily News*, Nov. 9, 1990.

79. Minutes, UT Board of Regents, Dec. 10, 1954. For diagrams of the administrative structures, see Appendices A-16, A-17 and A-18, WF441, CHP Archives. For views about the flip-flop arrangement, see letters exchanged between Wilson, Leake, Cappelmann, and Currie in box VF E/2, UT Chancellor's Records. Following the proposals of the Texas Research League, Currie appointed two assistant administrators by March 1955; see *Medi-Texan*, 2 (Mar., 1955), 1. Blocker believed that the shift in his appointment from that of dean of the medical faculty to that of dean of the medical school signified a need for a full-time dean who could devote all of his energies to managing the school. Blocker's clinical and teaching activities as a plastic surgeon were extensive, and he did not believe that he could adequately honor the requirements of a full-time deanship; see T. G. Blocker Jr. to Chauncey D. Leake, Jan. 7, 1955, letter, box VF E/2, UT Chancellor's Records.

80. Logan Wilson to all employees of the University of Texas, Jan. 11, 1955, memo, box 40, Charles Turner Stone Papers, Blocker Collections. Leake believed that "the Medical Branch suffered" after the new "System" arrangement started in 1950; see Chauncey D. Leake to John B. Truslow, Jan. 24, 1956, letter, box 68, Leake Papers, NLM. *Galveston Daily News*, Mar. 3 and 8, 1955; Chauncey D. Leake to Logan Wilson, June 8, 1955, letter, box VF E/2, UT Chancellor's Records. Leake believed that the actions of the regents had caused Hart to resign as chancellor. He commiserated with Hart: "The same circumstances and conditions which probably led you to resign from The University of Texas have finally forced my resignation"; Chauncey D. Leake to James P. Hart, June 25, 1955, letter, box 38, Leake Papers, NLM. A few weeks later Leake chastised the regents for their failure to honor "the advice of the experts whom

they hire to run the University." None of the regents, Leake added, have "any of the standards or ideals which are respected in academic circles"; Chauncey D. Leake to James P. Hart, July 15, 1955, letter, box 38, Leake Papers, NLM.

81. For tributes accorded at that time, see *Galveston Daily News*, July 13–14 and Aug. 7–8, 1955. Minutes, UT Board of Regents, July 8, 1955. For details about the decisions of this committee and the search for a new CEO, see folders 8 and 9, box 17, Department of Anatomy records, Blocker Collections.

82. *Galveston Daily News*, Dec. 1, 3, 7, and 10, 1955; Logan Wilson to Charles T. Stone Sr., Nov. 3, 1955; Logan Wilson to John B. Truslow, Dec. 9, 1955; letters, both in box VF E/2, UT Chancellor's Records. Stone was chair of this committee. *Galveston Daily News*, Jan. 24–25, 1956, and Apr. 1, 1956. A graduate of Harvard Medical School, Truslow had served in the U.S. Navy for five years before serving as an assistant dean at Columbia University's College of Physicians and Surgeons for six years, and dean at the Medical College of Virginia for five years. At UTMB Truslow received an appointment as professor of administrative medicine with tenure. For details, see *Medi-Texan*, 3 (Apr., 1956), 1–2.

83. Minutes, UTMB Faculty Meeting, May 17, 1956; John B. Truslow to Logan Wilson, June 7, 1956, letter, box VF G/5, UT Chancellor's Records; *Galveston Daily News*, May 9, 1957; and *Syndrome* (1958), 8–9. Truslow and the faculty also reorganized most committees; see list dated 10/2/56 in box VF G/1, UT Chancellor's Records.

84. Sailing the political waters with John McCullough produced some nausea for Truslow, especially after McCullough became adamant about using foundation dollars to build a new psychiatric hospital for UTMB. Truslow thought that McCullough had his own plan for developing UTMB; see John Truslow to Logan Wilson, Oct. 23, 1956, letter, box VF G/1, UT Chancellor's Records. In 1957 Wilson urged Truslow to renew his periodic luncheons with McCullough; see Logan Wilson to John Truslow, Nov. 27, 1957, letter, box VF G/1, UT Chancellor's Records. Whether he did or not is unknown, but perturbations continued between Truslow and McCullough; for examples, see John Truslow to Logan Wilson, Nov. 15, 1960, and John Truslow to Harry H. Ransom, July 17, 1961, letters, box VF L/6, UT Chancellor's Records.

85. See Melvin A. Casberg to Chester R. Burns, Sept. 7, 1989, interview, Blocker Collections (quotation), and *Galveston Daily News*, Feb. 19, 1956. For his views about administrative arrangements between universities and their medical schools, see Melvin A. Casberg, "The University and the School of Medicine," *Journal of Medical Education*, 35 (Jan., 1960), 56–61. To encourage cooperation and communication, on November 2, 1956, the regents approved the establishment of a Council on Medical Affairs that would meet at the call of Casberg, its chair. This council included the director of the M. D. Anderson Hospital and Tumor Institute, the dean of the Dental Branch, the director of UTMB, the dean of the Postgraduate School, and the dean of Southwestern Medical School. See Material Supporting the Agenda for Meetings of the UT Board of Regents, 4, no. 3. *Galveston Daily News*, July 15 and 21, 1956.

86. Melvin Casberg to Logan Wilson, Jan. 9, 1957, and Logan Wilson to John B. Truslow, June 7, 1957 (quotation), letters, box VF G/1, UT Chancellor's Records. Casberg claimed that Truslow "cow-towed to the authorities." Casberg also thought that the Truslows never really adapted to Texas and Texans in general; see Casberg to Burns, Sept. 7, 1989, interview. Kenneth Earle thought that Truslow experienced some trouble because of his "aggressive personality." But he also believed that Truslow was a "master" in supporting good faculty members; see Kenneth Earle to Chester R. Burns, Mar. 15, 1990, interview, Blocker Collections.

87. John B. Truslow to Logan Wilson, Dec. 23, 1957, letter, box VF G/5, UT Chancellor's Records (quotation). It is not easy to understand all of the political juggling that involved Roscoe Pullen, Jack Ewalt, Grant Taylor, and others who managed the UT Postgraduate School of Medicine. Some appeared to want control of all UT residency training programs as well as all UT continuing education programs. See Chauncey D. Leake to Roscoe Pullen, Mar. 19, 1952, letter, box VF A/3, UT Chancellor's Records; "Report of the Committee on the Postgraduate School of Medicine," Dec. 4, 1952, box VF C/1, UT Chancellor's Records; and "The University of Texas Postgraduate School of Medicine," June 30, 1955, Secretary's Files, Board of Regents, II, 123–126, 141–146. The management of this school became clearer after Casberg helped Wilson make important distinctions between residency training and continuing education; see Dr. Casberg to Dr. Wilson, Oct. 8, 1958, letter, box VF G/4, UT Chancellor's Records. In 1963 the regents transformed this school into the University of Texas Graduate School of the Biomedical Sciences at Houston; see "Activation of the Graduate School of Biomedical Sciences at Houston," box VF CC/5, UT Chancellor's Records.

88. Truslow probably thought that his anxieties were justified, considering the spectacular growth of institutions in the Texas Medical Center between 1946 and 1956. By the latter year, the major ones included the Baylor University College of Medicine (1948), a new Hermann Hospital and Hermann Professional Building (1949), the Methodist Hospital (1951), the Saint Luke's Episcopal Hospital (1954), the Texas Children's Hospital (1954), the Jesse H. Jones Library Building housing the Texas Medical Center Library (1954), a new building for the University of Texas M. D. Anderson Hospital and Tumor Institute (1954), and a new building for the University of Texas Dental Branch (1955).

Truslow's abiding fears of competition surfaced again in the early 1960s when the regents and system administrators began considering the addition of UT health units in San Antonio. In discussing a South Texas Medical Center, Truslow chided Ransom: "How, in the name of Heaven, can we look at each other in the face much longer and pretend either that we have such resources or that they will appear when needed?"; see John B. Truslow to Harry H. Ransom, Oct. 10, 1961, letter, box VF T/3, UT Chancellor's Records.

89. *Galveston Daily News*, June 28, 1958; John B. Truslow to Logan Wilson, July 10, 1958, and Melvin Casberg to Logan Wilson, Aug. 22, 1958, letters, box VF G/1, UT Chancellor's Records; *Galveston Daily News*, Aug. 2, 1958; and Melvin Casberg to Logan Wilson, Nov. 17, 1958, letter, box VF I/1, UT Chancellor's Records (quotation). In January 1957 the regents asked a committee of seventy-five Texas citizens to appraise the entire University of Texas. Their report was given to the regents in October 1958. On December 6, 1958, the regents distributed a printed version titled *The University of Texas Report of the Committee of 75*. The assessment of UTMB is on pages 35–37. A copy of this printed report is in RF165, CHP Archives. Affirmations of Truslow are in M. A. Casberg to Dr. Wilson, Dec. 2, 1958, memorandum, and Wilson, Dec. 2, 1958, press memorandum, both in box VF I/1, UT Chancellor's Records.

90. *Galveston Daily News*, Mar. 27, 1959, and Earle to Burns, Mar. 15, 1990, interview. For diagrams of the general administrative organization of UTMB, the hospitals, and the nursing school, see Appendices A-19, A-20, and A-21, WF441, CHP Archives.

91. Minutes, UTMB Faculty Meeting, Mar. 22, 1960.

92. *Galveston Daily News*, May 14, 1960. Ransom's father was principal of Ball High School when Harry was born in Galveston on November 22, 1908. For a biographical sketch and wonderfully provocative essays, see Harry Ransom, *The Conscience of the University and Other Essays* (Austin: University of Texas Press, 1982). For a quick summary of the ten-year plan, see "UT's Ten Year Plan," *University of Texas Record*, 6 (1960), 1–4. For a report on this plan about a year after its adoption, see "Status Report on the Ten Year Plan," Material Supporting the Agenda for Meeting of the UT Board of Regents, IXa, 1–14.

93. "Items suggested for discussion and decision at joint meeting of Regents' Medical Affairs Committee and Buildings and Grounds Committee at Galveston April 8, 1962," box VF P/3, UT Chancellor's Records. While in Galveston, Ransom and the regents met with John McCullough to plan their future collaborations. McCullough wanted Ransom and the regents to review all requests about UTMB before they were presented to the foundation's directors. Ransom agreed to this approach. He also agreed to prepare a new five-year development plan for UTMB and offer it to the foundation's directors for their review; see Harry Ransom to John W. McCullough, May 26, 1962, letter, box VF L/6, UT Chancellor's Records. Ransom and McCullough began negotiating directly, Truslow notwithstanding. For details, see Minutes, Sealy & Smith Foundation Board of Directors, Jan. 10, Jan. 26, and June 13, 1962.

94. John B. Truslow to Harry H. Ransom, Feb. 15, 1962, letter, box VF L/6, UT Chancellor's Records (quotation). Earle believed that Truslow "reversed his decisions often enough to make it hard for many to believe his promises." Truslow and Earle relieved some department chairs of their administrative roles. Earle believed that "John got the reputation of lopping off heads more than I did." The quotes are from Kenneth M. Earle to Truman G. Blocker Jr., May 4, 1964, letter, folder 24, box 3, Blocker Papers. See also Harry Ransom to the Board of Regents, Feb. 20, 1962, letter, box VF L/6, UT Chancellor's Records, and "Items suggested for discussion and decision at joint meeting of Regents' Medical Affairs Committee and Buildings and Grounds Committee at Galveston April 8, 1962," box VF P/3, UT Chancellor's Records.

95. *Galveston Daily News*, Apr. 26–27, 1964. Truslow did not accept the appointment as consultant; see Harry Ransom to Members of the Central Administration and Institutional Heads, Aug. 3, 1964, letter, box VF 33/A, UT President's Records. On April 27, 1964, Truslow told the Executive Committee that Ransom and the regents alleged that there had been "a complete breakdown in communications" between them and Truslow since April 1962; see Minutes, UTMB Executive Committee Meeting, box VF M/5, UT Chancellor's Records. Truman Blocker thought that Truslow failed as a CEO because "He talked down to the legislature. He didn't know how to handle people in the legislature. He made a lot of enemies in the financial committees and just was not acceptable to them." See Truman G. Blocker Jr. to Nonie Thompson, Mar. 4, 1980, typescript, p. 21, Galveston and Texas History Center (Rosenberg Library, Galveston). See also a news release from Office of the Chancellor, Apr. 25, 1964, box VF M/5, UT Chancellor's Records. In 1963 Ransom and two unidentified regents visited Blocker in Galveston. They told Blocker that they would move the schools to Houston and transform the hospitals into eleemosynary institutions if he refused to become UTMB's CEO; see Blocker to Thompson, Mar. 4, 1980, typescript, p. 21. One regent was probably Frank Connally, a former professor at UTMB. Connally lobbied mightily against lingering sentiments about moving UTMB; see Charles LeMaistre to Chester R. Burns, Dec. 18, 1989, and Jan. 31, 1990, interviews, Blocker Collections.

96. The richest source of information about Blocker is the collection of Truman G. Blocker Jr. Papers located in eighty-seven boxes in the Blocker Collections. Also see WF190, CHP Archives. For a short biographical overview, see Chester R. Burns, "Truman Graves Blocker Jr.," in Tyler, et al. (eds.), *The New Handbook of Texas*, I, 595–596. *Galveston Daily News*, Sept. 6, 1964 (quotation). For many congratulatory letters, see folder 24, box 3, Blocker Papers.

97. The committee included Bill McGanity, Donald Duncan, Mason Guest, Willard Verwey, Virgil Koenig, Bill Daeschner, John Middleton, Martin Towler, and Robert Cooley. They also prepared a list of responsibilities for a new dean; see William J. McGanity to Truman G. Blocker Jr., July 23, 1964, letter, folder 4, box 30, William C. Levin Papers, Blocker Collections. The regents approved a job description for each role, including explicit statements about lines of authority and accountability; see T. G. Blocker Jr. to Harry Ransom, Oct. 2, 1964; Material Supporting the Agenda for Meetings of the UT Board of Regents, Oct. 23, 1964, XIIa, 15–23, and Minutes, UT Board of Regents, Oct. 23–24, 1964. For the chart, see Appendix A-22, WF441, CHP Archives.

98. Minutes, UT Board of Regents, Oct. 7–8, 1965, and *Newsletter (UTMB)*, 1 (Oct. 21, 1965), 1.

99. Clifton McCleskey, Allan K. Butcher, Daniel E. Farlow, and J. Pat Stephens, *The Government and Politics of Texas* (Boston: Little, Brown, and Company, 1982), 311–312. Also see the first "Annual Report of the Coordinating Board, Texas College and University System" submitted to Gov. John Connally and the legislature on December 31, 1965 (CAH). The lack of coordination during the first half of the twentieth century is concisely reviewed in "Public Higher Education in Texas," 1950, 137–156 (CAH). During the 1960s the Texas Commission on Higher Education and its successor, the Coordinating Board of the Texas College and University System, developed comprehensive perspectives for expanding support of higher education in the state. For details, see Texas Commission on Higher Education, "Public Higher Education in Texas, 1961–1971," 1963, and "Challenge for Excellence—A Blueprint for Progress in Higher Education," 1971 (both at CAH). These overviews recommended two new medical schools (UT Houston and Texas Tech), subsidies to Baylor Medical School from state tax revenues, and increased enrollments (two hundred first-year medical students) at each of the three existing UT medical schools (Galveston, Dallas, and San Antonio).

100. See LeMaistre to Burns, Dec. 18, 1989 (quotation), and Jan. 31, 1990, interviews, Blocker Collections. A copy of LeMaistre's report is in WF260, CHP Archives. These folders also contain the self-study reports of UT Southwestern, the Graduate School of the Biomedical Sciences in Houston, and the Medical School in San Antonio.

101. For these reports, see WF260, CHP Archives.

102. Minutes, UT Board of Regents, June 16, 1967; Truman G. Blocker Jr. to Charles A. LeMaistre, Feb. 16, 1968, letter, and HJ to CAL, Feb. 21, 1968, memo, on reel 123, UT Chancellor's Office of Records Management; and Minutes, UT Board of Regents, Mar. 8, 1968. For organization charts, see Appendices A-23 and A-24, WF441, CHP Archives. *Newsletter (UTMB)*, 3 (Apr., 1968), 4. For White's view of his role, see *Alumni Bulletin (UTMB)*, 23 (Winter, 1968), 9–11. For comments about White, see Luther Travis to Chester R. Burns, Feb. 25 and Mar. 10, 1992, interviews, Blocker Collections.

103. *Newsletter (UTMB)*, 3 (Sept., 1968), 2–13.

104. See Joseph M. White to Chester R. Burns, Dec. 19, 1989, interview, Blocker Collections. After LeMaistre became executive vice chancellor for health affairs in 1968, Blocker reported directly to him. White established what he called a "working" relationship with LeMaistre.

105. In Aaron R. Schwartz to Chester R. Burns and Myles Knape, May 4 and June 25, 1990, interviews, Blocker Collections, "Babe" Schwartz declared that "Frank Erwin was the best friend that the Medical Branch ever had." Chancellor Walker thought that Erwin was "the best friend The University of Texas ever had"; see *Impact*, 4 (Oct. 10, 1980), 6. Mickey LeMaistre recognized Erwin as the "real strategist" in negotiating with key legislators; see LeMaistre to Burns, Dec. 18, 1989, and Jan. 31, 1990, interviews. Jack Thompson thought that Erwin deserved credit for reorganizing the UT System in a decentralized fashion so that it could really function as a system. He noted that five new UT institutions came into existence during Erwin's tenure as a regent: the Health Science Centers in Houston and San Antonio, and UT San Antonio, UT Dallas, and UT Permian Basin; see Vernon E. Thompson to Myles Knape, Feb. 26, Mar. 14, and Apr. 8, 1986, interviews, Blocker Collections. A native and lifelong resident of Galveston, Schwartz graduated from the UT Law School in 1951. He was elected to the Texas House of Representatives for two terms (1955–1959). After Sen. Jimmy Phillips resigned, Texans elected Schwartz as his replacement in a special election in 1959. Schwartz served as a senator from 1960 to 1981. For details, see Schwartz to Burns and Knape, May 4 and June 25, 1990, interviews. A. M. Aiken was the education leader in the senate and Schwartz was a member of all of Aiken's conference committees about education. When Blocker became CEO Schwartz viewed Blocker as someone who behaved in "the general's way," expecting everyone to come to his office for meetings. Schwartz convinced Blocker that he had to leave his office and travel to Austin and other cities to lobby for political and financial support. Courtney Townsend Sr. noted that Blocker

"flew all over the state, in each senatorial district, and each representative district and met each one of the legislators. He talked with them and made friends with them, and at the meetings he had one of the local doctors from that area to be with him. That's when his [Blocker] tenacity broke out; he really went to work on the legislators and it helped the school a lot"; see "T. G. Blocker Jr., M.D. Memorial Service May 22, 1984," 23–24, RF190, CHP Archives.

106. See William H. Knisely to Chester R. Burns, Oct. 19, 1989, interview, Blocker Collections.

107. For an organization chart of the UT System in 1970, see Appendix A-25, WF441, CHP Archives. For some meetings of the Health Affairs Council between 1972 and 1974, see RF172, CHP Archives. For a photo of Knisely attending a meeting of the University of Texas System Advisory Council on Allied Health Programs in Galveston, see "Council Meets," *University Medical*, 3 (Apr., 1972), 21.

108. For more details about the reorganization of the UT System in 1972 and 1973, see Kenneth E. Ashworth to Bevington Reed, Nov. 8, 1971, letter, folder 69, box 9, Blocker Papers. Organizational charts of each of the health science centers in the UT System accompany this letter.

109. For organization charts, see Appendices A-26, A-27, and A-28, WF441, CHP Archives; *University Medical*, 1 (Feb., 1970), 12–15. See Edward N. Brandt to Chester R. Burns, Oct. 29, 1989, interview, Blocker Collections. Robert Bing, the School of Allied Health Services dean, usually did not attend these sessions. Dorothy Damewood, the School of Nursing Dean, did not attend because she was accountable to Marilyn Williams, the president of the system-wide School of Nursing.

110. For examples of Blocker's efforts to communicate with the directors of the Sealy & Smith Foundation, see Minutes, Sealy & Smith Foundation Board of Directors, Feb. 10 and 29, 1971. In 1972 John W. McCullough, president of the Sealy & Smith Foundation board, praised Blocker: "You've been able to recruit young, promising faculty members, induced the Legislature to grant support more adequately, and, of great importance, gained and retained the respect and complete confidence of the Board of Regents"; see John W. McCullough to Truman G. Blocker Jr., June 8, 1972, letter, folder 76, box 10, Blocker Papers. For photos of Blocker hosting a reception in Galveston for Gov. and Mrs. Dolph Briscoe in 1972, see folder 13, box 2, Blocker Papers. This number of business trips was calculated from Virginia Blocker's diary for 1970, box 85, Blocker Papers. Most of these trips were in Texas: Austin (twenty), Houston (thirteen), College Station (five), Dallas (five), San Antonio (three), and one visit each to Beaumont, Corpus Christi, El Paso, Amarillo, and Lubbock. The number in parentheses indicates the number of trips to that city; Blocker visited more than one city on some trips. He also took eight trips to Washington, D.C., one each to Chicago and Panama, and a trip to Europe for an international burn society meeting.

111. *Galveston Daily News*, June 2, 1974. The first quotation is from the last page of a four-page tribute to Blocker included as an unnumbered insert between page 12 and page 13 of *University Medical*, July 5, 1974. This folio contains some superb photos. See also William C. Levin, "Truman G. Blocker, Jr.," *The Bookman*, 11 (July/Aug., 1984), 3–6 (2nd quotation).

112. For details about Levin's days as student, professor, and administrator, see William C. Levin to Myles Knape, Mar. 17, Apr. 4, and May 26, 1986, and William C. Levin to Chester R. Burns, May 2 and Nov. 7, 1989, interviews, Blocker Collections. Also see two family videotapes in the Blocker Collections and folders in box 1 of the Levin Papers. Interesting memories are also present in William C. Levin to Nonie K. Thompson, Mar. 19, 1980, interview (Galveston and Texas History Center, Rosenberg Library, Galveston). See also *Houston Post*, Sept. 2, 1974 (1st quotation). For details about his dreams for UTMB in 1974, see *University Medical*, 6 (Sept.–Oct., 1974), 4–7.

113. For photos, see *Impact*, 7 (Mar. 11, 1983), 5. Also see folders 1 and 2, box 54, Levin Papers. In 1977 Levin had hired Stevens to be a full-time liaison with various community groups, especially with elected officials in government agencies; see *Impact*, 1 (Jan. 21, 1977), 2. Stevens spent a great deal of time with legislators and their aides, who gave more attention to statewide issues in health care in addition to their recurring responsibilities for reviewing and approving budgets of state institutions. During the sixty-sixth session in 1979, for example, Texas legislators passed nine hundred House and Senate bills. One hundred related to health care; see *Impact*, 3 (June 19, 1979), 14. Stevens provided Levin and others with information about these bills.

114. William C. Levin to Chester R. Burns, Feb. 24, 1989, interview, notes in WF259, CHP Archives. For texts of several addresses given at the all-day meeting, see RF126, CHP Archives. Also see Levin to Knape, interview, May 26, 1986, Blocker Collections.

115. See Brandt to Burns, Oct. 29, 1989, Blocker Collections. For organization charts, see Appendices A-29 through A-32, WF441, CHP Archives. A fairly steady routine of executive meetings occurred during these years. The Executive Committee of the Faculty of Medicine met on the first Thursday of each month; the Executive Committee of the Hospital Staff met on the second Thursday; the Academic Council on the third Thursday; and the Medical

Service Research and Development Plan Board on the fourth Thursday. Brandt usually had weekly meetings with three associate deans: James Guckian (clinical affairs), George Bryan (curricular affairs), and David Eiland (student affairs). A graduate of UTMB, James Guckian was a professor in the Internal Medicine Department and served as acting associate dean for clinical affairs for one year (1973–1974). In 1963 Bryan came from the Clinical Endocrinology Branch of the National Heart Institute to be the associate director of UTMB's Clinical Research Center and professor of pediatrics. After a residency in UTMB's Department of Neurology and Psychiatry, Eiland became a member of the faculty in 1971. For details, see *University Medical*, 6 (Sept.–Oct., 1974), 20, and George Bryan to Myles Knape, Jan. 31, Feb. 6, 11, and 26, and Mar. 6, 1986; George Bryan to Chester R. Burns, July 26 and Oct. 10, 1989; and David Eiland to Myles Knape, Nov. 19, 1985, and Jan. 21, 1986, interviews, Blocker Collections. As School of Nursing dean, Damewood did not participate in this council until 1976, when the system-wide network of nursing schools was decentralized.

116. The regents changed Walker's title from acting chancellor to chancellor on October 19, 1978. After working at UTMB for ten years, Walker had served the UT System for twelve years, shifting from director of facilities planning and construction, to vice chancellor and executive vice chancellor for business affairs, to deputy chancellor for administration, and deputy chancellor. For photos, see *Impact*, 1 (Dec. 9, 1977), 1. Other pertinent comments about these appointments are in Brandt to Burns, Oct. 29, 1989; Bryan to Knape, Jan. 31, Feb. 6, 11, and 26, and Mar. 6, 1986; and Bryan to Burns, July 26, 1989, and Oct. 10, 1989, interviews, Blocker Collections. For the general administrative organization chart in 1980, see Appendix A-33, WF441, CHP Archives. LeBlanc chose seven executive directors and two directors to help him manage the hospital; Thompson promoted three employees to assistant vice president roles. For details, see *Impact*, 4 (Feb. 8, 1980), 1, 14–15, 18; WF258, CHP Archives; Alvin L. LeBlanc to Chester R. Burns, Oct. 24 and Nov. 19, 1989; and Thompson to Knape, Feb. 26, Mar. 14, and Apr. 8, 1986, interviews, Blocker Collections.

117. See Brandt to Burns, Oct. 29, 1989, interview, Blocker Collections.

118. The data are from Chancellor Walker's address to the UT Centennial Commission. For this address, see *Impact*, 5 (Aug. 14, 1981), 14–15.

119. Minutes, UT Board of Regents, Dec. 11, 1981; LeMaistre to Burns, Dec. 18, 1989, and Jan. 31, 1990, interviews, Blocker Collections.

120. Minutes, UT Board of Regents, June 12, 1981, and Feb. 12, 1982. They expected each plan to involve input from administrators, faculty, and community leaders; to include a consideration of all aspects of research, teaching, and service; to clearly interconnect budgetary resources and campus facilities with all academic programs; and to address ways to evaluate programs that would permit enhancement of strong programs and alterations or discontinuation of weak programs.

121. George T. Bryan to William C. Levin, Jan. 21, 1982, letter, folder 1, box 47, Levin Papers; Bryan to Knape, Jan. 31, Feb. 6, 11, and 26, and Mar. 6, 1986; Bryan to Burns, July 26, 1989, and Oct. 10, 1989, interviews, Blocker Collections. Ten other members of UTMB's staff and faculty also provided assistance. Staff members conducted interviews with each department head, resulting in more than one hundred interview summaries available for the work of the Steering Committee. See "Strategic Plan for 1983–1989, The University of Texas Medical Branch," UTMB Dean's Office Records, Active. Also see RF165 and WF261, CHP Archives. For comments about the strategic planning process by a professor, see Luther Travis to Chester R. Burns, Feb. 25 and Mar. 10, 1992, interview, Blocker Collections. Charles B. Mullins to William C. Levin, Apr. 25, 1983, letter, folder 6, box 47, Levin Papers. During the early 1980s, system administrators visited UTMB periodically to facilitate such coordination. Mullins visited for three days in late October 1982 and again in February 1984; see Charles B. Mullins to William C. Levin, Sept. 15, 1982, letter, UT Chancellor's Office of Records Management, reel HA3. Chancellor Hans Mark visited in November 1984. For details, see *Impact*, 8 (Oct. 19, 1984), 1, 19; (Nov. 2, 1984), 1, 21; and (Nov. 16, 1984), 1, 6–7.

122. For details, see the folders in box 51, Levin Papers. The system's office prepared colorful brochures about the UT System and its component institutions. Brochures for 1986 and 1988 are in WF247, CHP Archives. Another example of coordination involved the regental mandate for each institution to develop a Handbook of Operating Procedures. Liz Hermann prepared UTMB's first handbook in the summer of 1987. She organized the information into five volumes: general information, personnel, fiscal, academic, and medical/hospital. As appropriate to each area, sections included descriptions of the institution, general administrative policies and services, employment policies, fiscal policies, faculty policies, house staff and postgraduate education policies, medical/professional policies, and hospital policies. See *Impact*, 11 (June 26, 1987), 1, 4. A copy of the handbook for 1997 is in box 47, CHP Archives.

123. Bryan quickly developed an organizational framework for this role, assigning most of the associate deans of the medical school (Eiland, Kitay, LeBlanc, Russell, and Schottstaedt) joint appointments as associate vice presidents (Appendix B). Yvonne Russell, who had become associate dean for community affairs in 1982, guided the development of geriatric programs, continued the development of health education programs in South Texas, and coordinated other community oriented health projects; *Impact*, 8 (Aug. 24, 1984), 6. For details, see Bryan to Burns, July 26 and Oct. 10, 1989, interviews, Blocker Collections, and WF255, CHP Archives. For organization charts in 1984 and 1985, see Appendices A-34 through A-39, WF441, CHP Archives. Also see *Impact*, 9 (Aug. 9, 1985), 1 and 21.

124. For a profile of Levin's accomplishments and comments by faculty members, see *Impact*, 11 (Aug. 21, 1987), 5–9. For another summary of accomplishments, see the list in WF259, CHP Archives.

125. *Impact*, 11 (Feb. 6, 1987), 1, 4; *Galveston Daily News*, Jan. 25, Feb. 2, and Aug. 23, 1987.

126. *Impact*, 11 (Oct. 2, 1987), 1 (quotations). The Institute of Scientific Information had named James as one of the thousand contemporary scientists most cited between 1965 and 1978. Local reporters noted this legacy in presenting James as a researcher; see *Galveston Daily News*, Jan. 25 and Feb. 2, 1987. Before becoming UTMB's CEO, James had assumed management responsibilities that successively increased in size and scope: chair of a section on cardiovascular research at the Henry Ford Hospital in Detroit between 1959 and 1968; director of research for the University of Alabama's medical center for two years; director of the Cardiovascular Research and Training Center at the University of Alabama for seven years; and chair of Alabama's Department of Medicine for eight years. Throughout these years, James learned to manage his time maximally by opening his own mail and scheduling his own appointments. He was ever accessible but did not leave the door open for any "disturbance"; Thomas N. James to Chester R. Burns, Feb. 18, 1997, interview, notes in WF257, CHP Archives.

127. Don Stevens devoted many hours to the cultivation of cordial relationships with key members of the Texas legislature. James also met with Lloyd Bentsen and Phil Gramm to discuss programs the federal government supported.

128. For an organization chart of the UT System in 1991, see Appendix A-50, WF441, CHP Archives. For comments about these interactions, especially the preparation of strategic plans, see Thomas N. James to Chester R. Burns, Oct. 12 and 24, 1995, interview, Blocker Collections. UT Chancellor Mark visited Galveston a few times. Dolph Tillotson's report of his visit in 1990 stimulated considerable controversy; see *Galveston Daily News*, Feb. 22, 1990; Tom James to faculty, staff, and students, Mar. 2, 1990, letter, WF430, CHP Archives; and *Galveston Daily News*, Mar. 21–22, 25, 29–31, 1990; and Apr. 1 and 6, 1990. At the time of Mark's resignation, James observed that he was "one of the finest leaders I have ever had the pleasure of working with." See *Galveston Daily News*, Jan. 30, 1992.

129. Administrative directors who reported directly to James included Don Stevens, assistant to the president for governmental relations; Vicki Saito, executive director for public affairs; James P. Daniel, director of development; Laura Deerinwater, affirmative action officer; and Yvonne Russell as UTMB's legislative liaison to the federal government. For organization charts in 1988, 1990, and 1991, see Appendices A-41 through A-49, WF441, CHP Archives.

130. *Impact*, 14 (Aug. 31, 1990), 1. In 1988 Yvonne Russell became assistant vice president for student affairs and dean of students for the medical school; *Impact*, 12 (Aug. 5, 1988), 7. In 1991 Bryan named Walter J. Meyer III as vice dean of the medical school and Clifford W. Houston as assistant vice president for multicultural affairs; *Galveston Daily News*, Aug. 1, 1991. In the spring of 1990 James Arens succeeded Al LeBlanc as vice president for hospital affairs and Stephen Royal became the chief operating officer of UTMB hospitals; *Impact*, 14 (Apr. 6, 1990), 1; and *Galveston Daily News*, June 28, 1990. In the fall of 1990 Arens and Royal reorganized the administrative structure of the hospitals; *Impact*, 14 (Sept. 14, 1990), 1.

131. *Galveston Daily News*, Dec. 20, 1992, and May 26, 1991 (quotation). For comments about styles of leadership Blocker, Levin, and James exhibited, see James C. Thompson to Myles Knape and Chester R. Burns, June 27, July 3 and 13, 1989, and Byron Bailey to Chester R. Burns, Feb. 13, 1992, interviews, Blocker Collections.

132. See C. William Daeschner to Myles Knape and Chester R. Burns, July 13 and 20 and Aug. 3, 1988, interviews, Blocker Collections. Daeschner perceived this reality when he became chair of pediatrics in 1960 and he did not think it had changed much after twenty-eight years of service at UTMB.

133. Before 1915 one woman assisted the CEO with stenographic, secretarial, and librarian services. Among these were Magnenat and Hill; see Minutes, UT Board of Regents, Oct. 17, 1901, and May 30, 1906. In 1915 Dean Carter obtained salaries for two positions: a person who would be his secretary (Humphrey) and another who would be the librarian (Anabel Norwood); see Minutes, UT Board of Regents, June 7, 1915. Zinn was the "administrative secretary" during the 1920s; Massin during the 1930s (for specific years, see the operating budgets in Minutes, UT Board of Regents). By 1943 five women, including Massin, worked as secretaries and clerks in Chauncey Leake's office; see Minutes, UT Board of

Regents, July 17, 1943. Pomeroy was Blocker's executive assistant and Ray was White's executive assistant. Schaub and Hermann were Levin's executive assistants. Hermann was a secretary and administrative assistant for White, Brandt, and Bryan before beginning her work with Levin; see *Impact*, 1 (May 31, 1977), 7; and 3 (May 4, 1979), 2. By 1991 about twenty people exercised staff support roles for George Bryan; see Appendix A-47, WF441, CHP Archives. For a list of secretaries, senior secretaries, and administrative assistants who assisted UTMB's executives in 1991, see WF236, CHP Archives. Photos appear in most of the administration sections of the *Syndrome* between 1958 and 1991.

Chapter 3

1. Theophilus S. Painter to UT Regents, Feb. 8, 1946, letter, box VF 9/D, UT President's Records.

2. A native of Ireland, Thomas Nolan served three terms as a member of the House of Representatives from Galveston before assuming his role at UTMB. For a list of the legislators who represented Galveston between 1846 and 1991, see Appendix A-1, WF441, CHP Archives. John Nolan served UTMB as a bookkeeper for three years before succeeding his father in 1921. For details see *Medi-Texan*, 1 (Mar., 1954), 4–5, and RF138, CHP Archives.

3. The Sealys had given $525,000 by 1917. Edward Randall told UT President Vinson: "I think it may be said without fear of contradiction that but for the generosity of Mrs. Smith and Mr. Sealy, we could never have had a medical school of Class A, ranking with the very best in the country and second to none." See Edward Randall to R. E. Vinson, Jan. 10, 1917, letter, box 4Q21, UT President's Records.

4. Thirteen of Galveston's leading citizens were directors of the foundation before 1941 (Appendix T). Minutes of their meetings have been kept since their first meeting in 1922. These minutes are located in the Sealy & Smith Foundation Offices in Galveston. Patricia Jakobi prepared excerpts of these minutes, which are located in WF280 and WF281, CHP Archives. For a list of the annual contributions of the foundation between 1926 and 1991, see Appendix B-32 in WF442, CHP Archives. After John Sealy II died in 1926, Sen. T. J. Holbrook submitted a bill to the Thirty-ninth Legislature that allowed the Sealy & Smith Foundation to invest the inheritance tax on the Sealy estate (approximately $700,000) and use the interest for support of the hospital. The legislature approved this proposal; *Galveston Daily News*, Sept. 24, 1926, and Oct. 1 and 5, 1926. For an audited report of this special fund for the period from January 31, 1927, to August 31, 1942, see the report to Gov. Coke Stevenson, July 31, 1943, in box VF 9/A, UT President's Records. The bequest from the estate of John Sealy II and that of Jennie Sealy Smith after her death in 1938 substantially augmented the assets of the foundation; see *UTMB: Seventy-five Year History*, 131, and Sealy & Smith Foundation for the John Sealy Hospital, "Report 1922–1972," WF309, CHP Archives. The twentieth-century national context for health care financing is admirably discussed in Odin W. Anderson, *The Uneasy Equilibrium: Private and Public Financing of Health Services in the United States, 1875–1965* (New Haven: College & University Press, 1968) and Rosemary Stevens, *In Sickness and Wealth: American Hospitals in the Twentieth Century* (New York: Basic Books, 1989).

5. Minutes, UT Board of Regents, May 31, 1910; *Galveston Daily News*, Feb. 21, 27–28, 1915. For other examples of fund-raisers, see *Galveston Daily News*, Jan. 27, 1900; Mar. 9, 1913; Feb. 10, 12, 13, and Nov. 6, 1921; Feb. 12, and Nov. 5, 1922; June 3, 1923; and Dec. 22, 1937. For a photo of the Hospital Aid Society in 1916, see *Cactus*, 23 (1916), 416. This group evolved from the Young Ladies Hospital Aid Society that Margaret Sealy, later Mrs. Fred Burton, organized in 1898; *Galveston Daily News*, Feb. 11, 1899. Affectionately known as a "fairy godmother," Mrs. Burton was president for many years; *Galveston Daily News*, Apr. 7, 1929. She also organized a group of black women known as the Colored Hospital Aid Society. Both the John Sealy Hospital Aid Society and the Colored Hospital Aid Society were beneficiaries of Galveston's Community Chest, which began in 1924; *Galveston Daily News*, Dec. 9, 1926. See also *Galveston Daily News*, Oct. 26, 1919; Feb. 10, 1921; July 20, 1921, and Dec. 22, 1937.

6. Minutes, UT Board of Regents, Aug. 3, 1903; Oct. 31, 1905; May 30, 1906; May 30, 1907; May 31, 1910; Oct. 21, 1921; and Aug. 23, 1922; *Galveston Daily News*, Aug. 28, 1922. Titus Harris gave $500 for the purchase of EEG equipment; *Galveston Daily News*, Nov. 9, 1939. Former faculty and students also gave book collections to UTMB's library: Allen J. Smith in 1926; J. E. Thompson in 1927; and William MacKenzie in 1928; see *Galveston Daily News*, Nov. 17, 1940. See also Minutes, UT Board of Regents, Sept. 26, 1930; June 1, 1935; Jan. 5, 1931; Mar. 21, 1932; and Sept. 29, 1938; and *Galveston Daily News*, Nov. 29, 1936. In 1931 the Sealy & Smith Foundation provided capital to equip the John Sealy Memorial Research Laboratory in the John Sealy Hospital and to fund a stipend for a research fellow who worked with Bodansky, who directed the laboratory. Workers in this lab performed clinical tests for hospitalized patients as well as experiments associated with Bodansky's research. For details, see Bodansky's annual report for 1931 in box 16, UTMB Dean's Office Records, Inactive, Blocker Collections.

7. Dick Smith, "The Development of Local Government Units in Texas" (Ph.D. diss., Harvard University, 1938), 30; Burns, "The Development of Hospitals in Galveston During the Nineteenth Century," 248. The first entry regarding a

payment ($5) to UTMB is made in Minutes, Galveston County Commissioners Court, book 11, Nov. 14, 1921, p. 27 (Galveston County Courthouse, Galveston). Beginning in 1934, small amounts of money ($20 to $60 a month) were paid monthly to John Sealy Hospital. In the reports of the county's Charity Committee, there is evidence that John Sealy Hospital received money from the county for X-rays of indigents in 1939, 1940, and 1941 (for examples, see Minutes, Galveston County Commissioners Court, book 18: pp. 424, 440, 470, 496, 503, 505, 530, 536, 545, 562, 567, 625, and book 19: pages 22, 29, and 49). For examples of treatment at John Sealy without any reimbursement, see Minutes, Galveston County Commissioners Court, book 18: pp. 562 and 590, and book 19: pp. 22, 101, 104, 252, 306, 447, 480, 492, and 648. I am grateful to Patricia Jakobi for this data; she reviewed the minutes of the Galveston County Commissioner's Court between 1876 and 1968.

8. Minutes, UT Board of Regents, Sept. 17, 1900; Nov. 15, 1900; and Oct. 17, 1901; *UT Regents' Reports*, 9th biennial (1900), 25–27, 144–146.

9. *Rules and Regulations*, Nov. 11, 1912. In 1909 UT President Sidney Mezes used the phrase "scanty support" in characterizing legislative appropriations; see "Education in Texas," *University Record*, 9 (1909–10), 305. The most serious problem with state funding for universities involved the constitutional prohibition against the use of general revenue funds for construction of educational facilities on the campuses of state universities. In 1919 the legislature adopted a bill that permitted the regents to issue bonds for acquiring revenue for constructing new buildings; see *Galveston Daily News*, Feb. 15, 1919. In 1923 Governor Neff signed a revised bill that allowed the regents to borrow money for new buildings; see *Galveston Daily News*, Feb. 27, 1923. Though these were extremely important political events in support of higher education in Texas, the regents had to use Available University Fund dollars to begin repaying these loans in the early 1930s. The constitution did not forbid the use of tax dollars for constructing eleemosynary buildings that housed patients who could be used for teaching. Legislators also assigned dollars for operating these institutions. State contributions to operating funds for the children's hospital amounted to $50,000 in 1936, for example; see W. S. Carter to H. Y Benedict, Dec. 18, 1936, letter, box VF 9/C, UT President's Records. State contributions for operating the Psychopathic Hospital in fiscal years 1936 and 1937 totaled $311,184 plus $128,250 for constructing and equipping a new addition to the hospital; see *Galveston Daily News*, Mar. 29, 1935.

10. *Galveston Daily News*, Feb. 4, 1911; W. S. Carter to S. E. Mezes, Feb. 4, 1911 (1st quotation); and W. S. Carter to S. E. Mezes, Jan. 24, 1911 (2nd quotation), letters, box 4R82, UT President's Records. Another group visited in February 1913; see *Galveston Daily News*, Feb. 4, 20–21, 1913. W. S. Carter to R. E. Vinson, Dec. 17, 1917; W. S. Carter to I. E. Clark, Leonard Tillotson, and Oscar Davis, Dec. 21, 1917, letters, box 4Q22, UT President's Records; and *Galveston Daily News*, Dec. 14–15, 1917.

11. In 1913, for example, 31 senators and 142 representatives decided how many dollars each agency would receive; Henry Triplett and Ferdinand Hauslein, *Civics: Texas and Federal* (Houston: Rein & Sons, 1918), 25–28. The number of agencies continued to grow. By 1918 the state compensated twenty constitutionally appointed state officers and nine other statutory officers (most as heads of agencies). There were eighteen supervisory or managerial boards and twenty-nine examining boards or commissions; see Frank Mann Stewart, "Officers, Boards, and Commissions of Texas," *University of Texas Bulletin*, no. 1854 (Sept. 25, 1918), 5–58.

12. Caleb Patterson and James Hubbard, *A Civil Government of Texas* (Indianapolis: Bobbs-Merrill, 1927), 134; *Annual Report of the Comptroller of Public Accounts of the State of Texas* (1918–1919), 3–4 and (1919–1920), 3.

13. *Annual Report of the Comptroller of Public Accounts of the State of Texas* (1919–1920), 167–181; General Laws of the State of Texas (1919), 303, 392; *First Biennial Appropriation Budget Submitted by the State Board of Control of the State of Texas to the Governor and the Thirty-Seventh Legislature* (1920), 124–129, 240. For legislative debates about these recommendations, see *Galveston Daily News*, July 29–31; Aug. 2, 3, 5, 17, 21, 25; and Sept. 7, 1921.

14. The powerful finance committees were among the more than thirty legislative committees functioning by the 1920s; see Patterson and Hubbard, *A Civil Government of Texas*, 107; and *Galveston Daily News*, Mar. 27, 1929.

15. J. Alton Burdine, "Reorganizing the State Administration," in Arnold Foundation Conference on Public Affairs, *The Government of Texas: A Survey* (Dallas: Southern Methodist University, 1934), 42.

16. John C. Nolan to H. Y. Benedict, Mar. 15, 1934; John Nolan to Michael Little, Aug. 17, 1933 (quotation); and George E. Bethel to H. Y. Benedict, Sept. 6, 1933, letters, box VF 9/C, UT President's Records. Also see Nolan to Gay Eddy and Nancy Brown, Mar. 23, 1965, interview, folder 35, box 1, 75th Anniversary History Papers, Blocker Collections.

17. *Galveston Daily News*, Feb. 8 and July 30, 1939.

18. *Galveston Daily News*, Aug. 1, 1921. During the late 1920s, Nick Andronis (a 1918 UTMB graduate) attended USPHS–authorized patients housed on a twenty-bed first floor ward at John Sealy Hospital; see Cyril Black to Gwen Walker, Dec. 10, 1992, letter, WF358, CHP Archives. *Galveston Daily News*, Jan. 16, 1936.

19. Minutes, UT Board of Regents, May 29, 1903. For a detailed list of all expenditures for the schools and laboratories during fiscal years 1901 and 1902, see *UT Regents' Reports* (Oct. 1902), 120–164. This list includes repairs on the Medical College Building (Old Red) and University Hall after the hurricane of 1900.

20. Minutes, UT Board of Regents, Oct. 21, 1921. The total of salaries for all of these employees was $12,060. Other individuals employed by the hospital's board handled the business and building maintenance needs of the hospitals before 1941. Records of this board are not extant, but some insight into the occupational roles of these employees can be obtained from examining Minutes, Sealy & Smith Foundation Board of Directors, Dec. 21, 1932.

21. Minutes, UT Board of Regents, July 29, 1939. For a list of duties assigned in 1933 to Nolan and his assistant, Tony Smith, see the document dated Nov. 25, 1933 (signed by Sparenberg and Bethel) in RF138, CHP Archives. For a list of general and administrative expenses for each year between 1941 and 1968, see Appendix B-6, WF442, CHP Archives.

22. Cappelmann had been Nolan's assistant for four years. He resigned in October 1955; see *Medi-Texan*, 2 (Sept., 1955), 1, 10. Nolan continued as secretary for the faculty and registrar for the students until 1959; *Galveston Daily News*, Sept. 19, 1950, and *UTMB: Seventy-five Year History*, 269. A certified public accountant, Walker had earned degrees from Sam Houston State University and the University of Texas. Walker served UTMB until 1965, when he became director of facilities, planning, and construction for the UT System. See *Galveston Daily News*, Oct. 28, 1955; *Medi-Texan*, 3 (Dec., 1955), 3–4; and Walker's obituary in *Galveston Daily News*, May 3, 1991. Harding began his UTMB service in 1956 as registrar and assistant to the executive director; see *Medi-Texan*, 4 (Nov.–Dec., 1956), 2. *Newsletter (UTMB)*, 2 (Oct. 30, 1967), 11. Thompson came to Galveston from Austin, where he had replaced Don Walker as director of the office of facilities, planning, and construction when Walker became vice chancellor in 1966. Thompson had previously served as business manager at UT's Southwestern Medical School.

23. *Galveston Daily News*, Mar. 5–8, 13, 15, 19, 21, and 27, 1941; Apr. 3, 19, and 24, 1941; May 1, 9–10, 24, 27, and 30, 1941; June 2, 10, 12, 21, 26, and 29, 1941; July 1, 8, and 29, 1941; and Aug. 12, 1942. William Stone, the senator representing Galveston, was very influential in these events.

24. Leake's pleas for money are chronicled in *Galveston Daily News*, Feb. 5, 1943; Mar. 10, 19, 23–24, 1943; Apr. 7–8, 11, 17, 1943; and May 2–4, 6–7, 13–14, 16, 1943. See Minutes, Sealy & Smith Foundation Board of Directors, Oct. 14 and Nov. 20, 1942 (Sealy & Smith Foundation Offices, Galveston).

25. Chauncey D. Leake to T. S. Painter, Jan. 16, 1946, letter, box VF 10/C; Theophilus S. Painter to UT Regents, Feb. 8, 1946, letter, box VF 9/D (quotation), both in UT President's Records.

26. Painter also resented what he called Leake's "quasi autonomy," i.e., the freedom to "go to the Legislature and more or less independently present your request for money to run your institution"; see Theophilus S. Painter to C. D. Leake, Apr. 13, 1946, letter, box VF 9/D, UT President's Records.

27. Chauncey D. Leake, "Explanatory Statement Regarding Budget Estimates for the University of Texas Medical Branch, Galveston, Texas submitted March 1946 to the State Board of Control for the Biennial Beginning September 1, 1947," box VF 18/C, UT President's Records.

28. Theophilus Painter to Chauncey D. Leake, July 5, 1946, letter, box VF 10/C, UT President's Records. Painter wanted to cut UTMB's budget by $125,000. He recommended eliminating three new positions in the nursing school and the "technical apparatus shop." He wanted to reduce the number of assistants and technicians in all departments and he wished to "cut organized research down," relying on federal and private dollars for all research endeavors. Minutes, UT Board of Regents, July 13, 1946. Chauncey D. Leake to George W. Fraser, Sept. 18, 1946, letter, box VF 10/C, UT President's Records; *Galveston Daily News*, June 1 and Sept. 11, 1946; and Minutes, Galveston City Council/Commissioners, Sept. 5, 1946, and May 29, 1947. The new contract also relieved the Sealy & Smith Foundation of its legal obligation to contribute at least $60,000 annually for the care of indigents, an obligation incurred when the regents and the city's commissioners renegotiated their lease agreement in March 1941. At that time, some believed that the foundation's contribution was a supplement to the city's annual appropriation of $40,000, symbolically perpetuating the charitable sentiments of the Sealy family. In 1946 the foundation's directors wanted legal relief from this symbolic expectation, even though they informally agreed to give the hospital $60,000 per year; see G. A. W. Currie to Logan Wilson, Feb. 8, 1955, letter, box VF E/2, UT Chancellor's Records.

29. Chauncey D. Leake to T. S. Painter, July 8, 1946, and Aug. 9, 1946, letters, box VF 10/C, UT President's Records; D. K. Woodward Jr. to members of the Board of Regents of the University of Texas, Oct. 24, 1946, letter, box

VF 9/D, UT President's Records (quotation). Nineteen members of the Appropriations Committee of the House of Representatives visited UTMB in February and thirty-one senators visited in March; *Galveston Daily News*, Feb. 27–28, 1947; Mar. 11, 13–14, 1947; Apr. 1–2, 6, 1947; and May 4, 1947. Afterward, the legislators provided substantial increases in operating income. By the late 1940s legislators provided state dollars to twenty colleges and universities. These institutions and public schools (primary and secondary) received the largest share of the state's dollars; e.g. 33 percent or $106,013,331.77 for fiscal year 1947; see Frank M. Stewart and Joseph L. Clark, *The Constitution and Government of Texas* (Boston: D. C. Heath, 1949), 111, 125.

30. Theophilus Painter to D. K. Woodward Jr., Apr. 8, 1948 (quotation) and Apr. 27, 1948, letters, box VF 9/D and Painter to Woodward, June 21, 1948, letter, box VF 10/C, UT President's Records. Painter was annoyed by the lack of centralized control over Sealy & Smith Foundation gifts. Their directors and Leake—not Painter and the regents—made decisions about ways to spend these dollars. For a sample of the dialogues that took place between the foundation's directors and regents about using Available University Fund dollars for meeting deficits in hospital operations, see Minutes, Sealy & Smith Foundation Board of Directors, June 21, 1948.

31. *Galveston Daily News*, Dec. 19, 1948; Feb. 23, 1949; and Mar 7–8, 18–20, and 25–26, 1949. Minutes, UTMB Faculty Meeting, Apr. 2, 1949, Blocker Collections. In response, loyal alumni bombarded their elected officials with pleas for restoring these cuts; see G. V. Brindley to Dear Fellow Alumnus, April 1949, letter, box VF 10/D, UT President's Records.

32. D. K. Woodward Jr. to T. S. Painter, Apr. 4, 1949, letter, box VF 10/D, UT President's Records.

33. Theophilus S. Painter to Chauncey D. Leake, Apr. 5, 1949, letter, box VF 10/D, UT President's Records (quotations). Some legislators were distressed about the high cost of medical education at UTMB, estimated at $10,000 per student per year. One senator told Painter that this was too expensive. *Galveston Daily News*, June 27 and July 15 and 23, 1949.

34. *Galveston Daily News*, Jan. 24, 1951. The Legislative Budget Board (LBB) was created in 1949. The board includes the lieutenant governor as chair, the Speaker of the House as vice chair, four members from the house, and four members from the senate. Two members from the house are the chair of the House Appropriations Committee and the chair of the House Ways and Means Committee. Two members from the senate are the chair of the Senate Finance Committee and the chair of the Senate State Affairs Committee. The LBB employs a full-time staff of budget analysts who are assigned to particular state institutions. These analysts prepare recommendations the LBB uses to make decisions about the distribution of state funds. The governor also has a budget office and staff who prepare separate budget recommendations for the LBB to review.

35. For the hearings in Austin, see *Galveston Daily News*, Feb. 1 and 14, 1951. For the visits to Galveston, see *Galveston Daily News*, Feb. 10, 22–24, 1951, and Mar 3–4, 1951. For letters of support, see folder 16, H. Kempner Records. *Galveston Daily News*, Mar. 11, 14–15, 20–22, 24, 1951; Apr 4, 13, 15, 1951; and May 9, 1951.

36. James C. Dolley to Logan Wilson, July 6, 1956, letter, box VF E/2, UT Chancellor's Records; University of Texas News Release accompanying letter from Logan Wilson to members of the Texas Medical Association, July 16, 1955, box VF I/4, UT Chancellor's Records (quotation). During the preceding fiscal year, UTMB's doctors attended patients referred from 250 of the 254 counties in Texas. Logan Wilson to John W. McCullough, July 14, 1955, letter, box VF E/2, UT Chancellor's Records; and Minutes, Sealy & Smith Foundation Board of Directors, June 16, 1955.

37. *Galveston Daily News*, May 4–5 and Dec. 13–15, 1956. Ike Kempner was a key player in these events; see folder 21, H. Kempner Records. *Galveston Daily News*, Sept. 19 and 21, 1957, and Nov. 2, 1957; and Minutes, Galveston City Council/Commissioners, Mar. 7, 1957, Nov. 1, 1957, and Nov. 14, 1957.

38. *Galveston Daily News*, July 13, 1956; and Jan. 15 and 30, 1957. The administrative wheels had been greased by Truman Blocker and the interim administrative committee before Truslow moved to Galveston. Based on a detailed budget Don Walker prepared, Blocker urged Logan Wilson to support an increase in salaries, particularly for clinical faculty; see T. G. Blocker Jr. to Logan Wilson, Feb. 14, 1956, and Mar. 8, 1956, letters, box VF E/2, UT Chancellor's Records. For a copy of the budget request, see "The University of Texas Medical Branch Legislative Budget Requests Biennium 1958 and 1959," box VF S/3, UT Chancellor's Records. *Galveston Daily News*, Feb. 5 and June 30, 1957. Staff members of the Legislative Budget Board met with Truslow and others in Galveston on May 25, 1956. Their report provided a rationale for the successful outcome; see "Staff Report on the University of Texas Medical School at Galveston," box VF Y/4, UT Chancellor's Records. The Fifty-fifth Legislature approved a record spending budget of nearly $2.1 billion, including $186,420,735 for higher education during fiscal years 1958 and 1959; see Institute of Public Affairs, *The Fifty-fifth Texas Legislature: A Review of its Work* (Austin: University of Texas, 1957), 10–12.

39. John B. Truslow to Logan Wilson, Nov. 17, 1958; Logan Wilson to Members of the Legislative Budget Board, Dec. 1, 1958, letters, both in box VF I/1, UT Chancellor's Records. See also *Galveston Daily News*, Dec. 21, 1958; Aug.

8, 1959; and May 15 and Sept. 25, 1960. In 1959 the Fifty-sixth Legislature approved a general appropriation bill that included $15.7 million of general revenue funds for increasing the salaries of faculties at state-supported colleges and universities; see Institute of Public Affairs, *The Fifty-sixth Texas Legislature: A Review of its Work* (Austin: University of Texas, 1959), 5. Approving the first general sales tax in the state's history, the Fifty-seventh Legislature (1961) enacted a record spending bill of $2.74 billion for the biennium 1961–1963, including substantial increases of funds for public schools and higher education; see Institute of Public Affairs, *The Fifty-seventh Texas Legislature: A Review of its Work* (Austin: University of Texas, 1962), 1–7.

40. Blocker prepared himself thoroughly for budget hearings with the LBB; see notes and typescripts for 1964, 1966, 1968, and 1972 in the folders of unpublished speeches in boxes 78 and 79, Blocker Papers. Responding to Gov. John Connally's passionate commitment to improvements in education, the Fifty-eighth Legislature (1963) approved a biennial budget for higher education that was 27.8 percent more than that approved for the previous biennium; see Institute of Public Affairs, *The Fifty-eighth Texas Legislature: A Review of its Work* (Austin: University of Texas, 1963), 9–10; and *Galveston Daily News*, May 29, 1966.

41. The women of Galveston continued their fund-raising efforts for the hospitals. In 1956 seventy-five women belonged to a local chapter of the American Women's Voluntary Service (AWVS), led by Mrs. E. B. Krohn. Wearing blue uniforms with the red letters—AWVS—on their pockets, these women provided numerous services to patients. They rented television sets to patients and used the money to purchase a special "respiratory bed" for polio victims; see *Galveston Daily News*, Nov. 25, 1956.

42. *Galveston Daily News*, Mar. 16 and Apr. 29, 1941; Apr. 21, May 28, and Nov. 22, 1942; Mar. 30 and Oct 12, 1947.

43. Minutes, UT Board of Regents, Oct. 25, 1941, and Aug. 1, 1942; and *Galveston Daily News*, July 13, 1941, and July 16, 1942. For Poth, see Minutes, UT Board of Regents, Sept. 25, 1942; Nov. 26, 1943; Nov. 30, 1945; July 13, 1946; Nov. 29, 1946; Dec. 5, 1947; Sept. 18, 1948; and Oct. 22, 1949. For Herrmann, see Minutes, UT Board of Regents, Mar. 27, 1943; July 13, 1946; Jan. 23, 1948; Feb. 28, 1948; June 12, 1948; and Jan. 29, 1949. See also Minutes, UT Board of Regents, Mar. 27, 1943; July 15, 1944; July 13, 1945; Oct. 26, 1945; Jan. 11, 1946; July 13, 1946; Sept. 19, 1947; Jan. 23, 1948; Feb. 28, 1948; Sept. 18, 1948; and Jan. 29, 1949.

44. For the Kellogg grant, see *Galveston Daily News*, Oct. 18, 1951. For the NFME grant, see Minutes, UT Board of Regents, Sept. 21, 1951; Mar. 28, 1952; and *Galveston Daily News*, July 28, 1953.

45. *Galveston Daily News*, Jan. 11 and 26 and Aug. 14, 1952; L. J. Olson, "Activities Supported by James W. McLaughlin Fellowship Fund for the Study of Infection and Immunity, September 1, 1954–February 1, 1970," McLaughlin Fund Office, UTMB. For the annual income and expenses of this fund between 1955 and 1991, see Appendix B-35, WF442, CHP Archives.

46. Robert Sutherland was director of the Hogg Foundation for Mental Health when it began in 1940. In the early 1940s he met with Spies to discuss ways to develop mental hygiene programs at UTMB; see *Galveston Daily News*, Jan. 14, 17, 19, and 21, 1941. Chauncey Leake, Jack Ewalt, Titus Harris, John Otto, Lamar Ross, and Steven Weisz were professors at UTMB who participated in various educational programs sponsored by this foundation during the mid–1940s. See Robert L. Sutherland, "The Hogg Foundation Reports" (1944), 29–32, and other annual reports and correspondence in box VF 27/A, UT President's Records. The Hogg Foundation is an agency within the UT System. For a list of annual grants to UTMB from the Hogg Foundation between 1950 and 1991, see Appendix B-34, WF442, CHP Archives.

47. Hyman, *Oleander Odyssey*, 422–428. For comments about these gifts and styles of managing the Kempner Fund, see Leonora K. Thompson to Chester R. Burns, Dec. 12, 1994, interview, Blocker Collections. For the clause in Kempner's will, see R. Lee Kempner to John B. Truslow, Apr. 15, 1957, letter, box VF G/5, UT Chancellor's Records. Samuel Kolmen, later a UTMB professor, received the first Jeane B. Kempner scholarship.

48. Harris Kempner originally had offered Truslow a gift of $100,000 to support a program in gerontology. However, Blocker persuaded Kempner to support a genetics program instead. The grants were used to endow a professorship and to equip a laboratory. Blocker used these endowments to recruit Barbara Bowman, who became the first chair of a new Department of Human Genetics in 1967. For details, see T. G. Blocker Jr. to Harry Ransom, June 18, 1964, letter, box VF N/1, UT Chancellor's Records; T. G. Blocker Jr. to Harris L. Kempner, July 16, 1964; Harry Ransom to Harris L. Kempner, July 31, 1964; Harris Kempner to Harry Ransom, Aug. 21, 1964; Harris Kempner to T. G. Blocker Jr., Sept. 8, 1964, letters, all in box VF FF/2, UT Chancellor's Records; and T. G. Blocker Jr. to Harry H. Ransom, Feb. 22, 1967, letter, box VF EE/3, UT Chancellor's Records. For a list of annual grants to UTMB from the Kempner Fund between 1959 and 1991, see Appendix B-36, WF442, CHP Archives.

49. Moody was the son of Col. W. L. Moody and his wife, Pherabe Bradley Moody, who moved to Galveston after the Civil War. Colonel Moody became involved in banking, cotton, and railroad enterprises. W. L. Moody Jr. attended

school in Virginia and graduated from the University of Texas School of Law. He married Libbie Rice Shearn, a third-generation Texan, and they had four children who were born in the decade before the 1900 storm. These included Mary Elizabeth Moody (Mrs. E. C. Northen), William Louis Moody III, Shearn Moody, and Libbie Moody (Mrs. Clark W. Thompson). The family's financial interests included banks, hotels, newspapers, ranches, and the American National Insurance Company. See McComb, *Galveston: A History*, 171–174.

50. In 1964 the Moody Foundation gave $8 million to nine educational institutions in Texas. See W. W. Heath to Members of the Board of Regents, Apr. 16, 1964, letter, box VF M/5; and Robert E. Baker to Truman Blocker, Oct. 6, 1964, box VF FF/2, UT Chancellor's Records. For a list of annual grants to UTMB from the Moody Foundation between 1964 and 1991, see Appendix B-37, WF442, CHP Archives.

51. *Alumni Bulletin (UTMB)*, 19 (Feb., 1965), 1. For details about the Development Board see RF152, CHP Archives. See also *Faculty News (UTMB)*, 1 (Oct. 18, 1968), and *Alumni Bulletin (UTMB)*, 23 (Spring, 1969), 5–6.

52. For a background chapter (with a useful chronological table) on the fiscal federalism that steadily increased during the twentieth century, see George J. Gordon, *Public Administration in America* (New York: St. Martin's Press, 1982), 132–168. For a concise overview (with helpful statistical tables) of the monetary impact of federally sponsored research at universities in Texas by the early 1960s, see James Howard, *Federally Sponsored Research in Texas Higher Education* (Austin: Institute of Public Affairs, University of Texas, 1963).

53. *Galveston Daily News*, Feb. 4, Mar. 3, and Oct. 21, 1942; Feb. 14 and Sept. 19, 1943; *Newsletter (UTMB)*, 1 (July 21, 1966), 1; and 2 (Sept. 15, 1966), 1.

54. Minutes, UT Board of Regents, Jan. 27, 1945; July 13, 1945; Sept. 28, 1945; Feb. 22, 1946; Sept. 20, 1946; Dec. 5, 1947; and Sept. 17, 1949. David E. Price, *Research Grants Awarded by Public Health Service, Public Health Reports*, supplement no. 205, revised 1948, (Washington, D.C.: Government Printing Office, 1949), 1. For a list of U.S. Public Health Service research grants and contracts awarded to UTMB between 1946 and 1991, see Appendix B-33, WF442, CHP Archives.

55. *AAMC Datagram*, no. 9 (Mar., 1964), CHP Archives.

56. "Grants to States for Medical Assistance Programs Title XIX Social Security Act, Effect of Implementation on Medical Education in Texas, Report and Recommendations of Task Force of the University of Texas." Spencer Thompson, Joe Boyd, G. V. Brindley Jr., and G. T. Shires prepared this report, which was submitted to Charles LeMaistre in August 1966. Because UT health units relied on the medically indigent for teaching patients, administrators and faculty were especially concerned about the long-term impact of the new laws on the total number of patients available in the UT training institutions. The task force also hoped that their report would assist the state in preparing a plan for implementing the new federal laws. A copy of the report is in WF283, CHP Archives. For a succinct summary of the increasing role of the federal government in medicine between 1946 and 1976, see James Bordley III and A. McGehee Harvey, *Two Centuries of American Medicine, 1776–1976* (Philadelphia: W. B. Saunders, 1976), 417–444.

57. See Appendix B-6, WF442, CHP Archives.

58. Mrs. Dorothy Chionsini (formerly Dorothy Lynn McCoy) to Chester R. Burns, Oct. 27, 1997, untaped telephone interview. Minutes, UT Board of Regents, July 14, 1945.

59. *Medi-Texan*, 1 (Nov., 1953), 5; 2 (June, 1955), 6–7 ; 1 (Aug., 1954), 4–5; 3 (Nov., 1955), 6–7.

60. *Medi-Texan*, 1 (Feb., 1954), 4–5; 2 (Oct., 1954), 6–7; and *Galveston Daily News*, Oct. 29, 1959.

61. *Medi-Texan*, 1 (July, 1954), 4–5; 2 (Feb., 1955), 12.

62. J. Allen Scott and Peggy McDonough Brenkus, "The Functions and Methodology of a Hospital Statistical Division," *Texas Reports on Biology and Medicine*, 9 (Spring, 1951), 146; and *Medi-Texan*, 2 (Dec., 1954), 6–7, 11.

63. *Medi-Texan*, 3 (Dec., 1955), 3–4; 4 (Feb., 1957), 4–5, 8; and 5 (Nov., 1957), 4–5, 9.

64. *Newsletter (UTMB)*, 1 (Feb. 18, 1965), 3; *Medi-Texan*, 1 (Mar., 1954), 3. A 1949 graduate of UT Austin, Jannasch had been a civil service employee in hospital services at Camp Wallace and abroad, and then served as paymaster at Gray's Iron Works in Galveston. Jannasch had been UTMB's chief payroll clerk for three years and knew many of the faculty and staff. Jim Jannasch to Chester R. Burns, Aug. 2, 1995, untaped telephone interview, and James R. Jannasch to Megan Seaholm, July 20 and 27, 1989, interviews, Blocker Collections.

65. For copies of the 1987 and 1992 reports, see WF264, CHP Archives.

66. *University Medical Center News*, 1 (Summer, 1961), 8; *Newsletter (UTMB)*, 2 (May 4, 1967), 4. Also see Appendix B-6, WF442, CHP Archives.

67. Mary Jane Rogers to Chester R. Burns, July 25, 1995, untaped telephone interview; Mary Jane Rogers to Megan Seaholm, July 21, 1989, interview, Blocker Collections; and *Galveston Daily News*, Aug. 2 and 27, 1950.

68. *Medi-Texan*, 1 (Aug., 1954), 11.

69. Thompson to Knape, Feb. 26, Mar. 14, and Apr. 8, 1986, interviews, Blocker Collections.

70. Pederson came to UTMB from UT San Antonio, where he was vice president for business affairs. Pederson had served as a budget analyst for the Legislative Budget Board for seven years, and as business officers for the Texas College of Osteopathic Medicine, UT Dallas, and UT San Antonio. In 1987 Pederson appointed Moore as UTMB's assistant vice president for operations. Moore had been director of general services at the University of Texas at San Antonio for six years. See *Impact*, 14 (Aug. 31, 1990), 1.

71. The percentage from private foundations was calculated from the totals of two columns in Appendix Y (Sealy & Smith and Gifts & Grants). The percentage from private patients and insurance carriers was calculated from the totals of three columns in Appendix Y (Patient Services, Other Services, and Professional Fees).

72. These percentages were calculated from the annual totals listed in Appendix Z. With each passing year, the "Gifts and Grants" section in the reports of the regents grew longer and longer, reflecting private dollars received from individuals; businesses and industries; local community groups and foundations; professional societies; drug companies; and national foundations. Only a few of these are identified in the text. For more examples, see the reports.

73. See Appendix B-32, WF442, CHP Archives; "T. G. Blocker, Jr., M. D. Memorial Service May 22, 1984," p. 22, RF190, CHP Archives (quotation). The amount Shirley cited included both construction and operating dollars. Blocker and McCullough enjoyed a cordial relationship for many years. McCullough was a director of the Sealy & Smith Foundation for fifty years (1936–1986) and its president from 1949 to 1979. In 1974 the UT System gave McCullough its Santa Rita award; see Minutes, Sealy & Smith Foundation Board of Directors, June 12, 1974, and Jan. 11, 1978. McCullough died in 1986; see *Impact*, 10 (Oct. 17, 1986), 5. In 1947 Ballinger Mills Jr. succeeded his father, who was a director for seventeen years. Ballinger Mills Jr. was a director for forty-five years and president from 1979 to 1992, the year of his death. He believed that Blocker, Levin, and James established cordial and productive relationships with the board; see Ballinger Mills to Chester R. Burns, July 20, 1988, interview, Blocker Collections. Also see Minutes, Sealy & Smith Foundation Board of Directors, May 10, 1978, and Nov. 13, 1985, and the "In Commemoration" brochure about the foundation in WF279, CHP Archives.

74. Minutes, Sealy & Smith Foundation Board of Directors, Mar. 8, 1978; Nov. 14, 1984; Dec. 11, 1985; and Mar. 12, 1986. Because the foundation's charter stipulated support only for the John Sealy Hospital, legal changes were necessary before the foundation could provide dollars directly for research. For comments about these changes, see Mills to Burns, July 20, 1988, interview, Blocker Collections. Between 1987 and 1991, the professors receiving these awards attracted fifty-two grants from extramural sources worth more than $28 million. For details, see the April 1994 Grant Awards Program announcement in WF264, CHP Archives.

75. Minutes, Sealy & Smith Foundation Board of Directors, Dec. 13, 1989.

76. For a list of annual contributions from the Hogg Foundation and McLughlin Fund, see Appendices B-34 and B-35, WF442, CHP Archives. For the Kempner Fund, see Appendix B-36 in WF442, CHP Archives. For a list of annual contributions from the Moody Foundation, see Appendix B-37, WF442, CHP Archives. Truman Blocker nurtured a cordial relationship with Mrs. Mary Moody Northen, chair of the Moody Foundation's board of directors. For a profile of Mrs. Northen, see *University Medical*, 12 (Winter, 1980), 24–25. Among forty large foundations listed by total grants awarded in 1987, the Moody Foundation ranked twenty-sixth; see *Chronicle of Higher Education*, June 29, 1988.

77. Current Files, UT Board of Regents: Galveston Medical Branch: President's Club; Material Supporting the Agenda for Meetings of the UT Board of Regents, XVIIIc, July 30, 1971 (both at UT Regents' Offices, Ashbel Smith Hall, Austin).

78. See *University Medical*, 12 (Summer, 1981), 29. During fiscal year 1981, UTMB received more than $18.1 million in gifts from private donors, placing it second among UT System schools that year; see *University Medical*, 13 (Spring, 1982), 30, and 13 (Winter, 1982), 26–27. More than twenty individuals (including eleven professors or former professors) had each contributed at least $10,000, thereby becoming eligible for membership in the Chancellor's Council of the UT System; see folder 2, box 47, Levin Papers. Also see samples of minutes of Development Board meetings in boxes 45 and 46, Levin Papers. For details about the evolution of the development office between 1974 and 1985, see folders 5 and 6, box 46, Levin Papers.

79. *Impact*, 3 (Aug. 24, 1979), 5; and 6 (Aug. 20, 1982), 7. For other examples, see *Impact*, 4 (June 27, 1980), 3; and 20 (Mar. 18, 1996), 1.

80. Thomas N. James to UTMB faculty, Aug. 26, 1991, letter, WF429, CHP Archives, and the brochures in WF264, CHP Archives.

81. For an early statement of UT policy, see Material Supporting the Agenda of the UT Board of Regents, XIVa, Nov. 4, 1966. For important comments about the origins of this plan at UTMB, see Jay Fish to Chester R. Burns, Feb. 17, 1992; William J. McGanity to Myles Knape and Chester R. Burns, July 18 and Aug. 5, 1988; and Travis to Burns, Feb. 25 and Mar. 10, 1992, interviews, Blocker Collections. See also Charles B. Mullins to the UT Regents, Dec. 1, 1982, memo, UT Chancellor's Office of Records Management, Mullins Reading Files, reel HA3 (no. 198207). A shrewd and devoted CBO, Jack Thompson mastered the cumbersome bureaucratic regulations associated with Medicare and Medicaid. During the early 1980s, for example, he successfully negotiated with Blue Cross to obtain more than $7 million of reimbursements retroactively allowed by the Medicare regulations; see V. E. Thompson to Charles B. Mullins, Aug. 17, 1982, letter, UT Chancellor's Office of Records Management, reel HA3 (no. 198203). For other examples of Thompson's maneuvers, see letters and reports in RF154, CHP Archives.

82. *Impact*, 2 (Aug. 24, 1979), 8–9. For a list of annual totals, see Appendix B-33, WF442, CHP Archives.

83. The commissioners approved admission of indigents to the Mainland Hospital on June 25, 1956; Minutes, Galveston County Commissioners Court, book 25, p. 553, and book 29, p. 540. See the letters and reports in folders 24 and 25, box 28, H. Kempner Records, and John B. Truslow to Peter Lavalle, July 2, 1962, letter, Minutes, Galveston County Commissioners Court, book 30, pp. 539–540.

84. Minutes, Galveston County Commissioners Court, book 35, p. 120; book 46, pp. 421–425 (Jan. 5 1967); book 35, pp. 582 and 666; book 36, p. 518; and book 37, pp. 37 and 440. See also T. G. Blocker Jr. to Ray Holbrook, Dec. 13, 1967, letter, UT Chancellor's Office of Records Management, reel 123, no. 020702. County Judge Ray Holbrook was a key player in these transactions. For information about Holbrook and other county officials, see Mary Faye Barnes, *A History of the Leadership of Galveston County: Biographical Sketches of the County Judges, County Clerks, and County Commissioners: 1838–1996* (Galveston: Galveston County Historical Commission, 1996). A copy is in WF236, CHP Archives. For a list of annual contributions by Galveston County between 1969 and 1991, see Appendix B-38, WF442, CHP Archives.

85. *Galveston Daily News*, Oct. 9, 1991.

86. See Schwartz to Burns and Knape, May 4 and June 25, 1990, interview (quotation), Blocker Collections; and news release from the Office of the UT Chancellor, Aug. 11, 1972, UT Chancellor's Office of Records Management, reel 7, no. 021101.

87. Texas State Government Sourcebook (1978), 113, 87, 134, 81. Between fiscal years 1973 and 1978, Texas had a higher percentage increase in appropriations of state tax funds for higher education than any of the fifteen most populous states. The government of Texas increased its expenditures eightyfold between 1940 and 1980; from slightly less than $166 million in 1940 to slightly more than $10 billion in 1980. Education claimed the largest share of the total in 1980 (45.3 percent); see McCleskey, et al., *The Government and Politics of Texas*, 285.

88. "Instructions for Preparing Appropriation Requests for Fiscal Years 1978 and 1979 for Health Related Educational Units," UTMB Executive Vice President's Office, Inactive. Level One could not exceed 90 percent of the 1977 appropriated level of funding for that program. Level Two could be an amount in excess of Level One, but the total could not exceed the 1977 appropriated level. Level Three could exceed the 1977 appropriated level by 20 percent or more, but had to approximate 110 percent of the 1977 appropriated level. Level Four could be a request in excess of 120 percent of the 1977 appropriated level.

89. "State of Texas, Request for Legislative Appropriation, Fiscal Years Ending August 31, 1978 and 1979, The University of Texas Medical Branch at Galveston, Galveston, Texas," Oct. 15, 1976, UTMB Executive Vice President's Office, Inactive.

90. Minutes, UT Board of Regents, Apr. 11, 1986. Note that budget cycles required the preparation of a budget request almost two years before spending would be authorized. Moreover, budget officials had to use data from the preceding year as the basis for guesses about the realities of three years hence. In April 1986, for example, officials begin preparing the budget for fiscal year 1988 using data from 1985 as the basis for "best guesses" about 1987–1988. For guidelines issued by the regents and system officers, see Minutes, UT Board of Regents, Aug. 13, 1987. For examples of instructions, calendars, and approvals for most years between fiscal years 1980 and 1991, see the folders in RF154, CHP Archives.

91. During all these years, UTMB administrators and faculty developed strategic plans needed for the rituals determined by the budgeting calendars. By October 1986, for example, UTMB's strategic plan for three biennia (fiscal years 1988 through 1993) was completed. Atypical for the process, Gov. Bill Clements did not submit a separate set of recommendations in January 1989.

92. "Text of Conference Committee Report Senate Bill No. 222 and Governor's Veto Proclamation," Supplement to Senate Journal, Seventy-first Legislature, Regular Session, III–68 to III–70. Thus, in even-numbered years, UTMB's personnel are busy with two items: the first submission of a biennial budget request to the LBB in June and the creation and implementation of an operating budget for the fiscal year beginning in September. In the odd-numbered years, administrators experience a timetable crunch during late spring and summer because the operating budget for the fiscal year beginning in September is dependent on the actions of the legislators in adopting a final appropriations bill. Jere Pederson to Chester R. Burns, Feb. 28, 1989, untaped interview.

93. *Newsletter (UTMB)*, 3 (Sept., 1968), 10–12. Supervisors of other offices reported directly to these directors. In 1969, for example, Robert Walker and a staff of six operated the Payroll Office. They managed an incredible load of paperwork and an exquisitely timed transfer of computerized cards to Austin, all necessary for receiving checks from Austin worth about $1,700,000 for more than three thousand employees each month. This office also prepared and processed reports and checks required by institutional insurance carriers, agencies handling retirement funds, and federal agencies that maintained Social Security and IRS funds; see *Newsletter (UTMB)*, 4 (May, 1969), 6–7. Bonnie Rickleman, Thompson's administrative assistant, coordinated many of the transactions between the various business offices. By 1974 she had worked in these offices for twenty-seven years; see *Hospital News*, 7 (Nov. 25, 1974).

94. *Faculty News (UTMB)*, 2 (July 17, 1970). For organization charts, see Appendix A-27, Appendix A-29, and Appendix A-35, WF441, CHP Archives.

95. *Impact*, 10 (Mar. 7, 1986), 1, 17.

96. *Hospital News*, 6 (Jan. 22, 1973), 1; 9 (Feb. 13, 1976); *Impact*, 1 (Aug. 12, 1977), 1.

97. *Impact*, 4 (Aug. 29, 1980), 13; 5 (Mar. 20, 1981), 1; 5 (Sept. 11, 1981); 7 (Oct. 1, 1983), 8; 8 (Oct. 19, 1984), 7; 10 (Oct. 17, 1986), 6; and William C. Levin to David F. Winkler, Jan. 10, 1986, letter, folder 3, box 30, Levin Papers.

98. *Galveston Daily News*, Mar. 4, July 24, and Dec. 20, 1990.

99. These departments were: Accounting; Auxiliary Enterprises; Budget Office; Computing Services Center; Cost Reimbursements; Environmental Health and Safety; Facilities Planning; Finance; Financial Analysis and Reporting; Internal Audits; Mail and Telephone Services; MSRDP Plan; Patient Accounts; Payroll; Personnel; Physical Plant; Printing and Reproduction; Purchasing; Sponsored Research Business Affairs; University Police; and Workers Compensation Insurance. A copy of the plan is in folder 3, box 6, Levin Papers.

100. See the organization chart attached to Kathy J. Shingleton to Department Chairmen, Directors and Administrative Officials, May 4, 1988, memorandum, WF358, CHP Archives. UTMB, Office of the Comptroller, "Step by Step Handbook of Services" (1993). A copy of the Business Affairs Division Department Services Manual is in WF264, CHP Archives. For organization charts of business administration in 1988 and 1990, see Appendices A-42 and A-43, WF441, CHP Archives.

101. For a list of general and administrative expenses each year between 1969 and 1991, see Appendix B-18, WF442, CHP Archives.

102. *Medi-Texan*, 5 (Feb.–Mar., 1958), 3; *Galveston Daily News*, Aug. 31, 1991; and Kusnerik's retirement brochure, WF264, CHP Archives.

103. *Impact*, 2 (Oct. 20, 1978), 11.

CHAPTER 4

1. *Galveston Daily News*, June 1, 1932.

2. *Galveston Daily News*, May 17 and June 8, 1902; Allen J. Smith to W. L. Prather, Apr. 21, 1903, letter, box 4R82, UT President's Records.

3. Minutes, UT Board of Regents, Aug. 8 and Oct. 18, 1901; *Galveston Daily News*, July 13, 1901, Apr. 6, May 17 and June 29, 1902; and W. S. Carter to I. E. Clark, Leonard Tillotson, and Oscar Davis, Dec. 21, 1917, letter, box 4Q22, UT President's Records. Black citizens in Galveston collected more than $500 to help purchase furnishings for the new hospital. This hospital is incorrectly identified as an annex in a photo of the campus included in Ellen Beasley and Stephen Fox, *Galveston Architecture Guidebook* (Houston: Rice University Press, 1996), 121.

4. W. S. Carter to S. E. Mezes, May 3, 1911, letter, box 4R82, UT President's Records; Minutes, UT Board of Regents, May 31, 1911; *Galveston Daily News*, Sept. 28, 1911, and Dec. 3, 1911; and W. S. Carter to R. E. Vinson, Oct. 19, 1916, letter, box 4Q21, UT President's Records.

5. W. S. Carter to S. E. Mezes, Feb. 19, 1912, letter, box 4Q18, UT President's Records; and *Galveston Daily News*, July 17, 1912. Interns occupied three rooms on the second floor of this pavilion. In the mid-1920s, the legs of the seven beds for interns were set in cups of coal oil to keep bedbugs and ants out of the beds, and interns would dump cockroaches from their shoes before wearing them; see Cyril Black to Gwen Walker, Dec. 10, 1992, letter, WF358, CHP Archives. Black obstetrical patients were housed in this building during the 1920s. When this building began housing psychiatric patients in 1936, it was named Psycho One.

6. Minutes, UT Board of Regents, Nov. 11, 1912, and *Galveston Daily News*, Sept. 1 and 7, 1913. Acquiring considerable money with annual sales of Red Cross Christmas Seals, the Texas Anti-Tuberculosis Association agreed to pay UTMB $1.08 per child per day for charity patients who were not residents of Galveston. Minutes, UT Board of Regents, Oct. 26, 1915. After this transfer, legislators established a separate line appropriation for this hospital, including it with the state's other eleemosynary institutions.

7. *Galveston Daily News*, June 1, 1915, and *Alcalde*, 3 (1915), 823–824. See also Deed of Gift and Agreement, May 31, 1915, box VFF/3, UT Chancellor's Records; and *Galveston Daily News*, Feb. 15, 1914, and June 1, 1915.

8. W. S. Carter to R. S. Hyer, May 7, 1915, letter, box 4Q20, UT President's Records; *Galveston Daily News*, June 1, 1915.

9. W. S. Carter to W. J. Battle, Sept. 10, 1915, letter, box 4Q20, UT President's Records; Willard R. Cooke, "A Brief History of the Medical Department," *Alcalde*, 3 (1915), 751–765; W. S. Carter to R. E. Vinson, Apr. 28, 1921, letter, box 4R84, UT President's Records; W. Keiller to R. E. Vinson, May 2, 1922, letter, box 4R84, UT President's Records; Minutes, UT Board of Regents, May 31, 1922; M. L. Graves to Robert E. Vinson, Mar. 26, 1923, letter, box 16, UTMB Dean's Office Records, Inactive; and *Galveston Daily News*, Aug. 17 and Oct. 29, 1922.

10. *UT Regents' Reports* (1924), 61. The regents also expended some Available University Fund income for repairs, e.g. $12,700 authorized on July 12, 1922. During these same years they spent more than $250,000 for expansion on the Austin campus and slightly more than $37,000 for a dormitory at the College of Mines and Metallurgy in El Paso; *UT Regents' Reports* (1924), 61; Francis L. Fugate, *Frontier College: Texas Western at El Paso: The First Fifty Years* (El Paso: Texas Western Press, 1964), 42; *UT Regents' Reports* (Dec. 1922), 314–315. The exact total was $1,009,906, which included $82,481 for land, $744,700 for eleven buildings, and $182,725 for furniture and equipment. For photos of major buildings taken in 1920, see *Galveston Daily News*, Oct. 1, 1920. The buildings diagrammed in the schematics are numbered in order of their appearance on the campus. Throughout the history of UTMB, administrators, regents, citizens, and lawyers devoted countless hours to problems associated with acquiring land for an expanding campus. For an overview of these events, see Myles Knape, "Land Acquisition," WF297, CHP Archives.

11. For the power plant and laundry, see *Galveston Daily News*, Apr. 7, 1929. During the years of the Great Depression, the sale of oil and oil-related products from Texas brought considerable money into the state's coffers and those of the Sealy & Smith Foundation.

12. *Galveston Daily News*, Oct. 1, 1925. After the transfer of the Departments of Anatomy and Pathology to the new Laboratory Building, the regents spent $50,000 for remodeling Old Red; see W. Keiller to W. M. W. Splawn, Apr. 1925, letter, box 4Q25, UT President's Records, and *UT Regents' Reports* (1925), 36.

13. W. Keiller to R. E. Vinson, Mar. 20, 1923, and Mar. 21, 1923, letters, box 4R80, UT President's Records; and W. Keiller to W. S. Sutton, Dec. 7, 1923, letter, box 4Q23, UT President's Records. At the time of the move into the Laboratory Building, Keiller told UT President Splawn that the "new quarters" were "already too small," and that the faculty would "find relief" only with an eastern extension of the new building; see W. Keiller to W. M. W. Splawn, Aug. 31, 1925, letter, box 4Q24, UT President's Records. For details about the Sealy & Smith Foundation, see *Historical Review of the Medical Branch of the University of Texas and of the Sealy & Smith Foundation for the John Sealy Hospital at Galveston, Texas*, c. 1943, WF 309, CHP Archives. Before 1924 the Permanent University Fund of the University of Texas had received slightly more than $16,000 from oil, gas, and sulfur royalties. Between 1924 and 1934 the total grew to more than $17,000,000; see Haigh, *Land, Oil, and Education*, 332.

14. *Galveston Daily News*, Oct. 9 and 19, 1930. For a description of the building, see Edward Randall and Lucius R. Wilson, "Planning for Out-Patients in a Southern Teaching Hospital," *Modern Hospital*, 36 (Mar., 1931), 83–90. The laboratory of clinical pathology and the laboratory of experimental surgery moved into this new building. When the east half of the Keiller Building opened in 1932, the laboratory of experimental surgery moved to its top floor. See also George E. Bethel to H. Y. Benedict, Oct. 20, 1930, letter, box 4Q25, UT President's Records. In 1923 Keiller had argued that UTMB would not remain a first-class school without an improvement in the outpatient clinics. See W. Keiller to R. E. Vinson, Mar. 21, 1923, letter, box 4R80, UT President's Records; and W. Keiller to Herbert M. Greene, Oct. 26, 1923, letter, box 4Q23, UT President's Records. The Sealy & Smith

Foundation directors began discussing the need for a new outpatient clinic in 1927; Minutes, Sealy & Smith Foundation Board of Directors, Feb. 22, 1927.

15. For details about construction, see *Galveston Daily News*, June 24, July 9, and July 12, 1930, and Feb. 24, Mar. 3, and Sept. 1, 1931. In 1927 legislators authorized the creation of a state psychopathic hospital, but failed to make the necessary appropriations; see *Galveston Daily News*, May 8, 11, 12, and 15, 1927. After three years of fierce competition between physicians and other citizens in Dallas and Galveston, the Board of Control located the hospital in Galveston just west of Old Red; see *Galveston Daily News*, May 18–20, 24, and June 2, 5–6, 1927; Jan. 22, Feb. 4, June 4–5, July 1, 3, 5, and 11, Aug. 29, Sept. 8, 10, 17–18, 22, 28, Oct. 8, 15, Nov. 12, and Dec. 18, 1929; and Jan. 21, Feb. 25, 27, and Mar 2, 5–6, 1930. Sen. T. J. Holbrook and County Judge E. B. Holman spearheaded the political lobbying for Galveston, and the Galveston Chamber of Commerce pledged funds for purchasing the land. Galvestonians voted favorably for the issuance of bonds whose proceeds eventually reimbursed the chamber; see *Galveston Daily News*, Mar. 6, 8, 25, 28, and Apr. 24–27, 1930; George Bethel to H. Y. Benedict, Aug. 23, 1929, letter, box 4R85, UT President's Records; and A. O. Singleton to H. Y. Benedict, Sept. 3, 1929, letter, box 4R85, UT President's Records.

16. *Galveston Daily News*, July 21 and Aug. 12, 1936; Aug. 19, 1937; and *Texas State Journal of Medicine*, 33 (Oct., 1937), 467. Additional psychiatric beds had become available during the previous year when the old Isolation Pavilion became Psycho One. The State Psychopathic Hospital eventually became an integral part of UTMB's educational enterprise in 1945 when the legislature gave the hospital to the UT regents, thereby transforming its institutional status from eleemosynary to educational. For details, see *Galveston Daily News*, Apr. 27 and 29, May 30, and June 2, 1945, and July 8, 1956.

17. W. S. Carter to R. E. Vinson, Apr. 18, 1919, box 4Q21, UT President's Records. Though a few nurses were permitted to occupy rooms on the third floor of University Hall, conflicts developed between these students and the female pharmacy and medical students. Attempts to convert University Hall into a dormitory exclusively for nurses were unsuccessful. See Minutes, UT Board of Regents, July 18, 1927, and July 18, 1930. After the nurses moved into this new building, UTMB used the first Rebecca Sealy Nurses' Home for psychiatric patients and as sleeping quarters for interns and residents. Known today as Administration Annex I, it is the second oldest building on the campus.

18. "Report of the Auditor, 1932–33," *University of Texas Bulletin*, no. 3348 (Dec. 22, 1933), 49. In January 1951 the regents honored the legacy of William Keiller by changing the name of the Laboratory Building to the Keiller Building; see *Galveston Daily News*, Jan. 6, 1951.

19. *Galveston Daily News*, May 28–31 and June 1, 1932; *University Medical*, 36 (May, 1932), 7, 9; and *Galveston Daily News*, June 1 and Oct. 1, 1932.

20. When a U.S. Public Health Service Hospital opened in Galveston in November 1931, more federal dollars for medical care came to the island than ever before. The hospital had approximately eighty employees, including eight physicians, one dentist, and fifteen graduate nurses; *Galveston Daily News*, July 3, 1932.

21. Minutes, UT Board of Regents, June 1 and Aug. 3, 1935. Randall arrived in snowy, zero-degree Washington late in January 1936 to lobby with PWA officials and senators for the Negro Hospital; see Edward Randall to H. Y. Benedict, Jan. 29, 1936, letter, box VF 4/E, UT President's Records. Carter told Benedict: "Too much praise cannot be given to Dr. Edward Randall for his deep interest and untiring efforts in getting the appropriations for the new Negro Hospital and the Hospital for Crippled Children"; see W. S. Carter to H. Y. Benedict, Oct. 31, 1936, letter, box 4Q25, UT President's Records. The regents later named the hospital Randall Pavilion. For details about the funding, see *Galveston Daily News*, Aug. 7, Oct. 6–7, 10, 13, 18, Nov. 8–9, 11–13, Dec. 13–14, 1935; Jan. 16, 22–23, 31, 1936; Mar. 5, 15, Apr. 5, and May 31, 1936. See also Minutes, UT Board of Regents, Mar. 14, 1936; C. D. Simmons to Theophilus S. Painter, Jan. 30, 1947, letter, box VF 18/A, UT President's Records; *Galveston Daily News*, Aug. 31 and Oct, 20, 1937; and Minutes, UT Board of Regents, Oct. 23, 1937.

22. *Galveston Daily News*, Oct. 30, 1938.

23. "Financial Report of the University of Texas and its Branches, For the Year Ended August 31, 1942," *The University of Texas Publication*, no. 4248 (Dec. 22, 1942), 86, 89, 91, 97–99.

24. Chauncey D. Leake, "Needs of the University of Texas Medical Branch, Galveston," July 12, 1944, box 2, Leake Papers, Blocker Collections; and *Galveston Daily News*, Aug. 13, 1944.

25. Minutes, UT Board of Regents, Feb. 29, 1949; Theophilus S. Painter to Maco Stewart, Mar. 10, 1949; Theophilus S. Painter to D. K. Woodward Jr., Mar. 17, 1949; and Maco Stewart to Theophilus Painter, Mar. 20, 1949, letters, all in box VF 10/D, UT President's Records. Beginning in September 1949 the Leakes used this home as their personal residence; see Minutes, UT Board of Regents, Sept. 16, 1949. John and Georgia Truslow also lived in this home.

26. Chauncey D. Leake to T. S. Painter, Jan. 16, 1946 (quotation), and D. K. Woodward Jr. to J. C. Dolley, Mar. 26, 1946, letters, both in box VF 10/C, UT President's Records; and *Galveston Daily News*, Apr. 25, 1946. Robert Leon White, UT's architect, drew a plot plan of proposed development at UTMB dated March 29, 1946 (a copy is in box VF 10/D, UT President's Records).

27. T. S. Painter to C. D. Leake, Apr. 12, 1946; William B. Sharp to Chauncey D. Leake, May 23, 1947; and Theophilus S. Painter to D. K. Woodward Jr., June 9, 1947 (quotation), letters, all in box VF 9/D, UT President's Records.

28. C. D. Simmons to Theophilus S. Painter, Jan. 25, 1949, letter, box VF 10/D; Theophilus S. Painter to Medical Committee of the Board of Regents, Feb. 25, 1948, memorandum, box VF 10/C; Chauncey D. Leake to T. S. Painter, Apr. 20, 1948, letter, box VF 10/C; and E. N. Capplemann to S. A. Lauver, Apr. 24, 1948, letter, box VF 10/D, all in UT President's Records. See also *Galveston Tribune*, May 12, 1948; and C. D. Simmons to Theophilus S. Painter, Jan. 25, 1949, letter, box VF 10/D, UT President's Records.

29. See list of buildings showing insurance coverage accompanying C. D. Simmons to Theophilus S. Painter, Jan. 25, 1949, letter, box VF 10/D, UT President's Records.

30. Theophilus S. Painter to D. K. Woodward Jr., Apr. 8, 1948, letter, box VF 10/C, UT President's Records.

31. Theophilus Painter, "Remarks on Ground-Breaking Ceremony of the New Hospital, Galveston, Texas, May 11, 1949," box VF A/3, UT Chancellor's Records; *Galveston Daily News*, May 12, 1949; Minutes, Sealy & Smith Foundation Board of Directors, Aug. 3, Sept. 7, and Oct. 5, 1938; Current Files, UT Board of Regents, Buildings and Grounds, 200, Galveston Medical Branch: R. Waverley Smith Pavilion; and *Galveston Daily News*, Oct. 26, 1938.

32. Minutes, UT Board of Regents, July 15 and Sept. 29, 1944, Mar. 22, 1946, and July 9, 1948; John W. McCullough to Fred W. Catterall, et al., Feb. 25, 1949, Minutes, Sealy & Smith Foundation Board of Directors; *Galveston Daily News*, July 16, 1945; Mar. 24, 1946; Jan. 19, 1947; and Feb. 17, 1949; and Ballinger Mills Jr. to Chester R. Burns, July 20, 1988, interview, Blocker Collections. The foundation for the buildings required 1,658 twelve-inch, H-section, 53-pound steel piles driven to a depth of approximately 110 feet below sea level—a total of more than thirty-four miles of steel piling; see "Facts Concerning the New John Sealy Hospital and the Waverley Smith Memorial Pavilion," folder 63, box 6, School of Nursing Archives, Blocker Collections. Construction details are chronicled in *Galveston Daily News*, June 8, 1951; May 25, 1952; Sept. 20, 1953; and Dec. 13, 1953. See also Minutes, Sealy & Smith Foundation Board of Directors, May 14, 1952.

33. *Galveston Daily News*, Dec. 16, 1953; and Minutes, Sealy & Smith Foundation Board of Directors, July 14, 1954. Approximately 20 percent of the total represented federal dollars. Air conditioning the hospital and pavilion required three Carrier refrigeration units (capacity of approximately 1,250 tons) and five pumps that circulated 7,100 gallons of water per minute through the units. Scattered throughout these buildings at that time were 190 miles of wire in 55 miles of conduits, 350 telephones, 165 clocks, 4,850 lighting fixtures, and more than 45 miles of copper tubing in piping systems. For other details, see "Facts Concerning the New John Sealy Hospital and the Waverley Smith Memorial Pavilion," folder 63, box 6, School of Nursing Archives, Blocker Collections.

34. In August 1947 Texans boosted morale among educators by approving a constitutional amendment that permitted the issuance of bonds for funding permanent construction; see *Galveston Daily News*, Aug. 6, 12, 17, and 27, 1947. Dollars for the Gail Borden Building came from bond proceeds; see *Galveston Daily News*, Jan. 13, 20–21, 1949. See also *Galveston Tribune*, June 18, 1949; *Galveston Daily News*, Jan. 6, 1951, and June 7, 1952; and Current Files, UT Board of Regents, Buildings and Grounds, 200, Galveston Medical Branch: Laboratory Building, new 1949–1952. Documentary evidence explaining the naming of this building in honor of Gail Borden has not been found. Leake may have wished to honor the sentiments of Galvestonians who appreciated the legacy of Borden as a collector of customs, agent of the Galveston City Company, member of the first group of aldermen, inventor of the meat biscuit, and, later, of condensed milk; see Joe B. Frantz, *Gail Borden: Dairyman to a Nation* (Norman: University of Oklahoma Press, 1951). Surely he was thinking of soliciting funds for research from the Borden Company because their representatives attended the dedication ceremony. He did persuade officers of the Borden Company Foundation to establish the Borden Undergraduate Research Award at UTMB, a $500 award to a senior medical student who had done the most significant research as a student. See Chauncey D. Leake to James P. Hart, Aug. 16, 1952, letter, box VF C/1, UT Chancellor's Records; H. A. Ross to Chauncey D. Leake, June 20, 1955, letter, box VF E/3, UT Chancellor's Records; Chauncey D. Leake to H. A. Ross, June 24, 1955, letter, box VF E/3, UT Chancellor's Records; and *Galveston Daily News*, Sept. 21, 1952.

35. Minutes, UT Board of Regents, Jan. 23 and Feb. 4, 1954, and Jan. 24, 1948. For details about funding and construction see *Galveston Daily News*, Dec. 9, 1947; Feb. 5, 1948; Oct. 28, 1950; Feb. 2, June 28, and Sept. 20, 1952;

July 16, and Oct. 18, 1953; and Jan. 3 and 31, 1954. See also Current Files, UT Board of Regents, Buildings and Grounds, 200, Galveston Medical Branch: Ziegler Hospital.

36. Early discussions about air-conditioning took place in February 1950; see *Galveston Daily News*, Feb. 4 and 8, 1950. For a fascinating look at the ways that air conditioning affected ways of life in the South, see Raymond Arsenault, "The End of the Long Hot Summer: The Air Conditioner and Southern Culture," *Journal of Southern History*, 50 (Nov., 1984), 597–628. See also *Galveston Daily News*, Oct. 12, 1952, and Apr. 29, 1953; and Current Files, UT Board of Regents, Buildings and Grounds, 200, Galveston Medical Branch: Project Tex-41-CH-11 Housing and Home Finance Agency Loan Agreement. In the summer of 1948 the Sealy & Smith Foundation built four buildings with apartments that could be rented by personnel at UTMB; see *Galveston Daily News*, July 26–27, 1947.

37. Bethel Hall was named in honor of George Emmett Bethel, who had served as CEO between 1928 and 1935. Brackenridge Hall was named in honor of George W. Brackenridge, the regent who had provided funds for the construction of University Hall in 1897. Clay Hall was named in honor of Ethel D'Arcy Clay, who had served as director of nurses for the John Sealy Hospital and director of the John Sealy College of Nursing between 1905 and 1919. League Hall was named in honor of Nellie Bell League, one of the more active participants in the women's group that founded the John Sealy Hospital Training School for Nurses in 1890. Morgan Hall was named in honor of Jean Scrimgeor Morgan, who initiated the sale of Red Cross Christmas Seals in Galveston in 1908, thereby helping to raise funds that were used in constructing the first Children's Hospital. Nolan Hall was named in honor of Thomas H. Nolan, who had served as provost between 1903 and 1921. Vinsant Hall was named in honor of Wilma Rolena Vinsant, a 1940 nursing graduate who was killed in an airplane accident while helping to evacuate wounded servicemen in Germany during World War II. The Faculty House included a cafeteria, informal meeting places for students and faculty, and apartments for official visitors. When this building was later used as the fourth psychiatric inpatient facility on campus, it was named Unit D (1960). For more information about the honorees, see *Galveston Daily News*, Mar. 3, 1955, and John Truslow to Logan Wilson, Aug. 26, 1957, letter, box VF G/1, UT Chancellor's Records. For photos of Bethel Hall, Brackenridge Hall, Clay Hall, and Nolan Hall when they were first occupied in 1955, see *Medi-Texan*, 2 (Feb., 1955), 4; and (July, 1955), 13. For photos of the Faculty House in 1956 and 1957, see *Medi-Texan*, 3 (Aug., 1956), 1; and *Alumni Bulletin (UTMB)*, 11 (Oct., 1957), 1. As more students leased apartments off-campus, some of these dorms were used for other purposes. The School of Nursing was housed in Brackenridge Hall between 1959 and 1986. A Center for Audiology and Speech Pathology was housed in Bethel Hall. A Chronic Home Dialysis Center was housed in Clay Hall. Laboratories of the Marine Biomedical Institute were housed in League Hall. Beginning in late 1968, Unit D housed offices of a Vocational Rehabilitation Center and, in the 1980s, the Family Medicine Clinic and Department and a Geriatric Day Care Center.

38. *Galveston Daily News*, Aug. 3, 1949; and Aug. 2 and 27, 1950. A portion of this long building is still visible as the southwest portion of number 18 on the schematic for 1967. A substantial portion of this building was incorporated into the Surgical Research Laboratories when they were constructed in 1964. The warehouse was the long north section of building 18 on the schematic for 1967, building 7 on the schematic for 1991. For details, see Chauncey D. Leake to T. S. Painter, Feb. 16, 1950 (Galveston Medical Branch: Storage Building, Current Files, UT Board of Regents) and Chauncey D. Leake to James P. Hart, Jan. 16, 1951, letter, box VF A/3, UT Chancellor's Records.

39. This eleemosynary institution was located in Galveston after W. L. Moody Jr. gave a new building on Offats Bayou to the state. Originally Moody wanted this building used as a home for the indigent aged. The school was formally dedicated in March 1950 but did not open until the fall. For details, see *Galveston Daily News*, Jan. 15, 18, 20, 22, 25; Feb. 5–6, 26; Mar. 14–15, 28, 31; Apr. 1; July 11 and 26; Aug. 10; and Dec. 19, 1950.

40. "Annual Financial Report," fiscal year 1955, 218–219. The foundation's directors had also given several plots of land, including the east half of Block 604, as a site for a Student Union building, a project of the Medical Alumni Association. By 1955 alumni had not yet donated enough money for construction of this facility; see "Construction of Student Union, The University of Texas Medical Branch," box VF E/2, UT Chancellor's Office.

41. Minutes, UT Board of Regents, Dec. 6, 1955; and "Memorandum on the Building Program," Nov. 23, 1956, box VF G/1, UT Chancellor's Records.

42. *Galveston Daily News*, June 20 and 23, 1957; and Minutes, UT Board of Regents, June 29, 1957. A copy of the report is in RF45, CHP Archives.

43. For a sample of discussions with the Sealy & Smith Foundation directors, see Minutes, Sealy & Smith Foundation Board of Directors, Sept. 9, 1959. A diagram of a "Pilot Master Plan" appeared in *UTMB Catalog* (1958–1959), 8, and *Syndrome*, 7 (1959), 158–159. See also Minutes, Sealy & Smith Foundation Board of Directors, May 13, 1959, and John B. Truslow to Logan Wilson, Jan. 8, 1960, Feb. 25, 1960, and June 1, 1960, letters, box VF I/1, UT Chancellor's Records.

44. Minutes, UT Board of Regents, Sept. 23, 1960. Sketches of this plan appeared in *Syndrome*, 9 (1961), 184. For details, see "Status Report on the Ten Year Plan," Oct. 30, 1961, Material Supporting the Agenda for the UT Board of Regents, Vol. IXa, pp. 1–14.

45. "The University of Texas Medical Branch, Status of Certain Building Projects," box VF T/3, UT Chancellor's Records. Ransom had visited with the Sealy & Smith Foundation directors in January; Minutes, Sealy & Smith Foundation Board of Directors, Jan. 10, 1962. The accreditation team from the Liaison Committee on Medical Education that evaluated UTMB in January 1962 spurred continued interest in campus improvement by declaring that the physical facilities for research and teaching were inadequate. See "Report of Survey of the University of Texas Medical Branch, Galveston, Texas by the Liaison Committee on Medical Education . . .," Jan. 15–18, 1962, Office of the Liaison Committee on Medical Education, Association of American Medical Colleges, Washington, D.C. A copy is in WF178, CHP Archives. For many of these projects, negotiations occurred with the Sealy & Smith Foundation directors; see Minutes, Sealy & Smith Foundation Board of Directors, Sept. 14 and Nov. 9, 1960, and Jan. 11, Feb. 8, and Apr. 12, 1961. See also John B. Truslow to Harry H. Ransom, Jan. 25, 1962, letter, box VF L/6, UT Chancellor's Records. For a summary of Truslow's report to the faculty about the construction projects, see *University Medical Center News*, 2 (Feb., 1962), 1–2.

46. *Galveston Daily News*, Feb. 20, Mar. 11 and 23, and May 18, 1962; *University Medical Center News*, 2 (Summer, 1962), 2–3, 7–8; "Building Programs, The University of Texas Medical Center, Galveston, February 15, 1962," Material Supporting the Agenda of the UT Board of Regents, Mar. 8, 1962; and *University Medical Center News*, 2 (Dec., 1961), 8, and 2 (May, 1962), 6.

47. Minutes, UT Board of Regents, Feb. 3, 1962, and *Galveston Daily News*, Feb. 4, 1962. Between 1956 and 1962 the Sealy & Smith Foundation contributed $387,900 for remodeling several areas of the John Sealy Hospital. Until the Department of Anesthesiology was situated on 2A in 1959, for example, it had been housed in Old Red, a block away from the operating rooms. See John B. Truslow to Harry H. Ransom, Mar. 1, 1962, letter, box VF T/3, UT Chancellor's Records. Old Red was remodeled to provide "temporary" space for the Departments of Physiology, Pharmacology, and Microbiology. See "Report to the President: Basic Science Department Programs—The University of Texas–Medical Branch," June 1960, box VF I/1, UT Chancellor's Records; John B. Truslow to Harry H. Ransom, Nov. 14, 1962, letter, box VF M/5, UT Chancellor's Records; and "Report of the University of Texas Medical Branch Faculty Building Committee," Jan. 11, 1965, box VF CC/2, UT Chancellor's Records.

48. Minutes. UT Board of Regents, Apr. 27, 1962. For details of the meeting and Ransom's recommendations, see memos dated Apr. 8, 1962, and Apr. 19, 1962, in box VF L/6, UT Chancellor's Records. Ransom had already met with the Sealy & Smith Foundation directors; see Minutes, Sealy & Smith Foundation Board of Directors, Feb. 4, 1963. See also "Preliminary Report of The University of Texas Medical Branch Faculty Building Committee," Nov. 7, 1962, Minutes, UTMB Faculty Building Committees, RF155, CHP Archives. Between 1962 and 1968 this committee functioned in a remarkably cooperative and productive way; see minutes of their meetings in RF155, CHP Archives. Also see *Galveston Daily News*, July 17, 1964, and Minutes, UT Board of Regents, Apr. 4, 1963.

49. Minutes, UT Board of Regents, Oct. 6, 1962, and *Galveston Daily News*, Oct. 26, 1962. The Sealy & Smith Foundation owned and operated the Sealy & Smith Professional Building that housed the foundation's offices. Between 1964 and 2000 UTMB leased space in this building to accommodate specific needs at various times. See *Galveston Daily News*, June 24, 1964. In the summer of 1962 the Sealy & Smith Foundation directors learned that the Shriners of North America had decided to establish hospitals for burned children at three locations in the United States; Minutes, Sealy & Smith Foundation Board of Directors, Aug. 8, 1962. In 1963 Truslow, McCullough, Blocker, Ransom, and others negotiated with the Shriners about locating one of these hospitals in Galveston; *Galveston Daily News*, July 3 and 17, 1963. The Shriners were most impressed with Blocker's experience in the care of burned patients and UTMB's Division of Plastic Surgery. For details, see John B. Truslow to Harry H. Ransom, July 5, 1963, letter, box VF CC/5, UT Chancellor's Records; Lanier Cox, "Background Information Concerning Recent Developments Re Shriners Burns Institute," Aug. 7, 1963, box VF M/5, UT Chancellor's Records; and the extensive correspondence in box 14 of the Blocker Papers.

50. Supplemental Agenda Item for Board of Regents' Meeting, Sept. 18–19, 1964, box VF CC/4, UT Chancellor's Records, and *Alumni Bulletin*, 19 (Oct., 1965), 1–2.

51. In 1965 the federal government decided to close several USPHS hospitals including the one in Galveston. A committee of physicians from UTMB and the USPHS hospital prepared a lengthy report about the advantages of developing a strong affiliation between UTMB and the USPHS for providing care to USPHS clients (2,319 inpatients and 38,578 outpatient visits in Galveston during 1965). Using this data, Blocker and Nicholas C. Leone, the medical officer in charge of Galveston's USPHS hospital, recommended the construction of a 360-bed USPHS hospital on the

UTMB campus. This recommendation was not accepted and the USPHS hospital in Galveston closed in 1978; see *Galveston Daily News*, Dec. 8, 1982. A copy of the report is in RF180, CHP Archives. See also *UTMB: Seventy-five Year History*, 269. Don Walker was a key player in these developments, serving as UTMB's associate director for a year before becoming director of facilities, planning, and construction for the UT System. In January 1965 the building committee Truslow established gave Blocker an updated report that recommended a children's hospital, an additional basic science building, a library and conference center, a physical plant building, and a nursing school facility.

52. *Newsletter (UTMB)*, 2 (Nov. 3, 1966), 1. The $6 million needed for reconstruction came from the Sealy & Smith Foundation, the Babe Didrickson Zaharias Fund, Permanent University Fund bond proceeds, and state and federal agencies (a Hill-Burton grant via the Texas State Department of Health and a USPHS Health Research Facilities grant). For details, see Current Files, UT Board of Regents, Buildings and Grounds, 200, Galveston Medical Branch: "McCullough, John W. Outpatient Clinic." For the Babe Didrikson Zaharias Fund, see Susan E. Cayleff, "Mildred Ella Didrikson Zaharias," in Tyler, et al. (eds.), *The New Handbook of Texas*, VI, 1138–1139. For the dedication ceremony on March 10, 1967, see *Alumni Bulletin*, 21 (Apr., 1967), 2.

53. Harry Ransom to Truman Blocker, Hamilton Ford, Raymond Gregory, Willard F. Verwey, Daniel J. Bobbit, E. D. Waler, Lanier Cox, and G. W. Landrum, Feb. 10, 1964, memo, box VF CC/5, UT Chancellor's Records. Seven years earlier (May 1957), McCullough and the Sealy & Smith Foundation directors had offered to construct a 150-bed psychopathic hospital; Minutes, UT Board of Regents, May 3, 1957. Conflicts between Truslow and McCullough, as well as serious perturbations about ownership and responsibilities for daily management, sabotaged negotiations. The committee believed that UTMB should appoint the professional staff of the hospital and manage the hospital's operations; E. D. Walker to Harry H. Ransom, Mar. 4, 1964, letter, box VF M/5, UT Chancellor's Records. The Sealy & Smith Foundation directors proposed that the hospital be operated via a long-term agency contract with UTMB; see Minutes, Sealy & Smith Foundation Board of Directors, Apr. 6, 1964. A regental committee, UT administrators, and foundation directors changed many details during the ensuing months; see Minutes, UT Board of Regents, Apr. 24–25, 1964; Minutes, Sealy & Smith Foundation Board of Directors, May 13, 1964; Minutes, UT Board of Regents, May 16, 1964; and *Galveston Daily News*, Oct. 27, 1964. Developing acceptable architectural plans for the hospital was no easy matter, because it depended on discussions with the foundation's directors, the university's architect, the faculty in psychiatry and neurology, Walker, and Blocker. During a meeting on August 17, 1965, Blocker stated that he "really did blow my top to Mr. Byard," who was the executive director of the foundation. See the transcription of a recording made of this meeting in RF155, CHP Archives; and Minutes, Sealy & Smith Foundation Board of Directors, July 6 and 13; Aug. 11 and 17; and Sept. 8, 1965.

54. *Galveston Daily News*, Oct. 30, 1968; *Newsletter (UTMB)*, 4 (Jan., 1969), 9–11.

55. Minutes of their meetings between July 1963 and February 1964 are attached to Warren Harding to Harry H. Ransom, Feb. 28, 1964, letter, box VF P/e, UT Chancellor's Records. Members of the committee included Willard Verwey, Eric Hall, John Middleton, William Daeschner, Edgar Poth, and Abe Levy (director of the Animal Care Center). See also Minutes, UT Board of Regents, Mar. 10, 1967, and May 6, 1967.

56. Minutes, UT Board of Regents, Oct. 27, 1967; and News Release, UT News and Information Service, Oct. 28, 1967, box VF EE/3, UT Chancellor's Records.

57. Clark W. Thompson served the Ninth Congressional District in the U.S. House of Representatives for twenty-two years (1933–1934 and 1947–1967). Congressman Thompson met his wife, Libbie, while he was stationed at Fort Crockett in 1918. Mrs. Thompson provided an initial gift of $1 million and the building's two hundred-seat auditorium was named for the Thompson's daughter, Libbie; see T. G. Blocker Jr. to Harry H. Ransom, Mar. 26, 1969, letter, box VF BB/5, UT Chancellor's Records, and *University Medical*, 12 (Summer, 1981), 24–25. Additional dollars came from Permanent University Fund bond proceeds ($1,948,411), a NIH grant ($731,079), a Sealy & Smith Foundation gift ($673,200), and some Medical Service Research and Development Plan income ($110,000). See also *University Medical*, 3 (Oct., 1971), 4–7.

58. *University Medical*, 3 (Feb., 1972), 14–15. This new structure was integrated with the completely remodeled McCullough Outpatient Clinic Building.

59. For the Gorsline report, see RF155, CHP Archives. See also T. G. Blocker Jr. to Harry H. Ransom, Apr. 25, 1969, letter, GMB: Academic Planning, Current Files, UT Board of Regents; *Faculty News (UTMB)*, Sept. 26, 1969; and Joseph M. White to Chester R. Burns, Dec. 19, 1989, and Charles LeMaistre to Chester R. Burns, Dec. 18, 1989, and Jan. 31, 1990, interviews, Blocker Collections.

60. Minutes, UT Board of Regents, Dec. 12, 1969, and Oct. 22, 1971. For comments about this building, see C. William Daeschner to Myles Knape and Chester R. Burns, July 13 and 20 and Aug. 3, 1988, interviews, Blocker

Collections. See also Minutes, Sealy & Smith Foundation Board of Directors, Nov. 28, 1972. To retire these bonds, the Sealy & Smith Foundation pledged 80 percent of its net income for twenty-five years, estimated at $1,400,000 a year for the first ten years and $1,250,000 a year for the remaining fifteen years.

61. The incredible details required for grant applications for federal dollars for construction are fully exemplified in the application submitted for this grant. See WF300, CHP Archives, and the Child Health Center files in Current Files, UT Board of Regents, and UTMB Executive Vice President's Office, Active. See also Minutes, UT Board of Regents, Apr. 24, 1973, and *Hospital News*, 6 (July 23, 1973), 1.

62. For examples, see Minutes, Sealy & Smith Foundation Board of Directors, Jan. 12, 1972, and Nov. 28, 1972. This project was usually discussed during every monthly meeting of the foundation's directors. See three reports in RF155, CHP Archives. These were prepared by employees of G. Pierce, Goodwin, Flanagan (architects—engineers—planners); Ray S. Burns & Associates (mechanical engineers); Walter P. Moore & Associates (structural engineers); and Medical Planning Associates (hospital consultants). They submitted detailed specifications about the work site and schedule, concrete, masonry, metals, carpentry, moisture protection, doors, windows, finishes, equipment, furnishings, and the conveying, mechanical, and electrical systems. One report was a 2.5-inch-thick guide to the furnishings and equipment that could be installed in the new additions, such as cabinets, work counters, lockers, dividers, mirrors, toilet paper holders, and soap dispensers. See Minutes, UT Board of Regents, Oct. 26, 1973, and Feb. 1, 1974; and *Hospital News*, 8 (Feb. 18, 1974), 1.

63. "Summary of Proposal by Medical Branch Alumni Association for Construction of a Field House for the Benefit of Students and Faculty," Jan. 9, 1967, attached to excerpts from Minutes, UT Board of Regents, Mar. 10–11, 1967, in box VF EE/3, UT Chancellor's Records; and *Alumni Bulletin*, 22 (Winter, 1968), 3–5; (Spring, 1968), 2–3; and (Summer, 1969), 11.

64. UTMB's library had been inadequately housed almost as soon as it moved into the new Gail Borden Building in 1952. In the early 1960s the regents agreed to a new library building in principle, but insufficient state funds forced Truslow and others to seek dollars from private sources. For details, see W. F. Verwey to John B. Truslow, Feb. 27, 1963; John B. Truslow to Harry H. Ransom, Mar. 4, 1963; and Lanier Cox to Harry H. Ransom, Mar. 15, 1963, letters; Minutes, Meeting of the Faculty Building Committee, July 22, 1963, Feb. 24, 1964, and Aug. 3, 1964; and W. W. Heath to Board of Regents, Apr. 16, 1964, letter, all in box VF M/5, UT Chancellor's Records.

65. Minutes, UT Board of Regents, July 16, 1965, and Aug. 26, 1966. For details, see the correspondence in box 13 of the Blocker Papers. The architects met with the library committee in Galveston on November 22, 1966; see Minutes, Faculty Building Committee, Nov. 21, 1966. See also Minutes, UT Board of Regents, May 31, 1968. UTMB officials had applied for a federal grant soon after the U.S. Congress approved the "Library Assistance Act of 1965." See L. D. Haskew to E. D. Walker, Feb. 26, 1965, letter, box VF P/3, UT Chancellor's Records.

66. A typescript of the speeches given at the dedication ceremony is in RF155, CHP Archives. See also *University Medical*, 3 (June, 1972), 16–21. The library's history of medicine and rare book area was named in honor of Blocker after his death in 1984. See Larry J. Wygant (comp.), *The Truman G. Blocker Jr. History of Medicine Collections: Books and Manuscripts* (Galveston: University of Texas Medical Branch at Galveston, 1985), vii–xii.

67. Minutes, UT Board of Regents, July 26, 1968; and *Hospital News*, 5 (Nov. 1, 1971), 2.

68. Minutes, UT Board of Regents, Mar. 12, 1971.

69. For details about decisions pertaining to "surge" space, see V. E. Thompson to E. D. Walker, June 22, 1973, letter, Surge Facility files, UTMB Executive Vice President's Office, Inactive; Betty Anne Thedford to Eriksson Construction Company, Inc., June 12, 1972; R. L. Anderson to E. D. Walker, Aug. 14, 1972; and V. E. Thompson to E. D. Walker, June 22, 1973, letters, UTMB Executive Vice President's Office, Inactive; *Hospital News*, 6 (Sept. 18, 1972), 1; Minutes, UT Board of Regents, June 11, 1982, Aug. 11, 1983, Apr. 11, 1985, Aug. 8, 1985; and William C. Levin to Charles B. Mullins, Aug. 30, 1982, letter, "Pharmacology Bldg., Completion of Departmental Space (9/1/82–8/31/84)," Buildings and Grounds, Current Files, UT Board of Regents. See Cary Cooper to Myles Knape, Nov. 12, 1987, interview, Blocker Collections, for additional insights.

70. See V. E. Thompson to the members of the new planning committee, Mar. 4, 1974, letter, folder 2, box 20, Levin Papers. Possible projects included an addition to the Basic Sciences Building, an Allied Health Sciences Building, a facility for the School of Nursing, an extended care facility, a dormitory, additional outpatient facilities, a Student Activities Center, an auditorium, a Physical Plant Building, and additional facilities for parking, warehouse storage, and animal care.

71. The data presented in this paragraph were taken from Schedule C-11 (p. 46) and Schedule S-11b in UTMB's Financial Report for fiscal year 1974 (pp. 114–121). For a copy, see WF288, CHP Archives. These structures included

all major buildings, as well as several small ones used for the incinerator, a greenhouse, paint shop, tool shed, and gate houses. The total dollar value also reflected various cottages at Moody State School and four fraternity houses.

72. *Impact*, 1 (May 13, 1977), supplement; and *Impact*, 1 (Feb. 18, 1977), 8–9. For comments about the new Child Health Center, see Luther Travis to Chester R. Burns, Feb. 25 and Mar. 10, 1992, interviews, Blocker Collections.

73. For the North Addition, see *Hospital News*, 9 (Dec. 17, 1976), 1, 4; and *Impact*, 1 (May 13, 1977), supplement. For the South Addition, see *Impact*, 1 (Nov. 18, 1977), 1, 8–9; and 2 (June 30, 1978), 2. For dedication ceremonies, see *University Medical*, 9 (Mar.–June, 1978), 2–15.

74. Memorandum from Space Committee to John P. Poretto, Apr. 19, 1979, RF155, CHP Archives.

75. See George Bryan to Myles Knape, Jan. 31, Feb. 6, 11, and 26, and Mar. 6, 1986, interviews, Blocker Collections. During the mid-1980s, the Sealy & Smith Foundation gave much more for other renovation projects in the old John Sealy Hospital and the old Children's Hospital. Some of these are described in the letters attached to a proposed agenda item for the regents' meeting on June 10–11, 1982 in RF155, CHP Archives.

76. Minutes, UT Board of Regents, Nov. 1, 1974, and Jan. 31, 1975; "A Report to the Microbiology Department Faculty, Microbiology Building Committee," Oct. 29, 1975, box 3, folder 28, A. Packchanian Papers, Blocker Collections; and *Impact*, 2 (Aug. 25, 1978), 3. In 1982 George Bryan recommended that the open space adjacent to the stilts supporting the Microbiology Building could be closed to provide space needed by the rapid development of research on interferon in the Department of Microbiology. The regents eventually approved this request and, after a year of construction by Pat McMahon, Inc. of Houston, the ground floor area was occupied in August 1984. See George T. Bryan to William C. Levin, Mar. 5, 1982, and William C. Levin to Charles B. Mullins, Apr. 30, 1982, letters, Microbiology Building File, Current Files, UT Board of Regents; and Minutes, UT Board of Regents, June 10, 1982.

77. Minutes, UT Board of Regents, May 14, 1976; Feb. 11, 1977; and June 8, 1978; *Impact*, 2 (June 16, 1978), 1, 15; the Learning Center File in UTMB Executive Vice President's Office, Active; and *Impact*, Oct. 23, 1981, 1, 17. Only the interiors of the first two floors were ready for use at that time; the other floors were finished during the following two years.

78. Thomas N. James to Charles B. Mullins, Sept. 1, 1987, letter, William C. Levin Hall file, Current Files, UT Board of Regents; Minutes, UT Board of Regents, Oct. 9, 1987; and *Impact*, 11 (Oct. 30, 1987), 1.

79. Minutes, UT Board of Regents, Dec. 15, 1977. In 1976 the inspecting committee from the Joint Committee on Accreditation of Hospitals had recommended that the psychiatric program not be accredited because of inadequate life safety standards in both the Randall Pavilion and the Graves Hospital. See Minutes, UT Board of Regents, Aug. 3, 1978, and *Impact*, 6 (Apr. 23, 1982), 1, 14. For more on the Research Center plans, see Diane Hewell's memo from the Texas Health Facilities Commission dated Apr. 11, 1980, in RF155, CHP Archives. See also Minutes, UT Board of Regents, Oct. 7, 1982; *Impact*, 7 (June 3, 1983), 1, 16; and *University Medical*, 14 (Spring, 1983), 34–35. The Moody Foundation, the M.D. Anderson Foundation, and the Kempner Fund contributed dollars that augmented Permanent University Fund bond income the regents assigned; see *University Medical*, 15 (Fall, 1983), 38; *Impact*, 7 (June 3, 1983), 1, and (June 17, 1983), 18.

80. *Galveston Daily News*, Nov. 12, 1963. Committee members, administrators, and prison officials were "unanimously in favor of the project." See T. G. Blocker Jr. to John B. Truslow, May 6, 1964, Texas Dept. of Corrections Hospital folder, UTMB Executive Vice President' Office, Active. The regents agreed to support a request to the legislature by the Texas Department of Corrections (TDC) for funds to construct this hospital using prison materials and labor; see Minutes, UT Board of Regents, May 22–23, 1964. The hospital would be used for teaching and UTMB would operate the hospital via an interagency contract. But the timing for further development was not good because a master plan and a five-year construction plan had already been adopted for the UTMB campus.

81. Gene R. Branch to Don E. Kirkpatrick, Jan. 9, 1974, letter, Texas Dept. of Corrections Hospital File, UTMB Executive Vice President's Office, Active (quotation). There was only one physician for the entire prison system and no registered nurses at sixteen of the state's eighteen prisons; see McCleskey, et al., *The Government and Politics of Texas*, 241.

82. E. D. Walker to June Hyer, Dec. 30, 1976, letter, Texas Dept. of Corrections Hospital File, Current Files, UT Board of Regents. Prison officials selected an architectural firm in Fort Worth to conduct a "Feasibility Planning Study of a Multi-Program Treatment Facility for the Texas Department of Corrections." See Ronald L. Wilson to A. R. Schwartz, Feb. 28, 1977, letter, Texas Dept. of Corrections Hospital File, UTMB Executive Vice President's Office, Active. This letter has an attachment, which is a summary of the 508-page planning study that was completed in late March. See also William C. Levin, "Statement, Texas Department of Corrections Prison Hospital," Mar. 3, 1977, Texas Dept. of Corrections Hospital, UTMB Executive Vice President's Office, Active; and Minutes, UT Board of Regents, July 29, 1977.

83. Robert C. Hope to V. E. Thompson, Jan. 9, 1978, letter, Texas Dept. of Corrections Hospital File, UTMB Executive Vice President's Office, Active; and "TDC Program and Facility Requirements for the TDC-UTMB Hospital," [Technical Report 29], February, 1978, Texas Dept. of Corrections Hospital File, UTMB Executive Vice President's Office, Active. In February 1977 a prisoner escaped and raped a Galveston citizen. To provide an area secured by armed guards, the 9C ward on the ninth floor of John Sealy Hospital was remodeled in 1977 and 1978. It could accommodate thirty male and five female inmates; see A. R. Schwartz to John D. Hayes, Mar. 22, 1977, letter; "9C to House Prison Ward," News Releases of The University of Texas System, June 24 and July 29, 1977, in Texas Dept. of Correction Hospital File, UTMB Executive Vice President's Office, Active. Before this security ward was completed, it was not uncommon for prisoners to escape from the hospital; for an example, see *Galveston Daily News*, Jan. 23, 1978.

84. Minutes, UT Board of Regents, June 9, 1978; V. E. Thompson to E. D. Walker, Aug. 30, 1978, letter, Texas Dept. of Corrections Hospital File, UTMB Executive Vice President's Office, Active. Construction of a new health care facility in the state requires approval of a need for such a facility by the Texas Health Facilities Commission. Applications and hearings are part of this process. For a copy of the application form for the TDC hospital dated Nov. 3, 1978, see RF155, CHP Archives. See also Minutes, UT Board of Regents, June 1 and Oct. 12, 1979.

85. *Impact*, 7 (June 2, 1983), 1, 20; and *University Medical*, 15 (Fall, 1983), 38. For details, see the press release dated June 7, 1983, in RF155, CHP Archives, and items in RF175. In 1980 the regents approved plans for constructing an apartment complex that would house the guards employed in the prison hospital. The complex is located on a three-acre plot along Ferry Road, a short distance from the Bolivar Ferry landing and approximately six blocks northeast of the UTMB campus. It includes a warden's residence, 32 three-bedroom units, 48 two-bedroom units, 48 dormitory units, and parking space for 178 cars. For details, see letters and reports in Texas Dept. of Corrections Hospital File, UTMB Executive Vice President's Office, Active.

86. Prompted by a query from Regent Ed Clark during lunch one day, Ron Bailey, Bill Deiss, and Bill Levin told Clark that UTMB really needed a new ACC; see Byron Bailey to Chester R. Burns, Feb. 13, 1992, interview, Blocker Collections. For details, see the folders in box 24, Levin Papers. Thompson and Brandt prepared the rationale touting a new center; see the grant proposal dated Nov. 15, 1977, in RF155, CHP Archives.

87. "Memorandum to File, ACC-UTMB-PSP Project No. 7610-H," June 16, 1976, ACC File, UTMB Executive Vice President's Office, Active; Galveston Medical Branch: Ambulatory Care Center file, Current Files, UT Board of Regents; and *Impact*, 7 (Apr. 8, 1983), 1, 21.

88. For details and photos, see a sixteen-page *Impact* supplement dated Oct. 13, 1983, and *Impact*, 7 (Oct. 21, 1983), 12–13. A copy of the dedication brochure is in RF155, CHP Archives. The Sealy & Smith Foundation contributed $8 million and the regents assigned $14.7 million from Permanent University Fund bond proceeds.

89. Reports and letters are in folder 1, box 21, Levin Papers; *University Medical*, 4 (Sept., 1972), 4–17; and Minutes, UT Board of Regents, June 1, 1973.

90. The *New York Times* featured the Save Old Red project in its July 26, 1977, issue. See also Chester R. Burns, "The Historical Significance and Future Value of the Ashbel Smith Building—'Old Red'," *The Bookman*, 6 (Mar., 1979), 2–3. For an example of the hyperbole, see Ray Reece, "Endangered Species: Conduct Unbecoming a Superstate," *Texas Architect*, 26 (Sept./Oct., 1976), 29–31.

91. Minutes, UT Board of Regents, Oct. 19, 1978 (quotation). Also see the UT System news release in folder 1, box 22, Levin Papers; and Peter H. Brink to Bill Clayton; Peter H. Brink to William P. Hobby; and Peter H. Brink to Susan Fisher, letters, all dated May 3, 1979, folder 3, box 21, Levin Papers.

92. Peter H. Brink to William C. Levin, Sept. 5, 1980, letter, folder 4, box 21, Levin Papers (1st quotation). For the task force's letters and brochures, see folders 4 and 5, box 21, Levin Papers. See also V. E. Thompson to Joe E. Boyd Jr., June 8, 1982, letter, folder 6, box 21, Levin Papers; Minutes, UT Board of Regents, June 11, 1982; and *Impact*, 7 (July 1, 1983), 1, 12–13. See letters about the building's opening in folder 7, box 21, Levin Papers, and information about the dedication in *Impact*, 10 (Apr. 4, 1986), 1, 10. Blumberg's remarks are in folder 4, box 22, Levin Papers.

93. Minutes, Faculty Building Committee, Jan. 6, 1965, RF155, CHP Archives. In 1976, for example, the School of Nursing had 255 students and 31 faculty. Three years later, the school employed 42 faculty and enrolled 312 students. See William C. Levin to E. D. Walker, June 8, 1979, letter, reel 93, UT Chancellor's Office of Records Management.

94. William C. Levin to E. D. Walker, Sept. 16, 1980, letter, School of Allied Health Sciences and School of Nursing Building File, UTMB Executive Vice President's Office, Active; Galveston Medical Branch: School of Allied Health Sciences and School of Nursing—New Building, Current Files, UT Board of Regents; Minutes, UT Board of Regents, Oct. 24, 1980; and folder 4, box 28, Levin Papers. In 1980 Levin had listed this building as fifth among

thirteen priorities for capital improvements at UTMB; see Levin to Don Walker, Oct. 15, 1980, letter, folder 2, box 28, Levin Papers.

95. Minutes, UT Board of Regents, Oct. 9, 1981, and Feb. 8, 1984. Construction projects for new academic buildings also required approval of the Coordinating Board of the Texas College and University System. Their approval for this building occurred at a meeting on April 30, 1982; see Gordon Flack to Joe E. Boyd Jr., May 3, 1982, letter, Schools of Allied Health Sciences and Nursing Building File, UTMB Executive Vice President's Office, Active.

96. *Impact*, 10 (Sept. 19, 1986), 2, and *Galveston Daily News*, Oct. 3, 1986. A generous benefactor to both schools, Florence Marie Hall served on the advisory committees for each school when the regents approved this honor. See William C. Levin to Charles B. Mullins, Apr. 17, 1985, letter, RF155, CHP Archives.

97. *Impact*, 1 (June 24, 1977), 1, and folder 6, box 22, Levin Papers. See also *Impact* (Feb. 22, 1980), 5; (Nov. 21, 1980), 1, 12; (Sept. 12, 1980), 3; (Sept. 26, 1980), 1; and *University Medical*, 12 (Spring, 1981), 26–27.

98. *Impact*, 6 (Nov. 12, 1982), 1, 19, and (Dec. 3, 1982), 1. In June 1979 Levin had recommended construction of this new building as an efficient way to consolidate physical plant services then scattered in seven buildings.

99. See folder 2, box 28, Levin Papers. Between 1979 and 1985, prodigious energies were unsuccessfully expended by UTMB faculty and Moody Foundation officials to develop a Center for Health Promotion and Fitness. For details, see folders in box 27 of the Levin Papers. See also *Impact*, Sept. 4, 1987, 3.

100. The data presented in this paragraph were taken from Schedule B-12 (pp. 78–79) and Schedule S-12B (pp. 234–245) in UTMB's financial statement for fiscal year 1987.

101. *Impact*, 13 (Dec. 15, 1989), 5; *Galveston Daily News*, Mar. 7, and June 17, 1990.

102. *Impact*, 12 (Nov. 4, 1988), 1. In 1981 UTMB's building committee had recommended an additional basic science building; see committee reports in folder 5, box 19, Levin Papers. See also *Galveston Daily News*, Mar. 14, 1989; and *Impact*, 13 (Mar. 24, 1989), 2; 15 (Apr. 5, 1991), 3; and 19 (May 1, 1995), 3.

103. *Impact*, 13 (Aug. 18, 1989), 1; *Galveston Daily News*, Sept. 14, 1989; and *Impact*, 13 (Sept. 15, 1989), 1; 16 (Jan. 24, 1992), 3; and 15 (Sept. 13, 1991), 6.

104. *Impact*, 6 (Nov. 12, 1982), 1; *Galveston Daily News*, June 7, 1989. Boyce Tankersley refurbished this garden, which includes more than thirty varieties of oleanders.

105. *Impact*, 15 (Aug. 2, 1991), 7.

106. The data presented in this paragraph were taken from Schedule B-12 (pp. 96–97) and Schedule S-11B (pp. 312–329) in UTMB's Financial Statement for fiscal year 1991.

107. *UT Regents' Reports* (1900), 125, 142; Minutes, UT Board of Regents, May 29, 1903; *UT Regents' Reports* (1908), 56, (1910), 147, and (1920), 266; and Minutes, UT Board of Regents, Apr. 21, 1930.

108. Joseph T. Roberts to Homer P. Rainey and Chauncey D. Leake, Oct. 15, 1942, box VF 9/A, UT President's Records. Until 1941 the John Sealy Hospital Board of Managers employed caretakers for the hospital buildings. In September 1920, for example, these included a carpenter, two yardmen, two "cleaners," a "master mechanic," a housekeeper, and John Reiss as the "all around man." This information came from the hospital's payroll ledgers (September 1920 to June 1922), which are located in the Blocker Collections.

109. Minutes, UT Board of Regents, Aug. 8, 1942; Charles Sparenberg to Logan Wilson, Feb. 17, 1954, and May 27, 1954, letters, box VF A/3, UT Chancellor's Records. Names and salaries of these employees are included in this letter as well as a diagram of the department's organizational structure. A copy of this letter is in RF137, CHP Archives. See also *Medi-Texan*, 1 (Mar., 1954), 4–5.

110. *Medi-Texan*, 3 (Nov., 1955), 1, 4; Jimmy LeFevers to Myles Knape, Dec. 21, 1989, taped interview, box 47, CHP Archives.

111. *Hospital News*, 4 (May 11, 1970), 4. Regard for Gilliam was statewide. He was program chairman when about seventy-five members of the Texas Association of Hospital Engineers met in Galveston in 1966; see *Newsletter (UTMB)*, 2 (Nov. 17, 1966), 3; and *Impact*, 10 (Jan. 24, 1986), 11.

112. *Hospital News*, 4 (Aug. 9, 1971), 4, and 6 (Feb. 5, 1973), 1–2; *Impact*, 2 (July 14, 1978), 13, and 8 (May 18, 1984), 15.

113. "Physical Plant Department in Summary," March 1989, WF291, CHP Archives.

114. *Medi-Texan*, 4 (Mar., 1957), 4–5, 8; "Housekeeping," Annual Reports, 1960–1961, folder 8, box 1, 75th Anniversary History Papers, Blocker Collections; *Newsletter (UTMB)*, 4 (Feb., 1969), 7; and *Hospital News*, 9 (Apr. 23, 1976), 2. In 1974 three employees had been elected officers of the Houston Chapter of the National Executive

Housekeepers Association, a group of about eighty hospital and hotel executive housekeepers who were employed in supervisory or administrative positions. Cruz Cortez, director of UTMB's Laundry Department, was president; Kelly Carpenter, a Housekeeping Department supervisor, was recording secretary; and Bernita Duke, an in-service training specialist, was corresponding secretary; see *Hospital News*, 7 (Apr. 15, 1974), 1.

115. Myles Knape, WF437, CHP Archives, 16–19.

116. *Galveston Daily News*, June 20, 1954; George W. Carlson to Harry Ransom, June 11, 1968, letter, box VF EE/3, UT Chancellor's Records.

117. *Newsletter (UTMB)*, 3 (Oct., 1968), 2–3. Harr had been a member of Galveston's police department for eighteen years. *Hospital News*, 6 (Oct. 29, 1973), 1. In 1984 Lieutenant Singleton was one of 250 graduates of an eleven-week training program conducted by the Federal Bureau of Investigation's National Academy; see *Impact*, 8 (Oct. 19, 1984), 12.

118. *Impact*, 2 (Aug. 11, 1978), 7; the University of Texas System Police and Academy, 1984–1985 fiscal year report, 54–57. A copy is in WF358, CHP Archives, together with a summary of activities for fiscal year 1986 attached to a letter from William C. Levin to Maurice A. Harr dated March 5, 1987. Also see comments by Myles Knape in WF437, CHP Archives, 59–64.

119. For assistance with descriptions and interpretations in this section, I am grateful to Mary Winkler, Jimmy LeFevers, and Ken Steblein. Architectural information about some of the buildings is included in Beasley and Fox, *Galveston Architecture Guidebook*, 121–128.

120. Barrie Scardino and Drexel Turner, *Clayton's Galveston: The Architecture of Nicholas J. Clayton and His Contemporaries* (College Station: Texas A&M University Press, 2000), 95–99; Lawrence W. Speck and Richard Payne, *Landmarks of Texas Architecture* (Austin: University of Texas Press, 1986), 40 (quotation); and Jay C. Henry, *Architecture in Texas, 1895–1945* (Austin: University of Texas Press, 1993), 13–25; 97–101. Some of the exuberance of the Victorian era is present in the Rosenberg Library building in Galveston, designed in 1902 as a sophisticated example of Beaux-Arts Classicism; see Henry, *Architecture in Texas*, 85. See also Willard B. Robinson and Todd Webb, *Texas Public Buildings of the Nineteenth Century* (Austin: University of Texas Press, 1974), 188, and Howard Barnstone, *The Galveston That Was* (New York: Macmillan, 1966), 164–165, 182–189. For the marker dedication ceremony, see *Galveston Daily News*, Nov. 16, 1969.

121. See Henry, *Architecture in Texas*, 4, 194–195, and 227. The Etruscan motifs were common on theaters constructed during the 1930s.

122. Had their walk occurred at night, they would have noticed the accents of lighted areas: the "exposed aggregate" or brush concrete sidewalks; the multi-colored tiles on the Medical Research Building; the extra-bright lamps inside the Moody Medical Library; and the huge signs on the towers and TDCJ Hospital with their white letters (UTMB or John Sealy Hospital or Galveston) and bright green borders.

123. The really energetic visitor probably climbed the fifty-nine Texas pine steps of the grand staircase from the first to the third floor, touched the mahogany banisters, noted the pressed tin ceiling, and stopped to see the east end amphitheater on the second floor.

CHAPTER 5

1. "He didn't make up his mind," observed Dudgeon. See H. R. Dudgeon, "Random Undergraduate Recollections," *Alcalde*, 3, no. 8 (1915), 862.

2. Population growth also included immigrants. Between 1907 and 1914, for example, an estimated ten thousand Jewish immigrants were admitted to the United States via the port of Galveston. See Bernard Marinbach, *Galveston: Ellis Island of the West* (Albany: State University of New York Press, 1983). For a concise analysis of the acceptance of hospital care by middle-class Americans at the turn of the twentieth century, see Rosenberg, *The Care of Strangers*, 237–261.

3. Lists of gynecological operations performed between 1894 and 1914 are included in the statistical reports published in UTMB's annual catalogs; e.g. *UTMB Catalog* (1894–1895), 48, and (1913–1914), 65–66. The story of the changes in attitudes of American women toward physician specialists in obstetrics and gynecology is told in Judith Walzer Leavitt, *Brought to Bed: Child-Bearing in America, 1750–1950* (New York: Oxford University Press, 1986). See also William Keiller, "On Some Cases of Menorrhagia Requiring Hysterectomy," *Texas State Journal of Medicine*, 5 (Feb., 1910), 375–377. For treatment of specific diseases, see Willard Cooke, "Notes on the Treatment of the Toxemias of Pregnancy," *Texas State Journal of Medicine*, 21 (Oct., 1925), 372–374; and Willard Cooke, "Abruptio Placentae," *Texas State Journal of Medicine*, 23 (Nov., 1927), 448–454. Also see *Bulletin of the John Sealy Hospital and the School of Medicine of the University of Texas*, 2 (Jan., 1940), 1–8.

4. "Texas Vital Statistics," *Texas State Journal of Medicine*, 4 (Dec., 1908), 208; Marvin L. Graves, "Some Phases of Typhoid Fever," *Texas State Journal of Medicine*, 12 (Sept., 1916), 209–211; and G. C. Kindley, "Autopsy Findings in Galveston during a Period of Two Years," *Texas State Journal of Medicine*, 9 (Sept., 1913), 154–156. Between 1892 and 1932, UTMB doctors performed 2,960 autopsies. Lesions from tuberculosis were present in 533 bodies. See C. B. Sanders and J. T. Billups, "Tuberculosis: A Study of Necropsy Findings in the Southern Negro," *Texas State Journal of Medicine*, 28 (Sept., 1932), 364–366.

5. In 1916 about ten children had resided in the hospital for a year or more; see W. S. Carter to R. E. Vinson, Jan. 19, 1917, letter, box 4Q21, UT President's Records. Between twenty-five and thirty white children were inpatients each day.

6. J. E. Thompson, "Congenital Cysts of the Neck," *Texas State Journal of Medicine*, 2 (Nov., 1906), 198–202, and *UTMB: Seventy-five Year History*, 48. Thompson was delighted when the hospital's operating room was remodeled in 1906; see *Galveston Daily News*, Nov 18, 1906. Patients were wheeled to this room in "rubbered tired carriages to deaden sound." Carts with instruments also had rubber tires and "the floors and walls of the new operating theater were sterilized every morning." Lists of surgical operations performed between 1894 and 1914 are included in the statistical reports published in UTMB's annual catalogs; e.g. *UTMB Catalog* (1894–1895), 46, and (1913–1914), 60–62. See also *Galveston Daily News*, Oct. 27, 1921; and James E. Thompson, "Cystic Disease of the Breast," *Texas State Journal of Medicine*, 18 (Nov., 1922), 344–352.

7. On April 1, 1923, Thomas Mitchell Campbell, twice governor of Texas, died in the John Sealy hospital from complications associated with pernicious anemia; see *Galveston Daily News*, Apr. 2, 1923. No satisfactory treatment existed then, though Marvin Graves had witnessed some improvement in two patients who had been transfused with citrated blood five years earlier. See M. L. Graves, "Blood Transfusion in the Anemias," *Texas State Journal of Medicine*, 13 (Aug., 1917), 137–141. For valuable details about the changing patterns of diseases in the United States during the twentieth century, see Philip S. Lawrence, "The Health Record of the American People," in *Health in America: 1776–1976* (Washington, D.C.: U. S. Government Printing Office, DHEW Pub. no. HRA 76–616, 1976), 16–36, and Monroe Lerner and Odin W. Anderson, *Health Progress in the United States: 1900–1960* (Chicago: University of Chicago Press, 1963).

8. Georgia Jereleen Barnes, "Mortality in Texas: A Study of the Geographic Distribution of Twenty-Nine Selected Causes of Death, Exclusive of Stillbirths, in Texas Counties, 1930 and 1940" (M.A. thesis, University of Texas, 1946), 126; R. J. Brady, "Report of the Causes of Death in John Sealy Hospital Year 1938–1939," *Bulletin of the John Sealy Hospital and the School of Medicine of the University of Texas*, 1 (Dec., 1939), 136; and *Galveston Daily News*, Mar. 6, 1941.

9. By 1931 two dermatologists attended about fifty outpatients daily; see W. F. Spiller to president of the University of Texas, June 17, 1932, letter, box 17, UTMB Dean's Office Records, Inactive. By 1939 more than 250 outpatients came to night clinics in dermatology each week; see W. F. Spiller to president of University of Texas, c. 1939, letter, box VF 9/B, UT President's Records. At that time dermatologists were treating patients with venereal diseases. The building also contained administrative offices, a pharmacy, a room with the records of all patients, a mortuary and autopsy room, the emergency room, a teaching amphitheater, and an animal care facility. See *Galveston Daily News*, June 24 and Aug. 3, 1941.

10. *Galveston Daily News*, Mar. 3, 1919. Total salaries for all of these amounted to $3,500 monthly. In contrast, the hospital spent about $5,000 a month for food and beverages. Three cooks and three helpers prepared between 1,400 and 1,500 meals each day, which were served to patients, nurses, interns, students, faculty, and other employees. In 1920 the hospital's board increased the salary of the pupil nurses from five to ten dollars, which increased the total monthly costs of operating the hospital ($3,810.10 in September 1920, for example). This information came from the hospital's payroll ledgers dated September 1920 to June 1922, which are in the Blocker Collections.

11. Inpatient records were kept in the library that served students and faculty until 1913, when they were transferred to a room in the John Sealy Hospital; see Minutes, UTMB Faculty Meeting, Mar. 11 and Dec. 6, 1911, and Feb. 6, 1914. In 1920 Charles T. Stone Sr., Willard Cooke, A. O. Singleton, and Moise D. Levy organized the hospital records into the unit system; see Minutes, UTMB Faculty Meeting, May 30, 1919; and W. S. Carter to R. E. Vinson, Sept. 5, 1919, Feb. 10, 1920, and June 12, 1920, letters, all in box 4Q22, UT President's Records. McArdle began work in the fall of 1919, Hixon in the summer of 1920; see W. S. Carter to R. E. Vinson, June 12, 1920, letter, box 4Q22, UT President's Records.

12. Margaret McArdle to W. Sutton, Feb. 16, 1924; and Margaret C. McArdle to W. M. W. Splawn, Apr. 10, 1925, and Mar. 25, 1926, letters, box 4Q25, UT President's Records; and Margaret C. McArdle to H. Y. Benedict, June 7, 1929, letter, UTMB Dean's Office Records, Inactive, folder 6, box 17. The organizational meeting of the Junior Welfare League was held in the home of James Thompson on November 27, 1925. To raise funds for a Social Service

Department, a committee of league members sponsored a Valentine's Day dance; see *Galveston Daily News*, Feb. 5. 1928. For a photo of Miss Arnn, see page 36 in the Department of Surgery Scrapbook in the Blocker Collections.

13. Xilema Faulkner to L. R. Wilson, Sept. 24, 1929, letter, box 1, School of Nursing Archives, Blocker Collections; W. S. Carter to J. W. Calhoun, Nov. 1, 1937, letter, box 4Q18, UT President's Records; Dr. Gardner to Willard R. Cooke, June 24, 1940, letter, box VF 9/B, UT President's Records; and Willard R. Cooke to John W. Spies, Apr. 18, 1940, letter, box VF 9/B, UT President's Records (quotations).

14. *Galveston Daily News*, Jan. 17, 1932, and Feb. 21, 1932. As treatment protocols during the 1930s, doctors used work and play regimens, prolonged sleep induced by sodium phenobarbital, insulin coma, and metrazol-induced convulsions. See Giles W. Day, "Prolonged Continuous Sleep Treatment: Its Results in Psychiatry, with a Discussion of its Place in Modern Medicine," *Texas State Journal of Medicine*, 32 (Oct., 1936), 417–422; *Galveston Daily News*, Oct. 17, 1938; and Lewis Barbato, "Metrazol Therapy of Schizophrenia," *Texas State Journal of Medicine*, 34 (July, 1938), 220–227.

15. Titus H. Harris and Hamilton Ford, "The Management of Psychiatric Patients in a General Hospital," *Texas State Journal of Medicine*, 33 (Jan., 1938), 636–640. The building had three floors and a basement. The third floor housed agitated patients. The second floor housed patients with depression and psychoneuroses, as well as a tub bath, a room for treatment with sedative packs, and two large sun porches. The first floor contained offices for doctors and an occupational therapy room. The basement contained a physiotherapy facility and a woodwork shop.

16. Wilhelmena Beane, *Texas Thirties* (San Antonio: Naylor Co., 1963), 66–72.

17. *Galveston Daily News*, Mar. 18, 1938, and Oct. 6, 1938. For details about activities in the new State Hospital for Crippled and Deformed Children, see Estelle Greenwalt's scrapbook located in the Department of Orthopedic Surgery.

18. For the story of early clinical testing in American hospitals, see Joel D. Howell, *Technology in the Hospital: Transforming Patient Care in the Early Twentieth Century* (Baltimore: Johns Hopkins University Press, 1996), and Harry P. Smith, "Clinical Pathology: Its Creators and Practitioners," *American Journal of Clinical Pathology*, 31 (Apr., 1959), 283–292. See also *Galveston Daily News*, June 8, 1902.

19. As needed, inpatients were transported for exams and tests via a two-story arcade that connected the hospital and the outpatient building. In 1934 about five thousand X-ray exams were performed; see *Medi-Texan*, 3 (Aug., 1956), 5. In 1920 Marvin Graves asked Lee Rice to operate UTMB's first electrocardiograph, which had been placed in a basement room of the John Sealy Hospital; see M. L. Graves to Robert E. Vinson, Feb. 12, 1921, letter, box 4R81, UT President's Records. Charles Stone, Graves's successor, used the electrocardiograph extensively; see Joseph Kopecky, "Practical Uses of the Electrocardiogram," *Texas State Journal of Medicine*, 24 (Nov., 1928), 493. During the 1930s Meyer Bodansky was director of the clinical laboratory for patients as well as the director of the John Sealy Memorial Research Laboratory. The Sealy & Smith Foundation provided funds for the equipment and supplies Bodansky and his technicians used as they performed tests for patients, conducted biochemical tests for Bodansky's experiments, and performed tests for other experimental projects the faculty conducted. For a report about tests of blood for non-protein nitrogen, plasma proteins, carbon dioxide combining capacity, chloride, calcium, and phosphorus, see Meyer Bodansky, "A Summary of Some Chemical Procedures of Importance in Clinical Pathology," *Texas State Journal of Medicine*, 27 (Sept., 1931), 390–395. For a good example of Bodansky's multifaceted approach, see his letter discussed by the Sealy & Smith Foundation directors at their meeting on October 28, 1931; Minutes, Sealy & Smith Foundation Board of Directors. The foundation continued to provide funds for Bodansky's salary and for operating expenses for the research laboratory, which was housed in a separate facility by the late 1930s; for examples, see Minutes, Sealy & Smith Foundation Board of Directors, July 12, 1934, and July 13, 1938.

20. By 1930, EEG tracings had been used in diagnosing at least twenty-one neuropsychiatric patients who displayed various conditions including convulsive disorders, vascular disease, atrophy of the brain associated with general paresis, and brain tumors. See Titus Harris and A. Hauser, "Encephalography: A Review of the Subject with a Summary of Results in 21 Cases," *Texas State Journal of Medicine*, 26 (July, 1930), 246–255. James Greenwood of Houston reported that the first EEGs in Texas were done at UTMB; see S. R. Snodgrass, "The Electroencephalogram and its Abnormalities in Certain Clinical Disorders," *Texas State Journal of Medicine*, 37 (Dec., 1941), 536. In 1943 Jack Ewalt became director of the EEG lab; see *Galveston Daily News*, Oct. 3, 1943. In 1952 Martin Towler became the director; see *Newsletter (UTMB)*, 2 (Feb., 1966), 1–2. During the 1930s medical technologists—defined as trained and registered laboratory assistants to clinical pathologists—began to receive their training in schools accredited by the National Board of Registry of Medical Technologists established by the American Society of Clinical Pathologists in 1928. In 1932 there were no schools in Texas. By 1939 there were seven, including one at UTMB. For more details, see John J. Andujar, "The Training of Medical Technologists in Texas," *Texas State Journal of Medicine*, 36 (Nov., 1940), 503–507.

21. *UTMB Catalog* (1900–1901), 35; (1925–1926), 53; and (1937–1938), 61. A daughter of William Keiller, Violet graduated from UTMB in 1914. After James Thompson, her mentor, died in 1927, Violet moved to Houston and became a pathologist at the Hermann Hospital and a professor at Baylor. For a good photo, see page 14 of the Department of Surgery's scrapbook in the Blocker Collections.

22. Rothstein, *American Medical Schools and the Practice of Medicine*, 134–136. In 1914 the AMA published its first list of hospitals approved for internships. See *UTMB Catalog* (1911–1912), 48; (1922–1923), 48; and (1937–1938), 62.

23. Rothstein, *American Medical Schools and the Practice of Medicine*, 136–138. In 1923 the AMA promulgated its first standards for residency programs. See *Galveston Daily News*, July 14, 1949, and Minutes, Sealy & Smith Foundation Board of Directors, May 15, 1940.

24. *Galveston Daily News*, Feb. 13, 1905, and Mar. 3, 1919. Rates were $4 to $7 a day for a private room, $2 a day for private wards, and $1.50 per day for general wards. See *Galveston Daily News*, July 21, 1922.

25. Minutes, Sealy & Smith Foundation Board of Directors, June 30, 1931. Before 1941 private patients were usually not used as teaching subjects. Thus, the boards were always jockeying between the horns of a dilemma: How many charity patients should be admitted to honor the hospital's social mission and to have the number of patients needed for its educational mission? How many private patients should be admitted to provide supplemental income for the clinical professors as well as extra money needed by the hospital to offset losses assumed in caring for charity patients? For more examples of the conflicts generated by this dilemma, see RF44 and RF49, CHP Archives.

26. *Galveston Daily News*, May 14, 1916. The Rotary Club of Galveston and a local group of Shriners also staged parties and donated items for hospitalized children. See Estelle Greenwalt's scrapbook in the Department of Orthopedic Surgery and Dianne Treadaway Ozment, "Galveston During the Hoover Era, 1929–1933" (M.A. thesis, University of Texas, 1968), 161.

27. Minutes, Sealy & Smith Foundation Board of Directors, Dec. 21, 1932. There was more turnover among the nurses, especially during the depression years. In September 1937, for example, six nurses resigned and ten were employed at various times to help maintain a total of forty general duty nurses. This information came from the timekeeping ledgers of hospital employees for 1937, which are in the Blocker Collections. See also W. S. Carter to R. E. Vinson, Mar. 24, 1921, letter, box 4R81, UT President's Records.

28. For the organization in 1946, see "Bylaws, Rules and Regulations, Medical Staff, John Sealy Hospital," adopted in June 1946, vol. I, 26–40, Current Files, UT Board of Regents, and Chauncey D. Leake to T. S. Painter, June 7, 1946, letter, box VF 10/C, UT President's Records, and letters in RF56, CHP Archives. For concise overviews of four departments written by their chairs in the mid-1960s, see *Alumni Bulletin*, Dec. 1965 (Dermatology); Feb. 1966 (Neurology and Psychiatry); June 1967 (Pediatrics); and Fall 1967 (Ophthalmology). For the story of clinical specialization in the United States, see Rosemary Stevens, *American Medicine and the Public Interest: A History of Specialization* (Berkeley: University of California Press, 1998). For histories of the major clinical specialties in the United States, see Harold Speert, *Obstetrics and Gynecology in America: A History* (Chicago: American College of Obstetricians and Gynecologists, 1980); Charlotte G. Borst, *Catching Babies: The Professionalization of Childbirth, 1870–1920* (Cambridge: Harvard University Press, 1995); Thomas E. Cone Jr., *History of American Pediatrics* (Boston: Little, Brown and Company, 1979); Sydney A. Halpern, *American Pediatrics: The Social Dynamics of Professionalism, 1880–1980* (Berkeley: University of California Press, 1988); Russel C. Maulitz and Diana E. Long (eds.), *Grand Rounds: One Hundred Years of Internal Medicine* (Philadelphia: University of Pennsylvania Press, 1988); and Ira M. Rutkow, *American Surgery: An Illustrated History* (Philadelphia: Lippincott-Raven Publishers, 1998). For psychiatry, see James Bordley III and A. McGehee Harvey, *Two Centuries of American Medicine, 1776–1976* (Philadelphia: W. B. Saunders, 1976), 727–749; American Psychiatric Association, *One Hundred Years of American Psychiatry* (New York: Columbia University Press, 1944); and Daniel Blain and Michael Barton, *The History of American Psychiatry: A Teaching and Research Guide* (Washington, D.C.: American Psychiatric Association, 1979).

29. J. Allen Scott and Peggy McDonough Brenkus, "The Functions and Methodology of a Hospital Statistical Division," *Texas Reports on Biology and Medicine*, 9 (Spring, 1951), 170.

30. "The University of Texas–Medical Branch Trial Balance General Ledger and Appropriations Ledgers as of July 31, 1945," WF246, CHP Archives; *Medi-Texan*, 3 (Feb., 1956), 4–5, 9; *University Medical Center News*, 1 (Nov., 1960), 1.

31. By the fall of 1966 medical and surgical outpatients visited clinics in the new McCullough Building; orthopedic and urology patients went to the second floor of the reconstructed Outpatient Building; those with respiratory diseases went to the Ziegler Hospital; and children went to the Children's Hospital. Others visited the Rebecca Sealy Building, which housed the child development, dermatology, and ophthalmology clinics; and the university health services clinic for employees; see "Notes about Hospital Activities," 43. "Notes about Hospital Activities" refers to typescript pages

in WF311, CHP Archives. Chester Burns dictated these notes from documents stored in nine boxes at the Shearn Moody Plaza during the late 1980s. In 1996 it was not possible for the Department of Records Management to determine whether or not these boxes and their contents had been transferred from the Shearn Moody Plaza to the old Lipton Tea building on Harborside Drive when this new department was created in 1994.

32. *Newsletter (UTMB)*, 1 (Feb. 5, 1955), 5; and 1 (Nov. 5, 1964), 4; and *Hospital News*, 2 (Apr. 14, 1969), 2.

33. William O. Bohman to C. D. Leake, Sept. 29, 1945, letter, folder 17, box 2, Leake Papers, Blocker Collections. By early 1947 UTMB hospitals provided 653 inpatient beds, including 20 bassinets. The 447 ward beds (non-private) were assigned as follows: 20 for obstetrics; 22 for gynecology; 147 for pediatrics; 104 for medicine; 71 for surgery; and 83 for psychiatry. There were 63 semi-private and 143 private beds, with 110 assigned to psychiatry and the remaining 96 for all other services. See "University of Texas Medical Branch, Distribution of Hospital Beds by Buildings and by Services," Jan. 14, 1947, box VF 20/C, UT President's Records. For the distribution of inpatients by buildings and wards in fiscal year 1949, see Scott and Brenkus, "The Functions and Methodology of a Hospital Statistical Division," 162. For 1950, see the sheet titled "University of Texas Medical Branch, Galveston, 1948–1950," in box VF C/4, UT Chancellor's Records. For fiscal years 1957 and 1963, see "Notes about Hospital Activities," 16 and 35. For 1968 see *Hospital News*, 2 (Apr. 14, 1969), 2. Inpatient deaths numbered 671 in fiscal year 1957 and 678 in fiscal year 1963, or between 4 and 5 percent of those admitted.

34. William O. Bohman to C. D. Leake, Sept. 29, 1945, letter, folder 17, box 2, Leake Papers, Blocker Collections; NAHA, 12 and 35; *University Medical Center News*, 1 (Nov., 1960), 1; *Galveston Daily News*, Jan. 11, 1955, and Oct. 7, 1955.

35. *Galveston Daily News*, Dec. 13, 1942; June 15; Sept. 2 and 13, 1945. Children with post-polio paralysis and disabilities from other diseases received long-term care in the Margie B. Stewart Convalescent Home for Children, which functioned from February 1946 until February 1949. During the late 1940s two medical students died from polio; see *Impact*, 8 (Aug. 10, 1984), 16. See also *Galveston Daily News*, Feb. 11 and 13; Mar. 11, 20, and 22; Apr. 8 and 15; and July 6 and 22, 1955.

36. Jesse B. Johnson and W. S. Wallace, "Tuberculosis Among Medical School Personnel at the University of Texas from 1941 to 1944," *Texas State Journal of Medicine*, 40 (Dec., 1944), 428–432; and M. Thomsen and R. H. Rigdon, "Primary Disease Processes as Observed at Necropsy in 353 Pediatric Cases Examined Between 1948 and 1952 at the Medical Branch of the University of Texas," *Texas Reports on Biology and Medicine*, 12 (Spring, 1954), 182–186.

37. *Medi-Texan*, 1 (Feb., 1954), 1–2. The first floor of the new hospital housed offices, outpatient clinics, X-ray and clinical lab facilities, and sleeping quarters for residents; the second housed patients with various pulmonary diseases, and the top two floors housed patients with tuberculosis. See John Middleton to Chester R. Burns, Dec. 17, 1991, interview, Blocker Collections.

38. *Galveston Daily News*, Oct. 30, 1939; Nov. 9, 1938; Mar. 6, 1941; and Jan. 9, 1943. Of 1,107 patients examined in the ob-gyn clinic in 1941, 251 (22.7 percent) had gonorrhea; see Charles E. Lankford, "A Critical Study of the Laboratory Methods of Diagnosis of Gonorrhea in Women," *Texas State Journal of Medicine*, 37 (Dec., 1941), 553–556. About 85 percent of forty prostitutes arrested during the spring of 1942 were infected with syphilis or gonorrhea or both; see *Galveston Daily News*, Mar. 6–7, 10–-11, 1942.

39. *Galveston Daily News*, July 27, 1941; WF314, CHP Archives; E. E. Wilkinson, W. H. Saunders, A. E. Hansen, "Penicillin in Treatment of Congenital Syphilis," *Texas State Journal of Medicine*, 41 (Dec., 1945), 401–404; H. F. Johnson and C. N. Frazier, "Penicillin in Prenatal Syphilis," *Texas Reports on Biology and Medicine*, 6 (Winter, 1948), 427–435; and "Learning to Deal with Life and Death: The Story of Becoming a Doctor in Texas," *Texas Medicine*, 76 (May, 1980), 66.

40. Charles T. Stone, "Recent Advances in the Treatment of Pneumonia," *Texas State Journal of Medicine*, 37 (Oct., 1941), 396–400; G. W. N. Eggers and Maynard D. Knight, "Treatment of Osteomyelitis," *Texas State Journal of Medicine*, 39 (Sept., 1943), 297–301; and S. G. Thompson and Theodore C. Panos, "Shigellosis: Pediatric Aspects with Special Reference to Central Nervous System Manifestations," *Texas State Journal of Medicine*, 53 (May, 1957), 320–323. For a concise summary of the development of sulfa drugs and antibiotics, see Bordley and Harvey, *Two Centuries of American Medicine*, 447–464.

41. M. Finland, "Changing Patterns of Resistance of Certain Common Pathogenic Bacteria to Antimicrobial Agents," *New England Journal of Medicine*, 252 (Apr. 7, 1955), 570–580; *Galveston Daily News*, Mar. 21, 1958; and Harriet M. Felton, "Hospital Population Most Vulnerable to Staphylococcal Infection," *Texas State Journal of Medicine*, 55 (May, 1959), 335–339.

42. T. G. Blocker Jr., S. R. Lewis, H. S. Jacobson, and D. A. Grant, "Bacterial Contamination and Infection in the Severely Burned Patient," *Texas State Journal of Medicine*, 55 (May, 1959), 358–360.

43. See newspaper clippings in folder 6, box 1, Blocker Papers; *UTMB: Seventy-five Year History*, 178–181; Virginia Blocker and T. G. Blocker Jr., "The Texas City Disaster: A Survey of 3,000 Casualties," *American Journal of Surgery*, 78 (Nov., 1949), 756–771; and Hugh W. Stephens, *The Texas City Disaster, 1947* (Austin: University of Texas Press, 1997).

44. T. G. Blocker Jr. to T. S. Painter, July 5, 1949, letter, box VF 10/D, UT President's Records; and *Medi-Texan*, 3 (July, 1956), 6–8. Snodgrass had joined the faculty in 1937 as UTMB's first neurosurgeon. See Francis Garbade and T. G. Blocker Jr, "Management of Burns in Children: Newer Concepts," *Texas State Journal of Medicine*, 48 (Jan., 1952), 32–35. Steve Lewis joined the faculty in 1948 and eventually served as chief of the plastic surgery division; for important comments about the care of their patients, see Steve Lewis to Myles Knape, Oct. 2, 1986, interview, Blocker Collections. Blocker invited Joseph Paderewski, a sculptor and cellist with the Houston Symphony Orchestra, to design and create prostheses, such as plastic ears and noses, for patients who had experienced disfiguring burn injuries. Given a lab on the eighth floor of John Sealy Hospital, Paderewski became a full-time employee; see *University Medical Center News*, 1 (Sept., 1960), 7. Paderewski's talents were used at UTMB for more than thirty years; see *Galveston Daily News*, May 12, 1963; and *Impact*, 2 (Sept. 22, 1978), 12.

45. *Galveston Daily News*, Nov. 8, 1963; Dec. 25 and 27, 1963; Feb. 15, Aug. 11, and Dec. 1, 1964. Also see *Newsletter (UTMB)*, 3 (Dec. 1966), 1–2; *Newsletter (UTMB)*, 3 (July, 1968), 7–9; Duane L. Larson, Sally Abston, and Armond S. Goldman, "The Burned Child," *Texas Medicine*, 67 (Apr., 1971), 58–67; and Megan Seaholm, "Shriners Hospitals for Crippled Children, Galveston Burns Institute," in Tyler, et al. (eds.), *The New Handbook of Texas*, V, 1036–1037.

46. Albert O. Singleton and Norman Duren, "Tumors of the Salivary Glands," *Texas State Journal of Medicine*, 36 (Apr., 1941), 784–792; Robert E. Cone, "Diagnosis of Kidney Tumors and Cysts," *Texas State Journal of Medicine*, 48 (Apr., 1952), 223–230; Lewis W. Baldwin, Gardner Thomas Jr., and E. Burke Evans, "Primary Bone Tumors: Survey of 137 Cases," *Texas Medicine*, 63 (Dec., 1967), 63–74; and *Galveston Daily News*, Sept. 24 and 28, 1956. Also see the department's annual report in RF67, CHP Archives. The department was subdivided into eight divisions: general surgery, neurosurgery, oral surgery, orthopedic surgery, otorhinolaryngology, plastic surgery, thoracic surgery, and urology.

47. Mary Ellen Haggard and W. C. Levin, "Leukemia in Childhood," *Texas State Journal of Medicine*, 53 (Dec., 1957), 896–902; *Medi-Texan*, 3 (Feb., 1956), 1, 8. The first floor housed the outpatient clinic offices and examining rooms; the second floor contained offices of the Department of Pediatrics and several laboratories; the third floor housed inpatient beds and an isolation ward; and the fourth floor contained the premature nursery with twenty bassinets.

48. *Galveston Daily News*, Jan. 31, 1957. Camp Manison in Friendswood was the site of the summer camp for about a hundred diabetic children, ages six to sixteen. Luther Travis was the medical director. Pediatricians, residents, interns, medical students, nurses, and college-student counselors helped the children learn how to handle their chronic disease within a context of extensive social and recreational activities. For details, see *University Medical*, 1 (June, 1970), 4–7.

49. For examples, see Theodore C. Panos, "Adrenocortical Insufficiency in Infants Management," *Texas State Journal of Medicine*, 52 (Jan., 1956), 9–12; *Galveston Daily News*, Aug. 18, 1963, and Jan. 16, 1964; and Albert I. Hartley, "Identifying the Physically Abused Child," *Texas Medicine*, 65 (Mar., 1969), 50–55. In 1965 legislators in Texas adopted a law that gave civil and criminal immunity to physicians who reported child abuse. Also see a summary of the department's activities Bill Daeschner wrote in 1967 in *Newsletter (UTMB)*, 3 (June, 1966), 1–2; and Daeschner to Knape and Burns, July 13 and 20, and Aug. 3, 1988, interviews.

50. William F. Schmalstieg, "The Right to a Good Life: Moody State School for Cerebral Palsied Children," *Texas Historian*, 52 (Mar., 1992), 16–18. In September 1952 the Board for Texas State Hospitals and Special Schools designated Moody State School as an independent school district. In 1963 the legislature transferred the school to UTMB.

51. "The Galveston State Psychopathic Hospital of the University of Texas Medical Branch, Galveston, Texas," May 9, 1949–May 31, 1950, box VF 10/D, UT President's Records. Fifty beds were private pay; eighty-seven were part-pay or charity. Twenty of the latter beds were available for patients with neurological disorders. The fourth floor was a locked facility for agitated patients and those who were confined to beds. A growing number of older patients received psychiatric care. During the five years between 1950 and 1954, 950 patients over the age of sixty were admitted to hospitals for psychiatric care; see W. S. Williams, "Psychiatric Syndromes in Patients over 60," *Texas State Journal of Medicine*, 52 (Sept., 1956), 669–672.

52. Psychotherapeutic approaches were reinforced during the early 1950s with the appointment of clinical psychologists who performed diagnostic and clinical services, taught residents and graduate students in clinical psychology, and engaged in behavioral science research; see *Medi-Texan*, 2 (July, 1955), 6–7. Austin Foster was the first

clinical psychologist employed by the department (1949–1960). He introduced psychological testing of patients; see Austin Foster, transcript of self-directed audiotape recording, April 1989, box 24, CHP Archives. For the therapeutic viewpoints of psychiatrists then, see E. Ivan Bruce Jr., "Role of the Medical School in Psychiatry," *Diseases of the Nervous System*, 16 (Feb., 1955), 61–63, and E. Ivan Bruce Jr. (ed.), "Recent Developments in Neurology and Psychiatry: A Symposium from the University of Texas Medical Branch," *Texas State Journal of Medicine*, 52 (Sept., 1956), 665–689.

53. Irving M. Cohen, "Drugs Recently Introduced in the Treatment of Psychiatric Disorders," *Texas State Journal of Medicine*, 52 (Sept., 1956), 683–687. Cohen graduated from UTMB in 1945 and completed his residency at UTMB in 1952. Harry Davis recalled that he first prescribed thorazine in 1955; see Henry K. Davis to Chester R. Burns, Dec. 8, 1994, interview, Blocker Collections. See also *University Medical Center News*, 1 (Nov., 1960), 1, 7; and Titus H. Harris, "The Department of Neurology and Psychiatry," Annual Reports, 1960–1961, folder 8, box 1, 75th Anniversary History Papers, Blocker Collections.

54. *Galveston Daily News*, Mar. 7, 1943; Lloyd Gregory Jr. and Raymond L. Gregory, "Diseases of the Parathyroid Glands," *Texas State Journal of Medicine*, 48 (Nov., 1952), 741–748; Charles T. Stone, "The Anemias: Diagnosis and Treatment," *Texas State Journal of Medicine*, 53 (Aug., 1957), 635–639; Joe L. Koch, Mary E. Haggard, Lawrence Waterbury, and William C. Levin, "Hypoplastic Anemia Associated with Chloramphenicol Therapy," *Texas State Journal of Medicine*, 58 (May, 1962), 344–348; William C. Levin, "Diagnosis and Treatment of the Anemias," *Texas State Journal of Medicine*, 42 (Feb., 1947), 573–577; and Marcel Patterson, "Ulcerative Colitis: Recognition and Management," *Texas State Journal of Medicine*, 60 (Jan., 1964), 34–38.

55. *Medi-Texan*, 1 (Nov., 1953), 1–2.

56. *Medi-Texan*, 1 (May, 1954), 3. These employees included about 100 attending physicians, 125 residents, 25 interns, 200 registered nurses, 145 housekeeping employees, 200 dietary employees, 50 laundry workers, 180 buildings and grounds employees, and 900 others, such as clerks, pharmacists, therapists, aides, and technicians. By the spring of 1956, UTMB hospitals had 932 inpatient beds: John Sealy Main (387); Smith Pavilion private (96); Ziegler (60); Negro (131); Psychiatric (236); and Isolation (22); see "Staff Report on the University of Texas Medical School at Galveston," May 25, 1956, box VF Y/4, UT Chancellor's Records. In 1960, 5A and 5B opened with 54 beds. John Sealy Hospital then had 688 beds. Altogether the hospitals had 941 beds; see *University Medical Center News*, 1 (Feb., 1961), 1, 8. Even with the new beds, facilities were not sufficient to meet the needs of children and of blacks (children and adults). Moreover, there were no facilities for emotionally disturbed children under fourteen years of age or for any black patients needing psychiatric care; see *Galveston Daily News*, Jan. 1, 1955.

57. As they provided care to individual patients, many of these caregivers taught and trained a variety of students; 740 in 1957, for example. These included residents (143), interns (36), medical students (285), nursing students (226), X-ray technicians (26), lab technicians (6), students medical records librarians (5), operating room technicians (4), physical therapy students (4), occupational therapy students (3), one EEG technician, and one hospital administration resident. See "1957, A Year of Education and Service at The University of Texas Medical Branch Hospitals, Galveston," box VF S/3, UT Chancellor's Records. The particular mix of students varied from year to year as schools changed admission and curricular policies (see chapter six).

58. *Medi-Texan*, 2 (Feb., 1955), 6–7. For organization charts of nursing services, see Appendices D-5, D-6, and D-7 in WF444, CHP Archives. In January 1955 the hospital's nursing service included about seven hundred employees; see *Medi-Texan*, 2 (Jan., 1955), 6–7. The total number of nurses in each hospital building varied. In the spring of 1956, for example, about 130 registered nurses, licensed vocational nurses, aides, orderlies, and ward clerks attended 66 patients in Psycho Two and Three (former Nurses' Home) and Psycho One (old Negro hospital), and 183 patients in the State Psychopathic Hospital; see *Medi-Texan*, 3 (Apr., 1956), 4–5.

59. *University Medical Center News*, 1 (Apr., 1961), 7, and 1 (May, 1961), 3. There were sixty vacant positions. To deal with the shortage of nurses, UTMB recruited nurses from the Philippines, England, Ireland, Scotland, Australia, Canada, and Germany. Administrators also permitted staff nurses to accrue many hours of overtime work. For details, see Harry Ransom to Board of Regents, Apr. 25, 1961, memo, "GMB: School of Nursing," Current Files, UT Board of Regents.

60. *University Medical Center News*, 2 (Summer, 1962), 3–7. For a description (with photos) of the twelve-hour day of an intern, see *Galveston Daily News*, Oct. 4, 1964.

61. *Medi-Texan*, 3 (Sept., 1956), 4–6, and 3 (May, 1956), 4–6; and Roy D. Wilson, Billie Fern Strother, and Charles R. Allen, "A Study in the Effects of a Postanesthetic Recovery Room on Mortality and Morbidity in 9,212 Geriatric Patients," *Texas Reports on Biology and Medicine*, 25 (Spring, 1967), 35–47.

62. Elwood E. Baird and Vernie Stembridge supervised twenty-three full-time and twenty-two part-time technicians organized into five divisions: bacteriology, chemistry, urinalysis, hematology, and serology; see *Medi-Texan*, 2 (Mar., 1955), 6–7, 13. Some departments also supported technicians who performed specialized diagnostic tests. In the Department of Obstetrics and Gynecology, for example, Mrs. Julius Blackman annually examined microscopic smears from about 12,000 patients to detect changes in cells representing early stages in the development of cancer of the uterus. Her work as a cytologist enabled early diagnosis and curative treatment for many patients. See *Galveston Daily News*, Mar. 19, 1959. See also *University Medical Center News*, 1 (May, 1961), 2, 7–8, and Lamont Jennings, a summary of "Diagnostic Pathology Services," *Newsletter (UTMB)*, 3 (Feb., 1967), 1.

63. *Medi-Texan*, 3 (Aug., 1956), 4–7; and Robert N. Cooley, "The Department of Radiology," Annual Reports, 1960–1961, folder 8, box 1, 75th Anniversary History Papers, Blocker Collections.

64. *University Medical Center News*, 1 (Mar., 1961), 4–5.

65. *Medi-Texan*, 2 (Sept., 1955), 4–5, 7. Helen LeBeau Hedges was an OT in the State Psychopathic Hospital in 1931–32. In 1939 the OT division established a playroom and clinic for children on the fourth floor of the Children's Hospital. Occupational therapists later joined the team of caregivers in the rehabilitation clinic in the Special Surgery Unit. In 1954, the OT division moved from the Woman's Hospital into the new John Sealy Hospital. For details, see WF315, CHP Archives. See also *University Medical Center News*, 2 (Dec., 1961), 4–5; and *Galveston Daily News*, Dec. 17, 1961. Jointly financed with the Texas Education Agency, a vocational rehabilitation office opened at UTMB in 1965. This office provided workplace counseling to about fifty inpatients and eighty outpatients each day whose vocational pursuits had been compromised by injury or disease. Using information provided by occupational therapists, vocational counselors helped these patients find new forms of employment.

66. *Newsletter (UTMB)*, 3 (Oct., 1968), 4–5. John Jenicek was the first medical director of the respiratory therapy program.

67. *Medi-Texan*, 3 (Mar., 1956), 4–7; WF316, CHP Archives; and "Social Services," Annual Reports, 1960–1961, folder 8, box 1, 75th Anniversary History Papers, Blocker Collections.

68. *Medi-Texan*, 2 (May, 1955), 4–5, 11. McArdle worked at UTMB for thirty-eight years; see her obituary in *Galveston Daily News*, Oct. 6, 1957.

69. *Medi-Texan*, 2 (Aug., 1955), 6–7, 9. In 1956 this department issued UTMB's first formulary, a list of all drugs available for inpatients and outpatients; see *Galveston Daily News*, Feb. 25, 1960, and *Impact*, 10 (Nov. 14, 1986), 5. For a copy of this formulary, see WF303, CHP Archives. See also "Pharmacy," Annual Reports, 1960–1961, folder 8, box 1, 75th Anniversary History Papers, Blocker Collections.

70. *Galveston Daily News*, Mar. 15, 17, and 29, Apr. 5 and 22, and July 3, 1942; Mar. 28, 1943; *Medi-Texan*, 3 (Oct., 1955), 4–6.

71. Gwendolyn Charpentier, the chief dietitian, supervised five trained dietitians, three food service supervisors, two secretaries, and 143 food preparers and other personnel; see *Medi-Texan*, 3 (Feb., 1956), 2. See also "The Dietary Department," Annual Reports, 1960–1961, folder 8, box 1, 75th Anniversary History Papers, Blocker Collections; and *Newsletter (UTMB)*, 4 (Feb., 1969), 5–7.

72. *Medi-Texan*, 4 (Apr., 1957), 4–5, 9; and *Newsletter (UTMB)*, 4 (Feb., 1969), 5–7.

73. Jimmy Kessler, *Henry Cohen: The Life of a Frontier Rabbi* (Austin: Eakin Press, 1997), 29–30; *Newsletter (UTMB)*, 3 (Dec., 1968), 4–7; and Myles Knape, WF437, CHP Archives, 64-71. Some of these chaplains also coordinated educational programs for local clergy; for examples, see *Newsletter (UTMB)*, 1 (June 16, 1966), 4, and 2 (Jan. 19, 1967), 3.

74. In 1952 the Junior League gave its collection of books and magazines to UTMB; see *Galveston Daily News*, Mar. 22, 1952. See also *Galveston Daily News*, Dec. 8, 1946. For comments about the early years of the AWVS and the Red Cross, see Leonora K. Thompson to Chester R. Burns, Dec. 12, 1994, interview, Blocker Collections. AWVS members also organized health education programs for Galveston's schoolchildren; see *Galveston Daily News*, July 18, and Sept. 9, 11, and 18, 1945; Feb. 17 and 19 and May 2, 1946. For AWVS activities during the 1950s and 1960s, see *Galveston Daily News*, Jan. 25, 1953, Apr. 7, Sept. 16 and 18, and Nov. 3, 1955; Feb. 26 and Oct. 7, 1956; Feb. 3, 7, and 15, 1957; Feb. 1 and July 11, 1959; Jan. 3, Apr. 17, Oct. 20, and Dec. 11, 1960; Feb. 19, Mar. 23, Nov. 16 and 29, and Dec. 13, 1961; and July 5, Nov. 13, and Dec. 14, 1962. For Red Cross activities see *Galveston Daily News*, Feb. 3, Aug. 14, Nov. 10, and Dec. 20, 1955.

75. *Galveston Daily News*, Apr. 4, 1956; Mar 13, 1960; Mar. 4 and Oct. 24, 1962; and Mar. 13 and Oct. 22, 1963; *University Medical Center News*, 3 (Sept., 1962), 8; *Newsletter (UTMB)*, 2 (Oct., 20, 1966), 5; and 3 (Jan., 1968), 6–7; "Notes about Hospital Activities," 12 and 26; and *University Medical Center News*, 1 (Feb., 1961), 6.

76. For the expansion of hospital technology in the United States after 1950, see Rothstein, *American Medical Schools and the Practice of Medicine*, 210–213. For a critical overview and interpretation, see Stanley Joel Reiser, *Medicine and the Reign of Technology* (Cambridge: Cambridge University Press, 1978), 144–231.

77. *University Medical Center News*, 1 (Nov., 1960), 1, and 2 (Dec., 1961), 8; and *Galveston Daily News*, Nov. 17, 1960, and Dec. 20, 1961. See also Frank M. Rembert and Robert N. Cooley, "Implantable Cardiac Pacemakers: Radiologic Appearance," *Texas Medicine*, 63 (Sept., 1967), 72–78. For a concise summary of the development of cardiology and cardiovascular surgery, see Bordley and Harvey, *Two Centuries of American Medicine*, 481–514.

78. *University Medical Center News*, 2 (Oct., 1961), 3, and 2 (Jan., 1962), 4.

79. *Newsletter (UTMB)*, 2 (July 20, 1967), 1; 3 (Feb., 1968), 6–7; (Mar., 1968), 8–9; and (Jan., 1968), 2–3. For a concise historical summary of renal transplantation, see Bordley and Harvey, *Two Centuries of American Medicine*, 589–595.

80. *Galveston Daily News*, Nov 27, 1960; "Summary of Child Development Program," UT Chancellor's Office of Records Management, Vice Chancellor for Health Affairs, 1966–68, reel 123; *University Medical Center News*, 1 (Apr., 1961), 4–6; John B. Truslow to Harry H. Ransom, Oct. 3, 1962, letter, box VF N/1, UT Chancellor's Records; *University Medical Center News*, 2 (Jan., 1962), 1, 8; and *Galveston Daily News*, Feb. 29 and Aug. 23, 1964.

81. *Newsletter (UTMB)*, 3 (Mar., 1968), 6–7. The center had information about prescription and over-the-counter drugs, as well as files about the ingredients of more than ten thousand commercial products, such as household detergents and pesticides. A pharmacist or physician was "on-call" twenty-four hours every day.

82. When McGanity arrived at UTMB in 1960 there were two prenatal clinics, one for the city and one for the county; see William J. McGanity to Myles Knape and Chester R. Burns, July 28 and Aug. 5, 1988, interview, Blocker Collections. Also see *Newsletter (UTMB)*, 3 (Feb., 1968), 2–3; and (Apr., 1968), 14.

83. These decisions occurred throughout the nation, as hospital costs were the most rapidly increasing component of the steadily rising health care expenditures in the United States after 1950; see Rothstein, *American Medical Schools and the Practice of Medicine*, 184–186 and 207–219.

84. See Raymond L. Gregory to Myles Knape, Aug. 4, 1987, interview, Blocker Collections; Leake's annual report for fiscal year 1944 (p. 23) in folder 19, box 2, Leake Papers, Blocker Collections; and *Galveston Daily News*, Mar. 27 and Apr. 18, 1943. Part-pay patients were charged a registration fee of $2 and paid half of the usual private rates for tests and medicines. They paid $3.50 each day for hospitalization. They paid no fees to the doctors, nurses, or other professionals. Fully indigent patients had their fees paid by county governments and they were charged a registration fee of $1, one-fourth the usual rate for tests and medicines, and $1.75 per day for hospitalization.

85. *Galveston Daily News*, Jan. 27, 1956, and Sept. 1, 1955; "Notes about Hospital Activities," 18; and "Advantages of a University Hospital Associated with a Medical School Facility," 1966, WF303, CHP Archives.

86. In 1956, 90 percent of Southern hospitals were operated by whites and about one third of these did not admit black patients. For details, see E. H. Beardsley, "Good-Bye to Jim Crow: The Desegregation of Southern Hospitals, 1945–70," *Bulletin of the History of Medicine*, 60 (Fall, 1986), 367–386. See also Marjorie Bartholf to John B. Truslow, June 18, 1956, box 1, folder 9, School of Nursing Archives; RF69, CHP Archives; and "Notes about Hospital Activities," 15.

87. "Notes about Hospital Activities," 23 and 31; George Bryan to Myles Knape, Jan. 31, Feb. 6, 11, 26, and Mar. 6, 1986, interviews, Blocker Collections; Grace Jameson to Chester R. Burns, Feb. 21, 1991, untaped phone interview; and "Notes about Hospital Activities," 37 (quotation).

88. See the letters and reports in RF56 and RF64, CHP Archives. For details about the revised medical staff bylaws adopted in 1953, see folders 5 and 6, box 17, Department of Anatomy records, Blocker Collections. Officers of the medical staff included a chief, an assistant chief, and a secretary. Five committees met regularly: advisory, medical records, program, intern, and formulary; see "Notes about Hospital Activities," 1–3. The advisory committee became an executive committee in 1956 and met monthly to adopt policies, advise administrators, and prepare agendas for quarterly meetings of the entire medical staff; see "Notes about Hospital Activities," 10. For samples of minutes of quarterly staff meetings, see copies of meetings for January 26, 1960; January 31, 1961; and July 25, 1961. Other committees were added as needed; for examples, see "Notes about Hospital Activities," 7, 15, 20, 22, and 31.

89. "Notes about Hospital Activities," 24, 32–33, 42, and 46.

90. *Medi-Texan*, 1 (Feb., 1954), 1, 3 and letters in RF56, CHP Archives. On February 23 Currie held his first meeting at UTMB. It was attended by fifty-eight active members of the medical staff, forty-four members of the house staff, and six administrators; see "Notes about Hospital Activities," 4. See also *Galveston Daily News*, Mar. 5 and 13, 1955.

For charts depicting the administrative organization of the hospitals in 1954 and 1958, see Appendices A-16 and A-19, WF441, CHP Archives.

91. "Notes about Hospital Activities," 26. For an administrative organization chart in 1959, see Appendix A-20, WF441, CHP Archives. See also "Notes about Hospital Activities," 40 and 48.

92. One example involves the unit management system adopted in the 1960s. In late July 1965 four unit managers and seventeen ward clerks serving ob-gyn inpatients initiated UTMB's new unit management system; see "Notes about Hospital Activities," 38. A unit manager was responsible for coordinating all administrative functions in a specific patient care area, including food service, transportation, record keeping, visitor control, and housekeeping. A ward clerk worked with the unit manager in handling all clerical-secretarial activities for the nurses and others in a specific patient care area. Late in 1966 another group of 17 unit managers completed a thirteen-week training program and 108 ward clerks completed a ten-week training program; see *Newsletter (UTMB)*, 2 (Dec. 15, 1966), 1–2. As personnel completed training programs, the unit management system was adopted in all hospitals at UTMB.

93. "Feasibility Study Ambulatory Care Center, The University of Texas Medical Branch at Galveston," folder 1, box 24, Levin Papers; *Impact*, 1 (May 13, 1977), supplement; (Dec 9, 1977), 3; and 3 (May 4, 1979), 13.

94. "Notes about Hospital Activities," 55, 67, 85. Data for all tables in this chapter were obtained from the annual hospital reports of the University of Texas System. Copies are in WF312, CHP Archives.

95. *Impact*, 7 (May 20, 1983), 1; and 9 (May 3, 1985), 13; Myles Knape, WF437, CHP Archives, 44–46; and *Galveston Daily News*, May 17, 1989, and Sept. 10, 1990.

96. *Hospital News*, 4 (Aug. 17, 1970), 4. In 1969 St. Vincent's House, a recreation center owned by the Episcopal Church in a low-income black neighborhood on Post Office Street in Galveston, organized a free clinic staffed by Volunteers in Service to America nurses and students and staff from UTMB. During its first two years, these professionals attended 1,300 patients who made 1,910 visits; see "A Medical Oasis," *University Medical*, 4 (Nov., 1972), 4–6.

97. *Newsletter (UTMB)*, 4 (Dec., 1969), 14–15; *Impact*, 6 (Aug. 20, 1982), 8; McGanity to Knape and Burns, July 28 and Aug. 5, 1988, interviews, Blocker Collections; and *Impact*, 15 (May 3, 1991), 1, 5; and (Nov. 22, 1991), 4.

98. *Impact*, 10 (Apr. 18, 1986), 11 and Myles Knape, WF437, CHP Archives, 35–37. In 1981 the Department of Obstetrics and Gynecology established a teen pregnancy clinic in the 1700 Strand Building. By January 1984 the clinic's personnel had attended more than seven hundred pregnant teenagers. This clinic was needed because approximately 14 percent of the deliveries at UTMB occurred in women less than eighteen years old and nine out of ten of these women came from twelve counties within a hundred-mile radius of Galveston. See William J. McGanity to William C. Levin, Jan. 11, 1984, letter, folder 3, box 49, Levin Papers.

99. *Impact*, 1 (May 13, 1977), supplement; (Dec. 9, 1977), 3; and 3 (May 4, 1979), 13.

100. For a description of a day in the life of an obstetrician during these years, see Harry Little to Chester R. Burns, Jan. 27 and Feb. 10, 1992, interviews, Blocker Collections. See also *Impact*, 10 (Oct. 31, 1986), 1, 3; *Galveston Daily News*, May 10, 1987. UTMB's first "in vitro" baby girl was born in January 1986 and UTMB's first "in vitro" twin girls were born in August 1987. See *Impact*, 10 (Feb. 7, 1986), 1, 8; and 11 (Sept. 4, 1987), 1–2.

101. With more than two thousand babies born annually during the early 1970s, they were very busy in the newborn nursery, attending 25–30 normal neonates and 15–20 sick and premature neonates each day. In 1973, for example, the Nursery's Special Care Unit admitted 236 premature infants. There were 43 neonatal deaths that year. See *University Medical*, 6 (Sept.–Oct. 1974), 4–7. See also Michael H. Malloy, C. Joan Richardson, and C. W. Daeschner, "UTMB Infant Special Care Unit: Regional Function and Costs of Care for 1983," *Texas Medicine*, 82 (Oct., 1986), 31–34.

102. *University Medical*, 15 (Summer, 1984), 35; *Impact*, 8 (May 4, 1984), 21; and 9 (Sept. 6, 1985), 12–13. In addition to an increase in the number of mothers who had high-risk pregnancies because of diabetes, asthma, drug abuse, or HIV infection, there was also a significant increase in teenage pregnancies during the 1980s. Some parturients at UTMB were fifteen- and sixteen-year-old mothers who returned for their second or third delivery. Myles Knape, WF437, CHP Archives, 30–37. Normal babies were discharged within thirty-six hours of birth, but the average length of stay in the Infant Special Care Unit was 32.5 days.

103. Between 1969 and 1973, UTMB doctors attended 189 physically abused children; 22 of these were sexually abused. See Albert I. Hartley and Robert Ginn, "Reporting Child Abuse," *Texas Medicine*, 71 (Feb., 1975), 84–86. Also see Myles Knape, WF437, CHP Archives, 30–37. ECMO refers to extracorporeal membrane oxygenation, a technique made possible by a modified heart-lung machine similar to those used for open-heart surgery. The machine allows the baby's lungs and heart to develop until they are able to assume their normal functions, a process that usually occurs after five to ten days. Joseph Zwischenberger and Pat Allison directed the teams that could include a neonatologist, pediatrician,

cardiothoracic surgeon, perfusionist, respiratory therapist, and specially trained nurses. See *Impact*, 13 (Feb. 24, 1989), 1; and *Galveston Daily News*, Apr. 2, 1990.

104. *Newsletter (UTMB)*, 4 (May, 1969), 14–16; *University Medical*, 2 (Feb., 1971), 12–14; *Hospital News*, 5 (Apr. 5 1971), 1; and 10 (Sept. 17, 1976), 3. As an independent unit, the school closed in 1986, though the services continued as a part of pediatric rehabilitation services, which were eventually combined with adult rehabilitative services into a rehabilitation unit on the third floor of Jennie Sealy Hospital.

105. *Faculty News (UTMB)*, Jan. 20–24, 1975; *Hospital News*, 8 (Feb. 10, 1975), 2; and *University Medical*, 6 (Jan.–Feb., 1975), 4–7. Some children had dialysis in their homes; others in the hospital. Some had transplants. For an analysis of the management of twelve children with renal failure, see Ben H. Brouhard, Michael Berger, Luther B. Travis, Robert J. Cunningham III, and Hugo F. Carvajal, "Chronic Peritoneal Dialysis in Children," *Texas Medicine*, 72 (Jan., 1976), 84–89. Ryan Bell received one of his father's kidneys and was doing well in 1981; see *Impact*, 5 (May 22, 1981), 8.

106. The comprehensive care Travis's team provided attracted more outpatients; their visits increased from 330 in 1982 to 390 in 1984. See Luther Travis's report to Bill Levin, April 1985, p. 13, folder 3, box 26, Levin Papers. For an overview of the team concept, see Luther B. Travis, Ben H. Brouhard, Terry Johnson, Paula McMahon, Barbara Schreiner, Sue Ellen Bingham, Alok Kalia, Pam Fillebrown, and Susan Bullard, "Management of the Child with Diabetes," *Texas Medicine*, 79 (Mar., 1983), 55–61. More than 2,300 children had attended the camps (Friendswood and Kerrville) by the summer of 1977. In that year, 22 professionals from UTMB provided care for 167 children (ages six to sixteen) attending the camp in Kerrville. See *Impact*, 1 (Aug. 26, 1977), 8–9. In 1981 there were four summer camps for diabetic children in Texas. For important details about these camps and other educational efforts with diabetic children and their families, see Luther Travis to Chester R. Burns, Feb. 25 and Mar. 10, 1992, interviews, Blocker Collections. Also see Luther B. Travis, Terry A. Johnson, Paul McMahon, Ben H. Brouhard, and Robert J. Cunningham, "Camps for Children with Diabetes," *Texas Medicine*, 77 (Apr., 1981), 36–40.

107. *Galveston Daily News*, May 10, 1991.

108. *Hospital News*, 2 (Mar. 31, 1969), 1. The unit was located on ward 4-B of the John Sealy Hospital. By 1977 Steve Young coordinated an eighteen-member cardiac rehabilitation team that included a cardiologist, two nurse practitioners, four physical therapists, two occupational therapists, five counselors, two dietitians, a cardio-pulmonary resuscitation instructor, and a stress lab technician. The team provided comprehensive rehabilitative care to those who experienced heart attacks of varying severity; see *Impact*, 1 (Mar. 18, 1977), 7. For an analysis of the origins of coronary care units in American hospitals, see J. Roderick Kitchell and Lawrence E. Meltzer, "The Concept of Intensive Coronary Care," *Texas Reports on Biology and Medicine*, 24 (June, 1966), supplement, 309–316.

109. "Notes about Hospital Activities," 52, 64, 67, 71, 75–76, 79, and 86; *Hospital News*, 9 (Oct. 24, 1975), 1; *University Medical*, 9 (Nov.–Dec., 1977), 3–12; and *Impact*, 1 (May 13, 1977), 4.

110. See summary in "Proposal for the Provision of Tertiary Care Hospital Services," 1982, WF303, CHP Archives. The intensive care beds were allocated as follows: infant (25); pediatric (5); medicine (8); coronary care (5); surgery (16); burn (8); and neurosurgical (6). See Myles Knape, WF437, CHP Archives, 22–28 (quotation on 25).

111. *University Medical*, 4 (July, 1973), 10–13; and *Impact*, 1 (July 29, 1977), 7; and 2 (Apr. 21, 1978), 6.

112. *University Medical*, 5 (Nov., 1973), 7–9; *Impact*, 1 (May 13, 1977), 7; William D. Willis Jr. to William C. Levin, May 24, 1979, letter, box 17, Levin Papers; *Impact*, 4 (Mar. 21, 1980),16; (Apr. 18, 1980), 1; and Jon Mader to Myles Knape, Jan. 3, 1990, interview, box 47, CHP Archives. For a description of hyperbaric treatment by two patients, see *Galveston Daily News*, Feb. 24, 1991.

113. For valuable historical overviews, see James T. Patterson, *The Dread Disease: Cancer and Modern American Culture* (Cambridge, Mass.: Harvard University Press, 1987) and Patrice Pinell, "Cancer," in Roger Cooter and John Pickstone (eds.), *Medicine in the 20th Century* (Amsterdam: Harwood Academic Publishers, 2000), 671–686.

114. *University Medical*, 6 (Mar., 1975), 4–7; *Faculty News (UTMB)*, June 2–6, 1975; *Hospital News*, 9 (July 28, 1975), 1; and *Impact*, 1 (Aug. 12, 1977), 8. In May 1977, for example, the Cancer Center sponsored a postgraduate course entitled "Cancer: A Multidisciplinary Approach." The presentations were published. See Marvin H. Olson, "Current Concepts of Radiotherapy in Treatment of Carcinoma of the Cervix," *Texas Medicine*, 75 (Feb., 1979), 90–91; Frank J. Panettiere, "The Role of Adjuvant Therapy in Colorectal Carcinoma," *Texas Medicine*, 75 (Feb., 1979), 92–94; Frank J. Panettiere and John J. Costanzi, "Advances in the Therapy and Immunotherapy of Lung Cancer," *Texas Medicine*, 75 (Feb., 1979), 95–97; Kerry Ford and L. B. Morettin, "Special Radiologic Procedures in Diagnosis and Treatment of Cancer Patients," *Texas Medicine*, 75 (Feb., 1979), 69–74; and Robert E. Girtanner, "Ovarian Cancer:

Diagnosis, Staging, Treatment," *Texas Medicine*, 75 (Feb., 1979), 75–80. See also William C. Levin to Jack Brooks, Jan. 15, 1987, letter, folder 2, box 26, Levin Papers. For details, see the folders in boxes 25 and 26, Levin Papers.

115. For details, see folders 4 and 5 in box 7, Levin Papers. See also *Impact*, 10 (Oct. 3, 1986), 1, 4–5. As director of the Mount Royal National Research Institute of Gerontology and Geriatric Medicine in Melbourne, Australia, Prinsley had visited UTMB in November 1984. See "Geriatric Medicine, 1986–1987," RF74, CHP Archives.

116. The day hospital was a rehabilitation center for outpatients recovering from strokes or amputations, and for those learning how to deal with chronic diseases, such as arthritis and diabetes. Patients were transported by bus to the hospital, which was open from nine to five, Monday through Friday. Patients received whatever treatments (such as physical therapy and occupational therapy) and services they needed for effective adaptation; see *Impact*, 13 (Dec. 1, 1989), 1. See also "Report on Aging 1990–1991," WF303, CHP Archives; and *Galveston Daily News*, June 17 and July 5, 1991.

117. Eric Avery to Inci Bowman, May 10, 1996, letter, WF303, CHP Archives. David Paar thought that 721 cases had been reported by the end of 1991. The number of prisoners with appointments in the TDCJ Infectious Disease Clinic increased from 185 during fiscal year 1986 to 2,477 during fiscal year 1991 (data provided by Casey Peterson). For examples of AIDS-related research at UTMB, see *Galveston Daily News*, Oct. 29, 1991, and Jan. 5, 1992. For historical background, see Elizabeth Fee and Daniel M. Fox (eds.), *AIDS: The Making of a Chronic Disease* (Berkeley: University of California Press, 1992).

118. See RF175, CHP Archives. During six fiscal years (1971–1976), for example, UTMB expended $3,349,397 for the costs of care for prisoner inpatients. See V. E. Thompson to J. B. Pace, Oct. 4, 1976, letter, folder 1, box 58, Levin Papers. See also *Impact*, 2 (Feb. 10, 1978), 1, and 4 (Apr. 4, 1980), 1, 18.

119. Raymond Jarl to Carl E. Schow, Oct. 9, 1986, letter, folder 5, box 58, Levin Papers; and Myles Knape, WF437, CHP Archives, 3–9. About two hundred UTMB employees worked in this hospital. The TDCJ provided more than two hundred security officers. For a description of the hospital after five years of operation, see *Galveston Daily News*, June 4, 1988.

120. "Notes about Hospital Activities," 67, 71. Some of the decline in inpatients occurred because the Department of Surgery had opened a Day Surgery Unit on 7-C in the John Sealy Towers in 1981. This unit housed fifteen rooms for patients needing surgery who did not require overnight hospitalization; see *Impact*, 5 (June 5, 1981), 1, 12, and (Dec. 11, 1981), 9. During its first year, more than six hundred patients used this facility; see *Impact*, 6 (Aug. 6, 1982), 6; and James Tang, "Ambulatory Surgery," *Texas Medicine*, 80 (Jan., 1984), 39–42.

121. *University Medical*, 4 (Feb., 1973), 14–15; and *Impact*, 6 (Nov. 12, 1982), 8.

122. Stephen J. Blackwell, Ted T. Huang, and S. R. Lewis, "Intra-arterial Drug Abuse, *Texas Medicine*, 74 (Mar., 1978), 64–68; *Impact*, 2 (Mar. 23, 1978), 9; and David N. Herndon to Harris L. Kempner Jr., Mar. 29, 1984, letter, folder 5, box 17, Levin Papers. In 1980 Shriners Burns Institute and UTMB established a skin bank. Skin was obtained from people who had donated their skin before death. Skin was harvested from forty donors during the first year. By 1990 there were more than two hundred donors a year. The harvested skin, whose thickness varied from 1/5,000 to 1/15,000 of an inch, provided a temporary covering for a burned patient that helped maintain body heat, stopped loss of fluids, retarded or prevented infection, and relieved pain. These outcomes provided the environment needed for regeneration of the patient's own "harvested" skin. In 1989 UTMB also established a bone bank, storing harvested bone that could be used for spinal fusions and other surgical treatments. See Myles Knape, WF437, CHP Archives, 13–15.

123. *Impact*, 6 (Feb. 5, 1982), 1, 25; (Mar. 5, 1982), 1, 18; and 14 (Jan. 26, 1990), 1–2.

124. "Notes about Hospital Activities," 60; Jay Fish to Chester R. Burns, Feb. 17, 1992, interview, Blocker Collections; James C. Thompson to William C. Levin, Dec. 9, 1986, letter, folder 3, box 11, Levin Papers; *Impact*, 12 (May 13, 1988), 1–2; and *Galveston Daily News*, May 14, 1990.

125. *Hospital News*, 10 (Sept. 3, 1976), 1; and *Impact*, 1 (July 15, 1977), 5. Radiologists had established the new ultrasound division in December 1975. Technicians conducted sonic scans of the abdomen and pelvis, with pregnant women constituting 70 percent of the referrals; see *Faculty News (UTMB)*, Dec. 8–12, 1975; and *Impact*, 8 (Dec. 14, 1984), 1, 12–13.

126. *Impact*, 9 (June 14, 1985), 9–12. At birth, Maria had lacked a lower abdominal wall and portions of her urinary bladder and urethra. Other surgical specialists at UTMB developed new approaches during these years. The Department of Otolaryngology developed a team for treating patients with cancer of the head and neck (1979) and established a vestibular clinic (1981). For details, see *Galveston Daily News*, Jan. 5, 1972; *Hospital News*, 2 (Jan. 10, 1972), 1, 4; *Impact*, 3 (Sept. 7, 1979), 8; 5 (Feb. 20, 1981), 5; 9 (Jan. 11, 1985), 10–11; and WF317, CHP Archives.

127. In 1974 the department established a Division of Nuclear Medicine, whose members injected isotopes to obtain diagnostic information about the functions of various organs (95 percent of patients) or to treat a diseased organ, such as a hyperactive thyroid gland (5 percent of patients). See *University Medical*, 5 (Mar., 1974), 4–6; Minutes, Sealy & Smith Foundation Board of Directors, Apr. 14, 1976; *Faculty News (UTMB)*, July 21–Aug. 1, 1975; *Hospital News*, 9 (July 28, 1975), 2; and Mohammed Sawar, "Computed Cranial Tomography: Experience at The University of Texas Medical Branch," *Texas Medicine*, 73 (Sept., 1977), 42–61. By 1976 the department also had two ultrasound scanners, a new gamma camera that located radioactive tracers in body tissues, and a new 18,000,000 electron volt linear accelerator for treating various types of cancer; see *Faculty News (UTMB)*, Sept. 1–12, 1975; *Hospital News*, 9 (Sept. 22, 1975), 2; and *University Medical*, 8 (Nov.–Dec. 1976), 12–15.

128. Minutes, Sealy & Smith Foundation Board of Directors, Aug. 13, 1980; *Impact*, 6 (Feb. 5, 1982), 4; and *University Medical*, 15 (Summer, 1984), 26–29. The MRI's 5-kilogauss electromagnets contained radio frequency coils that sent signals into body parts and elicited responses from the protons in the nuclei of hydrogen atoms that were present in all bodily tissues. These responses were analyzed by spectroscopes that permitted radiologists to differentiate among soft tissues and evaluate functional and structural abnormalities. The data was transformed into computerized images that were recorded on photographic film. Physicians could thereby obtain more precise help in diagnosing small tumors, abscesses, localized areas of hemorrhage, and multiple sclerosis—to mention only a few conditions. For details, see *Impact*, 8 (Oct. 5, 1984), 1; and folder 5, box 10, Levin Papers. With a grant of $250,000 from the Sealy & Smith Foundation, the equipment was upgraded in the fall of 1988.

129. *Impact*, 10 (Mar. 21, 1986), 1, 19; and *Galveston Daily News*, Oct. 29, 1990, and June 21, 1991.

130. *Impact*, 6 (Sept. 3, 1982), 15. In 1979 Kuruse was president of the American Academy of Cardiovascular Perfusion and a member of the board of the American Board of Cardiovascular Perfusion, the accrediting agency in North America. See *Impact*, 8 (Mar. 9, 1984), 1, 13; *University Medical*, 15 (Summer, 1984), 34; *Impact*, 9 (June 14, 1985), 1, 17, and 11 (Nov. 13, 1987), 1; and *Galveston Daily News*, May 6, 1990, and Oct. 28, 1990.

131. *Impact*, 8 (June 29, 1984), 1, 17; (Aug. 10, 1984), 23; and 11 (Mar. 6, 1987), 1.

132. *Impact*, 12 (Nov. 18, 1988), 1; *Galveston Daily News*, Dec. 8, 1988, and May 5, 1989; *Impact*, 13 (June 30, 1989), 1; and *Galveston Daily News*, Jan. 22, 1990.

133. For family therapy, see *University Medical*, 4 (Mar., 1973), 14–15; for the drugs, see Harry K. Davis, "Updating Psychotropic Drug Therapy," *Texas Medicine*, 72 (Sept., 1976), 39–47. For the gender identification unit, see *Impact*, 1 (Apr. 1, 1977), 1. Sex-change operations were recommended to some of these patients. Between 1972 and 1991, about 160 men became women and about 50 women became men as part of the gender treatment program in Galveston; see *Galveston Daily News*, June 30, 1991. For the adult day program, see *Impact*, 7 (Mar. 25, 1983), 4; and for the eating disorder unit, see *Impact*, 12 (May 13, 1988), 1.

134. *Hospital News*, 7 (Apr. 2, 1973), 1–2; and Mike Ellis to Myles Knape, Nov. 13, 1989, interview, box 47, CHP Archives.

135. *University Medical*, 10 (Mar.–May, 1979), 8.

136. For a graphic description of the work of Judy Hays, an intensive care nurse in the Blocker Burn Unit at John Sealy Hospital, see *Galveston Daily News*, Feb. 26, 1989.

137. *Hospital News*, 3 (Aug. 18, 1969), 1; (Sept. 15, 1969), 3; and 4 (Feb. 16, 1970), 2; "Notes about Hospital Activities," 65, 88.

138. *Impact*, 3 (May 4, 1979), 17; *University Medical*, 10 (Sept.–Oct., 1979), 12–15; and V. E. Thompson to Charles B. Mullins, Nov. 13, 1981, letter, WF303, CHP Archives.

139. "Listing of Service Laboratories," Dorothy C. Felis to A. L. LeBlanc, Aug. 3, 1979, WF303, CHP Archives. Beginning in 1943, Juaneva Novak was the technical director of the EEG lab in the Department of Neurology and Psychiatry for more than thirty years. In conjunction with the School of Allied Health Sciences, she also trained four technicians each year. See *Hospital News*, 7 (Nov. 11, 1974), 2, and *Impact*, 3 (Jan. 12, 1979), 3. For instant evaluation of tissues received from the operating room, frozen sections were usually ready for microscopic evaluation ("reading") in ten minutes. Tissues received from clinics and wards not needing instant attention were embedded in paraffin, then cut, stained, and dried on slides that were ordinarily ready for "reading" within twenty-four hours. See *Impact*, 7 (Dec. 16, 1983), 12–15.

140. *Galveston Daily News*, June 21, 1986.

141. V. E. Thompson to Charles B. Mullins, Nov. 13, 1981, letter, WF303, CHP Archives; *Impact*, 9 (Apr. 5, 1985), 5; and Myles Knape, WF437, CHP Archives, 2–3.

142. V. E. Thompson to Charles B. Mullins, Nov. 13, 1981, letter, WF303, CHP Archives.

143. Myles Knape, WF437, CHP Archives, 53–59. For a profile of Martharein Brooks, a social worker on the internal medicine floors of Jennie Sealy in 1984, see *Impact*, 8 (Apr. 13, 1984), 20.

144. Minutes, Sealy & Smith Foundation Board of Directors, July 13, 1977; *Impact*, 3 (Mar. 9, 1979), 3; and Myles Knape, WF437, CHP Archives, 19–22.

145. V. E. Thompson to Charles B. Mullins, Nov. 13, 1981, letter, WF303, CHP Archives; and *Impact*, 6 (July 2, 1982), 16; and 10 (Nov. 14, 1986), 5.

146. *Impact*, 4 (Feb. 22, 1980), 17; Myles Knape, WF437, CHP Archives, 47–53; and *Galveston Daily News*, Oct. 15, 1990.

147. *Impact*, 8 (Feb. 24, 1984), 15. In 1988 Johnnie Mae James, food production manager for the Food and Nutrition Services Department, was president of the twelve thousand-member Dietary Managers Association. James had worked at UTMB for thirty-seven years; see *Impact*, 11 (June 26, 1987), 5.

148. V. E. Thompson to Charles B. Mullins, Nov. 13, 1981, letter, WF303, CHP Archives; *Impact*, 4 (Feb. 8, 1980), 17; 6 (July 2, 1982), 19; and 7 (Mar. 25, 1983), 11; and *Galveston Daily News*, June 21, 1986 (quotation).

149. *University Medical*, 6 (Nov.–Dec., 1974), 4–7. For details about the Moody Independent School District, see folder 5, box 23, Levin Papers. See also *Galveston Daily News*, Oct. 13, 1991.

150. *Newsletter (UTMB)*, 4 (June, 1969), 18. Members of this council included John DeForke and Joe Fiorenza (Catholic), Denton Bassett (Baptist), and Robert Wedergren (Lutheran).

151. For other examples, see *Faculty News (UTMB)*, Dec. 3, 1973, 4; *Hospital News*, 9 (Dec. 3, 1976), 2; *Impact*, 5 (Jan. 9, 1981), 4; 9 (Dec. 6, 1985), 6; and 11 (Jan. 23, 1987), 3.

152. In 1978 a small chapel was constructed on the first floor of the main hospital adjacent to the offices of the Department of Ministry. The group of eight chaplains included Nolen Holcomb, Denton Bassett, Bob Wedergren, Tom Law, Ralph Bucy, John Caskey, Timothy Curry, and John Reardon. UTMB received approximately $650,000 annually from the denominational judicatories who had authorized these chaplains. See Myles Knape, WF437, CHP Archives, 70. For details about the work of these chaplains between 1974 and 1985, see folder 8, box 19, Levin Papers.

153. The hospital funded this department in 1967 and Novella Cohen was the first director in 1968. For details, see WF368, CHP Archives. Also see *Impact*, 9 (Apr. 19, 1985), 10–11; (Nov. 15, 1985), 1, 17; and 10 (Apr. 18, 1986), 14; Myles Knape, WF437, CHP Archives, 80–86; *Galveston Daily News*, Apr. 25, 1990; Liz Payer to UTMB employees, Oct. 23, 1991, memo, WF303, CHP Archives.

154. *Impact*, 8 (Nov. 16, 1984), 20. The Pediatric Angels were volunteer members of the Junior League of Galveston County who played with hospitalized children for two or three hours each week; see *Impact*, 3 (Mar. 9, 1979), 15. Also see *Impact*, 11 (Oct. 16, 1987), 3; and 14 (Sept. 28, 1990), 9.

155. The Sealy & Smith Foundation allocated $1.6 million to UTMB for construction of this Ronald McDonald House, which is used by the families of seriously ill children who are inpatients at UTMB and Shriners Burns Institute; see *Impact*, 11 (Apr. 17, 1987), 1, 3.

156. For details, see folder 7, box 31, Levin Papers. See also *Impact*, 14 (Feb. 9, 1990), 3; and WF367, CHP Archives.

157. V. E. Thompson to Charles B. Mullins, Nov. 13, 1981, letter, CHP Archives WF303. The data in Appendix AD came from the annual hospital reports published by the University of Texas System; see WF312, CHP Archives. Because of the way that indirect income for patient care services was calculated, there are some differences between the totals in Appendix AD and those in the patient services column of Appendix U. Those in Appendix AD are a better indicator of income from direct patient care and those in Appendix U are a better indicator of revenue related to the total delivery of patient care services. For details, see WF282, CHP Archives.

158. William C. Levin to Sylvia Komatsu, Apr. 29, 1983, letter, folder 2, box 49, Levin Papers; and Alvin L. LeBlanc to Chester R. Burns, Oct. 24 and Nov. 29, 1989, interview, Blocker Collections.

159. For a copy of the final report, see folder 3, box 49, Levin Papers. As a member of this task force, Bill Levin spoke to the Committee on Urban Affairs of the Texas House of Representatives on November 16, 1983. He emphasized that most public teaching hospitals, like UTMB, had always been expected to earn a "significant portion of their operating funds" by providing services "for which reimbursement is received"; see "Testimony on Indigent Health Care," p. 6, folder 2, box 49, Levin Papers.

160. For a list of these laws, see the attachment of a letter from Helen Farabee to Bill Levin, June 18, 1985, folder 4, box 49, Levin Papers.

161. *Impact*, 9 (Jan. 11, 1985), 1, 6. For comments about UT-MED, see Harry Little to Chester R. Burns, Jan. 27 and Feb. 10, 1992, interviews, Blocker Collections. The Sixty-ninth Legislature adopted a law that made counties responsible for the medical care of indigents not covered by Medicaid and Medicare; see LeBlanc to Burns, Oct. 24 and Nov. 29, 1989, interviews, Blocker Collections; and *Galveston Daily News*, May 14, 1991.

162. "Notes about Hospital Activities," 95, 98.

163. Levin believed that there was a "new era in the Administration of the University Hospitals." See "Notes about Hospital Activities," 56 (quotation), 57, 60. See also *Hospital News*, 3 (Aug. 4, 1969); 4 (Jan. 19, 1970); 7 (May 28, 1974); and 7 (June 10, 1974). The Performance Appraisal System standardized evaluation of all hospital employees. New employees were evaluated by a supervisor after a ninety-day probationary period. All others were evaluated annually. Employees with ratings of excellent and good were eligible for merit increases if funds were available; see "Notes about Hospital Activities," 49.

164. For a chart of hospital administration in 1974, see Appendix D-8 in WF444, CHP Archives. For examples of the activities of medical staff committees during the 1970s, see "Notes about Hospital Activities," 52–93. For a list of the twenty-two medical staff committees in fiscal year 1986, see folder 1, box 20, Levin Papers.

165. *Impact*, 4 (Feb. 8, 1980), 1, 14–15, 18; LeBlanc to Burns, Oct. 24 and Nov. 29, 1989, interviews, Blocker Collections; and "Notes about Hospital Activities," 94. For a list of the appointments and committees, see "Notes about Hospital Activities," 95 (copied memo in WF311, CHP Archives). For comments about some of these committees, see Little to Burns, Jan. 27 and Feb. 10, 1992, and Travis to Burns, Feb. 25 and Mar. 10, 1992, interviews, Blocker Collections. For charts of hospital administration in 1977 and 1980, see Appendix D-9 and D-10, WF444, CHP Archives. Beginning in 1981, photos of these and other support staff appeared in every annual volume of the *Syndrome* (1981), 10–11; (1982), 10–11; (1983), 10–11; (1984), 18–19; (1985), 18–19; (1986), 64–65; (1987), 206–207; (1988), 30–31; (1989), 20–21; (1990), 21–22; and (1991), 27–28.

166. *Impact*, 6 (July 2, 1982), 5. Coordinated by Smith, teams of employees began "Environmental Rounds" in the hospital in September 1980 as a way of identifying deficiencies in the functions and appearances of hospital departments; see "Notes about Hospital Activities," 96 and 98. In 1986 UTMB hospitals began using a new quality assurance program titled medical management analysis (MMA). About ten nurses screened all inpatient records and assessed the quality of care rendered to these patients. Harry Little Jr. chaired the MMA task force that coordinated this program. Nurses and medical records personnel met weekly with physicians from each clinical service to review items signaled during the screening process. Monthly reports were sent to appropriate committees and administrators; see *Impact*, 10 (Jan. 10, 1986), 4.

167. For a copy of the handbook, see WF303, CHP Archives. During 1981 directors, nurses, department heads, unit managers, and others attended eight three-day management courses; see "Notes about Hospital Activities," 98. For comments, see LeBlanc to Burns, Oct. 24 and Nov. 29, 1989, interviews, Blocker Collections.

168. To address the problem of medical malpractice suits, the UT System developed a risk management program and UTMB's first risk management committee was established in the fall of 1982.

169. Myles Knape, WF437, CHP Archives, 71–75; and "Guest Relations Professional Program," WF358, CHP Archives.

170. For an organization chart, see Appendix D-11, WF444, CHP Archives. For the annual growth of these expenses between 1969 and 1991, see Appendix B-30, WF442, CHP Archives.

171. *Impact*, 14 (Apr. 6, 1990), 1; and *Galveston Daily News*, June 28, 1990. For an organization chart in 1991, see Appendix D-12, WF444, CHP Archives. See also *Impact*, 14 (Sept. 14, 1990), 1.

CHAPTER 6

1. *Texas State Journal of Medicine*, 39 (May, 1943), 41.

2. Among the eighty students admitted in 1905, for example, four had college degrees, eight had attended colleges, five had graduated from colleges of pharmacy or attended other medical schools, ten had graduated from officially recognized high schools or normal schools, nine had respectable credentials from other preparatory schools, seventeen had first-grade state teachers certificates, and twenty seven had passed the faculty's entrance examination. See W. S. Carter to S. E. Mezes, May 2, 1910, letter, box 4R85, UT President's Records.

3. Thirteen state university medical schools required two years of college work. See W. S. Carter to W. B. Collins, June 22, 1911, and R. O. Braswell to John T. Moore, June 21, 1911 (quotations), letters, box 4Q18, UT President's Records.

4. W. S. Carter to S. E. Mezes, May 3, 1912, letter, box 4Q25, UT President's Records.

5. In 1912 the AMA named as Class A medical schools only those that required not less than one year of college with satisfactory credits in chemistry, biology, physics, and a modern language. In 1913 the AAMC and the AMA specified that the preliminary education for admission to Class A schools would include two prescribed units in Latin and Greek and two in German or French among the fourteen high school units, and one college course each in physics, chemistry, biology, and German or French. UTMB's teachers adopted these requirements for students who entered after January 1, 1914; see Minutes, UTMB Faculty Meeting, Nov. 9, 1912.

6. W. S. Carter to S. E. Mezes, May 11, 1914, letter, box 4Q19, UTPR; Minutes, UTMB Faculty Meeting, Oct. 8, 1915. Four months later the AAMC required two years of college work for all member colleges. By that time, fifty-two of ninety-four U.S. medical schools honored this requirement. Carter was glad that UTMB had adopted this standard before it became "compulsory"; see W. S. Carter to W. J. Battle, Mar. 7, 1916, letter, box 4Q21, UT President's Records. These improvements occurred in all of the nation's medical schools; see Ludmerer, *Time to Heal*, 60–62.

7. *UTMB Catalog* (1914–1915), 2–3 and 22–38. Excellent photos of several professors are included in the seventy-fifth anniversary book; for a list, see *UTMB: Seventy-five Year History*, xix–xxii.

8. In January 1912 the faculty agreed to a six-year combined course leading to the B.S. and M.D. degrees, and a seven-year combined course leading to the B.A. and M.D. degrees; see Minutes, UTMB Faculty Meeting, Jan. 18, 1912. Students could study at UT Austin for two years in the College of Arts and then four years in the Medical School to acquire the combined B.S. and M.D. degrees. Or students could study three years in the College of Arts and four years in medical school to acquire the combined B.A. and M.D. degrees. These degree programs appealed to certain students. Between 1920 and 1942, 126 students earned combined B.S. and M.D. degrees, and between 1920 and 1946, 63 earned combined B.A. and M.D. degrees. See W. S. Carter to S. E. Mezes, May 11, 1914, letter, box 4Q19, UT President's Records.

9. The names of the graduates are in *UTMB: Seventy-five Year History*, 327–329.

10. W. S. Carter to S. E. Mezes, May 2, 1910, and May 3, 1912, letters, box 4R85, UT President's Records. See entry for November 26, 1922 (p. 57) in Bonnet's diary in folder 2, Edith Bonnet Papers, Blocker Collections (quotation). Bonnet's diary (1918–1969) is a valuable source of information about the life of a female medical student during the 1920s. Also see the typescript of her interview by Larry Wygant on Sept. 22, 1977, Blocker Collections. Megan Seaholm determined the attrition rate by dividing the annual number of graduates by the number of freshmen who had entered four years earlier. For her list, see WF358, CHP Archives. As a specific example, Dean Bethel reported that twelve students withdrew and nine failed during the first semester of the 1931–1932 academic year; see George E. Bethel to H. Y. Benedict, Feb. 13, 1932, letter, box VF 9/C, UT President's Records.

11. R. E. Vinson to W. S. Carter, May 12, 1920, letter, box 4Q22, UT President's Records; Minutes, UTMB Faculty Meeting, Sept. 25, 1920; Minutes, UTMB Executive Committee Meeting, Aug. 9, 1920; *Galveston Daily News*, Sept. 21, 1924; William Keiller to W. M. W. Splawn, Apr. 15, 1925, letter, box 4Q25, UT President's Records; William Keiller to W. M. W. Splawn, Dec. 14, 1925, letter, box 4Q24, UT President's Records; and *Galveston Daily News*, Apr. 15, 1927.

12. Thirty-six percent of those admitted in 1932 had bachelor's degrees, compared to 28 percent in 1925; see the chart prepared by Megan Seaholm in WF381, CHP Archives. Nationally, about one-half of the medical students had obtained bachelor's degrees; see Rothstein, *American Medical Schools and the Practice of Medicine*, 152. Also see Ludmerer, *Time to Heal*, 62; George E. Bethel to H. Y. Benedict, Aug. 13, 1932, letter, box 27, UTMB Dean's Office Records, Inactive. For more on the test, see Paul J. Sanazaro and Edwin B. Hutchins, "The Origin and Rationale of the Medical College Admission Test," *Journal of Medical Education*, 38 (Dec., 1963), 1044–1050.

13. George E. Bethel to H. Y. Benedict, Oct. 25, 1934, letter, box 4Q18, UT President's Records. For the class entering in 1935, 103 of 182 applicants were accepted. Forty-two matriculates had college degrees, thirty-one had credit for ninety or more semester hours, and thirty had credit for sixty or more but less than ninety semester hours. For this data, see W. S. Carter to H. Y. Benedict, Oct. 31, 1935, and W. S. Carter to H. Y. Benedict, Oct. 31, 1936, letters, box 4Q25, UT President's Records. More than two-thirds of the one hundred students admitted in 1937 had taken part or all of their pre-medical courses at UT Austin. UTMB's professors believed that students who had studied at UT Austin, Rice Institute, the Texas Colleges of Mines, Sam Houston State Teachers College, and Southern Methodist University made higher grade averages in medical school courses; see W. S. Carter to J. W. Calhoun, Nov. 1, 1937, letter, box 4Q18, UT President's Records.

14. W. S. Carter to R. E. Vinson, Mar. 24, 1921, letter, box 4R81, UT President's Records; Minutes, UTMB Faculty Meeting, Oct. 5, 1928; and "Comparison of Roster Hours at Pennsylvania and Texas, 1927–8," box 4Q24, UT President's Records. For notebooks kept by a student for both basic science and clinical courses between 1922 and 1926, see folders 4–7, Edith Bonnet Papers, Blocker Collections. For class notes taken between 1927 and 1931, see boxes 1–3

of the Francis A. Garbade Papers in the Blocker Collections. During the 1920s, students learned more gynecology than obstetrics, but most students did deliver a baby. In 1924, for example, students delivered a total of 244 patients (190 in the hospital and 54 in homes); see Willard R. Cooke to W. M. W. Splawn, Apr. 20, 1925, letter, box 4Q25; Willard R. Cooke to W. M. W. Splawn, Feb. 23, 1926, letter, box 4P263, UT President's Records; and RF28, CHP Archives. For comments about the teachers by a student who entered in 1929, see John L. Matthews to Myles Knape and Chester R. Burns, Aug. 25, 1989, interview, Blocker Collections.

15. *UTMB Catalog* (1928–1929), 7–9. In the proposed budget for fiscal year 1929, thirty-nine people are named with adjunct professor, associate professor, or professor appointments; ten as salaried part-time instructors; see Minutes, UT Board of Regents, Apr. 9, 1928.

16. *UTMB Catalog* (1928–1929), 30–44. John Sinclair, who began teaching histology and embryology in 1928, was listed in the Anatomy Department's budget until 1932, when Histology and Embryology became a separately budgeted department; see Minutes, UT Board of Regents, July 8, 1933. Five clinical departments emerged between 1919 and 1931: Dermatology and Syphilology; Otolaryngology; Pediatrics; Neurology and Psychiatry; and Radiology. In Appendix G, the years they were promoted to associate professor were designated as the "first" years of Earl Crutchfield's administrative leadership in Dermatology (1923) and Jesse Johnson's leadership in Radiology (1931). Crutchfield had been a faculty member since 1919, Johnson since 1925.

17. George E. Bethel to H. Y. Benedict, Oct. 15, 1930, letter, box 4Q25, UT President's Records; and Minutes, UTMB Faculty Meeting, June 2, 1931.

18. Bethel and the faculty were delighted that the forty-year practice of duplicating most of the basic science laboratory courses had finally ended; see George Bethel to H. Y. Benedict, Oct. 24, 1932, box 4Q25, UT President's Records.

19. George E. Bethel to H. Y. Benedict, Oct. 25, 1934, letter, box 4Q18, UT President's Records. John Middleton was a student between 1933 and 1937; William Seybold between 1934 and 1938. For delightful comments about their teachers, see John Middleton to Chester R. Burns, Dec. 17, 1991, and William D. Seybold to Chester R. Burns, Jan. 26, 1990, interviews, Blocker Collections. A medical student between 1932 and 1935, Mavis P. Kelsey Sr. provides numerous anecdotes about these teachers; see *Twentieth-Century Doctor: House Calls to Space Medicine* (College Station: Texas A&M University Press, 1999), 57–76. For lecture notes and tests taken during the 1930s, see the Philip A. Bergman Papers in the Blocker Collections. See also C. T. Stone to H. Y. Benedict, Aug. 31, 1935, letter, box 17, UTMB Dean's Office Records, Inactive, Blocker Collections; and W. S. Carter to H. Y. Benedict, Oct. 31, 1935, letter, box 4Q25, UT President's Records.

20. For a glimpse of the scope of teaching by basic science professors, see the teachers' reports for 1936 through 1940 in folder 5, box 16 of the Anatomy Department's records in the Blocker Collections. For a similar glimpse of teaching by clinical professors, see the reports for 1937 by five members of the Department of Medicine in RF107, CHP Archives. Bill Levin was a student between 1937 and 1941; for comments about School of Medicine teachers then, see Levin to Burns, Nov. 7, 1989, interview, Blocker Collections.

21. "Report of the Curriculum Revision Committee," appended to letter from John C. Nolan to H. Y. Benedict, July 2, 1936, box VF 9/C, UT President's Records; and W. S. Carter to H. Y. Benedict, Oct. 31, 1936, letter, box 4Q25, UT President's Records. For comments about his job as an instructor in pathology during this year, see Kelsey, *Twentieth-Century Doctor*, 87–92. During the late 1930s Spies and Carter received more dollars for adding new faculty; see *Galveston Daily News*, Sept. 20 and Oct. 6, 1936; Mar. 6 and Aug. 31, 1938; and July 18 and Oct. 7, 1939.

22. Rothstein, *American Medical Schools and the Practice of Medicine*, 173–174; *Galveston Daily News*, May 25 and 31 and June 1, 1941. Five Galvestonians, including Bill Levin, were among these graduates. The richest source of anecdotes about the professors during the late 1930s is in the compilation prepared by the class of 1940 for their fiftieth anniversary reunion in 1990. See "After 50 Years . . . Unreliable Memoirs by the Class of 1940," in WF401, CHP Archives. For the names of the 2,245 doctors, see *UTMB: Seventy-five Year History*, 327–334.

23. *Galveston Daily News*, Aug. 12, 1941 and "Report of the Curriculum Council," box VF 9/B, UT President's Records. A copy of the report is in RF4, CHP Archives. Also see Leake's Annual Report for fiscal year 1943 in folder 19, box 2, Leake Papers, Blocker Collections.

24. Calvin streamlined the admissions process. For details, see D. Bailey Calvin, "Procedure for Determining Weighted Average and Eligibility for Acceptance of Applicants to the University of Texas Medical School," box VF 10/B, UT President's Records; and D. Bailey Calvin to T. S. Painter, Dec. 2, 1946, letter, box VF 9/D, UT President's Records. For some comments about her husband's roles, see Novella V. Calvin to Myles Knape, Oct. 21, 1985, interview, Blocker Collections.

25. *Galveston Daily News*, Oct. 14, 1942; and Mar. 28, Sept. 9, and Dec. 15 and 18, 1943.

26. "A Message from Dr. Chauncey Leake," *University Medical*, 4 (Sept., 1972), 17 (1st quotation); and "Learning to Deal with Life and Death: The Story of Becoming a Doctor in Texas," *Texas Medicine*, 76 (May, 1980), 66 (2nd quotation). For other comments about teaching in these years, see Kenneth Earle to Chester R. Burns, Mar. 15, 1990, and Robert White to Chester R. Burns, Dec. 10 and 20, 1991, interviews, Blocker Collections.

27. *UTMB Catalog* (1945–1946), 11–19; and Minutes, UT Board of Regents, July 14, 1945. Beginning in 1928, the Department of Surgery established divisions that reflected continued specialization and subspecialization. These included Urology in 1928 with Robert Cone as chief; Orthopedics in 1929 with G. W. N. Eggers; Neurosurgery in 1937 with Sam Snodgrass; Thoracic Surgery in 1946 with Wilson Harrison; and Plastic Surgery in 1946 with Truman Blocker.

28. Raymond Blount, professor of anatomy, was a favorite. There are many stories about the antics he used to stimulate students. When they answered his questions with an "I don't know" or an incorrect answer, he would responded with such statements as "You haven't crossed the causeway yet"; or "You can't not know"; or "Are you here to be a carpenter, a ribbon merchant, or a physician?" Blount would scream or throw chalk at them. They would throw pennies at him and he would use the pennies to purchase items for the anatomy lab. On August 2, 1953, students presented him with a turkey and he immediately began lecturing about the anatomy of the turkey.

29. Helene Wioke, "Medschool Admission," *Daily Texan*, Sept. 26, 1944; D. Bailey Calvin, "Annual Report on Student and Curricular Affairs, Fiscal Years 1944–1945," box 2, Leake Papers, Blocker Collections; and *Galveston Daily News*, Sept. 13, 1945.

30. Chauncey D. Leake to T. S. Painter, Jan 10, 1946, letter, box VF 10/C, UT President's Records. For examples of the laboratory exercises in physiology, see the lab manual created for the course in 1947 by Howard Swann, Marshall Brucer, and Eric Ogden, box 3, vertical file A8, Blocker Collections. See also *UTMB Catalog* (1946–1947), 44–45, 51–71. To sample instructional guidelines in surgery, see the eighty-three-page "Notes on Surgical Anatomy and Operative Surgery" compiled by the Department of Surgery in 1941, box 5, vertical file A8, Blocker Collections. James C. Thompson and Spencer Thompson graduated in 1951; for comments about their teachers, see James C. Thompson to Myles Knape and Chester R. Burns, June 27, July 3 and 13, 1989, and Spencer Thompson to Chester R. Burns, July 1, 1986, interviews, Blocker Collections.

31. *University Medical* (May, 1946), 2 (1st quotation); *Galveston Daily News*, Nov. 27, 1949 (2nd quotation); and "Report on Fall-Outs Among Medical Students, The University of Texas Medical Branch, 1945–1954," box VF E12, UT Chancellor's Records.

32. Chauncey D. Leake to Edward C. Gould, Aug. 19, 1948, letter, box 36, Leake Papers, NLM; and D. Bailey Calvin to D. K. Woodward Jr., June 6, 1947, letter, box VF 10/C, UT President's Records.

33. D. Bailey Calvin to Howard Carney, Apr. 9, 1948, letter, box VF 10/D, UT President's Records. Improved standardization for all applicants had occurred after the AAMC developed a new standardized admissions test in 1946. Approximately 215 applicants for the class beginning in 1947 took this new test at UT Austin on January 11, 1947; see *Galveston Daily News*, Jan. 6, 1947. In 1948 this test was renamed the Medical College Admissions Test (MCAT).

34. D. Bailey Calvin to T. S. Painter, Mar. 28, 1949, letter, box VF 10/D, UT President's Records; Minutes, UTMB Faculty Meeting, May 4, 1948; Minutes, UTMB Executive Committee, Nov. 7, 1950; D. Bailey Calvin to Thomas G. Pollard, July 7, 1949,letter, box VF 10/D, UT President's Records; Chauncey D. Leake to cousins, Oct. 4, 1949, letter, box 2, Leake Papers, NLM; and *Galveston Daily News*, June 21 and July 5, 1949. Enrolled via a contract with Texas Southern University in Houston, Herman Barnett was expected to stay at UTMB until a medical school opened at TSU. That school never materialized.

35. AAMC Datagrams, "Physician Supply and the Talent Pool: A National Problem," June 1962, vol. 3, no. 12; *Galveston Daily News*, July 8, 1954; Minutes, UTMB Faculty Meeting, Apr. 3, 1956; and Melvin Casberg to Logan Wilson, Apr. 26, 1957, letter, box VF H/1, UT Chancellor's Records.

36. In the class beginning in 1961, for example, fourteen of the 139 freshmen were non-residents. Ten of these fourteen had master's degrees and two had doctorates; see *Galveston Daily News*, Oct. 1, 1961. In November 1957 the regents had authorized the UT medical schools to accept out-of-state residents as students, provided that none of these students would be admitted until all qualified Texas residents had been admitted. The number of non-resident students could not exceed 10 percent of the first-year class. Between 1958 and 1967 UTMB admitted fifty-five non-residents; see Charles A. LeMaistre to Harry Ransom, June 28, 1968, letter, box VF EE/3, UT Chancellor's Records.

37. Lanier Cox to John B. Truslow, June 18, 1962, box VF T/3; and L. D. Haskew to Don Walker, May 29, 1963, box VF P/3, letters, UT Chancellor's Records.

38. *Galveston Daily News*, July 4 and Nov. 16, 1952. For a list of students and their preceptors for the spring of 1953, see *Galveston Daily News*, Mar. 1, 1953. See also *Galveston Daily News*, Oct. 18, 1954. For comments about his student days (1951–1955) including a preceptorship, see Alvin L. LeBlanc to Chester R. Burns, Oct. 24 and Nov. 29, 1989, interviews, Blocker Collections.

39. "Minutes of Curriculum Committee Meeting," July 8, 1954, box 6, Duncan papers, Blocker Collections. To sample some of the deliberations of the Curriculum Committee during the 1950s, see minutes of their meetings in folder 7, box 17, Department of Anatomy records, Blocker Collections. The quotation was one comment in a litany of complaints from more than fifty members of the class of 1952. See "General Report on Medical Courses as Viewed by Senior Medical Students Interviewed by the Services and Development Committee," box VF C/1, UT Chancellor's Records. A copy is in RF36, CHP Archives. For comments about teaching by a member of the class of 1955 (Melvyn Schreiber), a member of the class of 1957 (Harry Little) and a member of the class of 1958 (Jay Fish), see Melvyn H. Schreiber to Chester R. Burns and Myles Knape, Aug. 9 and 23, 1989; Harry Little to Chester R. Burns, Jan. 27 and Feb. 10, 1992; and Jay Fish to Chester R. Burns, Feb. 17, 1992, interviews, Blocker Collections.

40. Dismissed from school because of cheating on exams, one student (in 1957) challenged this dismissal with court trials adjudicated in the Fifty-sixth District Court and the Tenth Court of Appeals. Both courts upheld the dismissal decision. For details, see *Galveston Daily News*, Apr. 3, 10–13, 15–16, 24, and 26, May 6–7, 15, and 17, June 14, and Oct. 4, 1957; and Jan. 13, 1962. See Mary Ellen Haggard to Megan Seaholm, Sept. 7, 1988, untaped interview, notes in "Student Life Interviews" folder, WF383, CHP Archives.

41. For their names, see *UTMB Catalog* (1955–1956), 75–87. Also see "Staff Report on the University of Texas Medical School at Galveston," May 25, 1956, box VF Y/4, UT Chancellor's Records.

42. Earle chaired the admissions committee. In January 1958 the regents adopted a formal admissions policy for all UT medical schools; see Minutes, UT Board of Regents, Jan. 11, 1958. This policy constituted eight members of the faculty as an admissions committee and permitted them to establish criteria for evaluating applicants. The faculty could translate their evaluations into a percentage rank for each student. Using a formula based on a total of one hundred, 60 to 70 percent of the total was determined by the college grades, 10 to 20 percent by MCAT scores, and the remainder from evaluations by college teachers and evaluations by medical school faculty, who interviewed the applicants.

43. Dr. Raymond R. Reese (class of 1961) provided this information in an untaped phone call to Chester R. Burns in April 2001.

44. For an extraordinary collection of dissection notes and exams given by professors of anatomy between 1928 and 1961, see the folders in boxes 11–16, Department of Anatomy records, Blocker Collections. Anatomy exam information from Mason Guest to Chester R. Burns, Feb. 21, 1991, telephone conversation. For a crisp, critical interpretation of changes in medical education at the national level after 1950, see Rothstein, *American Medical Schools and the Practice of Medicine*, 294–313.

45. M. Mason Guest to faculty of the School of Medicine, Mar. 16, 1960, memo, box 6, Duncan Papers, Blocker Collections; Glenn V. Russell to all members of the Faculty of Medicine, "Resolution Regarding a Revised Curriculum," Mar. 28, 1960, box 6, Duncan papers, Blocker Collections; Minutes, UTMB Faculty Meeting, Mar. 30, 1960; and *Galveston Daily News*, Mar. 31, 1960. For comments about the effects of the new curriculum on individual departments, see the annual reports in folder 8, box 1, 75th Anniversary History Papers, Blocker Collections. Reluctantly, Walther Hild "rolled with the punches" as the number of hours for anatomy were significantly decreased; see Walther Hild to Myles Knape, May 18 and July 6, 1987, and June 24, 1988, interviews, Blocker Collections. As an example of the impact of technological change on the teaching of a basic science subject during the 1960s, see Mason Guest's overview of changes in the teaching of physiology in *Newsletter (UTMB)*, 3 (June/July, 1967), 1–2.

46. The Department of Surgery had nine divisions including Ophthalmology and Otorhinolaryngology. For important details about the evolution of these nine divisions, see *UTMB: Seventy-five Year History*, 193–208, 265–266. For comments about the effects of the new curriculum on individual departments, see the annual reports in folder 8, box 1, 75th Anniversary History Papers, Blocker Collections. As an example of the impact of technological change on the teaching of a clinical subject during the 1960s, see Ed Ferguson's overview of ophthalmology in *Alumni Bulletin*, 22 (Fall, 1967), 4–9.

47. John B. Truslow to Logan Wilson, May 31, 1960, letter, box VF I/1, UT Chancellor's Records (a copy is in RF4, CHP Archives). For a diagrammatic representation of the new curricular schedules, see *UTMB Catalog* (1962–1963), 46–54. For a description of how one basic science department adapted, see "Annual Report of the Department of Anatomy September 1, 1960–August 31, 1961," folder 1, box 1, Department of Anatomy records, Blocker Collections.

48. "Proposed Curriculum Changes School of Medicine," undated, box VF T/3, UT Chancellor's Records; *Galveston Daily News*, Sept. 3, 1960, and Aug. 1, 1961. For a diagrammatic representation of all schedules available in the new

curriculum, see *UTMB Catalog* (1962–1963), 47–54. Some of the students who engaged in research had graduate degrees before entering medical school. The class entering in 1961, for example, included ten students with master's degrees, one with a Ph.D., and one with a doctorate in veterinary medicine; see *Galveston Daily News*, Oct. 1, 1961. With his research activities, Bryan Holland earned a master's degree while a medical student. In O. Bryan Holland to Chester R. Burns, Feb. 5, 1992, interview, Blocker Collections, Holland provides interesting glimpses of both basic science and clinical faculty during the 1960s.

49. *University Medical Center News*, 2 (May, 1962), 4, 8. Assisting with newborn deliveries was a major reason for the popularity of preceptorships because there were too few deliveries at John Sealy Hospital during the early 1960s; see William J. McGanity to Myles Knape and Chester R. Burns, July 28 and Aug. 5, 1988, interviews, Blocker Collections. Also see *University Medical Center News*, 2 (May, 1962), 4. For the names of UTMB graduates, see *UTMB: Seventy-five Year History*, 327–342.

50. The new faculty members' names are listed in *Galveston Daily News*, Oct. 8, 1964. Blocker appointed Bill McGanity as part-time dean and Warren Harding as dean of student affairs. See "The University of Texas Medical Branch at Galveston: Past, Present, Future," 1966, 14, WF260, CHP Archives. For an alphabetized list of the names of School of Medicine faculty through 1967, see *UTMB: Seventy-five Year History*, 360–373. Although she believed that they would be incomplete because of inconsistencies in the sources, Betty Grefenstette prepared two lists of the names of all School of Medicine faculty through 1991. An alphabetized list is in WF453, CHP Archives. A list by departments is in WF454, CHP Archives.

51. A copy of the letter inviting White to UTMB is in WF333, CHP Archives. See *Faculty News (UTMB)*, Oct. 10, 1969. To appreciate the expansion of the 1960s, compare the 1969 telephone directory with the 1959 directory; see *UTMB Campus Directories*, Blocker Collections.

52. To sample the flavor of discussions by members of one committee, see the minutes of the Behavioral Sciences Committee for the years 1970–1972 in WF334, CHP Archives.

53. *University Medical*, 6 (Nov.–Dec., 1974), 18–20. For a sample schedule of the new curriculum, see *UTMB Catalog* (1975–1976), 93–96. Family practice became an option after a new Division of Family Medicine began in the Department of Preventive Medicine and Community Health in 1969; see *Newsletter (UTMB)*, 4 (Oct., 1969), 5–7. Lamar Ross, a UTMB graduate (class of 1939) and longtime general practitioner in Galveston, became director of this division and later chair of the Department of Family Medicine until 1979. For important background documents about this program, see folder 170, box 23, Blocker Papers, Blocker Collections. For candid comments about the development of this program, see Marcus Lamar Ross to Myles Knape, Sept. 3, 1987, interview, Blocker Collections. Also see a one-page supplement to *Faculty News (UTMB)*, Dec. 5, 1969.

54. This was just one of the initiatives adopted by the federal government during the 1960s and 1970s to help medical schools increase the number of graduates; see Rothstein, *American Medical Schools and the Practice of Medicine*, 283–287. Fifteen new medical schools were established during the 1960s; see Ludmerer, *Time to Heal*, 212. To help manage applications to all UT health professional schools, the regents established a Central Application Center for the UT System in March 1969.

55. To increase the number of black and Spanish-surnamed applicants, the faculty began a Medical School Familiarization Program for college students in the summer of 1970. During the early 1970s twenty-two students attended special classes for eight weeks (later four weeks). These classes introduced them to the academic subjects and stressful demands of medical school. After attending this program, students could make better choices about what they needed to do during their college years to be more successful in gaining admission to a medical school. Of the 112 students who attended the first six summer sessions, 25 had been admitted to a medical school by January 1976. For details, see Harold G. Levine, Lafayette B. Williams Jr., and John G. Bruhn, "Six Years of Experience with a Summer Program for Minority Students," *Journal of Medical Education*, 51 (Sept., 1976), 735–742; John G. Bruhn, Raymond G. Fuentes Jr., Fernando M. Trevino, and Lafayette B. Williams Jr., "Follow-Up of Minority Premedical Students Attending Summer Enrichment Programs in a Medical Setting," *Texas Medicine*, 72 (Aug., 1976), 87–90; and John G. Bruhn, "A Response to History: A Review of One Medical School's Efforts to Graduate Minority Physicians," *Journal of National Medical Association*, 70, no. 11 (1978), 823–828.

56. In 1975 the committee offered admission to 90 women; 47 enrolled. Spanish-surnamed applicants numbered 143; 17 were accepted for admission; 4 enrolled. Seventy-three black students applied; 3 were accepted; 1 enrolled. Sixty-four Asian students applied; 8 were accepted; 6 enrolled. See E. Gene Powell, "Medical College Admission . . . A Special Report," in WF321, CHP Archives; and "Medical School Admission: It's Not What It Used To Be," *Texas Medicine*, 71 (Nov., 1975), 108–110. The data in most of the tables about medical students in this chapter were

obtained from the annual reports sent to the AAMC by the dean's office. For ethnic origins, Joyce Dryman provided the data by analyzing the reports sent to the coordinating board from the registrar's office at UTMB. In Table 6.5, the total for 1990–1991 is correct. The types of earned degrees were not known for three applicants.

57. For a sample policy, see "Policy and Procedures for the Admission of Students" adopted by the Committee on Admissions, 1981–1982, WF321, CHP Archives. Required college courses included two years of biology and chemistry, one year each of English and physics, and one-half year of calculus; see *UTMB Catalog* (1981–1983), 71; (1990–1992), 12. The mean GPA for those admitted in 1980 was 3.52. The combined MCAT mean for that year was 9.65. See Vernon K. Jenkins and David C. Eiland Jr., "Medical School Admissions at the University of Texas Medical Branch at Galveston," *Texas Medicine*, 78 (July, 1982), 42–46. Also see documents in "Medical Student: Admissions" folder in WF383, CHP Archives. For a comprehensive look at admission practices in U.S. medical schools, see the entire issue of *Academic Medicine*, 65 (Mar., 1990).

58. News Release, June 1, 1971, WF321, CHP Archives; and *Impact*, 7 (Jan. 14, 1983), 6. For details about the Area Health Education Center program, see folders 1 and 3, box 1, Area Health Education Center Archives, Blocker Collections. For the family medicine clerkship, see Wendy Wolf (chair of curriculum committee) to medical school faculty, Oct. 23, 1989, memo, WF321, CHP Archives. The family medicine clerkship was mandated by the Texas legislature as part of the Omnibus Health Care Rescue Act (House Bill 18) adopted in the spring of 1989. This was an attempt to encourage students to become family medicine physicians.

59. In 1970 Joe White named Harold Levine as director of the Office of Research in Medical Education. White wanted Levine to establish a "comprehensive, on-going evaluation of the new curriculum and its implementation"; see *Faculty News (UTMB)*, Nov. 6, 1970. Levine worked closely with course directors in shaping and evaluating all courses; see Harold Levine to Chester R. Burns, Jan. 7, 1992, interview, Blocker Collections. By 1974 Don Bosshart, Maury Mahan, and Billy Philips assisted Levine in several projects designed to improve teaching effectiveness; see *University Medical*, 6 (Sept.–Oct., 1974), 13–15. For example, Levine and his associates worked extensively with Bill Daeschner and the Department of Pediatrics to develop self-instructional modules for third-year medical students. By 1974 they were using twenty-seven modules. Most students praised their effectiveness, especially in helping them apply scientific information to clinical situations; see *Impact*, 1 (Mar. 18, 1977), 13. In 1982 this office was renamed the Office of Educational Development with Abdul Sajid as director of the work of twelve employees, who assisted faculty in designing and evaluating courses; see *Impact*, 6 (Oct. 15, 1982), 4. For activities in 1985, see Sajid's annual report in folder 2, box 31, Levin Papers.

60. In 1975, the dean's office established an academic reinforcement program for students who wanted to learn how to take better lecture notes, how to organize lecture materials, how to improve their memory skills, and how to prepare for course exams; see *Faculty News (UTMB)*, Mar. 10–14, 1975. Numerous students used and praised this program. For the course changes, consider three examples. In 1971 the regents approved a new Department of Human Biological Chemistry and Genetics with Barbara Bowman as chair. This department included three divisions: Human Genetics with Bowman as director; Biochemistry with Allan Goldstein as director; and Cell Biology with Bill Brinkley as director; see *University Medical*, 3 (Dec., 1971), 5–7, and three boxes of departmental records in the Blocker Collections. These professors and their colleagues reformed the cell biology and biochemistry courses in the new curriculum. In 1976 Edward S. (Ted) Reynolds came from Harvard Medical School to be chair of the Department of Pathology; see *University Medical*, 10 (Sept.–Oct., 1979), 2–5. In 1977 he hired Lester Grant to be professor and director of pathology education. Grant and colleagues developed a remarkable syllabus for the second-year course. About two thousand hours of effort were required for preparing the second edition first used in 1979; see *University Medical*, 10 (Sept.–Oct., 1979), 6–11. In 1978 Robert Rose came from Harvard Medical School to be UTMB's first full-time chair of the retitled Department of Psychiatry and Behavioral Sciences. More than ten new faculty members joined this department; see *University Medical*, 10 (Sept.–Oct., 1978), 2–7. These teachers not only reformed the teaching of psychiatry to junior and senior students, but they also participated in the introduction to patient evaluation course for first-year students.

61. In 1987 the faculty adopted a requirement that all senior students must satisfactorily complete a competency assessment exercise. Using simulated and real patients, each student took a clinical history and performed a physical examination that was witnessed by two faculty members (one basic science, one clinical). Each student then discussed diagnostic and therapeutic options with the professors. Self-evaluation and assessments from the faculty completed the exercise. For details, see "Summary Report to the Curriculum Committee Senior Student Competency Assessment Exercise 1987–1989," WF321, CHP Archives. In addition to evaluating the performance of students taking exams in specific courses, the faculty also established grading and promotion committees, which evaluated students according to their performance in all courses during a given term. When these committees recommended that a student be "dropped from the rolls," a separate Committee on Student Affairs painstakingly reviewed the student's record. This committee

interviewed the student and interviewed teachers who were responsible for assigning the failing grades. Extraordinary effort was expended to be certain that each student was handled fairly and judiciously. For the years 1987–1988 and 1988–1989, for example, these committees considered thirty-three students who had failed courses. Of eighteen who failed during their first year, six were reinstated (two by committee and four by the dean). Two failed during their second-year courses. The dean reinstated one. Twelve of thirteen who failed a course during their "clinical core" years were reinstated (nine by committee and three by the dean). See memo to the faculty from the ad hoc committee on grading and promotions, Sept. 6, 1989, WF321, CHP Archives.

62. See Edward N. Brandt to Chester R. Burns, Oct. 29, 1989, interview, Blocker Collections.

63. *Impact*, 2 (Sept. 22, 1978), 7, and (Oct. 6, 1978), 5. Although she believed that it would be incomplete because of inconsistencies in the sources, Betty Grefenstette prepared a list of the names of all School of Medicine graduates through 1991. This list is in WF447, CHP Archives.

64. *University Medical*, 10 (Nov.–Feb., 1979), 3–17; *Impact*, 3 (Mar. 9, 1979), 6–7; *Syndrome* (1979), 70–72; and George Bryan to Myles Knape, Jan. 31, Feb. 6, 11, and 26, and Mar. 6, 1986, interviews, and George Bryan to Chester R. Burns, July 26 and Oct. 10, 1989, interviews, Blocker Collections. For organization charts in 1984 and 1991, see Appendices A-34, A-37, and A-46, WF441, CHP Archives. Also see "Informational Handbook for Faculty of the School of Medicine," 1982, 8–23. A copy is in WF255, CHP Archives. Also see Appendix B for titles. For comments about some of these appointments, see Bryan's interviews. For comments about their roles as department chairs during these years, see William J. McGanity to Myles Knape and Chester R. Burns, July 28 and Aug. 5, 1988; C. William Daeschner to Myles Knape and Chester R. Burns, July 13 and 20 and Aug. 3, 1988; Melvyn H. Schreiber to Chester R. Burns and Myles Knape, Aug. 9 and 23, 1989; and James C. Thompson to Myles Knape and Chester R. Burns, June 27, July 3 and 13, 1989; interviews, Blocker Collections.

65. See Appendix B-20, WF442, CHP Archives.

66. During the late 1980s and 1990s, Delaney, for example, coordinated the distribution of several thousand letters of evaluation prepared by the dean's office for approximately two hundred graduates each year who applied for postgraduate positions. The expansion of these staff support groups from year to year can be appreciated quickly by viewing the excellent photos that began to appear in the *Syndrome* in 1986 (pp. 57–61). Secretaries of department chairs and professors also played key roles in the everyday life of the School of Medicine. Between 1956 and 1959, each *Syndrome* included photos of the principal secretary in each School of Medicine department. Unfortunately, these extremely important assistants were seldom pictured during the 1960s and 1970s. They reappeared in a few departmental photos during the 1980s.

67. Minutes, UTMB Faculty Meeting, May 29, 1912. The number of those seeking internships increased during the early decades. In 1904 six of twenty-three UTMB graduates obtained internships, four at John Sealy and two at St. Mary's in Galveston; see W. S. Carter to E. J. Mathews, c. 1910, letter, box 4R82, UT President's Records. In 1910 twenty-two of thirty-five graduates secured internships, seven at John Sealy or St. Mary's, six in other Texas hospitals, and nine in hospitals of other states; see Carter to Mathews, c. 1910, and *Galveston Daily News*, Sept. 16, 1910. See also *UTMB Catalog* (1900–1901), 35; (1903–1904), 69; (1904–1905), 69; and (1911–1912), 48.

68. *UTMB Catalog* (1922–1923), 48; and (1937–1938), 62. In 1926 the faculty selected Edith Bonnet and Frances Van Zandt as interns, overriding objections erroneously expressed by those who thought they would be the first women ever appointed as Sealy Hospital interns. A. O. Singleton wanted to exempt them from a six-week rotation in urology and Edward Randall did not believe that they should receive room and board during that exempted time; see *Galveston Daily News*, Jan. 27, 1926. For details, see RF56 and RF149, CHP Archives. See also *Galveston Daily News*, July 14, 1949. For the life of an intern at UTMB during 1941–1942, see William Gibson to Chester R. Burns, Oct. 7, 1988, interview, Blocker Collections. Also see *UTMB Catalog* (1950–1951), 118–119.

69. To obtain this approximate total, Heather Campbell reviewed lists of names available in the office of the associate dean for graduate medical education and those listed in annual catalogs. For many years, information about each intern and resident was placed on large cards. When he became associate dean for graduate medical education, Al LeBlanc inherited boxes of these cards plus chronologically arranged loose-leaf notebooks that list the names of house staff. These notebooks contain many penciled alterations that cannot be interpreted easily. During the 1990s Esther Koleng, Aurora Galvan, and others began entering this information into computer programs with the hope that more accurate data can be provided someday. As rotating internships disappeared and specialty boards no longer required an internship year, professors stopped using the label "intern" in the 1970s and began designating the first year of residency training as PGY-1 (postgraduate year one). Campbell's lists are in WF321, CHP Archives.

70. Ludmerer, *Time to Heal*, 79–101.

71. After graduating from UTMB in 1928, Barnes received postgraduate training in Baltimore and Philadelphia; see Johnson Peyton Barnes Jr. to Greg Diamond, Nov. 1, 1986, interview, Blocker Collections. For a photo, see Surgery Department scrapbook, Blocker Collections, 28. See also "A Brief History of the Department of Obstetrics and Gynecology of the University of Texas Medical Branch," typescript, p. 8, box 2, vertical file A8, Blocker Collections; *UTMB Catalog* (1932–1933), 59; (1933–1934), 60; and (1934–1935), 60; "History of the Department of Neurology and Psychiatry," typescript, p. 5, box 2, vertical file A8, Blocker Collections; and *Newsletter (UTMB)*, 2 (Feb., 1966), 1–2. For a biographical sketch of Ford, see Chester R. Burns, "Hamilton Ford," in Tyler, et al. (eds.), *The New Handbook of Texas*, II, 1072. Titus Harris believed that this department was the first in the Southwest to initiate residency training; see *UTMB: Seventy-five Year History*, 244. See also *UTMB Catalog* (1936–1937), 62; and Michael B. Shimkin, "A Year at Galveston—1937," *Impact*, 6 (May 7, 1982), 2, 18.

72. *Galveston Daily News*, July 14, 1949; Minutes, Sealy & Smith Foundation Board of Directors, May 15, 1940; and *UTMB Catalog* (1946–1947), 20–23. Lamar Ross was a resident in neuropsychiatry between 1940 and 1942; see Marcus Lamar Ross to Myles Knape, Sept. 3, 1987, interview, Blocker Collections. In 1943 and 1944 Bill Levin was the only resident in internal medicine; see William C. Levin to Myles Knape, Mar. 17, Apr. 4, and May 26, 1986, and Levin to Chester R. Burns, Nov. 7, 1989, interviews, Blocker Collections. Sources for Table 6.8 include Chauncey D. Leake to T. S. Painter, Apr. 8, 1948, letter, box VF 10/C, UT President's Records; The University of Texas Publication, School of Medicine, Galveston, Texas, Post-Graduate Program in Medicine, Announcements for 1948–1949, box VF 10/D, UT President's Records; and Chauncey D. Leake to T. S. Painter, Oct. 29, 1949, letter, box VF 10/D, UT President's Records. During the late 1940s and early 1950s there were two different training programs in neuropsychiatry. One was directed by Jack Ewalt at the State Psychopathic Hospital and the other was led by Titus Harris, who attended patients admitted to Psycho One, Two, and Three; see Austin Foster, transcript of self-directed audiotape recording done in April 1989, box 24, CHP Archives. For comments about his training as a neuropsychiatry resident during the 1940s, see Robert B. White to Chester R. Burns, Dec. 19, 1989, interview, Blocker Collections. For comments about his experiences as a surgical resident during the late 1940s, see Walter King to Greg Diamond, Apr. 7, 1987, interview, Blocker Collections.

73. *Galveston Daily News*, July 4, 1950; Chauncey D. Leake to cousins, July 15, 1953, letter, Leake Papers, NLM; *Medi-Texan*, 2 (July, 1955), 4–5, 11; and *Galveston Daily News*, July 7, 1955. In Table 6.9, FMG means foreign medical graduate. During the 1960s, Blocker was especially interested in the postgraduate training of Latin American doctors. By 1968 the chiefs of the plastic surgery services in the medical schools of four major cities (Mexico City, Lima, Buenos Aires, and Santiago) had completed residency and fellowship training at UTMB. See Truman G. Blocker Jr. to Harry Ransom, July 1, 1968, letter, box VF EE/3, UT Chancellor's Records.

74. Ludmerer, *Time to Heal*, 180–190. Internships disappeared after 1970. The specialty boards that accredited residency programs accepted new graduates directly into their programs without requiring any additional hospital training; see Rothstein, *American Medical Schools and the Practice of Medicine*, 314–318.

75. Robbie Loftin provided the data for internal medicine; David Rassin for pediatrics.

76. Truman G. Blocker Jr., "The Department of Surgery," Annual Reports, 1960–1961, folder 8, box 1, 75th Anniversary History Papers, Blocker Collections; Luther Travis to Chester R. Burns, Feb. 25 and Mar. 10, 1992, interviews, Blocker Collections. David Rassin provided the data about the residents trained in a list that is in WF321, CHP Archives. See *University Medical*, 3 (c. Sept., 1971), 13–15. The family medicine program was accredited in April 1972; see *Faculty News (UTMB)*, Apr. 27, 1973, 2; and *Impact*, 3 (June 29, 1979), 6. The totals of residents and fellows are rough estimates, as accurate lists do not exist. These estimates are based on the lists in Al LeBlanc's office, those in annual catalogs, and UTMB's annual reports to the AAMC. Heather Campbell also helped prepare these estimates.

77. For these and other letters, see folder 115, box 15, Blocker Papers, especially Thomas J. Baker to Truman G. Blocker Jr., Oct. 12, 1978 (quotation). For brochures about many of these training programs in 1991, see RF41, CHP Archives. For the brochures prepared by the Department of Surgery between 1970 and 1990, see RF26, CHP Archives. For a profile of Carmen Rocco, a third-year resident in pediatrics in 1985, see *Impact*, 9 (May 31, 1985), 13. For a profile of Jim Van Hook, chief resident in obstetrics and gynecology in 1986, see *Impact*, 10 (Mar. 7, 1986), 15. Information about the subsequent careers of residents is seldom available in any systematic way. One noteworthy exception is the "Salute to Our Chief Residents" that Marc Shabot assembled for distribution to those attending the alumni meeting of the Internal Medicine Department in 1999. Shabot provided profiles of fifty-four physicians who had been chief residents in this department between 1958 and 1999. A copy is in WF321, CHP Archives.

78. *University Medical*, 1, no. 7 (1896), 297; *Galveston Daily News*, Apr. 24, 1916; and May 13–14 and 27, 1916. The teachers began the course for its forty registrants on the day after the Texas Medical Association and State Board of

Health ended their annual meetings in Galveston. They lectured on a variety of topics in preventive medicine including immunizations and oral hygiene.

79. M. L. Graves, M. D. Levy, and W. C. Rose to Robert E. Vinson, May 22, 1921, letter , box 4R81, UT President's Records; *Galveston Daily News*, June 21, 27–28, and July 2, 1922. For a delightful description of the June 1922 course, see W. D. Jones, "A Week's Visit to the Medical Department and John Sealy Hospital," *Alcalde*, 10 (Nov., 1922), 1522–1526. See also *Galveston Daily News*, June 3, 6, 8, 12, and 24, 1923; and June 14, 1926; "Names and Addresses of Physicians Attending the 1926 Summer Course to Practitioners, Medical Branch, University of Texas, Galveston, Texas," box 4Q24, UT President's Records; and *Galveston Daily News*, May 17, 26–27, 1927. The third course was held in June 1925; see *Galveston Daily News*, June 8, 1925. Also see *Galveston Daily News*, May 20, 1928; May 12, June 3–4, 1929; and June 3, 1930; George E. Bethel to H. Y. Benedict, c. Oct. 1930, letter, box 4Q25, UT President's Records; and *Galveston Daily News*, May 13, 20–21, and June 11, 1940.

80. Chauncey D. Leake to T. S. Painter, Feb. 21, May 19, and May 29, 1945, letters, box VF 10/B, UT President's Records; and Chauncey D. Leake to David N. W. Grant, July 11, 1945, letter, box VF 10/C, UT President's Records. For the list of the courses held during 1945–1946, for example, see "Post-Graduate Program in Medicine, Announcements for 1945–46," box VF 10/C, UT President's Records.

81. *Galveston Daily News*, July 5, 1945, and Sept. 23, 1945. For pediatrics, see *Galveston Daily News*, May 13–15 and Nov. 13 and 16, 1945; Apr. 13, 15–16, 20, Oct. 27, 29–30, and Nov. 1–2, 4, 1946; and Apr. 8, 11, 14–17, Oct. 24, Nov. 4, 9–10, 12, 1948. For surgery, see *Galveston Daily News*, Nov. 11, 13–17, 1945; and Nov. 12, 17, 19–22, 1946. For internal medicine, see *Galveston Daily News*, Mar. 21, 24, 26–29, and 31, 1946. For physical medicine and rehabilitation, see *Galveston Daily News*, Feb. 10 and Mar. 3–6, 1946; Mar. 4, 1947; Mar. 3–6, 1948; Feb. 24 and Mar. 1, 1949. For courses on the diagnosis and treatment of cancer, see *Galveston Daily News*, June 20–22, Sept. 24, Nov. 5, 10, and 12, 1947; May 9 and 29, June 1, and Oct. 13, 21, 24, 1948; Jan. 23 and 30, Feb. 2–3, and Nov. 2, 1949. For obstetrics and gynecology, see *Galveston Daily News*, Mar. 9, 12–13, 17, 1946; Mar. 9–11, 14, 1948; and Mar. 21, 1949. For psychiatry, see *Galveston Daily News*, Nov. 3, 1948. Also see Truman Blocker Jr. to E. A. Rowley, Feb. 11, 1949, letter, folder 21, box 3, Blocker Papers. In notes for a talk about these courses (folder 19, box 3, Blocker Papers), Blocker noted that the postgraduate division also provided speakers for meetings of county and district medical societies, and other groups in the state.

82. For psychiatry, see *Galveston Daily News*, Feb. 12, 14–15, 1950; Jan. 23 and Feb. 6, 1959; Jan. 27, Feb. 3, 6–7, 1952. For the courses on cancer, see *Galveston Daily News*, Feb. 16, Oct. 27, Nov. 3, 7–9, 1950; Mar. 13, Oct. 28 and 30, Nov. 2, 1951; and Oct. 9–11, 1952. The Department of Pediatrics usually held a postgraduate course in the fall and in the spring; for examples, see *Galveston Daily News*, Nov. 14, 1950; Nov. 7, 18–21, 1952; Feb. 11–12, 1955; Jan. 31, Feb. 6, and 9, 1956; and Feb. 13, 1959. For obstetrics and gynecology, see *Galveston Daily News*, Feb 9–11, 1951; Apr. 21–22, 1952; Apr. 12 and 14, 1953; Apr. 23, 1954; and Mar. 19, 1959. For radiology, see *Galveston Daily News*, Oct. 26, 30, 1951. For heart diseases, see *Galveston Daily News*, Dec. 4, 11–15, 1951. For traumatic surgery, see *Galveston Daily News*, Jan. 6, 8, 10, 1952, and Feb. 27, 1953. For electrocardiography, see *Galveston Daily News*, Jan. 6, 13, and 15, 1952. For neurology and neurosurgery, see *Galveston Daily News*, Jan. 4, 8–10, 13, 1953. For dermatology, see *Galveston Daily News*, Jan. 17, 1953. For thoracic surgery, see *Galveston Daily News*, Jan. 31, 1953. For medical therapy, see *Galveston Daily News*, Aug. 17 and 26, 1954.

83. Four professors traveled to Tyler to give lectures during a postgraduate course sponsored by the Texas Academy of General Practice; see *Galveston Daily News*, Dec. 1, 1951. Seven professors participated in a postgraduate course for one hundred physicians in Longview; see *Galveston Daily News*, Jan. 18, 1952. In the spring of 1952 some faculty participated in a telephone network program of evening lectures carried to fifty-one communities in Texas; see *Galveston Daily News*, Feb. 12–13, 1952. Some participated in other postgraduate seminars sponsored by the Texas Academy of General Practice such as the one held in Beaumont in 1954; see *Galveston Daily News*, Feb. 21–22, 1954.

84. For pediatrics, see *Galveston Daily News*, Feb. 16, 1961; Jan. 21, 1962; Feb. 15, 1962; Feb. 14, 1963; Feb. 13, 1964; and *Newsletter (UTMB)*, 1 (Feb. 5, 1965), 3; 1 (Feb. 3, 1966), 1; and 2 (Feb. 2, 1967), 1. For obstetrics and gynecology, see *Galveston Daily News*, Mar. 9, 1961; Feb. 18, 1962; and *Newsletter (UTMB)*, 1 (Aug. 5, 1965), 1; and 1 (July 21, 1966), 1. See also *Newsletter (UTMB)*, 1 (Oct. 21, 1965), 3; 2 (Dec. 1, 1966), 1; 2 (May 4, 1967), 1; *Faculty News (UTMB)*, Sept. 6, 1968; "Status of Continuing Health Education at the Four University of Texas Health Science Centers," May 9, 1973, UT Chancellor's Office of Records Management, CHI reel 11; *Faculty News (UTMB)*, Feb. 6, 1970; Mar. 9, Dec. 3–7, and Dec. 10–14, 1973; Mar. 10–14, 1975; and *Impact*, 2 (Jan. 27, 1978), 2; and 3 (Jan. 26, 1979), 4. For examples and details, see the Area Health Education Center newsletter, *La Salud* (1973–1979) and the Area Health Education Center Archives in the Blocker Collections.

85. *Impact*, 8 (May 4, 1984), 16, and 1 (Apr. 15, 1977), 1.

86. For details, see WF335, CHP Archives. See also V. E. Thompson to Charles B. Mullins, Aug. 3, 1982, letter, UT Chancellor's Office of Records Management, reel 128; *Impact*, 4 (Sept. 26, 1980), 6–7; the supplement to the Sept. 11, 1981, issue of *Impact*; and Office of Continuing Education, Annual Report, 1983–1984.

87. Martyn O. Hotvedt and William W. Schottstaedt, "Tailoring Continuing Medical Education to the Individual Needs of Practicing Physicians," *Texas Medicine*, 79 (Dec., 1983), 51–52. For details about the academy, see *University Medical*, 6 (May–June, 1975), 5–7; *Impact*, 3 (Jan. 26, 1979), 6; and *University Medical*, 10 (May–June, 1980), 7–9. Also see *Impact*, 9 (Dec. 6, 1985), 8; 13 (Apr. 21, 1989), 4; and 15 (Apr. 5, 1991), 4.

88. "Pharmacy," *University Record*, 4 (July, 1902), 336; and R. R. D. Cline to Allen J. Smith, Apr. 27, 1903, letter, box 4R82, UT President's Records.

89. See *UTMB Catalog* (1908–1909), 121–123, and 99–100 for a schedule of courses.

90. *UTMB Catalog* (1909–1910), 88–89; (1919–1920), 57; and (1920–1921), 55–56.

91. After receiving a Ph.D. from Yale in 1921, Henze became adjunct professor of chemistry. See W. S. Carter to R. E. Vinson, June 15, 1921, letter, box 4R84, UT President's Records. Also see *UTMB Catalog* (1922–1923), 8, 57–63; Henry R. Henze to William Keiller, Apr. 1, 1922, letter; and "Report of Committee on Third Year Course in Pharmacy leading to Degree of Ph.C.," box 4R80, UT President's Records; and *UTMB Catalog* (1922–1923), 58, and (1923–1924), 61.

92. William Keiller to Chester A. Duncan, May 26, 1924, letter, box 26, UTMB Dean's Office Records, Inactive. For more about Cline, see *UTMB: Seventy-five Year History*, 69–71.

93. Minutes, UTMB Faculty Meeting, Dec. 8, 1924.

94. William Keiller to W. M. W. Splawn, Sept. 15, 1924, letter, box 4Q24, UT President's Records; and Minutes, UTMB Faculty Meetings, Oct. 10, 1924, and Feb. 26, 1925. UTMB's Executive Committee had recommended Gidley; see Minutes, UTMB Executive Committee Meeting, Oct. 8, 1926. See *Galveston Daily News*, Jan. 1, 1927, and the letters from 1926 and 1927 in RF5, CHP Archives. The pharmacy graduates' names are listed in *UTMB: Seventy-five Year History*, 352–353.

95. *UTMB Catalog* (1906–1907), 106–114; and *Galveston Daily News*, Apr. 11, 1902 and Mar. 26, 1903. For the first schedule of the three-year course that appeared in the annual catalogs, see *UTMB Catalog* (1910–1911), 104–106. See also Ethel Clay to S. E. Mezes, May 1, 1910, letter, box 4R82, UT President's Records.

96. These totals were found in the annual reports written by the directors of the school. The report for 1908 and the reports for 1910–1926 are in RF6, CHP Archives. Some of these students married; some left to provide care for their families; and some left because of poor health.

97. Ethel Clay to W. J. Battle, Mar. 1, 1916, and Ethel Clay to R. E. Vinson, Feb. 10, 1917, letters, box 4Q21, UT President's Records (copies are in R6, CHP Archives).

98. How members of the Advisory Board of Lady Managers might have influenced these conflicts is not known. Constituted by wives of faculty and prominent citizens, this board existed between 1896 and 1941. The names of the members are listed in the annual catalogs. Members of this advisory board were expected to support the directors of the school and the student nurses, and facilitate communication between the school and those serving on the hospital's boards of managers. More than anything else probably, they provided a network of female bonding that tempered the enthusiasms of the male physician-professors and the men who served on the hospital's boards.

99. Martha St. J. Eakins to R. E. Vinson, Mar. 1, 1920, letter, box 4Q23, UT President's Records (quotations). Eakins also wanted more graduate nurses, a "reasonable amount of equipment and supplies," and recreational facilities for the students. When her requests were ignored, she resigned. For details, see Martha St. J. Eakins to W. S. Carter, May 30, 1920; W. S. Carter to R. E. Vinson, June 10, 1920; Martha St. J. Eakins to W. S. Carter, June 13, 1920, letters, all in box 4Q22, UT President's Records.

100. Ella Read to R. E. Vinson, Mar. 31, 1921, letter, box 4R81, UT President's Records, copy in R6, CHP Archives (quotation); and *UTMB Catalog* (1920–1921), 60–63. The title "Clinical Instructor of Nursing" had been given to previous superintendents. In 1920 the school's name was changed to College of Nursing and the school began to give academic credit for college courses taken by students before matriculating (shortening the nursing school tenure by three months for each year of college).

101. These totals were cumulated from the annual reports of the directors. The originals are in box 4R82, UT President's Records; copies are in RF6, CHP Archives. Also see W. S. Carter to R. E. Vinson, Mar. 15, 1919, and W. S.

Carter to Robert E. Vinson, Dec. 16, 1919, letters, box 4Q22, UT President's Records; Minutes, UTMB Faculty Meeting, Feb. 12, 1920; *UTMB Catalog* (1921–1922), 65–66; and "Dean's Annual Report," April 1923, box 15, UTMB Dean's Office Records, Inactive. Zora McAnnelly Fiedler was one of the students who enrolled in 1922; see Zora McAnnelly Fiedler to Poldi Tschirch, Oct. 25, 1986, interview, Blocker Collections. The Rebecca Sealy Nurses' Home housed fifty-six students and others lived in nearby houses. Also see Chester R. Burns, "Health and Medicine," in Tyler, et al. (eds.), *The New Handbook of Texas*, III, 527.

102. Grace G. Grey to W. S. Sutton, Feb. 16, 1924, and Grace G. Grey to Marshall William Splawn, Apr. 11, 1925, box 4Q25; and Grace G. Grey to Marshall William Splawn, Feb. 27, 1926, box 4P263 (quotation), letters, UT President's Records. After the inspection nursing graduates could not practice in the state of New York. Reciprocity with the state had existed since 1910 when the school was approved for registration with the State Department of Education of the University of the State of New York.

103. Sadie N. Hausmann to H. C. Hartman, Oct. 2, 1926, letter, box 4Q23, UT President's Records. See also *UTMB Catalog* (1926–1927), 9–10. Remember that "adjunct" then was today's equivalent of "assistant." During the mid-1920s, the university began publishing separate catalogs of this school. These were among the items serially published as *University of Texas Bulletin* and they continued through the 1939–1940 year. There are some copies in box 2, vertical file A3, in the Blocker Collections and there are some copies in the Office of Student Affairs of the School of Nursing. Hereafter these separate "bulletins" are cited as *UT School of Nursing Catalog*.

104. For a sample schedule, see *UTMB Catalog* (1927–1928), 63–66. More complete schedules and excellent photos of classroom, laboratory, and hospital scenes were included in the separately published bulletins, the *UT School of Nursing Catalog*. Grace Decker was a student in the late 1920s; see Grace Decker to Poldi Tschirch, July 17, 1986, interview, Blocker Collections. See also Lucius R. Wilson to Dorothy Rogers, Mar. 9, 1931, letter, folder 17, box 2, School of Nursing Archives, Blocker Collections; and *UTMB Catalog* (1931–1932), 76. Insights into the teaching arrangements can be gleaned from the teachers' reports that were submitted to UT presidents between 1929 and 1942. These are deposited in boxes 4Q135, 4R106, 4R107, and 4R108, UT President's Records.

105. George Bethel to H. Y. Benedict, Nov. 3, 1931, letter, box 27, UTMB Dean's Office Records, Inactive, and W. S. Carter to H. Y. Benedict, Oct. 31, 1935, letter, box 4Q25, UT President's Records. For the names of the students who enrolled each month between January 1929 and September 1937, see folder 63, box 6, School of Nursing Archives, Blocker Collections. Also see Xilema Faulkner's annual report for 1930–1931 in folder 8, box 16, UTMB Dean's Office Records, Inactive, and Dorothy Rogers' annual report for 1931–1932, folder 1, box 17, UTMB Dean's Office Records, Inactive.

106. W. S. Carter to J. W. Calhoun, Nov. 1, 1937, letter, box 4Q18, UT President's Records.

107. Rogers had received a bachelor's degree from Wellesley, a master's degree from Columbia, and a nursing degree from Presbyterian Hospital in Chicago. To recognize the generous support of the Sealy family, the regents, in 1932, changed the school's name to the John Sealy College of Nursing of the University of Texas. In 1933 Rogers attended the organizational meeting of the Association of Collegiate Schools of Nursing; see Dorothy Rogers to H. Y. Benedict, Jan. 16, 1933, letter, box VF 9/C, UT President's Records. For insights into events of 1935–1940, see the letters of Dora Mathis in folders 14 and 15, box 2, School of Nursing Archives, Blocker Collections. For the best description of the nurses' home, see Dorothy Rogers, "Rebecca Sealy Nurses's Residence," *American Journal of Nursing*, 33 (May, 1933), 433–437. Excellent photos appeared in the bulletins issued between 1934 and 1939; the *UT School of Nursing Catalog*. For other details, see folder 64, box 6, School of Nursing Archives, Blocker Collections.

108. W. S. Carter to Edward Randall, Dec. 6, 1937, letter, box VF 9/C, UT President's Records. The hospital board and the foundation provided salaries for the following graduate nurses as supervisors: Olive Wilcox, Julia Ann Bartosh, Elsie Roberts, Bertha Boeker, Ellen Dick, and Ruby Howell. The regents provided salaries for the following graduate nurses as teachers: Dora Mathis, Dorothy MacLeod, Grace Collins, Cleo Parker, Pauline Wylie, Pauline Edmondson, and Mary Lou Smith. The regents also provided funds for Mrs. Rose Bowe, a graduate nurse who was the matron at the Rebecca Sealy Nurses' Home. See Minutes, UT Board of Regents, July 3, 1937, and *UTMB Catalog* (1937–1938), 12–13.

109. *UTMB Catalog* (1938–1939), 73–75. Of 715 students admitted to the school between 1935 and 1944, 408 (57 percent) graduated and 307 (43 percent) withdrew or failed; see list in folder 63, box 6, School of Nursing Archives, Blocker Collections. In 1923 the regents approved a five-year sequence that would allow a UT student to earn a bachelor of science in nursing degree; see *UTMB Catalog* (1923–1924), 74; (1924–1925), 75. In each annual UTMB catalog between 1923 and 1946, graduating nurses are listed as "Graduates in Nursing," with no indication that anyone earned a bachelor's degree. In 1933 Margaret Louise Hegler became the first student to complete the combined program, earning both a B.S. in nursing and a graduate nurse diploma; see Dorothy Rogers to H. Y. Benedict, June 8, 1933, letter, folder 2, box 17, UTMB Dean's Office Records, Inactive. Hegler was named in the list of

"Graduates of Nursing" for 1933, but there is no indication that she had earned a bachelor's degree; see *UTMB Catalog* (1933–1934), 72.

110. For some examples, see Special Session, UT Board of Regents, 789–812.

111. Dora Mathis to John W. Spies, Dec. 12, 1939, and John W. Spies to Homer P. Rainey, Dec. 19, 1939, letters, both in box VF 9/B, UT President's Records. Also see "Report from the Regents of the University of Texas to the Board of the Sealy and Smith Foundation, January 17, 1940," box VF 9/B, UT President's Records (quotations).

112. Elsa Kibbe to Titus Harris, Aug. 31, 1942, letter, box 1, School of Nursing Archives. Blocker Collections.

113. Homer Rainey offered the job to Bartholf before Leake was hired, but Bartholf did not accept it until after Leake agreed to be UTMB's CEO. See Homer P. Rainey to Chauncey D. Leake, Aug. 22, 1942, and Marjorie Bartholf to Homer P. Rainey, Sept. 8, 1942, letters, box VF 9/A, UT President's Records. Only ten student nurses received their caps after completing a six-month preliminary term in December 1942, for example; see *Galveston Daily News*, Dec. 17, 1942. To deal with the shortage of graduate nurses, hospital beds were closed, the nepotism rule was waived so that wives of employees at UTMB could be hired, medical students were employed as nurses, and more classes were admitted. For details, see Chauncey D. Leake to Homer P. Rainey, Apr. 1, 1943, and William O. Bohman to Chauncey D. Leake, May 13, 1943, letters, both in box VF 9/A, UT President's Records; and Chauncey D. Leake to T. S. Painter, June 6, 1945, letter, box 1, School of Nursing Archives, Blocker Collections.

114. *UTMB Catalog* (1942–1943), 53; and Chauncey D. Leake, John C. Noland, and E. M. Capplemann to Homer P. Rainey, Aug. 31, 1943, letter, box 2, Leake Papers, Blocker Collections.

115. Chauncey D. Leake to Homer P. Rainey, May 12, 1943, and Homer P. Rainey to Chauncey D. Leake, May 18, 1943, letters, box VF 9/A, UT President's Records; *UTMB Catalog* (1944–1945), 44–47; and Marjorie Bartholf to Homer P. Rainey, Feb. 18, 1944, letter, box VF 10/B, UT President's Records. The separate College of Nursing catalog for 1944–1945 identified a faculty of one professor, one associate professor, two assistant professors, and ten instructors; see *UT School of Nursing Catalog*, 10–11. This catalog also gives an outline of the curriculum and a description of twenty-one courses (pp. 15–18). See also A. Louise Dietrich to T. K. Brace, June 26, 1945, letter, box VF 26/D, UT President's Records; and Chauncey D. Leake to A. Louise Dietrich, Aug. 16, 1945, letter, box 1, School of Nursing Archives, Blocker Collections. For details, see the reports about nursing education on the UT Austin campus in 1941 in folder 13, box 1, School of Nursing Archives, Blocker Collections, and *UTMB Catalog* (1945–1946), 83–86. The program in Austin was situated in the Department of Physical and Health Education in the College of Education. The Department of Nursing Education had begun in 1930 as a joint project of the Texas Graduate Nurses Association and the Extension Division of the University of Texas.

116. Zora M. Fielder to Dudley K. Woodward, Nov. 12, 1946, letter, box VF 10/D, UT President's Records; *UTMB Catalog* (1946–1947), 23–25; Chauncey D. Leake to T. S. Painter, Oct. 14, 1946, and Marjorie Bartholf to D. K. Woodward Jr., Nov. 18, 1946, letters, both in box VF 10/D; and Chauncey D. Leake to T. S. Painter, Oct. 14, 1946, letter, box 1, School of Nursing Archives, Blocker Collections.

117. Chauncey D. Leake to T. S. Painter, June 10, 1948, letter, box VF 10/C, UT President's Records; and *UTMB Catalog* (1947–1948), 106. This total includes students who had received diplomas between 1892 and 1896 before UT managed the school.

118. Chauncey D. Leake to T. S. Painter, Dec. 10, 1948, letter; Theophilus S. Painter to members of the medical committee, June 27, 1949, memo; and Marjorie Bartholf to Chauncey D. Leake, June 27, 1949, letter; all in box VF 10/D, UT President's Records. A copy of Painter's memo is in folder 1, box 1, School of Nursing Archives, Blocker Collections, and a copy of Bartholf's letter is in folder 7, box 1, School of Nursing Archives, Blocker Collections. Bartholf's philosophy of nursing and nursing education is revealed in an address given to the Texas League of Nursing Education on November 3, 1949; typescript in folder 1, box 1, School of Nursing Archives, Blocker Collections.

119. For the first description of this dual route, see *UTMB Catalog* (1949–1950), 105–110. A good way to acquire insight into the faculty's approach to the education of student nurses is to examine the "Handbook for Headnurses, Supervisors, and Instructors" prepared in 1948. This handbook included detailed criteria used to evaluate student performance on the wards. A copy is in vertical file A3, box 1, Blocker Collections. For details about vocational nurse training programs, see folder 93, box 9; folder 155, box 14; and folders 156–157, box 15, School of Nursing Archives, Blocker Collections.

120. "The University of Texas Medical Branch, Galveston," March 1955, box VF I/4, UT Chancellor's Records; and *UTMB Catalog* (1954–1955), 144, 173–175. For names and ranks of the faculty during 1955 and other years between 1945 and 1959, see the lists in folder 99, box 10, School of Nursing Archives, Blocker Collections, and the catalogs for

those years available in the Office of Student Affairs, School of Nursing. It is notable that two UTMB catalogs included the following sentence: "All registered nurses in the Nursing Service Department of the Medical Branch Hospitals are assistants in instruction in the School of Nursing"; see *UTMB Catalog* (1953–1954), 114, and (1954–1955), 175. Outlines of courses taught during the 1940s and 1950s are in folders 158–161, box 15, School of Nursing Archives, Blocker Collections. For details about the affiliation programs, see folders 130–132, box 12, and folders 133–135, box 13, School of Nursing Archives, Blocker Collections. Designing effective lines of authority, responsibility, and communication challenged Bartholf and other members of the Nursing Service Council, who shaped policies for nursing care in the hospitals during the 1950s. For glimpses of these challenges, see the minutes and organizational charts in folder 114, box 11, School of Nursing Archives, Blocker Collections. During the 1950s Bartholf and her faculty also experimented with some off-campus continuing education courses known as "extension courses;" for some details, see folders 136 and 137, box 13, School of Nursing Archives, Blocker Collections. Elizabeth Knebel was a student in the baccalaureate program between 1954 and 1957; Anna Pearl Rains between 1955 and 1958. For comments about their days as students, see Elizabeth Knebel to Poldi Tschirch, June 12, 1986, and Anna Pearl Rains to Poldi Tschirch, July 17, 1986, interviews, Blocker Collections.

121. *UTMB Catalog* (1951–1952), 127–131; Marjorie Bartholf to James P. Hart, Oct. 16 and Dec. 15, 1952; John E. Ivey Jr. to Logan Wilson, Mar. 4, 1954; Chauncey D. Leake to Malcolm P. Aldrich, May 19, 1954; Emory W. Morris to Chauncey D. Leake, June 17, 1954, letters, all in box VF C/1, UT Chancellor's Records. In 1954 Catherine Ann Bane became the first student to earn a master's of science in nursing degree. Between 1957 and 1967 she was director of nursing services for UTMB's hospitals. For details about the graduate program, see folders 53–56, box 5; folders 57–59, box 6; folder 92, box 9; folder 101, box 10; folders 138–142, box 13; and folders 143–144, box 14, School of Nursing Archives, Blocker Collections.

122. For 1955, see the organization chart in folder 94, box 9, School of Nursing Archives, Blocker Collections. For 1962, see Appendix A-21, WF 441, CHP Archives. The institutional paths that produced different types of nurses significantly influenced the hierarchical arrangement of nurses who worked in the hospitals. In 1959, for example, the Department of Nursing Service expected a junior staff nurse, a licensed vocational nurse (LVN), a nurse aide, and an orderly to be accountable to a staff nurse, who was accountable to a head nurse, who was accountable to a supervisor, who was accountable to an assistant director of nursing service, who was accountable to the director of nursing service. For charts of these arrangements, see Appendices D-5, D-6, and D-7, WF444, CHP Archives. The "junior staff nurse" was a third-year diploma student who received a salary for forty hours of ward work each week. The legacies of the original training school lingered until 1960, when the final class of diploma students graduated.

123. For meetings of the Administrative Council between 1949 and 1963, see folders 76–79, box 8, School of Nursing Archives, Blocker Collections; for meetings of the Executive Committee between 1954 and 1960, see folder 94, box 9, School of Nursing Archives, Blocker Collections; and for the monthly faculty meetings between 1957 and 1962, see folders 95 and 96, box 9, School of Nursing Archives, Blocker Collections. In 1959 seven committees handled recruitment, library matters, special studies, curriculum, admissions, scholarships, and "faculty courtesy" (see "Standing Committees for the School of Nursing 1959–1960," folder 86, box 8, School of Nursing Archives, Blocker Collections). For meetings of some committees during the 1950s and 1960s, see folders 87–88, box 8; folders 89–91, box 9; folders 100, 103, 106, 109–110, box 10; folders 111–117, 119, and 121–123, box 11; and folders 124 and 129, box 12, School of Nursing Archives, Blocker Collections.

124. Deliberations of the faculty are found in the minutes of the curriculum committee meetings; see folders 89 and 90, box 9, School of Nursing Archives, Blocker Collections. Also see "The University of Texas School of Nursing Biennial Report 1959–1961," folder 6, box 14, Levin Papers. For the baccalaureate program, the faculty initially required 42 semester hours of pre-nursing courses at UT Austin (or another accredited college or university) and 151 quarter hours of courses in Galveston (total of four academic years and two summer sessions; *UTMB Catalog* (1957–1958), 152–153. For descriptions of the courses required on both campuses, see *UT School of Nursing Catalog* (1959–1961), 30–44; (1961–1962), 28–37, 42–46; and (1962–1963), 28–37, 41–44. By 1961, 154 semester hours (65 liberal arts courses, 89 nursing courses) were required. For descriptions, see "A Report of a Study of the School of Nursing The University of Texas by its Faculty," April 1961, vertical file A3, box 3, Blocker Collections.

125. Marjorie Bartholf, "The School of Nursing," Annual Report for 1961–62, folder 9, box 1, 75th Anniversary History Papers, Blocker Collections. See also *University Medical Center News*, 3 (Oct., 1962), 1. Thirty-seven graduate nurses (thirteen in Austin; twenty-four in Galveston) were taking courses toward a B.S. in nursing degree. Fifteen graduate nurses (six in Austin; nine in Galveston) were enrolled in the master's degree program. Marjorie Bartholf, "Confidential Report of the School of Nursing, 1955–1962," and Marjorie Bartholf to John B. Truslow, Dec. 5, 1962,

letter; both in folder 9, box 1, School of Nursing Archives, Blocker Collections. Also see John B. Truslow to Harry H. Ransom, Nov. 5, 1962, and J. R. Smiley to Harry Ransom, Nov, 19, 1962, letters, box VF 33/A, UT Chancellor's Records; and *UT School of Nursing Catalog* (1964–1966), 48.

126. Rudnick had graduated from the John Sealy College of Nursing in 1946. She earned her bachelor's degree in nursing from the University of Houston in 1954 and her doctorate of education from Columbia University in 1962. See John B. Truslow to Harry Ransom, May 28, 1963, letter, box VF N/1, UT Chancellor's Records. See also *UT School of Nursing Catalog* (1964–1966), 39–41; and *Galveston Daily News*, Oct. 8, 1964.

127. Betty R. Rudnick to John B. Truslow, Apr. 7, 1964, letter, folder 18, box 2, School of Nursing Archives, Blocker Collections. Some students worked as part-time ward nurses during evening shifts from 3 to 11 P.M.; see Mary Fenton to Myles Knape, Feb. 13 and 18 and Mar. 4, 1986, interviews, Blocker Collections.

128. Betty R. Rudnick to Truman G. Blocker, "Revision of Nursing Service Organization," May 6, 1964, folder 18, box 2, School of Nursing Archives, Blocker Collections.

129. Betty R. Rudnick, untitled position paper, c. Apr. 1964, box VF N/1, UT Chancellor's Records. In March 1964 an unknown author wrote a cogent analysis of Bobbitt's proposal to establish a diploma nursing school in the hospitals at UTMB; see "Memorandum on the proposal to establish a University of Texas Hospital School of Nursing in September, 1965," folder 4, box 30, Levin Papers; and Betty R. Rudnick to Harry Ransom, Apr. 27, 1964, letter, box VF N/1, UT Chancellor's Records (quotations). Sometime between 1963 and 1967, "Consultant X" (not Rudnick) prepared a succinct analysis of the grievances and goals that motivated those in Galveston who wanted to move the school to Austin; see "Report of Consultant X on the Nursing School," in folder 6, box 14, Levin Papers. Some of the agonies of the faculty are displayed in minutes of the meetings of the school's Administrative Council between 1964 and 1966; see folder 79, box 8, School of Nursing Archives, Blocker Collections.

130. Betty Rudnick, "The Graduate Program in Nursing: What it is, and What it Could Be," c. Nov. 1965, box VF 36/F, UT President's Records. In 1963 the master's degree program was lengthened from two to three semesters, with the first two in Austin and the third in Galveston. Students complained about the discomfort of moves between the cities, the relative absence of an academic atmosphere in Galveston, and the difficulties of completing theses during the semester in Galveston. See Truman G. Blocker Jr. to Harry H. Ransom, Jan. 3, 1966, letter, folder 19, box 2, School of Nursing Archives, Blocker Collections. Blocker continued to support the hospital's training program for vocational nurses. In February 1966 twelve vocational nurses graduated from this program and twenty students enrolled; see *Newsletter (UTMB)*, 1 (Feb. 17, 1966), 1; and (Mar. 3, 1966), 2.

131. These words were eliminated before Harry Ransom sent her report to Sen. Criss Cole in September 1965. The draft accompanied Marie Primm to Laurence Haskew, Sept. 21, 1965, letter, box VF R/2, UT Chancellor's Records. The final report accompanied Harry Ransom to Criss Cole, Sept. 22, 1965, letter, box VF R/2, UT Chancellor's Records.

132. Betty Rudnick, "The University of Texas School of Nursing, Past, Present and Future," paper prepared for Senate committee that accompanied the letter from Harry Ransom to Criss Cole, Sept. 22, 1965, box VF R/2, UT Chancellor's Records. For some names of graduates, see *UTMB: Seventy-five Year History*, 350. Although probably incomplete, School of Nursing graduates between 1898 and 1967 are listed in *UTMB: Seventy-five Year History*, 344–351. Although she believed that it would be incomplete because of inconsistencies in the sources, Betty Grefenstette prepared a list of the names of all School of Nursing graduates through 1991. This list is in WF448, CHP Archives.

133. Marie C. Primm, "The University of Texas Medical Branch School of Nursing," c. July 1966, accompanied letter to Truman G. Blocker, July 20, 1966, folder 19, box 2, School of Nursing Archives, Blocker Collections. Clinical assistants were BSN graduates who assisted the faculty in teaching the clinical courses. For an overview of the school Rudnick wrote earlier that year, see *Newsletter (UTMB)*, 2 (June, 1966), 1–2. For a list of alphabetized names of School of Nursing faculty between 1896 and 1967, see *UTMB: Seventy-five Year History*, 374–380. Although she believed that it would be incomplete because of inconsistencies in the sources, Betty Grefenstette prepared a list of the names of all School of Nursing teachers through 1991. This list is in WF455, CHP Archives. Resting on some shelves on the second floor of the Moody Medical Library are fifty-nine theses written by nurses who earned master's degrees between 1954 and 1967. Examining these theses, Cheryl Vaiani determined that forty students did their research at UTMB, fourteen at other institutions, and five were not specified. These theses provide invaluable insights into the development of nursing as a profession in Texas.

134. Marie C. Primm to Truman G. Blocker, July 22, 1966, folder 19, box 2, School of Nursing Archives, Blocker Collections.

135. Between 1954 and 1966, 346 women had graduated from the vocational nurse program operated by the hospital; see *Newsletter (UTMB)*, 2 (Apr., 1966), 1. In February 1967, for example, thirteen graduates of this training program

had passed their state board exams and nine were employed by the hospital; see *Newsletter (UTMB)*, 2 (May 4, 1967), 1. For the crises, see the letter from Lynn Schaff in the *Houston Chronicle*, Dec. 29, 1966, and "Proposals for the Improvement of Patient Care Recommended by the Local Unit of Registered Nurses Employed by the University of Texas Medical Branch, Galveston, Texas," Jan. 1967, "Vice Chancellor for Health Affairs, 1964–1970," reel 123, UT Chancellor's Office of Records Management. For the union, see Betty Rudnick to Charles LeMaistre, July 28, 1966, "Vice Chancellor for Health Affairs, 1964–1970," reel 123, UT Chancellor's Office of Records Management. Mary Fenton and some of her classmates would work afternoon and evening shifts after attending school during the day; see Mary Fenton to Myles Knape, Feb. 13 and 18 and Mar. 4, 1986, interviews, Blocker Collections.

136. Brown, "The Historical Development of the University of Texas System School of Nursing, 1890–1973," 306–322 (quotation on 319). In December 1966 Rudnick, Primm, and others urged Mrs. John T. Jones of Houston, chair of the coordinating board's subcommittee on nursing, to support the concept of a single UT School of Nursing managed by administrators in Austin. See Marie C. Primm and others to Mrs. John T. Jones, Dec. 16, 1966, folder 19, box 2, School of Nursing Archives, Blocker Collections. Letters to Mrs. Jones from Betty Rudnick are in the same folder. See also J. K. Williams to Harry Ransom, Jan. 20, 1967, "Vice Chancellor for Health Affairs, 1964–1970," reel 123, UT Chancellor's Office of Records Management; and Betty R. Rudnick to Charles A. LeMaistre, Jan 25, 1966, letter, box VF EE/3, UT Chancellor's Records. For details, see Brown, "The Historical Development of the University of Texas System School of Nursing, 1890–1973," 322–330.

137. Brown, "The Historical Development of the University of Texas System School of Nursing, 1890–1973," 330–335; Betty Rudnick to Truman G. Blocker Jr., Feb. 3, 1967 (1st quotation); and Betty Rudnick to Frank C. Erwin Jr., Feb. 3, 1967 (2nd quotation), letters, both in box VF EE/3, UT Chancellor's Records.

138. For details, see Brown, "The Historical Development of the University of Texas System School of Nursing, 1890–1973," 336–361; and "System-Wide: School of Nursing," Material Supporting the Agenda for Meetings of the UT Board of Regents, May 5, 1967. For some insights regarding Willman's administration before 1969, see the correspondence in folders 22 and 23 in box 2, School of Nursing Archives, Blocker Collections.

139. "UT News," Sept. 24, 1968, and "System Nursing School: Progress Report," Material Supporting the Agenda for Meetings of the UT Board of Regents, Mar. 6, 1970. For a concise overview of the new arrangement, see the report by Marilyn Williams in *Alumni Bulletin*, 23 (Winter, 1969), 6–11. For a comprehensive analysis of the school, see "Self-Evaluation Report, The University of Texas Nursing School (System-Wide), September, 1969," vertical file A3, box 1, Blocker Collections. For a profile of the school in 1971, see *University Medical*, 3 (Oct., 1971), 12–14. For pertinent comments by a member of the faculty then, see Elizabeth Knebel to Poldi Tschirch, June 12, 1986, interview, Blocker Collections. For details about the evolution of the six schools, see Brown, "The Historical Development of the University of Texas System School of Nursing, 1890–1973," 361–404. Also see the system-wide catalogs issued in Austin during these years and Chloe Floyd to Myles Knape, Jan. 16 and 22, 1986, interviews, Blocker Collections. For a chart of the new administrative organization, see Appendix A-28, WF441, CHP Archives.

140. When Damewood arrived in 1968, there were 135 students, 9 faculty, and 14 clinical assistants. Damewood thought that the school was at a "low ebb" then. See Dorothy Damewood to Myles Knape, Nov. 13 and Dec. 16, 1985, interviews, Blocker Collections.

141. In 1973–1974, for example, the faculty were members of twelve local committees and six system-wide committees; see folder 118, box 11, School of Nursing Archives, Blocker Collections. For some insights into the ones in Galveston between 1971 and 1975, see folder 86, box 8, School of Nursing Archives, Blocker Collections. For comments about the advantages and disadvantages of the system arrangement, see Donna Jean Barlow to Poldi Tschirch, June 16, 1986; Virginia A. Rahr to Poldi Tschirch, June 12, 1986; and Anna Pearl Rains to Poldi Tschirch, July 17, 1986, interviews, Blocker Collections. More than two hundred nurses from the six schools attended the meeting in Galveston in May 1974, for example; see *Faculty News (UTMB)*, May 6–10, 1974, 2. For a sample of local concerns, see the minutes of the meetings between 1972 and 1975; folder 97, box 9, School of Nursing Archives, Blocker Collections. For a sample of system-wide concerns in 1972 and 1973, see folder 98, box 9, School of Nursing Archives, Blocker Collections.

142. A glimpse of the new approach can be obtained by comparing descriptions of the courses taught in the "old" curriculum and those in the "new" curriculum; see *UT School of Nursing Catalog* (1972–1973), 40–42. See also Brown, "The Historical Development of the University of Texas System School of Nursing, 1890–1973," 260–264; and *UT School of Nursing Catalog* (1974–1975), 22, 51–57.

143. "The University of Texas System School of Nursing Fact Sheet," box 10, School of Nursing Archives, Blocker Collections; and folder 72, box 7, School of Nursing Archives, Blocker Collections.

144. Elizabeth Knebel, Helen Ptak, and Shirley Steele were assistant, then associate deans; see Appendix B. For a chart of the administrative organization, see Appendix A-31, WF441, CHP Archives. In 1977 the seven committees were continuing education; educational media; faculty affairs; public affairs; student affairs; research; and undergraduate curriculum; see "Self-Study Report, The University of Texas School of Nursing," 1977, 20. In 1981 the ten committees were: appointment, promotion, and tenure; continuing education; educational resources; evaluation; faculty affairs; public affairs; recruitment; research; student affairs; and undergraduate curriculum. Students were also appointed to these committees. For more details, see the Faculty Rules of Procedure, May 1981, folder 1, box 15, Levin Papers. In 1984 there were nine committees: academic appointment, promotion, and tenure; educational resources; evaluation; faculty affairs; research; student affairs; student recruitment; undergraduate admissions/progression; and undergraduate curriculum; see copy in folder 2, box 15, Levin Papers. As needed, ad hoc committees also functioned during these years.

145. For a chart of the administrative organization, see Appendix A-39, WF441, CHP Archives. In 1982 the regents approved Damewood's request to establish an Advisory Council for the nursing school. Jan Coggeshall, Judy Godinez, Marie Hall, Beth Jewett, Gail Rider, Marilyn Schwartz, Walter Sterling, and Clyde Verheyden attended the first annual meeting of this council on September 17, 1982. For details about this meeting and subsequent meetings through 1985, see folder 2, box 16, Levin Papers.

146. *University Medical,* 9 (Jan.–Feb., 1978), 2–11.

147. Excellent summaries of this program are in "Self-Study Report, The University of Texas School of Nursing," 1977, 95–138, and "Self-Study Report, The University of Texas School of Nursing," Fall 1980, vol. I, 130–261. Both are in vertical file A3, box 3, Blocker Collections. For details about the courses, see *UT School of Nursing Catalog* (1982–1983), 61–73; (1983–1985), 59–74; (1985–1987), 49–65; and *UTMB Catalog* (1989–1990), 151–155; (1990–1992), 72–75. Data about enrollment from Damewood's annual report to the State Board of Nurse Examiners, Sept. 26, 1977, folder 1, box 16, Levin Papers. The four semesters of the curriculum were staged in sequences as Level I, II, III, and IV. For details, see folders 104 and 105, box 10, School of Nursing Archives, Blocker Collections. In 1978, 93 percent of the graduates remained in Texas; 87 percent in 1979. Of these, 88.3 percent were staff nurses in hospitals in 1978; 80.7 percent in 1979. For details, see page 17 of the attachment to William C. Levin to Warren Harding, Apr. 24, 1981, letter, folder 5, box 47, Levin Papers.

148. By analyzing the reports sent to the coordinating board from the registrar's office at UTMB, Joyce Dryman provided these statistics. In the spring of 1978 the nursing school included twelve male students; see *Impact,* 2 (Apr. 21, 1978), 18. For a description of one male nursing student, see *Impact,* 7 (Feb. 25, 1983), 15.

149. *Impact,* 5 (Sept. 25, 1981), 9. Professor Linares provided the data for Table 6.11. In 1988 UTMB initiated a work-study program for its own employees that allowed them to become registered nurses and earn an associate degree in nursing from Galveston College. By 1991 seventy-eight employees were enrolled in this program, which was coordinated by Katie Matlack; see *Galveston Daily News,* Mar. 31, 1991.

150. Data from draft of "NLN Visitors Remarks" dated Nov 10, 1977 in folder 1, box 16, Levin Papers. For course descriptions, see the school's "Graduate Bulletin for 1977–1978." For summaries of the program, see "Self-Study Report, The University of Texas School of Nursing," 1977, 139–165; "Self-Study Report, Special Request Report for Graduate Program Accreditation, The University of Texas School of Nursing, 1978–79;" "Self-Study Report, The University of Texas School of Nursing," Fall 1980, vol. I, 262–369; and "Self-Study Report, University of Texas Graduate Nursing Program, Graduate School of Biomedical Sciences, Prepared for GSBS Graduate Program Review Committee," 1984. These self-study reports are in vertical file A3, box 3, Blocker Collections. Joyce Dryman provided the data in Figure 6.12.

151. Brown, "The Historical Development of the University of Texas System School of Nursing, 1890–1973," 356. For details about system-wide continuing education, see Attachment B accompanying Dorothy Damewood to William C. Levin, Mar. 29, 1976, memo, folder 6, box 14, Levin Papers. See also "Self-Study Report, The University of Texas School of Nursing," 1977, 168–169, and data taken from attachments to the agenda for the advisory council meeting, Sept. 17, 1982, folder 2, box 16, Levin Papers. For more on Floyd, see *Impact,* 9 (Feb. 22, 1985), 13. In 1973 some School of Nursing professors began a special four-month continuing education program to train pediatric nurse practitioners. Supported by a NIH grant, this program was a collaborative endeavor between the Department of Pediatrics in the medical school and faculty in the nursing school. By 1976, 58 nurses had completed this course and 9 were enrolled. A total of 118 nurses completed this program between 1973 and 1980, when it ended. See *Galveston Daily News,* May 13, 1973; and Dorothy M. Damewood, "The University of Texas School of Nursing at Galveston," April 1976, folder 6, box 14, Levin Papers. Billie Karacostas provided the total number of graduates.

152. Data taken from attachments to the agenda for the advisory council meeting, Sept. 17, 1982, folder 2, box 16, Levin Papers.

153. Fenton received a bachelor of nursing degree from the UT School of Nursing in 1966, a master's of science degree in medical-surgical nursing from the University of Michigan in 1968, and a doctor of public health degree from the UT School of Public Health in 1980. For more details, see the brochure about Fenton in WF338, CHP Archives. For her perspectives after becoming dean, see Mary Fenton to Myles Knape, Feb. 13 and 18 and Mar. 4, 1986, interviews, Blocker Collections. See also the University of Texas School of Nursing at Galveston, Bulletin (1988–1990), vii–xvii.

154. The rationale for what Fenton termed "decentralization" is succinctly stated in the request to Charles Mullins dated May 4, 1987, folder 5, box 15, Levin Papers. For organization charts, see Appendix A-40 and Appendix A-48, WF441, CHP Archives. The committees included academic appointment, promotion and tenure; educational resources; evaluation; research; student affairs; student recruitment; faculty affairs; undergraduate curriculum; and undergraduate admissions and progression. There were three task forces: faculty practice; strategic planning; and Southern Association of Colleges and Schools accreditation. Administrative groups included: Administrative Council; Undergraduate Nursing Program Council; Graduate Nursing Program Council; Flexible Option Coordinating Committee; Graduate Curriculum Committee; Graduate Admission and Progression Committee; Graduate Nominations Committee; and GSBS committees.

155. For a summary of the requirements and courses, see *UTMB Catalog* (1989–1990), 145–155, and (1990–1992), 62–75. Fenton and her colleagues developed proposals for a doctoral program in nursing. During the summer of 1987, a team of consultants from the Coordinating Board was "impressed with the vision and vitality of the dean and faculty" and recommended the continued recruitment of doctorally prepared faculty who could fully support a doctoral graduate program. See the comments on pages 51–52 of the report of the consultants accompanying William H. Sanford to Thomas N. James, Sept. 1, 1987, letter, folder 5, box 15, Levin Papers.

156. "1991–92 School of Nursing Operating Budget Request," 1–10, Dean's Office, School of Nursing; *Impact*, 9 (Oct. 4, 1985), 11; and 12 (Aug. 5, 1988), 3. To learn more about nursing and medical care, these students also visited homes of patients in Monterrey.

157. *Galveston Daily News*, Nov. 2, 1990. Endowed by the Sealy & Smith Foundation, this chair honored Rebecca Sealy, wife of John Sealy I.

158. John Bruhn asked Paula L. Levine to prepare a summary of historical highlights in the evolution of the School of Allied Health Sciences. In 1990 Paula generously gave me a copy of that summary, which is in WF336, CHP Archives; cited hereafter as Paula Levine, "SAHS," 1990. For a useful overview of the national status of five programs in the early 1950s, see F. H. Arestad, "Training and Utilization of Technical Personnel," *Texas Reports on Biology and Medicine*, 10 (Fall, 1952), 703–712.

159. During the World War I years, some professors trained lab technicians in the Laboratory of Clinical Pathology. See R. E. Vinson to Surgeon General, United States Army, Aug. 27, 1918, letter, box 4Q21, UT President's Records; Meyer Bodansky to W. D. Wilcox, Feb. 7, 1936, letter; and "List of Schools for Medical Technologists which meet the minimum essentials of Board of Registry of the American Society of Clinical Pathologists," June 1, 1938, both in box 2, Bodansky Papers; Minutes, UTMB Faculty Meeting, Feb. 6, 1942; *Galveston Daily News*, Apr. 24, 1943; and *UTMB: Seventy-five Year History*, 211. The names of those who received certificates between 1953 and 1955 are listed in *UTMB: Seventy-five Year History*, 358.

160. In the fall of 1942 Crook had visited four institutions that had programs approved by the American Association of Physiotherapists and the AMA; see G. W. N. Eggers to Chauncey D. Leake, Nov. 12, 1942, letter, box VF 9/A, UT President's Records. In January 1943 the faculty endorsed plans for the program; see Chauncey D. Leake to Homer P. Rainey, Jan. 6, 1943, letter, box VF 9/A, UT President's Records; and Minutes, UTMB Faculty Meeting, Jan. 6, 1943. The names of those who received certificates are listed in *UTMB: Seventy-five Year History*, 357. In 1949 the six graduates of the PT program made the highest grades in the exams given by the American Registry of Physical Therapy Technicians; see Chauncey D. Leake to T. S. Painter, Sept. 17, 1949, letter, box VF 10/D, UT President's Records.

161. For extensive comments about these PT programs, see Ruby Decker to Myles Knape, May 1 and 2, 1986, interviews, Blocker Collections. For more information about the courses taught between 1945 and 1965, see the lists in RF37, CHP Archives. See also *Medi-Texan*, 2 (Dec., 1954), 3.

162. Minutes, UTMB Faculty Meeting, Feb. 6, 1942; Robert N. Cooley, "The History of the Department of Radiology The University of Texas Medical Branch," c. 1986, 93. A copy is in WF472, CHP Archives. The names of those who earned certificates are listed in *UTMB: Seventy-five Year History*, 359.

163. *UTMB: Seventy-five Year History*, 211. The names of those who earned certificates are listed in *UTMB: Seventy-five Year History*, 357.

164. Chauncey D. Leake to James P. Hart, May 22, 1952 (quotation); and James P. Hart to Chauncey D. Leake, June 24, 1952, letters, both in box VF A/3, UT Chancellor's Records.

165. Minutes, UTMB Faculty Meeting, Feb. 5–6, 1952; Chauncey D. Leake to George Crosby, Feb. 6 and 14, 1952, letters, box 26, Leake Papers, NLM; Chauncey D. Leake to George H. Crosby, May 27 and June 6, 1952, letters, box 26, Leake Papers, NLM. Crosby also "supervised" other hospital employees: Margaret Otis in social work; Austin Foster in clinical psychology; and George Newman in medical illustration. The hospital served as a practical training site for "interns" in social work and clinical psychology. It is not known if Crosby had any managerial responsibilities for the EEG technicians, blood bank technicians, and audiometric technicians at UTMB.

166. George H. Crosby to C. D. Leake, Mar. 9, 1955, letter, box VF O/4, UT Chancellor's Records; and D. Bailey Calvin to Logan Wilson, Aug. 29, 1955, letter, box VF E/2, UT Chancellor's Records. The names of those awarded certificates and degrees are listed in *UTMB: Seventy-five Year History*, 357–358.

167. In 1957, for example, there were 45 students: X-ray (26); clinical lab (6); medical records (5); physical therapy (4); occupational therapy (3); and EEG (1). These numbers came from "1957—A Year of Education and Service at the University of Texas Medical Branch Hospitals, Galveston," box VF S/3, UT Chancellor's Records. See also *Medi-Texan*, 2 (May, 1955), 11; and *UTMB: Seventy-five Year History*, 357–359, for the names of those who earned certificates. For a description of the medical technology program, see *Galveston Daily News*, Nov. 17, 1963. Elwood Baird, its director, was chair of the Board of Schools of Medical Technology during the 1960s. Established by the American Society of Clinical Pathologists in 1949, this board was the accrediting agency for more than eight hundred schools of medical technology existing by the late 1960s; see *UTMB: Seventy-five Year History*, 211. Betty Grefenstette prepared an alphabetized list of the names of all Medical Services Curricula graduates that is in WF451, CHP Archives.

168. "Medical and Dental Schools—Degree Programs, the University of Texas Medical Branch at Galveston, July 19, 1965, box VF CC/2, UT Chancellor's Records; T. G. Blocker Jr. to Harry H. Ransom, Feb. 15, 1967, letters, box VF EE/3, UT Chancellor's Records; Current Files, Office of the Board of Regents, UTMB, GMB-6 School of Allied Health Sciences. For details, see the bound proposal in box 4, vertical file A2; the folder about the establishment of the SAHS in box 2, vertical file A2; and folder 1, box 13, Levin Papers, all in the Blocker Collections.

169. For details about the origins and growth of the School of Allied Health Sciences, see Robert K. Bing to Myles Knape, Sept. 10, 16, 23, and 30, 1987, and June 8, 1988, interviews, Blocker Collections. For the names of faculty members, see *UT School of Allied Health Sciences Catalog* (1968–1971), 76–79. Personnel in a variety of affiliated hospitals in Southeast Texas also served as tutors when students were assigned to these hospitals for clinical training. In March 1970, for example, the regents authorized affiliation agreements between the School of Allied Health Sciences and forty-five clinical centers (most in Texas; some in Oklahoma, Arkansas, and Kansas) for the purpose of training SAHS students in medical record administration, occupational therapy, and physical therapy; see the list in WF37, CHP Archives. For other affiliation agreements, see RF53, CHP Archives. For a copy of the first bylaws of the School of Allied Health Sciences, see RF37, CHP Archives. For a copy of the bylaws adopted in 1983, see folder 5, box 14, Levin Papers.

170. For the required courses, see *UT School of Allied Health Sciences Catalog* (1968–1971), 50 (medical record administration), 56 (medical technology), 62 (occupational therapy), 68 (physical therapy).

171. In a survey of allied health programs in Texas in 1974, the Coordinating Board of the Texas College and University System identified sixty-seven occupational roles in allied health. For a copy of this survey, see WF337, CHP Archives. In 1963 UTMB's hospitals had started a program to train inhalation (respiratory) therapists. Robert Weilacher was technical director and Edwin Elder was chief technical instructor in this School of Inhalation Therapy. Four students enrolled in the three-year course; see *Galveston Daily News*, Mar. 1, 1964. After the School of Allied Health Sciences began, Juaneva Novak continued to train four EEG technologists each year; see *Hospital News*, 7 (Nov. 11, 1974), 2.

172. The required college course are listed in *UT School of Allied Health Sciences Catalog* (1971–1973), 61. Descriptions of the courses in this two-year curriculum are on pages 63–65 of this catalog. Also see Robert K. Bing to Myles Knape, Sept. 10, 16, 23, and 30, 1987, and June 8, 1988, interviews, Blocker Collections. See also Charles C. Sprague to John W. Schermerhorn, June 11, 1974, letter, UT Chancellor's Office of Records Management, Chancellor's Office Subject Files, reel 16. John Young was named as the outstanding PA student in this first group of graduates. For a profile of Young's five years as a PA in Caldwell, Texas, see *Impact*, 3 (May 4, 1979), 10. See also *University Medical*, 8 (July–Aug., 1977), 13–15.

173. The 136 names are listed in *UT School of Allied Health Sciences Catalog* (1973–1976), 135–137. See Betty Anne Thedford to Carole Bryant, June 21, 1973, letter, Current Files, Office of the Board of Regents, UTMB, GMB-6, School of Allied Health Sciences. About 15 percent of the new students were not residents of Texas. See data sheets in WF336, CHP Archives. The number of baccalaureate students in the totals ranged from 193 (1975–1976) to 285 (1980–1981).

174. For an overview of all programs in 1974, see *University Medical*, 5 (Feb., 1974), 5–15. For the required courses, see *UT School of Allied Health Sciences Catalog* (1968–1971), 51–52 (medical records adminstration), 58 (medical technology), 64–65 (occupational therapy), 69–70 (physical therapy), and 74 (radiologic technology). For examples or training programs, see folder 12, box 2, Area Health Education Center Archives, Blocker Collections. For a historical overview of the entire program, see the last issue of *La Salud*, the Area Health Education Center newsletter that was issued in the spring of 1979. See also *Faculty News (UTMB)*, Aug. 16–27, 1976; *University Medical*, 9 (July–Aug., 1978), 6; and page 16 of the attachment to William C. Levin to Warren Harding, Apr. 24, 1981, letter, folder 5, box 47, Levin Papers.

175. For a chart of the administrative organization, see Appendix A-32, WF441, CHP Archives. During the 1981–1982 academic year, about twenty teachers and administrators developed a strategic plan for the School of Allied Health Sciences for the years 1983–1989. They developed specific goals for each of five major areas: faculty development; faculty governance; educational programs; student services; and public relations (external affairs). This plan provided a blueprint for the school during the 1980s. A copy of this Master Plan 1983–1989 is in box 3, vertical file A2, Blocker Collections. For details about administrative changes between 1973 and 1990, see Paula Levine, "SAHS," 1990, 9–10; and John Bruhn to Myles Knape, Dec. 3 and 5, 1985, interviews, Blocker Collections. For administrative organization charts in 1984 and 1991, see Appendices A-38 and A-49, WF441, CHP Archives.

176. *University Medical*, 9 (July–Aug., 1978), 8.

177. For their names, see *UT School of Allied Health Sciences Catalog* (1981–1983), 200–225. Photographs of faculty and students appear in the annual volumes of *Syndrome*.

178. For brief descriptions of the departments' curricula, see the supplement to the *Galveston Daily News*, Aug. 15, 1982. More than thirty courses were available for students in the Department of Allied Health Services. Descriptions of these courses are in *UT School of Allied Health Sciences Catalog* (1981–1983), 109–114. The Department of Health Related Studies was then subdivided into a Division of Health Related Professions, which offered baccalaureate degree programs in health administration and health education, and a Division of Health Related Occupations, which offered associate degree and certificates programs with Galveston College. See Paula Levine, "SAHS," 1990, 8–9.

179. The courses are described in *UT School of Allied Health Sciences Catalog* (1981–1983), 129–133.

180. For the courses, see *UT School of Allied Health Sciences Catalog* (1981–1983), 140–148.

181. For the standard courses, see *UT School of Allied Health Sciences Catalog* (1981–1983), 157–161; for the courses in cytotechnology, 167–169.

182. For occupational therapy courses, see *UT School of Allied Health Sciences Catalog* (1981–1983), 180–182; for physical therapy courses, 193–195.

183. For descriptions, see 1985 supplement to 1984–1986 Bulletin of The University of Texas School of Allied Health Sciences at Galveston, 1–2. A copy is in box 1, vertical file A-2, Blocker Collections.

184. For the new division, see *UT School of Allied Health Sciences Catalog* (1986–1988), 131–137.

185. A draft of the proposal for the master's degree program is in box 3, vertical file A2, Blocker Collections. Also see *Impact*, 11 (Sept. 4, 1987), 1, 6. For the graduate courses, see the brochure in WF336, CHP Archives.

186. Paula Levine, "SAHS," 1990, 11. Although she believed that it would be incomplete because of inconsistencies in the sources, Betty Grefenstette prepared an alphabetized list of the names of all SAHS faculty through 1991. This list is in WF457, CHP Archives. Appendix AF was taken from *UTMB Catalog* (1990–1992), 138. Although she believed that it would be incomplete because of some inconsistencies in the sources, Betty Grefenstette prepared a list of the names of all SAHS graduates through 1991. This list is in WF452, CHP Archives.

187. William C. Rose and W. T. Garbade to R. E. Vinson, Mar. 9, 1920, letter, box 4Q23, UT President's Records.

188. W. S. Carter to R. E. Vinson, Mar. 24, 1921, letter, box 4R81, UT President's Records. Although the regents authorized UT Austin to offer a doctor of philosophy degree in 1885, little interest developed in a graduate program until 1900, when the university created a Committee on Graduate Courses (later renamed Graduate Council), a small group of faculty headed by Harper, who was professor of chemistry. In 1910 the regents created the UT Graduate School and Harper became its dean in 1913, two years before the school awarded its first Ph.D.; see Gordon Whaley's historical summary attached to Logan Wilson to Ralph T. Green, Mar. 31, 1958, letter, box VF 30/A, UT President's

Records. The number of graduate students increased from about forty in 1910 to about three hundred in 1925. By 1934 the Graduate School had awarded 137 Ph.D.s; see "Ph.D. Degrees Granted by the University of Texas, 1915–1934," box 2R279, University of Texas file, Center for American History.

189. George E. Bethel to H. Y. Benedict, Oct. 31, 1933, letter, box 4Q25, UT President's Records.

190. A. P. Brogan to B. M. Hendrix, W. T. Dawson, and George Herrmann, Dec. 8, 1936, letter, box VF 9/C, UT President's Records. Brogan was dean of the Graduate School between 1936 and 1959. See *Galveston Daily News*, Oct. 19, 1939.

191. It has been very difficult to obtain reliable statistical data about the total number of students enrolled in graduate programs at UTMB and the total number of those graduating from these programs. The list of graduate degree students on page 356 of the *UTMB: Seventy-five Year History* is incomplete. It is highly probable that there were more students who received master's degrees for work in Galveston. Not infrequently, professors hired students who wanted to earn graduate degrees while working as research and teaching assistants (titled tutors or assistants in those years); for examples during the 1920s and 1930s, see the letters in RF86, CHP Archives. Using a variety of sources, Betty Grefenstette prepared a list of those receiving degrees from UT and from UTMB for graduate studies in Galveston. Her list is in WF451, CHP Archives. The number of ten earning master's degrees before 1941 is taken from her list.

192. Chauncey D. Leake to B. M. Hendrix, Aug 4, 1944, letter, folder 6, box 6, Duncan Papers. Eighteen professors (thirteen basic science and five clinical) are named on the list of those recommended as "supervisors." See B. M. Hendrix to A. P. Brogan, Jan. 6, 1947, letter, folder 8, box 6, Duncan Papers. The faculty in Austin and those in Galveston disagreed vigorously about such matters as the number of required courses at UT Austin, the ways in which UT Austin and UTMB would be represented on admission and dissertation committees, and the departments at UTMB that should be authorized to offer Ph.D.s. For details, see the correspondence in folders 6–9, Duncan Papers; the letters in RF87, CHP Archives; and the relevant folders in box 6 of the CHP Archives.

193. Theophilus S. Painter to C. D. Leake, June 6, 1947, letter, box VF 9/D, UT President's Records; American Medical Association Council on Medical Education and Hospitals, *Medical Education in the United States, 1934–1939* (Chicago: American Medical Education, c. 1940), 21, 36–38; Chauncey D. Leake to A. P. Brogan, June 4, 1947, and Chauncey D. Leake to T. S. Painter, July 7, 1947, letters, both in box VF 10/C; Chauncey D. Leake to T. S. Painter, Oct. 4, 1948, and Chauncey D. Leake to T. S. Painter, Jan. 4, 1949, both in box VF 10/D, letters, all in UT President's Records.

194. Minutes, UTMB Faculty Meeting, Jan. 4, 1949; James P. Hart to T. S. Painter, Jan. 3, 1951, letter, box VF B/4, UT Chancellor's Records; and Minutes, Meeting of the Graduate Faculty of the University of Texas at Austin, Jan. 9, 1951, box VF 25/A, UT President's Records. Brogan appointed an interim committee to oversee the collaborative venture. See also A. P. Brogan to James P. Hart, Aug. 1, 1952, letter, box VF B/1, UT Chancellor's Records; Whaley's historical summary (p. 2) attached to Logan Wilson to Ralph T. Green, Mar. 31, 1958, letter, box VF 30/A, UT President's Records. For a biographical sketch, see Chester R. Burns, "Donald Duncan," in Tyler, et al. (eds.), *The New Handbook of Texas*, II, 727. For valuable insights into Duncan's legacy, see the correspondence in boxes 32 and 33, Department of Anatomy records, Blocker Collections.

195. Mason Guest referred to these meetings as "hot sessions"; see M. Mason Guest to John Swann. Jan. 29, 1987, interview, Blocker Collections. For a biographical sketch, see Chester R. Burns, "Maurice Mason Guest," in Tyler, et al. (eds.), *The New Handbook of Texas*, III, 370–371. See also "Creation of a Graduate Legislative Council and Delegation of Authority to this Council," Jan. 19, 1953, box VF B/1, UT Chancellor's Records.

196. *UTMB Catalog* (1953–1954), 73. The names of the nineteen students are on a list attached to Patrick Romanell to Donald Duncan, Sept. 27, 1954, memo, folder 1, box 33, Department of Anatomy records, Blocker Collections.

197. Sources provide conflicting totals about the years 1942–1957. Compare the number in Whaley's report (attached to Logan Wilson to Ralph T. Green, Mar. 31, 1958, letter, box VF 30/A, UT President's Records) with the names listed in *UTMB: Seventy-five Year History*, 356. To obtain some insights about the students applying for graduate studies between 1955 and 1959, see box 31, Department of Anatomy records, Blocker Collections. Boxes 20, 21, and 22 of these records provide many details about this department's graduate students between 1948 and 1961. The 1959 number is from an enrollment sheet in folder 1, box 33, Department of Anatomy records, Blocker Collections. For 1964, see *Newsletter (UTMB)*, 1 (Nov. 5, 1964), 2.

198. The Graduate Legislative Council was renamed the Graduate Assembly and voting members were apportioned among all component institutions, with UTMB assigned two seats. The Graduate Assembly met three times a year to develop policies for graduate education in the UT System. The policies for each academic area were created by a Committee on Graduate Studies for that area and a faculty member was designated as the Graduate Adviser, serving as

the liaison between that graduate program and the chief administrator for each school. The Department of Pathology was approved for master's degree work only. Concise overviews of four of these departments were written by their chairs in 1965 and 1967, see *Newsletter (UTMB)*, 1 (June, 1965), 1–2 (biochemistry); (Aug., 1965), 1–2 (microbiology); 3 (Feb., 1967), 1–2 (pathology); and (Apr., 1967), 1–2 (physiology).

199. For minutes of these meetings between 1964 and 1968, see the Graduate Assembly folder, box 3, vertical file A4, Blocker Collections. To recognize Duncan's extraordinary accomplishments, students and faculty organized a testimonial dinner in 1968; see *Alumni Bulletin*, 22 (Summer, 1968), 4–6. The 1976 *Syndrome* and the 1981 *Syndrome* were dedicated to Duncan. For details between 1964 and 1969, see the folder of Graduate Faculty Minutes in box 3, vertical file A4, Blocker Collections.

200. *Faculty News (UTMB)*, Oct. 4, 1968. Also see Betty Grefenstette's list in WF451, CHP Archives.

201. Minutes, UT Board of Regents, Mar. 14, 1969. A member was a tenured teacher (professor, associate professor, or assistant professor) in a department conducting graduate studies. An associate member was a non-tenured or junior faculty member who could supervise master's degree work and, with authorized approval, a doctoral dissertation. A special member was someone acting in a part-time or visiting capacity who was qualified to teach or supervise graduate students.

202. See minutes of the April 30, 1969, meeting in box 3, vertical file A4, Blocker Collections. The regents expected each graduate faculty to elect a representative to the Graduate Council for the biomedical institutions in the UT System, a group that would advise the Health Affairs Council on all matters concerning biomedical graduate education.

203. Joe White recruited Brandt, who had earned an M.D. and a Ph.D. (biostatistics) at the University of Oklahoma Medical Center and had served in various teaching and administrative roles at his alma mater. For minutes of the February meeting and others between 1970 and 1974, see the Graduate Faculty Minutes folder, box 1, vertical file A4, Blocker Collections. For important comments, see Edward N. Brandt to Chester R. Burns, Oct. 29, 1989, interview. For samples of the committee's deliberations, see minutes of the Executive Committee Graduate Faculty for 1974, box 3, vertical file A4, Blocker Collections. The regents expected each graduate school to elect no fewer than four faculty members to serve with the graduate administrator as a Graduate Executive Committee that would be responsible for the overall academic policies of a particular school.

204. A copy of the bylaws is attached to the Graduate Faculty Minutes for August 30, 1970, box 1, vertical file A4, Blocker Collections. Minimum admission requirements included a bachelor's degree from an accredited institution, a satisfactory grade point average, a combined score of 1,000 on the verbal and quantitative sections of the Graduate Record Examinations Aptitude Test, adequate preparation for the proposed graduate major, and acceptance by the committee on graduate studies responsible for that scientific field. The graduate courses are described in *UT Graduate School of the Biomedical Sciences Catalog* (1971–1973), 76–115. For a sample of deliberations about courses in one program, see the minutes of the committee on graduate studies for the Human Biological Chemistry and Genetics department between 1972 and 1978 in folder 1, box 1 and folder 1, box 3, HBC&G records, Blocker Collections. Sample course outlines and exams are in folders 2, 3, and 4 in box 2 of these records.

205. For the names of the faculty, see *UT Graduate School of the Biomedical Sciences Catalog* (1973–1975), 122–130; for the students, 131. The numbers of graduate students were taken from the sheet titled "Graduate Education in the Sciences Basic to Medicine," c. 1976, RF87, CHP Archives. There are slight discrepancies with those in Table 6.15. The totals in Table 6.15 were those reported in the annual reports to the AAMC submitted by the office of the dean of the Medical School.

206. Minutes, UT Board of Regents, Sept. 14, 1973.

207. *University Medical*, 5 (July, 1974), 20–23. A native of London, England, Jack Palmer Saunders came to the United States at the age of fourteen and later earned a bachelor's degree in chemistry from the College of the City of New York, and a master's and Ph.D. in biochemistry from the University of Maryland. After ten years as a toxicologist and pharmacologist at the Chemical Corps Medical Laboratory, Saunders served in various administrative roles with the Division of Research Grants and the National Cancer Institute between 1956 and 1974. Saunders had worked with Bill Levin on various committees of the National Cancer Institute. For details about the evolution of the Graduate School of the Biomedical Sciences, see the relevant folders in box 6, CHP Archives, and J. Palmer Saunders to Myles Knape and John Swann, Nov. 5 and 14, 1985, interviews, Blocker Collections. The committee for 1978 included Blankenship as chair; David Bee, Gerald Callas, Charles (Pat) Davis, Joel Gallagher, Lester Grant, Viktor Holubek, Giuseppe Sant'Ambrogio, and Satish Srivastava as faculty members; and Jim Barnett and Linda Cole as student members. Blankenship became associate dean for curriculum in 1980, then associate dean in 1985.

208. Some details can be gleaned from the Graduate Faculty Minutes between 1975 and 1987 deposited in four folders in box 1, vertical file A4, Blocker Collections. For reports about the external reviews of specific programs and for a final

forty-six-page report of the entire external review process by the steering committee, see folders 1 and 2, box 12, Levin Papers. As an example of a review of a specific department, see folders 3, 4, and 5, HBC&G records, Blocker Collections.

209. For drafts and a final version of these bylaws, see the folder in box 3, vertical file A4, Blocker Collections. The new bylaws classified faculty as members or special members; the category of associate was eliminated. The bylaws specified two major liaison roles between departmental graduate programs and the dean's office: a director of each graduate program and a representative from each graduate program on the Graduate School of the Biomedical Sciences executive committee. Saunders urged each department to elect the same person to both roles, a policy adopted as an amendment to the school's bylaws in 1979. The initial group of program directors included Walther J. Hild (anatomy), Creed W. Abell (biochemistry), Barbara H. Bowman (human genetics and cell biology), Leroy J. Olson (microbiology), Lester H. Grant (pathology), Odd S. Steinsland (pharmacology and toxicology), John E. Remmers (physiology and biophysics), and Don W. Micks (preventive medicine and community health).

210. The names and ranks of these teachers are listed in the *UT Graduate School of the Biomedical Sciences Catalog* (1979–1980); a copy is in box 2, vertical file A4, Blocker Collections.

211. New chairs included Cary Cooper (1982), Brad Thompson (1984), Bill Willis (1985), Harold Sandstead (1985), Luis Reuss (1986), and David Walker (1987). For comments about the graduate programs in their departments, see Cary Cooper to Myles Knape, Nov. 12, 1987; Edward I. B. Thompson to Myles Knape and John Swann, Mar. 1, 1988; William Willis to Myles Knape, June 2, 9, and 23, 1986; Harold Sandstead to Myles Knape, May 11, 1988; Luis Reuss to Myles Knape and John Swann, May 13, 1988; and David Walker to Myles Knape and John Swann, Dec. 22, 1987; interviews, Blocker Collections. For other changes during these years, see the annual or biennial reports about the Graduate School of the Biomedical Sciences Saunders prepared. Some are in WF341, CHP Archives, as is a copy of the revised GSBS bylaws adopted in 1983. For additional details, see Don W. Micks to Myles Knape, Sept. 9, 1987, interview, Blocker Collections.

212. During the 1960s, a few students earned both an M.D. and Ph.D., including Earl Wilson Ferguson (class of 1970). Ferguson received an Ashbel Smith Alumnus Award in 1993; see *Impact*, 7 (Feb. 25, 1983), 5. For details about the program, see folder 4, box 12, Levin Papers.

213. In 1990 Aida Sacaan, a native of Bethlehem, received three student awards for her outstanding research endeavors; see *Galveston Daily News*, July 13, 1990.

214. Recognizing his outstanding accomplishments, the regents named Saunders as dean emeritus in 1990; see *Galveston Daily News*, Nov. 30, 1990.

215. Yielding received M.S. and M.D. degrees from the University of Alabama Medical Center and later served as a senior investigator at the National Institute of Arthritis and Metabolic Diseases (1958–1964). Yielding then served as professor of biochemistry, associate professor of medicine, and chief of the Laboratory of Molecular Biology at the University of Alabama Medical Center in Birmingham (1964–1980) and moved to Mobile to serve as professor and chair of anatomy and professor of medicine at the College of Medicine of the University of South Alabama (1980–1987). As a scientist Yielding focused on ways that environmental factors affected developmental processes at the molecular level. His studies involved enzyme regulation, DNA damage and repair, amino acid neurotransmitters, and the mechanisms of action of anticancer and antiparasitic drugs. Yielding continued his laboratory research at UTMB. For details, see the brochure about Yielding in WF341, CHP Archives and K. Lemone Yielding to John Swann, Sept. 18, 1989, interview, Blocker Collections.

216. Although she believed that it would be incomplete because of inconsistencies in the sources, Betty Grefenstette prepared an alphabetized list of the names of all Graduate School of the Biomedical Sciences faculty through 1991. This list is in WF456, CHP Archives.

217. *Galveston Daily News*, May 19, 1991. More than fifteen of these students received various awards and scholarships that recognized their outstanding talents as researchers. During these same years, at least 823 postdoctoral fellows also worked in the labs of many GSBS teachers, providing extremely important networks of support for students and faculty (Table 6.15). The totals in Table 6.15 were those reported in the annual reports to the AAMC submitted by the office of the dean of the Medical School. Computerized databases created in the office of the GSBS dean show 333 students earning master's degrees and 308 students earning doctorates during these years. From a variety of sources, Betty Grefenstette identified 422 students who earned master's degrees between 1922 and 1991 (not including nursing students) and 260 students who earned doctor of philosophy degrees in the biomedical sciences and humanities between 1942 and 1991. This list is in WF450, CHP Archives.

218. Marine Biomedical Institute members were scattered in several basic science departments. Institute of the Medical Humanities members were mostly in the Department of Preventive Medicine and Community Health.

219. For comments about the impact of the Marine Biomedical Institute on the basic science departments of the medical school, see Joseph M. White to Chester R. Burns, Dec. 19, 1989, interview, Blocker Collections.

220. These subjects were taught in other American schools. For a historical analysis of this teaching, see Genevieve Miller, "Medical History," in Numbers, *The Education of American Physicians*, 290–308; and Chester R. Burns, "Medical Ethics and Jurisprudence," in Numbers, *The Education of American Physicians*, 273–289. Descriptions of the lectures on law and jurisprudence are included in the annual catalogs. For example, see *UTMB Catalog* (1894–1895), 35. For Cerna's approach to the history of medicine, see *UTMB Catalog* (1893–1894), 13; (1894–1895), 36–37; and (1895–1896), 35–36. For Paine, see *University Medical*, 3 (Dec., 1897), 69.

221. For the national background, see Chester R. Burns, "Teaching the Humanities in American Medical Schools during the Twentieth Century: A Commentary on the Two Dominant Models," in David C. Thomasma and Judith Lee Kissell (eds.), *The Health Care Professional as Friend and Healer: Building on the Work of Edmund D. Pellegrino* (Washington, D.C., Georgetown University Press, 2000), 259–266. Graves made his claim about his lectures in remarks given during the annual meeting of the Texas Medical Association in 1927; see *Texas State Journal of Medicine*, 23 (June, 1927), 117–118. Graves may have taught an elective course on medical history and medical ethics during the 1927–1928 academic year; see *UTMB Catalog* (1927–1928), 41; and Minutes, UT Board of Regents, July 29, 1927, and Apr. 9, 1928.

222. For about fifteen years Lawrence gave seniors two lectures each week for nineteen weeks. For a description of this course, see *UTMB Catalog* (1915–1916), 41. The total of thirty-eight hours was the largest number of hours devoted to legal medicine in any American medical school at the time (see the survey list in RF22, CHP Archives). By the early 1920s this course involved three lectures a week for fifteen weeks. Harris continued this forty-five-hour course during the 1930s. For a sample listing, see *UTMB Catalog* (1931–1932), 37. See also *UTMB Catalog* (1945–1946), 55.

223. Chauncey D. Leake to James P. Hart, Apr. 9, 1952, and Chauncey D. Leake to James P. Hart, June 13, 1952, letters, box VF A/3, UT Chancellor's Records. In the mid-1940s Leake had unsuccessfully attempted to establish a Department of Medical Jurisprudence and Sociology. He wanted Hubert W. Smith to chair that department, but Smith wanted to establish a Law–Science Institute at UT Austin. For more on Smith, see RF22, CHP Archives. Romanell was probably the first professional philosopher to receive a full-time appointment to the faculty of a medical school in the United States. For comments about Romanell's first course in philosophy and ethics for medical students, see *Galveston Daily News*, Sept. 22, 1953. See also *UTMB Catalog* (1954–1955), 60–61.

224. *University Medical Center News*, 2 (Jan., 1962), 3. The Committee on Religion and Medicine included three full-time campus ministers (Bill Hailey, Carl Nighswonger, and Al Vastyan) and six members of the faculty and staff (Bill Daeschner, Donald Duncan, Hamilton Ford, John Johnson, Bill Ainsworth, and Warren Harding). The only exception was a course in the history of anatomy Donald Duncan taught to graduate students for many years.

225. *Alumni Bulletin*, 19 (Dec., 1965), 1. Leake repeated this series of lectures again in 1967 and in 1970. For the syllabus distributed during these three series, see folders 31 and 32, box 4, Leake Papers, Blocker Collections. For additional details, see RF23, CHP Archives.

226. Chester R. Burns, "IMH Celebrates Twenty Years: Some Reminiscences," *Medical Humanities Rounds*, 10 (Apr., 1993), 1–2. Chauncey Leake attended the April 1970 meeting at the Flagship Hotel and later gave his series of ten medical history lectures on the campus. Lester King, a senior editor of the *Journal of the American Medical Associaiton* and distinguished medical historian, gave the first Sam G. Dunn lecture endowed by the Dunn Family. Papers given during the meeting were published as John C. McGovern and Chester R. Burns (eds), *Humanism in Medicine* (Springfield, Ill.: Charles C. Thomas, 1973). For details about the meeting, see folders 15, 16, and 17, box 2, IMH Records, Blocker Collections.

227. The committee conducted its deliberations in four phases. The first was an analysis of the knowledge and skills associated with the disciplines of religion and medicine; philosophy and medicine; history and medicine; law and medicine; literature and medicine; and the creative arts and medicine. Students, other faculty, and patients were interviewed during Phase II. During Phase III the committee developed some behavioral objectives that could be used in teaching medical humanities. During Phase IV, the committee created some recommendations about developing teaching programs at UTMB. A copy of the final report is in folder 18, box 2, IMH Records, Blocker Collections.

228. Descriptions of these courses and other activities of the History of Medicine Division between 1969 and 1973 are included in the folders in boxes 1-3, IMH Records, Blocker Collections. Burns wrote the proposal Blocker used. For a copy, see "The Institute for the Medical Humanities at the University of Texas Medical Branch," box 1, vertical file A6, Blocker Collections. Because of the support given to the Marine Biomedical Institute, White thought that the "institute" rubric was still politically viable and Burns suggested the name Institute for the Medical Humanities. To honor Harris Kempner Sr., White persuaded the Kempner family to endow a professorship in the medical humanities.

See Harris L. Kempner, "Remarks on the Announcement of the Harris L. Kempner Professorship of Humanities at the University of Texas Medical Branch," *Texas Reports on Biology and Medicine*, 32 (Spring, 1974), 31–33.

229. The deliberations were published: Lorraine Hunt (ed.), *Proceedings of the Southwest Regional Institute* (Philadelphia: Society for Health and Human Values, 1974). A copy is in vertical file A6, box 1, Blocker Collections. For evaluations of this meeting, see folders 20–22, box 3, IMH Records, Blocker Collections. This spring 1974 issue of *Texas Reports on Biology and Medicine* was number 1 of volume 32. For samples of the responses, see folders 23 and 24, box 3, IMH Records, Blocker Collections.

230. The symposium's proceedings were published: H. Tristram Engelhardt Jr. and Stuart F. Spicker, *Evaluation and Explanation in the Biomedical Sciences* (Boston: D. Reidel, 1975). During 1973 Burns and Engelhardt prepared the grant proposal submitted to the NEH; for a copy, see vertical file A6, box 2, Blocker Collections. UTMB was the second academic medical center to receive an NEH development grant; the first was the Pennsylvania State University College of Medicine in Hershey where Al Vastyan was chair of the department of humanities, the first of its kind in an American medical school. When recruited for the position in Hershey, Vastyan was the Episcopal chaplain and director of the William Temple Community House in Galveston. Burns became the administrator for UTMB's NEH grant. For some letters regarding Bean's appointment, see folder 3, box 16, Levin Papers, Blocker Collections. Bean appointed Burns as the IMH's associate director.

231. Between 1974 and 1979, eight students were teaching assistants and forty-one teachers from other campuses were visiting lecturers or professors. For details about the IMH courses, see boxes 7–13, IMH records. For details on the NEH seminars for practitioners, see boxes 4 and 5, IMH records; H. T. Engelhardt Jr., "The History and Philosophy of Medicine: A Report on a Postgraduate Seminar on the Humanities in Medicine," *Clio Medica*, 10 (June, 1975), 205–211; and Chester R. Burns, "Continuing Education in the Humanities for Practicing Health Care Professionals: A Case Study," *Mobius*, 2 (July, 1982), 122–132.

232. NEH grant funds were available for seven years (1974–1981). For details about the use of these funds, see the annual reports sent to the NEH in boxes 14–18, IMH records, Blocker Collections.

233. Burns was acting director until January 1981; Bill Schottstaedt until Carson arrived. For Carson's goals for the institute, see Ronald A. Carson, "Institute for the Medical Humanities: Plans and Prospects," *Texas Medicine*, 79 (May, 1983), 61–62. For details, see Ronald A. Carson to Myles Knape, May 21 and 28 and June 11, 1986, interviews, Blocker Collections. Beverly DeVries was Carson's administrative assistant.

234. In 1986 Winslade and others created a self-study guide titled *The Texas Medical Jurisprudence Examination*. Designed to assist senior students at UTMB and elsewhere in preparing for licensure exams, this popular study guide has been revised several times.

235. These were Craig Braestrup, Jaclyn Low, and Suzanne Peloquin. Before 1988 Johanna Price and Susan Baker had earned Ph.D. degrees for work done in the Department of Preventive Medicine and Community Health with a concentration in the medical humanities. By 1991 the following foundations and agencies had awarded grants for support of IMH programs: Rockwell Fund, Charles E. Culpepper Foundation, Exxon Foundation, Greenwall Foundation, Florence Hall Endowment, Hogg Foundation for Mental Health, Houston Endowment, Kempner Fund, John P. McGovern Fund for the Behavioral Sciences, Moody Foundation, National Endowment for the Humanities, National Library of Medicine, Sid W. Richardson Foundation, Rockefeller Foundation, and the Texas Committee for the Humanities. For other details about the institute and its funding, see "The Institute for the Medical Humanities 1973–1993: Twentieth Anniversary Report" and "Inside The Institute for the Medical Humanities: Celebrating Twenty Years of Inquiry and Insight, 1973–1993." Copies are in boxes 1 and 2, vertical file A6, Blocker Collections. For an autobiographical account of the development of the IMH, see Chester R. Burns, "A Journey in the Borderlands of Medicine and the Humanities," *Medical Humanities Review*, 15 (Fall, 2001), 9–20.

CHAPTER 7

1. W. S. Carter to H. Y. Benedict, Oct. 31, 1935, letter, box 4Q25, UT President's Records.

2. These conflicts existed in most American medical schools then; see Ludmerer, *Time to Heal*, 49.

3. For the contents of this chapter, I am especially indebted to John Swann, who focused on this aspect of UTMB's history during his years as a research assistant on this project. See his typescript summaries in WF346, 347, and 348, CHP Archives. Also see RF85-124, CHP Archives, and the unnumbered files in boxes 6–8. For the history of research universities in the United States, see Roger L. Geiger, *To Advance Knowledge: The Growth of American Research Universities, 1900–1940* (New York: Oxford University Press, 1986) and Roger L. Geiger, *Research and Relevant*

Knowledge: American Research Universities Since World War II (New York: Oxford University Press, 1993). For a concise overview of the development of research in America's medical schools between 1920 and 1940, see Ludmerer, *Time to Heal*, 30–39. For a short historical overview of medical research in Texas during the twentieth century, see Chester R. Burns, "Medical Research," in Tyler, et al. (eds.), *The New Handbook of Texas*, IV, 599–600.

4. Allen J. Smith to W. L. Prather, Apr. 21, 1903, letter, box 4R82, UT President's Records.

5. The nine subjects were pathology, bacteriology, biology, histology, embryology, medical jurisprudence, mental and nervous diseases, medical climatology, and medicine for nurses.

6. Smith determined the conditions needed for formaldehyde to kill variously prepared cultures of bacteria that caused scarlet fever, typhoid fever, anthrax, and diphtheria. See Allen J. Smith, "Experiments to Determine the Disinfecting Value of the Morris Formaldehyde Generator," *Texas Medical Journal*, 19, no. 2 (1903–1904), 39–54. Smith also published case reports, essays about teaching pathology, and a textbook of bacteriology. For a summary of the teaching responsibilities of the faculty in 1903, for example, see Smith's annual report to UT President Prather in box 4R82, UT President's Records.

7. Minutes, UT Board of Regents, Jan. 15, 1907. Even the medical students wanted more support for research; for examples of their comments, see "The Medical Department: Retrospective and Prospective," *Cactus*, 9 (1902), 93–96; "Quotes and Appeal," *Cactus*, 11 (1904), 330–331; and "Want Column—Medical Department," *Cactus*, 10 (1903), 327.

8. Plant's publications were as follows: "Experiments on the Absorption of Fat from an Isolated Loop of Small Intestine in Healthy Dogs," *American Journal of Physiology*, 23, no. 1 (1908–1909), 65–80; "An Experimental Study of the Use of Nitrites in Accidents Occurring During Anaesthesia," *Texas State Journal of Medicine*, 5 (Sept., 1909), 179–184; and "Further Experiments on the Use of Drugs as Stimulants in Accidents Occurring During Anaesthesia," *Texas State Journal of Medicine*, 6 (Sept., 1910), 184–189. A copy of this latter paper is in RF93, CHP Archives. The *Journal of Experimental Medicine* was established in 1896 as America's first journal devoted to biomedical research. By 1906 about thirty medical schools had at least one faculty member engaged in experimental research; see Ludmerer, *Learning to Heal*, 103.

9. Flexner, *Medical Education in the United States and Canada*, 311; W. S. Carter to S. E. Mezes, May 19, 1910, letter, box 4R82, UT President's Records (quotation). The best source of insights into the values of American medical educators about the importance of research during this time is an anonymously edited book, *Medical Research and Education* (New York: The Science Press, 1913), which contains twenty-eight articles written by twenty-two medical academics at fifteen research universities and institutions.

10. W. Keiller to W. S. Sutton, c. Feb. 1924, letter, box 4Q23, UT President's Records (quotation). Keiller knew that teachers in his Department of Anatomy were unproductive as researchers because they were so busy with teaching; see William Keiller to R. E. Vinson, Jan. 24, 1920, letter, box 4Q22, UT President's Records. As dean, he did recognize the importance of hiring professors for other departments who would do experimental research. See also George E. Bethel to H. Y. Benedict, Nov. 21, 1929, letter, box 4R85, UT President's Records.

11. William C. Rose, "Experimental Studies on Creatine and Creatinine, V: Protein Feeding and Creatine Elimination in Pancreatic Diabetes," *Journal of Biological Chemistry*, 26 (1916), 331–338; William C. Rose, Frank W. Dimmitt, and Paul N. Cheatham, "Experimental Studies on Creatine and Creatinine, VI: Protein Feeding and Creatine Elimination in Fasting Man," *Journal of Biological Chemistry*, 26 (1916), 339–344; and William C. Rose and Frank W. Dimmitt, "Experimental Studies on Creatine and Creatinine, VII: The Fate of Creatine and Creatinine When Administered to Man," *Journal of Biological Chemistry*, 26 (1916), 345–353. See also William C. Rose and Walter T. Garbade to the president of the University of Texas, Feb. 26, 1916, letter, box 4Q21, UT President's Records (quotation).

12. Basic science departments with full-time Ph.D. researchers expanded steadily and significantly in American medical schools during the first half of the twentieth century; see Rothstein, *American Medical Schools and the Practice of Medicine*, 155–159.

13. For details, see RF99, CHP Archives. For the early history of microbiology in the United States, see Paul F. Clark, *Pioneer Microbiologists of America* (Madison: University of Wisconsin Press, 1961).

14. William B. Sharp to W. M. W. Splawn, Apr. 15, 1925; William B. Sharp to H. Y. Benedict, May 1929; and William B. Sharp to H. Y. Benedict, May 10, 1933, letters, box 17, UTMB Dean's Office Records, Inactive. Also see William B. Sharp and Elsie Urbantke, "Influenza Studies, XX: Identification of Fixed Type Pneumococcus Carriers: A Study of Technical Methods," *Journal of Infectious Diseases*, 37 (1925), 473–480; and William B. Sharp and Evelyn Kerans Taylor, "Interdigital Ringworm Control Among Students," *Journal of Preventive Medicine*, 2 (Nov., 1929), 485–491. Sharp also wrote three textbooks: *The Foundation of Health, a Manual of Personal Hygiene for Students* (1924); *Medical Biology, a Manual of Bacteriology, Mycology, Immunology and Parasitology* (1933); and *Practial Microbiology and*

Public Health,. a Textbook for Students of Medicine, Public Health and General Bacteriology (1938). See also William B. Sharp to H. Y. Benedict, May 7, 1930, and George E. Bethel to H. Y. Benedict, c. 1930, box 16; and George E. Bethel to H. Y. Benedict, Aug. 27, 1932, box 17, letters, UTMB Dean's Office Records, Inactive. Also see T. L. Johnson, "In Vivo Trypanolysis with Special Reference to Zones of Inhibition, Relapse Phenomena and Immunological Specificity," *American Journal of Hygiene*, 9 (Mar., 1929), 260–283.

15. William B. Sharp to H. Y. Benedict, May 10, 1933, and William B. Sharp to George Bethel, Aug. 5, 1932, letters, box 21, UTMB Dean's Office Records, Inactive. In 1922 Joseph Kass, a graduate of UTMB in 1913, began donating $150 a year to support a medical student who wanted to do research in this department. From three to five applications, a faculty committee selected one student as the J. B. Kass Fellow for an academic year. This student was expected to devote about 280 hours to research during that year. See *UTMB Catalog* (1923–1924), 14; and William B. Sharp to H. Y. Benedict, May 7, 1930, and William B. Sharp to H. Y. Benedict, May 25, 1932, letters, box 17, UTMB Dean's Office Records, Inactive. For reports of two fellows [George Horton (1928–1929) and Emile Zax (1930–1931)], see the Kass Fellowship Committee folder in box 24, UTMB Dean's Office Records, Inactive.

16. H. V. Atkinson to R. E. Vinson, Mar. 23, 1923, and H. V. Atkinson to W. M. W. Splawn, Apr. 20, 1925, letters, box 16, UTMB Dean's Office Records, Inactive. Atkinson did deliver a paper on the toxicity of impurities in wood alcohol at the meeting of the American Society of Pharmacology and Experimental Therapeutics in 1924; see "The Toxicity of Impurities in Wood Alcohol, I: Allyl Alcohol," *Journal of Pharmacological and Experimental Therapeutics*, 25 (Mar., 1925), 144. For reasons that are not clear, Atkinson was dismissed in 1925; see Minutes, UTMB Executive Committee, May 18, 1925; Henry Hartman to W. M. W. Splawn, Apr. 15, 1926, and H. V. Atkinson to W. M. W. Splawn, Apr. 15, 1926, letters, box 4Q24, UT President's Records. For the early history of pharmacology in the United States, see John Parascandola, *The Development of American Pharmacology: John J. Abel and the Shaping of a Discipline* (Baltimore: Johns Hopkins University Press, 1992).

17. W. T. Dawson, "Report of the Pharmacology Department of the Medical Branch, 1927–28"; and W. T. Dawson to H. Y. Benedict, June 14, 1929, and May 15, 1931, letters, box 16, UTMB Dean's Office Records, Inactive. For research reports, see W. T. Dawson and Oscar Bodansky, "Interruption of Perfusion of Isolated Rabbit Heart Upon Reaction of Coronary Flow," *Proceedings of the Society of Experimental Biology and Medicine*, 28 (Mar., 1931), 635–636; W. T. Dawson and Francis A. Garbade, "Idiosyncracy to Quinine, Cinchonidine and Ethylhydrocupreine and Other Levorotatory Alkaloids of the Cinchona Series: Further Chemical Delimitation of the Idiosyncracy: Alteration in Sensitiveness," *Journal of Pharmacological and Experimental Therapeutics*, 39 (Aug., 1930), 417–424; and J. P. Sanders and W. T. Dawson, "Efficacy of Quinidine in Malaria," *Journal of the American Medical Association*, 99 (Nov. 19, 1932), 1773–1777. Also see W. T. Dawson and E. L. Porter, "Barbiturate-Strychnine Antagonism in the Spinal Cat," *Proceedings of the Society of Experimental Biology and Medicine*, 31 (June, 1934), 1048–50. For more on Dawson's legacy, see Hans Ash, "Historical Development of the Department of Pharmacology and Toxicology," 36–56. Ash was the principal lab attendant in this department for many years. His scrapbook is in the Blocker Collections (MS 6). For a tribute to Dawson after his death in 1939, see *Bulletin of the John Sealy Hospital and the School of Medicine of the University of Texas*, 2 (Mar., 1940), 49. For details about research in the department before 1942, see Charles H. Taft, "Fifty Years of Pharmacology at the Medical Branch of the University of Texas," box 3, vertical file A8, Blocker Collections.

18. Eugene L. Porter to W. M. W. Splawn, Apr. 22, 1925, letter; Eugene L. Porter, "Annual Report for 1926–27"; Eugene L. Porter to Henry Hartman, Mar. 24, 1928, letter; and Eugene L. Porter to H. Y. Benedict, June 15, 1929, letter; all in box 16, UTMB Dean's Office Records, Inactive. Also see E. L. Porter, "The Tonic Contraction of Decerebrate Rigidity Compared With Nerve-Muscle Response in the Same Muscle," *American Journal of Physiology*, 81, no. 2 (1927), 504–505; and E. L. Porter, "Evidence that the Postural Tonus of Decerebrate Rigidity Increases in Amount by the Successive Innervation of Single Motor Neurones," *American Journal of Physiology*, 91, no. 1 ((1930), 345–361. Porter guided the research activities of several medical students and some master's degree candidates; see E. L. Porter to Henry Hartman, Mar. 24, 1928 and E. L. Porter to H. Y. Benedict, June 15, 1934, letters, box 16, UTMB Dean's Office Records, Inactive. For the early history of physiology in the United States, see W. Bruce Fye, *The Development of American Physiology: Scientific Medicine in the Nineteenth Century* (Baltimore: Johns Hopkins University Press, 1987).

19. Eugene L. Porter to H. Y. Benedict, June 15, 1929, June 6, 1930, and June 1, 1931; Eugene L. Porter to George Bethel, Sept. 17, 1931, box 21; and Eugene L. Porter to H. Y. Benedict, May 31, 1933, box 17, letters; all in UTMB Dean's Office Records, Inactive. Also see W. A. Selle and Meyer Bodansky, "Effect of Bromcaproic Acid on Rat Sarcoma 39," *American Journal of Cancer*, 23, no. 2 (1935), 289–296; W. A. Selle, "Progress in Cancer Research I Animal Experimentation and the Solution of the Cancer Problem," *Texas State Journal of Medicine*, 40 (June, 1944), 52–56;

Homer E. Prince, et al., "Molds in the Etiology of Asthma and Hay Fever: A Preliminary Report," *Texas State Journal of Medicine*, 30 (Sept., 1934), 340–344; and *Galveston Daily News*, Nov. 3, 1946.

20. Hendrix received his Ph.D. in biochemistry at Yale only a few years after Rose. Hendrix was a member of the faculty at the University of Pennsylvania when he accepted the offer to come to Galveston. He was chair for twenty-six years (1922–1948). For more details, see RF97, CHP Archives. For the early history of biochemistry in the United States, see Robert E. Kohler, *From Medical Chemistry to Biochemistry: The Making of a Biomedical Discipline* (Cambridge: Cambridge University Press, 1982). Bodansky's popular text, *Introduction to Physiological Chemistry*, appeared in 1926, the first of four editions. For more on the textbook, see B. M. Hendrix to W. M. W. Splawn, May 26, 1927, letter, box 16, UTMB Dean's Office Records, Inactive; and M. Bodansky to B. M. Hendrix, Jan. 13, 1939, letter, box 1, Bodansky Papers, Blocker Collections.

21. B. M. Hendrix to W. M. W. Splawn, May 26, 1927; B. M. Hendrix to H. Y. Benedict, May 30, 1929, and May 29,1930, box 16; B. M. Hendrix to H. Y. Benedict, June 15, 1934; and B. M. Hendrix to J. W. Calhoun, Aug. 30, 1937, box 17, letters; all in UTMB Dean's Office Records, Inactive. Also see B. M. Hendrix and Ava J. McAmis, "Alkalosis in Dogs Following Injection of Hydrazine," Proceedings, American Society of Biological Chemists, Eighteenth Annual Meeting, Dec. 27–29, 1923, in *Journal of Biological Chemistry*, 59 (1924), xxii; Byron M. Hendrix, "The Resorption of Copper and Ferrocyanide Ions By Coagulative Proteins," *Journal of Biological Chemistry*, 78 (Aug., 1928), 653–660; B. M. Hendrix to W. M. W. Splawn, May 26, 1927; B. M. Hendrix to H. Y. Benedict, May 30, 1929 and May 29, 1930; and B. M. Hendrix to H. Y. Benedict, Jul 5, 1932, letters, box 17, UTMB Dean's Office Records, Inactive; and Marion Fay, "Strontium as a Source of Error in Blood Calcium Determinations, *American Journal of Physiology*, 77, no. 1 (1926), 73–75. Fay later became dean of the Women's Medical College in Philadelphia; see *University Medical*, 3 (Mar., 1972), 16.

22. Between 1919 and 1922 Bodansky taught biochemistry to medical students and organic chemistry to pharmacy students and did enough research to earn a master's degree and write six published articles; see M. Bodansky to William Keiller, Aug. 1, 1922, letter, box 4R84, UT President's Records. For examples of Bodansky's subsequent research, see the following publications: "The Action of Hydrazine and Some of its Derivatives in Producing Liver Injury as Measured by the Effect on Levulose Tolerance," *Journal of Biological Chemistry*, 58 (Jan., 1924), 799–811; "The Distribution of the Unsaturated Fatty Acids, Cholesterol, and Cholesterol Esters In Experimental Anemia," *Journal of Experimental Biology*, 63 (Mar., 1925), 239–251; "Creatine Metabolism in a Case of Generalized Myositis Fibrosa," *Journal of Experimental Biology*, 85 (Dec., 1929), 307–325; and "The Permeability and Haemolytic Action of the Fatty Acids and Some of their Halogen Derivatives," *Journal of Experimental Biology*, 10 (Jan., 1933), 59–66. Also see M. Bodansky and Virginia B. Duff, "Influence of Glycine on Depleted Creatine Reserves of Skeletal and Cardiac Muscle in Experimental Hyperthyroidism," *Proceedings of the Society of Experimental Biology and Medicine*, 34 (Apr., 1936), 307–312; and Harry Levine, et al., "The Effect of Liver Damage on the Blood Level and Action of Paraldehyde," *Journal of Pharmacological and Experimental Therapeutics*, 67 (Nov., 1939), 299–306.

23. In the official budgets of the regents, this department is listed with the clinical departments and Bodansky is designated a part-time professor. I have found no evidence to indicate that the regents appointed Bodansky as "chair" or "head" of this department, but he did submit annual reports like the chairs of other departments. For details, see RF98, CHP Archives. See also Minutes, Sealy & Smith Foundation Board of Directors, Oct. 28, 1931. For a list of Brindley's publications before 1943, see the scrapbook for the Department of Pathology in the Blocker Collections. For a historical analysis of the evolution of pathology in the United States, see Esmond R. Long, *A History of American Pathology* (Springfield, Ill.: Charles C. Thomas, 1962). For more about Bodansky, see J. Andrew Grant, "Leaders of the University of Texas Medical Branch at Galveston," *Texas Medicine*, 87 (Dec., 1991), 44–45.

24. H. O. Knight to H. Y. Benedict, July 8, 1932; H. O. Knight to H. Y. Benedict, July 15, 1935; and H. O. Knight to H. Y. Benedict, July 14, 1936 (quotation), box 17, UTMB Dean's Office Records, Inactive. For a tribute to Knight after his death in 1939, see *Bulletin of the John Sealy Hospital and the School of Medicine of the University of Texas*, 2 (Mar., 1940), 51.

25. To sample Duncan's work, see "A Determination of the Number of Nerve Fibers in the Eighth Thoracic and Largest Lumbar Ventral Roots of the Albino Rat," *Journal of Comparative Neurology*, 59 (Feb., 1934), 47–60; "The Relation between Axone Diameter and Myelination Determined by Measurement of Myelinated Spinal Root Fibers," *Journal of Comparative Neurology*, 60 (Dec., 1934), 437–471; "The Incidence of Mild Degrees of Atrophy in the Fasciculus Gracilis," *Archives of Pathology*, 26 (Sept., 1938), 664–675; and "Some Effects of Anaesthetic Mixtures Dissolved in Oil on Motor Nerves in the Cat," *Proceedings of the Society of Experimental Biology and Medicine*, 42 (1939), 405–407. See also Donald Duncan, "The Importance of Diameter as a Factor in Myelination," *Science*, 79 (Apr. 20,

1934), 363; and W. T. Dawson, D. Duncan, E. D. Hollar, and C. H. Taft Jr., "Trauma in Strychnine Poisoning," *American Journal of Physiology*, 113, no. 1 (1935), 34–35. For a bibliography of Duncan's writings, see folder 1, box 1, Duncan Papers.

26. John G. Sinclair to H. Y. Benedict, May 21, 1929, and May 18, 1931, box 16; and John G. Sinclair to J. W. Calhoun, June 4, 1937, box 17, letters, UTMB Dean's Office Records, Inactive; and John G. Sinclair to Meyer Bodansky, Aug. 21, 1931, letter, box 1, Bodansky Papers. For details about Sinclair's work, see RF94 and RF95, CHP Archives.

27. The attitudes and activities of American clinicians interested in experimental research on humans are traced in A. McGehee Harvey, *Science at the Bedside: Clinical Research in American Medicine, 1905–1945* (Baltimore: Johns Hopkins University Press, 1981). See F. W. Aves, "The Hemorrhagic Tendency in Obstructive Jaundice and its Preoperative Treatment—with Experiments," *Texas State Journal of Medicine*, 12 (Feb., 1917), 382–385. A graduate of UTMB in 1911, Aves was an instructor in the Department of Surgery and chief of the Surgical Outpatient Clinic when he conducted these experiments.

28. M. D. Levy, "The Normal Differential Leucocytic Count as Determined by a Study of 114 Adults," *Texas State Journal of Medicine*, 13 (Sept., 1917), 179–181. He also thought that the 30 to 50 percent range of total white blood cells in cases of tuberculosis, pellagra, and syphilis represented normal variations and not the results of a disease process. A UTMB graduate in 1913, Levy was the hospital's clinical pathologist and instructor in the Department of Medicine.

29. For more about these and other studies in these departments, see the annual reports for the years 1922–1937 in UTMB Dean's Office Records, Inactive.

30. C. T. Stone to W. M. W. Splawn, July 5, 1926, letter, box 4Q23, UT President's Records. He visited departments at Tulane, Vanderbilt, Washington University, University of Iowa, University of Minnesota, University of Chicago, University of Michigan, Western Reserve University, and the University of Pennsylvania. He then spent several months in Europe, attending clinics and visiting research labs in Berlin, Vienna, Paris, Edinburgh, and London. For a biographical sketch of Stone, see Chester R. Burns, "Charles Turner Stone Sr.," in Tyler, et al. (eds.), *The New Handbook of Texas*, VI, 110–111.

31. C. T. Stone to H. Y. Benedict, Jan. 10, 1931, box 16; George Bethel to H. Y. Benedict, Nov. 12, 1931, box 27; and C. T. Stone to H. Y. Benedict, June 15, 1932, box 17, letter; all in UTMB Dean's Office Records, Inactive; and George E. Bethel to H. Y. Benedict, Oct. 24, 1932, letter, box 4Q25, UT President's Records. Herrmann's interest in UTMB may have been kindled by George Dock, who was professor of medicine and dean at Washington University School of Medicine between 1910 and 1922. Between 1918 and 1925 Herrmann was a resident, instructor, and assistant professor in internal medicine at this school. During these years he also completed work for a Ph.D. from the University of Michigan. Dock had been professor of pathology at the Texas Medical College and Hospital in Galveston between 1888 and 1891. For more details, see RF200, CHP Archives; Chester R. Burns, "George R. Herrmann," in Tyler, et al. (eds.), *The New Handbook of Texas*, III, 579; Harvey, *Science at the Bedside*, 280–281; and J. Andrew Grant, "Leaders of the University of Texas Medical Branch at Galveston," *Texas Medicine*, 87 (Dec., 1991), 47–48.

32. C. T. Stone to H. Y. Benedict, June 15, 1932; C. T. Stone to H. Y. Benedict, June 20, 1930, and C. T. Stone to H. Y. Benedict, June 10, 1931, letters, box 16, UTMB Dean's Office Records, Inactive. For examples of their investigative work, see George Herrmann, et al., "Diuresis in Patients with Congestive Heart Failure," *Journal of the American Medical Association*, 99 (Nov. 12, 1932), 1647–1652; and George Herrmann, et al, "Some Studies in the Mechanism of Diuresis in Patients with Congestive Heart Failure," *Transactions of the Association of American Physicians*, 47 (1932), 279–291. See also C. T. Stone to H. Y. Benedict, June 15, 1932, letter, box 16, UTMB Dean's Office Records, Inactive. As another example of collaborative research, see George Herrmann, et al., "On the Advantage of Altering the Vegetable and Metallic Diuretics in the Treatment of Edema of Congestive Heart Failure," *Journal of Laboratory and Clinical Medicine*, 18 (June, 1933), 902–915.

33. C. T. Stone to H. Y. Benedict, Aug. 30, 1934, Aug. 31, 1935, Aug. 20, 1936, and Aug. 31, 1937, box 17, letters, UTMB Dean's Office Records, Inactive. For samples of their work, see Charles T. Stone, "Peptic Ulcer: Benign or Malignant," *Southwestern Medicine*, 20 (Feb., 1936), 44–47; George Herrmann and George Decherd, "Creative Mobilization in Myocardial Damage," *Proceedings of the Society of Experimental Biology and Medicine*, 32 (Dec., 1934), 477–478; William Marr, "The Problem of the Diagnosis of the More Common Blood Dyscrasias," *Texas State Journal of Medicine*, 34 (Jan., 1939), 599–603; and Victor E. Schultze and Edward H. Schwab, "Arteriolar Hypertension in the American Negro," *American Heart Journal*, 11 (Jan., 1936), 66–74.

34. Robert M. Moore to A. L. Singleton, May 24, 1930, and June 4, 1930, box 21; and A. L. Singleton to H. Y. Benedict, May 27, 1931, box 16, letters, UTMB Dean's Office Records, Inactive. When offered the job at UTMB, Moore was a resident in surgery at Washington University in St. Louis. Before that, he had spent two post-internship

years at Harvard learning experimental techniques from Walter B. Cannon. See Robert M. Moore to George Bethel, Apr. 28, 1934, letter, box 17, UTMB Dean's Office Records, Inactive. For examples of his research, see Robert M. Moore, et al., "Vasoconstrictor Fibers: Peripheral Course as Revealed by a Roentgenographic method," *Archives of Surgery*, 26 (Feb., 1933), 308–322; and Robert M. Moore and C. W. Braselton Jr., "Experiments in Gas Embolism," *Bulletin of the John Sealy Hospital and the School of Medicine of the University of Texas*, 1 (May, 1939), 78–81. Moore collaborated with Singleton on a study of pain sensitivity, and with Singleton and Harris Williams on an investigation of the duration of vascular paralysis in relation to certain sympathetic nervous pathways. Moore also used the laboratory to teach a required course on operative surgery for senior medical students.

35. Willard R. Cooke to H. Y. Benedict, June 8, 1932, letter, box 17, UTMB Dean's Office Records, Inactive (quotation). Cooke attributed time consumed by clinical tests to an insufficient number of technicians. See Willard R. Cooke to H. Y. Benedict, Mar. 13, 1928, box 16; Willard R. Cooke to Benedict, Oct. 21, 1929, June 2, 1930, and May 23, 1931; W. R. Cooke to George E. Bethel, Aug. 30, 1930, box 21; and Willard R. Cooke to W. S. Carter, Sept. 1, 1937, box 17, letters, UTMB Dean's Office Records, Inactive; and *Galveston Daily News*, Oct. 11, 1942.

36. "News from the Medical Department," *Alcalde*, 5 (1916), 63. To control expenses, teachers of pharmacology and physiology shared the same equipment. See W. S. Carter to R. E. Vinson, Apr. 28, 1921, and R. E. Vinson to W. S. Carter, Apr. 29, 1921, letter, box 4R84, UT President's Records; H. V. Atkinson to R. E. Vinson, Mar. 23, 1923, and Charles A. Gault to Robert E. Vinson, Mar. 17, 1923, letters, box 16, UTMB Dean's Office Records, Inactive. After the Departments of Anatomy and Pathology occupied the Keiller Building, the Medical College Building (Old Red) housed labs and offices for Biochemistry (third floor), Bacteriology (second floor), Physiology and Pharmacology (first floor), and Pharmacy (basement). See William Keiller to W. S. Sutton, c. Feb. 1924, letter, box 4Q25, UT President's Records.

37. Elisabeth D. Runge to H. Y. Benedict, July 1, 1932, letter, box 17, UTMB Dean's Office Records, Inactive.

38. W. S. Carter to R. E. Vinson, Mar 15, 1919, letter, box 4Q22, UT President's Records (quotation); and William Keiller to W. S. Sutton, May 13, 1924, letter, box 27, UTMB Dean's Office Records, Inactive.

39. Eugene Porter to P. L. Gray, July 19, 1930, box 21 (quotation); and George Bethel to H. Y. Benedict, Dec. 7, 1932, box 27, letters, UTMB Dean's Office Records, Inactive.

40. William Keiller to W. S. Sutton, Apr. 7, 1924, box 27, UTMB Dean's Office Records, Inactive (quotation); W. S. Carter to R. E. Vinson, July 15, 1921, letter, box 4R84, UT President's Records; Minutes, UT Board of Regents, July 29, 1939.

41. W. S. Carter to J. W. Calhoun, Nov. 1, 1937, letter, box 4Q18, UT President's Records (quotation), and *Galveston Daily News*, May 13, 1937.

42. *Bulletin of the John Sealy Hospital and the School of Medicine of the University of Texas*, 1 (Oct., 1939), 96.

43. The other three were Sharp, Herrmann, and Bodansky.

44. Packchanian came to Galveston from the National Institutes of Health, where he studied trypanosomiasis and Weil's disease. Terry later became Surgeon General of the United State Public Health Service. See also *Galveston Daily News*, Feb. 9, 1941.

45. *Bulletin of the John Sealy Hospital and the School of Medicine of the University of Texas*, 1 (Feb., 1939), 37. When Spies became CEO he was the author or co-author (mostly) of no more than twenty-five journal articles, of which only nine involved experimental research. For a list of these, see RF223, CHP Archives. Spies wanted to retitle the publication as the "University of Texas Medical Journal" and make it a quarterly publication of the Alumni Association; see John W. Spies to Conn L. Milburn, Sept. 5, 1940, letter, box VF 9/B, UT President's Records. After eighteen months, however, it fell by the wayside, another victim of the political wars described in chapter two.

46. After Robert Moore left for military service, Spies and A. O. Singleton feuded over Moore's successor. Over Singleton's objection, Spies appointed Joseph Roberts as the director of the experimental lab. For more details, see A. O. Singleton to Robert M. Moore, June 27, 1942; Johns W. Spies to Homer P. Rainey, July 2, 1942; and A. O. Singleton to Homer P. Rainey, July 9, 1942, letters, all in box VF 9/A, UT President's Records.

47. Minutes, Meetings of the Research Council, Jan. 9 and 23, Feb. 6, Mar. 21 and 26, Apr. 9 and 26, 1941; and Luther L. Terry to John W. Spies, Feb. 11, 1941, letter, box 3, Bodansky Papers. See also Minutes, Meetings of the Research Council, Dec. 3 and 17, 1940, and Mar. 26, 1941, box 3, Bodansky Papers.

48. John E. Deitrick and Robert C. Berson, *Medical Schools in the United States at Mid-Century* (New York: McGraw-Hill, 1953), 37–42, and E. M. MacEwen and Fred C. Zapffe, "Report of Inspection of University of Texas School of Medicine," in box VF 18/C, UT President's Records (quotation).

49. *Galveston Daily News*, Nov. 13, 1942. For a list, see vertical file G3, box 1, Blocker Collections.

50. For the history and status of medical research in the United States during the years of Leake's tenure as CEO at UTMB, see Richard Harrison Shryock, *American Medical Research, Past and Present* (New York: Commonwealth Fund, 1947); and Esther Everett Lape, *Medical Research: A Midcentury Survey* (Boston: Little, Brown and Company, 1955).

51. During these four years, Leake hired other research-minded faculty. For the names of the fourteen employed in 1943–1944 alone, see pages 4 and 5 of Leake's annual report for that year in folder 19, box 2, Leake Papers, Blocker Collections. Leake identified one or more faculty in all fifteen medical school departments who were engaged in research that year (pages 16–20 of the annual report). The publications of the faculty between 1948 and 1962 are listed in five bound volumes published by the UT Graduate School: UT Publication no. 5707 covers 1948–1954; UT Publication no. 5821 covers 1955 and 1956; UT Publication no. 6019 covers 1957 and 1958; UT Publication no. 6312 covers 1959 and 1960; and UT Publication no. 6520 covers 1961 and 1962. In subsequent notes these numbers will be used to identify these volumes. Copies are in boxes 1 and 2 of vertical file G3 in the Blocker Collections.

52. John G. Sinclair, "Annual Report of the Department of Anatomy, 1944–1945," Oct. 26, 1945, folder 17, box 2, Leake Papers, Blocker Collections; and C. M. Pomerat, "Reticulo-Endothelial Immune Serum (REIS), *Texas Reports on Biology and Medicine*, 3 (Fall, 1945), 404–411. For titles of more than one hundred articles Pomerat authored and co-authored, see UT Publication no. 5707, 205–209; UT Publication no. 5821, 137–139; and UT Publication no. 6019, 166–168. Also see folder 11, box 9; folder 4, box 16; and folder 6, box 19, Department of Anatomy records, Blocker Collections. A tribute to Pomerat that includes a bibliography of his writings is in *Texas Reports on Biology and Medicine*, 23 (June, 1965), supplement I, 156–188.

53. In the summer of 1948, for example, twelve students worked in Pomerat's lab; see *Galveston Tribune*, July 5, 1948. For other details, see RF216, CHP Archives; *UTMB: Seventy-five Year History*, 225–229; *Biomedical Inquiry*, 3 (Autumn, 1991), 10; and J. Andrew Grant, "Leaders of the University of Texas Medical Branch at Galveston," *Texas Medicine*, 87 (Dec., 1991), 45–47. See T. C. Hsu and C. M. Pomerat, "Mammalian Chromosomes *in vitro*. II. A Method for Spreading the Chromosomes of Cells in Tissue Culture," *Journal of Heredity*, 44 (Jan.–Feb., 1953), 23–29. Also see Meyer Friedman and Gerald W. Friedland, *Medicine's 10 Greatest Discoveries* (New Haven: Yale University Press, 1998).

54. Glenn Drager, "Innervation of the Avian Hypophysis," *Endocrinology*, 36 (Feb., 1944), 124–129. For other articles by Drager, see UT Publication no. 5707, 202 and UT Publication no. 5821, 136. See also Leake, "Annual Report" (1943–1944), 18–19; Chauncey D. Leake to S. L. Bhatia, Mar. 30, 1945, box 19, and Chauncey D. Leake to George Gentry, Mar. 22, 1948, box 35, letters, Leake Papers, NLM. For titles of more than sixty publications by Emerson, see UT Publication no. 5707, 237–240; UT Publication no. 5821, 156; and UT Publication no. 6019, 188.

55. Leake, "Annual Report" (1943–1944), 19–20; J. Allen Scott, "Simplified Quantitative Methods for Hookworm Control Programs," *American Journal of Tropical Medicine*, 26 (May, 1946), 331–337; J. Allen Scott, "Hookworm Disease in Texas," *Texas Reports on Biology and Medicine*, 3 (Winter, 1945), 558–568; and *Galveston Daily News*, Dec. 1, 1946. For titles of more than thirty-five articles by Scott, see UT Publication no. 5707, 252–253; UT Publication no. 5821, 162–163; and UT Publication no. 6019, 195. Scott also established a statistical division that used IBM punch card machines to analyze research data for some faculty; see J. Allen Scott and Peggy McDonough Brenkus, "The Functions and Methodology of a Hospital Statistical Division," *Texas Reports on Biology and Medicine*, 9 (Spring, 1951), 146–147.

56. For a sample of Pollard's writings, see Morris Pollard and Mary S. Finegold, "The Concentration of Human Poliomyelitis Virus by Precipitation with Methanol," *Texas Reports on Biology and Medicine*, 6 (Summer, 1948), 200–205, and Morris Pollard, "Failure to Propagate Human Poliomyelitis Virus in Developing Avian Embryos," *Texas Reports on Biology and Medicine*, 7 (Fall, 1949), 480–483. For titles of more than thirty publications by Pollard, see UT Publication no. 5707, 251–252; UT Publication no. 5821, 161–162; and UT Publication no. 6019, 194. Also see *Galveston Daily News*, Oct. 27, 1946; Jan. 14, 1951, and Nov. 28, 1951; and Lape, *Medical Research: A Midcentury Survey*, II, 339–516.

57. See Frazier's report to Chauncey Leake in folder 17, box 2, Leake Papers, Blocker Collections. For an example of Frazier's approach, see H. F. Johnson and C. N. Frazier, "Penicillin in Prenatal Syphilis," *Texas Reports on Biology and Medicine*, 6 (Winter, 1948), 427–435. See also Chauncey D. Leake to George W. Cox, June 14, 1944, letter, folder 26, box 3, Leake Papers, Blocker Collections, and Chauncey D. Leake to William S. Middleton, May 25, 1943, letter, box 50, Leake Papers, NLM. Also see *Galveston Daily News*, May 26, and Aug. 29, 1943; and Apr. 7, 1944. With funding from the Office of Scientific Research and Development, Gingrich also tested chloroquine as an anti-malarial in canaries infected with malaria; see *Galveston Daily News*, Sept. 29, 1946.

58. Leake, "Annual Report," Aug. 31, 1944; Chauncey D. Leake to S. L. Bhatia, Mar. 30, 1945, letter, box 19, Leake Papers, NLM; and *Galveston Daily News*, Apr. 28, 1953. The Buchanan Foundation contributed $40,000 annually to

UTMB between 1943 and 1947. For examples of Hansen's research, see Arild E. Hansen and Hilda F. Wiese, "Fat in the Diet in Relation to Nutrition of the Dog. I. Characteristic Appearance and Gross Changes of Animals Fed Diets With and Without Fat," *Texas Reports on Biology and Medicine*, 9 (Fall, 1951), 491–515; Hilda F. Wiese and Arild E. Hansen, "Fat in the Diet in Relation to Nutrition of the Dog. II. Lipid Composition of Tissues from Animals Fed Diets With and Without Dietary Fat," *Texas Reports on Biology and Medicine*, 9 (Fall, 1951), 516–544; Hilda F. Wiese and Arild E. Hansen, "Fat in the Diet in Relation to Nutrition of the Dog. III. Spectral Analysis for Unsaturated Fatty Acid Content of Tissues From Animals Fed Diets With and Without Fat," *Texas Reports on Biology and Medicine*, 9 (Fall, 1951), 545–554; Arild E. Hansen, S. Grant Holmes, and Hilda F. Wiese, "Fat in the Diet in Relation to Nutrition of the Dog. IV. Histologic Features of Skin From Animals Fed Diets With and Without Fat," *Texas Reports on Biology and Medicine*, 9 (Fall, 1951), 555–570; Hilda F. Wiese, Reagan H. Gibbs, and Arild E. Hansen, "Essential Fatty Acids and Human Nutrition. I. Serum Level for Unsaturated Fatty Acids in Healthy Children," *Journal of Nutrition*, 52 (Mar., 1954), 355–365; and Arild E. Hansen and Hilda F. Wiese, "Essential Fatty Acids and Human Nutrition. II. Serum Level for Unsaturated Fatty Acids in Poorly-Nourished Infants and Children," *Journal of Nutrition*, 52 (Mar., 1954), 367–374. For titles of more than seventy publications by Hansen, see UT Publication no. 5707, 233–234; UT Publication no. 5821, 155; and UT Publication no. 6019, 186–187. For the award, see Lori E. Rogers, "The Need for Linoleic Acid is At Least Skin Deep," *Biomedical Inquiry*, 3 (Autumn, 1991), 8.

59. See Raymond Gregory to C. T. Stone Sr., Dec. 3, 1941, letter, folder 7, box 41, Stone Papers, Blocker Collections. For reports about Gregory's work, see *Galveston Daily News*, Dec. 20, 1942, and Sept. 15, 1943. For some of Gregory's publications, see UT Publication no. 5821, 143, 242–243 and UT Publication no. 6019, 173. Also see Lape, *Medical Research: A Midcentury Survey*, II, 223–258.

60. *Galveston Daily News*, May 25, 1943, and July 8 and 17, 1949. For a sample of his research, see Carl A. Nau, "The Accidental Generation of Arsine Gas in an Industry," *Southern Medical Journal*, 41 (Apr., 1948), 341. For titles of other articles, see UT Publication no. 5707, 251; UT Publication no. 5821, 161; and UT Publication no. 6019, 193.

61. *Galveston Daily News*, Nov. 10 and Dec. 5, 1943; and Oct. 13, 1946. For examples of his research, see Madero Bader and Ludwik Anigstein, "Specificity of Bullis Fever Rickettsia," *Texas Reports on Biology and Medicine*, 2 (Winter, 1944), 405–412; Charles M. Pomerat and Ludwik Anigstein, "Anti-Reticular Immune Serum: Its Action Demonstrated by Tissue Culture Technique," *Science*, 100 (Nov. 17, 1944), 456; and Charles Marc Pomerat and Ludwik Anigstein, "Reticulo-Endothelial Immune Serum (R.E.I.S.): I. Its Action on Spleen *in vitro*," *Texas Reports on Biology and Medicine*, 3 (Spring, 1945), 122–141. Between 1948 and 1958 Anigstein wrote or co-authored thirty articles; for their titles, see UT Publication no. 5707, 248–249; UT Publication no. 5821, 159; and UT Publication no. 6019, 192.

62. *Galveston Daily News*, Dec. 29, 1963. Between 1946 and 1956 Packchanian received more than $100,000 in research grants and contracts. For a list of these, see folder 92, box 10, Packchanian Papers, Blocker Collections. During the 1950s he went to Africa to supervise clinical tests of nitrofurazone, a drug used to treat sleeping sickness; *Galveston Daily News*, Aug. 13, 1963. For citations to more than forty of his publications, see UT Publication no. 5707, 213–214; UT Publication no. 5821, 149; and UT Publication no. 6019, 180. In 1983 the eighty-three-year-old scientist presented a paper at the fifty-eighth annual meeting of the American Society of Parasitology in San Antonio; see *Impact*, 8 (Feb. 10, 1984), 13. For details, see the thirteen boxes of Packchanian Papers in the Blocker Collections.

63. *Galveston Daily News*, July 8, 1943, and Minutes, Sealy & Smith Foundation Board of Directors, July 16, 1943. The faculty also published in numerous state, regional, and national journals. See Leake, "Annual Reports," Aug. 31, 1943, 8–9; Leake, "Annual Reports," Aug. 31, 1944, 14–15; Chauncey D. Leake to Molly Harrower, Sept. 21, 1954, letter, box 38, Leake Papers, NLM; John Sinclair, "Report to the Faculty," Oct. 4, 1955; and Chauncey D. Leake to John Sinclair, Sept. 20, 1957, letter, box 65, Leake Papers, NLM. For a tribute to Leake that includes a list of his publications between 1942 and 1955, see *Texas Reports on Biology and Medicine*, 13 (Winter, 1955), 707–711. That the University of Texas System attempted to take over *Texas Reports* in the late 1950s testifies to the journal's success. Early in 1958 Gordon Whaley, dean of the Graduate School in Austin, wanted the journal edited and produced in Austin. Whaley wanted a broader journal devoted to basic biology as well as the biomedical sciences and he wanted to eliminate clinical papers. The regents sided with Whaley, but they rescinded their decision after a strong protest by the faculty at UTMB. For details, see John G. Sinclair to Chauncey D. Leake, Jan. 3, 1958, May 23, 1958, June 18, 1958, and Oct. 24, 1958, letters, box 65, Leake Papers, NLM; [W. Gordon Whaley], "Proposal for an All-University Publication in the Biological Sciences and Medicine," four-page typescript, n.d., attached to W. Gordon Whaley to Melvin A. Casberg, et al., July 30, 1958, letter, box VF G/4, UT Chancellor's Records; W. Gordon Whaley to Logan Wilson, Jan. 5, 1952, letter, box VF 30/A, UT President's Records; Minutes, UT Board of Regents, Mar. 13–14, 1959;

Minutes, UTMB Faculty Meeting, May 14, 1959, and May 21, 1959; and [W. Gordon Whaley] to Donald Duncan, Aug. 7, 1959, letter, box VF 30/A, UT President's Records.

64. A campus-wide research seminar began meeting weekly in 1943, appealing not only to pre-clinical and clinical faculty, but also to residents, interns, and students. Leake, "Annual Reports," Aug. 31, 1944; Raymond Gregory, "Seminar Program," c. 1944, folder 19, box 2, Leake Papers, UTMB; and B. M. Hendrix to Chauncey D. Leake, Oct. 20, 1945, letter, folder 17, box 2, Leake Papers, UTMB. See also Minutes, UTMB Faculty Meetings, Oct. 10, 1949, and Nov. 7, 1950; and Chester R. Burns, "The Health Sciences," in *100 Years of Science and Technology in Texas*, 292.

65. Ella Sealy Newell to Chauncey D. Leake, Nov. 9, 1946, letter, box 53; Chauncey D. Leake to E. A. Fennel, Feb. 21, 1947, letter, box 32; Chauncey D. Leake to Morris Fishbein, Apr. 24, 1948, letter, box 32; folder "Pauling, Linus— 1948–77," box 55; C. M. Pomerat to C. D. Leake, Mar. 12, 1957, letter, box 56; and John G. Sinclair to Chauncey Leake, Oct. 4, 1958, letter, box 65, all in Leake Papers, NLM; and [Chauncey Leake] to all, June 1953, letter, folder 13, box 2, Leake Papers, Blocker Collections. In 1958 Hans Krebs, Whitley Professor of Biochemistry at Oxford University and the 1953 Nobel Laureate in Medicine, was the first Daniel W. Kempner Visiting Professor at UTMB; see John B. Truslow, "Daniel W. Kempner Visiting Professorship," *Texas Reports on Biology and Medicine*, 17 (Spring, 1959), 13–15 and H. A. Krebs, "The Regulation of Metabolic Processes," *Texas Reports on Biology and Medicine*, 17 (Spring, 1959), 16–28.

66. R. J. Valle, a professor of pharmacology from Sao Paulo, Brazil, worked for two months in 1946 as a traveling fellow of the Rockefeller Foundation; see *Galveston Daily News*, July 9, 1946. Werner Jacobson, a Cambridge University hematologist, worked with Pomerat during the summer of 1948; see *Galveston Daily News*, June 13, 1948. Nirur Raghavin from Delhi, India, worked with Scott and others during four months in the spring of 1953; see *Galveston Daily News*, Mar. 20, 1953.

67. *Galveston Daily News*, Sept. 9 and 11, 1944; [Titus] Harris, et al. to members of Texas Club of Internists, Feb. 19, 1943, letter; Minutes, Meeting of the Texas Club of Internists, Houston, Texas, Feb. 18, 1944, and "Annual Meeting: Texas Club of Internists," Feb. 18, 1944; all in folder 10, box 49, Stone Papers. See also *Galveston Daily News*, Sept. 28 and Nov. 2, 13–17, 19, 1952. For more on Dyer, see WF350, CHP Archives. For the 1954 meeting, see *Galveston Daily News*, Apr. 9, 1954.

68. *Galveston Daily News*, Sept. 3, 7, and Nov. 2, 1952.

69. Minutes, UTMB Faculty Meetings, July 17, Aug. 7, and Nov. 4, 1942; Nov. 7, and Dec. 5, 1945; June 4, 1946; and Oct. 5, 1948. Departmental research budgets were very modest. In fiscal year 1951, for example, slightly more than $50,000 of state funds were allocated to twelve labs for equipment and technicians; see "The University of Texas Medical Branch Budget for 1950–1951," box VF A/3, UT Chancellor's Records. Also see Minutes, Meeting of the UTMB Committee on Services and Development, Sept. 24, 1945, folder 17, box 2, Leake Papers, Blocker Collections, and Minutes, UTMB Faculty Meetings, Nov. 7, 1945, Dec. 5, 1945, June 4, 1946, and Oct. 5, 1948.

70. Leake, "Annual Report," Aug. 31, 1943, p. 21, Leake Papers, NLM; Chauncey Leake to F. J. L. Blasingame, Mar. 6, 1951, letter, box 19, Leake Papers, NLM (quotation).

71. Others shared Leake's fears. See James A. Shannon, "The Advancement of Medical Research: A Twenty-Year View of the Role of the National Institutes of Health," *Journal of Medical Education*, 42 (Feb., 1967), 97–108; and Stephen P. Strickland, *Politics, Science and Dread Disease: A Short History of United States Medical Research Policy* (Cambridge, Mass.: Harvard University Press, 1972), 24–25.

72. Rollo Dyer established the Division of Research Grants at the National Institutes of Health and helped design the peer-review system. For details, see Kenneth M. Endicott and Ernest M. Allen, "The Growth of Medical Research 1941–1953 and the Role of Public Health Service Research Grants," *Science*, 118 (Sept.. 25, 1953), 337–343, and James H. Cassedy, "Stimulation of Health Research," *Science*, 145 (Aug. 25, 1964), 897–902. Also see, "The Federal Government and Health Research, 1900–1960: A Symposium," *Bulletin of the History of Medicine*, 39, no. 3 (1965), 199–260. For a concise summary of the impact of federal and private funding on the research policies of all American medical schools, see Rothstein, *American Medical Schools and the Practice of Medicine*, 235–255.

73. *Galveston Daily News*, July 14, 1944. For other examples between 1944 and 1955, see *Galveston Daily News*, Dec. 23, 1944; Dec. 1, 1945; Jan. 20, July 4 and 6, 1946; Jan. 7 and 23, Mar. 11, Apr. 1–2, July 7, and Aug. 5, 1948; Jan. 7 and 11, Feb. 26, May 29, Aug. 10, Oct. 6 and 28, and Dec. 31, 1949; Feb. 24 and June 20, 1950; Jan. 6 and 14, Apr. 8, July 14–15, and Aug. 28, 1951; July 19, 1952; Jan. 6 and 26, 1953; Apr. 18, 1954; and Apr. 17 and July 2, 1955. For samples of support by drug companies during these years, see the relevant letters in RF125, CHP Archives.

74. *Galveston Daily News*, Oct. 30, 1947. For samples of contracts and grants involving federal agencies between 1947 and 1950, see the folders about contracts in boxes VF 9/D and VF 10/D, UT President's Records. Also see "Summarizing Report on Non-Governmental Gifts and Grants to the Medical Branch, 1946–47 through 1953–54," box VF I/4, UT Chancellor's Records. Leake also solicited private funds for students. In 1952 the Borden Company established an annual award of $500 for the senior medical student who had done the most significant research during his undergraduate years; see Chauncey D. Leake to James B. Hart, Aug. 16, 1952, letter, box VF C/1, UT Chancellor's Records. In 1954 Lederle Laboratories established two $600 research fellowships for medical students; see Chauncey D. Leake to Benjamin W. Carey, May 19, 1954, letter, box VF A/3, UT Chancellor's Records.

75. This expansion at UTMB mirrored the national experience. The financial support of research by governmental and private agencies caused unprecedented expansion of medical schools and transformed the attitudes of medical educators. Many became far more interested in research than teaching medical students. For an overview, see Ludmerer, *Time to Heal*, 139–161. In a summary of what he called "major research efforts" in UTMB's departments in 1945, Leake named twenty-nine basic science teachers and sixteen clinical teachers; see Chauncey D. Leake to S. L. Bhatia, Mar. 30, 1945, letter, box 19, Leake Papers, NLM.

76. B. M. Hendrix to A. P. Brogan, Jan. 6, 1947, letter, folder 8, box 6, Duncan Papers. The basic science teachers were Raymond Blount, D. Bailey Calvin, Donald Duncan, George Emerson, Wendell Gingrich, Byron Hendrix, Chauncey Leake, Eric Ogden, Charles Pomerat, Eugene Porter, Wilbur Selle, William Sharp, and John Sinclair. The clinical teachers were Raymond Gregory, Arild Hansen, George Herrmann, Robert Moore, and Edgar Poth. The summaries in folder 8, box 6, Duncan Papers, indicate the number of publications as follows: Blount (35), Calvin (45), Duncan (40), Emerson (120), Gingrich (12), Gregory (24), Hansen (68), Hendrix (40), Herrmann (200), Leake (200), Moore (25), Ogden (49), Pomerat (50), Porter (32), Poth (60), Selle (60), Sharp (31), Sinclair (2). See *Galveston Daily News*, Jan. 7, 1951.

77. For a list of research projects in all departments and laboratories in 1953, see "A Petition for a Charter to Form a Chapter of the Society of the Sigma Xi at the University of Texas Medical Branch, Galveston, Texas," September 1953, RF92, CHP Archives.

78. *Galveston Daily News*, Nov. 20, 1946; *Medi-Texan*, 4 (Jan., 1957), 4–5, 9. For citations to some publications, see UT Publication no. 5821, 140–141, 241–242; and UT Publication no. 6019, 204–205. Also see Lape, *Medical Research: A Midcentury Survey*, II, 3–67.

79. *Galveston Daily News*, July 4, 1947, Oct. 28, 1949, Oct. 14 and Dec. 14, 1950; and *Medi-Texan*, 1 (May, 1954), 4–5, 10. For examples of Rigdon's research, see R. H. Rigdon, "Tumors Produced by Methylcholanthrene in the Duck," *Archives of Pathology*, 54 (Oct., 1952), 469–475; and R. H. Rigdon, Jack Neal, D. Anigstein, and L. Anigstein, "Neoplasma in Mice Neonatally Inoculated with Rat Thymus Antiserum and Fed Benzo(a)pyrene," *Cancer Research*, 27 (Dec., 1967), 2318–2323. For references to one hundred publications by Rigdon (as author or co-author), see UT Publication no. 5707, 230–232; UT Publication no. 5821, 152–153; and UT Publication no. 6019, 184.

80. Levin thought that he had the largest amount of grant money of anyone on the campus during the 1960s; see William C. Levin to Chester R. Burns, Nov. 7, 1989, interview, Blocker Collections. As examples of collaborative research, see T. G. Blocker Jr., William C. Levin, S. R. Lewis, and C. C. Snyder, "The Use of Radioactive Sulfur Labeled Methionine in the Study of Protein Catabolism in Burn Patients," *Annals of Surgery*, 140 (Oct., 1954), 519–523; W. C. Levin, J. E. Perry, and T. G. Blocker Jr., "Adsorption of Sulfur-35 labeled L-Methionine by Serum Proteins *in vitro*," *Texas Reports on Biology and Medicine*, 14 (Fall, 1956), 372–375; and William C. Levin, John E. Perry, and T. G. Blocker Jr., "The Fate of the Chromium-51 Label of Autologous Hemoglobin and Plasma in Rabbits," *Texas Reports on Biology and Medicine*, 15 (Summer, 1957), 299–302. For references to publications by Levin between 1948 and 1958, see UT Publication no. 5707, 222–223; UT Publication no. 5821, 145; and UT Publication no. 6019, 175–176.

81. In 1949 the experimental laboratory in the Department of Physiology was named the Carter Physiological Laboratory in honor of William S. Carter, who had served UTMB as professor of physiology (1897–1922) and dean (1903–1922; 1935–1938). See *Medi-Texan*, 2 (Nov., 1954), 6–7, 11. For research publications by these faculty, see the citations in UT Publication no. 5707, 243–248; UT Publication no. 5821, 157–159; and UT Publication no. 6019, 189–191. Also see M. Mason Guest to John Swann, Jan. 29, 1987, interview, Blocker Collections.

82. *Medi-Texan*, 3 (Jan., 1956), 11. The lab assistants were Raymond Brown, Sam Perusina, and Betty Ann Hum. See *Medi-Texan*, 3 (Jan., 1956), 4–5, 7. For their publications between 1948 and 1958, see UT Publication no. 5707, 211–215; UT Publication no. 5821, 147–149, 244; and UT Publication no. 6019, 178–181. For comments about her experiences as a member of the faculty for more than thirty years, see Etta Mae MacDonald Davidson to Chester R. Burns, June 25, 1986, interview, Blocker Collections.

83. *Medi-Texan*, 4 (July, 1956), 4–5, 8–9. For their publications between 1948 and 1958, see UT Publication no. 5707, 215; UT Publication no. 5821, 140–141, 241–242; and UT Publication no. 6019, 170–172.

84. In 1955 the Sealy & Smith Foundation gave $16,000 to Raymond Gregory for support of his work as director of what he called the John Sealy Memorial Laboratory for Clinical Research; see Minutes, Sealy & Smith Foundation Board of Directors, Feb. 9, 1955. In 1957 the foundation gave Gregory money to buy an "artificial kidney"; see Minutes, Sealy & Smith Foundation Board of Directors, July 10, 1957, and Aug. 9, 1961. Also see Hugh P. Revely, George R. Herrmann, and Julio Ortiz, "Studies of Factors in Congestive Heart Failure During Effective Therapy," *Texas State Journal of Medicine*, 47 (Sept., 1951), 617–621; Belle Ruskin, Wiktor W. Nowinski, and Arthur Ruskin, "Effect of Mercurial Diuretics upon the Rat Heart and Kidney I. Effect of Mercuhydrin and its Fractions, *Texas Reports on Biology and Medicine*, 8 (Fall, 1950), 384–390 and B. Ruskin, Nowinski, and A. Ruskin, "Effect of Mercurial Diuretics upon the Respiration of Rat Heart and Kidney Slices II. The Effect of Thiomerin," *Texas Reports on Biology and Medicine*, 8 (Fall, 1950), 391–394. For other examples of experimental studies by UTMB's faculty between 1948 and 1958, see UT Publication no. 5707, 217–226; UT Publication no. 5821, 142–147, 242–243; and UT Publication no. 6019, 172–178.

85. *Galveston Daily News*, Jan. 30, 1949. For details, see G. W. N. Eggers, Thomas O. Shindler, and Charles M. Pomerat, "Pressure Studies on Bone Healing: A Preliminary Report," *Texas Reports on Biology and Medicine*, 7 (Spring, 1949), 125–128. Also see *Galveston Daily News*, Jan. 29, 1956, and May 6, 1957.

86. Reports from this research are in twenty-four bound volumes in the Blocker Papers.

87. In addition to the Blockers (Virginia was a research associate who wrote their reports), these projects involved six research fellows, ten faculty, six residents, twenty-two medical students, five lab aides, eight photographers, four technicians, three lab assistants, and two secretaries. Reports about these studies are in five bound volumes (black binders) in the Blocker Papers. For citations to Blocker's publications between 1948 and 1958, see UT Publication no. 5707, 256–258; UT Publication no. 5821, 168; and UT Publication no. 6019, 200–201. Also see two unpublished papers: "Experimental and Clinical Research on Burns: The University of Texas Medical Branch" (1951) and "Clinical Research on Burns and Related Problems" (1953), both in the folder of Unpublished Speeches, 1950–55, box 78, Blocker Papers.

88. Although John Spies and Edgar Poth were college roommates at UT Austin, Spies did not recruit Poth. A friend and teacher of Raymond Gregory, Poth accepted A. O. Singleton's invitation and arrived in Galveston on July 4, 1942. See Edgar J. Poth to Chester R. Burns, July 1 and 8, 1986, interview, Blocker Collections, and *Galveston Daily News*, Oct. 25, 1942. For a biographical sketch of Poth, see Chester R. Burns, "Edgar J. Poth," in Tyler, et al. (eds.), *The New Handbook of Texas*, V, 296. For samples of his research, see Edgar J. Poth, Stanley M. Fromm, Robert I. Wise, and Chinn Min Hsiang, "Neomycin, a New Intestinal Antiseptic," *Texas Reports on Biology and Medicine*, 8 (Fall, 1950), 353–360; Edgar J. Poth, "Intestinal Antisepsis," *American Journal of Surgery*, 88 (Nov., 1954), 803–806; and Edgar J. Poth, "A Critical Analysis of Intestinal Antisepsis," *Journal of the American Medical Association*, 163 (Apr. 13, 1957), 1317–1321. Also see *Galveston Daily News*, June 5, 1953. In 1982 Poth provided a useful summary: "Historical Development of Intestinal Antisepsis," *World Journal of Surgery*, 6 (Mar., 1982), 153–159. For citations to the research publications of Poth and Eggers between 1945 and 1962, see UT Publication no. 4812, 51; UT Publication no. 5103, 140–141; UT Publication no. 5707, 258, 260–262; UT Publication no. 5821, 165–168; UT Publication no. 6019, 198–200; UT Publication no. 6312, 253; and UT Publication no. 6520, 264, 268–269. See also *Galveston Daily News*, May 6, 1957.

89. The quotes are in a summary Micks sent to John Truslow on December 5, 1956. For this summary and other minutes of the Research Committee between 1956 and 1959, see folders 6–9, box 18, Department of Anatomy records, Blocker Collections.

90. *The University of Texas Report of the Committee of 75*, 35–36; and James A. Hamilton Associates, "Roles and Program of Physical Development: The Medical Branch of the University of Texas, Galveston, Texas," 1958, 23 (quotation).

91. *Galveston Daily News*, June 11, 1958. Also see Don W. Micks to Myles Knape, Sept. 9, 1987, and Spencer Thompson to Chester R. Burns, July 11, 1986, interviews, Blocker Collections.

92. H. W. Paley to Logan Wilson, Apr. 29, 1955; and H. W. Paley to L. D. Haskew, May 17, 1955, box VF O/3, letters, UT Chancellor's Records. Paley and J. E. Johnston Jr., faculty members in the Department of Internal Medicine, had attempted to establish this foundation within the UT System. But Paley balked when he realized that system officials would then control the foundation's decisions. See H. W. Paley to Logan Wilson, Oct. 11, 1954, box VF E/2; L. D. Haskew to [Logan] Wilson, Jan. 13, 1955, box VF O/3; and Hulon Black to Logan Wilson, June 6, 1955, box VF E/2, letters, UT Chancellor's Records; Minutes, UT Board of Regents, Jan. 28, 1955; and L. D. Haskew to H. W. Paley, May 13, 1955, letter, box VF E/2, UT Chancellor's Records.

93. Minutes, Meeting of the Board of Directors of the Medical Research Foundation of Texas, Oct. 9, 1955, box VF O/3, UT Chancellor's Records; "The Medical Research Foundation of Texas, Inc., By-laws as adopted October 9, 1955," Oct. 9, 1955, box VF E/2, UT Chancellor's Records. Also see *Galveston Daily News*, May 1, 1958; Mar. 23, 1958; July 12, 1959; and May 4, 1960.

94. *Galveston Daily News*, Sept. 23, 1954. A committee of representatives from the UT System and UTMB established the terms and administrative rules for these fellowships. Faculty fellowships were for those who had been at UTMB for at least three years. They could receive one-year awards for work at another institution. All of the other four types of fellowships involved funds for research done at UTMB. These included medical student fellowships for summer research with a faculty mentor (and renewable once); pre-doctoral fellowships for up to three years of work by a graduate student; post-doctoral fellowships for up to three years of work; and distinguished fellowships for established scholars in a field, ordinarily for one year. An advisory committee of faculty evaluated annual applications for these awards. For details, see Jack G. Taylor to Logan Wilson, May 14, 1954; and John B. Truslow to Logan Wilson, May 30, 1957, letters, box VF G/1, UT Chancellor's Records; and "Terms and Conditions Relating to the James W. McLaughlin Fellowship Fund for the Investigation of Infection and Immunity," July 1958, box VF I/1, UT Chancellor's Records. Nearly $100,000 were available for awards during the first year of the fellowships; see Jack G. Taylor to Chauncey D. Leake, July 14, 1954, letter, box VF I/1, UT Chancellor's Records.

95. *Galveston Tribune*, Dec. 1, 1955; W. F. Verwey, "The James W. McLaughlin Fellowship Fund: Report of the McLaughlin Committee, Fiscal Year 1957–58," c. Sept. 1958, box VF I/1, UT Chancellor's Records; and *Galveston Daily News*, Mar. 2, 1955. For the fellows' names and projects, see "Report of the McLaughlin Committee, Fiscal Year 1957–58," in box VF I/l, UT Chancellor's Records.

96. L. L. Salomon to Harry H. Ransom, Oct. 16, 1961, letter, box VF L/6, UT Chancellor's Records; "Annual Report of the James W. McLaughlin Fellowship Fund for the Investigation of Infection and Immunity, 1962–1963," c. Sept. 1963, box VF M/5; and L. J. Olson to Harry H. Ransom, Nov. 2, 1967, letter, box VF EE/3, UT Chancellor's Records. Fellowships were expanded in 1961 when residents became eligible for part-time research fellowships.

97. *Galveston Daily News*, July 21, 1957. The selection committee hoped that students receiving these awards would return to UTMB as junior faculty researchers; see H. L. Kempner to John B. Truslow, Apr. 15, 1957, letter, box VF G/1, UT Chancellor's Records; and Minutes, Meetings of the Special "Jeane B. Kempner Fund" Committee, May 17, and June 5, 1957, box VF G/1, UT Chancellor's Records.

98. For names of some professors receiving United States Public Health Service grants between 1950 and 1958, see the lists in WF352, CHP Archives. See also *Galveston Daily News*, Apr. 23, 1958, and Jan. 8, 1958; and *University Medical Center News*, 1 (Jan., 1961), 1, 7. For details about the management of the grant for training medical students, see boxes 23 and 24, Department of Anatomy records, Blocker Collections. Walther Hild recalled that about twenty-five students worked on various research projects in the Department of Anatomy each summer; see Walther Hild to Myles Knape, May 18 and July 6, 1987, and June 24, 1988, interviews, Blocker Collections.

99. In 1958 UTMB was one of thirteen medical schools receiving these training grants. See *Galveston Daily News*, Feb. 28, 1960, and Mar. 6, 1960. Jim Guckian, Ken Tyson, and Sally Abston (then students, later faculty) gave papers during the first Student Research Forum. Denton Cooley was a guest speaker. For details, see *Impact*, 3 (Apr. 20, 1979), 10, and *Galveston Daily News*, Mar. 11, 1962.

100. *University Medical Center News*, 1 (Sept., 1960), 1, 8, and *Galveston Daily News*, Sept. 11, 1960. For a list of the professors receiving grants, see D. Bailey Calvin to faculty and staff, Sept. 9, 1960, folder 71, box 7, School of Nursing Archives, Blocker Collections. Most of the grants to the School of Nursing faculty supported improvements in teaching and graduate training. See *University Medical Center News*, 3 (Nov., 1962), 1, 8; *Galveston Daily News*, Dec. 2, 1962; and *Newsletter (UTMB)*, Dec. 3, 1964. For lists of all externally funded research projects between 1956 and 1962, see the folder titled "Research Grant Data Individual Grants by Dept. 1957–1962," box 8, CHP Archives.

101. For details about research activities in each School of Medicine department during fiscal year 1961, see the Annual Reports in folder 8, box 1, 75th Anniversary History Papers, Blocker Collections. See also Ludmerer, *Time to Heal*, 148–151.

102. For citations, see UT Publication no. 5707, 202–210; UT Publication no. 5821, 136–139, 241; and UT Publication no. 6019, 166–169. See also *Medi-Texan*, 3 (July, 1956), 1. For a sample publication, see Donald Duncan, "Electron Microscope Study of the Embryonic Neural Tube and Notochord," *Texas Reports on Biology and Medicine*, 15 (Fall, 1957), 367–377. See Donald Duncan, "The Department of Anatomy," Annual Reports, 1960–1961, folder 8, box 1, 75th Anniversary History Papers, Blocker Collections.

103. *University Medical Center News*, 1 (Dec., 1960), 4–5; *Galveston Daily News*, May 17, 1960; and *University Medical Center News*, 2 (Summer, 1962), 1.

104. *University Medical Center News*, 1 (Jan., 1961), 4–6.

105. *University Medical Center News*, 1 (Sept., 1960), 2; *Galveston Daily News*, Dec. 11, 1960; *University Medical Center News*, 1 (Apr., 1961), 2; and *Galveston Daily News*, Apr. 15, 1960, and Apr. 6 and July 9, 1961.

106. *Galveston Daily News*, July 8, 1960, and Apr. 20, 1962.

107. In fiscal years 1960 and 1962, total research and training expenditures at UTMB were $1,190,088 and $1,658,352, respectively. The average per school expenditures from funds designated for research training and sponsored research in sixteen public medical schools were $1,601,800 for fiscal year 1960 and $2,625,800 for fiscal year 1962. See Office of Sponsored Programs—Academic, University of Texas Medical Branch," "Awards for Support of Research and Research Training," 1967–1968, 42; and Division of Operational Studies of the Association of American Medical Colleges, "Trends in Financing Medical Education According to Three Main Categories of Income, 1941–1962," *Datagrams* (AAMC), July 1964.

108. For details about these departments, see their annual reports for fiscal years 1961 and 1962 in folders 8 and 9, box 1, 75th Anniversary History Papers, Blocker Collections, and Liaison Committee on Medical Education representing the American Medical Association and the Association of American Medical Colleges, "Report on Survey of the University of Texas Medical Branch, Galveston, Texas," January 15–18, 1962. A copy is in RF178, CHP Archives.

109. *Galveston Daily News*, June 8, 1962; and "[Application for Research Grant: May 1, 1962–April 30, 1963]" n.d. [c. May 1, 1962], p. 22," Clinical Study Center—Application–01 Year," Records of the Clinical Research Center, UTMB (hereafter cited as CRC Records). See also Minutes, Meeting of the Advisory Committee of the Clinical Research Center, Apr. 16, 1963; William C. Levin and George T. Bryan to Departmental Chairman and Clinical and Basic Science Investigators, June 7, 1963, CRC Records; and William C. Levin to Myles Knape, Mar. 17, Apr. 4, and May 26, 1986; William C. Levin to Chester R. Burns, Nov. 7, 1989; and William J. McGanity to Myles Knape and Chester R. Burns, July 28 and Aug. 5, 1988, interviews, Blocker Collections. See *Galveston Daily News*, Aug. 20, 1964, and the folder titled Clinical Research Center 1960s, box 7, CHP Archives. For comments by a faculty member who used the CRC shortly after it opened, see Luther Travis to Chester R. Burns, Feb. 25 and Mar. 10, 1992, interviews, Blocker Collections.

110. *Galveston Daily News*, Dec. 9, 1963.

111. Truslow generally supported behavioral research, but he was not successful in negotiating with the Moody Foundation for funds to establish a gerontology/geriatrics institute. See John B. Truslow to Mary Moody Northern, Dec. 17, 1957, box VF G/1; and John B. Truslow to Logan Wilson, Nov. 14, 1959, box VF I/1, letters, UT Chancellor's Records; *Galveston Daily News*, Feb. 9 and 24, 1955; and Gartley Jaco, "Incidence of Psychoses in Texas, 1951–1952," *Texas State Journal of Medicine*, 53 (Feb., 1957), 86–91.

112. For a list of these projects in 1956, see Wayne Holtzman to John B. Truslow, June 26, 1956, letter, box VF G/4, UT Chancelor's Records. For more about Hogg Foundation support, see RF122 and Appendix B-34, WF442, CHP Archives.

113. United States Department of Health, Education, and Welfare, "Public Health Service Grants and Fellowships Awarded by the National Institutes of Health Fiscal Year 1958 Funds," 284; U.S.D.H.E.W., "Public Health Service Grants and Fellowships Awarded by the National Institutes of Health Fiscal Year 1960 Funds," 340; "Public Health Service Grants and Awards by the National Institute of Health Fiscal Year 1961 Funds Part I Health Research Facilities Construction and Research Projects," 338; U.S.D.H.E.W., "Public Health Service Grants and Awards Fiscal Year 1963 Funds Part I Research Grants," 400; U.S.D.H.E.W., "Public Health Service Grants and Awards Fiscal Year 1964 Funds Part I Research Grants,", 416; and U.S.D.H.E.W., "Public Health Service Grants and Awards Fiscal Year 1965 Funds Part I Research Grants," 486. For important comments about the evolution of research in the Department of Psychiatry and his own research during a long career at UTMB, see Ernest S. Barratt to Chester R. Burns, Jan. 8, 1992, interview, Blocker Collections.

114. U.S.D.H.E.W., "Research Grants and Fellowships Awarded by the Public Health Service Fiscal Year 1956 Funds," 87; U.S.D.H.E.W., "Research Grants and Fellowships Awarded by the Public Health Service Fiscal Year 1958 Funds," 284; U.S.D.H.E.W., "Research Grants and Fellowships Awarded by the Public Health Service Fiscal Year 1960 Funds," 340; and "The University of Texas School of Nursing Annual Report 1958–1959," box VF I/1, UT Chancellor's Records. Lane, Beaudry, and Moore were members of a Special Studies Committee charged with stimulating faculty interest in research (for samples of meetings, see the minutes for October 28 and November 4, 1959, meetings in folder 123,

box 11, School of Nursing Archives, Blocker Collections). They also supervised the growing number of master's students who conducted behavioral research for their master's theses. See U.S.D.H.E.W., "Public Health Service Grants and Awards Fiscal Year 1962 Funds Part I Research Grants," 378; U.S.D.H.E.W., "Public Health Service Grants and Awards Fiscal Year 1963 Funds Part I Research Grants," 400; U.S.D.H.E.W., "Public Health Service Grants and Awards Fiscal Year 1964 Funds Part I Research Grants," 416; and U.S.D.H.E.W., "Public Health Service Grants and Awards Fiscal Year 1965 Funds Part I Research Grants," 487.

115. For titles, see UT Publication no. 5707, 252; UT Publication no. 5821, 162; and UT Publication no. 6019, 194. For support of studies of John Locke's manuscripts in medical philosophy, Romanell received U. S. Public Health Service grants in 1961 and 1962; see U.S.D.H.E.W., "Public Health Service Grants and Awards by the National Institute of Health Fiscal Year 1961 Funds Part I Health Research Facilities Construction and Research Projects," 338; and U.S.D.H.E.W., "Public Health Service Grants and Awards Fiscal Year 1962 Funds Part I Research Grants," 379.

116. For the titles of Leake's publications, see *Texas Reports on Biology and Medicine*, 13 (Winter, 1955), 707–711. In volume one of *Texas Reports on Biology and Medicine* (1943), 93–94, Leake wrote a tribute to Vesalius celebrating the four hundredth anniversary of his book on anatomy. In volume 13 (1955), 1010–1026, Leake published "Leonardo Da Vinci as Anatomist and Physiologist: A Critical Evaluation," by J. B. de C.M. Saunders.

117. The total of 320 is based on the articles that were reported by ASCA between March 1968 and December 1969. These articles were listed at the end of each issue of *Newsletter* published during those months. See *Newsline*, 4 (July, 1990), 2. The top five departments included Surgery (sixty-eight publications), Human Biological Chemistry and Genetics (forty-five), Internal Medicine (thirty-seven), Physiology and Biophysics (thirty-one), and Pharmacology and Toxicology (twenty-nine). See Ludmerer, *Time to Heal*, 288–295. For a list of more than forty projects receiving federal funding between 1976 and 1981, see an attachment to William C. Levin to Warren Harding, Apr. 24, 1981, letter, folder 5, box 47, Levin Papers.

118. New chairs negotiated support for researchers before and after accepting their roles. Ron Bailey, for example, wanted Ph.D. researchers within his department. Joe White approved this during recruitment negotiations. See Byron Bailey to Chester R. Burns, Feb. 13, 1992, interview, Blocker Collections.

119. For an example of LeMaistre's beliefs about research, see his speech for the Research Day at UTMB on April 5, 1968 in RF46, CHP Archives. For comparative data on the total amount of federal grant dollars received by these institutions between 1946 and 1991, see Appendix B-33, WF442, CHP Archives. The data in these appendices were taken from the annual reports that were usually titled "Office of Sponsored Programs—Academic Awards for Support of Research Training," between 1967–1968 and 1987–1988 and "Awards for Support of Research and Research Training," September 1, 1989, through August 31, 1990. Some of these reports are in the Office of the Vice President for Research. Because these catalogs were not issued for fiscal years 1972–1974, data for those years were collected from Minutes, UT Board of Regents.

120. T. G. Blocker Jr. to Ralph W. Yarborough, Feb. 23, 1966, letter, box VF FF/2, UT Chancellor's Records.

121. J. Gordon Mills, "A History of the Department of Human Biological Chemistry & Genetics," May 5, 1990, unpublished typescript, WF469, CHP Archives; and *University Medical*, 1 (Mar., 1970), 4–7; and 4 (July, 1973), 8–9.

122. *Newsletter (UTMB)*, 2, no. 24. The date was probably September 14, 1967. See also *Newsletter (UTMB)*, 3 (Aug., 1968), 2–3; and *University Medical*, 2 (Oct., 1970), 14–15. For details, see Rose G. Schneider to Chester R. Burns, Dec. 12, 1985, interview, Blocker Collections, and volume 40 of *Texas Reports on Biology and Medicine* titled "Human Hemoglobins and Hemoglobinopathies: A Review to 1981."

123. "Memorandum of Understanding Concerning the Joint Participation by Texas A&M University and the University of Texas Medical Branch in the Marine Biomedical Program at Galveston," Oct. 11, 1968 (quotation). This memo and other documents pertaining to the origins of the Marine Biomedical Institute are in a folder titled "Marine Biomedical Institute Correspondence," box 7, CHP Archives. Sporadic attempts had been made to develop the marine sciences in Texas, the first as early as 1935 when John Sinclair attempted to interest the Texas Academy of Science in establishing a marine biological station in Galveston. During the 1940s, Chauncey Leake supported efforts to establish a marine biological laboratory in Galveston, but the development of the UT facility at Aransas Pass undermined further interest in Galveston. For details, see Chauncey D. Leake to Homer P. Rainey, June 12, 1944, box VF 10/B; and Chauncey D. Leake to T. S. Painter, June 25, 1946, box VF 10/C, letters, UT President's Records; and John G. Sinclair to John B. Truslow, Dec. 11, 1956, letter, box 1, folder 2, Sinclair Papers, Blocker Collections. UTMB did lease the Special Surgery Unit barracks to Texas A&M during the mid-1950s for an oceanographic laboratory, but there appears to have been no collaborative research between the two universities; see E. N. Capplemann to C. H. Sparenberg, Jan. 6, 1954, letter, box VF A/3, UT Chancellor's Records. In 1966 Donald Rappaport, a professor in the Department of

Pediatrics, wrote a detailed proposal for a Marine Biological Facility at UTMB. For details about the origins of the Marine Biomedical Institute, see folder 4, box 16, Levin Papers.

124. *University Medical*, 3 (Jan., 1972), 5. Ernie Barratt, Joe Tupin, Glenn Russell, John Calverly, and others were members of a committee who wanted a Brain and Behavior Institute. Further discussions, especially with Blocker, transformed these dreams into a research institute that combined the neurosciences and the marine environment surrounding Galveston. For details, see the notes in RF104, CHP Archives. For a biographical sketch of Wolf in 1970 and his vision for the Marine Biomedical Institute then, see the "Summary Statement of Purposes and Plans," folder 5, box 16, Levin Papers. Initially, a coordinating committee composed of both UTMB and Texas A&M representatives advised the Marine Biomedical Institute's director. During its early years, the institute included an earth and planetary sciences group that served as a major link between UTMB and NASA in Houston. But that tie was short-lived and UT administrators relocated these researchers to Austin. A prestigious National Advisory Committee began supporting the Marine Biomedical Institute in 1970.

125. "The Marine Biomedical Institute, 1969–1977," 6, 11–15. Beckman supervised the Tektite II undersea project in 1970; for details, see Edward L. Beckman and Elizabeth Miremont Smith, "Tektite II Medical Supervision of the Scientists in the Sea," *Texas Reports on Biology and Medicine*, 30, no. 3 (1972), 1–204. Robert Alderdice and others initiated studies of a coral reef 110 miles south of Galveston with the hope that a fixed platform could be constructed to house a Flower Gardens Ocean Research Center. For details, see the folders in box 2, vertical file A5, Blocker Collections.

126. For their names, see the Marine Biomedical Institute's progress report to the Moody Foundation, March 1, 1970, to February 28, 1973, folder 5, box 16, Levin Papers. Margie Watson, John Burr, and Ken Johnson provided excellent staff support during the early years. Financially, UTMB and Texas A&M each contributed $100,000 during the institute's first two years. In 1970 the state contributed $150,000 for each year of the next biennium, and the Moody Foundation contributed a three-year grant of more than $800,000. Though important dollars came from numerous research grants, the institute received more than half of its support from the state for every biennium during the 1970s and 1980s. For details, see Minutes, UT Board of Regents, July 10, 1970; documents in box 1, vertical file A5, Blocker Collections; and the annual reports and bulletins of the institute in box 4, vertical file A5. Texas A&M eventually withdrew its sponsorship.

127. Warren F. Dodge, Benjamin H. Spargo, Luther B. Travis, and Joseph A. Bass, "Acute Glomerulonephritis—Preliminary Report of Course and Prognosis in 44 Children," *Southern Medical Journal*, 60 (Dec., 1967), 1356; and G. Douglas Cain, Pruett Moore Jr., and Marcel Patterson, "A Ten-Year Review of Amebic Abscess of Liver: 1956–1966," *American Journal of Digestive Diseases*, 13, no. 8 (1968), 709–717.

128. *Galveston Daily News*, Aug. 16, 1964.

129. Harry E. Sarles, Sandra S. Hill, Alvin L. LeBlanc, Garland H. Smith, Carlos O. Canales, and August. R. Remmers Jr., "Sodium Excretion Patterns During and Following Intravenous Sodium Chloride Loads in Normal and Hypertensive Pregnancies," *American Journal of Obstetrics and Gynecology*, 102 (Sept. 1, 1968), 1–7; Jay C. Fish, Harry E. Sarles, August R. Remmers Jr., and Kenneth R. T. Tyson, "Lymphocyte Depletion and Prolonged Renal Allograft Survival," *Journal of the American Medical Association*, 204 (May 6, 1968), 537; Jay C. Fish, Marshal V. Ross, Harry E. Sarles, and August R. Remmers Jr., "Separation of Lymphocytes from Lymph by Continuous Flow Centrifugation," *Surgery*, 65 (May, 1969), 789–792; Jay C. Fish, Harry E. Sarles, August R. Remmers Jr., Kenneth R. T. Tyson, Carlos O. Canales, Gerald A. Beathard, Matsuo Fukushima, Stephen E. Ritzmann, and William C. Levin, "Circulating Lymphocyte Depletion in Preparation for Renal Allotransplantation," *Surgery, Gynecology and Obstetrics*, 128 (Apr., 1969), 777–787; *Newletter (UTMB)*, 4 (Nov., 1969), 6–7; and *University Medical*, 2 (Jan., 1971), 8–9. Verwey and Watanabe had been successful in isolating the immunizing substances from the two types of cholera organisms that produced the disease. With volunteers, they wanted to determine how serum antibodies protected immunized humans and how this protection could be prolonged.

130. Joe P. Tupin, George K. Schlagenhauf, and Daniel L. Creson, "Lithium Effects on Electrolyte Excretion," *American Journal of Psychiatry*, 125 (Oct., 1968), 536–543. For comments, see Harry K. Davis to Chester R. Burns, Dec. 8, 1994, interview, Blocker Collections.

131. For details, see *Houston Chronicle*, July 25, 1965; Ernest S. Barratt to Chester R. Burns, Jan. 8, 1992, interview, Blocker Collections; and U.S.D.H.E.W., "Public Health Service Grants and Awards Fiscal Year 1973 Funds Health Services and Mental Health Administration," Part VI, 422. For other examples, see the lists in WF354, CHP Archives.

132. *Galveston Daily News*, May 7, 1964; *Newsletter (UTMB)*, 4 (June, 1969), 14–15. Abstracts of these papers were published in *Texas Reports on Biology and Medicine*, 32 (Fall/Winter, 1974), 773–847.

133. *Newsletter (UTMB)*, 1 (July 1, 1965), 2; and Minutes, UTMB Faculty Meeting, Apr. 7, 1970.

134. See "Informational Handbook for Faculty of the School of Medicine," 1982, 143–155. A copy is in WF255, CHP Archives.

135. *Newsletter (UTMB)*, 1 (Sept. 16, 1965), 2; 2 (Sept. 28, 1967), 3; and 3 (Jan., 1968), 14.

136. *Newsletter (UTMB)*, 3 (Nov., 1968), 10–11. Levy had joined UTMB in 1960 as a research associate in the Department of Physiology. During the early years, the facility was named the Animal Care Center.

137. *Newsletter (UTMB)*, 4 (Feb., 1969), 12–13; and 3 (Feb., 1968), 8–9.

138. As an example, see Robert E. Roberts, George W. McBee, and Eleanor J. Macdonald, "Social Status, Ethnic Status, and Urban Mortality: An Ecological Analysis," *Texas Reports on Biology and Medicine*, 28 (Spring/Summer, 1970), 13–28.

139. Minutes, UTMB Faculty Meeting, Oct. 4, 1977. Between 1977 and 1981, Bryan sponsored monthly research conferences that showcased the work of researchers. Though the goals of recognition, communication, and cheerleading were laudable, most faculty and students were affixed to timetables that seldom allowed attendance at such campuswide conferences. For details, see Minutes, UTMB Faculty Meeting, Oct. 4, 1977, and Minutes, UTMB Research Council, June 2, 1981, RF89, CHP Archives.

140. "Report of the Ad Hoc Task Force to Evaluate Research in the School of Medicine," November 1983, folder 5, box 45, Levin Papers.

141. For comments about research in their departments, see their interviews in the Blocker Collections.

142. Minutes, UTMB Faculty Meeting, Dec. 2, 1975; and *University Medical*, 10 (May–June, 1980), 22. In fiscal year 1978 there were 193 awards for a total of $10,757,237; in fiscal year 1979, there were 244 awards for a total of $13,398,812. Issues of *Impact* contained lists of grants to faculty; for examples, see *Impact*, 3 (Feb. 23, 1979), 17; 6 (Feb. 5, 1982), 1; and 7 (Mar. 11, 1983), 1, 17.

143. For comparative data, see Appendix B-33, WF442, CHP Archives. Also see J. Palmer Saunders to Myles Knape and John Swann, Nov. 5 and 14, 1985, interviews, Blocker Collections (1st quotation); and K. Lemone Yielding to John Swann, Sept. 18, 1989, interview, Blocker Collections (2nd quotation). In 1988, for example, UTMB had about 3.5 percent of its salaries included in grants. Yielding believed that the proportion should be approximately 40 percent. See *Impact*, 12 (June 24, 1988), 8. These research grants exceeded $16 million in fiscal year 1983; $17 million in fiscal year 1984; see *Impact*, 8 (Feb. 10, 1984), 1, and 9 (Mar. 8, 1985), 1, 21. For annual totals, see Appendices B-34, B-35, B-36, and B-37, WF442, CHP Archives.

144. *Galveston Daily News*, Dec. 6, 1986; the letters in folder 6 and 7, box 43, Levin Papers; Ballinger Mills Jr. to Chester R. Burns, July 20, 1988, interview, Blocker Collections (quotation); Minutes, Sealy & Smith Foundation Board of Directors, Oct. 9, 1986; and *Impact*, 10 (Dec. 19, 1986), 1, and 12 (Apr. 29, 1988), 1.

145. An ad hoc Faculty Committee on Research evaluated proposals and selected awardees. For examples of this committee's work, see minutes of some meetings in RF89, CHP Archives. See also *Impact*, 6 (Oct. 29, 1982), 10. Between 1982 and 1987, the same professors attracted 146 external grants worth more than $14 million. See E. J. Pederson to Charles B. Mullins, Sept. 17, 1987, letter, folder 6, box 45, Levin Papers.

146. William C. Levin to Hans Mark, Feb. 11, 1987, letter, folder 6, box 45, Levin Papers.

147. *Impact*, 10 (Jan. 10, 1986), 1, 10; Craig B. McArdle, C. Joan Richardson, Deborah A. Nicholas, Mansour Mirfakhraee, C. Keith Hayden, and Eugenio G. Amparo, "Developmental Features of the Neonatal Brain: MR Imaging. Part I. Gray-White Matter Differentiation and Myelination," *Radiology*, 162 (Jan., 1987), 223–229; Craig B. McArdle, C. Joan Richardson, Deborah A. Nicholas, Mansour Mirfakhraee, C. Keith Hayden, and Eugenio G. Amparo, "Developmental Features of the Neonatal Brain: MR Imaging. Part II. Ventricular Size and Extracerebral Space," *Radiology*, 162 (Jan., 1987), 230–234; Craig B. McArdle, C. Joan Richardson, C. Keith Hayden, Deborah A. Nicholas, Marsha J. Crofford, and Eugenio G. Amparo, "Abnormalities of the Neonatal Brain: MR Imaging. Part I. Intracranial Hemorrhage," *Radiology*, 163 (Feb., 1987), 387–394; and Craig B. McArdle, C. Joan Richardson, C. Keith Hayden, Deborah A. Nicholas, and Eugenio G. Amparo, "Abnormalities of the Neonatal Brain: MR Imaging. Part II. Hypoxic-Ischemic Brain Injury," *Radiology*, 163 (Feb., 1987), 395–403.

148. See the following items in the Active Records file of the Office of Environmental Health and Safety: Committee on Ionizing Radiation, University of Texas Medical Branch, Galveston, Texas, "Handbook of Rules for the Use of Radioactive Material," Apr. 1969; "Radiation Safety Committee," 1989; "Biological Safety Committee," 1989; "Chemical Safety Committee," 1989; "UTMB Office of Environmental Health and Safety Training Catalog," June 1, 1989; and Bruce Schoenbucher to John P. Swann, Aug. 30, 1989, interview, Office of Environmental Health and Safety folder, box 7, CHP Archives.

149. The Institutional Review Board included clinical and basic science faculty, a citizen not employed by UTMB, a representative from the UTMB administration, a representative for prisoners, and a representative from the Institute for the Medical Humanities. The board met monthly to review research protocols. Key concerns included the extent to which a researcher had established the need for and relevance of a project, whether or not the use of non-human subjects could yield the same information, how risks to patients would be minimized, and how consent and confidentiality of human subjects would be secured. For details, see "Protection of Human Subjects: Policy and Administration Manual, University of Texas Medical Branch at Galveston," in folder titled "Office of Sponsored Research Human Research Subjects," box 7, CHP Archives. The Animal Care and Use Committee was composed of eighteen members (including a veterinarian, non-scientists, and a citizen not employed by UTMB), who reviewed research protocols to insure that investigators minimized the pain and distress of laboratory animals. This committee inspected all animal care facilities twice yearly, provided non-mandatory training for those using animals in their research, and submitted reports with the United States Department of Agriculture on compliance and non-compliance with the latest version of the Animal Welfare Act. For details, see "UTMB Handbook for Faculty and Staff: Regulation Concerning the Care and Use of Animals in Research and Training" and other documents in the folder titled "Office of Sponsored Programs Animal Research Subjects," box 7, CHP Archives.

150. For details, see the following documents in the Marine Biomedical Institute Records, "Marine Biomedical Institute, 1969–1977," "Marine Biomedical Institute, Galveston, Texas, First Annual Report, 1970–1971," T. G. Blocker Jr. to Maurice Ewing, Apr. 14 and June 9, 1972; Maurice Ewing to T. G. Blocker Jr., June 15, 1972; and *Impact*, 8 (Oct. 5, 1984), 14–15. With sixty-six lobes, the octopus brain is an excellent experimental model used throughout the world for research projects in biochemistry, physiology, toxicology, and pathology. Roger Hanlon, who joined the Marine Biomedical Institute in 1975, and John Forsythe began a lab for breeding octopuses in 1981, a project funded by a NIH grant. They created the National Resource Center for Cephalopods, the only facility in the world that provided cephalopods (squids, cuttlefishes, octopuses and the chambered Nautilus) for researchers. For details about Willis as director, see William Willis to Myles Knape, June 2, 9, and 23, 1986, interviews, Blocker Collections. From 1978 through UTMB's centennial year, Willis received superb administrative assistance from John Burr, Ken Johnson, Lori Del Buono, and Marion (Coy) Wilson. For historical summaries of research in the neurosciences until 1976, see Bordley and Harvey, *Two Centuries of American Medicine*, 705–726; and Robert J. Frank Jr., Louise H. Marshall, and H. W. Magoun, "The Neurosciences," in John Z. Bowers and Elizabeth F. Purcell (eds.), *Advances in American Medicine: Essays at the Bicentennial* (2 vols.; New York: Josiah Macy Jr. Foundation, 1976), II, 552–613.

151. For a list of the publications, see the Marine Biomedical Institute's 10th Anniversary Bulletin, 1970–1980, 87–102. See also William C. Levin to Charles W. Sprague, Jan. 20, 1986, letter, folder 6, box 45, Levin Papers.

152. *Impact*, 2 (Sept. 8, 1978), 13; and 10 (Oct. 31, 1986), 4.

153. *Impact*, 12 (Aug. 5, 1988), 4. This award had been won previously by three other UTMB professors: Harvey Levin, Arthur M. Brown, and William D. Willis.

154. *Impact*, 3 (Aug. 10, 1979), 16; and 5 (May 22, 1981), 3.

155. *Impact*, 5 (Feb. 20, 1981), 10; and 11 (Jan. 9, 1987), 1–2.

156. For the names of the fellows and the titles of the publications, see attachments to James C. Thompson to William C. Levin, Sept. 29, 1981, letter, folder 3, box 11, Levin Papers. At the beginning of his chairmanship, Thompson negotiated with Joe White for funds to support research fellows; see James C. Thompson to Myles Knape and Chester R. Burns, June 27, July 3 and 13, 1989, interviews, Blocker Collections. Many details about Thompson's research and administrative support for research are included in this interview.

157. *Impact*, 6 (Aug. 20, 1982), 5; and William C. Levin to Charles W. Sprague, Jan. 20, 1986, letter, folder 6, box 45, Levin Papers.

158. *Impact*, 4 (Jan. 25, 1980), 5. In 1980 the CRC moved to Unit 6 North of the Child Health Center. It became known as the General Clinical Research Center when the Psychiatric Clinical Research Center opened in 1984.

159. "Utilization by Department," photograph of bar graph, c. 1/9/68, "CSC—General—History"; "Agenda," Mar. 17, 1971, "Clinical Research Center—Thru 1977;" "Summary Statement," n.d., 23, attached to Jerry Gordon to P. L. Poffenbarger, Mar. 17, 1981; "Summary Statement," n.d., 26, attached to Barbara Menick to Walter J. Meyer, Aug. 12, 1983; and "Summary Statement," n.d., 47, attached to Judith L. Vaitukaitis to William C. Levin, Apr. 30, 1987. All of these are in box 7, CHP Archives. For samples of annual reports that include lists of publications, see the folders titled "Clinical Research Center 1970s" and "Clinical Research Center 1980s," box 7, CHP Archives. The Clinical Research Center was a venue for teaching research strategies to students and faculty. Medical students, junior

and senior faculty, Graduate School of the Biomedical Sciences students, residents and clinical fellows, and student and graduate nurses learned about clinical research by participating in various projects. During the 1970s the center sponsored a weekly seminar that attracted between thirty and forty faculty and staff members from both clinical and pre-clinical departments.

160. *Impact*, 2 (Mar. 23, 1978), 13; *University Medical*, 15 (Fall, 1983), 28–33; *Impact*, 6 (May 7, 1982), 16–17; and 7 (Nov. 18, 1983), 13–16. The faculty received invaluable help from the Clinical Research Center's staff of nurses, unit clerks, dietitians and metabolic cooks, laboratory and research technicians, and housekeepers.

161. *Impact*, 7 (June 17, 1983), 2; (Nov. 4, 1983), 1, 10; (Nov. 18, 1983), 1, 25, and pp. 13–16 of a separate insert in the same issue. Also see *Impact*, 11 (Mar. 10, 1989), 1–2.

162. For concise historical summaries of the development of immunology at that time, see Bordley and Harvey, *Two Centuries of American Medicine*, 601–634; and Lewis Thomas, "Immunology," in Bowers and Purcell (eds.), *Advances in American Medicine: Essays at the Bicentennial*, II, 459–483. For details about Baron's research group, see Samuel Baron to Myles Knape, Oct. 6, 1987, interview, Blocker Collections; and Samuel Baron, Dorian H. Coppenhaver, Ferdinando Dianzani, W. Robert Fleischmann Jr., Thomas K. Hughes Jr., Gary R. Klimpel, David W. Niessel, G. John Stanton, and Stephen K. Tyring, *Interferon: Principles and Medical Applications* (Galveston: University of Texas Medical Branch, 1992).

163. William C. Levin to Charles W. Sprague, Jan. 20, 1986, folder 6, box 45, Levin Papers. The last volumes of *Texas Reports on Biology and Medicine* were devoted to interferon studies. See Samuel Baron, Ferdinando Dianzani, and G. John Stanton, "The Interferon System: A Review to 1982—Part I and Part II," *Texas Reports on Biology and Medicine*, 41 (1981–1982). John J. Costanzi, director of the Cancer Center, also worked with these scientists in conducting clinical studies of interferon. See *Impact*, 9 (Dec. 6, 1985), 10–11.

164. For details, see *Impact*, 14 (Jan. 12, 1990), 1; *Galveston Daily News*, Jan. 8, 1990; Harold G. Levine, "History of Child Health Services at The University of Texas Medical Branch," 1992, 26–27, 63; and Armond S. Goldman, Sadhana Chheda, and Roberto Garofalo, "Evolution of Immunologic Functions of the Mammary Gland and the Postnatal Development of Immunity," *Pediatric Research*, 43, no. 2 (1998), 155–162. Goldman was one of the founders of the International Society for Research in Human Milk and Lactation. See also Frank C. Schmalstieg, Warren J. Leonard, Masayuki, Maria Berg, H. Elizabeth Rudloff, Richard M. Denney, Sanat K. Dave, Edward G. Brooks, and Armond S. Goldman, "Missense Mutation in Exon 7 of the Common Gamma Chain Gene Causes a Moderate Form of X-linked Combined Immunodeficiency," *Journal of Clinical Investigation*, 95 (Mar., 1995), 1169–1173.

165. *Impact*, 9 (June 14, 1985), 8. For a pathbreaking study, see J. E. Remmers, W. J. DeGroot, E. K. Sauerland, and A. M. Anch, "Pathogenesis of Upper Airway Occlusion During Sleep," *Journal of Applied Physiology*, 44 (1978), 931–938. For details, see Sam Kuna to Chester R. Burns, Nov. 25, 1991, memo, W349, CHP Archives. See also Harold G. Levine, "History of Child Health Services at The University of Texas Medical Branch," 1992, 62–63; and *Impact*, 12 (Apr. 29, 1988), 9.

166. Cecil G. Deming Jr. to V. E. Thompson, Feb. 14, 1980, "Mary Moody Northern Pavilion: Texas Health Facilities Commission Action," UTMB Executive Vice President's Office, Inactive; "Regents Approve Plans for Psychiatric Research Center," *Impact*, 7 (June 3, 1983), supplement, p. 3; and Minutes, UT Board of Regents, Oct. 8, 1982.

167. Eric M. Smith and J. Edwin Blalock, "The Hormonal Nature of the Interferon System," *Texas Reports on Biology and Medicine*, 41 (1981–1982), 350–358; Eric M. Smith, Walter J. Meyer, and J. Edwin Blalock, "Virus-induced Corticosterone in Hypophysectomized Mice: A Possible Lymphoid Adrenal Axis," *Science*, 218 (Dec. 24, 1982), 1311–1312; Walter J. Meyer III, Eric M. Smith, Gail E. Richards, Anita Cavallo, Audrey C. Morrill, and J. Edwin Blalock, "*In Vivo* Immunoreactive Adrenocorticotropin (ACTH) Production by Human Mononuclear Leukocytes From Normal and ACTH-Deficient Individuals," *Journal of Clinical Endocrinology and Metabolism*, 64, no. 1 (1987), 98–105; Allahyar Jazayeri and Walter J. Meyer, "Glucocorticoid Modulation of Beta-adrenergic Receptors of Cultured Rat Arterial Smooth Muscle Cells," *Hypertension*, 12 (Oct., 1988), 393–398; Geoffrey Leavenworth, "The Chemistry of Depression," *Biomedical Inquiry*, 1 (Fall/Winter, 1988), 11–13, 19; and Robert Nichols, "Hormones and Immunity: Parallel Worlds," *Biomedical Inquiry*, 3 (Autumn, 1991), 14–15. In 1989 alone these scientists published at least twenty papers about their research. For citations, see a report about the Psychiatric Clinical Research Center prepared by Walter Meyer and Eric Smith in 1992; a copy is in WF344, CHP Archives.

168. For examples, see Appendices B-34, B-36, and B-37, WF442, CHP Archives. See also U.S.D.H.E.W., "National Institutes of Health, Research Grants Fiscal Year 1980 Funds," NIH Publication no. 81–1042, 321; U.S.D.H.E.W., "National Institutes of Health, Research Grants Fiscal Year 1981 Funds," NIH Publication no. 82–1042, 337; and U.S.D.H.E.W., "National Institutes of Health, Research Grants Fiscal Year 1982 Funds," NIH

Publication no. 83–1042, 332; U.S.D.H.E.W., "National Institutes of Health, Research Grants Fiscal Year 1982 Funds," NIH Publication no. 83–1042, 333; U.S.D.H.E.W., "National Institutes of Health, Research Grants Fiscal Year 1984 Funds," NIH Publication no. 85–1042, 360; U.S.D.H.E.W., "National Institutes of Health, Research Grants Fiscal Year 1985 Funds," NIH Publication no. 86–1042, 376; U.S.D.H.E.W., "National Institutes of Health, Research Grants Fiscal Year 1988 Funds," NIH Publication no. 89–1042, 443; and U.S.D.H.E.W., "National Institutes of Health, Research Grants Fiscal Year 1989 Funds," NIH Publication no. 90–1042, 444. Lists of NIH research grants to faculty are in WF354, CHP Archives.

169. For samples of their research, see John G. Bruhn and F. David Cordova, "A Developmental Approach to Learning Wellness Behavior, Part I: Infancy to Early Adolescence," *Health Values*, 1 (Nov.–Dec., 1977), 246–254; John G. Bruhn and F. David Cordova, "A Developmental Approach to Learning Wellness Behavior, Part II: Adolescence to Maturity," *Health Values*, 2 (Jan.–Feb., 1978), 16–21; and *Galveston Daily News*, Oct. 3, 1986.

170. For details, see the memos and minutes in RF119, CHP Archives. For information about these and other projects conducted by School of Nursing faculty, see the attachment to William C. Levin to Warren Harding, Apr. 24, 1981, pp. 27–31, letter, folder 5, box 47, Levin Papers.

171. *Galveston Daily News*, Oct. 3, 1986. For details, see Jerry W. Lester to Chester R. Burns, Apr. 7, 1989, memo, WF349, CHP Archives.

172. Special Institute for the Medical Humanities fellowship programs resulted in important research contributions. In 1975 the institute received a grant from the Hogg Foundation for Mental Health to support a transdisciplinary symposium on philosophy and medicine and to provide support for twelve fellows and three visiting professors who were in residence at UTMB for varying periods of time. As a result of their work in Galveston, two fellows completed doctoral dissertations, and the other visitors in this program wrote five articles and two books that were published. The proceedings of the symposium were published as H. Tristram Engelhardt Jr. and Stuart Spicker (eds), *Mental Health: Philosophical Perspectives* (Dordrecht: Reidel, 1978). For details about the Hogg Foundation grant, see folders 137–40, box 18, IMH Records, Blocker Collections. See also *Impact*, 8 (Apr. 13, 1984), 1, 16–17.

173. See Appendices A-44 and A-45, WF441, CHP Archives.

174. *Galveston Daily News*, Apr. 15, 1988. As a public charitable foundation, the Sealy & Smith Foundation Board obtained some rulings that allowed it to expand its charitable purposes legally; for details, see Ballinger Mills to Chester R. Burns, July 20, 1988, interview, Blocker Collections. See also *Galveston Daily News*, Feb. 14, 1990, and Oct. 20, 1991.

175. For the names of previous and current fellows in 1988, see the Marine Biomedical Institute's Biennial Bulletin (1987–1988), 65–70. By that year, eighty-four postdoctoral fellows and forty-eight graduate students had completed their projects with institute members, who had also collaborated with more than seventy visiting scientists. For details about the labs, see UTMB Research Advisory Council, "Core Facility Review Final Reports," 1995/1996. For details and other examples of research activities, see WF349, CHP Archives, and the interviews with School of Medicine departmental chairs in the Blocker Collections.

176. For samples of their publications, see Stanley M. Hollenberg, Cary Weinberger, Estelita S. Ong, Gail Cerrilli, Anthony Oro, E. Brad Thompson, Michael G. Rosenfeld, and Ronald M. Evans, "Primary Structure and Expression of a Functional Human Glucocorticoid Receptor cDNA," *Nature*, 318 (Dec., 1985), 635–641; Karen W. Barbour, Sondra H. Berger, Franklin G. Berger, and E. Aubrey Thompson, "Glucocorticoid Regulation of the Genes Encoding Thymidine Kinase, Thymidylate Synthase, and Ornithine Decarboxylase in P1798 Cells," *Molecular Endocrinology*, 2 (Jan., 1988), 78–84; Paul H. Weigel, Benjamin L. Clarke, and Janet A. Oka, "The Hepatic Galactosyl Receptor System: Two Different Ligand Dissociation Pathways are Mediated by Distinct Receptor Populations," *Biochemical and Biophysical Research Communications*, 140 (Oct. 15, 1986), 43–50; Darrell Carney, David L. Scott, Eric A. Gordon, and Edward F. LaBelle, "Phosphoinositides in Mitogenesis: Neomycin Inhibits Thrombin-Stimulated Phosphinositide Turnover and Initiation of Cell Proliferation," *Cell*, 42 (Sept., 1985), 479–488; and Darrell Carney, David L. Scott, Eric A. Gordon, and Edward F. LaBelle, "Glucocorticoid Receptors: Evolution, Structure, Function and Abnormalities," supplement to *Cancer Research*, 49 (Apr. 15, 1989), 2199s–2303s.

177. Stephen J. Rinkus and Marvin S. Legator, "An Evaluation of *in vitro* Testing for Mutagens," in *Genetic Damage in Man Caused by Environmental Agents*, ed. K. Berg (New York: Academic Press, 1979), 343–362; and T. H. Connor, J. Meyne, L. Molina, and M. S. Legator, "A Combined Testing Protocol Approach for Mutagenicity Testing," *Mutation Research*, 64 (Feb., 1979), 19–26.

178. *Galveston Daily News*, Aug. 13, 1990, and July 4, 1991.

179. *Galveston Daily News*, Aug. 20, 1990.

180. Sung Yul Ahn, Kazuro Sugi, Pekka Talke, J. L. Thiessen, H. A. Linares, L. D. Traber, D. N. Herndon, and D. L. Traber, "Effects of Allopurinol on Smoke Inhalation in the Ovine Model," *Journal of Applied Physiology*, 68, no. 1 (1990), 228–234; and Kazuro Sugi, Josef L. Theissen, Lillian D. Traber, David H. Herndon, and Daniel L. Traber, "Impact of Carbon Monoxide on Cardiopulmonary Dysfunction After Smoke Inhalation Injury," *Circulation Research*, 66 (Jan., 1990), 69–75.

181. Kyriakos S. Markides and Charles H. Mindel, *Ethnicity and Aging* (Newbury Park, Calif.: Sage Publications, 1987).

182. "1991–92 School of Nursing Operating Budget Request," 1–10, Dean's Office, School of Nursing.

183. The following publications emerged from these conferences: Thomas R. Cole and Sally A. Gadow (eds.), *What Does it Mean to Grow Old?* (Durham, N.C.: Duke University Press, 1986); Anne Hudson Jones (ed.), *Images of Nurses: Perspectives from History, Art and Literature* (Philadelphia: University of Pennsylvania Press, 1988); Thomas R. Cole, W. Andrew Achenbaum, Patricia Jakobi, and Robert Kastenbaum, *Voices and Visions of Aging: A Critical Gerontolgy* (New York: Springer Publishing Company, 1993); and Mary G. Winkler and Letha Cole (eds.), *The Good Body: Asceticism in Contemporary Culture* (New Haven: Yale University Press, 1994).

184. Altogether during the Institute for the Medical Humanities' second decade, institute members wrote 11 books published as edited volumes or monographs; 184 essays published as journal articles or book chapters; and 70 other items published as book reviews, reports, and editorials. Details about these research activities can be found in the issues of the institute's newsletter, which began in 1982. A complete set of "The Chronicle: The Newsletter of the Institute for the Medical Humanities" is in the Blocker Collections. Between 1987 and 1991, nine scholars studied in Galveston in a fellowship program supported by a Rockefeller Foundation grant and directed by Mary Winkler. These fellows wrote a substantial number of publications based on their work in Galveston.

185. *Galveston Daily News*, Aug. 17, Sept. 6, 9, and 11, Nov. 29, and Dec. 2, 1990; and Apr. 8–10 and 16, 1991. In 1990, the National Student Research Forum attracted 184 participants from eighty-four medical schools, including 16 from UTMB (9 medical students, 6 graduate students, and 1 resident). Four of the students from UTMB won six of the forty-one awards. See *Impact*, 14 (Apr. 6, 1990), 3; and (May 4, 1990), 2.

186. For a photo of James at his microscope and a brief summary of his research, see *Galveston Daily News*, Feb. 28, 1988. James worked in his research lab every Saturday and on other weekdays as circumstances permitted. For details, see Thomas N. James to Chester R. Burns, Oct. 12 and 24, 1995, interviews, Blocker Collections. See also Thomas N. James, Thomas Geoghegan, and Conrad R. Lam, "Electrocardiographic Manifestations of Air in the Coronary Arteries of Dying and Resuscitated Hearts," *American Heart Journal*, 46 (Aug., 1953), 215–228. A reprint of this article is in box 28 of the CHP Archives, together with eighty-eight other articles that exemplify the research career of James between 1953 and 1994. Only a few of these are cited with the paragraphs in this chapter. For a more complete understanding of James's research, examine all of these reprints, read the transcript of James to Burns, Oct. 12, 1995, interview, and see the documents in WF257, CHP Archives.

187. Thomas N. James and Reginald A. Nadeau, "Direct Perfusion of the Sinus Node: An Experimental Model for Pharmacologic and Electrophysiologic Studies of the Heart," *Henry Ford Hospital Medical Bulletin*, 10 (Mar., 1962), 21–25. For samples of research using this technique, see Thomas N. James and Reginald A. Nadeau, "The Mechanism of Action of Quinidine on the Sinus Node Studied by Direct Perfusion Through its Artery," *American Heart Journal*, 67 (June, 1964), 804–811; and Thomas N. James, Edward S. Bear, Richard J. Frink, Klaus F. Lang, and John C. Tomlinson, "Selective Stimulation, Suppression, or Blockade of the Atrioventricular Node and His Bundle," *Journal of Laboratory and Clinical Medicine*, 76 (Aug., 1970), 240–256.

188. See Thomas N. James, *Anatomy of the Coronary Arteries* (Hagerstown, Md.: Harper Brothers), 1961; Thomas N. James, "Anatomy of the Human Sinus Node," *Anatomical Record*, 141, no. 2 (1961), 109–139; Thomas N. James, "Anatomy of the Sinus Node of the Dog," *Anatomical Record*, 143, no. 2 (1962), 251–265; and Thomas N. James, "Anatomy of the Conducting System of the Heart," *Heart Bulletin*, 12, no. 2 (1963), 21–25; Richard J. Frink and Thomas N. James, "Normal Blood Supply to the Human His Bundle and Proximal Bundle Branches," *Circulation*, 47 (Jan., 1973), 8–18; George K. Massing and Thomas N. James, "Anatomical Configuration of the His Bundle and Bundle Branches in the Human Heart," *Circulation*, 53 (Apr., 1976), 609–621; Thomas N. James, "Small Arteries of the Heart," *Circulation*, 56 (July, 1977), 2–14; and Thomas N. James, "The Sinus Node," *American Journal of Cardiology*, 40 (Dec., 1977), 965–986.

189. For examples, see Thomas N. James, Peter Froggatt, and Thomas K. Marshall, "Sudden Death in Young Athletes," *Annals of Internal Medicine*, 67 (Nov., 1967), 1013–1021; Thomas N. James, "Sudden Death in Babies: New Observations in the Heart," *American Journal of Cardiology*, 22 (Oct., 1968), 821–829; Thomas N. James, Robert C. McKone, and Allen S. Hudspeth, "De Subitaneis Mortibus. X. Familial Congenital Heart Block," *Circulation*, 51 (Feb.,

1975), 379–388; and Thomas N. James and LeRoy Riddick, "Sudden Death Due to Isolated Acute Infarction of the His Bundle," *Journal of the American College of Cardiology*, 15 (Apr., 1990), 1183–1187.

190. *Galveston Daily News*, Apr. 10–11, 1991. E. Donnall Thomas, the 1990 Nobel Laureate in Medicine or Physiology, gave the address of dedication for the $25 million, seven-story, 178,000-square-foot building.

CHAPTER 8

1. Virginia Stull to Chester R. Burns, Dec. 27, 1993, letter, WF380, CHP Archives.

2. Melvyn H. Schreiber, "The Art of Medicine," *Texas Reports on Biology and Medicine*, 27 (Spring, 1969), 1.

3. *University Medical*, 1 (Apr., 1970), 4–6; *Galveston County Daily News*, July 5, 1998; and *University Medical*, 4 (Mar., 1973), 14.

4. *Hospital News*, 8 (Mar. 24, 1975), 3; *Impact*, 8 (Aug. 24, 1984), 11; and 10 (Apr. 18, 1986), 5. To provide a summer camp experience for thirty children (ages six through seventeen) with terminal diseases, the Candlelighters organized the Rainbow Connection at a camp in Hitchcock during the summer of 1985. Mary Gordon Conner and Ruth Anne Herring coordinated this program; see *Galveston Daily News*, Jan. 20, 1985; and *Impact*, 9 (Apr. 19, 1985), 2; and 9 (Aug. 9, 1985), 10. In 1990 the Rainbow Connection used Camp Pine Tree, a YMCA camp near Spring, Texas; see *Impact*, 14 (Mar. 23, 1990), 1–2.

5. *American Journal of Nursing*, 4 (Feb., 1904), 403; and Myles Knape, WF437, CHP Archives, pp. 9–13.

6. Names and addresses for 1901 are in *University Record*, 3 (Dec., 1901), 490–496. The employees and students for 1928 were all named in the campus directory for 1927–1928. Located in the Blocker Collections, this is the first directory in a nine-volume set of bound UTMB directories that go through 1988. The totals in this year do not include employees of the hospital because those employees worked for the hospital, not the university. See the list for 1941 in box VF 9/B, UT President's Records.

7. *Galveston Daily News*, Oct. 2, 1956. The numbers are taken from a list in WF358 and UTMB's "Fact and Figures" brochures, which were published annually beginning in the 1970s. Some are in WF429, CHP Archives.

8. Minutes, UTMB Faculty Meeting, Apr. 12, 1977; and *Impact*, 1 (Dec. 22, 1977), 2. Also see the "Faculty (SOM): Special Issues re Women and Minorities" folder in WF383, CHP Archives. See also *Impact*, 3 (Feb. 9, 1979), 5. This advisory committee also supported the work of the other affirmative action programs at UTMB, especially the efforts of staff members in the Office of Special Programs situated in Bryan's network. These individuals provided many services related to the recruitment, admission, and retention of qualified minority students. See *Impact*, 3 (Jan. 26, 1979), 1; and 4 (June 13, 1980), 15. Through 1991, Guzman's successors included Henry Cavazos, Laura Derrinwater, Margaret Killough, Alan Chesney, and Dale Robinson. For many details, see Betty Grefenstette's summary in WF369, CHP Archives. For a concise summary of the national context, see Elizabeth R. McAnarney, "Women in Academic Medical Centers in the United States: An Update," in John Z. Bowers and Edith E. King (eds.), *Academic Medicine Present and Future* (North Tarrytown, N.Y.: Rockefeller Archive Center, 1983), 65–74.

9. The data were taken from "The Affirmative Action Program For Faculty The University of Texas Medical Branch at Galveston, 1981–1985." A copy is in folder 3, box 41, Levin Papers.

10. For more details, see Betty Grefenstette's short history of this group in WF366, CHP Archives and Betty Williams to Megan Seaholm, July 13, 1989, interview, Blocker Collections. Group members published a newsletter and held monthly meetings that featured animated discussions of many issues. For details, see the letters and newsletters in folder 10, box 34, Levin Papers. See also William C. Levin to Regent Beryl Buckley Milburn, July 31, 1985, folder 10, box 34, Levin Papers; and Minutes, UT Board of Regents, Aug. 9, 1985.

11. Nor were those at the other 123 academic health centers in the United States in 1983; see Rothstein, *American Medical Schools and the Practice of Medicine*, 225–227. The first systematic analysis of management in these centers was not published until 1984; see Marjorie Price Wilson and Curtis P. McLaughlin, *Leadership and Management in Academic Medicine* (San Francisco: Jossey-Bass Publishers, 1984). The first systematic analysis of the challenges of managing the complex hierarchy of academic territories in health centers was written by a former dean at UTMB; see John G. Bruhn, Harold G. Levine, and Paula L. Levine, *Managing Boundaries in the Health Professions* (Springfield, Ill.: Charles C. Thomas, 1993).

12. For comments about this loneliness, see George Bryan to Myles Knape, Jan. 31, Feb. 6, 11, and 26, and Mar. 6, 1986, interviews, Blocker Collections.

13. Harry Ransom, "Educational Resources in Texas," *Texas Quarterly*, 4 (Winter, 1961), 6.

14. How executives handled conflicts about their identities was extremely important for institutional stability and development. The rhetoric, behavior, and management style of a CEO generated images that provided comfort or discomfort, harmony or discord, optimism or pessimism, progress or regress. Their decisions and behaviors symbolized certain values and philosophies about an institution and its missions. If leaders understood and articulated these well, subordinates were motivated to do their best in fulfilling the institution's missions. If leaders failed to display their values in thoughtful and convincing ways, then subordinates were less enthusiastic and loyal. For a succinct summary of the tasks of administrative leadership, see George J. Gordon, *Public Administration in America* (New York: St. Martin's Press, 1982), 266–292. For an analysis of symbols in managing corporate culture, see Terrence E. Deal and Allan A. Kennedy, *Corporate Cultures: The Rites and Rituals of Corporate Life* (Reading, Mass.: Addison-Wesley Publishing Company, 1982), 141–155. For insights into the values of some CEOs at UTMB, see the documents in RF46, CHP Archives.

15. See "Notes from Bill McGanity's Talk at the Dinner for Bill Daeschner on February 24, 1989," WF356, CHP Archives; and William J. McGanity to Myles Knape and Chester R. Burns, July 28 and Aug. 5, 1988, interviews, Blocker Collections.

16. W. S. Carter to S. E. Mezes, May 14, 1913, letter, box 4Q19, UT President's Records. Carter was also concerned about salary differences among the basic science faculty and salary inequities among younger faculty members, especially those who served as demonstrators in the clinical specialties. Not only were their salaries different, but the amount of extra income allotted by their respective chiefs varied considerably. See W. S. Carter to S. E. Mezes, May 26, 1911, box 4R82; and W. S. Carter to S. E. Mezes, Aug. 15, 1911, box 4Q18, letters, UT President's Records.

17. W. Keiller to S. E. Mezes, Apr. 4, 1913, letter, box 4Q19, UT President's Records. Between 1911 and 1916 Carter persuaded the clinical faculty to accept a reduction in income that would allow the basic science faculty to receive more salary. The faculty formally agreed to this at a meeting in May 1913, but three more years elapsed before the salaries of clinical faculty were reduced and the salaries of younger faculty were increased. For details, see S. E. Mezes to W. S. Carter, May 15, 1911, letter, box 4R82, UT President's Records; Minutes, UTMB Faculty Meeting, May 9, 1913; and W. K. Battle to W. S. Carter, Apr. 13, 1916, letter, box 4Q20, UT President's Records.

18. W. S. Carter to R. E. Vinson, Mar. 15, 1919, box 4Q22, UT President's Records. In 1924 Keiller recommended higher salaries for Byron Hendrix and Meyer Bodansky because of their research accomplishments; see William Keiller to W. S. Sutton, May 13, 1924, letter, box 27, UTMB Dean's Office Records, Inactive. In that same year, Henry Hartman resigned as professor of pathology because his request for a salary increase was denied; see W. Keiller to W. S. Sutton, June 27, 1924, letter, box 4Q23, UT President's Records. Salaries were fairly modest in other American medical schools of this era; see Ludmerer, *Time to Heal*, 41–51.

19. "Facts on the University of Texas Medical Branch, Galveston," September 1944, box 2, Leake Papers, Blocker Collections; Chauncey D. Leake to Beverly H. Coiner, June 5, 1954, box VF 9/A; and Chauncey D. Leake to members of the clinical staff, June 8, 1945, box VF 10/C, letters, UT President's Records.

20. "Statement of Policy Regarding Clinical Appointments at the University of Texas Medical Branch," Jan. 1, 1946, box VF 10/C, UT President's Records. Full-time appointees were not permitted to accept retainer fees or any regular salaries for outside work unless authorized specifically by the regents. See the correspondence between Painter, Regent Chair Woodward, Leake, and others in December 1946 and January 1947, box VF 9/D and box VF 10/C, UT President's Records.

21. Chauncey D. Leake to James P. Hart, June 18, 1951, letter, box VF C/1, UT Chancellor's Records (quotation). In 1953 the Texas Medical Association appointed a committee to determine whether or not UTMB's physicians or physicians employed by other state agencies actually engaged in the "private practice of medicine." After reviewing letters and receiving testimony during two meetings, the committee "found no reason to censure any of our medical branches and found no infringement on private practice by any of our full-time medical staff members." For details, see Tom Sealy to T. G. Blocker Jr., Feb. 8, 1954, letter, box VF C/1, UT Chancellor's Records; the letters in "Practice of Staff" folder in this box; and Minutes, UT Board of Regents, Feb. 27, 1954.

22. John B. Truslow to Lanier Cox, Jan. 3, 1957, letter, box VF S/3, UT Chancellor's Records; "Full-time Clinical Faculty Program, University of Texas, Galveston," Jan. 26, 1957, box VF S/3, UT Chancellor's Records; "Augmentation Plan for the University of Texas Medical Branch," June 28, 1957, box VF S/3, UT Chancellor's Records. A copy is in RF129, CHP Archives. See also "Teaching Salaries, The University of Texas Medical Branch," Feb. 12, 1957, box VF S/3, UT Chancellor's Records. In addition to saving approximately $130,000 in the annual budget, Truslow and others made this decision because legislators were not willing to continue increasing the salaries of clinical faculty and because they wanted to continue replacing part-time faculty with full-time faculty. See John B. Truslow to Charles T. Stone Sr., July 29, 1959, letter, box 40, Stone Papers, Blocker Collections; and *Galveston Daily News*, Aug. 14, 1959.

23. See John Middleton to Chester R. Burns, Dec. 17, 1991, interview, Blocker Collections. For national changes in sources of salary income and titles designating part-time or full-time status, see Rothstein, *American Medical Schools and the Practice of Medicine*, 256–269. For the impact of Medicare and Medicaid, see Ludmerer, *Time to Heal*, 221–228.

24. Minutes, UT Board of Regents, July 18, 1967.

25. Minutes, UT Board of Regents, Sept. 20, 1968, and Dec. 13, 1968; and E. D. Walker to A. R. Schwartz, Mar. 26, 1969, letter, Medical Branch: Business and Budgetary Policies, Sept. 1, 1968–Aug. 31, 1970, UT Chancellor's Office of Records Management. In June 1969 the regents approved an amended MSRDP that had been adopted by the faculty during the previous month. The amendments permitted UTMB's vice president for academic affairs and dean of medicine to use some of the MSRDP funds for institutional development; see Minutes, UT Board of Regents, June 20, 1969. Also see the file titled "GMB: Augmentation," Current Files, UT Board of Regents.

26. The amount of income from professional fees was quite significant. For example, MSRDP income for fiscal year 1982 was $16,578,045; see V. E. Thompson to Thomas M. Keel, Oct. 29, 1982, letter, Chancellor Walker's subject files, reel 138, UT Chancellor's Office of Records Management. Many details about salary matters are located in RF129, CHP Archives. In 1982 the regents authorized UT System leaders to conduct a thorough review of MSRDP/PRS plans. During the next two years the system administration developed MSRDP/PRS handbooks, a standard format for institutional by-laws, and a centralized billing system. By September 1984 all UT Health Science Centers had adopted standardized bylaws for their MSRDP/PRS plans; see Minutes, UT Board of Regents, May 30 and June 14, 1984. For a list of the salaries of top executives and School of Medicine department chairs in 1991 see *Galveston Daily News*, Dec. 8, 1991.

27. W. S. Sutton to William Keiller, Dec. 17, 1924, box 4Q24; and John C. Nolan to H. Y. Benedict, Mar. 20, 1935; and W. S. Carter to J. W. Calhoun, Oct. 4, 1937, box VF 9/C, letters, UT President's Records. See also Minutes, UTMB Faculty Meeting, Feb. 19, 1958.

28. John B. Truslow to Logan Wilson, July 14, 1959, letter, box VF I/l, UT Chancellor's Records; *Newsletter (UTMB)*, 1 (Aug., 1965), 1; George T. Bryan to Robert W. Sappenfield, July 26, 1978, letter, in the "Faculty (SOM): Salaries and Fringe Benefits" folder, WF383, CHP Archives. Also see "Informational Handbook for Faculty of the School of Medicine" (1982), 68–69; 195–212. A copy is in WF255, CHP Archives.

29. Criteria for assigning titles, ranks, and tenure to teachers in American medical schools varied considerably by the early 1960s. There was variation in the minimum years of service required for promotion. Tenure could be granted to some assistant professors, though more institutions granted it to associate and full professors. See AAMC Datagrams, May 1963. See also Donald Duncan to Berwind N. Kaufmann, Mar. 6, 1969, letter, Duncan Papers, box 1, folder 12, Blocker Collections. Duncan knew of only one non-renewal of contract of a tenured professor at UTMB between 1932 and 1969. In 1955 Duncan had been a member of an ad hoc committee Mason Guest chaired that had recommended policies for promotion; a copy of its report is in RF130, CHP Archives.

30. Bill McGanity was the first dean at UTMB to use these ad hoc committees; see William J. McGanity to Myles Knape and Chester R. Burns, July 28 and Aug. 5, 1988, interviews, Blocker Collections. In 1964 faculty members below the rank of professor organized the Junior Faculty Association (JFA) as a forum for encouraging discussion about issues pertinent to career development. This group continued to flourish during the 1980s. For comments about the early years of the JFA, see Jay Fish to Chester R. Burns, Feb. 17, 1992, and Luther Travis to Chester R. Burns, Feb. 25 and Mar. 10, 1992, interviews, Blocker Collections. A copy of the JFA's constitution of 1985 is in the "Faculty (SOM): Organizations" folder, WF383, CHP Archives. For samples of letters recommending promotions written by Deans Joe White (1972), Ed Brandt (1974), and George Bryan (1980), see RF130, CHP Archives. See also Minutes, UTMB Faculty Meetings, Dec. 11, 1979, and Feb. 5, 1980. Also see "Informational Handbook for Faculty of the School of Medicine" (1982), 242–249. A copy is in WF255, CHP Archives.

31. The APC report was distributed to the faculty in December 1988. For a copy, see WF358, CHP Archives. Also see the "Faculty (SOM): Development, Tenure, Promotion" folder, WF383, CHP Archives. A variety of titles and ranks existed by the late 1980s. Criteria for their use were specified in the Handbook of Operating Procedures. For a copy of the Faculty Policies section, see the "Faculty: UTMB: Policies" folder, WF383, CHP Archives.

32. Minutes, UTMB Faculty Meeting, Oct. 5, 1965.

33. Warren G. Harding to E. D. Walker, Dec. 9, 1982, memo, reel HA3 (198207), UT Chancellor's Office of Records Management; and *Impact*, 8 (Aug. 24, 1984), 1, 21; 9 (Jan. 11, 1985), 1, 8; and (Feb. 8, 1985), 1.

34. *Faculty News (UTMB)*, Nov. 8–20, 1976; and list in "Faculty (SOM): Achievements" folder, WF383, CHP Archives.

35. For details, see "Faculty (SOM): Committees" folder, WF383, CHP Archives, and the pertinent items in RF128, CHP Archives.

36. Minutes, UTMB Faculty Meeting, Oct. 7, 1947; Minutes, Medical Staff of John Sealy and Affiliated Hospitals, Feb. 1, 1949, box VF 10/D, UT President's Records; and Minutes, John Sealy School of Nursing Faculty, Sept. 6, 1949, box VF 9/D, UT President's Records.

37. Minutes, UTMB Faculty Meeting, Oct. 2, 1956. One of the fourteen committees had three sub-committees; another had four. See also Minutes, UTMB Faculty Meetings, Dec. 3, 1957, and Feb. 18, May 6, and May 27, 1958. In 1958 the committees included Admissions; Animal Care; Curriculum; Executive; Fellowships and Research; Grading and Promotions (four committees); Intern Placement; Library; McLaughlin Fellowships; Nominating; Postgraduate Education; Retirement; Student Affairs; Student Scholarships and Loans; and *Texas Reports*. For the names of the committees in the 1960s, see Minutes, UTMB Faculty Meetings, Apr. 6, 1965; Apr. 4, 1966; Apr. 4, 1967; Apr. 2, 1968; and the revised bylaws adopted in October 1969. A copy of the bylaws is in WF371, CHP Archives, Blocker Collections.

38. The elected committees included Academic Planning; Admission; Curriculum; Executive; Grading and Promotion Committees A, B, and C; Nominating; and Student Affairs. Committees appointed by the dean included nine course committees (Cell Biology, Endocrinology, Immunology, Introduction to Clinical Medicine, Integrated Functional Laboratory, Introduction to Patient Evaluation, Medical Ethics, Medical Jurisprudence, Neuroscience); two joint committees with the GSBS (Committee on Research and M.D./Ph.D. Combined Degree Program); and thirty with the following names: Academic Computing Advisory; Academic Scholarship; Affirmative Action; Animal Care and Use; Appointment, Promotion and Tenure; Biological Safety; Budget Advisory; Chemical Safety; Scientific Misconduct; Continuing Education Advisory; Coordinating Center on Aging Advisory; Evaluation for 3–Year Graduates; Faculty Advisory; Faculty Awards; Faculty Coordinating; Fellowship; Herman Barnett Award; Hispanic Health Studies; Institutional Review Board; Intellectual Property; Kempner Visiting Professorship; McLaughlin Fellowship; Moody Medical Library Advisory; Radiation Safety; Radioactive Drug Research; Residency Advisory; School Health Programs Advisory; Senior Student Competency Assessment; Medical Student Honors Program; and UTMB Concert Series.

39. Betty Grefenstette prepared a short history of this group; see WF363, CHP Archives. In the Blocker Collections, there are two scrapbooks about this group for the years 1946 to 1988. Mrs. John Middleton recalled the many pleasures of these events; see John Middleton to Chester R. Burns, Dec. 17, 1991, interview. For examples, see *Galveston Daily News*, Oct. 14, 1951; Feb. 21, and Nov. 6, 1952; Apr. 25, 1954; Jan. 23, May 14, and Sept. 25, 1955; Feb. 7, Apr. 1, May 6, and Oct. 2, 1956; Feb. 17, and Sept. 22, 1957; Sept. 20, 1959; and Feb. 7, Mar. 20, May 15, and Sept. 19, 1960.

40. Opening in 1965, the Caduceus Room on the seventh floor of the Sealy & Smith Professional Building was the site of many social events. Bobbie Jackson and Gertie Mavis provided service during many luncheons, dinners, and parties—150 in December 1968, for example. See *Newsletter (UTMB)*, 4 (Jan., 1969), 17. For photos and songs from Faculty Follies, see volume I of the Faculty Women's Club Scrapbook in the Blocker Collections. Also see *Alumni Bulletin*, 14 (June, 1960), 3. The play "Sawbones on a Sandbar" was written to celebrate UTMB's seventy-fifth anniversary. About thirty employees and wives staged the first performance at St. Mary's Cathedral School on April 1, 1967; see *Newsletter (UTMB)*, 2 (Apr. 6, 1967), 1. Photos are in the second volume of the UTMB Women's Faculty Club Scrapbook in the Blocker Collections. The production in 1973 was an effort to raise funds for "Saving Old Red."

41. *Impact*, 3 (Feb. 23, 1979), 13; (Jan. 26, 1979), 3; 4 (Feb. 8, 1980), 3; 9 (Mar. 22, 1985), 6; and 10 (Feb. 7, 1986), 5.

42. Between 1931 and 1940, for example, 246 women began medical studies at UTMB. Megan Seaholm calculated the percentages from the annual reports of the regents. For details, see the appendices in WF381, CHP Archives. Recognizing the significant increases of the 1980s, some students participated in behavioral science research about female students. Shelley Sekula worked with two faculty members on a study involving the personality characteristics of women entering medical school. See Patricia Blakeney, Mary Frances Schottstaedt, and Shelley Sekula, "Personality Characteristics of Women Entering Medical School Over a 10–Year Period," *Journal of Medical Education*, 57 (Jan., 1982), 42–47.

43. See Virginia Irvine Blocker to Myles Knape, Aug. 18, 1986, interview, Blocker Collections; and Grace Jameson to Megan Seaholm, Sept. 13, 1988, unrecorded interview, notes in folder titled "Student Life Interviews UTMB Faculty," WF 383, CHP Archives. As more female medical students were admitted, the anxieties of men about competing with women were expressed in relentless teasing and crude jokes as well as the use of naughty nicknames for the female students. On the other hand, the female students named more than one male student who was willing to study with them and provide assistance in numerous ways. For examples, see Larry Wygant's interviews with ten female graduates in Larry Wygant, "Women Medical Students at the University of Texas Medical Branch: An Oral History Project,"

1978, Blocker Collections. Also see the items in the "Women Students" folder in WF383, CHP Archives. Before their marriage in October 1943 two classmates, Caroline Webster and Ed Rowe, experienced unique challenges during their courtship. Some are described in letters Caroline sent to her mother. See Caroline Webster Rowe, *The War Years Time Capsule: Letters Home* (Galveston: ePelican Press, 2002).

44. *Galveston Daily News*, Nov. 27, 1949; C. D. Leake to D. Bailey Calvin, Aug. 2, 1955, box VF E/2, UT Chancellor's Records; and *Galveston Daily News*, May 13, 1962; May 18 and 19, 1961.

45. *Galveston Daily News*, Feb. 17, 1944; Oct. 21, 1945; Aug. 27, Oct. 13, 14, 16, 1946; Jan. 12, 1947; Jan. 16, Nov. 14, 18, 21, 1948; Feb. 18, Mar. 10, May 12, 1949; Jan. 24, Mar. 12, 16, 17, and Oct. 8, 1950. For examples of events, see *Galveston Daily News*, Feb. 11, Mar. 17, Oct. 19, and Dec. 9, 1951; Mar. 30 and May 4, 9, 15, 1952; Feb. 11 and Mar. 10, 1953; Mar. 14, 1954; Feb. 23, Mar. 17, May 8, and Oct. 12–13, 1955; Feb. 8, Mar. 10, Oct. 5, Oct. 12, and Dec. 9, 1956; Jan. 13, Feb. 10, Mar. 16, Apr. 28, May 14, Oct. 6, and Nov. 24, 1957; Feb. 12, Mar. 30, Apr. 13, and Oct. 12, 1958; Feb. 11, Mar. 5, and Oct. 14, 1959; Jan. 13, Feb. 10, Apr. 12, and Oct. 12, 1960; Feb. 24, Apr. 19, and Oct. 26, 1961; Jan. 8, Nov. 17, and Dec. 8, 1963; and Apr. 9 and May 14, 1964. For "Chapter of the Year" award, see *Galveston Daily News*, May 13, 1961.

46. *University Medical*, 3 (June, 1972), 12. For anecdotes about the life of a married student who attended medical school between 1971 and 1975, see Joanne Mallett to Megan Seaholm, Oct. 20, 1989, interview, Blocker Collections. For examples of the group's activities during the early 1980s, see folder 6, box 34, Levin Papers, Blocker Collections, and WF364, CHP Archives.

47. In 1959 forty-six interns and residents were married; see *Galveston Daily News*, Sept. 20, 1959. See also *Galveston Daily News*, Nov. 17, 1963; Feb. 16, July 12, Sept. 13, and Dec. 29, 1964. For examples of activities between 1961 and 1974, see the Resiterns Scrapbook in the Blocker Collections. Also see WF365, CHP Archives. With 146 members in 1986, the Resiterns published a monthly newsletter, sponsored two large parties, provided guidance to newcomers about housing and other services in Galveston, and initiated a story-reading service in the Child Health Center. See Yvette M. Broocks to William C. Levin, Jan. 5, 1987, letter, folder 3, box 34, Levin Papers, Blocker Collections.

48. Manuel D. Hornedo, summary from self-directed audiotape of memories sent in August 1986, box 24, CHP Archives, Blocker Collections.

49. In 1964, 24 Hispanic students applied to the School of Medicine; 8 were accepted and 6 enrolled. In 1983, 214 Hispanics applied to the School of Medicine, 58 were accepted, and 14 enrolled. For details, see the list prepared by the Office of Admissions and Student Personnel Services in WF369, CHP Archives, and the "Medical Students: Minority Recruitment & Retention" folder in WF383, CHP Archives. See also *Impact*, 3 (Dec. 7, 1979), 4; "School of Medicine: Student Organizations, 1967–1991" folder in WF383, CHP Archives; *Syndrome* (1981), 254, and (1982), 264; and *Impact*, 5 (Jan. 9, 1981), 7.

50. In 1949 the Texas Legislature had appropriated money for a "Negro medical school," but it had not been constructed. See Minutes, UT Board of Regents, Sept. 10, 1949, and Sept. 3 and 29, 1950. Barnett did have some problems in the community. During his internship year at John Sealy Hospital, he was once stopped for speeding near La Marque and was beaten by the officer, who believed that Barnett was lying to him when he said that he was a physician; see *Galveston Daily News*, July 14–17, 22, and Aug. 5, 1953.

51. *University Medical Center News*, 3 (Oct., 1962), 6; Virginia Stull to Chester R. Burns, Dec. 27, 1993, letter, WF380, CHP Archives; *University Medical*, 2 (Jan., 1971), 5; and *Newsletter (UTMB)*, 3 (June, 1968), 2.

52. See the list in RF150, CHP Archives. For comments about the number of ethnic minority and women students in the School of Medicine in the early 1970s, see *University Medical*, 2 (June, 1970), 7–8. In 1964, 11 blacks applied, two were accepted, and one enrolled. In 1983, 105 blacks applied, 15 were accepted, and 7 enrolled. See the list prepared by the Office of Admissions and Student Personnel Services in WF369, CHP Archives, and the "Medical Students: Minority Recruitment & Retention" folder in WF383, CHP Archives. Supported in part by a three-year grant from the Robert Wood Johnson Foundation, John Bruhn and others expended enormous energies in successful attempts to recruit more minority students between 1976 and 1979. In 1970 only 3 black students were enrolled in the School of Medicine; in 1979, 22 blacks were enrolled. In 1970, 23 Hispanic students were enrolled in the School of Medicine; in 1979, 60 Hispanics were enrolled. By 1978, 62 of 225 students who had attended UTMB's summer Familiarization Programs were enrolled in medical schools; 20 at UTMB. For many important details, see Bruhn's "Final Report to the Robert Wood Johnson Foundation." A copy is in folder 6, box 42, Levin Papers. Also see RF153 and WF369, CHP Archives. Key players in implementing this grant included Bill Levin, Ed Brandt, George Bryan, Raymond Fuentes Jr., Fernando Trevino, Raymond Lewis Jr., Raquel Bauman, Martha Torres, and Michael Bowie. For more details about the

Medical School Familiarization Program between 1977 and 1986, see folder 3, box 40, Levin Papers. See also *Syndrome* (1981), 255, and (1982), 265.

53. Marjorie Bartholf to Chauncey D. Leake, Aug. 31, 1949, letter, folder 7, box 1, School of Nursing Archives, Blocker Collections; *Syndrome* (1957), 160–162; and *Galveston Daily News*, Mar. 11, 1990.

54. In 1915–1916, two were from China and one each from England, Germany, Greece, Italy, Russian, and Scotland; see Carter's report in box 4Q21, UT President's Records. In 1936–1937, there was one student each from Canada, China, Cuba, Germany, Mexico, Poland, and the Philippines; see W. S. Carter to H. Y. Benedict, Mar. 1, 1937, letter, box 4Q18, UT President's Records. For details, see RF139, CHP Archives. See also Betty McAshan to George Bryan, Apr. 16, 1987, UTMB Dean's Office Records, Active; *Galveston Daily News*, June 7, 1991; and the "School of Medicine: Student Organizations, 1967–1991" folder in WF383, CHP Archives.

55. Megan Seaholm compiled the data for these statistics. See "Student Life at the University of Texas Medical Branch, 1901–1941," pp. 7–9, WF381, CHP Archives.

56. W. S. Carter to W. D. Collins, June 22, 1911, letter, box 4Q18, UT President's Records. Using data in the annual reports of the regents, Seaholm calculated these percentages. See the appendices in WF381, CHP Archives. In 1940 and 1941, about forty students received $15 a month from the federal government via the National Youth Administration for performing a variety of clerical, library, research, stenographic, and hospital jobs; see *Galveston Daily News*, Sept. 5, 1940, and Aug. 21, 1941. For details, see RF143, CHP Archives.

57. As a student between 1906 and 1910, J. Gordon Bryson had jobs as a church janitor, clothes salesman, streetcar conductor and co-op manager. See J. Gordon Bryson, *One Hundred Dollars & A Horse: The Reminiscences of a Country Doctor* (New York: William Morrow, 1965), 55–59. When he graduated in 1927, Jap Custer gave Cyril Black his job as the night manager at John Sealy Hospital. Black received meals and ten dollars a week. See Cyril Black to Gwen Walker, Dec. 10, 1992, WF358, CHP Archives. Kenneth Earle (class of 1945) worked as a blood bank technician and Bill Daeschner (class of 1945) was the switchboard operator at John Sealy Hospital every other night from 1 A.M. until 7 A.M.; see Kenneth Earle to Chester R. Burns, Mar. 15, 1990, and C. William Daeschner to Myles Knape and Chester R. Burns, July 13 and 20 and Aug. 3, 1988, interviews, Blocker Collections. Daeschner also earned income as an extern at the U.S. Public Health Service Hospital and he received free room and board while managing the Phi Chi fraternity house.

58. For a comment by a student, see *University Medical*, 18, no. 4 (1914), 22. For other examples, see *UTMB: Seventy-five Year History*, 282–291; a letter from C. M. Phillips (class of 1931) in folder 4, box 1, 75th Anniversary History Papers, Blocker Collections; and James C. Thompson to Myles Knape and Chester R. Burns, June 27, July 3 and 13, 1989, interviews, Blocker Collections. Thompson matriculated in 1946, married the following year, and earned about $200 a month from several jobs. He punched meal tickets and stuffed envelopes in the dean's office. He also managed three colonies of experimental animals (ducks for Rigdon in pathology, mice for Blount in anatomy, and rats for Sinclair in histology). See also *Galveston Daily News*, May 18 and 19, 1961.

59. Jarrett E. Williams to the Board of Directors of the Will C. Hogg Loan Fund, Nov. 14, 1940, box VF 9/B, UT President's Records; RF143, CHP Archives; Minutes, UTMB Faculty Meeting, Oct. 4, 1960; and *UTMB Catalog* (1966–1968), 36–49.

60. *Galveston Daily News*, May 18 and 19, 1961.

61. Sadie N. Hausmann to Henry C. Hartman, Dec. 6, 1926, letter, box 6, folder 64, School of Nursing Archives, Blocker Collections (quotation); and Chloe Floyd to Myles Knape, Jan. 16 and 22, 1986, interviews, Blocker Collections.

62. *Impact*, 4 (Jan. 25, 1980), 14. Also see John Bruhn's final report to the Robert Wood Johnson Foundation in folder 6, box 42, Levin Papers; and see page 11 of the attachment to William C. Levin to Warren Harding, Apr. 24, 1981, letter, folder 5, box 47, Levin Papers.

63. *Galveston Daily News*, Apr. 13, 1913. The dining club had officers. The president and secretary received their meals free. The vice president and "cop" received all the milk each wanted. The "cop" was the doorman who kept the hungry students outside until the food was ready. The student who managed the "cigar store" received a free cigar each week; see *Galveston Daily News*, Oct. 17, 1914. For more details, see the "Dining Club" folder in WF383, CHP Archives.

64. Though many students ate meals in fraternity houses, others headed off-campus. During the mid-1930s, for example, students rushed to "Gus's" or the "Greeks" as they nicknamed a restaurant on Tenth and Mechanic operated by Gus Saras, an uncle of George Mitchell. Students drank coffee between classes and played the slot machines. This restaurant later became the College Inn, a popular place for meals and coffee breaks. During the early 1960s students would eat at Giusti's on Fifteenth and Seawall and then ride the adjacent wooden roller coaster. For details, see the notes

from Virginia Blocker and comments by alumni during public presentations by Chester Burns in 1991 and 1993; these are in WF358, CHP Archives.

65. *Galveston Daily News*, Dec. 27, 1914; and Virginia Irvine Blocker to Myles Knape, Aug. 18, 1986, interview, Blocker Collections (quotation).

66. Marjorie Bartholf to D. Bailey Calvin, Apr. 3, 1946, letter, folder 5, box 1, School of Nursing Archives, Blocker Collections.

67. *Syndrome* (1961), 112 (quotation); *UTMB Catalog* (1966–68), 66; and RF146, CHP Archives.

68. See Schedule I-C 3 of application for loan under Title IV of the Housing Act of 1950, Sept. 23, 1952, box VF A/3, UT Chancellor's Records.

69. Sixty percent lived with one other person; 20 percent alone; 15 percent with two or three people; and 5 percent with four or more people. The survey results are attached to George T. Bryan to William C. Levin, Apr. 22, 1982, letter, folder 7, box 34, Levin Papers.

70. *Galveston Daily News*, June 26, 1952. For Runge's reports between 1922 and 1937, see UTMB Dean's Office Records, Inactive, boxes 16 and 17. Also see Elisabeth Runge to Myles Knape, Oct. 24, 1985, interview, Blocker Collections; *University Medical Center News*, 1 (Feb., 1961), 4–5; *Galveston Daily News*, Jan. 28, 1962, and Jan. 31, 1964; and *Newsletter (UTMB)*, 3 (Aug., 1968), 4. Also see the typescript of an interview with Miss Runge conducted in April 1965 in folder 35, box 1, 75th Anniversary History Papers, Blocker Collections; *Alumni Bulletin*, 22 (Fall, 1967), 13; and *Newsletter (UTMB)*, 3 (Aug., 1968), 4.

71. For a profile of Jones, see *Newsletter (UTMB)*, 4 (Apr., 1969), 2–4. For the new library, see *University Medical*, 3 (June, 1972), 15–21; and Larry J. Wygant, "Moody Medical Library," in Tyler, et al. (eds.), *The New Handbook of Texas*, IV, 814. For Frey, see Emil Frey to Myles Knape, Jan. 29 and 30 and Feb. 4, 1987, interviews, Blocker Collections. See also *Impact*, 8 (May 18, 1984), 13; and 10 (Apr. 18, 1986), 7; and *Galveston Daily News*, Oct. 8, 1990. For important details about the library, see vertical file A10 in the Blocker Collections. Elisabeth Runge died on November 28, 1990; see *Galveston Daily News*, Nov. 30, 1990.

72. See petition by students dated May 30, 1919; W. S. Carter to R. E. Vinson, July 17, 1919, letter; and R. E. Vinson to W. S. Carter, July 23, 1919, letter; all in box 4Q22, UT President's Records. See also Chauncey D. Leake to J. Edward Johnson, Sept. 27, 1945 (quotation) and C. D. Simmons to Theophilus Painter, May 24, 1950, letters, box VF 10/C, UT President's Records. After the fraternities created a political monopoly with the caucus in 1934, they were able to determine which students would have bookstore jobs. By the 1940s a large number of students objected to the arrangements. When elections were held in February 1947, a student poll indicated increasing disfavor. Although 171 students voted to continue the status quo, 147 students voted to abolish the current form of management. The student-managed cooperative was dissolved in the spring of 1950, when UTMB purchased the inventory of the bookstore from three senior medical students. For details, see D. Bailey Calvin to Drs. C. D. Leake (and others), Feb. 4, 1947, letter, Duncan Papers, no. 25, box 6, F. 96; "Minutes of a Meeting of the Bookstore Committee," Jan. 24, 1950; and letters about the bookstore in folder 1, box 1, School of Nursing Archives, Blocker Collections.

73. *Syndrome* (1961), 124; (1964), 92–93; and (1965), 82–83. See also *University Medical Center News*, 1 (Sept., 1960), 8; and *Impact*, 4 (Sept. 12, 1980), 13.

74. W. S. Carter to S. E. Mezes, May 28, 1910, letter, box 4R85, UT President's Records; *UTMB Catalog* (1931–1932), 30–31; Minutes, UTMB Faculty Meeting, Apr. 7, 1915; May 28 and 30, 1919; and June 6, 1933; folder 2, box 29, UTMB Dean's Office Records, Inactive; and RF148, CHP Archives.

75. *UTMB Catalog* (1959–1960), 165–170; and Minutes, UTMB Faculty Meeting, May 13, 1960. A copy of this constitution is in RF141, CHP Archives. Generally, there were few disciplinary problems. Early in 1960, for example, the Student Affairs Committee recommended that a freshmen be expelled because he had "conducted himself in a manner unbecoming a medical student and [had] exhibited judgment deficient to that required of the practicing physician"; see Minutes, UTMB Faculty Meeting, Oct. 2, 1960. The student was expelled. For examples of the Honor Council's actions between 1959 and 1963, see folder 164, box 15, School of Nursing Archives, Blocker Collections. For the 1970s and 1980s, see Minutes, UTMB Faculty Meetings, Oct. 2, 1973; Apr. 2 and Dec. 3, 1974; Oct. 7 and Dec. 2, 1975; and Apr. 12 and Dec. 13, 1977. Details about appeals are included in the constitution; a copy is in the "Medical Students: Student Government" folder in WF383, CHP Archives. See also Minutes, UTMB Faculty Meetings, Feb. 3 and Apr. 7, 1981; and Oct. 1, 1985; and letters and surveys in the "Medical Students: Student Government" folder in WF383, CHP Archives.

76. When the students revised the constitution of the Students' Association in the fall of 1912, fifteen female students lobbied unsuccessfully for a clause that would have compelled the students to elect a woman as secretary-treasurer every year.

Though the clause was defeated, the students unanimously elected Violet Keiller as the incoming secretary-treasurer; see *Galveston Daily News*, Oct. 26–27, 1912. For other details, see the Student Government folder in WF383, CHP Archives.

77. Some fraternities encouraged male interns to bring dates from the "red-light district," which occasionally resulted in sexual intercourse on the dance floor. These so-called "Annual Rat Dances" were held on the first floor of Psycho One. *University Medical* ceased publication after the June 1946 issue. By that year, it was merely a gossip journal and a forum for advertising Galveston's businesses. In April Leake told the regents and the Chamber of Commerce that the journal was not sanctioned by the administration and should not be supported. For details, see "Report to the Students," *University Medical* (June, 1946), 2–5. See also "The Agenda of the Meeting of the Faculty Committee on Student Affairs," Oct. 23, 1946, folder 12, box 6, Duncan Papers, Blocker Collections.

78. William D. Baird to Walter H. Kemp, Oct. 28, 1951, letter, folder 12, box 1, Duncan Papers, Blocker Collections; Minutes, UTMB Faculty Meetings, May 19, 1952, and Oct. 7, 1952 (quotation); *UTMB Catalog* (1953–1954), 54; and *Syndrome* (1956), 58.

79. Between 1897 and 1952, UTMB students were included in the *Cactus*, the UT Austin yearbook. See *Galveston Daily News*, Oct. 26 and Dec. 14, 1952; and Apr. 9 and 16, 1953.

80. Minutes, UTMB Faculty Meeting, May 6, 1958.

81. *Syndrome* (1960), 120–21.

82. Short-lived groups appeared in 1918 and 1941; see Megan Seaholm, "Student Life at the University of Texas Medical Branch 1942–1966," 63–67, WF382, CHP Archives. See also *Syndrome* (1956), 152; (1957), 150; (1958), 162; (1961), 111 and 119, as well as notes from meetings of School of Nursing Honor Council between 1959 and 1963 in RF141, CHP Archives.

83. Minutes, UTMB Faculty Meeting, May 24, 1963. A copy of this constitution is in RF141, CHP Archives.

84. *University Medical*, 2 (Nov., 1970), 7–10.

85. For more details, see *University Medical*, 2 (Jan., 1971), 10–11. For a copy of the new constitution, see "Medical Students: Student Government" folder in WF383, CHP Archives. See also *University Medical*, 3 (June, 1972), 10–11; and *Syndrome* (1979), 112, and (1980), 251.

86. See *Syndrome* (1981), 249, and (1982), 258. For student safety, see George T. Bryan to Diane Simpson, May 5, 1983, memo, "Medical Students: Student Issues" folder, WF383, CHP Archives. Also see *Impact*, 8 (Apr. 13, 1984), 19; and D. C. Eiland Jr. to V. E. Thompson, Dec. 10, 1982, letter, folder 6, box 34, Levin Papers.

87. Before mid-century, fraternities held numerous "smokers" and banquets honoring their faculty members. The Epsilon chapter of Phi Alpha Sigma hosted an eight-course dinner at the Galvez in March 1915; see *Galveston Daily News*, Mar. 12, 1915. For other examples, see *Galveston Daily News*, Dec. 12, 1914; Mar. 18, 1915; and Mar. 13, 1917.

88. For the Jolly Bone Jugglers and Sigma Ribbon, see *Cactus*, 7 (1900), 161–163; and 8 (1901), 128, 130–131. The Jolly Bone Jugglers appeared for the last time in *Cactus*, 10 (1903), 312, and Sigma Ribbon appeared for the last time in 11 (1904), 316–317. For Alpha Mu Pi Omega, see *Cactus*, 7 (1900), 159; 8 (1901), 128; and *Alumni Bulletin*, 17 (June, 1963), 4. Megan Seaholm calculated the 1916 percentage. See the appendices in WF381, CHP Archives.

89. See letter dated Oct. 1, 1922, in the Felix Butte letters, Blocker Collections (quotation). Butte pledged Alpha Kappa Kappa. See also *Galveston Daily News*, Sept. 29, 1934.

90. *Galveston Daily News*, Sept. 22, 1940, and June 15, 1941. Megan Seaholm calculated the percentages by counting the number of students in the photos of annual volumes of the *Cactus* and *Syndrome*. See the appendices in WF381, CHP Archives.

91. *Galveston Daily News*, Feb. 26, 1938; and May 30–31 and June 1, 1941. For details, see the Phi Chi publications in the "School of Medicine: Student Fraternities, 1967–1991" folder in WF383, CHP Archives; C. William Daeschner to Myles Knape and Chester R. Burns, July 13 and 20 and Aug. 3, 1988, interviews, Blocker Collections; and Jacob E. Reisch (ed.), *The History of the Phi Chi Medical Fraternity*, reprinted from the *Phi Chi Quarterly*, 50 (1953), 54–55. For details about the convention, see the January 1950 issue of *Phi Chi Quarterly*; a copy is in the "School of Medicine: Student Fraternities, 1967–1991" folder in WF383, CHP Archives.

92. *UTMB: Seventy-five Year History*, 285; and *Galveston Daily News*, Feb. 19, 1938.

93. *Galveston Daily News*, Sept. 5–8, 1951. Several essays in the November 1951 issue of *The Centaur* (the fraternity's monthly publication) reveal the excitement, fraternalism, and outreach spirit of this convention. See also James Oates, "A History of Alpha Theta Chapter," *The Centaur*, 56 (Mar., 1951), 227–231; and *Syndrome* (1966), 128–131 (quotation on 128).

94. *Galveston Daily News*, Mar. 12, 1938, and Dec 20, 1949. In WF378, CHP Archives, there is an excellent history of Theta Kappa Psi that was written by James Scott Buie (class of 1975).

95. See a history of this chapter in Will Walter and Stuart Graves, *A Half-Century of Nu Sigma Nu, 1882–1932* (Louisville, Ky.: The Nu Sigma Nu Fraternity, c. 1935), 1375–1397. See also *Galveston Daily News*, Mar. 19, 1938, and Nov. 20 and 27, 1954.

96. *Galveston Daily News*, Mar. 26, 1938.

97. Unlike the male fraternities, AEI did include at least one black student in 1958 (Marjorie Roberts). See *Syndrome* (1958), 110–111. See also *Galveston Daily News*, Apr. 2, 1938, and Oct. 1 and 7, 1950.

98. *Galveston Daily News*, Aug. 10, 1941. For other examples of fraternity parties and dances, see *Galveston Daily News*, July 23, Aug. 2 and 10, Oct. 2–5, 12, 19, 30–31, Nov. 14, 16, 18, 22–26, Dec. 21, 1941; Jan. 16, 31, Feb. 8, 15, 18, 22, 26, 27, July 12, Aug. 2, 16, 23, Oct. 25, Nov. 1, 24, 1942; Jan. 16, 17, 24, 29, Feb. 21, 27, Mar. 7, 14, 16, 20–21, 28, Apr. 4, Oct. 6, 24, Nov. 26, 1943; and Jan. 26, Feb. 23, and Dec. 9, 1945. For comments by former students, see Harry K. Davis to Chester R. Burns, Dec. 8, 1994, and James C. Thompson to Myles Knape and Chester R. Burns, June 27, July 3 and 13, 1989, interviews, Blocker Collections.

99. See *UTMB: Seventy-five Year History*, 285–286; and *Galveston Daily News*, May 31, 1917; Oct. 30, 1942; and Jan. 24, 1947. Also see the diary in folder 5 of the William Seybold Papers in the Blocker Collections.

100. Minutes, Sealy & Smith Foundation Board of Directors, May 13 and June 9, 1953; and July 11, Aug. 8, and Oct. 10, 1973. See also V. E. Thompson to E. D. Walker, Sept. 11, 1973, letter, folder 7, box 34, Levin Papers.

101 See D. C. Eiland Jr. to Frank J. Borrelli, June 8, 1977, and other items in the "School of Medicine: Student Fraternities, 1967–1991" folder, WF383, CHP Archives; and Gene D. Forrester to Chester R. Burns, Nov. 27, 1989, letter, WF378, CHP Archives.

102. *Galveston Daily News*, Sept. 25, 1910.

103. *Galveston Daily News*, June 23 and Aug. 28, 1951; and *University Medical*, 2 (Mar., 1971), 12–14.

104. For details about events between 1957 and 1961, see folder 2 in box 6, Duncan Papers, Blocker Collections. For Vastyan, see *University Medical Center News*, 1 (Dec., 1960), 6. For Jarrell, see *Newsletter (UTMB)*, 3 (Jan., 1968), 5.

105. For their names, see "William Temple Foundation History," WF358, CHP Archives. For details about the foundation's activities between 1963 and 1974, see folder 7, box 7, UTMB Alumni Association Records, Blocker Collections.

106. *Galveston Daily News*, June 3, 1960; and *Impact*, 9 (Sept. 20, 1985), 7.

107. *Syndrome* (1964), 86.

108. *Galveston Daily News*, Nov. 3, 1908; Nov. 17, 1940; Mar. 3, 1941; Oct. 3, 1941; Mar. 3, Apr. 9, and Dec. 3, 1942; *University Medical Center News*, 1 (Dec., 1960), 1; *Syndrome* (1960), 120–121; and *Impact*, 2 (Oct. 6, 1978), 19; and 3 (Nov. 2, 1979), 5. For a list of performers in 1987–1988, see *Impact*, 11 (Sept. 4, 1987), 5.

109. W. S. Carter to S. E. Mezes, May 2, 1910, letter, box 4R85, UT President's Records. For examples of Athletic Council events, see *Syndrome* (1956), 59; (1957), 107; and (1961), 179–183. See also *Newsletter (UTMB)*, 4 (Mar., 1969), 10–11.

110. Minutes, UTMB Faculty Meeting, Apr. 7, 1970; *Newsletter (UTMB)*, 4 (Jan., 1969), 2–3; and *Impact*, 9 (Aug. 23, 1985), 13.

111. *Impact*, 8 (Oct. 5, 1984), 7; and 10 (Mar. 21, 1986), 10–11.

112. *Alcalde*, 10 (1922), 1368. For details, see the AOA records in the Blocker Collections.

113. *Galveston Daily News*, Feb. 13, 1948; *Cactus*, 56 (1948), 550; "School of Medicine: Student Organizations, 1967–1991" folder, WF383, CHP Archives; and *Syndrome* (1979), 213; (1980), 252; (1981), 250; and (1982), 259.

114. *Galveston Daily News*, Oct. 15, 1944; *Alumni Bulletin*, 9 (Mar., 1954); *University Medical Center News*, 1 (May, 1961), 3; and *Syndrome* (1965), 89.

115. *Syndrome* (1966), 147; (1972), 126; (1975), 154–155; and (1980), 254. Also see the "School of Medicine: Student Organizations, 1967–1991" folder, WF383, CHP Archives, and the AMWA file in the Office of Student Life.

116. In 1930, for example, a new rule forbade student nurses to own or keep automobiles during their years as students; see Lucius R. Wilson to L. Gwynn Adams, Aug. 18, 1930, letter, folder 11, box 1, School of Nursing Archives, Blocker Collections.

117. For examples, see *Galveston Daily News*, Sept. 22, 1940; Apr. 25, May 30, and Sept. 27, 1941; Mar 3 and 7, 1942; Apr. 21, 1944; Oct. 28, 1949; Feb. 11, 1950; and May 16, 1952. For a photo of the officers of the Student Nursing Organization in 1954, see *Galveston Daily News*, Apr. 30, 1954. For examples of activities, see the answers to the questionnaire in WF378, CHP Archives.

118. *University Medical Center News*, 2 (Dec., 1961), 3. Graduate students had acquired some recognition when they were invited to be members of the Society of Sigma Xi after UTMB's chapter was organized in 1954. A few students were among the society's forty-three members in 1960; see *Syndrome* (1960), 123. Student representatives were also selected for the Curriculum Committee and the Program Review Committee.

119. A copy of its constitution is in "The Official Survival Guide for SAHS Students, 1982–83," pp. 78–81. A copy of the guide is in WF358, CHP Archives. Also see *Impact*, 1 (Dec. 9, 1977), 4; and 3 (Oct. 19, 1979), 5.

120. *Impact*, 4 (Sept. 26, 1980), 8; and 12 (June 10, 1988), 3. For examples of activities, see the answers to the questionnaire in WF378, CHP Archives.

121. For a complete list, see WF378, CHP Archives. Also see the "School of Medicine: Student Organizations, 1967–1991" folder, WF383, CHP Archives.

122. For their names, see *University Record*, 3 (1901), 496–498. This list also includes the names of the student editors of *University Medical* and the members of the Sigma Ribbon Society, the Jolly Bone Jugglers, and the Alpha Mu Pi Omega Medical Fraternity.

123. Minutes, UTMB Faculty Meeting, Apr. 19, 1956; *Galveston Daily News*, Apr. 17, 20, 1958; *Syndrome* (1964), 155; *Impact*, 8 (Feb. 24, 1984), 7; and 12 (Oct. 7, 1988), 8.

124. *Galveston Daily News*, May 8, 1961; *Impact*, 9 (May 3, 1985), 8; (Aug. 23, 1985), 5; 2(Jan. 13, 1978), 3; 5 (Apr. 24, 1981), 2; 8 (Feb. 24, 1984), 2; 10 (Mar. 7, 1986), 2; and 14 (Jan. 12, 1990), 5.

125. Most of the nicknames came from the interviews in the Blocker Collections. The one for Dean Carter came from Bryson, *One Hundred Dollars & a Horse*, 49.

126. *Galveston Daily News*, Apr. 9–10, and May 28, 1927; Feb. 23 and 26, 1931; and Apr. 18–20, 1935.

127. *University Medical Center News*, 1 (Mar., 1961), 1; *Newsletter (UTMB)*, 1 (Apr. 7, 1966), 3; 2 (Mar. 16, 1967), 3; and *Faculty News (UTMB)*, Mar. 9, 1973, 2.

128. For this and other incidents, see the list prepared by Megan Seaholm in WF383, CHP Archives.

129. Minutes, UTMB Faculty Meetings, Dec. 3, 1974; Oct. 7, 1975; Apr. 4, 1978; and Aug. 17, 1978.

130. *Faculty News (UTMB)*, June 23–July 4, 1975, 1. For Blakeney, see *Impact*, 3 (Jan. 26, 1979), 5. See also *Impact*, 3 (June 29, 1979), 2; 4 (June 27, 1980), 8–9; (Nov. 7, 1980), 5; and *Syndrome* (1980), 28, and (1981), 26. Also see "Informational Handbook for Faculty of the School of Medicine" (1982), 90–95. A copy is in WF255, CHP Archives. By the late 1980s some of the programs were titled Peer Tutorial Program, Study Skills Workshops, Test-Taking Strategies, and Relaxation Training.

131. See "Report of Activities of Student Affairs Office from September 1976 to Present and Proposed Priorities through August 1979," Jan. 13, 1978, in "Medical Students: Student Affairs Committee" folder in WF383, CHP Archives. Camille King and Gene Powell were key players in the Student Personnel Office during the 1970s; see Camille King to Myles Knape, Oct. 16, 1985, and Eugene Powell to Myles Knape, Oct. 15, 1985, interviews, Blocker Collections. In 1984 Eiland appointed Betty McAshan as UTMB's registrar; see Betty McAshan to Myles Knape, Oct. 23, 1985, interview, Blocker Collections.

132. For details, see David Eiland to Myles Knape, Nov. 19, 1985, and Jan. 21, 1986, interviews, Blocker Collections.

133. For examples, see *Galveston Daily News*, Nov. 16, 1900; Sept. 25, 1910; and Oct. 2, 1914. Some speeches were printed in the newspaper; for examples, see *Galveston Daily News*, Oct. 1, 1912 and 1922; Oct. 2, 1906–1909, 1913, 1915, 1926–1938, 1940; Oct. 3, 1911, 1939, and 1941; and Oct. 21, 1921. The Young Men's Christian Association (YMCA) hosted welcoming parties for incoming and returning students. In addition to "food and smoking," the dining club, bookstore, honor system, student council, and *University Medical* were explained to new students; see *Galveston Daily News*, Sept. 22, 1912. For Rainey's address, see *Galveston Daily News*, Oct. 3, 1941. The only extant photo of an opening ceremony appeared in the preceding year when Raymond Gregory gave the opening address; see *Galveston Daily News*, Oct. 2, 1940. For the informal welcoming speeches, see *Galveston Daily News*, Sept. 12–13, 17, 1950; and Sept. 18–20, 1951. For some of Leake's receptions, see *Galveston Daily News*, Jan. 13 and Nov. 15, 1952; and July 9 and Oct. 3, 1954.

134. *Newsletter (UTMB)*, 3 (Nov., 1968), 15; *Impact*, 2 (Aug. 25, 1978), 1, 13; 6 (Aug. 20, 1982), 6; and 15 (Aug. 16, 1991), 6.

135. For examples, see *Galveston Daily News*, May 13, 1900; and June 16, 1901; and the commencement brochures in the three boxes of vertical file E3 in the Blocker Collections. There are a few brochures for the years between 1893 and 1930, and a fairly complete set for the years between 1930 and 1982.

136. *Galveston Daily News*, May 29 and June 1, 1910; and May 15, 28, 31, and June 5, 1927. The last ceremony for pharmacy students in Galveston was in 1927, as the school moved to Austin during the summer. For the fiftieth commencement, see *Galveston Daily News*, May 25 and 31, and June 1, 1941. Bill Levin was one of five Galvestonians in this graduating class; see *Galveston Daily News*, May 31, 1941.

137. *Galveston Daily News*, Mar. 19–21, 1942; and Dec. 17–18, 1942. Also see the brochures in box 1, vertical File E3, Blocker Collections. See also *Galveston Daily News*, Mar. 1 and 3, 1946. Betty Rudnick was one of the nurse graduates in 1946. The two students who received physical therapy certificates in 1946 were probably UTMB's first "allied health" graduates. For the last accelerated class, see *Galveston Daily News*, Feb. 14, 1948.

138. For examples, see the commencement brochures in the 1940–1949 folder, box 1, vertical file E3, Blocker Collections. For a fascinating description of the capping ceremony, see "At the University of Texas School of Nursing," *American Journal of Nursing*, 31 (Apr., 1931), 491–492. For a photo of forty-five students attending this ceremony at the Rebecca Sealy Nurses' Home in May 1941, see *Galveston Daily News*, May 9, 1941. For programs and letters about the capping ceremonies between 1932 and 1955, see folder 61, box 6, School of Nursing Archives, Blocker Collections.

139. *Galveston Daily News*, May 27 and June 1–2, 1951; and *Alumni Bulletin*, 6 (July 1951), 1. James C. Thompson was one of the graduates in 1951. See also *Galveston Daily News*, May 13 and June 3, 7, 1952; *Alumni Bulletin*, 7 (July–Aug., 1952), 1–3; and *Galveston Daily News*, June 4–6, 1953.

140. *Galveston Daily News*, May 29, 1955. Melvyn Schreiber was one of the physician graduates in 1955. See also *Medi-Texan*, 3 (June, 1956), 1, 3; *Alumni Bulletin*, 11 (July, 1956), 1–2; and *Galveston Daily News*, May 27, 31, and June 1–2, 1956.

141. *Galveston Daily News*, May 22, 29–30, 1957; and June 1 and 3, 1958. The winner of the Gold-Headed Cane Award keeps the cane until the next graduation, when another student is selected. See *Galveston Daily News*, May 27, 1960 (quotation); *Alumni Bulletin*, 14 (Aug., 1960), 1; and *UTMB: Seventy-five Year History*, 295. For the seventy-fifth commencement, see *Alumni Bulletin*, 19 (Aug., 1965), 1.

142. As an example, see the 1973 brochure in the collection of commencement brochures in the Dean's Office of the School of Nursing.

143. Information about School of Allied Health Sciences commencements was obtained from the brochures in the Dean's Office of the School of Allied Health Sciences.

144. For a list of names of award and scholarship winners, see *Impact*, 2 (June 2, 1978), 3, 14. Also see the commencement brochures for the 1970s in box 3, vertical file E3, Blocker Collections. The names of those receiving the awards in 1991 are in a list in WF341, CHP Archives.

145. T. C. Thompson to T. D. Wooten, Feb. 18, 1895, letter, Wooten Papers; W. S. Carter to W. J. Battle, June 2, 1915, box 4Q20; and W. S. Carter to S. E. Mezes, Nov. 12, 1912, box 4Q19, letters, UT President's Records. When Elbert died in 1927, after thirty years of service, classes were suspended so that students and faculty could attend his funeral; see *Galveston Daily News*, Feb. 2–3, 1927.

146. See Keiller's Annual Report for 1917–1918, box 4Q22, UT President's Records. John Sinclair told H. Y. Benedict that his janitor was expected to "raise" a family of five on $65 a month, which was less than he had received twelve years ago; see Sinclair to Benedict, Aug. 18, 1933, letter, box VF 9/C, UT President's Records. During the early 1930s, Sinclair and Paul Brindley contributed personal funds to pay the salaries of their technicians. See John Sinclair to H. Y. Benedict, May 18, 1931, letter, box 16, UTMB Dean's Office Records, Inactive. Hiring suitable employees was also a challenge because of the anti-nepotism rule that made it difficult to hire wives, daughters, and sons. After receiving a special waiver in 1916, Dean Carter was permitted to hire John Nolan's daughter as an administrative secretary; see R. E. Vinson to W. S. Carter, Aug. 12, 1916, letter, box 4Q21, UT President's Records.

147. H. O. Knight to H. Y. Benedict, July 8, 1932, letter, box 16, UTMB Dean's Office Records, Inactive. In fiscal year 1932 Beissner prepared photographs, slides, and motion pictures for ten academic departments and the John Sealy Hospital Memorial Laboratory. See also Chauncey D. Leake to T. S. Painter, Sept. 19, 1949, and Chauncey D. Leake to T. S. Painter, Aug. 9, 1950, letters, both in box VF 10/D, UT President's Records.

148. Minutes, UT Board of Regents, Sept. 19, 1947; and James P. Hart to Mrs. Jack C. Buchanan, Apr. 11, 1952, letter, box VF C/1, UT Chancellor's Records. For details about the discount on hospital charges and services, see "Policy

Statements" in box VF I/4, UT Chancellor's Records. See also Charles T. Clark to James P. Hart, Dec. 17, 1953, letter, box VF 20/B, UT President's Records.

149. *Galveston Daily News*, Mar. 15, 1955; *Galveston Tribune*, Mar. 29, 1955; and Chauncey D. Leake to Logan Wilson, Mar. 2, 1955, letter, box VF E/2, UT Chancellor's Records. For these and other "classified salary" categories, see the table accompanying Truman Blocker Jr. to Logan Wilson, Sept. 9, 1955, letter, box VF E/2, UT Chancellor's Records.

150. Charles T. Clark to Logan Wilson, Dec. 18, 1956, box VF G/1; and Arthur Hennings to John B. Truslow, c. June 1958, box VF S/3, letters, UT Chancellor's Records; "The University of Texas Medical Branch Hospitals, 1965–67," box VF FF/2, UT Chancellor's Records; and *Newsletter (UTMB)*, 1 (Aug., 1965), 1.

151. *Impact*, 1 (July 29, 1977), 5; 2 (June 2, 1978), 8–9; and supplement to *Impact*, 3 (June 29, 1979), 3.

152. For details about the improved coverage, see *Impact*, 4 (June 13, 1980), 5. See also Department of Human Resources, "Benefits in Brief," undated copy, and the Employee Handbook titled "High Tech High Touch," 1986, pp. 8–12, both in WF358, CHP Archives.

153. Chauncey D. Leake to T. S. Painter, June 23, 1949, letter, box VF 10/D, UT President's Records; *Medi-Texan*, 4 (June, 1957), 4–5; and *University Medical*, 2 (Dec., 1970), 12–13.

154. *Hospital News*, 7 (Oct. 14, 1974), 3; and *Impact*, 11 (June 26, 1987), 1.

155. *Hospital News*, 4 (Mar. 2, 1970), 4, and (Mar. 16, 1970), 4; *Impact*, 6 (Dec. 17, 1982), 1, 10; 12 (Dec. 2, 1988), 1; and 13 (Dec. 1, 1989), 1.

156. *Medi-Texan*, 1 (Oct., 1953), 4; 2 (Aug., 1955), 11; and 3 (June, 1956), 8–9. See also *Newsletter (UTMB)*, 3 (Mar., 1968), 11; *University Medical*, 2 (Nov., 1970), 11–13; *Faculty News (UTMB)*, Sept. 14, 1973, 2; Sept. 16–20, 1974, 1; and Aug. 12, 1983, 3.

157. *Impact*, 3 (Sept. 7, 1979), 13, 15, 19. The softball leagues continued each year through the centennial year. See *Impact*, 4 (Oct. 10, 1980), 11; 6 (Oct. 1, 1982), 18; 7 (Mar. 25, 1983), 20; 8 (Apr. 13, 1984), 26; 9 (Mar. 22, 1985), 8; 10 (Apr. 18, 1986), 13; 11 (May 15, 1987), 4; 12 (Mar. 4, 1988), 7; and 15 (Mar. 8, 1991), 11. Also see *University Medical*, 1 (Jan., 1970), 22. For the volleyball league, see *Impact*, 5 (June 18, 1981), 16.

158. *Medi-Texan*, 3 (Sept., 1956), 1–2, 7. Betty Grefenstette prepared a short history of the club in 1991; see WF362, CHP Archives. For other details, see folder 5, box 33, Levin Papers. Diane Wonio was an active member during the 1980s; for comments, see Diane Wonio to Megan Seaholm, July 27, 1989, interview, Blocker Collections.

159. For details, see RF135, CHP Archives; *Impact*, 3 (Mar. 23, 1979), 2; and V. E. Thompson to all department heads and administrative officials, May 25, 1984, memo, WF358, CHP Archives.

160. *Impact*, 4 (Jan. 11, 1980), 6; 5 (Mar. 20, 1981), 7; 6 (Sept. 3, 1982), 7; 7 (Sept. 9, 1983), 24; and 9 (May 3, 1985), 5.

161. *Impact*, 6 (Oct. 29, 1982), 1; 7 (May 20, 1983), 12. For details, see Chesney's letter and reports in WF358, CHP Archives.

162. See the section on Annual Personnel Evaluations dated November 19, 1985, in the Handbook of Operating Procedures.

163. *Impact*, 12 (June 24, 1988), 3. For details, see WF370, CHP Archives.

164. See the supplement to *Impact*, 3 (June 29, 1979); and the supplement to *Impact*, 5 (Jan. 9, 1981); *Impact*, 6 (Oct. 1, 1982), 14–15; (Dec. 3, 1982), 13–16; and 9 (Dec. 20, 1985), 9–11.

165. *Galveston Daily News*, Feb. 3 and 5, 1941; Oct. 5, 1961; and *Newsletter (UTMB)*, 1 (Aug. 18, 1966), 2–3.

166. *Hospital News*, 4 (July 6, 1970), 4; and *Impact*, 2 (Feb. 10, 1978), 11.

167. *University Medical*, 3 (Feb., 1972), 17; *Impact*, 5 (Aug. 28, 1981), 11; and 3 (Apr. 6, 1979), 13; and *Galveston Daily News*, Feb. 15, 1962.

168. *Impact*, 8 (Aug. 24, 1984), 12–13; 14 (Sept. 14, 1990), 4; and 11 (Dec. 18, 1987), 5.

169. For more details, see the typescript by Myles Knape, "The University of Texas Medical Branch: A Media Event," pp. 1–7. A copy is in WF420, CHP Archives. For other details, see RF152, CHP Archives.

170. Meyer was an experienced newspaper reporter and publicist. For details, see Myles Knape, "The University of Texas Medical Branch: A Media Event," pp. 24–26. The first number of volume one of *University Medical Center News* was issued in mid-September 1960. In number ten of volume one (summer 1961) the title changed to *The University of Texas Medical Center News*. Usually called *Medical Center News* by most employees, this newsletter ended

with number three of volume three in November 1962. For additional details, see Minutes, UTMB Faculty Meeting, Feb. 7, 1961; and Myles Knape, "The University of Texas Medical Branch: A Media Event," pp. 26–28.

171. *Newsletter (UTMB)*, 2 (Oct. 16, 1966), 6. For some of Knape's correspondence, see the Office of External Affairs Records in the Blocker Collections. See also *Newsletter (UTMB)*, 3 (Nov., 1968), 13.

172. Myles Knape, "The University of Texas Medical Branch: A Media Event," p. 42. During the 1980s, marketing values loomed larger and larger in the perspectives of storytellers and imagemakers in UTMB's "publicity" offices. In *Impact*, for example, advertisements occupied spaces that had been filled previously by stories and photos about the richly diverse contributions of different employees who worked at UTMB during the late 1970s.

173. *Alumni Bulletin*, 21 (Feb., 1967), 3; and *University Medical*, 3 (Nov., 1971), 6–9. A few copies of the *Synapse* are in the Blocker Collections.

174. For details, see WF421, CHP Archives.

175. *Galveston Daily News*, Oct. 4, 1979.

176. *Impact*, 7 (July 1, 1983), 2.

177. For details about these administrative changes, see Myles Knape, "The University of Texas Medical Branch: A Media Event," pp. 44–56; and *Impact*, 10 (Apr. 18, 1986), 8.

CHAPTER 9

1. *UTMB: Seventy-five Year History*, 51.

2. A substantial number of alumni remained in Texas. Of those still practicing in 1989, these included approximately 67 percent of School of Medicine alumni; 75 percent of School of Nursing alumni; 80 percent of School of Allied Health Sciences alumni; and 62 percent of Graduate School of the Biomedical Sciences alumni. For these tabulations, see Betty Grefenstette's memo in WF389, CHP Archives.

3. Allen J. Smith to William L. Prather, Apr. 21, 1903, letter, box 4R82, UT President's Records; *Galveston Daily News*, Sept. 16, 1910; and W. S. Carter to the Honorable Board of Regents and the President of the University of Texas, c. May 1915, letter, box 4R85, UT President's Records. Accompanying this letter was a list of internships awarded to UTMB graduates for all of the sessions between 1904 and 1915.

4. *Galveston Daily News*, May 8, 1922, and June 1, 1926. In 1925 the Texas State Board of Medical Examiners began requiring an internship for a medical license. See W. S. Carter to J. W. Calhoun, Nov. 1, 1937, letter, box 4Q18, UT President's Records. By 1937 the AMA's Council on Medical Education and Hospitals had approved more than seven hundred hospitals for the training of more than seven thousand interns, though schools then only produced between five and six thousand graduates each year. During the 1930s many teaching hospitals systematized their acceptance patterns for interns, with most selecting them before January of the year in which the internship would begin. In January 1938, for example, eighty-one members of the senior class had accepted internships; ninety-one in January 1939; see *Galveston Daily News*, Jan. 19, 1938, and Jan, 19, 1939. For examples of appointments in the 1940s, see *Galveston Daily News*, Mar. 16, 1940; Jan. 29 and Dec. 15, 1942; June 6, 1943; Feb. 24, 1946; and Nov. 8, 1946.

5. Chauncey D. Leake to James P. Hart, Mar. 16, 1953, letter, box VF A/3, UT Chancellor's Records; and *Galveston Daily News*, Apr. 1, 1960.

6. *University Medical Center News*, 2 (Apr., 1962), 5; Edward N. Brandt Jr., Frances Holmstrom, and Elizabeth L. Fitzsimmons, "A Study of UTMB Graduates: 1967–1976," *Texas Medicine*, 75 (June, 1979), 54–58; William C. Levin to Warren Harding, Apr. 24, 1981, p. 13 of attachment in letter, folder 5, box 47, Levin Papers. During these same years, between 50 and 60 percent of the graduates remained in Texas for their residencies and between 72 and 92 percent were accepted into university-based residencies. For details about 1980–1991, see the reports in WF329, CHP Archives.

7. *University Record*, 2, no. 4 (1900), 400–402. For other examples, see *UTMB: Seventy-five Year History*, 299–303.

8. For examples of alumni meetings, see *Galveston Daily News*, June 1, 1904; May 30, 1908; May 31, 1910; and May 31, 1914. For examples of banquets during TMA meetings, see *Galveston Daily News*, May 26, 1903; Apr. 28, 1905; May 12, 1909; May 16, 1914; and May 13, 1923; and *Alcalde*, 4 (May, 1916), 637–641 and 706–708; and 10 (June, 1922), 1448–1453. For the May 1909 meeting see *Galveston Daily News*, May 12, 1909. For 1914, see W. S. Carter to S. E. Mezes, May 16, 1914, letter, box 4Q20, UT President's Records; and for the 1930s see *Galveston Daily News*, May 9, 1931, and May 12, 1938; and *Alcalde*, 20 (Mar., 1932), 136–137.

9. *University Medical*, 2, no. 5 (1897), 197; 4, no. 6 (1899), 255; 5, no. 7 (1900), 224; 6, no. 3 (1901), 56; 6, no. 5 (1902), 129; 7, no. 3 (1902), 88; 9, no. 1 (1904), 11; 13, no. 1 (1908), 17; and 14, no. 3 (1909), 12. For Speed, see *Impact*, 4 (Nov. 21, 1980), 13. From volume 1 in 1905 through volume 62 in 1966, the *Texas State Journal of Medicine* included superb obituaries. In these volumes, the names of those physicians are listed in an index to each volume. Thus,

if a reader knows the name of a physician and the year of death, it is easy to determine if the *Texas State Journal of Medicine* published an obituary. Many of these physicians were UTMB graduates. For example, four graduates were included in volume 36, August 1940, pp. 339–342: Robert Lee Yeager (class of 1898); Ralph S. Jackson (class of 1900); Summerfield M. Taylor (class of 1913); and John Harold Turner (class of 1919). Yeager practiced in Mineral Wells; Jackson in San Antonio; Taylor in Austin; and Turner in Houston. It would be possible for an enterprising scholar to obtain much more biographical information about the careers of UTMB's graduates by studying these obituaries. From 1967 to the present, the practice of publishing obituaries of some physicians continued in *Texas Medicine*, but their names are not listed in an index or table of contents.

10. *Galveston Daily News*, Nov. 3, 1954; J. W. Young Sr., *It All Comes Back* (Sweetwater, Texas: Watson-Focht Company, 1962); and Bryson, *One Hundred Dollars & a Horse*.

11. Elizabeth Silverthorne, "Claudia Potter," in Tyler, et al. (eds.), *The New Handbook of Texas*, V, 297–298; and *Galveston Daily News*, Feb. 29, 1964.

12. *Texas State Journal of Medicine*, 34 (June, 1938), 65–66; *UTMB: Seventy-five Year History*, 300; Randy J. Sparks, "Ernst William Bertner," in Tyler, et al. (eds.), *The New Handbook of Texas*, I, 505–506; and Jeanette Barry, *Notable Contributions to Medical Research by Public Health Service Scientists* (Washington, D.C.: U.S. Department of Health, Education, and Welfare Public Health Service, 1960), 19–22. Also see WF350, CHP Archives; and *Alumni Bulletin*, 22 (Fall, 1967), 2. Victoria Harden provided details about Dyer's work at NIH. Leake knew that Dyer was an alumnus; see Chauncey D. Leake to Rollo E. Dyer, Aug. 5, 1948, letter, box VF 10/C, UT President's Records.

13. *Texas State Journal of Medicine*, 39 (Oct., 1943), 359; and *Galveston Daily News*, Jan. 20, 1944. For information about alumni who served during World War I, see *UTMB: Seventy-five Year History*, 109–110.

14. For details, see the book prepared mostly by Robert Moore titled, *The 127th General Hospital*; the World War II Alumni Collection of newspaper clippings; and Mildred Robertson's "Overseas Letters," all in the Blocker Collections.

15. Born in 1907, Mildred Robertson began work at UTMB in 1930 as an assistant to her cousin, Elisabeth Runge, who directed the library. In the summer of 1944 Robertson began writing a series of "Overseas Letters" to those alumni who were serving with the 127th General Hospital Unit. When "Millie" served with the American Red Cross between May 1945 and February 1946, Margaret McArdle, UTMB's medical record librarian, wrote the "Overseas Letters." Millie edited the *Alumni Bulletin* for many years, coordinated alumni tours of Europe during the 1960s and 1970s, and organized a host of alumni reunions and dinners. For details, see *UTMB: Seventy-five Year History*, 303–304; Mildred Robertson to Myles Knape, May 8 and 29 and June 18, 1986, interviews; *Alumni Bulletin*, 17 (Aug., 1963), 5; (Oct., 1963), 3; and (Dec., 1963), 3; and twelve boxes of the UTMB Alumni Association Records in the Blocker Collections. For profiles of Millie after her retirement, see *Impact*, 2 (Oct. 6, 1978), 14; and 6 (Aug. 6, 1982), 18–19.

16. In 1965, 60 percent of School of Medicine alumni were general practitioners; see *UTMB: Seventy-five Year History*, 303. In 1990 M. T. Pepper Jenkins, McDermott Professor Emeritus of Anesthesiology at UT Southwestern, assembled a unique collection of memorabilia about himself and thirty-four classmates who graduated from the School of Medicine in 1940. Twelve of the ninety-one graduates in this class were still practicing; ten solo, one in a partnership, and one a professor. Twenty-five children of the graduates had become doctors or dentists. The profiles of thirty of these classmates revealed a broad spectrum of specialty interests that included general practice (five), internal medicine (five), general surgery (three), pediatrics (three), EENT (three), urology (two), thoracic surgery (two), anesthesiology (two), and one each in ob-gyn, pediatric surgery, and psychiatry. One was a U.S.P.H.S. physician and one was a V.A. chest physician. See "After 50 Years . . . Unreliable Memoirs by the Class of 1940," WF401, CHP Archives.

17. Steven M. Spencer, "We Need More Country Doctors," *Saturday Evening Post*, Oct. 9, 1954, p. 54 (quotation). Schulze attended many patients from the German-speaking towns in Central Texas, admitting some to the LaGrange Hospital, others to the Renger Hospital in Hallettsville. For details about his practices, see his book titled *Yesterday's Seasons* (New York: Hawthorn Books, 1978). For information about Franks, see *Impact*, 11 (May 1, 1987), 7.

18. *Alumni Bulletin*, 6 (June, 1951), 1; 7 (June, 1952), 1; and 8 (June, 1953), 1; *Alumni Bulletin*, 9 (July, 1954), 1; *UTMB: Seventy-five Year History*, 297; and *Alumni Bulletin*, 11 (June, 1957), 1.

19. For a copy of the revised constitution and bylaws, see *Alumni Bulletin*, 20 (Apr., 1966), 3–4. See also T. G. Blocker Jr. to Harry H. Ransom, Apr. 28, 1965, letter, box VF FF/1; and Truman G. Blocker Jr. to Harry H. Ransom, May 16, 1968, letter, box VF EE/3, UT Chancellor's Records; *Alumni Bulletin*, 19 (Aug., 1965), 1–2; and *UTMB: Seventy-five Year History*, 295–297. For biographical information about each of the award winners, see WF400, CHP Archives. For details about awards between 1976 and 1985, see folder 8, box 29, Levin Papers.

20. For samples of Levin's reports, see folders 4 and 5, box 29, Levin Papers.

21. More than thirty additional examples are given later in this chapter.

22. For source citations in the *Alumni Bulletin*, see the list in WF399, CHP Archives. Although incomplete, this list does contain the names of other alumni who served as officers in societies. When the Texas State Medical Association

changed its name to the Texas Medical Association in 1951, Allen T. Stewart was president; see *Texas State Journal of Medicine*, 47 (May, 1951), 263. For more on Holland Jackson, see *Galveston Daily News*, Mar. 7, 1957. For other examples, see *UTMB: Seventy-five Year History*, 299–303.

23. *Alumni Bulletin*, 17 (June, 1963), 3; and (Dec., 1963), 2–3; 18 (Feb., 1964), 2–3; (Apr., 1964), 4–5; and (June, 1964), 4–5; 20 (Oct., 1966), 4; 21 (Feb., 1967), 4–5; (Apr., 1967), 4–5; and (June, 1967), 4–5. For the names of other alumni who served in various official roles during these years, see the list in WF399, CHP Archives.

24. *University Medical*, 2 (Oct., 1970), 16; 2 (Nov., 1970), 17; 2 (Jan., 1971), 17; 2 (Mar., 1971), 17; 3 (Oct., 1971), 19; 3 (Dec., 1971), 19; 4 (Oct., 1972), 17; 5 (Apr., 1974), 20; 8 (June, 1977), 17; and 9 (Dec., 1977). 16. For the names of other alumni who served in various official roles during these years, see the list in WF399, CHP Archives.

25. *Impact*, 4 (Oct. 24, 1980), 1, 17.

26. *Alumni Bulletin*, 14 (Apr., 1960), 2; Elizabeth Silverthorne and Geneva Fulgham, *Women Pioneers in Texas Medicine* (College Station: Texas A&M University Press, 1997), 127–139; *Impact*, 6 (May 21, 1982), 11; and *Texas Medicine*, 78 (June, 1982), 32–33. Also see Ruth Bain, *Doors Will Open For You* (Denton: Texas Woman's University Printing Services, 1997).

27. *Alumni Bulletin*, 16 (Dec., 1962), 2; and the biographical sketch in WF400, CHP Archives.

28. Clotilde P. García, "José Antonio García," in Tyler, et al. (eds.), *The New Handbook of Texas*, III, 85; *Impact*, 9 (Aug. 9, 1985), 12. Also see García's contributions to "After 50 Years . . . Unreliable Memoirs by the Class of 1940," WF401, CHP Archives; Hercilia X. Toscano, "Edward Treviño Ximenes," in Tyler, et al. (eds.), *The New Handbook of Texas*, VI, 1103; *Impact*, 8 (June 1, 1984), 11; and (Mar. 23, 1984), 13.

29. *Galveston Daily News*, July 10, 1949; and *Texas State Journal of Medicine*, 50 (May, 1954), 275.

30. *UTMB: Seventy-five Year History*, 299–300; Chauncey D. Leake to Kenneth L. Lynch, Dec. 14, 1949, letter, box VF 10/D, UT President's Records; and "Dr. Kenneth M. Lynch," *Southern Medical Journal*, 51 (Feb., 1958), 248–249. One of the earliest diplomates of the American Board of Pathology, Lynch was president of two organizations in 1930: the American Society of Clinical Pathologists and the American Society of Tropical Medicine. See also *Alumni Bulletin*, 16 (June, 1963), 6; *University Medical*, 1 (Jan., 1970), 18; 6 (Sept.–Oct., 1974), alumni folio between pages 12 and 13; 2 (Nov., 1970), 16; and 4 (June, 1973), 18.

31. *Galveston Daily News*, Nov. 23 and 26, and Dec. 2 and 4, 1952; Aug. 23 and Dec. 7, 1959; and Jan. 22 and 24, 1954; *Alumni Bulletin*, 9 (Feb., 1954), 2. For a biographical sketch of Singleton, see Chester R. Burns, "Albert Olin Singleton," in Tyler, et al. (eds.), *The New Handbook of Texas*, V, 1060. See also *Impact*, 5 (Sept. 25, 1981), 4–5.

32. *Galveston Daily News*, Nov. 15, 1959, and Sept. 7, 1960. See also *Impact*, 2 (Feb. 10, 1978), 2, and (Feb. 24, 1978), 2; *Galveston Daily News*, Jan. 29, 1962; and *Impact*, 3 (May 18, 1979), 6.

33. *Impact*, 2 (Mar. 10, 1978), 8–9; *University Medical*, 10 (Mar.–May, 1979), 23; *Impact*, 6 (Apr. 23, 1982), 9; 11 (May 1, 1987), 5–12; and 10 (Apr. 4, 1986), 11.

34. See the minutes in folder 5, box 19, School of Nursing Archives, Blocker Collections. The names of the 103 members are listed in the minutes for December 1, 1925. See also *Galveston Daily News*, May 12, 1927; and the minutes of meetings in folders 6 and 6a, box 19, School of Nursing Archives, Blocker Collections.

35. See the annual report of the association's secretary and treasurer for 1933–1935 in folder 6a, box 19, School of Nursing Archives, Blocker Collections.

36. For details, see the minutes in folders 6b and 6c, box 19, School of Nursing Archives, Blocker Collections; folder 6, box 22, School of Nursing Archives, Blocker Collections; *Alumni Bulletin (School of Nursing)*, 1 (June, 1953), 2–3; and *Galveston Daily News*, May 26, 1940.

37. *Galveston Daily News*, June 1, 1950; *Alumni Bulletin (School of Nursing)*, 2 (July, 1954), 1; and *Galveston Daily News*, June 3, 5, 1954. For reports about other reunion dinners and the activities of graduates during the 1950s, see the quarterly *Bulletin* that Annie Lee Shaw, a secretary in the School of Nursing, edited. Some are in the Blocker collections. See also *Newsletter (UTMB)*, 1 (Apr. 1, 1965), 1; and (Apr. 15, 1965), 1–2. By the late 1960s several committees did the work of the School of Nursing Alumni Association: archives, finance, membership, nominating, program, publicity, and social. For copies of the bylaws as they evolved through the years, see folder 1, box 20, School of Nursing Archives, Blocker Collections. Important insights into the activities of the SONAA can be gleaned from correspondence that extends from 1949 to 1989; see folders 2–6, box 20, School of Nursing Archives, Blocker Collections. Also see issues of the *Bulletin* for the late 1960s in folder 3, Box 21, School of Nursing Archives, Blocker Collections. When the system-wide School of Nursing existed between 1967 and 1976, a system-wide Alumni Association functioned; for some details see folder 9, box 21 and folder 3, box 22, School of Nursing Archives, Blocker Collections.

38. For details, see minutes of meetings and related materials in folders 4, 4a, and 5–9, box 22, School of Nursing Archives, Blocker Collections.

39. *Impact*, 2 (July 28, 1978), 13; 10 (Oct. 3, 1986), 1; and (Oct. 17, 1986), 3.

40. *Texas State Journal of Medicine*, 4 (Apr., 1909), 326–327. For more information about the attractions of Galveston, see David G. McComb, "Galveston as a Tourist City," *Southwestern Historical Quarterly*, 100 (Jan., 1997), 330–360.

41. For examples, see the photos on the unnumbered page of section 9 of Linda Macdonald, *A Pattern of Love* (Houston: Sisters of Charity of the Incarnate Word Health Care System, 1996). The social and financial changes of the late twentieth century fostered some conflicts and tensions, though Sister M. Anastasia Enright and Tom James respectfully interacted to maintain a spirit of cooperative harmony during the early 1990s before UTMB acquired St. Mary's in 1996. For comments by Enright, see Macdonald, *A Pattern of Love*, unnumbered page in section 3. Also see Reza Jahadi's presidential address to the Galveston County Medical Society (1991) in WF389, CHP Archives.

42. *Galveston Daily News*, July 6, 1903; and *Texas State Journal of Medicine*, 1 (July, 1905), 36–37. For examples of meetings before 1955, see *Texas State Journal of Medicine*, 2 (Feb., 1907), 283; 4 (Jan., 1909), 235–236; 5 (Feb., 1910), 393; and *Galveston Daily News*, Dec. 17, 1903; Feb. 1 and Apr. 25, 1908; Jan. 9 and Oct. 30, 1909; Jan. 10, 1914; Mar. 10 and Apr. 14, 1917; Nov. 29, 1919; Jan. 31, 1920; Oct. 28, 1921; Nov. 14, 1931; Apr. 8, 1938; May 3 and Dec. 15, 1940; Nov. 2, 1941; Dec. 24, 1946; and Feb. 26, 1953. Wives of faculty members were active in the Galveston County Medical Society Auxiliary and attended meetings of the various auxiliaries during the TMA's annual meetings; see *Galveston Daily News*, May 3, 1942, and Mar. 14, 1951. Extensive archival records about the society and its auxiliaries are deposited in the Blocker Collections. These include minute books from 1927 to 1975, annual reports from 1923 to 1969, and yearbooks from 1945 to 1974. These items include many references to professors and alumni who supported the GCMS.

43. *Galveston Daily News*, Jan. 10, 1901. See also *Galveston Daily News*, May 19, 1904; Apr. 3, 1912; and Apr. 11, 1915. Some of the women in the Women's Health Protective Association were wives of faculty members. For an overview, see Jane A. Kenamore, "Women's Health Protective Association," in Tyler, et al. (eds.), *The New Handbook of Texas*, VI, 1056. See also *Galveston Daily News*, Feb. 24, Mar. 9, 11, 18, 21, and Apr. 7, 1913. A series of eight articles about UTMB's role in preventive medicine and public health appeared serially in the *Galveston Daily News* between January 11 and 18, 1914. Also see an editorial in *Galveston Daily News*, Jan. 22, 1914; Jane A. Kenamore, "Women's Health Protective Association," in Tyler, et al. (eds.), *The New Handbook of Texas*, VI, 1056; and Chester R. Burns and Heather Campbell, "Sanitizing Galveston: Politics, Policies, and Practices Before 1915," *Houston Review*, 19, no. 1 (1997), 5–26.

44. For the Nursing Service, see *Galveston Daily News*, Oct. 27, 1936; May 5, 1939; June 11, 1939; Jan. 14, 1940; and Nov. 3, 1944. More information can be found in the Jean Scrimgeour Morgan Papers at the Texas and Galveston History Center of the Rosenberg Library. Jean Morgan (Mrs. George D. Morgan) was a founder and third president of the Women's Health Protective Association, a founder of the American Red Cross Chapter (1916), a secretary of the Anti-Tuberculosis Association of Galveston County, and first president of the Galveston Public Health Nursing Service when that group separated from the American Red Cross in 1936. For Leake's role, see *Galveston Daily News*, Dec. 15, 1944, and Jan. 5, 1945.

45. For a copy of the EMS program plan, see WF411, CHP Archives. For the new services, see *University Medical*, 7 (Nov.–Dec., 1975), 1–13. For comments by Bailey, see Byron Bailey to Chester R. Burns, Feb. 13, 1992, interview, Blocker Collections. See also *University Medical*, 8 (Sept.–Oct., 1976), 2–7. For an example of volunteer surgery efforts, see *Impact*, 10 (May 16, 1986), 1, 7. Four professors were presidents of the Rotary Club of Galveston: D. Bailey Calvin (1944–1945); Charles T. Stone Sr. (1961–1962); Chester R. Burns (1980–1981); and John Bruhn (1990–1991). See Chester R. Burns, "The Rotary Club of Galveston, Texas: Eighty Years of Service, 1913–1993," 34–35. A copy is in WF389, CHP Archives.

46. For a succinct historical overview of medical societies in Texas, see Chester R. Burns, "Medical Societies," in Tyler, et al. (eds.), *The New Handbook of Texas*, IV, 600–601.

47. *Galveston Daily News*, June 16–19, 1908; June 17–20, 1913; and June 12–15, 1923.

48. *Galveston Daily News*, June 4–5, 1907. Also see John Levis Brown, "Texas Nurses Association," in Tyler, et al. (eds.), *The New Handbook of Texas*, VI, 382–383; and *Galveston Daily News*, Apr. 24 and May 4–6, 1910; Apr. 27 and May 4–6, 1921; May 16–17, 19, 1934; and Apr. 8, 12–14, 1948.

49. *Galveston Daily News*, Oct. 16–17, 19, 1955; Dec. 28, 1958; and Apr. 13, 1959. For examples of other School of Nursing faculty who served as committee chairs and officers in state associations, see the list in WF399, CHP Archives. See also *Galveston Daily News*, Apr. 14, 1963; *Newsletter (UTMB)*, 1 (Apr. 15, 1965), 5; and *Impact*, 9 (Apr. 5, 1985), 19; and 11 (May 1, 1987), 13.

50. James E. Thompson was president of the Texas Academy of Science (TAS) during fiscal year 1908. However, TAS annual meetings no longer occurred in Galveston after 1900 and medically oriented papers were seldom given. The group ceased functioning in 1912. See also *Galveston Daily News*, Apr. 5, 11, 13, 1936; Oct. 19, 23, and Nov. 5, 10–12, 1944; and Dec. 18, 1946.

51. *Galveston Daily News*, Jan. 28, 1950; Nov. 22 and Dec. 3–6, 1953; and Dec. 7, 1955. See also *University Medical Center News*, 2 (Nov., 1961), 7; *Galveston Daily News*, Nov. 30, 1962; and *Newsletter (UTMB)*, 1 (Dec. 16, 1965), 2.

52. For a brief historical overview of the TMA, see Megan Seaholm and Chester R. Burns, "Texas Medical Association," in Tyler, et al. (eds.), *The New Handbook of Texas*, VI, 358. See also *Galveston Daily News*, Apr. 23–27, 1901; May 9, 11–14, 1909; Apr. 24 and May 7–11, 1916; Apr. 20, 22, 30, and May 1, 3, 5–12, 1928; May 9–13, 1938; May 6–9, 1946; Apr. 28–30 and May 1–3, 1951; Apr. 21–23 and 25–26, 1956; and Apr. 16, 22, 25, 1961. For three poignant speeches welcoming those doctors who attended the annual meeting in April 1901, only seven months after the devastating hurricane of the previous year, see *Transactions, Texas State Medical Association* (1901), 9–14. See also Nixon, *A History of the Texas Medical Association*, 395. For some details about these meetings, see pages 220–226 (1901), 267–270 (1909), 296–299 (1916), 338–341 (1928), 369–371 (1938), 395–399 (1946), and 421–426 (1951). The TMA became so large that only the largest cities in Texas had suitable meeting and housing facilities. By 1970, for example, the 103rd session in Dallas was expected to attract five thousand physicians, spouses, and guests; see *Faculty News (UTMB)*, Apr. 3, 1970.

53. *Galveston Daily News*, Jan. 1, 1904, and Apr. 27, 1904; *UTMB: Seventy-five Year History*, 276; and *Galveston Daily News*, May 9, 1913. When the TSMA held its seventy-fifth annual meeting in May 1941, Taylor was serving his thirty-second year as its secretary-treasurer; see *Galveston Daily News*, May 16, 1941. See names of delegates in a list dated December 15, 1986, in WF389, CHP Archives. For examples, of presentations see *Texas State Journal of Medicine*, 5 (Apr., 1910), 438–443; *Galveston Daily News*, May 7, 1939; May 10, 1942; Apr. 27, 1948; Apr. 27, 1949; May 2, 1954; Apr. 14, 1957; Feb. 26, 1960; and Apr. 23, 1962. For examples of committee and section membership, see *Texas State Journal of Medicine*, 3 (July, 1907), 87–88; 9 (Nov., 1913), 206–207; 19 (Sept., 1923), 267–268; 36 (Aug., 1940), 285–286; and *Galveston Daily News*, Oct. 17, 1955.

54. The Texas Radiology Society was initially named the Texas Roentgen Ray Society. For some details about the evolution of medical societies in Texas, see Chester R. Burns, "Medical Societies," in Tyler, et al. (eds.), *The New Handbook of Texas*, IV, 600–601.

55. *Galveston Daily News*, Nov. 10–12 , 1914; Oct. 19–20 and Nov. 1, 1915; Oct. 14, 17, 1916; Oct. 18, 25–26, 1932; Oct. 6, 8–9, 1935; Oct. 4–8, 1941; Sept. 19 and Oct. 1, 4, 1944; Oct. 5, 7–8, 1947; Apr. 3, 1951; and Oct. 3–5, 1954. See also "Newsline," 5, p. 2, in *Impact*, 15 (Jan. 11, 1991).

56. *Galveston Daily News*, Nov. 2, 1930; Sept. 25 and 30 and Oct. 6–7, 1934; Sept. 28, 30, and Oct. 1, 1941; Oct. 20, 27, and Nov. 3, 1946; and Feb. 12, 1958. See also *Faculty News (UTMB)*, Feb. 25–Mar. 1, 1974, 5; *Alumni Bulletin*, 9 (Apr., 1954), 1–2; and 21 (Apr., 1967), 2; *University Medical*, 4 (Oct., 1972), 17; *Galveston Daily News*, Mar. 15, 1991; Jan. 2 and 19, 1936; and Jan. 19–20, 1951; and *Impact*, 11 (Apr. 17, 1987), 3.

57. *Galveston Daily News*, May 9, 11–12, 1942; Oct. 21 and 23, 1954; and *Alumni Bulletin*, 9 (Nov., 1954), 2.

58. *Galveston Daily News*, Feb. 14, 1940; Feb. 19, 1941; Feb. 18, 1942; Feb. 21, 26–27, 1943; Mar. 11, 1949; Feb. 25–27, 1954; Jan. 13, 20, 1952; Dec. 10–12, 1954; Dec. 4, 1958; and Dec. 5, 1961.

59. *Galveston Daily News*, Sept. 5, 7–11, 1954; and Oct. 4, 1959. Actively involved in orchestrating these meetings were members of the Galveston chapter of the American Academy of General Practice, which had been organized in 1950; see *Galveston Daily News*, July 18, 21, 1950. See also *Alumni Bulletin*, 9 (Oct., 1954), 2; and 18 (Feb., 1964), 3; and *Faculty News (UTMB)*, Nov. 4–8, 1974, 1; and Nov 18–22, 1974, 1. The Department of Family Medicine hosted an open house for its clinic, whose personnel had attended about sixteen hundred patients during its first year of operation.

60. *Galveston Daily News*, Sept. 26 and Oct. 5–6, 1940; and Oct. 21, 1955; *Alumni Bulletin*, 18 (Dec., 1964), 3; 8 (Aug., 1953), 2; and *Galveston Daily News*, Jan. 17, 20, 1958.

61. For minutes and programs of meetings, see the archival records of the Texas Society of Pathologists in the Blocker Collections. See also *Galveston Daily News*, Jan. 26, 1948; Jan. 25, 1957; Jan. 27, 1962; and *Impact*, 4 (Jan. 25, 1980), 7; and 11 (Mar. 20, 1987), 3.

62. *Alumni Bulletin*, 6 (June, 1951), 2; 11 (June, 1956), 3. See items about Jenkins and Withers in "After 50 Years . . . Unreliable Memoirs by the Class of 1940," WF401, CHP Archives. For Lewis, see *Alumni Bulletin*, 18 (June, 1964), 1.

63. *Galveston Daily News*, Aug. 2, 14, 23, 30–31, 1908; Sept. 24, 25, 28–29, 1908; Oct. 2, 5, 8, 13, 22, 1908; and *Texas State Journal of Medicine*, 4 (Nov., 1908), 181. This association held its twenty-fourth annual meeting in Galveston in 1933; see *Galveston Daily News*, May 13–14, 1933; and Sept. 12 and Oct. 3–5, 1939. See also *Galveston Daily News*, Feb. 15, 18, 21, 1951; Feb. 15, 17–20, 1952; Feb. 17, 1953; Feb. 14–17, 1954; and Feb. 13–16, 1955; and *Alumni Bulletin*, 9 (Apr., 1954), 3.

64. *Galveston Daily News*, Nov. 2, 1934; Mar. 6, 1943; Jan. 17, 1946; Mar. 4, 7, 1951; and *Alumni Bulletin*, 21 (Apr., 1967), 4.

65. *Texas State Journal of Medicine*, 37 (June, 1941), 144; *Galveston Daily News*, Apr. 30, 1953; *Faculty News (UTMB)*, May 2, 1969; *Alumni Bulletin*, 18 (Feb., 1964), 2; and *University Medical*, 5 (Oct., 1973), 21.

66. *Galveston Daily News*, Mar. 6, 1991.

67. *Galveston Daily News*, Oct. 30–31, 1937; *Texas State Journal of Medicine*, 33 (Dec., 1937), 589; and *Impact*, 14 (Aug. 17, 1990), 4.

68. *Galveston Daily News*, Apr. 5, 1945; Feb. 25 and Apr. 14, 1949; Feb. 26 and Mar. 5, 1950; and May 12–14, 1953. For a preview of the twentieth meeting with good photos of Galveston, including the Marine Room of the Pleasure Pier and the Buccaneer Hotel, see *Texas Hospitals*, 4 (Mar., 1949), 6–9.

69. *Galveston Daily News*, Apr. 5–7, 1951; and Apr. 22, 1961; *Newsletter (UTMB)*, 2 (Apr. 20, 1967), 1; *Faculty News (UTMB)*, Apr. 14–18, 1975, 1; and *Impact*, 4 (May 30, 1980), 9.

70. *Galveston Daily News*, Nov. 26, 30 and Dec. 5, 7, 1952; and Apr. 29, 1953; *Newsletter (UTMB)*, 1 (May 19, 1966), 1; *Faculty News (UTMB)*, May 18, 1973, 2; *Impact*, 6 (Sept. 3, 1982), 9; *Faculty News (UTMB)*, July 21–Aug. 1, 1975, 3; and *Impact*, 2 (Sept. 8, 1978), 5.

71. *Impact*, 4 (June 13, 1980), 6; and 8 (Oct. 5, 1984), 12.

72. *Galveston Daily News*, Dec. 7, 9–10, 1903; June 10, 14, 1905; Dec. 9–10, 1909; Apr. 11, 1913; Oct. 4, 8–10, 1914; Oct. 10–11, 1919; Oct. 9, 15, 1921; Apr. 9, 11–12, 1924; Apr. 12–13, 1928; and Apr. 13, 17–18, 1941. See also *Galveston Daily News*, Dec. 16, 1904; Dec. 9–10, 1909; and Oct. 12, 15, 1917. Boyd Reading and Titus Harris were directors and H. Reid Robinson was vice president in 1937; see *Galveston Daily News*, Oct. 31, 1937. C. S. Sykes was first vice president in 1958; see *Galveston Daily News*, July 25, 1958.

73. *Galveston Daily News*, Dec. 20, 1918; Dec. 9, 1938; and Dec. 8, 1961. During its organizational meeting in January 1947, the founders of the Southern Society for Clinical Investigation elected Moore as a councilor. For details, see James A. Pittman Jr. and Donald M. Miller, "The Southern Society for Clinical Investigation at 50: The End of the Beginning," *American Journal of the Medical Sciences*, 311 (June, 1996), 248–253. See also *Galveston Daily News*, Nov. 12, 1941; Oct. 12, 1943; and Mar. 23 and Dec. 22, 1960. Harold Goolishian, Foster's colleague at UTMB, was president of the Texas Psychological Association in 1965. See *Alumni Bulletin*, 16 (Dec., 1962), 2; 19 (June, 1965), 2; and 21 (Feb., 1967), 2; and *University Medical*, 2 (Dec., 1970), 22; and 4 (Jan., 1973), 17.

74. *Galveston Daily News*, Oct. 5, 16, 18, 1947; Mar. 23, 1960; Oct. 7, 1962; and Nov. 20, 1963.

75. *Faculty News (UTMB)*, Apr. 5–9, 1976, 1; June 7–18, 1976, 1; and *Impact*, 1 (Nov. 4, 1977), 3; 10 (Dec. 5, 1986), 2; and 11 (Apr. 2 and 3, 1987), 1, 4. This group included deans of forty-seven medical schools in fourteen southern states and was one of the regional divisions of the Council of Deans of the Association of American Medical Colleges.

76. *Galveston Daily News*, May 8, 1903; Mar. 23, 1922; Apr. 7, 12, 18–21, 23, 1926; and May 19, 1939.

77. *Galveston Daily News*, Aug. 13, 1952; John B. Truslow to Charles Stone, June 30, 1959, letter, box VF I/1, UT Chancellor's Records; items about Jenkins in "After 50 Years . . . Unreliable Memoirs by the Class of 1940," WF401, CHP Archives; and *Faculty News (UTMB)*, July 2, 1971; and Mar. 23, 1973, 3.

78. For the names of those attending the AAAS meeting, see *Galveston Daily News*, Dec. 24, 28–30, 1941. For the titles of papers presented by the faculty and staff, see *Texas State Journal of Medicine*, 37 (Dec., 1941), 558. For examples of speeches, see *Galveston Daily News*, Apr. 19–20, 1942; and Apr. 5, 1953. See also *Newsletter (UTMB)*, 1 (Feb. 3, 1966), 2. Members of the Department of Pediatrics gave twenty presentations during the 1985 meeting of the Southern Society for Pediatric Research; see *Impact*, 9 (Feb. 8, 1985), 17.

79. *Galveston Daily News*, Apr. 28 and May 2–3, 1942; Nov. 3–4, 1944; and Apr. 10–13, 1949. Luther Evans, the director of the Library of Congress, gave a dinner address in 1949. See also *Galveston Daily News*, Feb. 3–4, 1951; Sept. 28, Nov. 2, 13–17, 19, 1952; Apr. 4, 7–8, 10, 1954; Apr. 21–23, 1954; and Feb. 8, 16–18, 1955.

80. *Galveston Daily News*, Mar. 31, 1964; and *Faculty News (UTMB)*, May 10–14, 1976, 3. For a copy of the 1990 Society of University Surgeons program, see WF389, CHP Archives.

81. *Galveston Daily News*, Sept. 21, 26–28, 1941; June 9–10, 1945; Oct. 25, 1946; Mar. 10, 1951; May 11, 16–17, 1952; Jan. 13, 1953; Jan. 7, 17–19, 1955; and Feb. 6, 1959.

82. *Galveston Daily News*, Nov. 22, 1962. Other groups meeting in the same venue included the Texas Rheumatism Association, the Texas Academy of Internal Medicine, and the Texas Society of Internal Medicine. During this meeting, George Herrmann became president of the Texas Academy of Internal Medicine; see *Galveston Daily News*, Dec. 2, 1962. See also *Faculty News (UTMB)*, Dec. 1, 1972; Sept. 16–20, 1974, 3; and Jan. 27–31, 1975, 4; and *Impact*, 4 (Oct. 10, 1980), 5; and 6 (Oct. 1, 1982), 5.

83. C. R. Burns and H. G. Campbell, "The Extraordinary Influences of Two British Physicians on Medical Education and Practice in Texas at the Turn of the 20th Century," *Vesalius*, 5 (Dec., 1999), 82. By 1915 at least nine School of Medicine graduates were fellows of the American College of Surgeons; see *Galveston Daily News*, Nov. 23, 1920. Also see

Proceedings, AAMC (1917), 58; W. S. Carter to R. E. Vinson, Nov. 3, 1919, letter, box 4Q22, UT President's Records; *Texas State Journal of Medicine*, 10 (Dec., 1914), 336; *Galveston Daily News*, Apr. 10, 18, 1928; and Oct. 20, 1939; and Chauncey D. Leake's annual report about UTMB, 1942–1943, box 2, Leake Papers, Blocker Collections.

84. *Galveston Daily News*, May 4, 1940. The other Texans admitted to the American Surgical Association were James E. Thompson and A. O. Singleton. See *Galveston Daily News*, Oct. 22, 1948; June 16 and Aug. 9, 1942; May 13, 23, 1944; and Nov. 10, 1946. Cooke was a director of the American Board of Obstetrics and Gynecology for twenty years; see *UTMB: Seventy-five Year History*, 136. Singleton was one of four professors listed in the 1940–1941 edition of "Who's Who in America." The others were Paul Brindley, George Herrmann, and John Spies; see *Galveston Daily News*, May 28, 1940.

85. *Galveston Daily News*, Apr. 3, 1954; and June 17, 1956; *Alumni Bulletin*, 9 (June, 1954), 3; *Galveston Daily News*, Feb. 16, 1955; *Alumni Bulletin*, 10 (June, 1955), 2; and RF190, CHP Archives.

86. For Snodgrass, see *Galveston Daily News*, Oct. 27, 1960. For Eggers, see "Minutes of the Quarterly Meeting of the Medical Staff, Tuesday, July 16, 1960," WF399, CHP Archives; and *Galveston Daily News*, June 2, 1962. Eggers was the first surgeon of the southwestern section of the association to become president. For Middleton, see *Galveston Daily News*, May 22, 1962. For Hooks, see *Newsletter (UTMB)*, 1 (Nov. 5, 1964), 6. For Robison, see *Newsletter (UTMB)*, 1 (Nov. 5, 1964), 1. Sixteen faculty and graduate students in the Department of Anatomy delivered research papers at the seventy-ninth annual meeting of the American Association of Anatomists in San Francisco in 1966 when Duncan became president; see *Newsletter (UTMB)*, 1 (Apr. 7, 1966), 1–2.

87. *Newsletter (UTMB)*, 1 (Mar. 18, 1965), 3. In 1965 the office of the National Board of Schools of Medical Technology was on the fifth floor of John Sealy Hospital and Mrs. Paul Brindley was its secretary. For Lewis and Mullins, see *Newsletter (UTMB)*, 1 (May 19, 1966), 1; and 3 (May, 1968), 14. Mullins had been elected to the board of directors of the American Academy of Dermatology in 1961 and selected as a member of the Residency Review Committee for Dermatology by the AMA's Council on Medical Education and Hospitals; see *Galveston Daily News*, Dec. 14, 1961; and *Newsletter (UTMB)*, 2 (June 2, 1966), 1. For Wilson, see *Newsletter (UTMB)*, 3 (Aug., 1968), 10. At that time, there were forty-seven approved schools of inhalation therapy and 515 registered inhalation therapists.

88. *Newsletter (UTMB)*, 1 (Dec., 1964), 3; 3 (June, 1968), 12; and 3 (Oct., 1968), 17.

89. *Faculty News (UTMB)*, Mar. 14, 1969; and May 2, 1969; *University Medical*, 1 (Jan., 1970), 21; and 6 (Sept.–Oct., 1974), 20; *Faculty News (UTMB)*, Nov. 24–28, 1975, 1; *Hospital News*, 9 (Dec. 17, 1976), 1, 3; *Faculty News (UTMB)*, Dec. 7–21, 1976, 1; *Texas Medicine*, 73 (Sept., 1977), 101; list accompanying William C. Levin to Warren Harding, Apr. 24, 1981, letter, folder 5, box 47, Levin Papers; and *Impact*, 4 (Nov. 21, 1980), 16.

90. *Hospital News*, 5 (Oct. 30, 1972), 1; and 6 (July 9, 1973), 2.

91. *Impact*, 5 (Feb. 20, 1981), 3. During that same year, Bowman was president of the Texas Genetic Society. See also *Impact*, 6 (Feb. 5, 1982), 21; 7 (Jan. 14, 1983), 19; 5 (June 18, 1981), 6; 9 (June 14, 1985), 2; and 12 (Oct. 21, 1988), 3. Bailey had already served as president of the Association of Academic Departments of Otolaryngology, the Texas Otolaryngological Association, and the Society of University Otolaryngologists. See *Impact*, 12 (Jan. 22, 1988), 5; 13 (Mar. 10, 1989), 3; and *Newsline*, 5 (May 3, 1991), 1.

92. *Impact*, 9 (Dec. 20, 1985), 4; 11 (May 1, 1987), 15; and 10 (Dec. 5, 1986), 2; *Galveston Daily News*, May 3, 1991.

93. *Impact*, 10 (Nov. 14, 1986), 7; and 12 (Dec. 2, 1988), 3; and *Galveston Daily News*, July 12, 1990.

94. *Impact*, 3 (Nov. 2, 1979), 10; and 14 (June 29, 1990), 3. For other examples, see the list in WF399, CHP Archives. For more physician examples, see the list accompanying William C. Levin to Warren Harding, Apr. 24, 1981, letter, folder 5, box 47, Levin Papers; and the responses of thirty-five members of the class of 1940 on pages 20–22 of "After 50 Years . . . Unreliable Memoirs of the Class of 1940," WF401, CHP Archives.

95. *Impact*, 4 (Jan. 25, 1980), 11; (Aug. 15, 1980), 8; (Nov. 21, 1980), 16; 5 (Sept. 25, 1981), 2; and 6 (Mar. 19, 1982), 4. In 1983, Daeschner became chair of the National Board of Medical Examiners; see *Impact*, 7 (June 3, 1983), 10. See also *Newsline*, 4 (July, 1990), 3.

96. William Keiller to Grace Grey, Oct. 31, 1924, box 4Q24, UT President's Records; and George Bethel to H. Y. Benedict, Mar. 14, 1929, box 27, UTMB Dean's Office Records, Inactive, Blocker Collections.

97. *Galveston Daily News*, Feb. 12 and Apr. 27, 1944; Jan. 9, 1945; May 24, 1946; and Oct. 20, 1946. See also Chauncey D. Leake to Gov. Beauford H. Jester, Aug. 14, 1948, letter, box VF 10/C, UT President's Records. For other examples of faculty travel in foreign countries, see RF186, CHP Archives. For Eggers' award, see *Galveston Daily News*, Oct. 14, 1949.

98. Chauncey D. Leake to Theophilus Painter, Aug. 12, 1950, Dec. 8, 1949, and June 5, 1950, letters, boxes VF 10/C, VF 10/D, and VF 10/C, UT President's Records. For details about Blocker's activities in Japan, see the reports in folder 493, box 67, Blocker Papers. For the conference in Amsterdam, see *Galveston Daily News*, Aug. 12, 1954.

99. For details about Blocker's activities, see folders 505 and 509, box 68, Blocker Papers. For Hansen and Wiese, see *Galveston Daily News*, July 5, 1956; and for Nowinski, see H. F. Connally to Logan Wilson, Sept. 10, 1958, box VF I/1, UT Chancellor's Records.

100. See Harry Ransom to members of the Executive Committee, May 19, 1961, and John B. Truslow to Harry H. Ransom, Aug. 10, 1962, memos, both in box VF L/6, UT Chancellor's Records; John B. Truslow to Harry H. Ransom, Mar. 11, 1964, memo, box VF N/1, UT Chancellor's Records; *Galveston Daily News*, Oct. 12, 1962; and Oct. 14, 1963. For details about the exchanges with the University of Nuevo Leon Medical School, see the letters in RF186, CHP Archives. See also Truman G. Blocker Jr. to Harry H. Ransom, July 1, 1968, letter, box VF EE/3, UT Chancellor's Records.

101. Emile Holman, Wilder Penfield, and Wilburt C. Davison—all former pupils of Osler—gave presentations at the 1970 conference; see *University Medical*, 2 (Oct., 1970), 18. For the immunology symposium, see *Impact*, 4 (June 27, 1980), 1. Co-chaired by Palmer Saunders and Jerry Daniels, this meeting provided a forum for interdisciplinary exchange among cancer immunologists from the states, England, Switzerland, France, Israel, Sweden, and Norway. A copy of the program is in WF389, CHP Archives. Several papers from the 1982 injury control and prevention conference were published in *Texas Medicine*, 79 (Aug., 1983), 5–52. For details, see folder 5, box 53, Levin Papers. A second conference was held in October 1985; see folder 6, box 53, Levin Papers.

102. *Impact*, 12 (Mar. 4, 1988), 1; and (Sept. 23, 1988), 1, 3. Leading researchers in geriatrics and nutrition from Australia, Canada, Sweden, the United Kingdom, and the United States participated in the Global Nursing conference. For the symposia on gastrointestinal hormones, see *Galveston Daily News*, Apr. 4, 1989; and *Impact*, 13 (Apr. 21, 1989), 1.

103. *Impact*, 1 (Oct. 7, 1977), 2; 5 (June 5, 1981), 10; and 13 (June 2, 1989), 3; and *Galveston Daily News*, Mar. 1 and Oct. 18, 1991.

104. *Impact*, 9 (Sept. 20, 1985), 14; and (Dec. 6, 1985), 17.

105. *Impact*, 9 (Apr. 19, 1985), 1, 16; (Sept. 20, 1985), 1, 16; (Nov. 1, 1985), 8; and (Nov. 15, 1985), 1, 3.

106. *Impact*, 12 (Jan. 8, 1988), 1–2; and *Galveston Daily News*, Feb. 12, 1988; Apr. 7, 1990; and Mar. 28, 1991.

107. For comments about these departmental reviews, see Luther Travis to Chester R. Burns, Feb. 25 and Mar. 10, 1992, interviews, Blocker Collections.

108. *University Record*, 2, no. 4 (1900), 384 (quotation). UTMB no longer supported the ASMC; see *Texas State Journal of Medicine*, 3 (Jan., 1908), 242. For details about UTMB's relationships to the AMA between 1912 and 1950 and to the AAMC between 1909 and 1989, see RF177 and RF178, CHP Archives.

109. Ludmerer, *A Time to Heal*, 166–173. The AMA established its Council on Medical Education in 1904, renaming it Council on Medical Education and Hospitals in 1920. In this chapter, "AMA Council" refers to this group. See also Flexner, *Medical Education in the United States and Canada*, 312 (quotation); and *Galveston Daily News*, Sept. 11, 16, 25, 1910.

110. *Collier's*, 45 (June 11, 1910), 16.

111. *Journal of the American Medical Association*, 55 (Aug. 20, 1910), 680–681; W. S. Carter to E. J. Mathews, Sept. 1910, letter, box 4R82, UT President's Records; and *UT Regents' Reports* (1910), 10 (quotation); (1912), 25.

112. *Galveston Daily News*, Apr. 11, 1913; Feb. 27, Mar. 2, and Sept. 18, 1913; and *UT Regent's Reports* (1914), 40.

113. Minutes, UT Board of Regents, Oct. 28, 1912; Proceedings, AAMC (1913), 42–45; and *Galveston Daily News*, Feb. 27 and Mar. 2, 1913. In 1910 Flexner discovered that thirty-five of the fifty member colleges in the AAMC were not meeting the association's minimal standards. In 1914 the AAMC began enforcing its standards by terminating a member school; see Ludmerer, *Learning to Heal*, 313.

114. Proceedings, AAMC (1914), 78–80, 116; (1915), 73–77; (1916), 108; and (1917), 58; and *Galveston Daily News*, Feb. 9, 1918. The AAMC required periodic re-inspections for continuing status as an approved member. During 1920–1921, Fred Zapffe, the AAMC's secretary-treasurer, apparently re-inspected UTMB; see Proceedings, AAMC (1921), 81.

115. In RF178, CHP Archives, there are pertinent notes created from a review of the minutes of all of the annual meetings of the AAMC through 1987. See Proceedings, AAMC (1922), 107; (1923), 64–75, 147–155; (1924), 38; (1925), 17–21, 124–128; (1926), 6; and (1927), 6. There were two meetings in 1925. Bethel experienced ill health and also had limited funds for travel during the depression years. He attended the meetings in 1928, 1929, 1931, and 1934. Carter left Galveston in the late summer of 1938 and UTMB was not represented at the forty-ninth annual AAMC meeting in Syracuse in October 1938.

116. It is important to emphasize that this AMA-sponsored inspection in 1936 was not part of a formal re-accreditation process. When Herman Weiskotten (dean of the Syracuse medical school) and James Baker (the state health

officer for Alabama and a member of the National Board of Medical Examiners) inspected UTMB in January 1936 they were gathering data for a statistical profile of the school. In April 1937 Carter was annoyed that he had not yet received a report about this inspection. W. D. Cutter, secretary of the AMA's Council on Medical Education, provided Carter with a brief summary of the inspection report; see W. S. Carter to H. Y. Benedict, Apr. 4, 1937, and William D. Cutter to W. S. Carter, Apr. 21, 1937, letters, both in box VF 9/C, UT President's Records. Finally published in 1937, the AMA survey report was a collection of statistical charts about all of the surveyed schools and not a profile of each individual school. Only a few political authorities in Texas ever read any written reports about UTMB based on the inspections of Weiskotten and Baker.

117. As part of the re-inspection requirement for continuing status as an AAMC member, UTMB was visited by Maurice H. Rees (dean at Colorado) and C. W. M. Poynter (dean at Nebraska) in January 1941. Although they acknowledged "jurisdictional problems" at UTMB, they did not recommend probation; see C. W. M. Poynter and Maurice Rees to Russell H. Oppenheimer, Feb. 13, 1941, letter, box VF 18/C, UT President's Records. Their report was discussed with Dean Spies at a meeting of the AAMC's Executive Council in October 1941. This council decided to re-inspect UTMB in January 1942. Fred Zapffe (secretary for the AMA Council) and E. M. MacEwen (dean at Iowa) visited UTMB for five days and submitted a twenty-eight-page report; see E. M. MacEwen and Fred Zapffe, "Report on Inspection of University of Texas School of Medicine," January 1942, box VF 18/C, UT President's Records. On February 15, 1942, the AAMC's Executive Council reviewed this report and recommended that UTMB be placed on probation by a vote of the members during the annual business meeting of the AAMC in October of that year; see Fred Zapffe to Homer P. Rainey, Feb. 17, 1942, letter, box VF 18/C, UT President's Records. The AMA's Council sent J. H. Musser and H. G. Weiskotten to inspect UTMB in May 1942 (remember that Weiskotten had been a member of the survey team in 1936). After reviewing their eighty-eight-page report, the AMA's Council placed UTMB on probation during their meeting in Atlantic City on June 6, 1942; see J. H. Musser and H. G. Weiskotten, "University of Texas Medical Branch," May 8–11, 1942, and H. G. Weiskotten to Homer P. Rainey, June 7, 1942, both in box VF 18/C, UT President's Records. For copies of these reports and more details about these events, see RF45, RF177, and RF178, CHP Archives.

118. Inspections of the School of Medicine occurred in November 1947; see *Galveston Daily News*, Nov. 7, 19, and 23, 1947, and in September 1950; see *Galveston Daily News*, Aug. 23 and Sept. 19, 24, 26, and 30, 1950. Begun in 1942, the LCME was a collaborative effort of the AMA's Council on Medical Education and the Association of American Medical Colleges; see Ludmerer, *Time to Heal*, 214. Fred Zapffe, who was secretary of the AMA's Council on Medical Education and Hospitals for forty-five years, liked the local scene so much that he vacationed in Galveston in 1949; see *Galveston Daily News*, May 20, 1949.

119. Elsa Kibbe to Titus Harris, Aug. 31, 1942, folder 13, box 1, School of Nursing Archives, Blocker Collections. In November 1946 a nurse consultant for the American Psychiatric Association commended the School of Nursing's psychiatric training program; see *Galveston Daily News*, Nov. 15, 1946. See also Brown, "The Historical Development of the University of Texas System School of Nursing, 1890–1973," 49, and *Galveston Daily News*, Feb. 2, 1949. By this date, the National League of Nursing Education had accredited only 117 of 1,100 nursing schools in the United States. For the ranking, see Marjorie Bartholf to Chauncey Leake, Sept. 10, 1949, letter, folder 7, box 1, School of Nursing Archives, Blocker Collections. For accreditation, see *Galveston Daily News*, Dec. 5, 1950. This accrediting group included the Association of Collegiate Schools of Nursing, the National League of Nursing Education, the National Organization of Public Health Nurses, and the National Association of Industrial Nursing.

120. Stevens, *American Medicine and the Public Interest*, 90–92, 119. For samples of public recognition of these rankings during the 1920s, see *Galveston Daily News*, Nov. 23, 1920; Oct. 30, 1921; Oct. 24, 1922; Oct. 21, 1924; and Oct. 27, 1925. UTMB became a member of the American Hospital Association in 1928; see *Impact*, 2 (Oct. 6, 1978), 6. St. Mary's Hospital in Galveston also received a Class A ranking throughout these years. See also *Galveston Daily News*, Nov. 3, 1941. For samples of local recognition, see *Galveston Daily News*, Oct. 14, 1930; Oct. 14, 1931; Oct. 15, 1934; Oct. 18, 1938; Oct. 21, 1940; Nov. 3, 1941; Jan. 4, 1943; Feb. 1, 1946; and Jan. 22, 1947. In 1939 three of the nine ACS-approved hospitals in Texas were in Galveston: John Sealy, St. Mary's, and the U.S.P.H.S. Hospital; see *Galveston Daily News*, Oct. 17, 1939.

121. Chauncey D. Leake to T. S. Painter, Oct. 29, 1949, letter, box VF 10/D, UT President's Records; and *Galveston Daily News*, Oct. 11–12, 1949.

122. "Notes About Hospital Activities," 5, 7, 12, 16, 21, 26, 27, and 35; and RF56, CHP Archives.

123. "Notes About Hospital Activities," 44, 68, 70, 74, 76, 77, 81, 82, 87, 88, 92, 93, 96, 103, and 104; folders 3–7, box 32, Levin Papers; *Impact*, 4 (Aug. 29, 1980), 1, 15; 7 (Mar. 11, 1983), 1, 17; and Ann Smith to Chester R. Burns, Dec. 8, 1998, untaped interview. For a photo of the JCAH survey team at UTMB in December 1982, see *Impact*, 6 (Dec. 3, 1982), 2. Some reports are available in UTMB's Quality Management Office.

124. E. D. Walker to William C. Levin, June 6, 1977, letter, folder 3, box 32, Levin Papers.

125. *Impact*, 8 (Nov. 2, 1984), 13.

126. *Impact*, 3 (Dec. 7, 1979), 1, 15; and 4 (Nov. 7, 1980), 10. The accreditation program of the College of American Pathologists had existed for twenty years. This inspection at UTMB was the largest one the college had ever conducted.

127. "Report of Survey of The University of Texas Medical Branch Galveston, Texas, (1962), 4 (1st quotation), and 54–55 (other quotations). This report is in folder 3, box 33, Levin Papers.

128. "Report of the Survey of The University of Texas Medical Branch at Galveston" (1970), 27. Specific recommendations were included in the final report. A copy is in folder 3, box 33, Levin Papers.

129. *Impact*, 1 (Feb. 18, 1977), 6. Also see oral summary by LCME Committee on February 1, 1977, folder 4, box 33, Levin Papers (1st quotation); and *Impact*, 1 (Apr. 29, 1977), 1 (2nd quotation).

130. For details, see folder 5, box 33, Levin Papers.

131. *Impact*, 16 (Mar. 20, 1992), 1, 4 (quotation). For a copy of the Self-Study Summary Report and other details about the 1991 survey, see WF434, CHP Archives.

132. In 1982 seven School of Medicine professors were members of national specialty boards who accredited residency training programs throughout the United States. They included James Arens, American Board of Anesthesiology; Paul Young, American Board of Family Practice; William Deiss, American Board of Internal Medicine; Byron Bailey, American Board of Otolaryngology; William Daeschner Jr., president, American Board of Pediatrics; John Calverly, secretary, American Board of Neurology; and James C. Thompson, American Board of Surgery. Calverly also chaired the Psychiatry/Neurology Residency Review Committee and Young chaired the Family Medicine Residency Review Committee. In addition to these, Burke Evans was a member of the Orthopaedic Residency Review Committee and Al LeBlanc was chair of the Advisory Committee on Graduate Medical Education of the American Medical Association; see *Impact*, 6 (Feb. 5, 1982), 21. These roles signaled judgments of very high regard by peers.

133. See the list attached to Al LeBlanc's response to a memo from Chester R. Burns dated Aug. 20, 1991, WF416, CHP Archives. The umbrella association of the twenty-four specialty boards was the American Board of Medical Specialties, one of the five member organizations of the Accreditation Council for Graduate Medical Education (ACGME). The other four were the American Hospital Association, the American Medical Association, the Association of American Medical Colleges, and the Council of Medical Specialty Societies. By the early 1990s the ACGME, using its twenty-four Residency Review Committees, accredited more than six thousand residency training programs in then United States.

134. For a copy of the 1961 report, see RF125, CHP Archives. In 1981 the accrediting agencies included the National Medical Record Association, the National Accrediting Agency for Clinical Laboratory Sciences, the American Occupational Therapy Society, the American College of Radiology, the American College of Chest Physicians, the American Society of Anesthesiology, the American Thoracic Society, the American Electroencephalography Society, and the American Physical Therapy Association. The data mentioned in this paragraph were taken from summaries that accompanied William C. Levin to Warren Harding, Apr. 24, 1981, letter, folder 5, box 47, Levin Papers. For a list of these agencies in 1990 (some with new names), see the sheet in WF416, CHP Archives.

135. Details about UTMB's membership in the SACS and the accreditation visits may be found in WF417, CHP Archives; folders 7 and 8, box 64, Levin Papers; and the SACS folders in the UTMB Dean's Office Records. Organized in 1895, the SACS is a voluntary regional association that uses specific standards and methods for assessing and improving the educational programs of schools and colleges in the southern United States. Copies of the SACS standards used for university institutions during the 1980s are in WF417, CHP Archives. See also "Report of the Evaluation Committee of the Commission on Colleges of the Southern Association of Colleges and Schools" (1973), 1 (quotation). This report is in folder 7, box 64, Levin Papers.

136. For a photo of the eleven-member committee, see *Impact*, 2 (Feb. 24, 1978), 7; "SACS Final Report," *Impact*, 2 (Mar. 22, 1978), 1, 6 (quotations); "Report of the Visiting Committee of the Reaffirmation of Accreditation by the Southern Association of Colleges and Schools," March 21–24, 1978, 2; *Impact*, 2 (Mar. 23, 1978), 1, 6; folder 8, box 64, Levin Papers; and *Impact*, 2 (Apr. 6, 1978), 3, 17.

137. See "The University of Texas Medical Branch at Galveston Fifth Year Report for the Southern Association of Colleges and Schools," Aug. 31, 1983, which accompanied William C. Levin to Gordon W. Sweet, Nov. 11, 1983, letter, SACS Files, UTMB Dean's Office Records, Active; and Gordon W. Sweet to William C. Levin, Dec. 19, 1983, letter, SACS Files, UTMB Dean's Office Records, Active.

138. *Impact*, 12 (Apr. 15, 1988), 1–2.

139. For a useful overview of accreditation in American higher education, see W. H. Cowley, *Presidents, Professors, and Trustees* (San Francisco: Jossey-Bass, 1980), 145–162.

140. For details, see Myles Knape, "The University of Texas Medical Branch: A Media Event," pp. 1–7, in WF420, CHP Archives; and RF152, CHP Archives. For an index to articles about UTMB in the *University*

Record, see WF423, CHP Archives. For articles about UTMB in the *Alcalde* between 1913 and 1951, see WF424, CHP Archives.

141. Volume 25, no. 1 of the *Alumni Bulletin* combined with volume 4, no. 8 of the *UTMB Newsletter* in September 1969. Subsequent numbers of the *Newsletter* included alumni news and descriptions of the annual meetings of the School of Medicine Alumni Association. Issues of *Impact* often included a page or two with photos about the alumni meetings held during the annual TMA convention. For example, about three hundred physicians and spouses attended the meeting in Dallas in May 1979; see *Impact*, 3 (May 18, 1979), 12. Issues of *Impact* often included photos about the homecoming meetings of the SOMAA in March of each year. For examples, see *Impact*, 4 (Apr. 4, 1980), 10; 5 (Apr. 24, 1981), 8; 6 (Apr. 2, 1982), 12–13; 7 (Mar. 25, 1983), 1, 13; 8 (Apr. 13, 1984), 10–11; 9 (Apr. 5, 1985), 17; 10 (Mar. 21, 1986), 1, 16; and 11 (May 1, 1987), 5–12.

142. As examples during Leake's first three months as CEO, see *Galveston Daily News*, Sept. 27, Oct. 11, and Nov. 13, 1942.

143. As reflected in the many citations in this book, much of what is known today about UTMB before 1942 came from the daily columns of Galveston's newspapers. Leake also shared newsworthy items with William Keys, director of the UT News and Information Service in Austin, and flirted with the idea of employing a publicity director in Galveston. See Chauncey D. Leake to all, Jan. 21, 1943, letter, folder 12, box 2, Leake Papers, Blocker Collections; and Chauncey D. Leake to Lillian Herz, Sept. 22, 1952, and Sept. 21, 1953, letters, box VFA/3, UT Chancellor's Records. For more details, see the typescript by Myles Knape, "The University of Texas Medical Branch: A Media Event," pp. 20–22. For an example of outstanding local coverage, see "A City Within a City" in the *Galveston Tribune*, Mar. 29, 1955.

144. *Houston Post*, Jan. 15, 1961. A copy is in RF152, CHP Archives.

CHAPTER 10

1. Allen J. Smith, "The Medical Department and the Galveston Storm," *University Record*, 3 (Mar., 1901), 66–67.

2. Robert M. Crunden, *Ministers of Reform: The Progressives' Achievement in American Civilization, 1889–1920* (New York: Basic Books, 1982).

3. *Texas State Journal of Medicine*, 5 (May, 1909), 12 (quotation); and 5 (June, 1909), 41–42.

4. Allen J. Smith, "The First Decade," *University Medical*, 6 (Oct., 1901), 1–15 (1st quotation); J. F. Y. Paine, "History of Medical Teaching in Texas," *Texas Medical Journal*, 22 (Nov., 1906), 173–184. The lecture was also printed in *Galveston Daily News*, Oct. 2, 1906. Also see *Galveston Daily News*, Nov. 18, 1906; and W. S. Carter, "A Decade of Progress in the Medical Department," *Alcalde*, 2 (Mar., 1914), 447–459 (2nd quotation).

5. Willard R. Cooke, "Dr. J. F. Y. Paine," *Alcalde*, 3 (June, 1915), 739 (1st quotation); *Alcalde*, 3 (July, 1915), 736–773; 823–826; and 853–866, including J. J. Terrill, "Dr. William Keiller," *Alcalde*, 3 (July, 1915), 772–773 (2nd quotation); and H. R. Dudgeon, "Random Undergraduate Recollections," *Alcalde*, 3 (July, 1915), 856–863. In the early 1950s, Dudgeon prepared a more extensive set of recollections about his years as a student. These recollections were transformed into a sixty-page typescript by his son, Howard R. Dudgeon Jr. It is titled, "My Recollections of the Medical Department of the University of Texas at Galveston" and is in the Blocker Collections. See also Allen J. Smith, "Some Memories of the Medical Department in its Beginning," *Alcalde*, 3 (July, 1915), 742 (3rd quotation), 745, and 749 (4th quotation).

6. Willard R. Cooke, "A Brief History of the Medical Department," *Alcalde*, 3 (July, 1915), 751–765.

7. Bixel and Turner, *Galveston and the 1900 Storm*, 157.

8. Flexner, *Medical Education in the United States and Canada*, 279–282 (North Carolina); 289–291 (Oklahoma); 314–316 (Virginia); and 309–312 (Texas).

9. Rosemary Stevens, *American Medicine and the Public Interest: A History of Specialization*, 85–92. In 1920, all of the other schools in Texas no longer functioned. See "Texas Medical Schools," *University Medical*, 23 (Feb., 1919), 1–3.

10. *Galveston Daily News*, June 1, 1923.

11. *Galveston Tribune*, June 5, 1925.

12. The first native Texan to be the university's CEO, Splawn received degrees from Baylor, Yale, and the University of Chicago. He was professor and chair of UT's economics department when he became CEO; see *Galveston Daily News*, July 6, 1924, and Mar. 15 and 22, 1925.

13. *Galveston Daily News*, July 15, 1926.

14. The professors were delighted that the Texas Supreme Court supported their legal right to enforce rigorous requirements for promotion and graduation. In 1932 the faculty had dismissed a student who had failed certain exams during his first year. In December 1932 the court upheld a judgment by the Commission of Appeals that validated the

legal right of the UT regents to sanction such rules adopted by the faculty of the university. For details, see the attachments to Douglas J. Glasscock to Chester R. Burns, Jan. 27, 1987, letter, WF321, CHP Archives.

15. *Texas State Journal of Medicine*, 23 (Apr., 1928), 808–809 (1st quotation). This article included thirteen marvelous photos. See also Meyer Bodansky, "The Historical Background of Modern Medicine and Modern Medical Education," *University Medical*, 33 (Oct., 1928), 8–25 (2nd quotation).

16. S. C. Griffin, *History of Galveston, Texas, Narrative and Biographical* (Galveston: privately printed, 1931), 115 (quotation). Griffin also included biographical sketches of twenty physicians, mostly UTMB professors, and one dentist. Griffin's obituary appeared in *Galveston Daily News*, Feb. 21, 1945.

17. *Galveston Daily News*, Nov. 12, 1933.

18. Diane Treadaway Ozment, "The Port City of Galveston," in Willena C. Adams (ed.), *Texas Cities and the Great Depression* (Austin: Texas Memorial Museum, 1973), 140, 143, 139.

19. *University Medical*, 41 (Nov., 1936), 4–10; and (Dec., 1936), 4–14. For a photo of Roosevelt's calvacade passing in front of the John Sealy Hospital, see *UTMB: Seventy-five Year History*, 157.

20. *Texas State Journal of Medicine*, 33 (Apr., 1938), 836 (quotation); and *Galveston Daily News*, May 10, 1938.

21. In his address about UTMB's past, present, and future to UT alumni meeting in Galveston in March 1940, Spies used only tiny amounts of the past as an introduction to the present and future; see *Galveston Daily News*, Mar. 3, 1940. See also *Galveston Daily News*, Dec. 6, 1940; and C. W. Sanders, "History of the Medical Department of the University of Texas, Galveston, Texas," *Phi Chi Quarterly*, 38 (May, 1941), 281–296.

22. This article was in Section E, page 8 of the supplement for April 11, 1942. UTMB's hospitals were described in another article about Galveston's hospitals in Section E, page 6.

23. John G. Sinclair to chairmen of departments, Nov. 10, 1942, memo, folder 7, box 40, Stone Papers, Blocker Collections. Other departmental histories may have been written at this time, but only nine are extant. The author's name is not included on some of these histories. The departments and probable authors were Anatomy (John Sinclair); Bacteriology and Preventive Medicine (William Sharp); Biochemistry (Byron Hendrix); Dermatology (Earl B. Ritchie); Internal Medicine (Charles Stone); Neurology and Psychiatry (Titus Harris); Obstetrics and Gynecology (Willard Cooke); Otolaryngology (George S. McReynolds); and Pharmacology (Charles H. Taft). These typescripts are in vertical files A8 in the Blocker Collections. Whether these histories were distributed in typescript form is not known. Some information in these typescripts became public for the first time in *UTMB: Seventy-five Year History*. For an example, see "A Brief History of the Department of Obstetrics and Gynecology of the University of Texas Medical Branch," pp. 3–4 (quotation).

24. *Galveston Daily News*, Dec. 19, 1942 (1st quotation), and *Galveston Daily News*, Dec. 18, 1942 (2nd quotation). For details, see *Galveston Daily News*, Dec. 8–9 and 17–19, 1942.

25. *Galveston Daily News*, Feb. 25, 1943. A copy is in WF309, CHP Archives.

26. *Medi-Texan*, 2 (June, 1955), 14.

27. Chauncey D. Leake, "A Century of Internal Medicine in Texas," *Texas State Journal of Medicine*, 49 (May, 1953), 282–287.

28. Emmett N. Wilson, "History of Medical Education in Galveston," *The Centaur of Alpha Kappa Kappa*, 56 (Mar., 1951), 215–221; and W. J. Battle, "University of Texas, Medical Branch of," in Walter Prescott Webb and H. Bailey Carroll (eds.), *The Handbook of Texas* (2 vols.; Austin: Texas State Historical Association, 1952), II, 823.

29. Mildred M. Robertson, "Faculty Sketches: The University of Texas Medical Branch," Alumni Association, 1951. Robertson's "Overseas Letters" and *Alumni Bulletins* were rich sources of information about UTMB as the institution evolved between 1944 and 1970. *Handbook of Texas* entries included George Bethel, Meyer Bodansky, Paul Brindley, Albert Clopton, Marvin Graves, Titus Harris, William Keiller, James McLaughlin, Edward Randall, Edward Randall Jr., Allen Smith, and James E. Thompson. A copy of Brindley's history is in box 2, vertical file A8, Blocker Collections. Anne Brindley was president of the TSHA in 1973–1974.

30. *Texas State Journal of Medicine*, 47 (Mar., 1951), 166.

31. Lait and Mortimer, *U.S.A. Confidential*, 213; and McComb, *Galveston: A History*, 150–163. Houston had become the state's largest city by 1930.

32. McComb, *Galveston: A History*, 184–187 and 212–214. Dean Truslow probably talked about these social changes when he took Sen. and Mrs. Lyndon B. Johnson on a tour of UTMB two years later; for a photo, see *UTMB: Seventy-five Year History*, 234.

33. John S. Chapman, *The University of Texas Southwestern Medical School Medical Education in Dallas, 1900–1975* (Dallas: Southern Methodist University Press, 1976); R. W. Cumley and Joan McCay (eds.), *The First Twenty Years of the University of Texas M.D. Anderson Hospital and Tumor Institute* (Houston: M. D. Anderson Hospital and Tumor Institute,

1964); and E. W. D'Anton, *Memories: A History of the University of Texas Dental Branch* (Houston: U.T. Dental Branch, 1991). Also see M. O. Rouse, "Medical Education in Texas," *Texas State Journal of Medicine*, 49 (May, 1953), 320–322.

34. Mary Ellen Haggard and Arild E. Hansen, "Development of Pediatrics at the University of Texas School of Medicine in Galveston," *Texas Reports on Biology and Medicine*, 15 (Summer, 1957), 269–282; a copy of Abreu's history is in box 3, vertical file A8, Blocker Collections; and William B. Sharp, "Microbiology at the Medical College," undated manuscript, WF470, CHP Archives. Even professional historiographers not directly connected with UTMB focused narrowly. Ralph W. Jones, a historian at the University of Alabama, prepared a carefully researched article about the propriety medical schools in Galveston that preceded the establishment of UTMB. See Ralph W. Jones, "The First Roots of the University of Texas Medical Branch at Galveston," *Southwestern Historical Quarterly*, 45 (Apr., 1962), 465–474.

35. T. G. Blocker Jr., "Albert O. Singleton," *Surgery*, 24 (Sept., 1948), 587–588; and "G. W. N. Eggers 1896–1963," *Transactions of the Southern Surgical Association*, 75 (1963), 429–431. The history of the Department of Surgery is in the folder titled Unpublished Speeches, 1956–60, box 78, Blocker Papers. For much of the information in his speech, Blocker used an unpublished autobiographical review of surgery at UTMB that was delivered as the presidential address to the Texas Surgical Society in 1955 by C. B. Carter (School of Medicine class of 1919). A copy of this speech is in box 5, vertical file A8, Blocker Collections. See also Charles T. Stone, "Internal Medicine," *Texas Medicine*, 63 (Mar., 1967), 74–77. In this issue, two professors analyzed the careers of Ashbel Smith and Edward Randall Sr. See Alvin E. Rodin and Albert O. Singleton Jr., "Two Early Leaders: Medical Branch," *Texas Medicine*, 63 (Mar., 1967), 112–116.

36. John Truslow had first suggested the preparation of a UTMB history. See John B. Truslow to Harry H. Ransom, Dec. 20, 1963; John B. Truslow to Harry H. Ransom, Apr. 30, 1964; and Harry Ransom to John B. Truslow, May 8, 1964, letters, all in box VF M/5, UT Chancellor's Records. One of the earliest articles on medical history published in the *Southwestern Historical Quarterly* was written by Harry Ransom, then professor of English and assistant dean of the Graduate School at UT Austin. See Harry Ransom, "Sherman Goodwin—Texas Physician, 1814–1884," *Southwestern Historical Quarterly*, 55 (Jan., 1952), 325–340. Transcripts of eight interviews are in folder 35, box 1, 75th Anniversary History Papers, Blocker Collections. Audiotapes of interviews with Willard Cooke, Chauncey Leake, and Titus Harris are also in the Blocker Collections. For additional details, see four folders of correspondence in box 2 of the 75th Anniversary History Papers. Blocker had also supported the preparation of an anniversary issue of *Texas Reports on Biology and Medicine*. Eleanor Porter and Charles G. Tucker edited this 401-page supplement to volume 34, which was published in June 1966. It included twelve scientific/clinical articles by alumni and more than fifty pages of artwork, poems, cartoons, short essays, drawings, and photos submitted by students, faculty, and staff. Lise Darst's watercolor of Old Red was particularly haunting.

37. *Newsletter (UTMB)*, 3 (Jan., 1968), 14; and *UTMB: Seventy-five Year History*, foreword (quotations).

38. *Southwestern Historical Quarterly*, 72 (Oct., 1968), 269–270.

39. The label was used by Al LeBlanc in LeBlanc to Chester R. Burns, Oct. 24 and Nov. 29, 1989, interviews, Blocker Collections.

40. Also see the annual reports for fiscal years 1980–1985 in WF436, CHP Archives, and those for fiscal years 1986–1991 in WF429, CHP Archives.

41. See Vernon E. Thompson to Myles Knape, Feb. 26, Mar. 14, and Apr. 8, 1986, interviews, Blocker Collections. After 1950 the state legislature authorized new medical schools for UT San Antonio, UT Houston, Texas Tech, and Texas A&M; a new UT Health Center at Tyler; and the allocation of state dollars to Baylor Medical School in Houston after it separated from Baylor University (1969). State expenditures for health care in 1975 were estimated to be $946 million, with $123 million assigned to education and research (13 percent). In 1986 they were $3.6 billion, with $652 million for education and research (17.9 percent). For details, see D. Clayton Brown, "Medical Education in Texas: the Growth of Schools," *Texas Medicine*, 82 (May, 1986), 49–53; Charles E. Begley and Douglas A Mains, "Health Care Spending in Texas, 1975–1984," *Texas Medicine*, 83 (Sept., 1987), 30–35; and Charles E. Begley and Douglas A. Mains, "Health Care Spending in Texas, 1980–1986," *Texas Medicine*, 85 (Sept., 1989), 25–30. For histories of two of the new schools, see Robert McCartor and George Tyner, *Eye of the Storm* (Lubbock: Texas Tech University Press, 1986), and Bryant Boutwell and John P. McGovern, *Conversation with a Medical School: The University of Texas–Houston Medical School, 1970–2000* (Houston: University of Texas–Houston Health Science Center, 1999).

42. "Economic Impact: The University of Texas Medical Branch at Galveston: A Report to the Community," (Galveston, UTMB Office of Public Affairs, 1988), 6 (1st quotation). A copy is in vertical file B7, Blocker Collections. See also *Galveston Daily News*, June 26, 1988 (2nd quotation). A second report in 1989 revealed that 95 percent of UTMB's 8,200 employees lived in Galveston County (69 percent in the city). In Galveston alone, they contributed $16.8 million in revenues to the Galveston taxing authorities and school district; see *Galveston Daily News*, June 25, 1989.

43. *Galveston Daily News*, Feb. 26, 1989.

44. Walter B. King Jr., "James E. Thompson: Texas' First Professor of Surgery," *Texas Medicine*, 64 (Feb., 1968), 82–87; and Joseph P. McNeil, "Albert Olin Singleton, M.D.: Contributions to Surgery," *Texas Medicine*, 76 (May, 1980), 40–42.

45. Brown "The Historical Development of the University of Texas System School of Nursing, 1890–1973"; and Burlage, Henry M. and Margot E. Beutler, *Pharmacy's Foundation in Texas: A History of the College of Pharmacy, 1898–1976* (Austin: Pharmaceutical Foundation of the College of Pharmacy of the University of Texas at Austin, 1978).

46. Ash's unpublished manuscript (MS 6.1.3) is in box 6, Miscellaneous Manuscripts, Blocker Collections. See also Donald Duncan, "A Commentary on Eighty Years of Anatomy at the University of Texas Medical Branch Part I, 1891–1932," *Texas Reports on Biology and Medicine*, 32 (Spring, 1974), 89–105. Also see folders 1–3, box 10, Duncan Papers, Blocker Collections; Don W. Micks, "Historical Highlights of the Department of Preventive Medicine and Community Health," n.d., 27 pages, box 4, vertical file A8, Blocker Collections; Robert N. Cooley, "The History of the Department of Radiology, The University of Texas Medical Branch," typescript, WF472, CHP Archives; and Charles R. Allen, "A History of the Department of Anesthesiology, 1942–1990," typescript, WF468, CHP Archives.

47. "University of Texas Medical Branch at Galveston," *The Handbook of Texas: A Supplement* (Austin: Texas State Historical Association, 1976), 1046–1047; McComb, *Galveston: A History*, 191; Chester R. Burns, "Medicine in Texas: The Historical Literature," *Texas Medicine*, 82 (Jan., 1986), 60–63; Kathleen M. Stephens, "Old Red: a Legacy Lives On," *Texas Medicine*, 82 (Apr., 1986), 50–53; D. Clayton Brown, "Medical Education in Texas: The Growth of Schools," *Texas Medicine*, 82 (May, 1986), 49–53; and Susan E. Cayleff, "'Babe' Didrikson Zaharias: Her Personal and Public Battle with Cancer," *Texas Medicine*, 82 (Sept., 1986), 41–45.

48. *Impact*, 13 (Dec. 1, 1989), 2; 14 (Jan. 12, 1990), 3–4; (Mar. 9, 1990), 5–8; (Nov. 9, 1990), 6; and (Nov. 30, 1990), 1–2; and *Galveston Daily News*, Nov. 10, 1989, and Oct. 27–28, 1990. For details, see WF431, CHP Archives. For photos, see *Centennial Reflections: The University of Texas Medical Branch*, 6–13. Beginning in the fall of 1985, Chester Burns directed a research team that eventually included (among others) Myles Knape, Megan Seaholm, and John Swann. In 1988 and 1989, Burns, Knape, Seaholm, and Swann gave some Centennial Preview lectures on campus. Burns and Knape gave additional ones in 1990 and 1991.

49. *Galveston Daily News*, Jan. 10–12 and 15 (quotation), 1990; *Impact*, 14 (Jan. 12, 1990), 3–4; and Robert B. Nichols, *A Bridge to a Better World* (Galveston: The Sealy & Smith Foundation for the John Sealy Hospital, 1989).

50. *Impact*, 14 (Mar. 9, 1990), 5–8; and *Galveston Daily News*, Jan. 26 and 30, Mar. 10–11, and May 8, 1990. A copy of the brochure is in WF338, CHP Archives.

51. *Galveston Daily News*, Jan. 24 and 26, 1991, and *Impact*, 15 (Feb. 22, 1991), 4–6. For photos of this event and other celebrations during 1991, see *Centennial Reflections: The University of Texas Medical Branch at Galveston*.

52. Watts also prepared a summary of this brochure, which was published in *Texas Medicine*, 87 (Apr., 1991), 61–64. Copies of these items are in the Centennial Year Memorabilia boxes in the Blocker Collections. See "A Century of Service: The University of Texas Medical Branch at Galveston, 1891–1991," 1 (quotation). A copy is in WF431, CHP Archives. Also see *Impact*, 15 (Feb. 22, 1991), 2. The School of Medicine Alumni Association focused its energies on acquiring funds for a Student Center building; see *Impact*, 15 (Mar. 22, 1991), 1.

53. *Impact*, 14 (Aug. 31, 1990), 1, and (Nov. 9, 1990), 6. Copies of the calendars are in the Centennial Year Memorabilia boxes in the Blocker Collections.

54. *Galveston Daily News*, Mar. 17, 21–22, 1991; and *Impact*, 15 (Apr. 19, 1991), 5.

55. *Impact*, 15 (May 17, 1991), 6; and *Galveston Daily News*, June 11 and 18, 1991. A sample of the postcard and samples of other printed items issued during the year are in the Centennial Year Memorabilia boxes in the Blocker Collections. See also *Impact*, 15 (May 17, 1991), 1, 6; (June 14, 1991), 5–6; and (June 28, 1991), 10.

56. Chester R. Burns, "The University of Texas Medical Branch at Galveston: Origins and Beginnings," *Journal of the American Medical Association*, 266 (Sept. 11, 1991), 1400–1403; *Impact*, 15 (Sept. 13, 1991), 1–2; and *Galveston Daily News*, Sept. 11, 1991 (quotation).

57. *Impact*, 15 (Oct. 11, 1991), 1, 6–7. A copy of the cachet is in WF431, CHP Archives.

58. *Texas Medicine*, 87 (Dec., 1991), 40–80; and Byron J. Bailey and Thomas N. James, "Commentary: UTMB celebrates 100 years of service to Texans," *Texas Medicine*, 87 (Dec., 1991), 43 (quotation).

59. *Impact*, 15 (Dec. 13, 1991), 3.

60. *Impact*, 19 (Mar. 6, 1995), 4; 17 (Sept. 3, 1993), 5; 16 (Aug. 7, 1992), 2; 17 (May 14, 1993), 2; 19 (Sept. 4, 1995), 1; 11 (Feb. 7, 1992), 2; 19 (June 12, 1995), 1; 17 (Mar. 19, 1993), 1, 5; and 20 (Aug. 5, 1996), 6. After serving as dean of medicine for eighteen years and vice president for academic affairs for twelve years, George Bryan relinquished those positions in 1995; see *Impact*, 18 (May 2, 1994), 1 and; 19 (Aug. 7, 1995), 7–10.

61. A copy of "Vision 2020: The University of Texas System Strategic Plan, 1991–1997, Preparing Texans for a Changing World" is in WF429, CHP Archives. See also *Impact*, 15 (Apr. 17, 1991), 1; 21 (Apr. 21, 1997), 1; (May 5, 1997), 2; (May 21, 1997), 2; and (June 5, 1997), 2.

62. For accolades about James, see *Galveston County Daily News*, Oct. 8–9, 13, 1996. In the summer of 1997, the Sealy & Smith Foundation, the Houston Endowment, and the John S. Dunn Research Foundation provided funds to establish the Thomas N. and Gleaves T. James Distinguished Chair in recognition of the leadership and contributions of Dr. and Mrs. James; see *Impact*, 21 (Aug. 4, 1997), 1. See also *Impact*, 21 (Aug. 22, 1997), 1; *Galveston County Daily News*, Aug. 14 and 24, and Oct. 5, 1997; and *Impact*, 21 (Oct. 20, 1997), 1, 4. For other insights about Stobo, see *Galveston County Daily News*, Sept. 14 and Nov. 17, 1997.

63. *Impact*, 22 (Feb. 16, 1998), 3.

64. *Impact*, 22 (Jan. 6, 1998), 3. These meetings were videotaped and made available to anyone who could not attend. As a follow-up to these meetings, Stobo also wrote a column in *Impact* entitled "Our Town." In these columns he expanded on items introduced during town meetings and addressed related topics. In 1998, for example, these appeared in the following issues: Feb. 2, 1998, 6–7; Mar. 2, 1998, 2–3, 6; Apr. 6, 1998, 8–9; May 18, 1998, 8–9; June 15, 1998, 8–9; and Aug. 17, 1998, 8–9. A web site (www.utmb.edu/townmeeting) allowed employees to communicate their concerns directly to him.

65. *Impact*, 18 (Mar. 4, 1994), 4; and 17 (Aug. 6, 1993), 2; *Galveston County Daily News*, Jan. 29, 1994, and June 10, 1998. To recognize and honor individuals and groups who made donations to UTMB, Tom James and development officers established the Sealy Society, the President's Cabinet, and the Heritage Council. See *Impact*, 18 (Sept. 19, 1994), 2; 17 (Jan. 13, 1997), 7; and 22 (Aug. 3, 1998), 3; and *Galveston County Daily News*, June 11, 1995.

66. *Galveston Daily News*, Jan. 17, 1992 (quotation); and *Impact*, 20 (Sept. 16, 1996), 1.

67. *Impact*, 17 (June 11, 1993), 13; and *Galveston County Daily News*, July 3, 4, and 19, 1997. After ten years of service, the Life Flight helicopters had transported seven thousand patients. See also *Texas Medicine*, 91 (Oct., 1995), 28–35, and 93 (May, 1997), 30–33. For one professor's analysis of the managed-care era, see James C. Thompson, "Seed Corn Impact of Managed Care on Medical Education and Research," *Annals of Surgery*, 223 (May, 1996), 453–463. This was Thompson's presidential address to the Southern Surgical Association.

68. *Galveston County Daily News*, Oct. 10 and Dec. 9 and 27, 1998; Jan. 15, Mar. 7, June 4, and July 18, 1999.

69. *Impact*, 16 (Aug. 7, 1992), 1; 21 (Sept. 15, 1997), 3; (Oct. 6, 1997), 5; (Oct. 20, 1997), 5; and (Nov. 3, 1997), 3; 22 (Jan. 6, 1998), 9; (Jan. 20, 1998), 3; and (Feb. 2, 1998), 9. These employees had previously been part of seven departments: Biocommunication Services; Fleet Planning and Administration; Mail Services; Materials Management; Accounts Payable; Purchasing; and Records Management.

70. *Impact*, 18 (June 27, 1994), 9; 19 (May 1, 1995), 3; (June 26, 1995), 2; 20 (Aug. 19, 1996), 1; and 21 (Feb. 3, 1997); *Galveston County Daily News*, May 10, 1995, May 16, Aug. 10, and Sept. 28, 1996; and Dec. 10, 1997.

71. *Impact*, 16 (Jan. 24, 1992), 3; *Galveston Daily News*, Jan. 10, Apr. 15, and Oct. 28, 1992; *Impact*, 17 (June 25, 1993), 2; (Aug. 6, 1993), 3; and 20 (Nov. 18, 1996), 4. See also *Galveston County Daily News*, Jan. 25, 1997; and *Impact*, 21 (Feb. 3, 1997), 5–7.

72. *Impact*, 22 (May 18, 1998), 4.

73. *Impact*, 21 (Jan. 13, 1997), 8; and *Galveston County Daily News*, July 20, 1997.

74. *Impact*, 17 (June 25, 1993), 1, 4. For photos of children whose lives were saved by the ECMO team, see *Galveston County Daily News*, Sept. 29, 1997. See also *Impact*, 19 (Sept. 4, 1995), 5. For an example of outstanding success with one patient in the Victoria clinic, see *Impact*, 20 (Aug. 19, 1996), 4. See also *Impact*, 17 (Feb. 5, 1993), 5; 18 (Aug. 22, 1994), 9; (Nov. 14, 1994), 1–2; and 22 (Nov. 16, 1998), 1–2.

75. *Impact*, 16 (Feb. 21, 1992), 1; 18 (Feb. 21, 1994), 2; and 20 (Mar. 18, 1996), 6.

76. Albert Rosenfeld, "Open Gates Dream and Reality," copy in WF429, CHP Archives. See also *Impact*, 19 (Aug. 7, 1995), 1; and *Galveston County Daily News*, Nov. 25, 1997.

77. *Impact*, 16 (Apr. 3, 1992), 4; and (May 1, 1992), 1. In 1997, after thirty years, Jay Fish and colleagues had performed sixteen hundred transplants; see *Galveston County Daily News*, Mar. 30, 1997; and *Impact*, 21 (Apr. 7, 1997), 6. Also see Luther B. Travis, Alok Kalia, Kristene K. Gugliuzza, and Rajendra N. Srivastava, "Renal Transplantation in Children: Experience of 23 Years at the Children's Renal Center at the University of Texas Medical Branch at Galveston," *Texas Medicine*, 87 (Dec., 1991), 50–55; *Impact*, 17 (Apr. 2, 1993), 2; and 18 (Nov. 14, 1994), 3. For a dramatic report about one heart transplant patient, see *Galveston County Daily News*, May 24–27, 1998. Also see *Galveston County Daily News*, Oct. 16, 1999; and *Impact*, 19 (Jan. 23, 1995), 1; (Oct. 16, 1995), 3; and 21 (Mar. 5, 1997), 1.

78. *Impact*, 21 (Apr. 7, 1997), 4; 18 (Aug. 22, 1994), 1; and *Galveston County Daily News*, Feb. 17, 1997.

79. *Impact*, 18 (June 27, 1994), 1–2, and 20 (Sept. 3, 1996), 1; *Galveston County Daily News*, Jan. 1 and Feb. 18, 1996. Also see Larry Besaw, "Hats Off to Texas Medical Schools," *Texas Medicine*, 92 (Nov., 1996), 36–42; and *Impact*, 20 (May 20, 1996), 5.

80. *Impact*, 19 (June 26, 1995), 8; and 22 (Oct. 19, 1998), 7.

81. *Impact*, 22 (Aug. 3, 1998), 13.

82. *Impact*, 16 (Aug. 21, 1992), 8; 20, (Aug. 5, 1996), 3; and Graduate School of Biomedical Sciences, University of Texas Medical Branch at Galveston, Report of Internal Review Committee, May 5, 1995; a copy is in WF429, CHP Archives.

83. *Impact*, 22 (Mar. 2, 1998), 5.

84. See several documents in WF429 and WF435, CHP Archives. These include minutes of the Research Advisory Council between 1995 and 1998 and two important reports issued in the spring of 1996: the "Directory of Research Resources" and the "Catalog of Research Expertise."

85. See *Newsline* in *Impact*, 16 (Aug. 20, 1993), 1–2. See also *Impact*, 19 (Apr. 17, 1995), 7; and *Newsline* in *Impact*, 16 (Dec. 4, 1992), 1–2. For a profile of a volunteer research subject, see *Impact*, 20 (Aug. 19, 1996), 3.

86. See *Newsline* in *Impact*, 16 (Oct. 2, 1992), 1; *Galveston Daily News*, Apr. 19, 1992, and Mar. 12, 1995; *Newsline* in *Impact*, 17 (Feb. 5, 1993), 1; *Impact*, 17 (Oct. 15, 1993), 4; 19 (Jan. 23, 1995), 4; (Oct. 2, 1995), 1; and 22 (June 15, 1998), 6–7. By 1998 the Endowment Fund totaled $100 million. For more details about research during the 1990s, see the newsletter *Catalyst* issued for a few years during the mid-1990s and *Biomedical Inquiry* issued twice a year. Some of the centers distributed reports about their work. In 1996 Brad Thompson replaced Samuel Wilson as director of the Sealy Center for Molecular Science and issued periodic newsletters about this center. In 1998 Stratford May and colleagues prepared a splendid report about the Sealy Center for Oncology and Hematology; see a copy in WF429, CHP Archives.

87. *Galveston County Daily News*, Sept. 6, 1998. For details about the work of Carney and others at UTMB and the Shriners Burns Institute interested in trauma, infection, and wound healing, see a report titled "An Integrated Approach to Trauma, Infection, and Repair at UTMB," March 1997; a copy is in WF429, CHP Archives.

88. For glimpses into the extent of these influences, see "UTMB in the News" for 1993 and 1994, collections of articles about UTMB personnel published in numerous newspapers and newsletters during those years. Copies are in WF429, CHP Archives. See also *Galveston County Daily News*, Apr. 9, 1999.

89. *Galveston County Daily News*, Mar. 22, 1997.

90. All citations are in *Impact*. For Herndon, see 16 (Mar. 20, 1992), 2; for Belli, 16 (Apr. 3, 1992), 5; for Bailey, 16 (May 29, 1992), *Newsline*; for Blankenship, 17 (June 26, 1992), *Newsline*; for Linda Philips, 17 (Feb. 5, 1993), *Newsline*; for Nusynowitz, 20 (Feb. 5, 1996), 15; for Billy Philips, 17 (Jan. 22, 1993), 6; and for Rahr, 17 (Sept. 17, 1993), *Newsline*.

91. *Impact*, 16 (Jan. 24, 1992), 1; (Dec. 1992), *Newsline*; and 19 (Jan. 9, 1995), 3. See also *Galveston Daily News*, Jan. 18, 1992, and Jan. 31, 1992; and *Impact*, 22 (Dec. 7, 1998), 6; and 23 (Nov. 9, 1999), 3.

92. For specific examples, see *Impact*, 20 (June 3, 1996), 6–7; and (June 17, 1996), 10–11.

93. *Impact*, 22 (Apr. 6, 1998), 11.

94. *Galveston Daily News*, Apr. 9, 1991. Two years earlier the city of Galveston had celebrated Medical Researchers Day at UTMB; see *Galveston Daily News*, Jan. 13, 1989.

95. J. Andrew Grant, "Leaders of the University of Texas Medical Branch at Galveston," *Texas Medicine*, 87 (Dec., 1991), 44–49; Harold G. Levine, *History of Child Health Services at the University of Texas Medical Branch, Galveston, Texas* (Galveston: University of Texas Medical Branch, 1992); Chester R. Burns, "The Development of Hospitals in Galveston During the Nineteenth Century," *Southwestern Historical Quarterly*, 97 (Oct., 1993), 238–263; and Chester R. Burns, "A Brief History of the Graduate School of Biomedical Sciences at the University of Texas Medical Branch at Galveston" (Galveston: UTMB Biomedical Communication Services, 1994).

96. For details, see Chester R. Burns, "The New Handbook of Texas," *Medical Humanities Rounds*, 14 (Sept., 1996). As advisory editor, Burns coordinated all of the health and medicine entries. He wrote thirty-three biographical entries and eight non-biographical essays (Epidemic Diseases; Health and Medicine; John Sealy Hospital; Medical Quackery; Medical Research; Medical Societies; Texas Medical Association [with Megan Seaholm]; and UTMB). Also see Campbell, "A Note on the First Nursing School in Texas and its Role in the Nineteenth Century Experience," 49–58.

97. Burns and Campbell, "The Extraordinary Influences of Two British Physicians on Medical Education and Practice in Texas at the Turn of the 20th Century," 79–84; Vernie A. Stembridge, "Training the Healers," *Heritage*, 17 (May, 1999), 8–12; Kelsey, *Twentieth-Century Doctor*; and Harry K. Davis (ed.), "University of Texas Medical Branch Class of 1949 Recollections," 1999. A copy of the class of 1949's recollections is in WF429, CHP Archives.

Selected Bibliography

ARCHIVAL AND MANUSCRIPT COLLECTIONS

Birmingham, Alabama
  JCMS/UAB Health Sciences Archives
    Tom D. Spies Papers and Spies Nutrition Clinic Collection (1902–1960)
Austin, Texas
  Center for American History, UT Austin
    J. R. Parten Papers
    Harry Ransom Papers
    Ashbel Smith Papers
    Transcripts Relating to the Medical History of Texas
    Thomas D. Wooten Papers
  Legislative Reference Library
    Proceedings of the Senate Committee Investigating the
    University of Texas Controversy
  Texas State Archives, Texas State Library
    General Laws of the State of Texas
    Special Laws of the State of Texas
    Journals of the House and Senate, State of Texas
    Warrant Registers, Treasurer's Office, State of Texas
  Texas Medical Association Library
    Archival Records, Texas Medical Association
    Transcripts Relating to the Medical History of Texas
  UT Board of Regents' Offices, Ashbel Smith Hall
    Unpublished Minutes, published Reports, and other archival records about the
    University of Texas.
Bethesda, Maryland
  History of Medicine Division, National Library of Medicine
    Chauncey D. Leake Papers
Galveston, Texas
  City Secretary's Office, City Hall
    Unpublished Minutes, Galveston City Council
    Unpublished Ordinances, Galveston City Council
  District Clerk's Office, Galveston County Courthouse
    Registers, Galveston County
    Unpublished Minutes, Galveston County Commissioners Court

Truman G. Blocker Jr. History of Medicine Collections, Moody Medical Library, University of Texas Medical Branch
  Archives, Area Health Education Center
  Archives, Galveston County Medical Society
  Archives, Galveston Medical College
  Archives, Singleton Surgical Society
  Archives, Texas Medical College and Hospital
  Archives, Texas Occupational Therapy Association
  Archives, Texas Society of Pathologists
  Archives, Texas Society of Plastic Surgeons
  Archives, Texas Surgical Society
  Archives, University of Texas Medical Branch
  Benedict E. Abreu Papers
  Ludwik Anigstein Papers
  Kenneth Hazen Aynesworth Papers
  Philip A. Bergman Papers
  F. J. L. Blasingame Papers
  Truman G. Blocker Jr. Papers
  Raymond Frank Blount Papers
  Meyer Bodansky Papers
  Edith Marguerite Bonnet Papers
  Donald Duncan Papers
  A. W. Fly Papers
  Walter T. and Francis A. Garbade Papers
  M. Mason Guest Papers
  George R. Herrmann Notebooks
  Thomas Terrell Jackson Papers
  Chauncey Depew Leake Papers
  William C. Levin Papers
  Ardzroony Packchanian Papers
  F. Hermann Rudenberg Papers
  Glenn V. Russell Papers
  William Dempsey Seybold Papers
  John G. Sinclair Papers
  Charles Turner Stone Papers
  James Edwin Thompson Papers
  Fred J. Wolma Papers
  UTMB Centennial History Research Files
  UTMB Centennial History Writing Files
Sealy & Smith Foundation, Sealy & Smith Professional Bldg.
  Minutes, Sealy & Smith Foundation
Texas and Galveston History Center, Rosenberg Library
  Ordinances of the City of Galveston

City Directories of Galveston
H. Kempner Records
Houston, Texas
Texas Medical Center/ Houston Academy of Medicine Library
Archival Collections
San Francisco, California
School of Medicine, University of California
Chauncey D. Leake Papers
Washington, D.C.
Association of American Medical Colleges Archives

INTERVIEWS

Interviews with eighty-five individuals were recorded at various times between 1985 and 1994. Unless indicated otherwise, the following interviews were audiotaped in Galveston. A topical outline of most interviews was typed and written materials were solicited from some of the interviewees. This printed information is enclosed in a folder for each interviewee that is deposited in the Centennial History Archives at the Moody Medical Library in Galveston. The audio portion of each interview is available in streaming audio format (http://ar.utmb.edu/centennial/) from the Truman G. Blocker Jr. History of Medicine Collections of the UTMB Academic Resources web site (http://ar.utmb.edu/). This list is alphabetized according to the interviewee's last name.

Bailey, Byron. Interview by Chester Burns. Feb. 13, 1992.

Barlow, Donna Jean. Interview by Poldi Tschirch. June 16, 1986.

Barnes, Johnson Peyton Jr. Interview by Greg Diamond in Houston. Nov. 1, 1986.

Baron, Samuel. Interview by Myles Knape. Oct. 6, 1987.

Barratt, Ernest S. Interview by Chester Burns. Jan. 8, 1992.

Bing, Robert K. Interview by Myles Knape. Sept. 10, 16, 23, 30, 1987 and June 8, 1988.

Blocker, Virginia Irvine. Interview by Myles Knape. Aug. 18, 1986.

Brandt, Edward N. Interview by Chester Burns in Washington, D.C. Oct. 29, 1989.

Bruhn, John. Interview by Myles Knape. Dec. 3 and 5, 1985.

Bryan, George. Interview by Myles Knape. Jan. 31, Feb. 6, 11, 26, and Mar. 6, 1986. Interview by Chester Burns. July 26, 1989 and Oct. 10, 1989.

Calvin, Novella V. (Mrs. Dea Bailey). Interview by Myles Knape. Oct. 21, 1985.

Carson, Ronald A. Interview by Myles Knape. May 21 and 28 and June 11, 1986.

Casberg, Melvin A. Phone interview by Chester Burns. Sept. 7, 1989.

Cooper, Cary. Interview by Myles Knape. Nov. 12, 1987.

Daeschner, C. William. Interview by Myles Knape and Chester Burns. July 13 and 20, and Aug. 3, 1988.

Damewood, Dorothy. Interview by Myles Knape. Nov. 13, and Dec. 16, 1985.

Davidson, Etta Mae MacDonald. Interview by Chester Burns. June 25, 1986.

Davis, Harry K. Interview by Chester Burns. Dec. 8, 1994.

Decker, Grace. Interview by Poldi Tschirch. July 17, 1986.

Decker, Ruby. Interview by Myles Knape. May 1 and 2, 1986.

Earle, Kenneth. Interview by Chester Burns. Mar. 15, 1990.

Eiland, David. Interview by Myles Knape. Nov. 19, 1985, and Jan. 21, 1986.

Fenton, Mary. Interview by Myles Knape. Feb. 13 and 18 and Mar. 4, 1986.

Fiedler, Zora McAnelly. Interview by Poldi Tschirch. Oct. 25, 1986.

Fish, Jay. Interview by Chester Burns. Feb. 17, 1992.

Floyd, Chloe. Interview by Myles Knape. Jan. 16 and 22, 1986.

Foster, Austin. Self-directed audiotape. April 1989.

Frey, Emil. Interview by Myles Knape. Jan. 29 and 30 and Feb. 4, 1987.

Gibson, William. Interview by Chester Burns. Oct. 7, 1988.

Gregory, Raymond L. Interview by Myles Knape. Aug. 4, 1987.

Guest, M. Mason. Interview by John Swann. Jan. 29, 1987.

Hardwicke, Charles. Interview by Chester Burns. Nov. 1, 1988.

Hild, Walther. Interview by Myles Knape. May 18 and July 6, 1987; June 24, 1988.

Holland, O. Bryan. Interview by Chester Burns. Feb. 5, 1992.

Hornedo, Manuel D. Self-directed audiotape. August 1986.

James, Thomas N. Interview by Chester Burns. Oct. 12 and 24, 1995.

Jannasch, James R. Interview by Megan Seaholm. July 20 and 27, 1989.

Jennings, F. Lamont. Interview by Guy Lindberg. Jan. 29, 1990.

King, Camille. Interview by Myles Knape. Oct. 16, 1985.

King, Walter. Interview by Greg Diamond. Apr. 7, 1987.

Knebel, Elizabeth. Interview by Poldi Tschirch. June 12, 1986.

Knisely, William H. Interview by Chester Burns. Oct. 19, 1989.

LeBlanc, Alvin L. Interview by Chester Burns. Oct. 24 and Nov. 29, 1989.

LeMaistre, Charles. Interview by Chester Burns. Dec. 18, 1989, and Jan. 31, 1990.

Levine, Harold. Interview by Chester Burns. Jan. 7, 1992.

Levin, William C. Interview by Myles Knape, Mar. 17, Apr. 4, and May 26, 1986. Interview by Chester Burns, Nov. 7, 1989.

Lewis, Steve. Interview by Myles Knape. Oct. 2, 1986.

Little, Harry. Interview by Chester Burns. Jan. 27 and Feb. 10, 1992.

Mallett, Joanne. Interview by Megan Seaholm. Oct. 20, 1989.

Matthews, John L. Interview by Myles Knape and Chester Burns. Aug. 25, 1989.

McAshan, Betty. Interview by Myles Knape. Oct. 23, 1985.

McGanity, William J. Interview by Myles Knape and Chester Burns. July 28 and Aug. 5, 1988.

Micks, Don W. Interview by Myles Knape. Sept. 9, 1987.

Middleton, John. Interview by Chester Burns. Dec. 17, 1991.

Mills, Ballinger. Interview by Chester Burns. July 20, 1988.

Poth, Edgar J. Interview by Chester Burns. July 1 and 8, 1986.

Powell, Eugene. Interview by Myles Knape. Oct. 15, 1985.

Rahr, Virginia A. Interview by Poldi Tschirch. June 12, 1986.

Rains, Anna Pearl. Interview by Poldi Tschirch. July 17, 1986.

Reuss, Luis. Interview by Myles Knape and John Swann. May 13, 1988.

Robertson, Courtney. Interview by Chester Burns. Mar. 27, 1993.

Robertson, Mildred. Interview by Myles Knape. May 8 and 29 and June 18, 1986.

Rogers, Mary Jane. Interview by Megan Seaholm. July 21, 1989.

Ross, Marcus Lamar. Interview by Myles Knape. Sept. 3, 1987.

Runge, Elisabeth. Interview by Myles Knape. Oct. 24, 1985.

Sandstead, Harold. Interview by Myles Knape. May 11, 1988.

Saunders, J. Palmer. Interview by Myles Knape and John Swann. Nov. 5 and 14, 1985.

Schneider, Rose G. Interview by Chester Burns. Dec. 12, 1985.

Schreiber, Melvyn H. Interview by Chester Burns and Myles Knape. Aug. 9 and 23, 1989.

Schwartz, Aaron R. Interview by Chester Burns and Myles Knape. May 4 and June 25, 1990.

Seybold, William D. Interview by Chester Burns. Jan. 26, 1990.

Singleton, Edward B. Interview by Greg Diamond. Jan. 18, 1987.

Stephen, W. W. Interview by Greg Diamond. Dec. 19, 1986.

Thompson, Edward I. B. Interview by Myles Knape and John Swann. Mar. 1, 1988.

Thompson, James C. Interview by Myles Knape and Chester Burns. June 27 and July 3 and 13, 1989.

Thompson, Leonora K. Interview by Chester Burns. Dec. 12, 1994.

Thompson, Spencer. Interview by Chester Burns. July 1, 1986.

Thompson, Vernon E. Interview by Myles Knape. Feb. 26, Mar. 14, and Apr. 8, 1986.

Travis, Luther. Interview by Chester Burns, Feb. 25 and Mar. 10, 1992.

Walker, David. Interview by Myles Knape and John Swann. Dec. 22, 1987.

White, Joseph M. Interview by Chester Burns. Dec. 19, 1989.

White, Robert B. Interview by Chester Burns. Dec. 10 and 20, 1991.

Williams, Betty. Interview by Megan Seaholm. July 13, 1989.

Willis, William. Interview by Myles Knape. June 2, 9, and 23, 1986.

Wonio, Diane. Interview by Megan Seaholm. July 27, 1989.

Yielding, K. Lemone. Interview by John Swann. Sept. 18, 1989.

Unpublished Theses and Dissertations

Barnes, Georgia Jereleen. "Mortality in Texas: A Study of the Geographic Distribution of Twenty-Nine Selected Causes of Death, Exclusive of Stillbirths, in Texas Counties, 1930 and 1940." M.A. thesis, University of Texas, 1946.

Brown, Billye J. "The Historical Development of the University of Texas System School of Nursing, 1890–1973." Ed.D. diss., Baylor University, 1975.

Cox, Alice Carol. "The Rainey Affair: A History of the Academic Freedom Controversy at the University of Texas, 1938–1946." Ph.D. diss., University of Denver, 1970.

Giles, Mary Louise. "The Early History of Medicine in Dallas, 1841–1900." M.A. thesis, University of Texas, 1951.

Ozment, Diane Treadaway. "Galveston During the Hoover Era, 1929–1933." M.A. thesis, University of Texas, 1968.

Smith, Dick. "The Development of Local Government Units in Texas." Ph.D. diss., Harvard University, 1938.

Wygant, Larry James. "Women Medical Students at the University of Texas Medical Branch: An Oral History Project," M.A. thesis, University of Houston at Clear Lake City, 1978.

Newspapers

Dallas Weekly Herald
Flake's Bulletin
Galveston County Daily News
Galveston Daily News
Galveston Tribune
Houston Chronicle
Houston Post
San Antonio Daily Express

Books and Pamphlets

Association of American Medical Colleges. *AAMC Directory of American Medical Education 1990–91.* Washington, D.C.: Association of American Medical Colleges, 1990.

American Medical Association Council on Medical Education and Hospitals. *Survey of Medical Schools 1934–1937.* Chicago: American Medical Association, 1937.

American Medical Association Council on Medical Education and Hospitals. *Medical Education in the United States, 1934–1939.* Chicago: American Medical Education, c. 1940.

Anderson, Odin W. *The Uneasy Equilibrium; Private and Public Financing of Health Services in the United States, 1875–1965.* New Haven: College & University Press, 1968.

Arnold Foundation Conference on Public Affairs. *The Government of Texas: A Survey.* Dallas: Southern Methodist University, 1934.

Bain, Ruth M. with Marilyn Miller Baker. *Doors Will Open For You*. Denton: Texas Woman's University Printing Services, 1997.

Barkley, Roy R. and Mark F. Odintz, eds. *The Portable Handbook of Texas*. Austin: Texas State Historical Association, 2000.

Barnstone, Howard. *The Galveston That Was*. New York: Macmillan, 1966.

Barr, Alwyn. *Reconstruction to Reform: Texas Politics, 1876–1906*. Austin: University of Texas Press, 1971.

Beane, Wilhelmena. *Texas Thirties*. San Antonio: Naylor Co., 1963.

Beasley, Ellen. *The Alleys and Back Buildings of Galveston: An Architectural and Social History*. Houston: Rice University Press, 1996.

Beasley, Ellen and Stephen Fox. *Galveston Architecture Guidebook*. Houston: Rice University Press, 1996.

Becker, Howard S., Blanche Geer, Everett C. Hughes, and Anselm L. Strauss. *Boys in White: Student Culture in Medical School*. Chicago: University of Chicago Press, 1961.

Berry, Margaret C. *The University of Texas: A Pictorial Account of Its First Century*. Austin: University of Texas Press, 1980.

Biographical Encyclopedia of Texas. New York: Southern Publishing Co., 1880.

Bixel, Patricia Bellis and Elizabeth Hayes Turner. *Galveston and the 1900 Storm: Catastrophe and Catalyst*. Austin: University of Texas Press, 2000.

Bonner, Thomas Neville. *American Doctors and German Universities*. Lincoln: University of Nebraska Press, 1963.

Bonner, Thomas Neville. *Becoming a Physician: Medical Education in Great Britain, France, Germany, and the United States 1750–1945*. New York: Oxford University Press, 1995.

Bordley, James, III and A. McGehee Harvey. *Two Centuries of American Medicine 1776–1976*. Philadelphia: W. B. Saunders, 1976.

Bowers, John Z. and Elizabeth F. Purcell, eds. *Advances in American Medicine: Essays at the Bicentennial*. 2 vols. New York: Josiah Macy Jr. Foundation, 1976.

Bowers, John Z. and Edith E. King. *Academic Medicine: Present and Future*. North Tarrytown, N.Y.: Rockefeller Archive Center, 1983.

Branda, Stephen, ed. *The Handbook of Texas: A Supplement*. Austin: Texas State Historical Association, 1976.

Brands, H. W. *The Reckless Decade: America in the 1890s*. New York: St. Martin's Press, 1995.

Bruhn, John G., Harold G. Levine, and Paula L. Levine. *Managing Boundaries in the Health Professions*. Springfield, Ill.: Charles C. Thomas, 1993.

Bryson, J. Gordon. *One Hundred Dollars & a Horse: The Reminiscences of a Country Doctor*. New York: William Morrow, 1965.

Burlage, Henry M. and Margot E. Beutler. *Pharmacy's Foundation in Texas: A History of the College of Pharmacy, 1898–1976.* Austin: Pharmaceutical Foundation of the College of Pharmacy of the University of Texas at Austin, 1978.

Burns, Chester R. "A Brief History of the Graduate School of Biomedical Sciences at the University of Texas Medical Branch at Galveston." Galveston: UTMB Biomedical Communication Services, 1994.

"By-Laws and Rules of the John Sealy Hospital. Medical Department of the University of Texas, Galveston, Texas." Galveston: Clarke & Courts, 1891.

Calvert, Robert and Arnoldo De Leon. *The History of Texas.* Arlington Heights, Ill.: Harlan Davidson, Inc., 1990.

Carleton, Don E. *A Breed So Rare: The Life of J. R. Parten, Liberal Texas Oil Man, 1896–1992.* Austin: Texas State Historical Association, 1998.

Clarke, Edward H., Henry J. Bigelow, Samuel D. Gross, T. Gaillard Thomas, and J. S. Billings. *A Century of American Medicine, 1776–1876.* Reprint. Brinklow, Md.: Old Hickory Book Shop, 1962.

Coordinating Board, Texas College and University System. "Challenge for Excellence—A Blueprint for Progress in Higher Education." Austin: Coordinating Board, Texas College and University System, 1971.

Cooter, Roger and John Pickstone, eds. *Medicine in the 20th Century.* Amsterdam: Harwood Academic Publishers, 2000.

Cowley, W. H. *Presidents, Professors, and Trustees.* San Francisco: Jossey-Bass, 1980.

Crowder, Eleanor McElheny. *Nursing in Texas: A Pictorial History.* Waco: Texian Press, 1980.

Cummins, Light Townsend and Alvin R. Bailey Jr., eds. *A Guide to the History of Texas.* New York: Greenwood Press, 1988.

Daniell, L. E. *Personnel of the Texas State Government, with Sketches of Representative Men of Texas.* San Antonio: Maverick Pub. Co., 1892.

Deal, Terrence E. and Allan A. Kennedy, *Corporate Cultures: The Rites and Rituals of Corporate Life.* Reading, Mass.: Addison-Wesley Publishing Company, 1982.

Deitrick, John E. and Robert C. Berson, *Medical Schools in the United States at Mid-Century.* New York: McGraw-Hill, 1953.

Evans, C. E. *The Story of Texas Schools.* Austin: Steck Co., 1955.

Flexner, Abraham. *Medical Education in the United States and Canada.* New York: The Carnegie Foundation for the Advancement of Teaching, 1910.

Fornell, Earl Wesley. *The Galveston Era: The Texas Crescent on the Eve of Secession.* Austin: University of Texas Press, 1961.

Frantz, Joe B. *Gail Borden: Dairyman to a Nation.* Norman: University of Oklahoma Press, 1951.

Friedman, Meyer and Gerald W. Friedland. *Medicine's 10 Greatest Discoveries.* New Haven: Yale University Press, 1998.

Fugate, Francis L. *Frontier College: Texas Western at El Paso: The First Fifty Years*. El Paso: Texas Western Press, 1964.

Gantt, Fred Jr. *The Chief Executive in Texas: A Study in Gubernatorial Leadership*. Austin: University of Texas Press, 1964.

Geiger, Roger L. *To Advance Knowledge: The Growth of American Research Universities, 1900–1940*. New York: Oxford University Press, 1986.

Geiger, Roger L. *Research and Relevant Knowledge American Research Universities Since World War II*. New York: Oxford University Press, 1993.

Gordon, George J. *Public Administration in America*. New York: St. Martin's Press, 1982.

Griffin, S. C. *History of Galveston, Texas, Narrative and Biographical*. Galveston: Privately printed, 1931.

Haigh, Berte R. *Land, Oil, and Education*. El Paso: Texas Western Press, 1986.

"Handbook for Members of Texas State Boards and Commissions." Austin: Texas Advisory Commission on Intergovernmental Relations, 1984.

Harvey, A. McGehee. *Science at the Bedside: Clinical Research in American Medicine 1905–1945*. Baltimore: Johns Hopkins University Press, 1981.

Hayes, Charles W. *Galveston: History of the Island and the City*. 1879. Reprint. Austin: Jenkins Garrett Press, 1974.

Hegarty, Sister Mary Loyola. *Serving with Gladness: The Origin and History of the Congregation of the Sisters of Charity of the Incarnate Word Houston, Texas*. Houston: Bruce Publishing Co., 1967.

Henry, Jay C. *Architecture in Texas, 1895–1945*. Austin: University of Texas Press, 1993.

Horowitz, Helen Lefkowitz. *Campus Life: Undergraduate Cultures from the End of the Eighteenth Century to the Present*. New York: Knopf, 1987.

Howard, James. "Federally Sponsored Research in Texas Higher Education." Austin: Institute of Public Affairs, University of Texas, 1963.

Howell, Joel D. *Technology in the Hospital: Transforming Patient Care in the Early Twentieth Century*. Baltimore: Johns Hopkins University Press, 1996.

Hudson, Robert P. *Disease and its Control: The Shaping of Modern Thought*. New York: Praeger, 1983.

Hyman, Harold M. *Oleander Odyssey: The Kempners of Galveston, Texas. 1854–1880s*. College Station: Texas A&M University Press, 1990.

Institute of Public Affairs. "The Fifty-fifth Texas Legislature: A Review of its Work." Austin: University of Texas: 1957.

Institute of Public Affairs. "The Fifty-sixth Texas Legislature: A Review of its Work." Austin: University of Texas, 1959.

Institute of Public Affairs. "The Fifty-seventh Texas Legislature: A Review of its Work." Austin: University of Texas: 1962.

Institute of Public Affairs. "The Fifty-eighth Texas Legislature: A Review of its Work." Austin: University of Texas, 1963.

Kalisch, Philip A. and Beatrice J. Kalisch. *The Advance of American Nursing.* Boston: Little, Brown and Company, 1986.

Kaufman, Martin, Stuart Galishoff, and Todd L. Savitt, eds. *Dictionary of American Medical Biography.* Westport, Conn.: Greenwood Press, 1984.

Kelsey, Mavis P. Sr. *Twentieth-Century Doctor: House Calls to Space Medicine.* College Station: Texas A&M University Press, 1999.

Kessler, Jimmy. *Henry Cohen: The Life of a Frontier Rabbi.* Austin, Eakin Press, 1997.

Kiple, Kenneth F., ed. *The Cambridge World History of Human Disease.* New York: Cambridge University Press, 1993.

Klosterman, Leo J., Loyd S. Swenson Jr., and Sylvia Rose, eds. *100 Years of Science and Technology in Texas.* Houston: Rice University Press, 1986

Lape, Esther Everett. *Medical Research: A Midcentury Survey.* 2 vols. Boston: Little, Brown and Company, 1955.

Lane, J. J. *History of the University of Texas.* Austin: Hutchings, 1891.

Lane, J. J. *History of Education in Texas.* Washington, D.C.: Government Printing Office, 1903.

Leavitt, Judith Walzer. *Brought to Bed: Child-Bearing in America, 1750–1950.* New York: Oxford University Press, 1986.

Lerner, Monroe and Odin W. Anderson. *Health Progress in the United States 1900–1960.* Chicago: University of Chicago Press, 1963.

Ludmerer, Kenneth M. *Learning to Heal: The Development of American Medical Education.* New York: Basic Books, 1985.

Ludmerer, Kenneth M. *Time to Heal: American Medical Education from the Turn of the Century to the Era of Managed Care.* Oxford: Oxford University Press, 1999.

Macdonald, Linda. *A Pattern of Love.* Houston: Sisters of Charity of the Incarnate Word Health Care System, 1996.

Marinbach, Bernard. *Galveston: Ellis Island of the West.* Albany: State University of New York Press, 1983.

McCleskey, Clifton, Allan K. Butcher, Daniel E. Farlow, and J. Pat Stephens. *The Government and Politics of Texas.* 7th edition. Boston: Little, Brown and Company, 1982.

McComb, David G. *Galveston: A History.* Austin: University of Texas Press, 1986.

McComb, David G. *Texas: A Modern History.* Austin: University of Texas Press, 1989.

McComb, David G. *Galveston: A History and a Guide.* Austin: Texas State Historical Association, 2000.

McCullough, William Wallace, Jr. *Doctor William Dennis Kelley, 1825–1888: Texas Physician and Surgeon.* Galveston: Privately printed, 1961.

McGovern, John P. and Chester R. Burns. *Humanism in Medicine.* Springfield, Ill.: Charles C. Thomas, 1973.

Nichols, Robert B. *A Bridge to a Better World*. Galveston: The Sealy & Smith Foundation for the John Sealy Hospital, 1989.

Nimmo, Dan and William Oden. *The Texas Political System*. Englewood Cliffs, N.J.: Prentice-Hall, 1972.

Nixon, Pat Ireland. *A History of the Texas Medical Association, 1853–1953*. Austin: University of Texas Press, 1953.

Numbers, Ronald L., ed. *The Education of American Physicians*. Berkeley: University of California Press, 1980.

Patterson, Caleb Perry and James B. Hubbard. *A Civil Government of Texas*. Indianapolis: Bobbs-Merrill, 1927.

Patterson, James T. *The Dread Disease: Cancer and Modern American Culture*. Cambridge, Mass.: Harvard University Press, 1987.

"Public Higher Education in Texas." Austin: Texas Legislative Council, 1950.

Rainey, Homer P. *The Tower and the Dome: A Free University versus Political Control*. Boulder, Colo.: Pruett, 1971.

Ransom, Harry Hunt. *The Conscience of the University and Other Essays*. Austin: University of Texas Press, 1982.

Rauch, John H. *Illinois State Board of Health. Report on Medical Education, Medical Colleges and the Regulation of the Practice of Medicine in the United States and Canada, 1765–1890*. Springfield, Ill.: Roker Pub. Co., 1890.

Reiser, Stanley Joel. *Medicine and the Reign of Technology*. Cambridge: Cambridge University Press, 1978.

Reverby, Susan M. *Ordered to Care: The Dilemma of American Nursing, 1850–1945*. Cambridge: Cambridge University Press, 1987.

Rice, Bradley Robert. *Progressive Cities: The Commission Government Movement in America, 1901–1920*. Austin: University of Texas Press, 1977.

Richardson, Rupert Norval, Ernest Wallace, and Adrian N. Anderson. *Texas: The Lone Star State*. 4th edition. Englewood Cliffs, N.J.: Prentice-Hall, 1981.

Robinson, Willard B. and Todd Webb. *Texas Public Buildings of the Nineteenth Century*. Austin: University of Texas Press, 1974.

Rogers, David E. *American Medicine Challenge for the 1980s*. Cambridge, Mass.: Ballinger Publishing Company, 1978.

Rodriquez, Louis J. *Dynamics of Growth An Economic Profile of Texas*. Austin: Madrona Press, 1978.

Rosenberg, Charles E. *The Care of Strangers: The Rise of America's Hospital System*. New York: Basic Books, 1987.

Rothstein, William G. *American Medical Schools and the Practice of Medicine: A History*. New York: Oxford University Press, 1987.

Scardino, Barrie and Drexel Turner. *Clayton's Galveston: The Architecture of Nicholas J. Clayton and His Contemporaries*. College Station: Texas A&M University Press, 2000.

Schulze, Gene. *Yesterday's Seasons.* New York: Hawthorn Books, 1978.

Sealy & Smith Foundation. "Historical Review of the Medical Branch of the University of Texas and of the Sealy & Smith Foundation for the John Sealy Hospital at Galveston, Texas. Galveston: n.d. (c. 1943).

Shryock, Richard Harrison. *American Medical Research: Past and Present.* New York: Commonwealth Fund, 1947.

Shryock, Richard Harrison. *Medical Licensing in America, 1650–1965.* Baltimore: Johns Hopkins University Press, 1967.

Sibley, Marilyn. *George Brackenridge: Maverick Philanthropist.* Austin: University of Texas Press, 1973.

Silverthorne, Elizabeth. *Ashbel Smith of Texas: Pioneer, Patriot, Statesman, 1805–1886.* College Station: Texas A&M University Press, 1982.

Silverthorne, Elizabeth and Geneva Fulgham. *Women Pioneers in Texas Medicine.* College Station: Texas A&M University Press, 1997.

Smith, Henry Nash. *The Controversy at the University of Texas, 1939–1945: A Documentary History.* Austin: Students' Association of the University of Texas, 1945.

Sonnedecker, Glenn. *Kremers and Urdang's History of Pharmacy.* Philadelphia: J. B. Lippincott, 1976.

Speck, Lawrence W. and Richard Payne. *Landmarks of Texas Architecture.* Austin: University of Texas Press, 1986.

Splawn, W. M. W. *The University of Texas: Its Origin and Growth to 1928.* Austin: University of Texas: 1956.

Spratt, John S. *The Road to Spindletop: Economic Change in Texas, 1875–1901.* Dallas: Southern Methodist University Press, 1955.

Starr, Paul. *The Social Transformation of American Medicine.* New York: Basic Books, 1982.

Stevens, Rosemary. *American Medicine and the Public Interest: A History of Specialization.* Berkeley: University of California Press, 1998.

Stewart, Frank. "Officers, Boards, and Commissions of Texas," *University of Texas Bulletin,* no. 1854, Sept. 25, 1918.

Stewart, Frank M. and Joseph L. Clark. *The Constitution and Government of Texas.* Boston: D. C. Heath, 1949.

Texas Commission on Higher Education. "Public Higher Education in Texas, 1961–1971." Austin: Texas Commission on Higher Education, 1963.

Texas. Governor's Budget and Planning Office. *Texas State Government Sourcebook.* Austin: Budget and Planning Office, 1978.

Texas Research League. "To Make Texas State Government Modern, Viable, Responsive." Austin: Texas Research League, 1975.

Texas Research League. "Texas State & Local Government: A Financial Handbook." Austin: Texas Research League, 1975.

Tindall, George Brown and David E. Shi. *America: A Narrative History*. 3rd edition. New York: W. W. Norton, 1992.

Triplett, Henry F. and Ferdinand A. Hauslein. *Civics: Texas and Federal*. Houston: Rein & Sons, 1918.

Turner, Elizabeth Hayes. *Women, Culture, and Community: Religion and Reform in Galveston, 1880-1920*. New York: Oxford University Press, 1997.

Turner, Paul Venable. *Campus: An American Planning Tradition*. Cambridge, Mass.: The MIT Press, 1984.

Tyler, Ron, Douglas E. Barnett, Roy R. Barkley, Penelope C. Anderson, and Mark F. Odintz, eds. *The New Handbook of Texas*. 6 vols. Austin: Texas State Historical Association, 1996.

The University of Texas Medical Branch at Galveston: A Seventy Five Year History by the Faculty and Staff. Austin: University of Texas Press, 1967.

Vernon's Annotated Constitution of the State of Texas. St. Paul, Minn.: West Publishing Co., 1993.

Vernon's Texas Codes Annotated (Education). St. Paul, Minn.: West Publishing Co., 1991.

Webb, Walter Prescott, ed. *The Handbook of Texas*. 2 vols. Austin: Texas State Historical Association, 1952.

Wheeler, Kenneth W. *To Wear a City's Crown: The Beginnings of Urban Growth in Texas, 1836–1865*. Cambridge, Mass.: Harvard University Press, 1968.

Whisenhunt, Donald W. *The Encyclopedia of Texas Colleges and Universities: An Historical Profile*. Austin: Eakin Press, 1986.

Wilkinson, C. H. "A Short History of St. Mary's Infirmary," in *Souvenir of the Golden Jubilee of the Sisters of Charity of the Incarnate Word*. Galveston, 1916.

Wilson, Marjorie Price and Curtis P. McLaughlin. *Leadership and Management in Academic Medicine*. San Francisco: Jossey-Bass Publishers, 1984.

Wygant, Larry, comp. *The Truman G. Blocker Jr. History of Medicine Collections: Books and Manuscripts*. Galveston: University of Texas Medical Branch at Galveston, 1985.

Young, Sr., J. W. *It All Comes Back*. Sweetwater, Tex.: Watson-Focht Company, 1962.

ARTICLES AND CHAPTERS

Abercrombie, Maggie. "Sketch of Galveston County." *American Sketch Book*, 6, no. 5 (1881), 325–345.

Arsenault, Raymond. "The End of the Long Hot Summer: The Air Conditioner and Southern Culture." *Journal of Southern History*, 4, no. 4 (1984), 597–628.

Beardsley, E. H. "Good-Bye to Jim Crow: The Desegregation of Southern Hospitals, 1945–70." *Bulletin of the History of Medicine*, 60 (Fall, 1986), 367–386.

Blakeney, Patricia, Mary Frances Schottstaedt, and Shelley Sekula. "Personality Characteristics of Women Entering Medical School Over a 10-Year Period." *Journal of Medical Education*, 57 (Jan., 1982), 42–47.

Bowman, Inci. "James Wharton McLaughlin (1840–1909)." *The Bookman*, 7, no. 5 (1980), 3–8; no. 6 (1980), 3–8.

Bowman, Inci. "John Sealy Hospital Training School for Nurses." *The Bookman*, 9, no. 8 (1982), 3–5.

Bowman, Inci. "Beginnings of Medical Journalism in Texas." *Texas Medicine*, 82, no. 2 (1986), 51–55.

Brandt, Jr., Edward N., Frances Holmstrom, and Elizabeth L. Fitzsimmons. "A Study of UTMB Graduates: 1967–1976." *Texas Medicine*, 75 (June, 1979), 54–58.

Brandt, Jr. Edward N. "Medical Education: The Past 80 Years." *Texas Medicine*, 76 (May, 1980), 4–5.

Brown, D. Clayton. "Medical Education in Texas: the Growth of Schools." *Texas Medicine*, 82 (May, 1986), 49–53.

Bruhn, John G., Raymond G. Fuentes Jr., Fernando M. Trevino, and Lafayette B. Williams Jr. "Follow-Up of Minority Premedical Students Attending Summer Enrichment Programs in a Medical Setting." *Texas Medicine*, 72 (Aug., 1976), 87–90.

Bruhn, John G. "A Response to History: A Review of One Medical School's Efforts to Graduate Minority Physicians." *Journal of the National Medical Association*, 70, no. 11 (1978), 823–828.

Brunet, Lesley Williams. "Alan Gregg and the Early Years of the Texas Medical Center." *Houston Review*, 12, no. 2 (1990), 97–112.

Burns, Chester R. "The Historical Significance and Future Value of the Ashbel Smith Building—'Old Red.'" *The Bookman*, 6 (Mar., 1979), 2–3.

Burns, Chester. R. "Medicine in Texas: The Historical Literature." *Texas Medicine*, 82, no. 1 (1986), 60–63.

Burns, Chester R. "The Health Sciences." In Leo J. Klosterman, Loyd S. Swenson Jr., and Sylvia Rose, eds. *100 Years of Science and Technology in Texas*. Houston: Rice University Press, 1986, 286–296.

Burns, Chester R. "The University of Texas Medical Branch at Galveston: Origins and Beginnings." *Journal of the American Medical Association*, 266, no. 10 (Sept. 11, 1991), 1400–1403.

Burns, Chester R. "The Development of Hospitals in Galveston During the Nineteenth Century." *Southwestern Historical Quarterly*, 97 (Oct., 1993), 238–263.

Burns, Chester R. "Health and Medicine." In Ron Tyler, Douglas E. Barnett, Roy R. Barkley, Penelope C. Anderson, and Mark F. Odintz, eds. *The New Handbook of Texas*. 6 vols. Austin: Texas State Historical Association, 1996, III, 524–532.

Burns, Chester R. and Heather G. Campbell. "Sanitizing Galveston: Politics, Policies, and Practices Before 1915." *Houston Review*, 19, no. 1 (1997), 5–26.

Burns, Chester R.. "Traditions and Transformations: How Texas Medicine Changed in the 20th Century." *Texas Medicine*, 96 (Jan., 2000), 45–47.

Burns, Chester R. "Teaching the Humanities in American Medical Schools during the Twentieth Century: A Commentary on the Two Dominant Models" In David C.

Thomasma and Judith Lee Kissell, eds. *The Health Care Professional as Friend and Healer: Building on the Work of Edmund D. Pellegrino*. Washington, D.C.: Georgetown University Press, 2000, 259–266.

Burns, C. R. and H. G. Campbell. "The Extraordinary Influences of Two British Physicians on Medical Education and Practice in Texas at the Turn of the 20th Century." *Vesalius*, 5 (Dec., 1997), 79–84.

Campbell, Heather G. "A Note on the First Nursing School in Texas and its Role in the Nineteenth Century Experience." *Houston Review*, 19, no. 1 (1997), 49–58.

Carson, Ronald D. "Institute for the Medical Humanities: Plans and Prospects." *Texas Medicine*, 79 (May, 1983), 61–62.

Cassedy, James H. "Stimulation of Health Research." *Science*, 145 (Aug. 25, 1964), 897–902.

Dudgeon, H. R. "Random Undergraduate Recollections." *Alcalde*, 3, no. 8 (1915), 856–863.

Dyer, Isadore. "A Note on the Medical Relief Work Done in Galveston after the Storm." *New Orleans Medical & Surgical Journal*, 53, no. 5 (1900), 261–265.

Endicott, Kenneth M. and Ernest M. Allen. "The Growth of Medical Research 1941–1953 and the Role of Public Health Service Research Grants." *Science*, 118 (Sept. 25, 1953), 337–343.

Gammon, William. "A Brief Sketch of the John Sealy Hospital and the Medical Department of the University of Texas." *University Medical*, 1, no. 3 (1895), 77–89.

Grant, J. Andrew. "Leaders of the University of Texas Medical Branch at Galveston." *Texas Medicine*, 87 (Dec., 1991), 44–49.

"The Great Storm at Galveston—From a Medical Standpoint." *Texas Medical Journal*, 16, no. 4 (1900), 164–169.

"The Great Storm at Galveston." *Texas Medical News*, 9, no. 12 (1900), 699–716.

Griffin, Roger A. "To Establish a University of the First Class." *Southwestern Historical Quarterly*, 86 (Oct., 1982), 135–160.

Jenkins, Vernon K. and David C. Eiland Jr. "Medical School Admissions at the University of Texas Medical Branch at Galveston." *Texas Medicine*, 78 (July, 1982), 42–46.

Jones, Ralph W. "The First Roots of the University of Texas Medical Branch at Galveston." *Southwestern Historical Quarterly*, 65 (Apr., 1962), 465–474.

Levine, Harold G., Lafayette B. Williams Jr., and John G. Bruhn. "Six Years of Experience with a Summer Program for Minority Students." *Journal of Medical Education*, 51 (Sept., 1976), 735–742.

"Looking Back on the Millenium of Medicine." *New England Journal of Medicine*, 342 (Jan. 6, 2000), 42–49.

Miller, Edmund Thornton. "A Financial History of Texas." *University of Texas Bulletin*, no. 37 (1916), 1–449.

Overbeck, Ruth Ann. "Alexander Penn Wooldridge." *Southwestern Historical Quarterly,* 67 (Jan., 1964), 317–349.

Ozment, Diane Treadaway. "The Port City of Galveston." In Willena C. Adams, ed. *Texas Cities and the Great Depression.* Austin: Texas Memorial Museum, 1973, 135–151.

Paine, J. F. Y. "Status of Medical Education in the United States, Being the Annual Report of the Dean to the Board of Regents at the Commencement Exercises of the First Session of the Medical Department of the University of Texas." *Transactions, Texas State Medical Association* (1892), 235–244.

Pittman, James A. Jr. and Donald M. Miller. "The Southern Society for Clinical Investigation at 50: The End of the Beginning." *American Jounral of the Medical Sciences,* 311 (June, 1996), 248–253.

Randall, Edward and Lucius Wilson. "Planning for Out-Patients in a Southern Teaching Hospital." *Modern Hospital,* 36 (Mar., 1931), 1–8.

Ransom, Harry H. "Educational Resources in Texas." *Texas Quarterly,* 4 (Winter, 1961), 5–12.

Rogers, Dorothy. "Rebecca Sealy Nurses's Residence." *American Journal of Nursing,* 33 (May, 1933), 433–437.

Schmalstieg, William F. "The Right to a Good Life: Moody State School for Cerebral Palsied Children." *Texas Historian,* 52 (Mar., 1992), 16–18.

Schroeder, Steven A., Jane S. Zones, and Jonathan A. Showstack. "Academic Medicine as a Public Trust." *Journal of the American Medical Association,* 262 (Aug. 11, 1989), 803–812.

Smith, Allen J. "The Medical Department and the Galveston Storm." *University Record,* 3, no. 1 (1901), 53–67.

Smith, Allen J. "Some Memories of the Medical Department in its Beginning." *Alcalde,* 3, no. 8 (1915), 741–750.

West, H. A. "Further Observations on the Medical Aspects of the Galveston Storm." *Transactions, Texas State Medical Association* (1901), 128–136.

West, H. A. "Medical and Sociological Aspects of the Galveston Storm." *Transactions, Texas State Medical Association* (1901), 118–127.

White, Elizabeth Borst. "Patterns of Development in Texas Hospitals, 1836–1935: Preliminary Survey." *Texas Medicine,* 82 (Dec., 1986), 55–60.

Wilson, R. L. "Recollections of School Days '95–'99, Medical Department, University of Texas." *Alcalde,* 3, no. 8 (1915), 853–855.

Wooldridge, A. P. "A History of the Location of the University of Texas at Austin, Texas." *Alcalde,* 2, no. 1 (1913), 26–41.

Wygant, Larry. "The John Sealy Hospital: A Study of Late 19th Century Hospital Design." *Texas Architect,* 30 (Sept./Oct., 1980), 52–55.

Wygant, Larry. "A Note on the Early Medical Education of Women at UTMB." *The Bookman,* 7, no. 3 (1980), 3–5.

Index

Photographs, maps, and tables are indicated by bold face page numbers

A

AAMC. *See* Association of American Medical Colleges (AAMC)

Abell, Creed: 230, 559n209

Abreu, Benedict: 368

Abston, Sally: 285, 333, 345, 572n99

Academic Council: 68

Academic Planning Committee: 284

academic reinforcement program: 543n60

Academy of Continuing Medical Education: 205

accreditation: 207, 209, 346–52, 384–85

Acosta, Michelle: 100

acute diseases: 138–44. *See also* therapies and therapeutics; specific diseases

Adams, Perrie: 262

Administration Annex I: 134, 514n17

Administration Annex II: 120, 126, 134

Administration Building: 98, 115, 120, 134

Administrative Advisory Committee: 63–64, **64**

Administrative Council: 61, 62, 64, 68, 71

Admissions Committee: 296

Adrian, Earl Jr.: 229

Adriance, Carroll: 320

Advisory Board of Lady Managers: 206, 547n98

Advisory Council: 322

aerospace medicine: 382

Aetna Life Insurance Company: 283

Affirmative Action Advisory Committee: 70, 278–79

Affirmative Action Office: 70

affirmative action plan: 352

Aging and the Human Spirit: 271

AIDS: 164

AIDS Clinical Trial Group: 380

AIDS Education Organization: 303

AIDS Research Center: 380

Ainsworth, William: 320, 560n224

Albrecht, Thomas: 164

Alcalde: 353

Alchier, Alma: 219

Alderdice, Robert: 575n125

Allen, Charles: 312, 373

Allen, G. W. Jr.: 318

Allen, N. N.: 10

Allensworth, Dan: 201

Allied Health Services Department: 223, 225, 556n178

allied health staff. *See* hospital staff

Allison, Pat: 532–33n103

Alperin, Lynn: 314

Alpert, Arthur M.: **91**

Alpha Epsilon Iota: 299

Alpha Eta: 303

Alpha Kappa Kappa: 298, 299, 300, 366

Alpha Mu Pi Omega: 36, 298

Alpha Omega Alpha: 302

alumni: 317–32. *See also* Graduate School of the Biomedical Sciences; School of Allied Health Alumni Association; School of Medicine Alumni Association; School of Nursing Alumnae Association; specific schools

Alumni Bulletin: 353

Alumni Committee on Minority Affairs: 70, 326

Alumni Field House: 119, 125, 298, 302, 379

Alumni News: 315, 353

Ambulatory Care Center: 122, 123, 134, 160

Ambulatory Pediatric Association: 343

American Academy of Cerebral Palsy: 342

American Academy of Dermatology: 343, 599n87

American Academy of General Practice: 597n59

American Academy of Neurological Surgery: 342

American Academy of Orthopedic Surgery: 253, 342, 366

American Academy of Otolaryngology—Head and Neck Surgery: 343

American Academy of Pediatrics: 248, 342

American Academy of Physicians' Assistants: 303, 304

American Academy of Tropical Medicine: 250, 340

American Association for the Advancement of Science: 339

American Association for the History of Medicine: 341

American Association for the History of Nursing: 374

American Association for the Surgery of Trauma: 342

American Association of Anatomists: 250, 340, 342

American Association of Blood Banks: 349

American Association of Colleges of Pharmacy (AAPC): 205–6

American Association of Inhalation Therapy: 342

American Association of Medical Record Librarians: 342

American Association of Obstetrics, Gynecology, and Abdominal Surgery: 341

American Association of Pediatric Department Chairmen :342

American Board of Anesthesiology: 602n132

American Board of Dermatology: 342

American Board of Family Practice: 204, 345, 602n132

American Board of Internal Medicine: 343, 376, 602n132

American Board of Neurology: 602n132

American Board of Orthopedic Surgery: 342

American Board of Otolaryngology: 376, 384, 602n132

American Board of Pathology: 595n30

American Board of Pediatrics: 343, 602n132

American Board of Plastic Surgeons: 341

American Board of Plastic Surgery: 341, 342

American Board of Radiology: 342

American Board of Surgery: 341, 602n132

American Cancer Society: 85, 337

American College of Chest Physicians: 342

American College of Nuclear Physicians: 384

American College of Nutrition: 345

American College of Physicians: 341, 376

American College of Surgeons: 341, 348, 358, 376, 384

American Conference of Pharmaceutical Faculties: 205–6

American Diabetes Association: 343

American Federation for Clinical Research: 340

American Heart Association: 342

American Hospital Association: 154

American Laryngological Association: 384

American Medical Association: Council on Medical Education and Hospitals: 44, 47, 53, 182, 204, 346–47, 376; peer reviews 55, 184, 188, 258, 347–48, 351–52; research grants 76; faculty participation 339, 343, 384, 599n87, 602n132

American Medical College Association: 12

American Medical EEG Society: 342

American Medical Record Association: 343

American Medical Student Association: 303

American Medical Women's Association: 299, 302–3

American Medical Writers Association: 343

American National Insurance Company: 364

American Orthopedic Association: 342

American Ortho-Psychiatric Association: 341

American Physical Therapy Association: 341

American Physiological Society: 250

American Psychiatric Association: 340, 342

American Red Cross: 153, 154

American School Health Association: 343

American Society for Clinical Investigation: 244

American Society for Microbiology: 341

American Society for Pharmacology: 250

American Society for Psychosomatic Obstetrics and Gynecology: 343

American Society for Rickettsiology and Rickettsial Diseases: 376

American Society of Allied Health Professions: 343

American Society of Anesthesiologists: 343

American Society of Anesthetists: 340

American Society of Clinical Pathologists: 343, 555n167, 595n30

American Society of Hospital Pharmacists: 349

American Society of Human Genetics: 343

American Society of Microbiology: 341

American Society of Ophthalmologic and

Otolaryngologic Allergy: 342

American Society of Plastic Surgeons: 340

American Society of Plastic Surgery: 342

American Society of Tropical Medicine: 250, 340, 595n30

American Society of X-Ray Technicians: 340

American Society on Aging: 345

American Speech-Language-Hearing Association: 343

American Surgical Association: 341, 342, 343, 384

American Surgical Society: 341–42

American Trauma Society: 337

American Urological Association: 338, 341, 342

American Women's Voluntary Services: 154, 508n41

Amon G. Carter Foundation: 272

Anatomy Department: 47, **197**, 243, 256, 258, 372

Anderson, Elizabeth: 384

Anesthesiology Department: 90, 152, 155–56, 162, **163**, 186, 373

Anigstein, Ludwik: 246, **247**, 248–49, 251, 344

Animal Care and Use Committee: 577n149

Animal Care Center: 112, 115, 117, 121, 263

"Annual Rat Dances": 588n77

antibiotics: 147

Apolinar, Ruth: 223

Appel, Doris: 134

Appointments, Promotions, and Tenure Committee: 284

Area Health Education Center: 194, 204, 223, 314, 382

Arens, James: 72, 167, 178, 343, 602n132

Arledge, Shirley: 198

Armstrong, John: 325

Armstrong, T. D.: 158, 367

Arnn, Rosa Lee: 140

Arnold, Hiram: 335

Artz, Curtis: 262, 338

Ash, Hans: **241**, 312, 372

Ashbel Smith Building. *See* Old Red

Ashbel Smith Distinguished Alumni: 322, **323–25**

Ashbel Smith Professors: 285, **285**

Asian American Student Association: 291

Associated Health Occupations Department: 222, 225

Association of Academic Departments of Otolaryngology: 599n91

Association of American Medical Colleges (AAMC): standards 12, 39, 184, 185, 188, 346; peer reviews 53, 55, 247, 258, 347; faculty participation 341, 343, 358–59, 376

Association of American Physicians: 244

Association of American Universities: 56

Association of Collegiate Schools of Nursing: 210, 348

Association of Neurosciences Departments and Programs: 384

Association of Physician Assistant Programs: 384

Association of Southern Medical Colleges: 39, 346

Association of Women Surgeons: 343, 384

Asthma Support Group: 277

Athletic Council: 302

Atkinson, Harry: 241–42, 245

Audiovisual Services: 117, 119

Austin, Arthur: 205, 282

Austin, Kathy: 72

Available University Fund: regent allocation 16, 25, 43, 77; projects 63, 84, 107, 110, 115, 116, 121, 126, 128; hospitals 75, 82, 83, 112; operating expenses 81; Nurses' Home 106; Keiller Building 109, 362

Ave Maria Hall: 120, 125, 126

Aves, F. W.: 243

Axelsen, Sunny: 311

Aynesworth, K. H.: **40**, 47–48, 49, 52, 318, 492n27, 493n38

B

Babe Didrickson Zaharias Fund: 518n52

Backe, Gale: 72

Bacterial Metabolism Lab: 253

Bacteriology Department: 113, 185, 228, 240, 241, 242, 253

Bader, Madero: **247**

Baha'i Club: 303

Bahr, Judy: 381

Bailey, Byron: professional networks 333, 342, 343, 384, 602n132; centennial celebration 375, 376; research 574n118

Bain, Ruth: 326

Baird, Elwood: 152, 336, 342, 530n62, 555n167

Baird, Jim: 333

Baker, James: 600–601n116

Baker, John: 262
Baker, Susan: 561n235
Baker, Tom: 201–2
Baldwin, Louise: 328
Ballard, Billy: 197, 306
Ball High School: 484n95
Ballinger, Thomas: 233, 478n51
Bane, Catherine: 334, 550n121
Baptist General Convention of Texas: 154
Baptist Student Union: 301
Baranowski, Tom: 269
Barber, Jessica: **161**
Barker, Lewellys: 109
Barlow, Donna: 216
Barnes, J. Peyton: 199
Barnett, Donald: 229, 261
Barnett, Herman: 187, 290–91, 308, 540n34, 585n50
Barnett, Jim: 558n207
Baron, Sam: **238**, 267–68
Barr, H. Buford: 322
Barranco, Sam: 230
Barratt, Bobbye: 313, 369
Barratt, Ernest: 230, 259, 262, 345, 575n124
Barrett, James: 88
Bartholf, Marjorie: political networks 55, 61, 210–11, 334, 348, 495n56; teaching 209; research 259; professional networks 353
Barton, Clara: 3
Bartosh, Julia Ann: 548n108
Basic Science Building: 115, 117, 122, 131
Basic Science Core Committee: 190
basic science departments: 185, 189. *See also* specific departments
Bass, Joe: 263
Bassett, Denton: 154, 536(nn150,152)
Baum, Alan: 384
Bauman, Raquel: 585–86n52
Baxter Construction Company: 117
Beall, Frank: 336
Bean, William: 68, 234, 235
Beathard, Gerald: 229
Beauchamp, Robert: **356**
Beaudry, Betty: 259, 308
Beck, Carol: 266
Beckman, Edward: 261

Becton, E. P.: 37
Bee, David: 558n207
Beecherl, Louis Jr.: 374
Behavioral Sciences Committee: 190
Beissner, J. E.: 309
Belcher, Edgar Jr.: 98
Bell, Ryan: 162, 533n105
Belli, James: 166, 270–71, 343, 384
Benecke, Henry: 87
Benignus, Vernon: 263
Bennett, James: 339
Bennett, Robert: 232, 306
Bernhard, Adolph: 480n61
Bernier, George Jr.: 376
Bertner, Ernst: 320
Bessey, Otto: 254
Beta Phi Sigma: 298
Betatron: **151**, 152
Bethel, George **46**; political networks 46, 78, 79; death of 47, 305; teaching 184, 185, 241; professional networks 341
Bethel Hall: 114
Bettis, Moody: 325
Beutler, Margot: 372
Beverly, Alfred: 79
Bickett, John Jr.: 57
Bieri, John: 344
Billiot, Linda: 100
Bing, Robert: 68, 221, 223
Biochemistry Department: 113, 117, 189, 228, 240, 242, 253, 258
Biological Chemistry Department: 185
biomedical communications office: 122
Biomedical Engineering Shop: 263
Biomedical Inquiry: 315
"Birth" (sculpture): 125, 133
Bixler, Elizabeth: 328
Black, Cyril: 586n57
Black, Gordon: 325
Blackert, E. J.: **40**
black health care: 26, 105, 140, 157–58, 481n72. *See also* Negro Hospital
Blackman, Mrs. Julius: 530n62
Blackshear, Joe: 74
Blackwell, Steven: 165
Blailock, H. F.: 318

Blakeney, Patricia: 167, 197, 306

Blalock, J. Edwin: 268

Blankenship, James: 230, 231, 233, 261, 384, 558n207

Blanton, Jack: 373

Blasingame, F. J. L.: 60, 326

Blocker, Truman Jr.: **64, 316, 321, 340**; political networks 60, 61, 63–67, 84, 211–13, 233–34, 302, 497n79, 499n95, 500–501n105, 501n110; economic resources 86, 90, 91, 94; campus development 116–21, 124; patient care 147–48, 158, 540n27; professional networks 246, 337, 341, 342, 344, 345; research 253–54, 257–63; family 289; reminiscences 369; teaching 545n73

Blocker, Virginia: 571n87

Blocker Burn Unit: 535n136

Blocker-Lewis Society: 201

Blood Bank: 116, 153, 171–72

blood bank technology program: 220–21, **221**

Blount, Raymond: 186, 540n28, 570n76

Blumberg, Jane Weinert: 124

Blume, Dorothy: 216

Board of Regents. *See* University of Texas Board of Regents

Bobbitt, Daniel: 61, 62, 64, 158, 211–12

Bodansky, Meyer: research 76, 242–43, 244, 246, 525n19, 582n18; teaching 205, 219, 226, 245; professional networks 336, 339; reminiscences 363; biography 385

Bodansky, Oscar: **241**

Boeker, Bertha: 548n108

Boelsche, Nell: 156, **200**

Boesser, Mark: 301

Bohman, William: **147**

Bondurant, William: 244, 335

bone bank: 534n122

Bonnet, Edith: 183, **289**, 544n68

Bookman: 314

Bookstore: 295, 296

Borden, Gail: 113

Borden Milk Company: 307, 570n74

Boring, Jesse: 10

Borucki, Michael: 164

Bosshart, Don: 543n59

Botany Department: 205

Bowe, Rose: 548n108

Bowen, Ray: 57

Bowie, Michael: 197, 585–86n52

Bowling League: 310

Bowman, Barbara: political networks 120, 230, 279, 559n209; teaching 190, 543n60; research 260–62; professional networks 343

Bowman, T. H.: 15

Box, Edith: 253

"Boys Choir": 310

Brackenridge, George: 27, 43, 76, 110

Brackenridge Hall: 114, 125, 211

Braestrup, Craig: 561n235

Bramel, Sue: 198

Brandt, Edward Jr.: **336**; dean of graduate school 66, 230, 558n203; dean of medicine 68, 119, 120, 264, 285, 351; professional networks 339; vice chancellor 370; teaching 585–86n52

Braswell, R. O.: 182

Brautigan, Albert: 87, 128

Bray, Juanita Phipps: 229

Breckenridge, Joe: 253

Brenkus, Peggy: **70**, 197

Brenner, Manon: 201

Brents, W. R.: 44

Brick, Rosalie: 312

Briggs, J. R.: 38

Brindley, Anne: 367, 599n87

Brindley, G. V.: **316**

Brindley, George Jr.: **316**, 325, 338

Brindley, Hanes: **316**

Brindley, Paul: 184, 242–43, 336, 344, 367, 591n146, 599n84

Brink, Peter: 124

Brinkerhoff, Ann: 373, 376

Brinkerhoff, James: 376

Brinkley, Bill: 543n60

Briscoe, Dolph: 67

Brogan, A. P.: 227

Brooks, Martharein: 536n143

Brown, Arthur: 120, 577n153

Brown, B. S.: 318

Brown, Billye: 334, 372

Brown, M. B.: 12

Brown, Nancy: 369

Brown, Raymond: 570n82

Bruce, Ivan Jr.: 203, 335

Bruhn, John: 71, 133, 197, 223, 268–69, 350, 351, 596n45

Bryan, Beauregard: 3

Bryan, George: political networks 68, 69–70, 71, 97, 121, 307, 606n60; research 258, 262, 263–64; professional networks 339; peer reviews 346, 351; teaching 585–86n52

Bryant, Cleo: 215

Bryson, J. Gordon: 320, 586n57

Buckner, John: 205

Bucy, Ralph: 536n152

budget. *See* economic resources

buildings. *See* campus development

Bulletin of the Alumnae Association of the John Sealy College of Nursing: 328

Bulletin of the John Sealy Hospital and the School of Medicine: 246, 313

Bullington, Orville: 57

Bunce, Harvey: 197

Bureau of Health Manpower: 119

Burke, John: 26

Burks, Henry: 156

Burks, Larry: 127

Burlage, Henry: 372

Burns, B. I.: 158, 366

Burns, Chester: teaching 234, 236, 561n233; professional networks 342, 345, 596n45; research 385, 606n48, 608n96

burn treatment: 147–48, 534n122. *See also* Shriners Burns Institute

Burnworth, Lucille: 223

Burr, John: 98, 575n126, 577n150

Burroughs, Sam: 12

Burton, Margaret Sealy: 504n5

business offices: organization and personnel 75, 79, 80, 87–90, 96–100, 379; budget process 94–98; Administration Annex II 120, 126, 134; Administration Annex I 134. *See also* Appendix J; economic resources

Busy Bees Club: 381

Butte, Felix: 245, 298

C

Cactus: 25, 290, 296, 313

Cadaver Ball: 301

Caduceus Room: 116, 120, 584n40

Cafe-on-the-Court(yard): 134

Calhoun, J. W.: **40**

Calhoun, Jason: 376

Calhoun, John: 48

Callan, Chester: 321, 336

Callan, Walter: 321

Callas, Gerald: 197, 229, 558n207

Callaway, J. M.: 12, 474–75n16

Calverly, John: 575n124, 602n132

Calvin, D. Bailey: political networks 51, 60, 62; teaching 186, 227, 305; research 254, 570n76; professional networks 334

Calvin, Novella: 289

Campbell, Clarke: 474–75n16

Campbell, Heather: 385

Campbell, Thomas: 524n7

Camp Manison: 528n48

Campus, Anthony: **223**

campus development: pre-1902 **8**, **27**; 1943–1955 **102**, **110**, 110–14; 1902–1922 **104**, **105**, 105–7, **107**; 1923–1942 107–10, **108**; 1956–1964 114–16; 1965–1974 116–21, **118**; 1975–1987 121–26; 1988–1991 126–28, **132**. *See also* Appendix N; individual buildings

Campus Life Office: 383

Camp Wallace: 112, 146, 148

cancer: 138, 148, 149, **151**, 166–67

Cancer Center: 164, 204, 315

Cancer Clinic: 50

Cancer Perspective: 315

Candlelighters of Galveston: 277

candy stripers: 155, **155**

Canterbury House: 301

Cantwell, James: 222

Capplemann, Edgar N.: 60, 80, **80**, 81, 87, 88, 89

Cardiac Catheterization Unit: 167

Cardiovascular Research Lab: 251

cardiovascular surgery: 155, 167

Cardiovascular Surgical Care Unit: 167

Carlson, John: 79, 128

Carnegie Foundation: 346

Carnes, James: 304

Carney, Darrell: 270, 383

Carpenter, Kelly: 522–23n114

Carrier, Judy: 197, 352

Carson, Ronald: 71, 235–36, 343

Carter, Earl: 325

Carter, William: 205

Carter, William S.: **42**; teaching 24, 182, 185, 226, 295, 305; political networks 34–35, 41, 42–45, 47, 106; campus development 105–7; research 239, 240, 245, 246; professional networks 337, 339, 341, 358; peer reviews 347; reminiscences 359

Carter Physiological Lab: 253

Cary, Edward H.: 109

Casberg, Melvin: 61, 62, 498(nn85,86,87)

Caskey, John: 301, 536n152

Caskey, Juanita: 338

Catholic Church: 301

Cato, Arthur: 52

Cavazos, Henry: 581n8

centennial anniversary: 373–76

Centennial Capital Campaign: 91, 92, 271, 374, 378

Centennial Chorus: 374, 376

Centennial Commission: 373

Center for Cardiovascular Diseases: 384

Center for Environmental Toxicology: 272, 385

Center for Home Dialysis: 156

Center for International Health: 218, 345–46, 384

Center for Molecular Cardiology: 383

Center for Molecular Science: 126, 383

Center for Nursing Development: 218, 374, 384

Center for Oncology and Hematology: 383

Center for Psychosocial Factors in Health: 345

Center for Structural Biology: 383

Center for Tropical Diseases: 272, 384, 385

Center on Aging: 315, 383

Central Neuropsychiatric Association: 338

Central Services Department: 154

Central Supply: 172, **172**

Cerna, David: 31, 34, 37, 38, 233, 487n111, 488n125

Chadwick, Charles: 86

Chaney, Harriett: 269

chaplains: 154, 173, 234, 301

Chapman, L. E.: 233

Charity Hospital: 9–10, 13, 37, 43–44, **105**

Charles E. Culpepper Foundation: 561n235

Charles T. Stone Society: 327

Charpentier, Gwendolyn: 530n71

Chauncey Leake History of Medicine Society: 302

Chemistry Lab: 106, 244

Chesney, Alan: 311, 581n8

chief executive officers: 278–81. *See also* Appendix A; individual CEOs

Child Development Clinic: 156

Childers, John: 336

Child Health: 314

Child Health Center: 95, 119, 121, 133, 160, 163, 379. *See also* Children's Hospital

Child Health Program: 248

Child Psychiatry Division: 5, 156

Children's Diabetes Management Center: 162

Children's Hospital: 76, 109, **141**, 143, 146, 148–49, 162, **200**

Chinese Student Association: 291, 303

Chiriboga, David: 226, 269

Christensen, Jandee: 72

Christiansen, Charles: 377

chronic diseases: 138–44, 149. *See also* therapies and therapeutics; specific diseases

Chronic Home Dialysis Center: 277, 278

Chrysalis BioTechnology: 383

City Hospital: 9, 10, 16, 17, 26, 103

Clark, Ed: 124

Clark, I. E.: 78

Claude Pepper Award: 270

Clay, Ethel: 206, 207, 334, 516n37

Clay Hall: 114

Clayton, Bill: 124

Clayton, Nicholas: 18, 127, 477n37

Cleander, David: 253

Clements, Bill: 67

Cleveland, Mark: 231

Cline, Joseph: 246

Cline, R. R. D.: 32, 38, 205

clinical departments: **176**, 185, 189. *See also* specific departments

Clinical Lab: 142, 168–69, **169**

Clinical Microbiology Update: 315

Clinical Pathology Lab: 106, 142, 554n159

Clinical Research Center: 157–58, 258, 262, 267, 368, 383, 577–78(nn158–160)

Clinical Science Core Committee: 190

Clinical Sciences Building: 115, 117, 119, 134

Clopton, Albert: 20, 21, 22, 23, 31, 34, 480n60

Clough, George: 84
Coastal Area Health Education Center: 382
Cochran, J. Layton: 322
Coggeshall, Jan: 553n145
Coggeshall, Richard: 233
Cohen, Henry: 154, 307
Cohen, Irving: 529n53
Cohen, Novella: 536n153
Cole, Linda: 558n207
Cole, Tom: 236
College Inn: 586–87n64
College of American Pathologists: 343, 349
Collins, Grace: 548n108
Colored Hospital Aid Society: 504n5
Colquitt, Oscar: 106
Colquitt, Walter: 106
Colwell, N. P.: 44, 347
Committee of 75: 62, 254
Commonwealth Fund: 210
Comparative Neurobiology Division: 265
Compendium: 314
competency assessment exercise: 543n61
Comprehensive Health Manpower Training Act: 93
Computing Center: 89, 98, 256–57, 263
Conant, James Bryant: 249
Cone, Robert: 336, 338, 540n27
conjoined (Siamese) twins: 166
Connally, H. Frank Jr.: 62, 499n95
Connally, John: 84, 158, 370
Conner, Mary Gordon: 581n4
Conner, Patrick: 314
"Consultant X": 551n129
Conti, Vincent: 167
Continuing Medical Education Office: 122, 204
Cook, Ann: 256
Cook, Kay: 177
Cooke, Henry: 24, **24**, 28, 34, 37, 478n43, 478n51
Cooke, Mrs. Willard: 289
Cooke, Willard: 140, 244, 339, 341, 359, 360
Cooley, Denton: 494n47, 572n99
Cooley, Robert: 262, 327, 342, 372
Cooper, Cary: 264, 377, 382, 559n211
Cooperative (bookstore): 295, 296
Coordinating Board of the Texas College and University System: 64

Copado, Lila: 198
Copado, Theresa: 232
Corbett, Linda: 100
Cordova, David: 225, 226, 269, 343
Coronary Care Unit (CCU): 162
corporate executives: 278–81. *See also* Appendices A and B; individual CEOs
Correia, Manning: 261, 266, 270
Cortez, Cruz: 522–23n114
COSMOS: 266
Costanzi, John: 164
Coulter, Susan: 377
Council of Health Institutions: 68, 71
Council of Hospital Chaplains: 173
Council on Medical Affairs: 498n85
Council on Medical Education and Hospitals: 44, 47, 53, 182, 204, 346–47, 376
Council on Religious Ministries: 173
Cranial Tomography (CT): 166
Crawford, Stanley: 327
Creson, Dan: 167–68, 278
Crews, Barbara: 374, 384
Critchfield, A. S.: 88
Cronin, Thomas: 325
Crook, Billie Louise: 219
Crosby, George: 220
Crow, Jim: 129
Crow, T. J.: 491n14
Crutchfield, Earl: 243, 539n16
Cuenod, Marc: 74
Culberson, Charles A.: 33
Cunningham, A. W. B.: 256–57
Cunningham, William: 376
Currie, George: 59–60, 61, 158
Currie, John: **91**
Curry, Timothy: 536n152
Custer, Jap: 586n57
Cutter, William: 600–601n116
Cytology Lab: 253

D

Daeschner, William: political networks 115, 119, 281; teaching 186, 301, 560n224; research 257, 258; professional networks 342, 343, 602n132; student life 586n57
Daily, Ray Karchmer: 325

Dale, Sandra: 269

Damewood, Dorothy: 213, 215, 218, 552n140

Daniel, James: 92

Daniel, Price: 84

Daniels, Jerry: 229, 600n101

Daniel W. R. Lee, and Stanley Kempner Laboratory of Human Genetics: 86

Darst, Lise: 605n36

Davidson, Donald: 338

Davis, Charles: 558n207

Davis, Harry: 385, 387, 529n53

Davis, John M.: 121

Davis, Maradee: 269

Davis, Oscar: 78

Davison, Wilburt: 600n101

Dawson, Wilfred: 184, 227, **241,** 242, 243, 493n31

Dean's Advisory Committee: 61

Dean's Award for Academic Excellence: 235

Decherd, George Jr.: 203, 244

Decker, Grace: 320, 548n104

Decker, Ruby: 133, 219, 220

Decker, William: 233

Deer, Toni: 303

DeForke, John: 536n150

DeGroot, William: 258, 262, 268

Deiss, William: 119, 120, 343, 602n132

Delalondre, Marie: 37

Delaney, John: 335

Delaney, Roxanne: 198, 544n66

Del Buono, Lori: 577n150

DeLoach, Jane: 269

Deming, Cecil: 121

Dennis, Joe: 227

Dermatology Department: 185, 189, 243, 524n9

Derrick, John: 155, 262, 277, 337

Derrinwater, Laura: 581n8

De Santo, John: 169, 172

Developmental Nutrition and Metabolism Lab: 268

Development and Alumni Affairs Office: 314

Development Board: 86, 91, 92, 322

Development Office: 70, 91, 92

DeVries, Beverly: 561n233

diabetic children: summer camps for 162, 528n48, 533n106

Diagnostic Virology Lab: 169

Dialysis: 156, 162, 163, 277, 278

Dick, Ellen: 548n108

Dickenson, John: 14

Dietary Department: 153–54, 172, **172,** 310

Dietary Managers Association: 536n147

Diseases: 138–44. *See also* therapies and therapeutics; specific diseases

Diseases of Children Department: 185

Dobson, Vera: 232

Dock, George: 2, 472n5, 478n43, 565n33

Dodge, Warren: 222, 257, 258, 261, 267

Domingo, Emma: 290

Donnenwirth, Richard: 301

Donovan, Claire: 72

Donovan, Jim: 123

Douard, John: 236

Dougherty, W. H.: 44

Dowd, L. E.: 51

Dowell, Greensville: 2, 10, 11, 12, 17, 474–75n16

Downs, James: 359

Drager, Glenn: 248

Drayton, Harold: 384

Dryden, Virginia: 306

Dudgeon, Howard Sr.: 137, 359–60

Duffy, John: 370

Duggan, Malone: 319

Duke, Bernita: 522–23n114

Dunaway, Jim: 229

Duncan, Donald: political networks 61, 64, 230, 254; teaching 228, 243, 245, 285, 305, 372, 560n224, 570n76; research 255–56; professional networks 334, 342

Dunham, Mearl: 328

Dunn, Sam: 322

Duren, Norman: 320

Durkee, Josephine: 28, 33

Dyer, Rollo: 250, 320, 322, 569n72

E

E. Burke Evans Plaza: 379

E. S. Levy & Co.: **288**

Eakins, Martha: 207

Earle, Kenneth: 62, 63, 188–89, 255, 498n86, 499n94, 586n57

eating disorder unit: 168

Echoflow II Doppler Imaging Unit: 167

Eckel, John: **74**

economic impact: 364, 372

economic resources: state resources 3, 19, 23, 26, 77–79, 80–84, 94–98, 174, 247, 250, 264, 360, 378, (*See also* Available University Fund; Permanent University Fund); student fees 23, 80, 90; patient care 26, 90, 93, 121, 126, 143, 157, 174, 178, 283, 479n57; local governments 44, 76–77, 84, 93–94, 143, 157, 174; private resources 76, 84–86, 90–92, 143, 174, 251, 255, 264, 268, 270; federal resources 79, 86–87, 93, 109, 174, 250–51, 255–56, 260, 264, 268, 270, 378; commercial partnerships 265, 383. *See also* Appendices K, L, M, U, V, W, X, Y, Z, AD, AG, and AH; business offices; campus development

Eddy, Gay: 369

Eden, Avrim: 266

Edmondson, Pauline: 548n108

Educational Development Office: 543n59

educational television: 119

EEG Lab: 142, 169, 535n139

EEG technician program: 220

Eggers, G. W. N.: teaching 185, 219, 540n27; research 253, 366; professional networks 336, 342, 344

Eiland, David: 197, 300, 306, 307, 351

Elbert, August: 79

Elbert, Gus: 309, 591n145

Elder, Edwin: 555n171

electrocardiography: 142, 525n19

Electrocardiography Lab: 142

Electroencephalographic (EEG) Lab: 142, 169, 535n139

Elliott, Fred: 56

Ellis, Mike: 168

Emergency Medical Services (EMS): 333

Emergency Room: 112, 116, 126, 145, 159, 379

Emerson, George: 186, 248, 570n76

Employee Assistance Program: 311

"Employee of the Month": 311

Engelhardt, H. Tristram Jr.: 234

Enright, Anastasia: 374, 596n41

Entrance Examinations for Admission to the School of Pharmacy Committee: 25, 286

Environmental Health and Safety Office: 265

Environmental Toxicology Division: 270

Episcopal Church: 301, 532n96

Eriksson Construction Company: 120

Erwin, Frank: 65, 213, 370, 500–501n105

Esther, Brenda: 198

Evans, E. Burke: 379, 602n132

Evans, Luther: 598n79

Everett, Eva: **251**

Everhart, Edgar: 38

Ewalt, Jack: 342, 545n72

Ewing Hall: 126, 265

Executive Committee: 25, 46, 47, 49, 52, 55, 206, 284. *See also* Appendix I

Executive Committee, Hospital: 62

Executive Council: 63, 64, 297

Experimental Medicine Lab: 106, 244, 245

Experimental Pathology Lab: 251, 252

Experimental Surgery Lab: 244, 245

External Affairs Office: 315, 353, 373, 374, 385

Extracorporeal Membrane Oxygenation (ECMO): 162, 379

Exxon Foundation: 561n235

Eye Lab: 253

Ezell, Edgar: 335

F

facilities, physical. *See* campus development; individual buildings

faculty: 113–14, 281–87. *See also* individual faculty

Faculty Advisory Committee: 61

Faculty and Admissions Committee: 55, 58, 111–12

Faculty Committee on Research: 576n145

Faculty Coordinating Council: 381

Faculty Follies: 287

Faculty House: 114, 149, 516n37

Faculty News: 314

Faculty Prom: 287

Faculty Senate: 382

Faculty Women's Club: 287

Fairchild, Mrs. I. D.: **40**, 495n54

Familiarization Program for Minority Students: 235, 542n55, 585–86n52

Family Medicine Department: 67, 160, 194, 201, 381–82, 542n53

Family Physician Review: 204

Family Practice Review: 205

Family Practice Student Association: 303

Family Therapy programs: 277

Faulkner, Xilema: 328

Fay, Marion: 242

Federal Credit Union: 310

Federal Housing Authority: 113–14

Federation of American Societies for Experimental Biology: 340

fellowships: 572n94

Felton, Harriet: 253

Fenton, Mary: 71, 218, 219, 383, 552n135, 554n153

Ferguson, Earl: 559n212

Feuille, Kate: 79, 295

fever cabinet therapy: 146, **147**

Fick, Dorothea: 477n41

Field House: 119, 125, 298, 302, 379

Fiftieth Anniversary Committee: 365

Final Ball: 300, 305

financial management and resources. *See* business offices; economic resources

Finerty, John: 306, 334, 344

Finney, J. M. T.: 20

Fiorenza, Joe: 536n150

First Methodist Church: 301

Fish, Jay: 156, 162, 166, 262, 285, 341, 607n77

Fishbein, Morris: 249

Fisher, Lewis: 43

Fishman, Harvey: 383

Fitzsimmons, Bettylu: **70**, 72, 197

Flavin, Thomas: 22, 30, 31, 35, 38, 318

Fleischmann, Robert: 268

Fletcher, Joseph: 233

Flewellen, Eugene: 267

Flexner, Abraham: 42, 44, 240, 346–47, 361

Florence and Marie Hall Endowment: 92, 561n235

Florence Marie Hall Community Room: 125

Flower Gardens Ocean Research Center: 575n125

Floyd, Chloe: 216, 292

Fly, A. W.: 12, 307, 478n43

Ford, Hamilton: 199, 285, 335, 337, 338, 339, 560n224

Ford, Laura: 100

Ford, O'Neil: 120

Ford, Ruth: 312

Forster, Marjorie: 263

Forsythe, John: **260,** 577n150

Fort Crockett: 146

Foster, Austin: 259, 338, 529n52, 555n165

Foster, J. H.: 109

Foundation Advisory Council: 86

Fowler, M. Lake: 337

Framer, Annie: 87

Franklin, Bob: 187

Franklin, Sandra: 162

Franks, Edwin: 321

fraternities: 36, 120, 291, 296, 298–300, 302, 492n23. *See also* individual fraternities

Frazier, Chester: 86, 186, 248

Freund, A. P.: 87

Frey, Emil: 295

Friddel, Patricia: 305

Fritz, Richard: 229

Froggatt, Peter: 374

Fuentes, Raymond Jr.: 585–86n52

Fuller, Sara: 269

Furman, McIver: 322

G

Gadow, Sally: 236

Gail Borden Laboratory Building: 113, 114, 115, 120, 133, 307, 515n34

Gallagher, Joel: 352, 558n207

Galvan, Aurora: 544n69

Galveston, medical heritage of: 9–15, 114

Galveston Chamber of Commerce: 45–46, 57, 58, 83, 84, 93

Galveston Chorale: 310

Galveston City Commissioners: 84

Galveston City Council: 16–17, 18

Galveston City Hospital. *See* City Hospital

Galveston College: 222, 225, 553n149

Galveston County Bicentennial Committee: 124

Galveston County Commissioners: 11, 77, 93–94

Galveston County Medical Society: 10, 37, 52, 56–57, 333, 473n4

Galveston County Medical Society Auxiliary: 84

Galveston County Welfare Department: 93

Galveston Daily News: 353

Galveston Fund. *See* Kempner Fund

Galveston Health Council: 333

Galveston Independent School District: 292, 333

Galveston Medical College: 10–11, 475n21

Galveston Office of Civilian Defense: 153

Galveston Society for Crippled Children: 143

Galveston State Psychopathic Hospital: evolution 5, 57, 108, 141, 149, 528n51; economic resources 77, 362; walking tour 131. *See also* Graves Psychopathic Hospital

Gambrell, William: 322

Gamel, William: 384

Gammon, William: teaching 26, 28, 30, 31, 37, 38, 233, 319; patient care 29; history by 39; professional networks 341

Gantt, W. H.: 10

Garbade, Francis: 336

Garbade, Walter: 205

Garbage House: 110

Garcia, Alfonso: 290

García, Hector Perez: 326

García, José Antonio: 326

gardener's shop: 112

Gardner, Frank: 267

Garrett, Henry: 325

Gates, Don: 189–90

Gatson, Wilina Iona: 291

gender identification unit: 168, 535n133

General Clinical Research Center: 577n158

General Education Board: 44

General Intensive Care Unit (GICU): 162, **163**

General Stores Warehouse: 112, 114, 125

George and Magnolia Willis Sealy Conference Center: 127

George Sealy Jr. Oleander Garden: 127, 522n104

Geriatric Day Hospital: 164, 278

geriatric medicine: 164

Geriatrics Division: 164

Gidley, W. F.: 205, 206, 491n19

Gillespie, Charles: 325

Gilliam, Louis: 98, 119, 120, 129

Gilmer, P. Ridgeway Jr.: 336, 343

Gingrich, Wendell: research 86, 242, 246, 248, 253; teaching 185, 570n76; professional networks 342

Girardeau, Dorothy: 88

Girtanner, Robert: 164

Giusti's: 586–87n64

Gleaves T. James Centennial Rose Garden: 127–28, 133, 379

Glee Club: 301

Global Nursing Conference: 374

Godinez, Carlos: 326

Godinez, Judy: 553n145

Goldblum, Randy: 268

Gold-Headed Cane Award: 296–97, 308

Goldman, Armond: 156, **198**, 268, 383, 578n164

Goldstein, Allan: 543n60

Goleman and Rolfe Architects: 119

Golibart, Ernestine Schumann: 328

gonorrhea: 146, 527n38

Goodall, Van Doren: 322, 336

Goodwin, James: 383

Goolishian, Harold: 190, 259, 277, 598n73

Gordon, Glenn: 325

Gorenstein, David: 383

Gottschalk, Janet: 345

Grabar, Pierre: 255

Graduate Assembly: 557–58n198

Graduate Council: 230, 558n204

Graduate Legislative Council: 228

Graduate Nurses' Association of Texas: 333–34

Graduate School of the Biomedical Sciences: evolution 226–32, 233, 385; M.D.–Ph.D. program 231, 233, 559n212; faculty 279, 286; students 291, 297, 303, 382; commencement ceremonies 308; peer reviews 351. *See also* Appendices B,G,K,M, and P; specific departments

Graduate Student Organization: 297, 303

Graduate Studies Department: 226

Graham, Barbara: 177

Grant, Adah: 364

Grant, J. Andrew: 267, 268, 385

Grant, Lester: 543n60, 558n207, 559n209

Grant, Silas: 325

Grants and Contracts Office: 254

Graves, Marvin: 43, 45, 76, 203, 233, 334–35

Graves Psychopathic Hospital: 112, 114, 122, 131, 349. *See also* Galveston State Psychopathic Hospital

Gray, Phillip: 245

Gray Ladies: 154

Gready, Donald: 325

Greater Houston AHEC: 382

Green, Blye: 155

Green, Eddie: 153

Greenwall Foundation: 561n235

Gregg, F. C.: 318

Gregory, Raymond: **203**; teaching 61, 157, 227, 285, 305, 570n76; research 248, 251, 253, 571n84

Gregory, Ulloa: **251**

Gresham, Walter: 1, 17

Grey, Grace: 207, 344

Griffin, Samuel: 363

Groner, Hilda: 304

Guckian, James: 70, 71, 190, 263, 285, 572n99

Guest, Mason: teaching 189, 228, 230, 285, 557n195, 583n29; research 253, 258

Guest Services Office: 177–78

Guillet, Glen: 262

"Gus's" or "Greeks": 586–87n64

Gustafson, Arene: 337

Guzman, Lucia: 279, 306

Gwyn, Charles: 38

Gynecological and Obstetrical Pathology Lab: 244

H

Haber, Bernard: 233, 261

Haden, Henry: 341

Hadra, B. E.: 478n43

Haggard, Mary Ellen: 188, 279, 368

Hailey, Bill: 560n224

Hall, Charles Eric: 115, 253, 258, 287

Hall, Florence: 92

Hall, George: 24, 28, 34, 478n43

Hall, Granville T.: 92

Hall, Harvey: 87, 98

Hall, Marie: 92, 553n145

Hall, Octavia: 253

Halsted, Bruce: 38

Hamilton, Ann: **91**

Hamilton, Mrs. William: 155

Hanlon, Roger: 577n150

Hansen, Arild: **180**; teaching 186, 227; research 248, 368, 570n76; professional networks 342, 344

Harding, Warren: 61–66, 80, **81**, 115, 306, 560n224

Harmon, William: 88

Harper, Henry W.: 226

Harr, Maurice: 98, 130

Harrell, George: 234

Harris, Brantley: 233

Harris, Leonard: 155

Harris, Titus: political networks 61, 108; research 243; professional networks 322, 335, 337, 338, 339, 598n72; teaching 545n72

Harris and Eliza Kempner Fund. *See* Kempner Fund

Harrison, Dan: 57

Harrison, Wilson: 540n27

Hart, James: 59, 220, 233

Hartford, Lyle S.: 158

Hartgraves, Ruth: 326

Hartman, Albert: 322

Hartman, Henry: 45–46, **46**, 184, 246, 335, 582n18

Harwood, T. M.: 18

Hasselmeier, Joy: 198

Hausmann, Sadie: 207

Hawkins, Dorothy: 198

Hawkins, Hattie: 328

Hawkins, Marvin: 87, 89, 98

Hay, Jess: 70

Hayden, Charles: 223

Haynes, Leo C.: **40**

Hays, Judy: 535n136

Health Affairs Council: 68, 71, 558n204

Health Care Administration Division: 226

Health Care Sciences Department: 222, 225

Health Information Management Department: 226

Health Manpower Act: 93

Health Professions Educational Assistance Act: 87, 93

Health Promotion and Gerontology Department: 226

Health Related Occupations Division: 556n178

Health Related Professions Division: 556n178

Health Related Studies Department: 225, 226

heart disease: 138, 155

Hedges, Helen: 530n65

Heermans, Mary Frances: 221

Hegler, Margaret Louise: 548–49n109

Heidt, Pam: 374

Hejtmancik, Milton: 253, 254

helipads: 126

Hematology Division: 252

Hematology Research Lab: **150,** 251

Hendrick, Jesse: 28, 30, 37

Hendrix, Byron: teaching 184, 227, 305, 564n20; research 242, 245, 570n76, 582n18

Hennings, Arthur: 158

Henze, Henry: 205, 242

Heritage Council: 607n65

Hermann, Liz: **70,** 72, 197, 502n122

Herndon, David: 384

Herring, Ruth Anne: 581n4

Herrmann, George: research 85, 244, 245, 251, 253; teaching 184, 227, 285, 570n76; professional networks 335, 337, 339, 342, 344, 598n82, 599n84; biography 385

Herz, B. J.: 173

Hild, Ursula: **174**

Hild, Walther: 541n45, 559n209, 572n98

Hill, Addie: 72

Hill, Alice: 352

Hill, Freddie: **356**

Hilliard, Robert: 326

Hilton, Betty: 287

Hilton, James: 230

Hirschfeld, Robert: 271

Histology and Embryology Department: 185

History of Medicine Division: 234

Hixon, Miss D. B.: 140

Hobby, William: 44

Hobby–Clayton Commission: 122

Hodges, R. C.: 28, 34, 478n51

Hogg, Will C.: 76

Hogg Foundation: 85, 91, 258–59, 262, 264, 268, 561n235, 579n172

Holbrook, Ray: 124, 511n84

Holcomb, Nolen: 301, 536n152

Holland, Bryan: 229, 267, 542n48

Holle, Henry: 337

Holley, Atmar: 480n65

Holliday, E. S.: 363

Holman, Emile: 600n101

Holubek, Viktor: 558n207

Honor Council: 295–96, 297

Honor Education Council: 296

Hooks, Charles: 338, 342

Hooper, John: 128, 309

Hoover, Cindy: 198

Hope, Robert: 122

Hopps, Howard: 257

Hopson, Jennie: 312

Hornedo, Manuel: 290

Horton, Kathy: 171

Hospital Advisory Committee: 61

Hospital Aid Society: 142

Hospital Auxiliary: 173–74, **174**

Hospital News: 314

Hospital Nursing Advisory Committee of Directors of Nursing: 219

hospitals: organization 158–59, **175, 176,** 176–78; peer reviews 348–49; history about 385. *See also* Appendices F,U,W,Y,AA,AB,AC,and AD; economic resources; specific hospitals

hospital staff: 28, 140–44, 148–54, 156, 158, 168–73, 198–99, 198–200, **199,** 286. *See also* nursing staff; support staff; volunteer services; specific occupations

Hotchkiss, William: 325, 326

Hotvedt, Marty: 205

House Appropriations Committee: 98

House Councils: 297

House Higher Education Committee: 98

Housekeeping Department: 130

house staff. *See* hospital staff

House Staff Committee: 158

Houston, Forrest Gish: 253

Houston Chamber of Commerce: 57

Houston Endowment: 85, 122, 271, 561n235, 607n62

Houston–Galveston Area Council Health Systems Agency: 349

Howard, Kathy: 304

Howell, Ruby: 548n108

Hoxie, David: 66, 119, 120, 176

Hsu, T. C.: 248

Huang, Becky: **174**

Huang, Ted: 165

Hubely, Shirley: 87

Hull, Edgar: 348

Hum, Betty Ann: 570n82

Human Biological Chemistry and Genetics

Department: 260–61, 270, 543n60

Human Genetics Lab: 86

Humanities and Basic Sciences Department: 226

Human Resources Department: 88–89, 98, 99, 309, 311, 312, 378

Humphrey, Ruth: 72

hurricane, 1900: 2–3, 42, 77, 105

Huvelle, Rene: 322

Hyde, Robert: 325

Hyperbaric Facility: 126, 163–64

I

I. H. Kempner Professorship in Human Genetics: 85–86, 284

Immunology Division: 268

Impact: 314, 315, 353, 354

indigent health care: clinical education and 11, 13, 18, 20, 143, 157, 526n25; funding 26, 77, 82, 83–84, 87, 93–94, 490n12; patient load 174–76. *See also* economic resources

Industrial Hygiene Lab: 251

infantile paralysis: 85, 142, 146, 219, 258, 527n35

Infant Special Care Unit (ISCU) : **161**, 162, 532(nn101,102)

infectious diseases: 29, 113. *See also* specific diseases

Information Services Office: 313–15

inhalation therapy: 555n171

Institute for the Medical Humanities: evolution 5, 232–36, 259, 315; interdisciplinary programs 193–94; research 269, 271, 378, 385; professional networks 341

Institutional Review Board: 265, 577n149

Institutional Services Division: 314

Integrated Medical Curriculum: 382

intensive care units: 162–63

Interactive Learning Tract: 382

Interdisciplinary Studies Division: 226

Interfraternity Council: 300, 302

Internal Medicine Department: faculty 90, 281; patient care 144; residents and fellows 168, 201, 381, 545n77; research 253, 258; professional networks 340

International Cancer Research Foundation: 85

International Center for Health: 345

International Congress of Physiology: 242

International Forum: 305

International Health Division: 345

International Pediatric Nephrology Association: 345

International Society for Research in Human Milk and Lactation: 578n164

International Society for the History of Medicine: 345

International Society for the Study of Individual Differences: 345

International Society of Surgery: 253

International Surgical Society: 366

Internet: 385

Intramural Research Grants Program: 264

Introduction to Clinical Medicine Committee: 190

Introduction to Patient Evaluation: 306

Irvine, Virginia: **274**, 289, 294

Isenberg, J. Nevin: 267

Ishizeka, Jin: **356**

Isolation Hospital: 112, 141, 146, 294

Ives, Kirk: **380**

J

J. W. Bateson Company: 123

Jackson, Bobbie: 584n40

Jackson, Dudley: 322

Jackson, Holland: 322, 336

Jackson, Lillian: 311

Jackson, R. S.: 318

Jackson, Ralph: 594n9

Jackson, Thomas: 28, 30, 319

Jaco, Gartley: 258–59

Jacob K. Javits Award: 266

Jacobson, Werner: 569n66

James, Gleaves: 126, 127

James, Johnnie Mae: 536n147

James, Thomas: **71**; political networks 70–72, 90–91, 372, 607n62; campus development 122, 126–28; research 271, 272, 384, 503n126, 580n186; centennial celebration 373, 374, 376

James A. Hamilton Associates: 114–15, 254

Jameson, Grace: 289

Janek, Doris: 177

Jannasch, James: 88–89, **89**, 98, 99, 313, 509n64

Jarl, Ray: 121

Jarrell, Gammon: 234, 301

Jenicek, Alice: 173, **174**

Jenicek, John: 530n66

Jenkins, Dan: 322

Jenkins, David: 271

Jenkins, M. T.: 326, 337, 339, 594n16

Jenkins, Marion: 325

Jennie Sealy Smith Chair in Obstetrics and Gynecology: 285

Jennie Sealy Smith Hospital: 90, 116–17, 134

Jennings, Lamont: 336

Jesse H. Jones Research Endowment: 271

Jewett, Beth: 553n145

Jewish Student and Faculty Organization: 303

Jinkins, Julius: 335

John and Mary R. Markle Foundation: 85

John P. McGovern Fund: 561n235

John P. McGovern Hall of Medical History: 134

John S. Dunn Research Foundation: 607n62

John Sealy Annex: 379

John Sealy Biomedical Endowment: 378

John Sealy Centennial Chair in Radiation Therapy: 91

John Sealy Centennial Chair in Rehabilitation Sciences: 91

John Sealy Centennial Chair of Neonatology: 91

John Sealy College of Nursing: 47, 49, 55, 86, 548n107

John Sealy Hospital: **104, 105, 136, 139, 145, 150;** administration 18, 24, 42, 43, 45, 46, 49, 51, 106; construction 21, 27–28, 83, 134, 149–50, 328; renovations 78, 105, 115, 119, 121; Christmas celebration **277,** 278; peer reviews 348–49; centennial celebration 373; prison ward 521n83. *See also* Appendices E,F,K,L, and O; John Sealy Towers; Sealy & Smith Foundation

John Sealy Hospital Aid Society: 504n5

John Sealy Hospital Training School for Nurses: 18, **32,** 33

John Sealy Memorial Endowment: 90, 264, 270, 350, 383

John Sealy Memorial Research Lab: 242, 245, 251, 504n6, 571n84

John Sealy Towers: 95, 119, 121, 125, 126, 160, 163, 379

Johnson, Daniel Jr.: 326, 384

Johnson, James: 26, 35, 75, 79

Johnson, Jesse: 143, 539n16

Johnson, Jim: 253

Johnson, John: 560n224

Johnson, Ken: 575n126, 577n150

Johnson, Lyndon: 158, 604n32

Johnson, Thurston: 242

Johnston, J. E. Jr.: 571n92

Johnston, MacKenzie: 474–75n16

Johnston, Vurtis: 88

John W. McCullough Building: 87, 115, 116, **144,** 159, 379

Joint Commission on Accreditation of Hospitals (JCAH): 348–49

Joint Commission on Healthcare Organizations: 385

Jolly Bone Jugglers: **35,** 36, 298

Jones, Anne Hudson: 236, 271, 279, 343

Jones, Edwin: 319

Jones, J. Guy: 322

Jones, J. S.: 318

Jones, James: 319

Jones, L. Bonham: 322

Jones, Lee: 295

Jones, W. D.: 359

Jorizzo, Joseph: 267

Joseph–Levy, Marion: 233

Josie, Earnie: 312

Josie, Joe Jr.: 312

Junior Faculty Organization: 583n30

Junior League: 154, 173

Junior Welfare League: 140, 143, 154

K

Kaiser, Ann: 198

Karacostas, Billie: 218

Kass, Joseph: 563n15

Keiller, Violet: 142, 587–88n76

Keiller, William: **45, 183;** teaching 20, 22, 31, 182, 184; patient care 37, 138; professional networks 38, 335, 338, 339, 347; political networks 45, 106, 107–8, 240–41, 245–46, 282, 480n60; death of 305; reminiscences 359, 361–62; biography 385

Keiller Building: 87, 107, 109, 115, 131, 361–62, 379

Kelley, William: 10, 474–75n16

Kelsey, Mavis: 385

Kelso, John: 74

Kemp, John: 205

Kempen, Rene: **375**

Kempner, Dan: 52, 85

Kempner, Harris Jr.: 92

Kempner, Harris Sr.: 560–61n228

Kempner, Hetta T.: **91**

Kempner, I. H.: 57, 58, 77, 83, 93

Kempner, Jeane: 85, 255

Kempner, Mrs. Dan: 154

Kempner, Ruth: 367

Kempner Fund: Kempner family 85; project support 91, 561n235; trustees **91**; scholarships 255, 378; research support 262, 264, 268, 508n48; public information office 313

Kennedy, James: 32

Kennedy, Thomas: 28, 31, 484n94

Kenny, Alexander: 230

Kent, James: 262

Kerr, C. Denton: 322

Kevetter, Golda: 266

Kibbe, Elsa: 209

Killough, Margaret: 581n8

Kimbro, Robert: 322

Kimbrough, Billy: 89

Kimpel, Gary: 268

Kindbom, Hanna: 33, 34, 38, 480n64

Kindley, Eugene: 133

King, Camille: 72, 198

King, Charles: 98

King, Lester: 560n226

King, Walter Jr.: 372

Kirkpatrick, Brett: 295

Kirksey, Thomas: 277

Kitay, Julian: 197, 343, 352

Knape, Myles: 314, 353, 606n48

Knebel, Elizabeth: 306, 550n120, 553n144

Knight, Harry: 184, 205, 243, 245, 335, 493n31

Knisely, Bill: 66

Knox, R. W.: 478n51

Koenig, Virgil: 228

Koeppe, Patsy: 164

Kolb, Weldon: 325, **336**

Koleng, Esther: 177, 198, 544n69

Kolmen, Samuel: 193, 255, 263

Kopeckey, Joseph: 344

Krause, Neal: 269

Krebs, Daisy: 206

Krebs, Hans: 249, 569n65

Krohn, Mrs. E. B.: 508n41

Kronenberg, Marvin: 271

KTP/532 Laser: 167

Kubala, Mark: 384

Kuna, Sam: 268

Kuruse, Mark: 167, 535n130

Kusnerik, John: 99, **99**, 100

L

laboratories: 152, 168–69, **169**, 251, 265, 569n69. *See also* specific laboratories

Laboratory Building. *See* Basic Science Building; Gail Borden Laboratory Building; Keiller Building; Medical Research Building

Ladd, Alan: 121

Lady Board of Managers, John Sealy Hospital Training School for Nurses: **32**

Lamar, Jules: 85, 244

Lambert, Curtis: 92

landscaping: 127–28, 133, 134, 379, 522n104

Langer, Betty: 381

Langley, Weldon: 154

Larson, John Jr.: 98

La Salud: 314

Lasker, Mary: 249

Latimer, Truett: 124

laundry facility: 110, 112, 115, 116

Law, Tom: 536n152

Lawrence, Charles: 315

Lawrence, David: 233

Lawrence, Harry: 128

LCME: 348, 349–50

League, Nellie: 516n37

League Hall: 114, 125

Leake, Chauncey: **55**; political networks 41, 54–61, 80–83, 307, 497–98n80; campus development 110–14, 278; research 227, 247–51, 259; teaching 233–34, 570n76; professional networks 341, 342

Leake, Elizabeth: 54, 153, 287, 289

Learning Center: 122, 133

Learning Resources Center: 125

Leaton, Robert: 322

LeBlanc, Al: political networks 68, 158, 176–78, 197, 373; research 262; professional networks 344, 602n132; peer reviews 350

Lederman, Regina: 306, 343

Lee, George: teaching 20, 21, 22, 28, 31, 478n43, 480n63; political networks 24; research 34; professional networks 341

Lee, Sheldon: 156

Lee Hage Jamail Student Center: 379, 606n52

Legator, Marvin: 270

Legislative Budget Board: 83, 84, 95, **95**, 96, 97, 122

LeMaistre, Charles: 64, 65, 66, 68, 370

Lemmons, Marion: 304

Leonard, J. J.: 256

Leonard, Lisa: 133

Leone, Nicholas: 517n51

Leslie, Paul: 130

Lester Gorsline Associates: 119

Lett-Brown, Michael: 268

Levetown, Marcia: 379

Levin, Edna: 125

Levin, Harvey: 269, 577n153

Levin, William: **67**; political networks 67–70, 90, 92, 93, 176; campus development 121–26; blood bank 153; research 164, 251, 252, 257–58, 262–64, 570n80; teaching 190, 585–86n52

Levine, Harold: 230, 543n59

Levine, Harry: 344

Levy, Abe: 263

Levy, Louis: 322

Levy, Moise: 203, 243, 336, 565n28

Lewellyn, Jo: 328

Lewis, Gibson: 337

Lewis, Raymond Jr.: 197, 306, 585–86n52

Lewis, Stephen: 62, 188–89, 203, 262, 337, **340**, 342

Liaison Committee on Graduate Medical Education: 351

Liaison Committee on Medical Education (LCME): 348, 349–50

Libbie Moody Thompson Basic Science Building: 115, 117, 122, 131

library: librarians 79, 294–95, 503n133; location 107, 115, 119, 245, 519n64; collections 249, 365, 519n66. *See also* Moody Medical Library

Library Committee: 47, 286

Life Flight: 126, 159–60, 378

Linares, Aletta: 216

Litchfield, William: 278

lithotripter, non-immersion: 167

Little, Harry: 205

Little, Harry Jr.: 335, 537n166

Little, Michael: 79, 128, 129

Lockerman, Robert G.: 130

Lockhart, Lillian: 260, 279, 302

Lokey, J. P.: 318

Loney, Judy: 72

Lopez, Simona: 290

Loukas, Demitrius: 164

Lovelady, Carl: 57

Low, Jaclyn: 561n235

Lucas, Walter: 128

Ludmerer, Ken: 2

Lundberg, George: 375

Lunsford, Joyce: 311

Lynch, John: 262

Lynch, Kenneth: 326, 595n30

Lynch, Robert: **91**

M

M. D. Anderson Foundation: 122

McAmis, Ava: 205

McAnelly, Zora: 207, 328

McArdle, Margaret: 140, 153

McAshan, Betty: 352

MacBeth, Thomas: 312

McClendon, K. T.: 263

McComb, David: 373

McCombs, Michael: 260

McCoy, Dorothy Lynn: 87

McCready, Donald: 325

McCullough, John: 61, 119, 498n84, 499n93, 501n110, 510n73

McCutchon, Percival: 475n19

MacDonald, Etta Mae: 253

MacDonald, Linda: 315

MacEwen, E. M.: 601n117

McGanity, William: 64, 120, 190, 281, 285, 343, 583n30

McGovern, John P.: 134–35, 234

McGraw, Pat: 223

Machles, Fannie: 320

McKay, James A.: 263

McLarty, Ewing: 322

McLaughlin, Andrew: 85

McLaughlin, James: 24, 85

McLaughlin Fellowship Fund: 85, 91, 253, 255, 264

McLean, C. J.: 128

McLeary, J. H.: 15

MacLeod, Dorothy: 548n108

McMahan, Joe: 129

McMahon, Robert L.: 31

McMillan, Francis: 187

McMillan, Madie: 312

McMullen, Heather: **381**

MacNeill, Joseph: 372

Maco Stewart Home: 114

McPhail, Susan: 338

McReynolds, George: 106

Maden, J. M.: 12

Magliolo, Andrew: 325

Magnenat, Florence: 72, 79

Magnenat, Louis: 31, 319

Magnetic Resonance Imager (MRI): 166

Mahan, Maury: 543n59

Mainland Hospital: 93

malaria: 482n81

Malaria Research Lab: **252**, 253

Mann, Cindy: 100

March of Dimes Birth Defects Foundation: 343

Mardi Gras Rugby Tournament: 302

Margie B. Stewart Convalescent Home: 57, 111, 277, 527n35

Marie B. Gale Professor of Psychiatry: 285

Marine Biology and Resources Division: 265

Marine Biomedical Institute: evolution 5, 232–33, 261, 266; interdisciplinary courses 193–94; research **260**, 265, 270, 385

Marine Medicine Division: 265

Markides, Kyriakos: 269, 271, 383

Markwell, Russell: 233

Marr, William: 242–43, 244, 338, 339

Marshall, Richard: 230

Martin, Janice: 269

Martinez, Maria: 166

Mary Moody Northen Pavilion: 122, 131, 133

Massin, Esther: 72, 294

Materials Management Department: 99, 120

Mathis, Dora: 49, 208, 209, 548n108

Matlack, Katie: 553n149

Maurice Ewing Hall: 265

Mavis, Gertie: 584n40

May, Stratford Jr.: 383

McArdle, Margaret: 594n15

Mead, Johnson, and Company: 76

Medicaid and Medicare: 87, 93, 159, 174, 378, 511n81

Medical Association of the Southwest: 335

Medical Center News: 313, 353

Medical College Building. *See* Old Red

Medical Dames: 287, 289–90, 297

Medical Electronics: 117

Medical Humanities Committee: 234

Medical Humanities Review: 271

Medical Illustrations: 117

Medical Intensive Care Unit (MICU): 163

medical library. *See* library; Moody Medical Library

Medical Library Association: **339**, 340, 341

medical licensure: 474–75n16

medical management analysis (MMA): 537n166

Medical Photography: 88, 117

Medical Records Department: 116, 153, 171, 225

Medical Research Building: 71, 126, 131, 133, 272, 379

Medical Researchers Day: 608n94

Medical Research Foundation of Texas: 255

Medical School Familiarization Program: 235, 542n55, 585–86n52

Medical Services Curricula Division: 220, 297

Medical Services Research and Development Plan (MSRDP): 93, 121, 126, 178, 283

medical staff. *See* hospital staff

Medical Student Research Training Program: 256

Medical Student's Forum: 302

Medical Technology Department: 220, 225, 554n159

Medicare and Medicaid: 87, 93, 159, 174, 378, 511n81

Medicine Department: 91, 116, 187, 243, 244, 248, 267

"The Medics": 301

Medi-Texan: 313

meetings and societies. *See* professional networks

Mendle, Lois: 308

mental illness: 141, 149

Merritt, Gary: 92, 315

Messer, Darlene: 369

Methodist Church: 301

Meunier, Lana: 72, 381

Meyer, Ralph: 313, 353

Meyer, Walter: 197, 267, 268

Mezes, S. E.: 43

Micks, Don: 230, 254, 305, 372–73, 559n209

Microbiology Building: 120, 265, 520n76

Microbiology Department: 189, **238,** 257, 267–68, 341, 368

Microbiology Lab: **238, 249,** 251, 253, **257**

Middleton, John: 115, 146, 253, 342

Middleton, Mrs. John: 584n39

Mills, Ballinger Jr.: **74,** 264, 373, 374, 510n73

Mills, Gordon: 230, 253

Ministry Department: 173

Minter, Merton: 322

Miss Mary's Boarding House: 293

Mitchell, George: 586–87n64

Mitchell, Robert: 325

Montagu, Ashley: 56

Moody, Harriet: 198

Moody, Libbie: 117

Moody, Robert: **92**

Moody, Ross: **92**

Moody, W. L.: 508–9n49

Moody, W. L. Jr.: 86, 117, 508–9n49

Moody Foundation: Moody family 86; projects 91; trustees **92;** library 119–20, 378; restoration of Old Red 124; research support 264, 268, 345, 573n111; project support 561n235; Marine Biomedical Institute 575n126

Moody Independent School District: 173

Moody Medical Library: collections: 67, 233, 245; construction 86, 119–20, 133; librarians 295; publications 314; peer review 350; endowment 378

Moody State School: 114, 149, 162, 277, 516n39

Moore, J. Fain: 322

Moore, John: 129

Moore, John T.: 31, 334, 338

Moore, Lucille: 259

Moore, Richard: 72, 90, **90,** 99

Moore, Robert: political networks 61; teaching 185; research 244, 251, 565–66n34, 570n76; World War II 320; professional networks 338, 341, 342, 598n73

Moore, Samuel Jr.: 322

Moore, William: 129

More, Ellen: 236

Morgan, Jean: 516n37, 596n44

Morgan Hall: 114, 294, 297

Morris, Ruth: 133, 221–22, 343, 345

Morris, Seth: teaching 20, 22, 31, 32, 35, 182, 184; professional networks 38, 341; reminiscences 364; research 482–83n85

Morrow, W. Grady Jr.: 325

Mount, Sally: 133, 222, 342, 343

Moursund, W. H.: 326

Moya, Frances: 173

MSRDP: 93, 121, 126, 178, 283

Mu Delta: 296, 301, 302, 303

Mulherin, Charles: 200

Mullins, Charles: 69, 72, 373, 374, 377

Mullins, Fred: 342

Musser, J. H.: 601n117

Myklebust, James: 306

N

Nader, Philip: 333, 343

NASA: 266

Nash, Joe: 156

National Board of Medical Examiners: 341, 599n95

National Board of Schools of Medical Technology: 342

National Cancer Institute: 267, 270

National Center for Chronic Disease Control: 156

National Committee for the Improvement of Nursing Services: 348

National Council for International Health: 345

National Endowment for the Humanities: 234, 235, 271, 561n235

National Executive Housekeepers Association: 522–23n114

National Foundation for Infantile Paralysis: 85, 258

National Fund for Medical Education: 85

National Institute of Allergy and Infectious Disease: 380

National Institute of Neurological Disorders and Stroke: 266, 383

National Institute on Deafness and Other Communication Disorders: 270

National Institutes of Health: 86, 93, 261, 262, 266, 267, 268–69

National Intern Matching Program: 318

National League of Nursing: 351

National League of Nursing Education: 209, 348

National Malaria Society: 342

National Nursing Accrediting Service: 348

National Register of Historic Places: 5, 124

National Research Council: 85

National Resource Center for Cephalopods: 577n150

National Student Nurses' Association: 304

National Student Research Forum: 256, 262–63, 269

National Youth Administration: 586n56

Nau, Carl: 246, 248, 251, 305

Neal, Jean: **70**, 72, 173, 197

Negro Hospital: 3, 79, **104**, 105, 109, 114, **199**, 512n3, 514n21. *See also* black health care

Neighbors, DeWitt: 205

Nelson, Thomas: 267

Nesbitt, Bob: 364

Neurological Intensive Care Unit: 162–63

Neurology and Psychiatry Department: 5, 116, 117, 156, 162–63, 185, 189

Neuropsychiatry Department: 187, 545n72

Neurosurgery Division: 148, 162–63, 167

Neville, W. R.: 205

Newell, Ella Sealy: 58, 477n41

Newlands, Shawn: 231, 270

Newman, Frances Moody: **92**

Newman, George: 555n165

Newman, Ken: 119, 120, 350

Newman Club: 301

Newsletter: 313, 353

Newsletter/Alumni Bulletin: 314

Newsline: 315

New York City Chamber of Commerce: 105

Ni, Ming-Duenn: 266

Nichols, Myron: **375**

Nichols, Robert: 373

Nighswonger, Carl: 154, 301, 560n224

1902 Harborside Drive Building: 379

Nixon, Richard: 366

Nixon, Sam: 325, 326, 384

Nolan, John: 75, 79, 80, **80**, 87, 591n146

Nolan, Thomas: 75, 516n37

Nolan Hall: 114, 294

Norcross, Karyl: 352

Northen, E. C.: **293**, 487n116

Northen, Mary Moody: 86, 124, 487n116

Norton, Charles: 319

Norwood, Anabel: 503n133

Novak, Juaneva: 220, 535n139, 555n171

Nowinski, Wiktor: 251, 252, 253, 255, 344

Now Nursing: 314

Nuclear Magnetic Resonance Chemical Shift Imaging Unit: 265

Nuclear Medicine Division: 535n127

Nurses' Home: 27, 78, **104**, **105**, 142, 360. *See also* Rebecca Sealy Nurses' Home

Nurses Notes: 313

Nursing Education Department: 210

Nursing School Committee: 206

Nursing Service Department: 550(nn120,122)

Nursing Services Council: 550n120

nursing staff: staffing and duties 140–41, 151–52, 168, 480n64; student nurses 206; graduate nurses 208, 209; staff shortages 208, 211, 212, 529n59, 549n113; continuing education 219. *See also* hospital staff

Nursing Student Association: 297

Nu Sigma Nu: 298, 299, 300

Nusynowitz, Martin: 384

O

O'Brien, John: 474n15

Obstetrics and Gynecology Department: 156–57, 160, 199, 244, 258, 281, 379

occupational medicine: 382

occupational therapy: 152–53, 170, **170**, 220, 530n65

Occupational Therapy Department: 226

O'Daniel, W. Lee: 51

O'Donell, Alice Anne: 328

Ogden, Eric: 85, 186, 227, 248, 570n76

Oldani, Dan: **70**, 197

Old Mess Hall: 293

Old Red: **104**; description 5, 109, 131, 134, 186, 360, 481–82n74; construction 18–19, 21, 27, 484n93; renovations 107, 120, 123–24; centennial logo 374

oleander garden: 127, 522n104

Olson, Leroy: 230, **257**, 559n209

Omni: 383

127th General Hospital: 320–21

Open Forum: 315

Open Gates: 126, 127, 379, 380

Ophthalmology Department: 167, 185, 253

Organization of Hispanic Medical Students: 290, 303

Ormsby, Andrew: 305

Orthopedic Surgery Department: 376

Osler, William: 234, 345

O'Steen, Keith: 256

Osteon: 300

Otis, Margaret: 555n165

Otolaryngology Department: 261, 266, 270, **381**, 534n126

Otology, Rhinology, and Laryngology Department: 185

Otorhinolaryngology Division: 156

Otto, John: 335

Ousley, Clarence: 43

Outpatient Clinic Building: 108, 109, 133–34, 139, 142, 145. *See also* John W. McCullough Building

Overall, John: 263

P

Packchanian, Ardzroony: 246, 248, 249, 251, 253, 344, 566n44

Paderewski, Joseph: 528n44

Page Southerland Page Architects: 123

Paine, J. F. Y.: **21**; political networks 1, 23, 33, 39, 480n60; Texas Medical College 12; teaching 20, 28, 233, 317, 478n43, 484n94, 489n131; nursing school 30, 206; professional networks 37, 38; retirement 307; reminiscences 359, 365

Painter, Joseph: 326, 384

Painter, Theophilus: political networks 57, 58, 59; economic resources 75, 81, 82, 83; campus development 111, 112

Paley, H. W.: 571n92

Pan American Health Organization: 345, 384

Pan-American Medical Congress: 38

Panisset, Ulysses: 384

Panos, Theodore: 254

Parcel, Guy: 269, 333

Pardue, Stephanie: 306

Parker, Belinda: 198

Parker, Cleo: 548n108

Parker, Tim: 121

parking facilities: 116, 120, 125

Parr, David: 534n116

Parsons, Ann: 223

Parsons, John: 310

Parten, J. R.: **40**, 48, 49, 50, 51, 57–58

Partners in Caring: 177

pastoral care: 154, 173, 233, 234, 301

"The Path I Choose": (poem) **386**

Pathological Chemistry Department: 242

Pathology Department: 121, 185, 189, 257, 258, 367, 558n198

Patient Relations Department: 177

patients: 276–78. *See also* Appendices O, AA, AB, AC, and AD; black health care; economic resources; indigent health care; therapies and therapeutics

Patterson, Marcel: 261

Patton, Larry: 310, 374

Pauling, Linus: 249

Payne, Brittain: 322

Peckham, C. K.: 233

Pederson, E. J. "Jere": 71–72, **81**, 90, 99, 100, 510n70

Pediatric Alumni Foundation: 314

Pediatric Angels: 173

Pediatric HIV Clinic: 380

Pediatrics Department: teaching 90, **198**, 201, 381; patient care 162–63; research 243, 258, 267, 268, 383; professional networks 340; history about 368, 385

peer reviews: 207, 209, 346–52, 384–85

Peloquin, Suzanne: 561n235

Pena, Dolores: 177

Penfield, Wilder: 600n101

penicillin: 146

Penny, William: 12

Perachio, Adrian: 266, 270, **381**

Perachio, Elaine R.: **91**

Perez, Pat: 72, 198

Perez-Polo, J. Regino: 266

Performance Appraisal System: 176, 537n163

Permanent University Fund: 16, 63, 115, 116, 120–22, 124–26, 128

Perry, William K.: 152

Personnel Office: 88–89, 98, 99, 309, 311, 312, 378

Personnel Recruitment Office: 314

Perusina, Sam: 570n82

Peters, Leo Sr.: 322

Peterson, A. J.: 51

Peterson, Ethelyn: 210

Peterson, Gene: 304

Pharmaceutical Chemistry Department: 205

Pharmacology and Physiology Lab: 245

Pharmacology and Toxicology Department: 189

Pharmacology Building: 133, 265

Pharmacology Department: 120, 228, 240, 241–42, 246, 368, 372

Pharmacology Lab: 106, **241**

pharmacy: 116, 171, **171**

Pharmacy Department: 153

Phi Alpha Sigma: 298, 299, 300, 588n87

Phi Beta Pi: 298, 299, 300

Phi Chi: 293, 298, 300

Phi Delta Chi: 298

Phi Delta Epsilon: 299, 300

Philips, Billy Jr.: 337, 343, 384, 543n59

Philips, Rose Marie: 352

Phillips, Frances: 320

Phillips, Jimmy: 83

Phillips, Linda: 343, 384

Phi Rho Sigma: 299, 300, **300**

Physical Plant Department: 115–16, 116, 125, 128–30

physical therapy: 152, **152**, 169–70, **170**

Physical Therapy Alumni Association: 332

Physical Therapy Department: 5, 219, 226

Physician's Assistant Studies Department: 225

physician staff. *See* hospital staff

Physiology and Biophysics Department: 382–83

Physiology Department: 106, 228, 242, 244, 245, 253, 255

Pierce, Goodwin and Flanagan Architects: 119

Pilcher, John: 336

Pineda, Alice: 223

Piney Woods AHEC: 382

Plant, Oscar: 205, 240

plants and landscaping: 127–28, 133, 134, 379, 522n104

Plastic and Maxillo-facial Surgery Division: 148

pneumonia: 138

poems: 277, **386**

Poffenbarger, Phillip: 267

Poison Control Center: 126, 156, 168

Polansky, Donna: 198

Police Department: 130–31

polio: 85, 142, 146, 219, 258, 527n35

Polk, Janie: 232

Pollard, Morris: 248, 251

Pollard, Richard: 164, 169

Pomerat, Charles: teaching 186, 227, 570n76; research 248–49, 251, 253, 254, 255, 256; professional networks 334, 344; biography 385

Pomeroy, Patricia: 72

Poretto, John: 98, 121

Porter, Eugene: 184, 242, 245, 570n76

Port Holiday Mall: 125, 379

Post, Joyce: **238**

Postgraduate Medical Training Program: 203–5

Poth, Edgar: research 85, 253, 254, 570n76; campus development 115; teaching 285, 305, 571n88; professional networks 344

Potter, Claudia: 320, 322

Powell, Gene: 197, 302, 306

Powell, Geraldine: 267

Powell, L. C. Jr.: 156, **375**, 384

Power Plant: 110

Poynter, C. W. M.: 601n117

Practice of Medicine Department: 185

Prather, William: 42, 346

preceptor program: 188, 189–90

President's Cabinet: 607n65

President's Club: 91, 374

Preventive Medicine and Community Health Department: graduate program 228, 231, 382; humanities courses 233; research 246, 270, 271, 383; professional networks 345; history about 372–73

Price, Johanna: 235, 561n235

Primary Care Pavilion: 379

Primm, Marie: 212–13

Prinsley, Derek: 164

print shop: 112, 125

prison hospital: 5, 67, 122–23, 164, 350, 370–71

professional networks: 38, 332–46. *See also* specific societies

professorial chairs: 85–86, 90–91, 219, 284, 285, 342, 343, 384, 607n62

professors. *See* faculty

Protein Chemistry Lab: 270

Protz, Ed: 124

Prough, Donald: 376

Psychiatric Adult Day Program: 168

Psychiatric Clinical Research Center: 122, 268

Psychiatry Department: 5, 144, 164, 167–68, 258, 268

Psycho One, Two, and Three: 110, 112, 114–15, 115, 141

Psychopathic Hospital. *See* Galveston State Psychopathic Hospital; Graves Psychopathic Hospital

Ptak, Helen: 553n144

Public Affairs Office: 315

publications: 313–15, 352–54, 383. *See also* specific publications

Public Health Nursing Service: 333

Public Information Office: 313–15, 353, 354, 369

Public Works Administration (PWA): 79, 109, 112

Pulkingham, Graham: 301

Purcell, Ian: **381**

Purvis, Reuel S.: 129

Putegnat, Fanny: 486n108

Pyle, Bonnie: **174**

Q

quality assurance program: 177

"Quest" orientation program: 307, 383

Quinn, Houston T.: 30

R

R. Waverley Smith Pavilion: 112–13, 126, 146, 150, 379

Rabbi Henry Cohen Humanitarian Award: 384

Radiation Research Society: 343, 384

Radiation Therapy Department: 91, 166–67

radiological exams: **167**

Radiologic Health Sciences Division: 226

Radiology Department: **151**, 152, 155, 166, 244, 372, 380, 534n122

Radkey, O. H.: 318

Raghavin, Nirur: 569n66

Rahr, Richard: 225, 343, 384

Rainbow Connection: 581n4

Rainey, Homer: 49, 51–58, 79, 80, 246

Rains, Anna Pearl: 304, 334, 550n120

Randall, Edward Jr.: 146, 181, 344

Randall, Edward Sr.: teaching 20, 22, 32, 182, 205, 478n43; professional networks 37, 38, 474–75n16; research 37, 38; campus development 43–45, 107–9, 112; political networks 46–54, 78, 107, 113, 333, 480n60, 493n39, 514n21

Randall Pavilion: 115, 149

Rankin, Billy: 306

Rankin, J. D.: 12

Ransom, Harry: 63, 64, 65, 86, 119, 212, 499(nn92,93)

Rassin, David: 268

Ray, Betty: 72, 198

Rayford, Philip: 197, 278

Reach to Recovery program: 173

Read, Ella: 207

Reading, Boyd: 243, 341, 598n72

Reading, William: 480n65

Reardon, John: 536n152

Rebecca Sealy Centennial Chair: 219

Rebecca Sealy Hospital: 379

Rebecca Sealy Nurses' Home: **339**; Sealy family 43; addition to 57, 110; opening of 106, 108, 109, 206, 208, 514n17; renovation of 112, 115, 141, 145, 294; walking tour 134. *See also* Nurses' Home

Recombinant DNA Lab: 270, 383

Red Cross nurses: 140

Redus, Nell: 219, 220

Rees, Maurice: 601n117

Reese, Raymond: 541n43

Regional Maternal/Child Health Center: 160

Reis, John: 312, 522n108

Reitzel, Raymond: 341

Religion and Medicine Committee: 233

relocation controversies: 42–45, 55–58

Remmers, John: 267, 268, 559n209

Remmers, Ray: 156, 262

Renal Dialysis and Transplantation Unit: 162

Renal Dialysis Center: 163

Renal Transplant Center: 156, 162, 166, 380

Renger, Harvey: 322

Rennels, Edward: 228, 258

research: 1890s 34; 1900–1942 240–47; 1942–1964 247–59; 1964–1991 259–72; after 1991 382–83. *See also* Appendices AG and AH; economic resources; specific departments; specific laboratories

Research Advisory Council: 263, 264, 382

Research Committee: 250, 254

Research Computation Center: 256–57, 263

Research Council: 246, 250

Research Grants and Contracts Office: 254

Research in Medical Education Office: 194, 543n59

residents and interns. *See* hospital staff

Resiterns: 290

Respiratory Care Department: 376

Respiratory Therapy Division: 153, 170, **171**, 226

Retirees' Association: 313

Reuss, Luis: 264, 559n211

Reynolds, Edward: 543n60

Rhew, Bonnie: 198

Rice, Lee: 525n19

Richards, Ann: **161**, 375

Richardson, C. Joan: **161**

Richardson, Charles: 87, 98

Richmond, Shirley: **223**

Rickelman, Bonnie: 89, 100, 311

Rickettsial Research Lab: **247**, 251

Rickleman, Bonnie: 512n93

Rider, Gail: 553n145

Rigdon, Raymond: 251, 252, 336

Ripley, Fitz: 88

Ripperton, Clara: 328

Robert E. McKee, Inc.: 125

Robert J. Kleberg Jr. and Helen C. Kleberg Foundation: 271–72

Robert N. Cooley Radiological Society: 327

Roberts, Diane: 223

Roberts, Elsie: 548n108

Roberts, Harry: 312

Roberts, Joseph: 85, 128, 246, 566n46

Roberts, Marjorie: 589n97

Roberts, Oran: 15

Robertson, Hunt: 301

Robertson, Mildred: 321, **321**, 353, 367, **369**, 594n15

Robertson, Sybil: 328

Robert Wood Johnson Foundation: 381

Robinson, Dale: 581n8

Robinson, H. Reid: 598n72

Robison, J. M.: 342

Robson, Martin: 166

Rocco, Carmen: 545n77

Rockefeller, John: 44

Rockefeller Foundation: 76, 561n235, 580n184

Rockwell, James Wade: 234

Rockwell Fund: 234, 561n235

Rodriquez, Belinda: 177

Rogers, Dorothy: 208

Rogers, Mary Jane: 72, 89, 198

Rogers, W. S.: 474–75n16

Romanell, Patrick: 233, 259, 338

Ronald McDonald House: 173, 302

Roosevelt, Franklin: 364

Rose, Earl: 301

Rose, Robert: 263–64, 268, 281, 543n60

Rose, William: 203, 205, 226, 241, 242

rose garden: 127–28, 133, 379

Rosenberg, Henry: 128

Rosenberg, Letitia: 128

Rosenberg House: 126, 379

Rosenberg Library: 292

Rosenbloom, Charles: 153

Ross, Lamar: 542n53

Ross, Larry: 229

Rostow, Elspeth: 375

Rotary Club: 333, 526n26

Rounding, Gary: 376

Rowe, Ed: 585n43

Royal, Stephen: 178

Royston, Mart: 45, 51, 493n39

Rudnick, Betty: 64, 211–13, 259, 591n137

rugby team: 311

Runge, Anita: 127

Runge, Elisabeth: 127, 295, 344, **369**

Runge, Louis: 127

Runge, Marshall: 383

Runge House: 126, 127

Ruskin, Arthur: 253

Russell, Glenn: 256, 259, 575n124

Russell, John: 266

Russell, Mrs. Glenn: **155**

Russell, Rosemary: 312

Russell, Yvonne: 197, 306

Russell Sage Foundation: 258

Ryan, Doyle: 301

S

Saavedra, Rebecca: 383

Sacaan, Aida: 559n213

Saenz, Daniel: 290

St. Christopher's Church: 301

St. John, Camellia: 338

St. Luke's Chapel: 301

St. Mary's Hospital: 77, 93, 301, 379

St. Mary's Hospital Nursing School: 120

St. Mary's Infirmary: 9–10, 13, 37, 43–44, **105**

St. Vincent's House: 532n96

Saito, Vicki: 315

Sajid, Abdul: 345, 543n59

Salk vaccine: 146

Salomon, Lothar: 253

Sam G. Dunn Lectureship: 560n226

Sampson, Jacob: 488n125

Sanders, C. W.: 364

Sandstead, Harold: 264, 559n211

Sant'Ambrogio, Giuseppe: 558n207

Santos, Ray: 326

Sapire, David: 162

Saras, Gus: 586–87n64

Sarles, Harry: 156, 262

Sasser, Barbara: **91**

Saunders, Palmer: political networks 68, 558n207; teaching 230, 231–32, 308; research 263, 264; peer reviews 351; professional networks 600n101

"Sawbones on a Sandbar": 287, 375, **375**

Schaefer, Charlotte: 305, 318

Schaub, Jeanne: 72

Schenck, Jeanne: 222

Schmalstieg, Frank: 268, 383

Schmidt, Bill: 88

Schneider, Rose: 252, 261, 279, 287, 375

School Health: 314

School Health Advisory Committee: 314

School of Allied Health Alumni Association: 332

School of Allied Health/School of Nursing Building: 120, 124–25, 133, 218

School of Allied Health Sciences: evolution 5, 94, 219–26; graduates 223, **225**, 226, **331**, 332; students **224**, 290, 291; humanities courses 235; research 269; faculty 279, 284, 286; commencement ceremonies 308; peer reviews 351. *See also* Appendices B, G, K, M, P, and AF; students; specific departments

School of Allied Health Sciences Student Organization: 303

School of Inhalation Therapy: 555n171

School of Medicine: evolution 5, 29–32, 34, 122, 181–205, 233, 245, 382; faculty 22, 24, 251, 279–85, 478n51; students 35, 36, **274**, 275, 288–92; World War II 186–87; M.D.–Ph.D. program 231, 233, 559n212; humanities courses 233, 235, **235**, 236; administration 281–82; opening ceremonies 306, 317; commencement ceremonies 307–8; graduates **316**, 317–28, **319**, **327**, 329–30, 384. *See also* Appendices B, G, K, M, P, and Q; students; specific departments

School of Medicine Alumni Association: formation 37; Field House 119, 125, 302; annual banquets 319, **321**; M. Robertson 321–22, 353, 367, **369**; presidents **329–30**; publications 353, 367; centennial homecoming 374–75

School of Nursing: evolution 5, 18, 25, 29–30, **32**, 33–34, 47, 49, 55, 206–19; graduates 36, 328, **330**, 331; J. Spies 49–50, 54, 209; graduate program 71, 382; research 85, 86, 259, 269, 271; nursing shortage 211–12; humanities courses 235; faculty 279, 284, 286; commencement ceremonies 308; history about 372; centennial celebration 374. *See also* Appendices B, G, K, M, P, Q, and AE; John Sealy College of Nursing; John Sealy Hospital Training School for Nurses; students

School of Nursing Advisory Council: 553n145

School of Nursing Alumnae Association: 328, **330**, 331–32, 353

School of Nursing Committee: 25, 286

School of Nursing/School of Allied Health Building: 120, 124–25, 133, 218

School of Pharmacy: evolution 5, 23, 29, 30, 45, 205–6, 479n58, 491n19; admission policies 25,

32, 286, 485n100; graduates 32–33, 36; history about 372. *See also* students

School Services Department: 172–73

Schottstaedt, William: 68, 197, 205, 561n233

Schreiber, Melvyn: 263, 276, 308, 335, 343, 591n140

Schultz, Steve: 89

Schulze, Gene: 321, 594n17

Schuster, Karl: 87

Schwab, Edward: 48, 49, 243, 244, 319

Schwartz, Aaron: 65, **65**, 94, 124, 158, 370, 500–501n105

Schwartz, Marilyn: 553n145

Scott, J. Allen: 248, 250, 344

Seaholm, Megan: 606n48

Sealy, George: 1, 16, 77, 127, 373

Sealy, George III: **74**

Sealy, George Jr.: 51, 52, 77, 127

Sealy, John I: 16, **16**, 76, 476n31

Sealy, John II: John Sealy Hospital 43, 44, 77, 105; UTMB relocation 45; establishes foundation 76; Medical College Committee 78; Woman's Hospital 106; death of 108, 365

Sealy, Magnolia: 18

Sealy, Rebecca: 106, 554n157

Sealy, Tom: 83–84

Sealy Centers: 91, 126, 270, 272, 383, 385

Sealy Conference Center: 127

Sealy Hospital. *See* John Sealy Hospital

Sealy & Smith Foundation: establishment 3, 76, 77; E. Randall 46–47, 51, 107–9, 110; John Sealy Hospital 57, 82, 112, 121; J. McCullough 61, 499n93, 501n110; trustees 74; patient care 80, 84, 161, 166, 167; professorial chairs 90–91, 607n62; campus development 98, 116–17, 119, 120, 125, 126, 127, 128, 171; C. Leake 114; salaries 142, 208; research 264, 270, 504n6, 510n74, 525n19; fraternities 300; public information office 313; history about 365, 373; centennial 373, 378. *See also* Appendix T; campus development; economic resources; Jennie Sealy Smith Hospital; John Sealy Hospital; R. Waverley Smith Pavilion

Sealy & Smith Professional Building: 116, 120, 134, 517n49

Sealy Society: 607n65

Seaman, Gerald: 253, 257

seawall: **104**, 134

Secretary's Club: 311

Seeley, Elyda: 220

Seinsheimer, J. Fellman III: 74

Sekula, Shelley: 584n42

self-help groups: 277–78

Selle, Wilbur: 76, 242, 245, 570n76

Senate Finance Committee: 83, 98

Service Computation Center: 89, 98

Services, Development, and Space Committee: 114

Sessums, John V.: 199

1700 Strand Building: 125, 160, 379

seventy-fifth anniversary: 369–70

Sexual Dysfunction Clinic: 168

Seybold, William Jr.: 300, 322, 337

Shackford, Clara: 206, 334

Sharp, Amber: **257**

Sharp, John: 378

Sharp, William: 184, 241, 368, 570n76

Shaver, Elvie: 140

Shaw, Annie Lee: 595n37

Shearn Moody Plaza: 131

Shelton, Steve: 382

Shepard, Seth: 18

Sheppard, Louis: 269

Shieh, Jell: **380**

Shimkin, Michael: 200

Shingleton, Kathy: 99

Shirley, Preston: 90, 373

Shoemake, Myra: 162

Shriners Burns Institute: 5, 126, 148, 165, 271, 385, 517n49

Shriners of North America: 148, 371, 526n26

Sid W. Richardson Foundation: 561n235

Siegel, Harry: 306

Sigel, Bernard: 327

Sigma Ribbon Society: 36, 298

Sigma Xi: 249, 308, 590n118

Sigtenhorst, Mary Louise: 253

Simmons, Sheila: 100

Simon, Adam: 171–72

Simonds, J. P.: 333

Simons, David: 201

Simpson, A. D.: 57

Simpson, Rosemary: 382

Sinclair, John: **386**; teaching 184, 365, 539n16; research 243, 263, 570n76, 574n123, 591n146; professional networks 334

Singh, I. P.: **238**

Singh, Rajendra: 305

Singleton, A. O. Sr.: political networks 45, 47, 50, 51, 54, 78; teaching 184; research 244, 566n34; professional networks 327, 338, 339, 341–42, 599n84; peer reviews 348; biography 372

Singleton, Barbara: 130

Singleton, Edward: 325

Singleton Surgical Society: 327, **327**

Sininger, Rollin: 306

Sisters of Charity of the Incarnate Word: 9, 10

skin bank: 534n122

Slocumb, Judy: 71, 72

Smith, Allen: teaching 20, 22, 25, 28, 33, 203, 233; political networks 23, 24, 41, 357, 488n125; professional networks 37, 38, 339; research 240; reminiscences 359, 360

Smith, Ann: 177, 349

Smith, Ashbel: **12**, 12–13, 14, 15, 131, 474n14, 476(nn26,30)

Smith, Ben: 343

Smith, C. Wayne: 268

Smith, Clifton: 229

Smith, Eric: 268

Smith, Howard: 322

Smith, Hubert: 560n223

Smith, Irma: 205

Smith, Jack: 325

Smith, Jennie Sealy: 41, 43, 76, 77, 106, 112, 365

Smith, Lottie Bursey: 328

Smith, Mary Lou: 548n108

Smith, R. Waverley: 41, 77, 112

Smith, Tony: 87

Smyth, Roger: 325

Smythe, D. P.: 10

Snodgrass, Samuel: 148, 339, 342, 540n27

Social Security: 310

Social Service Department: 140, 152, 153, 170–71

societies and meetings. *See* professional networks

Society for Experimental Biology: 250, 341

Society for Health and Human Values: 342, 343

Society for Surgery of the Alimentary Tract: 343–44, 345

Society for Surgical Chairmen: 384

Society of Academic Anesthesia Chairmen: 343

Society of American Bacteriologists: 340, 341

Society of Chairmen of Academic Radiology Departments: 343

Society of Experimental Biologists: 341

Society of Experimental Biology and Medicine: 341

Society of University Otolaryngologists: 342, 599n91

Society of University Surgeons: 341, 376, 384

Sociomedical Sciences Division: 271

Soule University: 10, 11, 473n5

South Central Urological Association: 338

South District Medical Association: 38, 338

Southeast Surgical Congress: 338

Southeast Texas Poison Control Center: 126, 156, 168

Southern Association of Colleges and Schools (SACS): 351

Southern Group on Medical Education: 339

Southern Psychiatric Association: 338

Southern Regional Education Board: 210

Southern Region Council of Deans: 339

Southern Society for Clinical Investigation: 340, 598n73

Southern Society for Pediatric Research: 340

Southern Surgical Association: 338, 384, 607n67

South Texas District Medical Association: 347

South Texas Medical Association: 38

Southwest Allergy Forum: 338

Southwestern Association of Medical Psychologists: 338

Southwestern Association of Toxicologists: 339

Southwestern Construction Company: 119

Southwestern Medical Foundation: 55

Southwestern Psychological Association: 338

Southwest Philosophy Society: 338

Southwest Regional Institute on Human Values in Medicine: 234

Spanish-American War: 37

Spann, Stephen: 271

Special Programs Office: 581n8

Special Surgical Unit (SSU): 112, 148

speech therapy: 156

Speed, Harry: 319

Spence, Mary John: 127

Spence, Ralph: 127

Spencer, Frank: 23, 41, 479n56

Spies, John: 48–54, **49**, 80, 209, 246, 338, 566n45, 599n84

Spies, Tom: 48, 50–51

Spiller, William: 243, 339

Spitler, James: 221, 226, 352

Splawn, Walter: 184, 207, 362

Sprague, Charles: 326–27

Srivastava, Deepak: 304

Srivastava, Satish: 558n207

Stalnaker, Paul: 319–20, 322

Stanley, Wendell: 249

Stanton, John: 268

Stark, H. J. Lutcher: **40**, 51

Starkey, John: 290

Starkey, L'Nell: 290

Starley, W. F. Jr.: 31, 37

State Board of Control: 78, 79, 81, 82–83

State Board of Education: 149

State Board of Health: 113

State Board of Medical Examiners: 52, 68, 182, 474–75n16, 491n14

State Board of Nurse Examiners: 348

State Cancer Institute: 50

State Department of Health: 113

State Hospital for Crippled and Deformed Children: 77, 106

Steding, Mary Jane: 311

Steele, Shirley: 306, 553n144

Stegall, Fred: 256

Steinsland, Odd: 559n209

Stembridge, Vernie: 220, 385, 530n62

Sterling, Walter: 553n145

Stevens, Don: 67, 71, 501n113

Stevenson, Coke: 57

Stewart, Allen: 322

Stewart, Maco: 111

Stinebring, Warren: 253

Stinson, Ray: 263

Stobo, John: **377**, 377–78

Stone, Charles Sr.: political networks 61; teaching 184, 185, 308; research 242, 243–44; professional networks 327, 337, 339, 341, 596n45; reminiscences 369

Stone, Ed: 301

Stone, Mrs. Charles Sr.: 154

Stone, William: 58

strategic planning: 64, 69

Stream, Richard: 343

Street, Robert: 233

Strickland, D. F.: 57–58

stroke: **139, 152**

Stroke Club: 277

Stubbins, Jean: 153, 220–21, **221**

Stubbs, Don: 229, 258

Stubbs, James B.: 13

Stubbs, Mary Catherine: 220

Student Advisory and Counseling Service Center: 306

Student Affairs Committee: 296, 297, 306, 543–44n61, 587n75

Student American Medical Association: 262, 290, 296, 297, 301, 304

Student Association of Health Information Managers: 303

Student Center: 379, 606n52

student clubs and fraternities. *See* fraternities; individual clubs

Student Financial Aid Office: 306

Student Government Association: 297–98, 301, 306, 383

Student Honor Council: 47

Student National Medical Association: 291, 303

Student Newspaper: 314

Student Nurses Organization: 303

Student Occupational Therapy Association: 303

student personnel offices: 124

Student Personnel Services: 117

Student Physical Therapy Association: 303

Student Research Forum: 256, 262–63, 269

students: housing 3, 113–14, 120, **293**, 293–94, (*See also* fraternities; Nurses' Home; Rebecca Sealy Nurses' Home; University Hall); demographics 27, 30, 32, 35, 76, 187, 191–93, 275, 288–92; expenses and financial aid 28, 80, 84–85, 90, 306; student-faculty relationships 36, 305, 306–9; honor system 47, 295–96, 297, 305, 541n40. *See also* Appendix P

Students' Association: 295, 296, 587–88n76

Students Cooperative Bookstore: 295, 296

Students' Council: 25, 296, 297, 304

Student's Honor Council: 305

Student Social Organization Committee: 47
Stull, Virginia: 275, 291
Sugar Research Foundation: 85
sulfa drugs: 147
Sullivan, John: 312
support staff: 309–13. *See also* business offices; hospital staff
"surge" building: 120
surgery: 29, 112, 155, **165**, 165–66, 167, 524n6. *See also* transplant surgery
Surgery Department: J. Spies 50; professorial chairs 90; patient care 148; clinical fellows 201; research 244, 253–54, 258, 267; history about 369; divisions 540n27; postgraduate training 545n73. *See also* specific divisions
Surgical Biochemistry Lab: 266–67, **356**
Surgical Pathology Lab: 169, **169**
Surgical Research Lab: 115, 116, 125, 251, 254, 260, 262, 265
Surgical Suite: 126
Swann, Howard: 251, 253, 254, 258–59
Swann, John: 606n48
Sweeney, Mary Anne: 269
Sweet, Gordon: 351
Sweets, Henry: 219
Swicegood, Henry: 158–59
Swinnea, Antoinette: 173
Swinnea, Jim Jr.: 65, 98, 352
Swinney, Bowen Jr.: 325
Synapse: 298, 314
Syndrome: 290, 296, 297, 313
syphilis: 146, 527n38

T

Tabaracci, David: 263
Tabaracci, Maria Mancuso: 100, **100**
Tandy, Charles: 69, **70**, 121, 197
Tankersley, Boyce: 127, 522n104
Tansey, Zelcer Jr.: 312
Task Force for the Preservation and Restoration of Old Red: 124
Task Force on Indigent Health Care: 175
Tau Phi Gamma: 298
Taylor, Agnes: 140
Taylor, Holman: 335
Taylor, Judson: 365

Taylor, Summerfield: 594n9
Teacher of the Year Award: 285
teachers: 113–14, 281–87. *See also* individual teachers
Teachers Retirement System: 283
Technical Training Curricula Division: 220
teen pregnancy clinic: 160, 532n98
Tektite II undersea project: 575n125
telemedicine program: 127, 380
Tellespen Construction Company: 119, 120
Tenery, Robert Jr.: 384
Terrell, A. W.: 14
Terrill, James: 205, 359
Terry, Luther: 246, 566n44
Texas Academy of Family Physicians: 336, **336**
Texas Academy of General Practice: 188, 190, 336, 546n83
Texas Academy of Internal Medicine: 335, 598n82
Texas Academy of Science: 38, 334
Texas Anti-Tuberculosis Association: 106, 337, 513n6
Texas Association of Blood Banks: 338
Texas Association of Medical Record Librarians: 342
Texas Association of Mexican-American Medical Students: 290
Texas Association of Obstetricians and Gynecologists: 335
Texas Association of Occupational Therapists: 337
Texas Cancer Council: 337
Texas City disaster: 148
Texas Club of Internists: 250, 335
Texas Commission on Higher Education: 64
Texas Committee for the Humanities: 561n235
Texas Dental College: 54
Texas Department of Corrections Women's Unit: 160
Texas Department of Criminal Justice Hospital: 5, 67, 122–23, 164, 350, 370–71
Texas Dermatological Society: 376
Texas Genetic Society: 599n91
Texas Health Facilities Commission: 123
Texas Heart Association: 337
Texas Higher Education Coordinating Board: 126, 221
Texas Historical Society: 488n125

Texas Hospital Association: 122, 337

Texas League of Nursing Education: 334

Texas Medical and Surgical Record: 13

Texas Medical Association: 68, 304, 319, 334–35, 384, 582n21. *See also* Texas State Medical Association

Texas Medical Center: 54, 58, 61, 81

Texas Medical College and Hospital: 11–13, 17, 19, 20, 26, 475n19, 478n43

Texas Medical Record Association: 338

Texas Mental Health Association: 337

Texas Neurological Society: 335

Texas Neuropsychiatric Association: 335

Texas Nurses Association: 333–34

Texas Nursing Students Association: 304

Texas Occupational Therapy Association: 338

Texas Ophthalmological Association: 336–37

Texas Organization of Public Health Nursing: 334

Texas Orthopedic Association: 336

Texas Otolaryngological Association: 337, 599n91

Texas Pathological Society: 246

Texas Pediatric Society: 336

Texas Pharmaceutical Association: 45, 333

Texas Physical Therapy Association: 338

Texas Psychological Association: 598n73

Texas Public Health Association: 337

Texas Radiological Society: 335

Texas Regional Medical Program: 333

Texas Reports on Biology and Medicine: 234, 247, 249, 259, 263, 295, 313, 568n63

Texas Research League: 60, 61

Texas Rheumatism Association: 598n82

Texas Society for Electron Microscopy: 338

Texas Society for Gastrointestinal Endoscopy: 338, 376

Texas Society for Histotechnology: 376

Texas Society for Medical Technology: 338, 376

Texas Society for Mental Health: 337

Texas Society for Mental Hygiene: 337

Texas Society of Allied Health Professions: 343, 384

Texas Society of Anesthesiologists: 337, 376

Texas Society of Internal Medicine: 341, 376, 598n82

Texas Society of Medical Technicians: 337

Texas Society of Medical Technologists: 337

Texas Society of Pathologists: 336

Texas Society of Plastic Surgeons: 337, **340**

Texas Society of X-Ray Technicians: 338

Texas Speech and Hearing Association: 338

Texas State Medical Association: 10, 13–14, 17, 37–38, 52, 332, 358, 488n126. *See also* Texas Medical Association

Texas Student Nurses Association: 303

Texas Surgical Society: 335, 358

Texas Urological Society: 336

therapies and therapeutics: 1890s 28–29; 1901–1940 138–44; 1941–1968 144–59; 1969–1991 159–78. *See also* Appendices O, AA, AB, AC, and AD; black health care; economic resources; indigent health care; patients

Theta Kappa Psi: 298, 299, 300

Theta Nu Epsilon: 298

30th Evacuation Hospital: 320

Thomas, E. Donnall: 581n190

Thomas, June: 100

Thomas, Lyda Ann Quinn: **91**

Thomas Construction Company: 119

Thomas N. and Gleaves T. James Distinguished Chair: 607n62

Thompson, Aubrey: 270

Thompson, Barbara: 164

Thompson, Brad: 264, 270, 559n211, 608n86

Thompson, Clark: 117, 122, 518n57

Thompson, E. R. Jr.: **91**

Thompson, James C.: **356**; research 266–67; professional networks 335, 343, 344, 345, 384, 602n132, 607n67; student life 586n58

Thompson, James E.: teaching 20, 22, 28, 182, 206; patient care 29, 138; research 34; professional networks 37, 38, 335, 338, 341, 358, 596n50, 599n84; peer reviews 39; death of 305, 307; reminiscences 362; biography 372, 385; political networks 480n60

Thompson, June: 125

Thompson, Karen Sevier: 232

Thompson, Leonora "Nonie": **91**, 153, 499n95

Thompson, Libbie Moody: 117, 122, 518n57

Thompson, Spencer: 64, 65, 156, 197, 255, 260, 263

Thompson, T. C.: 1, 17, **17**, 18, 19–20, 23, 30, 477n38

Thompson, Vernon: **81**; political networks 65, 66, 68; economic resources 80, 90, 511n81; business offices 95, 98, 100, 176; campus development 119, 120, 121, 125

Thorek, Phil: **336**

Thrasher, B. O.: 76

Thueson, David: 268

Tillotson, Leonard: 78

"time office": 112

Timmer, Richard: 119

Tinney, Dick: 130

Tipple, Doreen: 72

Tips, Walter: 14

Tipton, Sharon: 198

Tissue Culture Lab: 251, **251, 380**

Tissue Metabolism Lab: 251, 252

Titus Harris Society: 327

Tolston, Leroy: 129

Torres, Martha: 585–86n52

Towler, Martin: 200, 220, 342

Townsend, Courtney Jr.: 267, 337, 376–77, **380**

Townsend, Courtney Sr.: 322, 500–501n105

Traber, Dan: 193, 229, 258, 271

Track Program Committee: 190

Trahen, Jennifer: **161**

transplant surgery: 156, 162, 166, 167, 380

Trauma Center and Emergency Department: 112, 116, 126, 145, 159, 379

trauma injuries: 29, 165–66

Travis, Luther: 162, 201, 261, 267, 343, 345, 528n48

Trevino, Daniel: 306

Trevino, Fernando: 197, 585–86n52

Troutman, Edwin: 61, 62, 115

Trueheart, Charles: 10, 474–75n16, 476n32, 477n38

Truslow, John: **62**; political networks 61–63, 498(nn82,85,86,87), 499n95; economic resources 84, 93; business offices 89; campus development 114–16; teaching 188, 220; research 254–55, 573n111; professional networks 344

Truslow, Mrs. John: 154

Tschirch, Poldi: 374

tuberculosis: 113, 138, 143, 146, 149

Tunnel, Ira: 262

Tupin, Joe: 65, 262, 575n124

Tupper, John: 375

Turner, John: 594n9

Turner, Robert: 257

Tyler, Patsy: 72, 198

typhoid fever: 138

Tyson, Ken: 572n99

U

Un-American Activities Committee: 52–53, 494n46

Unit D: 114, 149, 160, 516n37

United Methodist Campus Ministry: 301

U.S. Air Force: 253

U.S. Army: 186–87

U.S. Army Medical Research and Development Command: 253–54

U.S. Department of Health, Education and Welfare: 349

U.S. Department of Commerce: 379

U.S. Department of Health and Human Services: 383

U.S. Navy: 186–87

U.S. Public Health Service: 79, 86, 93, 119, 120, 251, 253, 258, 259

U.S. Public Health Service Hospital: 116, 514n20, 517–18n51

University Advancement Office: 385

University Hall: **105**; repairs 3, 76; construction 27; dining club 36, 293, 304; reminiscences 294

University Medical: 25, 296, 313, 314, 315, 353, 354

University Medical Branch Cooperative Society: 295, 296

University of Texas Board of Regents: 15, 20, 22, 24, **40**, 43, 47, 78, 478–79n54. *See also* Appendix C; economic resources

University of Texas Graduate Council: 227–28

University of Texas M. D. Anderson Hospital for Cancer Research: 55, 57, 59

University of Texas Medical Branch: "firsts" 5; Galveston as site for 9, 13–15, 476(nn26,30); delay in establishment 15–21, 477n34; first decade 21–39; reputation 38–39, 47, 57–58, 346–52, 383–84; relocation 42–45, 55–58, 75–76, 78; administrative organization 60, 61, 63–64, 68, 71–72, (*See also* Appendices R and S); comprehensive planning 114–16, 120, 377;

walking tour 131–35; century overview 358–73; historical accounts of 359–73; fiftieth anniversary 365; seventy-fifth anniversary 369–70; centennial anniversary 373–76; home page 385; school name 473n2

The University of Texas Medical Branch at Galveston: A Seventy-five Year History by the Faculty and Staff. 369–70

University of Texas Medical Branch Foundation: 86, 91, 92, 322

University of Texas Medical Department. *See* University of Texas Medical Branch

University of Texas Pharmaceutical Association: 304

University of Texas Record: 353

University of Texas School of Nursing: 213, 215

University of Texas School of Public Health: 59

University of Texas Student Association: 297

University of Texas System: 59, 69, **95, 96, 97,** 121–22

UT-MED: 70, 175, 178, 302, 350

V

Vaiani, Luisa: 197

Valle, R. J.: 569n66

Vanacek, Bill: 87

Vanderpool, Harold: 236

Vanderpool, Nathalie: 333

Van Hook, Jim: 545n77

van Lier, Johannes: 229

Van Zandt, Frances: 544n68

Vanzant, Thomas: 336

Varsity Club: 84–85

Vastyan, Elmer Arthur "Al": 301, 560n224, 561n230

Venable, John: 325

venereal diseases: 146

Verheyden, Clyde: 553n145

Verret, Lynn: 343

Verwey, Willard: 115, 256, 262, 575n129

Vinsant, Wilma: 516n37

Vinsant Hall: 114, 294, 297

Vinson, Robert: 43, 44–45, 226

Virus Research Lab: 248, 251

Visitor's Center: 125

Vo, Thuy: **223**

Vogel, Edward Jr.: 327

volleyball league: 311

volunteers, hospital: 142, 143, 154–55, 173–74, 381, 504n5, 508n41

Volunteer Services Department: 173

Volunteers in Service to America (VISTA): 532n96

W

W. K. Kellogg Company: 84

W. K. Kellogg Foundation: 85, 210

Waggener, Leslie: **40,** 50

Waite, F. C.: 347

Wakeman General Hospital: 148

Walker, David: 264, 384, 559n211

Walker, Don: **80;** business offices 61, 62, 80, 89; political networks 63, 64, 65, 68, 69, 370; campus development 114–16, 119

Walker, Gwen: 328

Walker, Kenneth: 306

Walker, Paul: 168

Walker, Robert: 512n93

Wall, Dick: 184, 233

Wallace, Anyce: 209, 328

Walsh, Jean: 353

Walter Colquitt Memorial Children's Hospital: 77, 106

Ware, Ella: 320

Warmoth Professorship of Neurology: 285

Warner, Henry: 319

Warren, James: 256, 281

Warren, Michael: 310, 345

Watanabe, Yoshikazu: 262, 575n129

Watkins, John: 10

Watson, Margie: 575n126

Watson, Marjorie: 72, 198

Watts, Edwin: 474–75n16

Watts, Leslie: 374

Webb, Charley: 200

Webb, John: 10

Webb, Mary Jane: 337

Webster, Caroline: 585n43

Wedergren, Bob: 154, 536(nn150,152)

Weeks, Julius: 87

Wegner, Mildred: 253

Weidenmeier, Leni: **174**

Weigel, Paul: 270

Weilacher, Robert: 342, 555n171

Weinert, H. H.: **40**, 57

Weinert, Herman Jr.: 322

Weiskotten, Herman: 600–601(nn116,117)

Weiss Chair of Otolaryngology: 284

Welch, Dennis: 304

Welford, Norman: 263

Well Baby Clinic: **180**

Weller, Susan: 271

Wells, Rose Marie: 152

Werrbach-Perez, Karin: 266

West, H. A.: 478n43, 480n60, 488n125

West, Hamilton: **19**; teaching 12, 20, 21, 28, 31, 33; patient care 29; research 34; professional networks 37, 38, 334

West End Chilled Water Plant: 379

Western Surgical Association: 339

Weston, Dee: 72

Weston, Harris K.: **91**

Whitby, Bob: 385

White, Ed: 129

White, Joseph: teaching 65, 66, 190, 194, 234, 307; campus development 119; professional networks 339

White, Mark: 67, 175

White, Robert: 285

White, Stanford: 127

Whiteside, Emily: 124

Whitfield, Dennis: 297

Whitney, Harvey Jr.: 156

Whorton, Elbert: 230

Who's Who in American Colleges and Universities: 304–5

Wichlep, Fred: 72

Wiese, Hilda: 344

Wilcox, Olive: 548n108

Wilkenfeld, Byron: 229

Wilkinson, Cary: 13, 14

Willard R. Cooke Obstetrical and Gynecological Society: 327

Will C. Hogg Loan Fund: 292

William Buchanan Foundation: 248

William C. Levin Hall: 122, 133

William Osler Society: 302

Williams, Arthur: 125, 133

Williams, Betty: 279, 285

Williams, Harris: 566n34

Williams, Jan: 173

Williams, Jim: 333

Williams, Lafayette Jr.: 291

William Temple Foundation: 234, 301

Willis, William, Jr.: political networks 71; teaching 231, 233, 285, 559n211; research 261, 264, 265, 577n153

Willman, Marilyn: 213

Wilson, Crain, Anderson, and Reynolds, Inc.: 124

Wilson, Dorothea: 269, 382

Wilson, Elijah: 153

Wilson, Emmett: 366

Wilson, Logan: 60, 61, 62, 63, 83–84, 84

Wilson, Louis: 103, 109, 114

Wilson, Lucius: 49, 51, 339

Wilson, Marion: 577n150

Wilson, R. L.: 359

Wilson, Roy: 342

Wilson, Samuel: 383

Wilson, Weta: 304

Winkler, Mary: 236, 580n184

Winn, James: 262

Winslade, Bill: 236

Winston, George: 23, 37, 42

Wise, George: 12

Withers, Ben: 337

Witherspoon, John: 347

Wolf, Stewart: 68, 261

Wolfe, Robert: 267

Wolfram, Joydelle: 72

Woman's Auxiliary to the Student American Medical Association: 290

Woman's Hospital: 43, 106, 110, 138, 140, 146

Women's Club of San Antonio: 76

Women's Faculty Association: 279, 315

Women's Health Protective Association: 333

Wonio, Diane: 592n158

Wood, Thomas: 383

Woodard, Paul: 244

Woodward, D. K. Jr.: 82, 83

Woolridge, A. P.: 14, 15

Wooten, Thomas: 15, 17, 19–20, 22, 477n34

World Health Organization Collaborating Centers: 218, 345–46, 374, 384

World War I: 554n159